Veterinary Immunology

Veterinary Immunology

11TH EDITION

Ian R. Tizard, BVMS, PhD, ACVM (Hons), DSc (Hons)
University Distinguished Professor of Immunology Emeritus
Department of Veterinary Pathobiology
Texas A&M University
College Station, Texas

ELSEVIER

ELSEVIER
3251 Riverport Lane
St. Louis, Missouri 63043

VETERINARY IMMUNOLOGY, ELEVENTH EDITION   ISBN: 978-0-443-10975-1

Notice

Practitioners and researchers must always rely on their own experience and knowledge in evaluating and using any information, methods, compounds or experiments described herein. Because of rapid advances in the medical sciences, in particular, independent verification of diagnoses and drug dosages should be made. To the fullest extent of the law, no responsibility is assumed by Elsevier, authors, editors or contributors for any injury and/or damage to persons or property as a matter of products liability, negligence or otherwise, or from any use or operation of any methods, products, instructions, or ideas contained in the material herein.

Previous edition copyrighted 2018, 2013, 2009, 2004, 2000, 1996, 1992, 1987, 1982, 1977.

Executive Content Strategist: Lauren Willis
Content Development Manager: Somodatta Roy Choudhury
Content Development Specialist: Sneha Kashyap
Publishing Services Manager: Deepthi Unni
Senior Project Manager: Kamatchi Madhavan
Book Designer: Brian Salisbury

Printed in India

Last digit is the print number: 9   8   7   6   5   4   3   2   1

Working together
to grow libraries in
developing countries

www.elsevier.com • www.bookaid.org

To Claire

PREFACE

Its complicated but its not sorcery! Since the last edition of this text was published, immunology has been in the headlines. Specifically, a debate has raged over the effectiveness and safety of coronavirus disease (COVID) vaccines. As in so many such arguments, it has been a battle between facts and opinions. Those who believe that vaccines are useless and unsafe demonstrate their total lack of understanding of immunology. They have never had to suffer through an immunology course. As a result, most individuals know nothing about immunology or its importance. Veterinarians do. To those who do not believe that vaccines are effective, consider the use of vaccines in the beef, swine, and poultry industries. Not one vaccine would be used by these industries if they could be avoided. Vaccines cost money to purchase and, more significantly, cost money to administer. These livestock industries would not consider not vaccinating. Vaccines keep animals alive and healthy. They make a difference between profit and loss. Vaccines work despite the efforts of vaccine skeptics.

It is also relevant to note that COVID vaccine skeptics are increasingly reluctant to vaccinate their dogs—many worry about autism! The consequences of this remain to be seen but one may reasonably expect a resurgence in cases of canine viral diseases once herd immunity drops below an effective level. It may not happen soon or suddenly, given the current high level of canine vaccination coverage in the United States, but undoubtedly dogs will suffer the consequences.

This textbook was first published in 1977, at a time when veterinary immunology was relatively undeveloped and very poorly understood. Nevertheless, it was recognized, even then, that the immune system held the key to solving many significant problems in veterinary medicine. Beginning in the 1960s it entered an era of exciting new discoveries and insights. The science grew exponentially. New vaccines became available. New treatments were developed. Diagnosis became easier. Nevertheless, in the decades since then, we have seen the prevalence of immunologic diseases such as allergies and autoimmunity grow, not just in humans but also in their pets. Vaccines have evolved and remain the most important tools in solving infectious disease problems, despite skepticism. The importance of immunodeficiencies, both primary and secondary, is increasingly recognized. Tumor immunotherapy, after years of frustration, is beginning to show significant progress. Immunology remains central to our understanding and solving many major animal health issues.

Over the many years that this textbook has been published, we have seen many changes in the science of immunology. In most cases, these changes have been gradual as investigators add detail to existing knowledge. Occasionally, however, major leaps have revolutionized the discipline—so-called paradigm shifts. For example, in the late 1990s, the concept of innate immunity was accepted. Inflammation and other processes were finally recognized as being essential components of the immune system. I recall that inflammation was ignored in the first editions of this text because I considered it to be pathology, not immunology! It is important to note that this was not a new discovery but a new way of looking at well-recognized processes.

We have known about the commensal bacteria in the intestine since the dawn of microbiology. They, too, were ignored for many years. We did not know how they fit in, and besides, they were far too complex for past technologies. New methodologies have changed all that. Much of immunology has had to be reassessed in light of this new knowledge. Many previously unexplained phenomena have now been shown to depend on the normal microbiota.

Since the previous edition was published, *Veterinary Immunology* has continued to advance. There have been no revolutionary paradigm shifts such as those described above. However, gaps continue to be filled, and previously unknown details added.

Some of these described in this new edition include the critical role of inflammasomes, the relevance of new antibacterial peptides, the roles of neutrophil extravascular traps, the development of immunothrombosis, and trained immunity in innate lymphoid cells. New cytokines have been shown to be of greater importance than previously thought. As have new dendritic cell populations, new DNA vaccines, new adjuvants, and new parasite vaccines. RNA vaccines have assumed greater importance than previously imagined and may well revolutionize the animal vaccine industry. After many years of frustration, human cancer immunotherapy is beginning to yield significant results. These include antitumor vaccines as well as chimeric antigen receptor–T cell and immune checkpoint therapy. Hopefully, effective animal treatments will not be far behind. Autoinflammatory diseases, new immunosuppressive drugs, and monoclonal antibodies, as well as new, rapid, and sensitive serologic assays and their practical applications all have a direct impact on animal health.

For all these reasons, this book has continued to grow. Veterinarians need to know much of this new information if they have to practice cutting-edge medicine in the 21st century. I make no apologies for the size and complexity of this text. Immunology is a complex subject since it encompasses so many aspects of modern veterinary medicine. Veterinary students as well as graduate veterinarians ignore it at their peril. Read it, study it, and enjoy its wonderful complexity.

Visit Elsevier eBooks+ (eBooks.Health.Elsevier.com) to access the Flash Cards and Animations *included with print purchase.*

Ian R. Tizard

ACKNOWLEDGMENTS

As always, a book such as this could not be written without the support of colleagues and family. I am grateful especially to the Department of Veterinary Pathobiology at Texas A&M University for providing me with an office with easy access to the current literature, free coffee, and a photocopier! I would especially like to thank my colleague Dr. Brian Porter for providing many excellent photomicrographs of normal and diseased tissues.

I would also like to acknowledge the professionalism and assistance provided by the staff of Elsevier, especially my content development specialist, Sneha Kashyap, and my content strategist, Lauren Willis.

Finally, of course, I must thank my wife, Claire, for her continuous encouragement and support, without which none of this would have been possible.

Ian R. Tizard

CONTENTS

Surviving in a Microbial World

CHAPTER OUTLINE

The mammalian body contains all the components necessary to sustain life. It is warm, moist, and rich in nutrients. As a result, animal tissues are extremely attractive to microorganisms that attempt to invade the body and exploit these resources for themselves. The magnitude of this microbial attack can be readily seen when an animal dies. Within a few hours, especially when warm, a dead body decomposes rapidly as bacteria invade its tissues. On the other hand, the tissues of living, healthy animals are highly resistant to attack as their survival depends on preventing this microbial invasion. The defense of the body is encompassed by the discipline of immunology and is the subject of this book. Without an immune system, we would simply be eaten alive.

Because effective resistance to infection is critical, the body cannot rely on a single defense mechanism alone. To ensure reliability, multiple flexible defense systems must be available. Some may be effective against many different invaders. Others may destroy specific organisms. Some act at the body surface to exclude invaders. Others act deep within the body to destroy organisms that have breached the outer defenses. Some defend against bacterial invaders, some against viruses that live inside cells, and some against larger invaders such as fungi or parasitic worms and insects. The defense of the body therefore depends upon a complex system of overlapping and interlinked networks using cells and molecules that can collectively destroy or control almost all invaders. Any failure in these defenses that permits invading organisms to overcome or evade them will result in disease and possibly death. An effective immune system is therefore not simply a useful system to have around but is essential to life itself.

The immune system can be thought of as a set of interacting cellular and molecular networks where the presence of foreign invaders triggers changes in cell behavior and generates an expanding set of responses that eventually results in the elimination of the invaders and increased resistance to infection. Most of the complexity of the immune system stems from the fact that it has to be able to respond appropriately to thousands of diverse bacteria, viruses, and parasites. To do this, pathways must interact and intersect. Microbial invasion must therefore trigger multiple responses involving many different cell types and producing many different molecules. Collectively, these responses keep us alive in a microbial world.

THE MICROBIAL WORLD

Historically, our concerns regarding infectious diseases have caused us to regard all microbes as potential enemies. Dangerous microbial invaders include not just bacteria and viruses but also fungi, parasitic protozoa, arthropods, and helminths (worms). Nevertheless, the real situation is much more complex. Bacteria find animal bodies to be a rich source of nutrients and a great place to shelter. As a result, enormous numbers of bacteria colonize our body surfaces, especially within the intestine, in our airways, and on our skin. Most of these bacteria—our normal microbiota—do not even try to invade the body and do not normally cause damage. They share resources with us and so are regarded as commensal organisms.

The presence of this commensal microbiota must either be tolerated or ignored if an animal is to remain healthy. An animal cannot afford to act aggressively toward its own microbiota. Any such response must be carefully regulated and must not happen unless necessary for the defense of the body. The immune system is aware of the intestinal microbiota. Numerous bacterial molecules can cross the intestinal epithelium, enter the body, and influence the immune system. They do not however automatically trigger strong defensive responses unless tissue damage occurs. The response is measured, proportional, and carefully controlled. The immune system has to watch them warily, but they rarely cause trouble. In fact, the commensal microbiota is needed for the proper digestion of food and acts as a stimulus that keeps our defenses in peak operating condition.

A small number of more aggressive bacteria may try to invade animal tissues and hence cause damage. This is normally prevented, or at least controlled, by our immune defenses. If these organisms succeed in invading the body and overcoming the immune defenses, they may cause sufficient damage to result in disease or death. On the other hand, organisms such as viruses are intracellular parasites that can survive for only a limited time outside the animal body. These invaders will only survive if they can avoid the host's defenses for a sufficient time to replicate and transmit their progeny to a new animal host. While it is essential for an animal to control invading organisms (or at least minimize damage), viruses are under even more potent selective pressure. They must find a host or die. Viruses that cannot evade or overcome the immune system's defenses will not survive and will be eliminated. Fungi, like bacteria, are opportunistic invaders that can take advantage of local circumstances to invade the host. They commonly exploit situations where the host's immune system is defective or suppressed in some way. Parasitic worms and protozoan parasites, like viruses, must be able to survive within a host or be eliminated. They too have evolved numerous and complex strategies to evade immune destruction.

An organism that can cause sufficient damage to result in disease is said to be a pathogen. Remember, however, that only a small proportion of the world's microorganisms are associated with animals, and a very few of these can overcome the body's defenses and act as pathogens. Pathogenic microorganisms vary greatly in their ability to invade the body and cause damage. This ability is termed virulence. Thus a highly virulent organism has a greater ability to cause damage than an organism with low virulence. If a bacterium can cause significant damage almost every time it invades a healthy individual, even in low numbers, then it is considered a primary pathogen. Examples of primary pathogens include canine distemper virus, feline panleukopenia virus, and *Brucella abortus* that causes contagious abortion in cattle. Other pathogens may be of such low virulence that they will only cause disease if administered in very high doses or if the immune defenses of the body are first impaired. These are considered opportunistic pathogens. Examples of opportunistic pathogens include bacteria such as *Mannheimia hemolytica* and fungi such as *Pneumocystis canis*. These organisms rarely cause disease in healthy animals.

THE DEFENDERS

The defenses of the body, collectively called the immune system, consist of interacting networks of cells and molecules. For descriptive purposes, it is convenient to divide these networks into two discrete pathways (Fig. 1.1). Nevertheless, the reader should be aware that these biochemical and cellular pathways are extensively interlinked. No immune response is restricted to a single biochemical mechanism or pathway. The invasion of the animal body by microbes alters the behavior of many different cell types and results in the production of many different protective molecules. Understanding immunity requires an understanding of these dynamic immunological networks. These networks possess redundancies, regulatory mechanisms, and multiple simultaneous responses working together to ensure microbial destruction. In addition, the immune responses must be adaptable and adjust their mechanisms depending on the nature and severity of the threat.

Physical Barriers

Because the successful exclusion of microbial invaders is essential for survival, it is not surprising that the animal body employs multiple, overlapping layers of defense (Fig. 1.2). Thus a microbe that has succeeded in breaking through the first layer of defenses is then confronted with the need to overcome a second, higher barrier, and so forth. The first and most obvious of these defenses are the physical barriers to invasion. Thus intact skin provides an effective barrier to invading microbes. If the skin is broken, microbes may invade, but wound healing ensures that breaks are repaired promptly. On other body surfaces, such as in the respiratory and gastrointestinal tracts, simple physical defenses include the "self-cleaning" processes: coughing, sneezing, and mucus flow in the respiratory tract; vomiting and diarrhea in the gastrointestinal tract; and urine flow in the urinary system. The presence of huge populations of commensal bacteria on the skin, respiratory tract, and in the intestine also excludes many potential invaders. Well-adapted commensal organisms adapted to living on body surfaces can easily outcompete poorly adapted pathogens. The microbiota thus plays an essential role in resistance to invasion.

Innate Immunity

Physical barriers, though essential in excluding invaders, cannot be totally effective in themselves. Given time and persistence, an invading microorganism will eventually overcome mere physical obstacles. Nevertheless, most microbial attempts at invasion are rapidly blocked before they can result in disease. All animals and plants, even the least evolved, need to detect and eliminate microbial invaders as fast and as effectively as possible. This immediate response is the task of the innate immune system. Many different innate defense mechanisms have evolved over time, and the mammalian innate immune system consists of a diverse collection of subsystems that work through many different

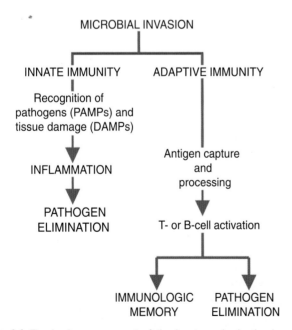

Fig. 1.1 The basic arrangement of the innate and adaptive immune systems. Innate immunity is the initial line of defense, and adaptive immunity is a more permanent defensive system and provides long-term disease resistance through the establishment of immunologic memory. *DAMPs*, Damage-associated molecular patterns; *PAMPs*, pathogen-associated molecular patterns.

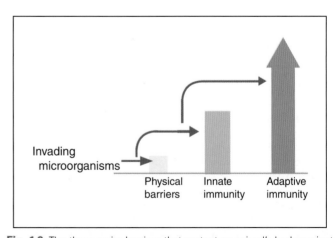

Fig. 1.2 The three major barriers that protect an animal's body against microbial invasion. Each barrier provides a more effective defense than the previous one. The adaptive immune system also improves with experience so that, over time, it presents a progressively greater barrier to invading microbes.

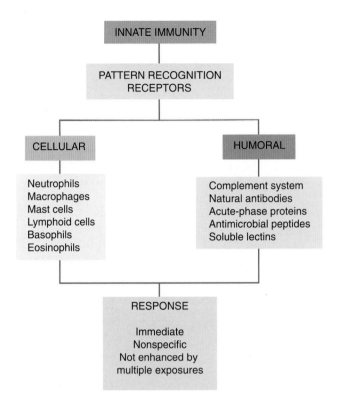

Fig. 1.3 The innate immune system consists of a collection of subsystems. They can be divided into the cellular mechanisms where populations of specialized cells, detect, eat, and kill invaders, and the humoral mechanisms where diverse soluble molecules bind and kill the invaders.

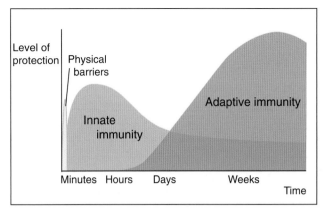

Fig. 1.4 The time course of innate and adaptive immunity. Surface barriers provide immediate protection. Innate mechanisms provide rapid protection that keeps microbial invaders at bay until adaptive immunity can develop. It may take several days or even weeks for adaptive immunity to become effective.

TABLE 1.1	A Comparison of Innate and Adaptive Immunity	
	Innate Immunity Always "on"	Adaptive Immunity Turned on by Antigens
Cells engaged	Macrophages, dendritic cells neutrophils, NK cells	T and B cells
Evolutionary history	Ancient	Recent
Onset	Rapid (minutes–hours)	Slow (days–weeks)
Receptor specificity	Common microbial structures	Unique antigens
Potency	May be overwhelmed	Rarely overwhelmed
Memory	None	Long lasting
Effectiveness	Does not improve	Improves with exposure

pathways. Collectively, they all respond rapidly to block microbial invasion and minimize tissue damage (Fig. 1.3). Innate immune responses can be divided into constitutive defenses that are present in all animals and induced defenses that are activated immediately after a pathogen penetrates the epithelial barriers. They can detect microbes such as bacteria and viruses because they differ structurally and chemically from normal animal tissues. Once the invaders are recognized, alarms go off, and multiple innate responses are immediately activated. These induced defenses are activated in response to the presence of bacteria, viruses, or cell and tissue damage.

The major innate pathways rely on rapid cellular responses to invasion. Thus the body employs sentinel cells that can detect molecules associated with invading bacteria and viruses. Sentinel cells sound the alarm! This attracts white blood cells, called leukocytes, that converge on the invaders and destroy them in the process we call inflammation. Inflammation is central to the innate defense of the animal body. Once the invaders have been eliminated, some of these cells may also help repair damaged tissues. The presence of a combination of microbial-induced tissue damage and the body's response to inflammation results in the set of animal behaviors that we call sickness.

The innate immune system is thus a mixture of "hard-wired" subsystems that act automatically, and as a result, each episode of infection tends to be treated identically. The intensity and duration of innate responses such as inflammation therefore remain largely unchanged, no matter how often a specific invader is encountered. These innate responses also come at a price, causing the pain of inflammation or the development of sickness, which largely result from the activation of innate immune pathways. On the other hand, the multiple subsystems of the innate immune system are "on call" and ready to respond immediately when invaders are detected.

Adaptive Immunity

Inflammation and other innate defenses are critical to the defense of the body. Animals that fail to mount innate responses will die from overwhelming infections. Nevertheless, these responses cannot offer the ultimate solution to the problem of invasive microorganisms. A defense system is needed that can recognize and destroy specific invaders, and then learn from the process so that if (or when) they invade a second time, they will be destroyed even more effectively. In this system, the more often an individual encounters an invading bacterium or virus, the more effective its defenses against that organism will be. This type of "smart" response is the function of the so-called adaptive immune system as it adapts itself to ongoing threats to an animal (Fig. 1.4). Although it develops slowly, when an animal eventually develops adaptive immunity, the chances of successful invasion by that organism decline precipitously, and the animal is said to be immune. The adaptive immune system provides the ultimate defense of the body. Its essential nature is readily seen when its loss leads inevitably to uncontrolled infections and death.

A key difference between the innate and adaptive immune systems lies in their use of cell surface receptors to recognize foreign invaders (Table 1.1). The cells of the innate system use a limited number of preformed receptors that recognize molecules expressed by many different

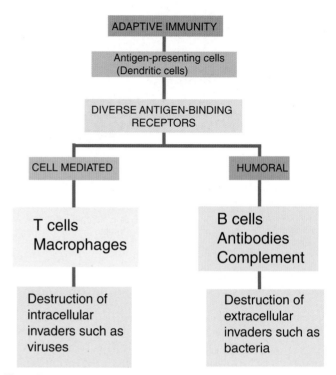

Fig. 1.5 A simple flow diagram showing the essential features of the humoral and cell-mediated adaptive immune responses.

microbes, and their response is therefore generic in nature. In contrast, the cells of the adaptive immune system can generate enormous numbers of completely new, structurally unique receptors that bind specifically to those foreign molecules that induce them. Because the binding repertoire of these receptors is generated randomly, they are assured of recognizing at least some of the molecules found on almost any invading microorganism.

The adaptive immune system not only recognizes invading microbes but also destroys them and retains the memory of the encounter. If the animal encounters the same organism a second time, the adaptive immune system responds more rapidly and very much more effectively. Such a sophisticated system must of necessity be complex.

Another reason for this complexity is the great diversity of potential invaders including bacteria, viruses, fungi, protozoa, and helminths (worms). These invaders may be classified into two broad categories. One category consists of the organisms that normally live and grow outside cells—extracellular invaders. This includes most bacteria and fungi, as well as many protozoa and invading helminths. The second category consists of organisms that originate or live within the body's own cells—the intracellular invaders. These include viruses and some intracellular bacteria or protozoa. Each category of invader requires a different defensive strategy.

The adaptive immune system thus consists of two major branches. One branch is directed against the extracellular invaders. The other is directed against intracellular invaders. Both branches depend on the use of specialized cells called lymphocytes. The body employs two major lymphocyte populations, called B and T cells. Immunity to extracellular invaders is mainly the function of B cells. They produce proteins called antibodies that promote microbial destruction. This B-cell-mediated immune response is sometimes called the "humoral immune response" as antibodies are found in body fluids (or "humors") (Box 1.1).

Because antibodies do not work inside cells, immunity to intracellular invaders is the function of T cells. T cells can destroy infected or abnormal cells. This type of response is therefore called a "cell-mediated immune response" (Fig. 1.5). T cells themselves have to be flexible and adjust their functions as needed. As a result, there are three major types of T cells. One is responsible for killing abnormal cells and hence consists of cytotoxic T cells. Another type provides the signals that activate the adaptive immune responses and hence are called helper T cells. The third cell type regulates immune responses and hence is called regulatory T cells. In addition, and most importantly, both types of adaptive immune responses generate long-lived populations of memory T and B cells that ensure that this immunity persists for a long time, perhaps even as long as the animal's lifetime.

Antibody-Mediated Immunity

Soon after it was discovered that animals could be made immune to infectious agents by vaccination (see Chapter 25), it was recognized that the substances that provided this immunity could be found in

blood serum. For example, if blood is taken from an immune horse that has been previously vaccinated against tetanus toxin (or has recovered from tetanus), its serum separated and then injected into a normal horse, the recipient animal will become temporarily resistant to tetanus (Fig. 1.6).

These protective molecules found in the serum of immune animals are proteins called antibodies. Antibodies against tetanus toxin are not found in normal horses but are produced following exposure to the toxin as a result of infection or vaccination. Tetanus toxin is an example of a foreign substance that stimulates an adaptive immune response. The general term for such a substance is an antigen. When an antigen enters an animal, the animal's B cells are stimulated to produce antibodies that bind to that antigen and ensure its destruction. Antibodies are highly specific and bind only to the antigen that stimulates their production. For example, the antibodies produced in response to tetanus toxin bind only tetanus toxin. When the antibodies bind, they "neutralize" the toxin so that it is no longer toxic. In this way, these antibodies protect animals against lethal tetanus.

The time course of the antibody response to tetanus toxin can be examined by taking blood samples from a horse at intervals after the injection of a low dose of the toxin. The blood is allowed to clot, and the clear serum is removed. The amount of antibody in the serum may be estimated by measuring its ability to neutralize a standard amount of toxin. Following a single injection of toxin into an unexposed horse, no antibody is detectable for several days (Fig. 1.7). This lag period lasts for about 1 week as responding B-cell populations grow and begin to produce antibodies. When antibodies eventually appear, their levels climb to reach a peak by 10 to 20 days before declining and disappearing within a few weeks. The amount of antibody formed, and therefore the amount of protection conferred, during this first, or primary, response is relatively small as there are few antibody-producing B cells. However, memory B cells are produced in large numbers.

If, sometime later, a second dose of toxin is injected into the same horse, it is recognized by this much larger population of memory B

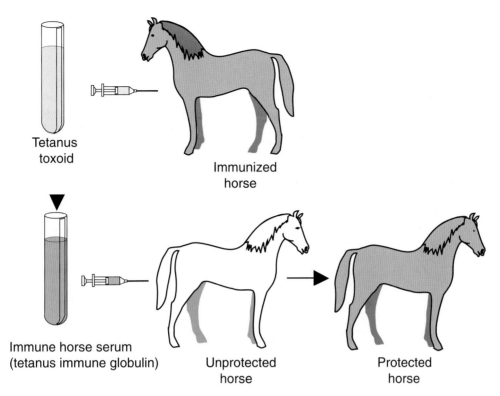

Tetanus toxoid

Immunized horse

Immune horse serum (tetanus immune globulin)

Unprotected horse

Protected horse

Fig. 1.6 Immunity to tetanus can be transferred to a normal horse by means of serum derived from an immunized horse. This clearly demonstrates that antibodies in serum are sufficient to confer immunity to tetanus in horses.

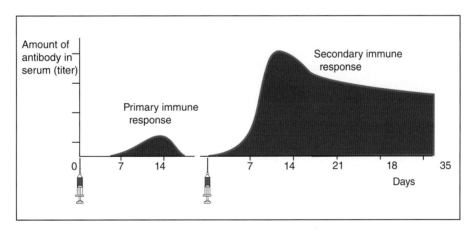

Fig. 1.7 The characteristic time course of the adaptive immune response to an antigen as measured by serum antibody levels. Note the differences between a primary and a secondary immune response. These are the reasons why the adaptive immune responses are so successful.

cells. As a result, the lag period lasts for no more than 2 or 3 days. The amount of antibody in serum then rises rapidly to a high level before declining slowly. Antibodies may be detected for many months or years after this injection. A third dose of the antigen given to the same animal results in an immune response characterized by an even shorter lag period and a still higher and more prolonged antibody response. As will be described later, the antibodies produced after repeated injections are better able to bind and neutralize the toxin than those produced early in the immune response. This progressive improvement in the adaptive immune responses following repeated injections of antigen effectively generates memory cells and is the basis of vaccination.

The response of an animal to a second dose of antigen is very different from the first in that it occurs much more quickly, antibodies reach much higher levels, and it lasts for much longer. This secondary B-cell response is specific in that it can be provoked only by a second dose of the same antigen. A secondary response may be provoked many months or years after the first injection of antigen, although its size tends to decline as time passes. A secondary response can also be induced even though the response of the animal to the first injection of antigen was so weak as to be undetectable. These features of the secondary response indicate that memory B cells possess the ability to "remember" previous exposure to an antigen. For this reason, the secondary immune response is sometimes called an anamnestic response (*anamnesko* is Greek for "memory").

A similar situation is seen when using antiviral vaccines such as those directed against the coronavirus that causes COVID-19 in humans. Multiple doses of vaccine may be required to induce sufficient memory cells to provide prolonged, strong immunity.

Cell-Mediated Immunity

If a piece of living tissue such as a kidney or a piece of skin is surgically removed from one animal and grafted onto another of the same species, it only survives for a few days before being rejected and destroyed by the recipient. This process of graft rejection is significant because it demonstrates a mechanism whereby foreign cells, differing only slightly from an animal's own normal cells, are rapidly recognized and destroyed. Even cells with minor structural abnormalities may be recognized as foreign by the immune system and destroyed. These abnormal cells include aged cells, virus-infected cells, and some cancer cells. The immune response to foreign cells as shown by graft rejection is mediated by cytotoxic T cells that identify and destroy the "abnormal" cells.

If a piece of skin is transplanted from one dog to a second, unrelated dog, it will survive for about 10 days. The grafted skin will initially appear healthy, and blood vessels will connect the graft and its host. By 1 week, however, these new blood vessels will begin to degenerate, the blood supply to the graft will be cut off, and the graft will eventually die and be shed (Fig. 1.8). If the experiment is repeated and a second graft is taken from the original donor and placed on the same recipient, then the second graft will survive for no more than a day or two before being rejected. Thus the rejection of a first graft is relatively weak and slow and analogous to a primary antibody response, whereas a second graft stimulates very rapid and powerful rejection, similar in many ways to a secondary antibody response. Graft rejection, like antibody formation, is a specific adaptive immune response in that a rapid secondary reaction occurs only if the second graft is from the same donor as the first. Like antibody formation, the graft rejection process involves the generation of long-lived memory cells, because a second graft may be rapidly rejected many months or years after the loss of the first.

However, graft rejection differs from antibody-mediated immunity in that it cannot be transferred from a sensitized to a normal animal by serum. The ability to mount a secondary reaction to a graft can only be transferred between animals by living T cells. These T cells are found in the spleen, lymph nodes, or blood, and they are responsible for organ graft rejection. It is a good example of a cell-mediated immune response.

Mechanisms of Adaptive Immunity

In some ways, the adaptive immune system may be compared to systems in a totalitarian state in which foreigners are expelled, citizens who behave themselves are tolerated, but those who "deviate" are eliminated. While this analogy must not be carried too far, clearly such regimes possess a number of characteristic features. These include border defenses and a police force that keeps the population under surveillance and promptly eliminates dissidents. In the case of the adaptive immune system the antibody-mediated responses would be responsible for keeping the foreigners out, whereas the cell-mediated responses would be responsible for stopping internal dissent. Organizations of this type also tend to develop a pass system, so that invading foreigners or dissidents not possessing certain identifying features are rapidly detected and dealt with.

Similarly, when foreign antigens enter the body, they first must be trapped and processed so that they can be recognized as being foreign. If so recognized, then this information must be conveyed either to the antibody-forming B cells or to the T cells of the cell-mediated immune system. These cells must then respond by producing specific antibodies and/or cytotoxic T cells that can eliminate the antigen. The adaptive immune system must also generate long-lived B or T memory cells that can remember this event so that the next time an animal is exposed to the same antigen, these cells will respond faster and with greater efficiency. In our totalitarian state analogy the police force would be trained to recognize selected foreigners or dissidents, keep a file on them, and respond more promptly when they reappear.

It must be emphasized, however, that just as human societies and responses are very complex and involve the interactions of thousands of individuals, so too is the immune system. While, for reasons of simplicity we discuss discrete cells, processes, and pathways, the immune system should be thought of as a huge, very complex interactive network. Thousands of different cells interact in many ways and are subject to multiple influences. The cells involved interact with each other, sometimes in a very complex fashion. Likewise, the invading microbe, its virulence, its ability to evade defenses, and its interactions with other microbes all result in variations in a host's immune response.

For introductory purposes, we can consider that adaptive immunity proceeds by a series of steps (Fig. 1.9). Thus it is triggered by cells that can recognize, trap, and process antigens. The most important of these cells are dendritic cells and macrophages. These cells then present the processed antigen to the T and B cells of the immune system. The T and B cells can recognize and respond to this processed antigen as they possess specific antigen receptors on their surface. The B cells, once activated, will produce specific antibodies, while the T cells participate in the cell-mediated immune responses. Long-lived B and T memory cells are generated at the same time. These cells retain the memory of these events and will react very rapidly to each specific antigen if it is encountered again. They are thus responsible for the enhanced immunity that develops in secondary immune responses. Finally, helper and regulatory T cells control these responses and ensure that they function at an appropriate level.

In subsequent chapters, we will first review the mechanisms involved in innate immunity. Following that, we will review adaptive immunity and examine each of its basic components in turn. We will then examine the role of the immune system in protecting animals against microbial invasion. Finally, we will look at the diseases that result when the immune system functions either excessively or inadequately.

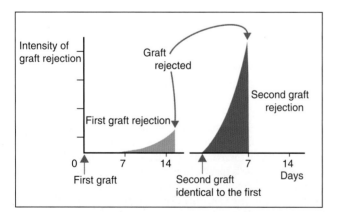

Fig. 1.8 The time course of the rejection of a foreign skin graft. The rejection of a first graft is slow and relatively mild. The rejection of a second graft is rapid and accompanied by severe inflammation. This accelerated rejection is due to the presence of memory cells. Notice the similarity of this response to that in Fig. 1.6.

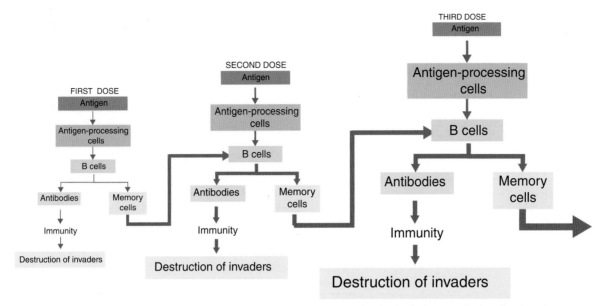

Fig. 1.9 In adaptive immunity, on first exposure to a foreign invader the body destroys the invaders but, in addition, generates memory cells. On second and subsequent exposures to that invader, these memory cells act to mediate a very much stronger immune response that results in much faster destruction of the invader. Thus the adaptive immune response strengthens over time.

WHERE TO GO FOR ADDITIONAL INFORMATION

Many veterinary journals carry articles of interest to immunologists. Some of the most important ones used in this book include *Animal Genetics, Australian Veterinary Journal, BMC Veterinary Research, Developmental and Comparative Immunology, Frontiers in Immunology (Comparative Immunology), Journal of Comparative Pathology, Journal of Veterinary Internal Medicine, Research in Veterinary Science, Trends in Parasitology, Vaccine, Veterinary Dermatology, Veterinary Immunology and Immunopathology, The Veterinary Journal,* and *Veterinary Pathology.*

For information on new developments in basic immunology (with occasional papers on subjects of veterinary interest), the reader should review journals such as *Cell, Cell Host and Microbe, Infection and Immunity, Immunity, Immunogenetics, Immunology, Journal of Immunology, Journal of Leukocyte Biology, Molecular Immunology, Nature, Nature Immunology, Nature Reviews Immunology, Proceedings of the National Academy of Sciences, Science, Trends in Immunology, Trends in Microbiology, Trends in Molecular Medicine,* and *Vaccine.*

As in many scientific fields, the World Wide Web can be a very useful source of information about veterinary immunology although care should be taken to verify the information provided. Some important sites include PubMed at http://www.ncbi.nlm.nih.gov/sites/entrez, which provides rapid access to scientific journals. You may also wish to look at the website of the American Association of Veterinary Immunologists at http://www.theaavi.org/, or your national Immunology organizations such as the American Association of Immunologists at www.aai.org/, or the British Society for Immunology at https://www.immunology.org.

2

Innate Immunity: How to Detect Invaders

The body needs an alarm system that can detect invaders and immediately activate its defenses. These must work fast as bacteria and viruses multiply incredibly rapidly. A single bacterium with a doubling time of 50 minutes can produce about 500 million offspring within 24 hours. When these microbes invade the body, they must be destroyed before they can overwhelm its defenses. Time is, therefore, of the essence, and delay can be fatal. The body must, therefore, employ fast-acting responses as its first line of defense against invaders. These response mechanisms need to be on constant standby and respond immediately to the first signs of microbial invasion and tissue damage. They constitute the first components of the innate immune system.

Because all multicellular organisms are subject to microbial attack, innate immunity has evolved over millions of years in animals and plants, vertebrates, and invertebrates. These innate immune mechanisms have evolved in different ways and at different times in response to different threats. As a result, the innate immune system can respond by using diverse subsystems or modules. The most important of these responses is inflammation.

Inflammation is the process whereby defensive cells and antimicrobial molecules rapidly converge on sites of microbial invasion and tissue damage. These defensive cells consist of the white blood cells (leukocytes) that circulate constantly in the bloodstream. Invasion triggers their migration from the bloodstream into tissues where they attack and destroy invaders. Similarly, many protective proteins, such as antibodies and complement components, are normally found only in the blood. They also enter tissues during inflammation. These defensive cells and antimicrobial proteins together destroy the invaders and repair any subsequent tissue damage. But before that happens, the alarm must go off!

HOW INVADERS ARE DETECTED

Innate immunity is activated when the body detects that it is under attack. It uses alarm signals generated either by the presence of invading microorganisms or by cellular injury. Microbial invaders express

a diverse mixture of molecules that can be recognized by the body as foreign. Collectively, these are called pathogen-associated molecular patterns (PAMPs). Similarly, molecules released from damaged and broken cells, collectively called damage-associated molecular patterns (DAMPs), also generate alarm signals. Together, the PAMPs and DAMPs bind to pattern-recognition molecules (PRMs) found on sentinel cells located throughout the body. Inflammation is triggered when PAMPS and/or DAMPs bind to their specific PRMs, and the sentinel cells respond by releasing a flood of proteins called cytokines (Fig. 2.1).

Pattern-Recognition Molecules

The innate immune system is activated when sentinel cells sense that they are under attack. Alarm signals are generated either by the presence of invading microorganisms or by dead, damaged, and dying cells. Together, the released PAMPs and DAMPs bind to PRMs expressed on or in sentinel cells located throughout the body. This binding triggers a cascade of reactions that culminate in local tissue inflammation and a systemic response that we call sickness.

Microbes not only grow very fast but also are highly diverse and can alter their surface molecules very rapidly. For this reason, the PRMs of the innate immune system do not try to recognize all possible microbial molecules. Rather, PRMs recognize abundant, essential microbial components. Because they are essential, these components are structurally conserved and are shared by entire classes of pathogens. They form, in effect, conserved molecular patterns. For example, the walls of gram-positive bacteria are largely composed of peptidoglycans and lipoteichoic acids. Similarly, the walls of gram-negative bacteria consist of peptidoglycans covered by a layer of lipopolysaccharide (LPS) (Fig. 2.2). Acid-fast bacteria are covered in glycolipids. Yeasts have a mannan- or β-glucan-rich cell wall. Viruses have unique nucleic acids. Mammals use many diverse PRMs to ensure the detection of as many of these PAMPs as possible. Most PRMs are cell-associated receptors located on cell membranes, within the cytosol and cytoplasmic vesicles (endosomes). However, others such as pentraxins, collectins, and

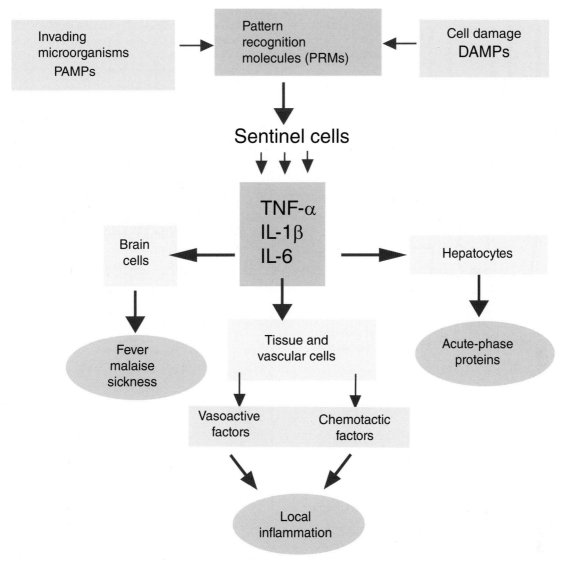

Fig. 2.1 The essential features of acute inflammation, an innate mechanism for focusing cells and other defensive molecules at sites of microbial invasion. Inflammation is triggered by microbial invasion and tissue damage. The resulting pathogen-associated molecular patterns (PAMPs) and damage-associated molecular patterns (DAMPs) signal through pattern-recognition receptors to sentinel cells that then respond by secreting a cytokine mixture that, in turn, triggers local inflammation, fever, and sickness. *IL,* Interleukin; *PRMs,* pattern-recognition molecules; *TNF-α,* tumor necrosis factor–alpha.

ficolins are soluble PRMs that circulate in the bloodstream (Fig. 2.3; Thompsen et al., 2011).

Toll-Like Receptors

The most important family of PRMs are the toll-like receptors (TLRs) (Box 2.1). Some TLRs are located on external cell surfaces, where they can bind PAMPs from extracellular invaders such as bacteria and fungi. Other TLRs are found inside cells, where they bind PAMPs from intracellular invaders such as viruses. When activated, they turn on genes involved in producing pro-inflammatory molecules. Thus they trigger a response immediately as they sense the presence of invaders or tissue damage (Akira, 2003).

TLRs are mainly expressed on the cell types most likely to encounter invaders. These include neutrophils, monocytes, macrophages, and dendritic cells. However, dendritic cells and macrophages consist of multiple subpopulations, and their TLR expression may differ between subpopulations and their degree of activation. TLRs are also expressed on T and B cells, in addition to some nonimmune cells such as the epithelial cells that line the respiratory and intestinal tracts. For example, in pigs, B cells express high levels of TLR1, TLR6, TLR9, and TLR10 (Osvaldova et al., 2017). TLR11 differs from the others in that it is found only on the dendritic cells, macrophages, and epithelial cells in the mouse urinary tract, where it binds PAMPs from bacteria and protozoan parasites. TLRs are also expressed on the bone marrow stem cells, the source of blood leukocytes. Bacterial LPS binding to TLR4 on these stem cells stimulates them to divide, thus increasing leukocyte production. An increase in leukocyte numbers in the blood (the white cell count) is, therefore, a consistent feature of mammalian infectious diseases (Baldridge et al., 2011).

All TLRs are transmembrane glycoproteins. Most are homodimers formed by paired peptide chains. They may also, however, form heterodimers by combining two different chains. For example, a TLR2 chain can associate with a TLR6 chain, and this dimer can then bind bacterial diacylated lipopeptides. TLR2 can also associate with TLR1

Gram-negative

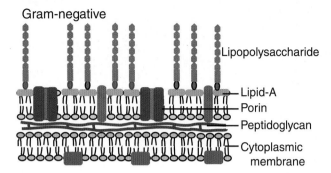

Lipopolysaccharide

Lipid-A
Porin
Peptidoglycan

Cytoplasmic
membrane

Gram-positive

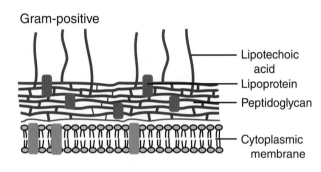

Lipotechoic
acid
Lipoprotein
Peptidoglycan

Cytoplasmic
membrane

Acid-fast

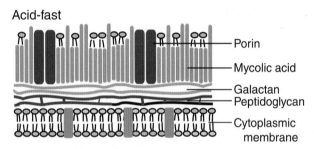

Porin

Mycolic acid

Galactan
Peptidoglycan

Cytoplasmic
membrane

Fig. 2.2 The major structural features of the cell walls of gram-negative, gram-positive, and acid-fast bacteria. It is these conserved structural molecules that serve as pathogen-associated molecular patterns and are recognized by pattern-recognition receptors such as the toll-like receptors.

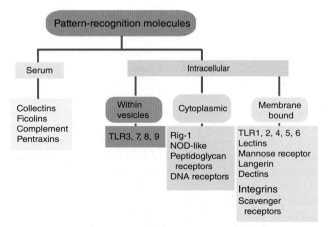

Fig. 2.3 There are many different pattern-recognition molecules used by mammals. Most are found on or within cells. Others are soluble molecules that are present in the blood serum. *NOD,* Nucleotide-binding oligomerization domain; *TLR,* toll-like receptors.

TABLE 2.1   Pathogen-Associated Molecular Patterns and the Functions of the Major Mammalian Toll-Like Receptors (TLR)

TLR	Cell Location	Ligand	Pathogens Recognized
TLR1	Cell surface	Triacylated lipoprotein	Bacteria
TLR2	Cell surface	Lipoproteins	Bacteria, viruses, parasites
TLR3	Intracellular	dsRNA	Viruses
TLR4	Cell surface	LPS	Bacteria, viruses
TLR5	Cell surface	Flagellin	Bacteria
TLR6	Cell surface	Diacylated lipoprotein	Bacteria, viruses
TLR7	Intracellular	ssRNA, guanosine	Viruses, bacteria
TLR8	Intracellular	ssRNA	Viruses, bacteria
TLR9	Intracellular	CpG DNA, dsDNA	Viruses, bacteria, protozoa
TLR10	Intracellular	Regulates TLR2 responses	Suppresses inflammation

CpG, Cytosine-guanosine; *LPS,* lipopolysaccharide.

to recognize mycobacterial triacylated lipopeptides. Given the number of possible TLR chain combinations, it is believed that the currently known TLRs can collectively bind all the major PAMPs.

Mammals possess 10 or 12 different functional TLRs (TLRs 1–10 in humans, sheep, and cattle and TLRs 1–9 and 11–13 in mice) (Table 2.1). The cell-surface TLRs (TLR1, 2, 4, 5, 6, and 11) mainly bind bacterial and fungal proteins, lipoproteins, and LPSs. For example, TLR4 on the cell surface binds LPSs from gram-negative bacteria. TLR2 binds peptidoglycans, lipoproteins, from gram-positive bacteria, and a glycolipid called lipoarabinomannan from *Mycobacterium tuberculosis.* TLR5 binds flagellin, the major protein of bacterial flagella.

The intracellular TLRs (TLR3, 7, 8, 9, and 10) bind viral and bacterial nucleic acids. For example, TLR9 senses bacterial DNA. It is, therefore, triggered by intracellular bacteria. Other intracellular receptors, such TLR3, bind viral double-stranded (ds) ribonucleic acid (RNA), whereas TLR7 and TLR8 bind viral single-stranded RNA (Fig. 2.4; Wagner, 2004; Blasius and Beutler, 2010).

Toll-Like Receptor Signaling

When a PAMP binds to its corresponding TLR, signals are passed to the cell. As a result, multiprotein signaling complexes called inflammasomes form, signal transduction cascades are initiated, and proinflammatory molecules are produced by the cell. Each step in the process involves multiple biochemical reactions involving many

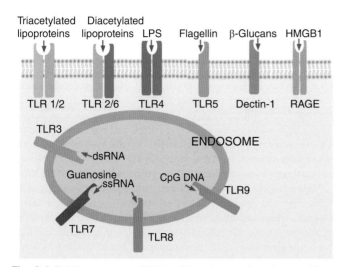

Fig. 2.4 Toll-like receptors (TLRs), either alone or in pairs, can bind a diverse array of microbial molecules. The TLRs expressed on the outer cell membrane are generally optimized to bind bacterial molecules. The TLRs expressed inside the cell in endosomes are optimized to bind viral and bacterial nucleic acids. *LPS,* Lipopolysaccharide.

different proteins. Additionally, the cell-surface TLRs use different signaling pathways than do the intracellular TLRs. All extracellular TLRs except TLR3 use an adaptor protein called MyD88 to activate the transcription factors, nuclear factor kappa-B (NF-κB), and IRF3 (Fig. 2.5). NF-κB activates the genes for three proteins, interleukin-1 (IL-1), IL-6, and tumor necrosis factor–alpha (TNF-α). IRF3 activates the gene for interferon-β (IFN-β). (For additional details on these signal transduction pathways, see Chapter 9.) (Kawasaki and Kawai, 2014).

The proteins produced in response to TLR ligation on sentinel cells are known as cytokines—proteins that regulate the behavior of cells involved in the defense of the body. The three primary inflammatory cytokines are IL-1, IL-6, and TNF-α. These cytokines are produced as inactive precursors and then activated by an enzyme called caspase-1. The production of caspase-1 is triggered by a protein complex called an inflammasome (see Chapter 4). Caspases are proteases (*c*ysteinyl *asp*artate-*s*pecific protein*ases*). Many, such as caspase-1, -4, -5, and -12, are activated by signals generated by the TLRs. Caspase-1 is most important because it acts on inactive precursors to generate the active cytokines (see Chapter 9).

Different TLRs trigger the production of different cytokine mixtures, so that different PAMPs trigger distinctly different responses from even a single cell type. For example, TLRs that bind bacterial PAMPs tend to trigger the production of cytokines optimized to combat bacteria, while those that bind viral PAMPs produce antiviral cytokines, and so forth. Activated TLRs not only trigger innate responses such as inflammation but also begin the process of "turning on" the adaptive immune system. For example, DAMPs binding to TLR4 trigger macrophages and their close relatives, the dendritic cells, to produce cytokines that are potent stimulators of lymphocytes (see Chapter 11). The intracellular TLRs detect the presence of viral nucleic acids. When triggered, they synthesize antiviral cytokines called interferons (IFNs). These IFNs turn on antiviral pathways and so "interfere" with viral growth (Fitzgerald and Kagan, 2020).

The TLRs of the major domestic mammals have been examined in detail. They appear to be similar to the TLRs of humans and rodents. They also vary in structure (they are "polymorphic"), and these variations can influence an animal's resistance to infections. Thus some bovine TLR polymorphisms are associated with increased resistance to mastitis and Johne disease (Box 2.2; Netea et al., 2012).

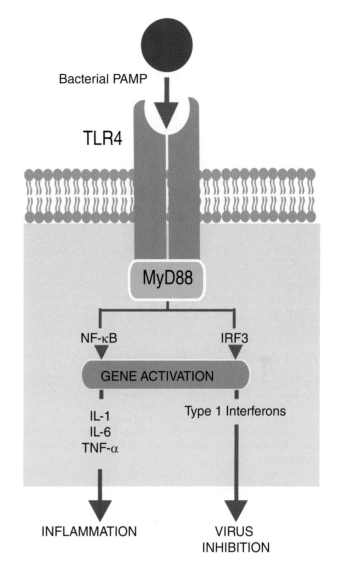

Fig. 2.5 Binding of a pathogen-associated molecular pattern such as lipopolysaccharide to a toll-like receptor (TLR) generates a signaling cascade through the signal transduction factor MyD88 that eventually activates two transcription factors, nuclear factor kappa-B (NF-κB), and IRF3. The NF-κB activates the genes for the three major cytokines, interleukin (IL)-1, IL-6, and tumor necrosis factor–alpha (TNF-α). IRF3 activates the gene for interferon-β. *PAMP,* Pathogen-associated molecular pattern.

BOX 2.2   Toll-Like Receptors (TLRs) and Diarrhea in German Shepherd Dogs

TLRs trigger the initial steps in resistance to microbial invaders. If they are ineffective, an animal may show increased susceptibility to infections. For example, chronic enteric disease is especially common in German Shepherd dogs. Genetic analysis of a large number of affected dogs showed that several single-nucleotide polymorphisms in their *TLR4* and *TLR5* genes were associated with the occurrence of this disease. It is likely that in German Shepherd dogs, changes in their TLR4 and TLR5 reduced their ability to defend against intestinal bacterial invasion. This predisposes to enteric infections, as shown by diarrhea and vomiting.

From Kathrani, A., House, A., Catchpole, B., et al., 2010. Polymorphisms in the TLR4 and TLR5 gene are significantly associated with inflammatory bowel disease in German shepherd dogs. PLOS One 5, e15740.

TABLE 2.2 Other Mammalian Pattern-Recognition Receptors

Receptor	Location	Ligand	Source of Ligand
RLRs			
RIG-1	Intracellular	Short dsRNA	RNA viruses
NLRs			
NOD1	Cytoplasm	Peptidoglycans	Bacteria
NOD2	Cytoplasm	Muramyl dipeptide	Bacteria
CLRs			
Dectins	Cell surface	Glucans	Fungi
Mannose receptor (CD206)	Cell surface	Glycoproteins	Bacteria
Others			
CD14	Cell surface	LPS	Bacteria
Peptidoglycan recognition proteins	Cell surface	Peptidoglycans	Bacteria
CD1	Cell surface	Glycolipids	Bacteria
CD36	Cell surface	Lipoproteins	Bacteria
CD48	Cell surface	Fimbria	Bacteria

CD, Cluster of differentiation; *CLR*, C-type lectin receptors; *LPS*, lipopolysaccharide; *NLR*, nucleotide-binding oligomerization domain, leucine-rich repeat (receptor); *NOD*, nucleotide-binding oligomerization domain; *RIG*, retinoic acid–inducible gene; *RLR*, retinoic acid–inducible gene–like receptor.

RIG-1-Like Receptors

TLRs are not the only pattern-recognition molecules expressed by sentinel cells (Table 2.2). Retinoic acid–inducible gene (RIG)–like receptors are a family of PRMs expressed within cells and, as a result, are important sensors of viral RNA. They can detect viral ds RNA molecules. Because dsRNA molecules do not occur in uninfected cells, their interaction with RLRs activates caspases and triggers the production of IFNs (Loo and Gale, 2011).

Nucleotide-Binding Oligomerization Domain–Like Receptors

Nucleotide-binding oligomerization domain (NOD), leucine-rich repeat receptors (NLRs) can also detect intracellular PAMPs. Although TLRs and NLRs differ in their location and function, they both react to microbial PAMPs and trigger innate responses to invaders. NOD1 and NOD2 have been most extensively studied. NOD1 binds bacterial peptidoglycans, whereas NOD2 binds muramyl dipeptides and serves as a general sensor of intracellular bacteria. Ligand binding to the NLRs activates the NF-κB pathway and triggers the production of pro-inflammatory cytokines. NOD2 binding also triggers the production of antibacterial proteins called defensins. NOD3 binds diverse ligands including many viral nucleic acids as well as inorganic particles such as silica, asbestos, and alum (Elinav et al., 2011).

AIM2 Receptors

AIM2 is a pattern-recognition receptor expressed within the cytosol of hematopoietic cells that recognized dsDNA and activates IFN responses. In humans, there are four members of the AIM2 family. It plays an important role in host defense against intracellular bacteria and viruses. Nevertheless, it is absent from dogs and cats.

Cyclic Guanosine Monophosphate–Adenosine Monophosphate Synthase

Another important DNA-binding PRM is cyclic guanosine monophosphate–adenosine monophosphate synthase (cGAS). This receptor initiates a response mediated by a downstream adaptor molecule, known as stimulator of interferon genes (STING). dsDNA activates cGAS that then binds and activates an adaptor molecule, known as STING. STING then activates the IRF3 and NF-kB pathways. The activation of these pathways by bacterial and viral dsDNA leads to the production of large quantities of IFNs, especially IFN-β as well as the NF-κB-mediated expression of inflammatory cytokines (Motwani et al., 2019).

Macrophages, mast cells, and dendritic cells express many other PRMs that can recognize microbial molecules and trigger innate responses. These include C-type lectin receptors (CLRs) that bind carbohydrates, a molecule called CD36 that binds lipoproteins, and CD1 that binds glycolipids. CD1 is an important ligand-binding molecule that is also used for the presentation of selected lipid antigens to T cells and thus triggers an adaptive response (see Chapter 20).

PATHOGEN-ASSOCIATED MOLECULAR PATTERNS

As described earlier, PAMPs are common, essential, conserved molecules that are consistently present in diverse microbial invaders. They include structural proteins such as flagellae as well as bacterial LPS, peptidoglycans, and their critical genetic material, nucleic acids.

Bacterial Lipopolysaccharides

LPS are major structural components of the cell walls of gram-negative bacteria. They are recognized by TLR4 (Vaure and Liu 2014). TLR4 does not bind LPS directly but only when linked to three other proteins. These proteins are MD-2 (myeloid differentiation factor-2), LBP, and CD14. The CD14 interacts with TLR4 in such a way that it decreases the specificity of these reactions and enables both rough and smooth strains of bacteria to be recognized. Binding of LPS to the CD14/TLR4/MD-2 complex activates macrophages and triggers cytokine production (Fig. 2.6). CD14 also binds many other bacterial molecules, including lipoarabinomannans from mycobacteria, mannuronic acid polymers from *Pseudomonas*, and peptidoglycans from *Staphylococcus aureus* (Vaure and Liu, 2014).

Bacterial Peptidoglycans

Peptidoglycans are polymers of alternating *N*-acetyl glucosamine and *N*-acetyl muraminic acid that are major constituents of the cell walls of both gram-positive and -negative bacteria (Fig. 2.2). PRMs that can bind these peptidoglycans, include some TLRs, NODs, and CD14. Peptidoglycan recognition proteins (PGRPs) are PRMs that respond by inducing the production of pro-inflammatory and antimicrobial peptides. They are found in humans, mice, cattle, and pigs. In pigs, PGRPs are expressed constitutively in the skin, bone marrow, intestine, liver, kidney, and spleen. Bovine PGRP-S (short) can kill microorganisms in which the peptidoglycan is either buried (gram-negative bacteria) or absent (*Cryptococcus*), raising questions about its precise ligand. PGRP-S also binds bacterial LPS and lipoteichoic acids (Tydell et al., 2006). It is found in bovine neutrophil granules, and these neutrophils release PGRP-S when exposed to bacteria. Thus PGRP-S probably plays a significant role in the resistance of cattle to bacterial infections.

Bacterial DNA

Bacterial DNA can stimulate innate immunity because it is structurally different from eukaryotic DNA. Much of it contains large amounts of the dinucleotide, unmethylated cytosine-guanosine (CpG). (The cytosine in eukaryotic DNA is normally methylated.) Unmethylated CpG dinucleotides bind and activate TLR9. Bacterial DNA also contains deoxyguanosine (dG) nucleotides. These dG nucleotides form molecular structures that differ from the usual mammalian DNA double helix. They also bind to TLR9 and trigger production of cytokines such as TNF-α, IL-6, and IL-12.

Viral Nucleic Acids

Viruses are simple structures, usually consisting of a nucleic acid core surrounded by a layer of proteins, the capsid, and possibly a lipid envelope (see Fig. 10.2). Viruses have few characteristic molecular signatures. However, their nucleic acids are structurally different from those in mammals, so they also bind to intracellular PRRs. TLR9 binds DNA from viruses and intracellular bacteria, whereas TLR7 and TLR8 bind ssRNA from viruses. TLR3, in contrast, mainly binds viral dsRNA, but it can also recognize some ssRNA and some dsDNA viruses. Intracellular RLRs also bind and respond to viral dsRNA. TLR7 and TLR9 activate the MyD88-mediated signaling pathways and trigger production of inflammatory cytokines and type I IFNs. TLR3 uses another signaling molecule, the "TIR-domain-containing adaptor protein inducing IFN-β" (TRIF). The TRIF pathway activates the transcription factor IRF3 that then activates the genes for inflammatory cytokines and IFN-β.

DAMAGE-ASSOCIATED MOLECULAR PATTERNS

Inflammation and sickness are triggered not only by microbial infection but also by physical trauma and tissue damage. Thus the TLRs recognize not only PAMPs from invading microorganisms but also molecules escaping from dead, dying, and damaged tissues. These molecules, collectively called DAMPs or "alarmins," are released when cells die (intracellular) or generated when connective tissue is damaged (extracellular). Other DAMPs may be produced by stimulated sentinel cells. Some of these DAMPs recruit and activate cells of the innate immune system and thus promote adaptive immunity (Fig. 2.7).

Mitochondria provide a link between PAMPs and DAMPs. Mitochondria are cytoplasmic organelles that generate energy for cells. They evolved from intracellular bacteria and hence retained many of their original bacterial features. Indeed, in many respects, they act like intracellular bacteria. For example, they have their own DNA that is rich in unmethylated CpG. When cells die, broken mitochondria may release large amounts of this DNA that can bind TLR9 and trigger inflammation. Mitochondria, like bacteria, also contain proteins with a formyl group at their amino termini. When these formylated proteins escape, they bind and attract neutrophils.

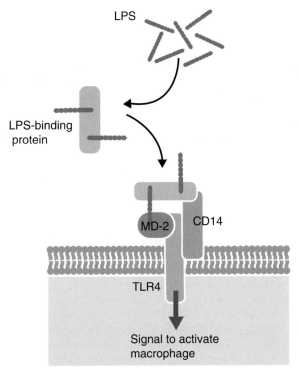

Fig. 2.6 Bacterial lipopolysaccharides cannot bind toll-like receptor (TLR) 4 directly. They must first bind to lipopolysaccharide (LPS)-binding protein and then to two other proteins, myeloid differentiation factor-2 (MD-2) and CD14, before they can bind and activate cells such as macrophages.

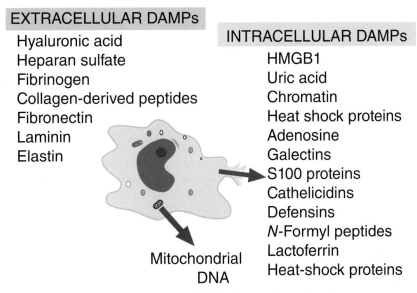

Fig. 2.7 Damage-associated molecular patterns (DAMPs) that can trigger innate immune responses such as inflammation. They are derived from both intracellular and extracellular sources.

These neutrophils leave blood vessels and move into tissues such as the lung where they release their proteases and cause damage. Thus, in animals with severe trauma, mitochondrial DNA and formyl peptides are released from damaged tissues and flood into the bloodstream. The resulting inflammatory cascade is an initiating factor for the life-threatening systemic inflammatory response syndrome (see Chapter 8).

One of the most important intracellular DAMPs is high-mobility group box protein–1 (HMGB1). HMGB1 normally binds DNA molecules and ensures that they fold correctly. However, HMGB1 is also a potent trigger of inflammation (Yanai et al., 2009). It is secreted by macrophages that have been activated by LPS or by cytokines such as IFN-γ. HMGB1 also escapes from broken cells. HMGB1 binds both TLR2 and TLR4 and thus sustains and prolongs inflammation (Sha et al., 2008). It stimulates the secretion of inflammatory cytokines from macrophages, monocytes, neutrophils, and endothelial cells. Administration of HMGB1 causes fever, weight loss, anorexia, acute lung injury, arthritis, and even death. HMGB1 stimulates the growth of new blood vessels and tissue repair. It also has potent antimicrobial activity (Yanai et al., 2009). The cytokine IL-33 is also stored within cell nuclei and released when cells die. It, too, is a potent DAMP (see Chapter 30; Andersson et al. 2002; Brown et al., 2009).

Many other molecules released from broken cells act as DAMPs. These include adenosine and adenosine triphosphate, uric acid, S100 proteins (a family of calcium-binding proteins involved in cell growth and tissue injury), and heat shock proteins. An important extracellular DAMP is heparan sulfate. This molecule is normally found in cell membranes and the extracellular matrix but is shed into tissue fluids following injury. Heparan sulfate binds and triggers TLR4 as well as some NK cell receptors.

SOLUBLE PATTERN-RECOGNITION MOLECULES

While the TLRs, NLRs, and RLRs are expressed on cell surfaces, soluble PRMs also bind PAMPs (Fig. 2.3). They promote the destruction of any organisms they encounter by causing them to be eaten by cells, a process called phagocytosis. In general, soluble PRMs do not induce the expression of inflammatory cytokines. That task is accomplished by the cell-surface PRMs (Werling and Coffey, 2007). It appears that soluble PRMs may have a special role to play on body surfaces such as the epithelial mucosa of the airways. Epithelial cells at these sites produce large quantities of these molecules that contribute to the defenses of the respiratory tract (Smole et al., 2020).

Because many bacterial PAMPs are glycoproteins and polysaccharides, circulating carbohydrate-binding lectins play important roles in innate immunity. Three extracellular lectin families, the S-, C-, and P-type lectins, are involved in this process.

C-type lectins (CTLs) are a family of carbohydrate-binding proteins with many different roles. (At least 1000 have been identified.) All require calcium to bind to their carbohydrate ligands. Each end of a CTL peptide chain has a distinct function; the C-terminal domain binds to carbohydrates, whereas the N-terminal domain interacts with cells or complement components, thereby exerting their biological effect. CTLs may be both soluble and membrane-bound. The most important of the soluble CTLs is mannose-binding lectin (MBL). MBL is found in large amounts in the blood. It has multiple sites that bind oligosaccharides, such as N-acetylglucosamine, mannose, glucose, galactose, and N-acetylgalactosamine. MBL thus binds strongly to bacteria such as Salmonella enterica and Listeria monocytogenes. It binds to Escherichia coli with moderate affinity. It binds strongly to yeasts such as Candida albicans and Cryptococcus neoformans. MBL can also bind to viruses such as influenza A as

well as parasites such as Leishmania. Bacteria coated by MBL are readily ingested by phagocytic cells. MBL plays an important role in activating the complement system. There are two forms of MBL in pigs: MBL-A and MBL-C. These can bind to Actinobacillus suis and Haemophilus parasuis. Some European pig breeds may express very low levels of MBL-C and hence suffer from increased disease susceptibility.

Multiple CTLs such as the surfactant proteins SP-A and SP-D are produced in the lungs. Six different soluble CTLs (conglutinin, MBL, pulmonary surfactant proteins [SP-A, SP-D], and collectins-46 [CL-46 and CL-43]) have been identified in mammals. However, conglutinin, CL-46, and CL-43 are restricted to cattle and their relatives, the Bovidae (see Chapter 5).

Some CTLs are expressed on cell surfaces where they can bind bacteria, fungi, and some viruses. The most important are the dectins. The dectins bind β-glucans on fungal cell walls and play an important role in antifungal defense by promoting their intracellular destruction. Dectin-1 is expressed by bovine macrophages, monocytes, and dendritic cells. Bovine dectin-2 is expressed on Langerhans cells in the skin. DEC-205 is expressed on bovine dendritic cells. Selectins are CTLs expressed on vascular endothelial cells and play a key role in the emigration of leukocytes from the bloodstream into the tissues during inflammation. Galectins are extracellular S-type lectins. Their name derives from their binding specificity for galactosides. They play a role in inflammation by binding leukocytes to the extracellular matrix. Other soluble collectins include the ficolins (H-, L-, and M-ficolins), produced by the liver and some lung cells. These, too, can bind bacterial carbohydrates and activate the complement system. There are also many cell-associated lectins. DC-SIGN, for example, is a lectin expressed on macrophages and dendritic cells. Not only does DC-SIGN recognize bacterial carbohydrates, but it also recognizes T cells and thus is used by dendritic cells to interact with T cells. The collectins are especially important in the defense of young animals whose immature adaptive immune system is not yet capable of mounting an efficient response (Thompson et al., 2011).

P-type lectins are also called pentraxins. Pentraxins are formed by five protein subunits arranged in a flat disk. They serve as pattern-recognition molecules. One face of the disk recognizes diverse molecular patterns. The opposite face interacts with complement component C1q in addition to several immunoglobulin Fc receptors. Pentraxins have multiple biological functions, including activation of complement and stimulation of leukocytes. They bind bacterial LPS in a calcium-dependent manner and activate the classical complement pathway by interacting with C1q. They also interact with Fc receptors on neutrophils, monocyte macrophages, and NK cells and augment their activities (Yang et al., 2022).

Two important pentraxins are C-reactive protein (CRP) and serum amyloid P (SAP). CRP (Pentraxin-1) is the major acute-phase protein produced in primates, rabbits, hamsters, and dogs and is important in pigs. CRP has a pentameric structure (five 20-kDa units arranged in a disk) with two faces. One face binds phosphocholine, a common side chain found in all cell membranes and many bacteria and protozoa. The other face of the disk binds to the antibody receptors FcγRI and FcγRIIa on neutrophils. CRP thus promotes the phagocytosis and removal of damaged, dying, or dead cells in addition to microorganisms. CRP can bind to bacterial polysaccharides and glycolipids and to necrotic cells, where it activates complement C1q. (Its name is derived from its ability to bind and precipitate the C-polysaccharide of Streptococcus pneumoniae.) CRP also has an antiinflammatory role as it inhibits neutrophil superoxide production and degranulation and blocks platelet aggregation. CRP stimulates fibrosis and may promote healing by enhancing the repair of damaged tissue. In lactating cows, serum CRP rises two- to fivefold. The reasons for this are unknown (see Chapter 8).

SAP is also a pentraxin (Pentraxin-2) and the major acute-phase protein in rodents (Cox et al., 2014). Like CRP, it is a PRM, where one face of the disk can bind nuclear constituents such as DNA, chromatin, and histones, as well as cell membrane phospholipids. The other face binds and activates C1q and thus triggers the classical complement pathway. A major function of SAP is to regulate innate immune responses. It interacts with macrophage Fc receptors, reduces binding of neutrophils to the extracellular matrix, reduces the differentiation of macrophages into fibroblasts thus inhibiting fibrosis, and promotes phagocytosis of cell debris. Other soluble PRMs that act as acute-phase proteins include LBP in cattle, humans, and rabbits; CD14 in humans, horses, and mice; and CTLs such as MBL and conglutinin in other species. LPS-binding protein (LBP) is an acute-phase protein that presents LPS to CD14 and TLR4 on phagocytic cells and enhances their pro-inflammatory activity up to 1000-fold. It can also bind lipotechoic acids on the cell wall of gram-positive bacteria and trigger inflammation through TLR2 activation.

SENTINEL CELLS

The cells whose primary function is to recognize and respond to invading microbes are considered sentinel cells. The major sentinel cell types, namely, macrophages, dendritic cells, and mast cells, are scattered throughout the body but are found in highest numbers just below body surfaces where invading microorganisms are most likely to be encountered. Each of these cells is equipped with multiple, diverse PRMs, so they can detect and respond rapidly to both PAMPs and DAMPs. Other cell types, such as epithelial cells, endothelial cells, neutrophils, monocytes, and fibroblasts, may also serve as sentinel cells when opportunity arises.

Macrophages

The most important sentinel cells are the macrophages. These cells are produced by the bone marrow, spend a short period of time circulating in the bloodstream where they are called monocytes, and then move into tissues where they are called macrophages. Macrophages scattered throughout the body can capture, kill, and destroy microbial invaders. When activated, they can differentiate into two populations: pro-inflammatory M1 cells and antiinflammatory M2 cells (see Chapter 19).

Dendritic Cells

The second major population of sentinel cells consists of dendritic cells, so called because many possess long, thin cytoplasmic processes called dendrites that can trap invaders. Dendritic cells encompass several distinct cell types, many of which are closely related to, or derived from, macrophages. They are discussed in detail in Chapter 11.

Mast Cells

A third population of professional sentinel cells are the mast cells. These cells, strategically located close to epithelial and endothelial surfaces, are among the first to detect pathogens and danger signals. They express multiple PRRs and are packed with cytosolic granules that store a complex mixture of inflammatory mediators. When released in response to appropriate stimuli, these mediators promote the clearance of pathogens. Long known to play a key role in allergies, it has now been recognized that they also trigger inflammation in conventional situations. Mast cells are described in detail in Chapter 30.

SPECIES DIFFERENCES

Pigs

Pigs have 10 functional TLRs. TLR2 is expressed in the thymus, spleen, Peyer's patches, mesenteric lymph nodes, and palatine tonsils. It is expressed on M cells and macrophages but not on lymphocytes (Mair et al., 2014). Other pattern-recognition receptors such as NOD1 and NOD2 have also been cloned and characterized. Similarly, pigs possess and express RIG-1, MDA5, and LGP2. These appear to be functionally similar to their human counterparts. Several porcine CLRs have also been characterized including CD69, CD205, CD207 (Langerin), DC-SIGN, and Dectin-1. Pig lungs are rich in pulmonary surfactant proteins such as the CTLs, SP-A, and SP-D. Porcine SP-D appears to have activity against influenza viruses. Porcine MBL concentrations are highly heritable in some pig breeds.

Bovine

Cattle express 10 different TLR genes. They have the usual overlapping PAMP recognition profiles, and it is clear that their primary role is to detect bacterial and viral invaders. They are all type I transmembrane proteins with a large extracellular domain (Du et al., 2021). Both *Bos taurus taurus* and *Bos taurus indicus* share haplotypes at all the TLR loci (Baldridge et al., 2011).

Cattle also possess the cytosolic PAMP recognition receptors such as RIG-1 and MDA5, and they activate sentinel cells through the NF-κB, IRF3, and IRF pathways. These, in turn, activate the inflammasomes that generate the inflammatory cytokines, TNF-α, IL-1β, and IL-6.

Dogs and Cats

Dogs possess a complete set of TLRs (TLR 1–9). They express two NOD receptors (NOD1 and NOD2). Feline TLRs have also been quantified in normal cat lymphoid tissues. Different expression patterns are found in the spleen, mesenteric lymph nodes, retropharyngeal lymph nodes, thymus, intestinal intraepithelial lymphocytes, and lamina propria lymphocytes (Ignacio et al., 2005). For example, TLR1 was detected in the spleen but not in any other lymphoid organ. TLR6 could not be detected in any of the organs tested. In the thymus TLR7 and TLR9 predominated. Feline B cells, CD4+ and CD8+ T cells all express TLR2, 5, and 7–9.

Horses

Equine TLRs, TLR2, 3, 4, 5, 7, and 8, have been fully sequenced (Jungi et al., 2011).

REFERENCES

Akira, S., 2003. Mammalian toll-like receptors. Curr. Opin. Immunol. 15, 5–11.

Andersson, U., Erlandsson-Harris, H., Yang, H., Tracey, K.J., 2002. HMGB1 as a DNA-binding cytokine. J. Leukoc. Biol. 72, 1084–1091.

Baldridge, M.T., King, K.Y., Goodell, M.A., 2011. Inflammatory signals regulate hematopoietic stem cells. Trends Immunol. 32, 57–65.

Blasius, A.L., Beutler, B., 2010. Intracellular toll-like receptors. Immunity 32, 305–315.

Brown, M.P., Trumble, T.N., Merritt, K.A., 2009. High-mobility group box chromosomal protein 1 as a potential inflammatory biomarker of joint injury in thoroughbreds. Am. J. Vet. Res. 70, 1230–1235.

Cox, N., Pilling, D., Gomer, R.H., 2014. Serum amyloid P: a systemic regulator of the innate immune response. J Leukoc. Biol. 6 (5), 739–743.

Du, X., Poltorak, A., Wei, Y., Beutler, B., 2021. Three novel mammalian toll-like receptors: gene structure expression, and evolution. Eur. Cytok. Network 1, 362–371.

Elinav, E., Strowig, T., Henao-Mejia, J., Flavell, R.A., 2011. Regulation of the antimicrobial response by NLR proteins. Immunity 34, 665–679.

Fitzgerald, K.A., Kagan, J.C., 2020. Toll-like receptors and the control of immunity. Cell 180, 1044–1066.

Ignacio, G., Nordone, S., Howard, K.E., Dean, G.A., 2005. Toll-like receptor expression in feline lymphoid tissues. Vet. Immunol. Immunopathol. 10, 229–237.

Jungi, T.W., Farhat, K., Burgener, I.A., Werling, D., 2011. Toll-like receptors in domestic animals. Cell Tissue Res. 343, 107–120.

Kawasaki, T., Kawai, T., 2014. Toll-like receptor signaling pathways. Front. Immunol. https://doi.org/10.3389/fimmu.2014.00461

Loo, Y.M., Gale, M.J.R., 2011. Immune signaling by RIG-I-like receptors. Immunity 34, 680–692.

Mair, K.H., Sedlak, C., Käser, T., Pasternak, A., Levast, B., et al., 2014. The porcine innate immune system: an update. Dev. Comp. Immunol. 45, 321–343.

Motwani, M., Pesiridis, S., Fitzgerald, K.A., 2019. DNA sensing by the cGAS-STING pathway in health and disease. Nat. Rev. Genet. https://doi.org/10.1038/s41576-0151-1

Netea, M.G., Wijimenga, C., O'Neill, L.A.J., 2012. Genetic variation in toll-like receptors and disease susceptibility. Nat. Immunol. 13, 535–542. 2012

Osvaldova, A., Stepanova, H., Faldyna, M., Matiasovic, J., 2017. Gene expression pattern-recognition receptors in porcine leukocytes and their response to Salmonella enterica serovar Typhimurium infection. Res. Vet. Sci. 114, 31–35.

Sha, Y., Zmijewski, J., Xu, Z., Abraham, E., 2008. HMGB1 develops enhanced proinflammatory activity by binding to cytokines. J. Immunol. 180, 2531–2537.

Smole, U., Kratzer, B., Pickl, W.F., 2020. Soluble pattern recognition molecules: guardians and regulators of homeostasis at airway mucosal surfaces. Eur. J. Immunol. 50, 624–642.

Thomsen, T., Schlosser, A., Holmskov, U., Sorensen, G.L., 2011. 2011. Ficolins and FIBCD1: soluble and membrane bound pattern recognition molecules with acetyl group selectivity. Mol. Immunol. 48, 369–381.

Tydell, C.C., Yuan, J., Tran, P., Selsted, M.E., 2006. Bovine peptidoglycan recognition protein-S: antimicrobial activity, localization, secretion, and binding properties. J. Immunol. 176, 1154–1162.

Vaure, C., Liu, Y., 2014. A comparative review of toll-like receptor 4 expression and functionality in different animal species. Front. Immunol. https://doi.org/10.3389/fimmu.2014.00316

Wagner, H., 2004. The immunobiology of the TLR9 subfamily. Trends Immunol. 25, 381–386.

Werling, D., Coffey, T.J., 2007. Pattern recognition receptors in companion and farm animals: the key to unlocking the door to animal disease? Vet. J. 174, 240–251.

Yanai, H., Ban, T., Wang, Z., et al., 2009. HMGB proteins function as universal sentinels for nucleic-acid-mediated innate immune responses. Nature 462, 99–103.

Yang, R., Hu, J., Zeng, B., Yang, D., et al., 2022. Structural characterization of immune receptor family short pentraxins, C-reactive protein and serum amyloid P component, in primates. Dev. Comp. Immunol. https://doi.org/10.1016/j.dci.2022.104371

Humoral Innate Immunity: Inflammation

Acute inflammation develops within minutes after tissues are damaged by invading microorganisms. Broken cells release alarmins (or damage-associated molecular patterns [DAMPs]). Invading microbes provide pathogen-associated molecular patterns (PAMPs). Both types of signals trigger sentinel cells to make and release three cytokines, interleukin-1 (IL-1), IL-6, and tumor necrosis factor–α (TNF-α) from sentinel cells (Fig. 2.1) This primary cytokine cascade in turn activates nearby target cells, causing them to release a mixture of secondary mediators—small, bioactive molecules that cause the vascular and cellular responses associated with inflammation. In addition, pain due to tissue damage causes sensory nerves to release bioactive peptides. This complex mixture of bioactive molecules collectively attracts defensive white blood cells (leukocytes) and at the same time acts on blood vessels, resulting in increased local blood flow leading to redness, swelling, and pain. These responses amplify innate resistance and eventually result in tissue repair and the restoration of homeostasis.

INFLAMMASOMES

The first steps in inflammation occur when PAMPs and DAMPs bind to pattern recognition receptors on sentinel cells and initiate the assembly of large multiprotein complexes called inflammasomes (Fig. 3.1). Inflammasomes are molecular machines that assemble within the cell cytosol after exposure to PAMPs and DAMPs. They initiate and then regulate the inflammatory response through the release of a flood of cytokines.

Each inflammasome chain consists of three subcomponents. A C-terminal ligand-binding domain that recognizes PAMPs and DAMPs. A central nucleotide-binding adaptor domain and an N-terminal effector domain (Fig. 3.2). There are two major types of inflammasome (Lamkanfi and Dixit, 2014). One type employs ALR (AIM2-like receptors) proteins such as AIM2 in its ligand-binding domain. The other type of inflammasome uses one of a family of NLR proteins (NLRP or NLRC) as its ligand-binding sensors. (The NLRP and NLRC inflammasomes differ in their N-terminal effector domains.) Once the inflammasome complex is assembled, its effector domain is activated, and cytokines such as TNF-α, IL-1β, IL-6, and IL-18 are produced, activated, and released. Although some inflammasomes require toll-like receptor

(TLR)–mediated activation and downstream nuclear factor kappa B (NF-κB)–mediated transcription of pro-IL-1 and pro-IL-18, others do not require this transcriptional activation step (Vrentas et al., 2018).

Inflammasome-mediated responses are important in controlling microbial infections as well as in regulating some metabolic processes and immune responses. Inflammasomes can be generated by many different stimuli. Thus dsDNA activates the AIM2 complex; anthrax toxin activates NLRP1, while bacterial flagellin activates NLRC4. As a result, inflammasomes are assembled and pro-caspase-1 activated. This activated caspase-1 acts on pro-IL-1 and pro-IL-18, to generate the active forms of these cytokines (Bryant and Fitzgerald, 2009).

Interestingly, cats lack both AIM2 and NLRP1 inflammasomes. Dogs also lack AIM2 and have only a truncated form of NLRC4. It has been suggested that this may serve to reduce the severity of some inflammatory responses in these species (Cui and Zhang, 2021). Caspase-1-deficient mice are more susceptible to bee and snake venoms, suggesting that inflammasomes also play a role in defense against envenomation.

PRODUCTS OF SENTINEL CELLS

Sentinel cells thus synthesize and secrete the cytokines that trigger inflammation and inhibit microbial growth. They also initiate the first steps in adaptive immunity. The cytokines diffuse to other nearby cells, bind to their specific receptors, and trigger secondary responses.

Cytokines

Sentinel cell signaling pathways activate the genes that result in inflammasome activation and the synthesis and secretion of the three major cytokines. These are called TNF-α, IL-1, and IL-6. TNF-α is produced very early in inflammation and is followed by waves of IL-1 followed by IL-6. At the same time, stimulated sentinel cells synthesize enzymes, such as nitric oxide synthase 2 (NOS2), that in turn generate nitric oxide (NO), a powerful and lethal antimicrobial oxidant. They also make the enzyme cyclooxygenase-2 (COX-2) that generates inflammatory lipids such as prostaglandins and leukotrienes. If these molecules enter the circulation and reach the brain and liver, they cause a fever and sickness (see Chapter 7). If the sentinel cells detect the presence

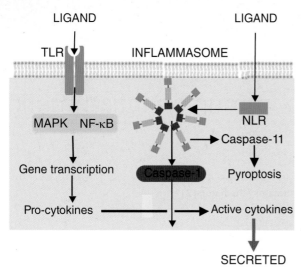

Fig. 3.1 Pathogen-associated molecular patterns signaling through NOD-like receptors generate large, star-shaped, multiprotein complexes called inflammasomes. Inflammasomes generate caspase-1 that activates cytokines such as interleukin (IL)-1 and IL-18. Inflammasomes mediate the production of inflammatory cytokines as well as their activating caspases. *NF-κB,* Nuclear factor kappa B; *TLR,* toll-like receptor.

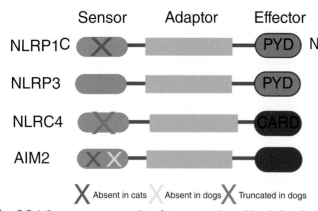

Fig. 3.2 Inflammasomes consist of aggregated peptide chains that form a star-shaped structure. These chains consist of three components. A sensor domain that receives signals by binding ligands such as pathogen-associated molecular patterns and damage-associated molecular patterns, an adaptor domain, and an effector domain. This can be a pyrin domain (PYD) or a caspase activating domain (CARD). This activates a pro-caspase that, when activated, activates interleukin (IL)-1, IL-18, and tumor necrosis factor–α. There are multiple forms of inflammasome, each triggered by different ligands. Interestingly, dogs and cats do not possess all the components found in other mammals.

of damaged or foreign DNA or RNA, such as that from viruses, they will also secrete the antiviral molecules called interferons (IFNs) (see Chapter 9).

Tumor Necrosis Factor-α

TNF-α is a protein of 17 kDa produced by macrophages, monocytes, mast cells, endothelial cells, T cells, B cells, and fibroblasts in response to TLR stimulation (Fig. 3.3). It is initially membrane-bound but is subsequently cleaved from the cell surface by a protease called TNF-α convertase. TNF-α acts through two receptors: TNFR1 is found on diverse cell types, where it can bind both soluble and membrane-bound

TNF-α, while TNFR2 is restricted to the cells of the immune system and responds only to membrane-bound TNF-α.

Soluble TNF-α in turn triggers the release of chemokines and cytokines from nearby cells and promotes the adherence, migration, attraction, and activation of leukocytes such as neutrophils.

TNF-α is an essential mediator of inflammation because, in combination with IL-1, it triggers changes in small blood vessels. A local increase in TNF-α causes the classic signs of inflammation, including heat, swelling, pain, and redness. Circulating TNF-α can depress cardiac output, induce microvascular thrombosis, and cause capillary leakage. TNF-α acts on neutrophils to enhance their ability to kill microbes. It attracts neutrophils to sites of tissue damage and increases their adherence to the vascular endothelium. It stimulates macrophage phagocytosis and oxidant production. It amplifies and prolongs inflammation by promoting macrophage synthesis of important enzymes such as NOS2 and COX-2, and it also activates mast cells. TNF-α induces macrophages to increase its own synthesis together with that of IL-1. As its name implies, TNF-α can kill some tumor cells as well as virus-infected cells. In high doses, TNF-α can cause septic shock. Mast cell-derived TNF is required for neutrophil recruitment to inflamed skin because it activates endothelial cells and triggers chemokine release. Mast cells are situated around blood vessels, and the TNF causes them to release their TNF-containing granules in a specific direction, directly into the blood vessels, thus sensitizing any circulating neutrophils and specifically attracting them to the degranulation sites (Dudeck et al., 2021).

TNF-α is a member of a family of related cytokines. Other important members of this family include TNF-β (or lymphotoxin) (see Chapter 9), CD40L (see Chapter 20), and FasL (CD95L) (see Chapter 19).

Interleukin-1

When stimulated through CD14 and TLR4, sentinel cells such as macrophages also synthesize cytokines belonging to the IL-1 family. The most important of these are IL-1α and IL-1β. IL-1β is synthesized as a large precursor protein that is cleaved by caspase-1 to form the active 17.5-kDa molecule. Ten- to 50-fold more IL-1β is produced than IL-1α, and whereas IL-1β is secreted, IL-1α remains attached to the cell surface. As a result, IL-1α only acts on cells that directly contact macrophages (Fig. 3.4). (This is known as juxtacrine signaling.) Like TNF-α, IL-1β acts on nearby cells to initiate and amplify inflammation. For example, it acts on vascular endothelial cells to make them adhesive for neutrophils. IL-1 also acts on macrophages to stimulate their synthesis of NOS2 and COX-2 (Dinarello, 2018). Transcription of IL-1β messenger RNA occurs within 15 minutes of ligand binding. It reaches a peak 3 to 4 hours later and levels off for several hours before declining.

During severe infections, IL-1β circulates in the bloodstream where, in association with TNF-α, it is responsible for sickness behavior. Thus it acts on the brain to cause fever, lethargy, and malaise. It acts on muscle cells to mobilize amino acids, causing pain and fatigue. It acts on liver cells to induce the production of new proteins, called acute-phase proteins, that also assist in the defense of the body (see Chapter 8).

The most important IL-1 receptors are CD121a and CD121b. CD121a is a signaling receptor, whereas CD121b is not. CD121b thus binds IL-1, but nothing more happens. IL-1 activity is also regulated by IL-1 receptor antagonist (IL-1RA), a protein that binds and blocks CD121a. IL-1RA is therefore an important regulator of IL-1 activity and inflammation. It reduces mortality in septic shock and graft-versus-host disease and has antiinflammatory effects (see Chapter 8).

IL-1 is a member of a large family of cytokines that regulate innate immune responses. Other important family members include IL-1RA,

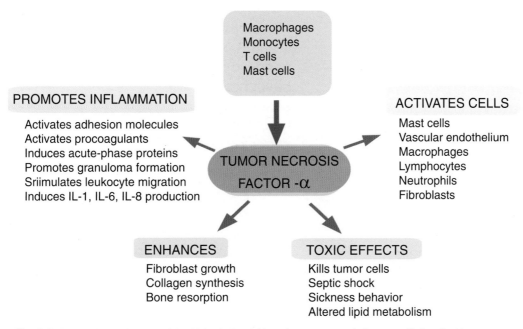

Fig. 3.3 The origins and some of the biological activities of tumor necrosis factor–α. *IL*, Interleukin.

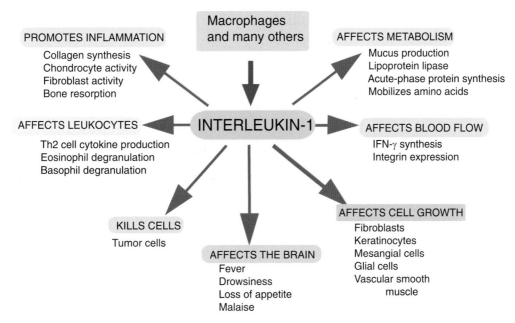

Fig. 3.4 The origins and some of the biological activities of interleukin-1. *IFN*, Interferon.

IL-18, IL-33, IL-36, IL-37, and IL-38 (see Chapter 9 and Appendix 3). Some, like IL-36, have a proinflammatory effect, while others such as IL-37, have antiinflammatory effects.

Interleukin-6

The third of the major cytokines produced by sentinel cells is IL-6. IL-6 is a glycoprotein of 21 kDa produced by macrophages, T cells, and mast cells (Fig. 3.5). Its production is triggered by bacterial endotoxins, as well as by IL-1 and TNF-α. IL-6 promotes inflammation, especially in response to tissue damage, and it is a major mediator of fever, the acute-phase response, and septic shock. IL-6 receptors are found on T cells, neutrophils, macrophages, hepatocytes, and neurons. IL-6 also

has an antiinflammatory role in that it inhibits some of the activities of TNF-α and IL-1 and promotes the production of the suppressive cytokine IL-10. It has been suggested that IL-6 regulates the transition from a neutrophil-dominated process early in inflammation to a macrophage-dominated process later (Kaplanski et al., 2003).

IL-6 signals to target cells through a heterodimeric receptor with a cytokine-binding antigen-binding chain (IL-6Rα) and a signal transducing chain, gp130. IL-6R can form soluble complexes with IL-6, and these can then act on target cells that only express gp130 (gp130 is ubiquitous, so many cell types can respond to IL-6). IL-6 is released by skeletal muscle cells in response to exercise where it exerts an antiinflammatory role.

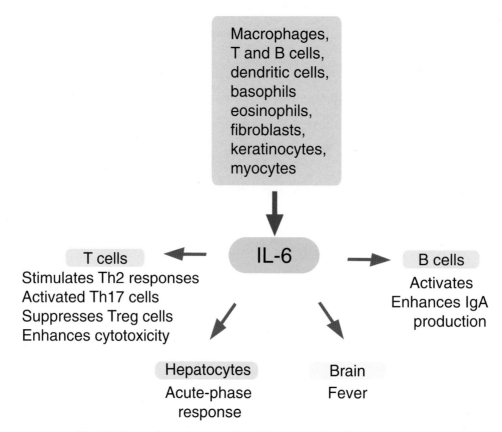

Fig. 3.5 The origins and some of the biological activities of interleukin-6 (IL-6).

Interleukin-18

The first cytokine wave triggers the production of IL-18. IL-18 is an IL-1 family member of 17 kDa that is constitutively produced by all cells but especially by macrophages, monocytes, keratinocytes, and other epithelial cells. Like IL-1β, it is synthesized as an inactive precursor and then activated by the actions of caspase-1. IL-18 promotes inflammation by promoting nitric oxide and chemokine production. However, it does not induce a fever. IL-18 also activates Th1 and NK cells to promote the production of IFN-γ, TNF-α, IL-1, CD95L, and several chemokines. This can lead to positive feedback where the IL-18 and IFN-γ reinforce each other's activities (see Chapter 9). IL-18 activity is controlled by a naturally occurring, high-affinity, IL-18-binding protein (Dinarello et al., 2013).

Interleukin-31

IL-31 is a protein of 18 kDa and a member of the IL-6 family. It is produced by activated Th2 cells, mast cells, macrophages, basophils, and dendritic cells. Its receptors are expressed on keratinocytes and other epithelial cells, eosinophils, activated macrophages, and especially on dorsal root ganglia neurons and peripheral neurons. When activated, they signal to cells through the Janus kinase pathway. IL-31 is a potent inducer of itch and skin inflammation. IL-31 is released by Th2 cells partially in response to histamine acting through H2 receptors. IL-31 activity can be blocked by the monoclonal antibody, Lokivetmab (see Chapter 31).

Chemokines

Once activated by the initial cytokine wave, sentinel cells also secrete a mixture of small chemotactic proteins called chemokines. These chemokines attract leukocytes to sites of microbial invasion. Chemokines are a large family of at least 50 small (8–10 kDa) proteins (Baggiolini, 1998). They coordinate the migration and position of leukocytes at inflammatory sites and in lymphoid tissues and hence dictate the course of many inflammatory and immune responses (Table 3.1; Luster, 2019). Chemokines are produced by sentinel cells, including macrophages and mast cells. They are classified into four subfamilies based on their amino acid sequences (Fig. 3.6). For example, the alpha (or CXC) chemokines have two cysteine (C) residues separated by another amino acid (X), whereas the beta (or CC) chemokines have two contiguous cysteine residues. (Chemokine nomenclature is based on the following classification: each molecule or receptor receives a numerical designation, and in addition, ligands have the suffix "L" [e.g., CXCL8], whereas receptors have the suffix "R" [e.g., CXCR1].)

In addition to structural criteria, chemokines may be classified functionally. Thus, inflammatory chemokines are upregulated in inflammation and are mainly involved in leukocyte recruitment. Other chemokines promote new blood vessel growth. Some are found in normal tissues where they regulate cellular migration and homing, and many have overlapping functions (Baggiolini, 2001).

One of the most important chemokines is CXCL8 (also called IL-8). CXCL8 attracts and activates neutrophils, releasing their granule contents and stimulating their respiratory burst (see Chapter 6). Another important CXC chemokine is CXCL2 (also called macrophage inflammatory protein–2, MIP-2), which is secreted by macrophages and also attracts neutrophils.

CC chemokines act predominantly on macrophages and dendritic cells. Thus CCL3 and CCL4 (MIP-1α and -1β) are produced by macrophages and mast cells. CCL4 attracts CD4+ T cells whereas CCL3 attracts B cells, eosinophils, and cytotoxic T cells. CCL2 (monocyte chemotactic protein-1, MCP-1) is produced by macrophages, T cells,

TABLE 3.1 Nomenclature of Some Selected Chemokines, Their Receptors, and Their Targets

Current Names	Receptor	Target Cells
α Family		
CCL2/MCP-1	CCR2	Monocytes, memory T cells, dendritic cells
CCL3/MIP-1α	CCR1, CCR5	Neutrophils, macrophages, T cells, NK cells
CCL4/MIP-1β	CCR5	NK cells, monocytes
CCL5	CCR1, CCR3, CCR5	T cells, eosinophils, basophils
CCL7/MCP-3	CCR3	Monocytes, eosinophils
CCL8	CCR3	Monocytes
CCL11/Eotaxin 1	CCR3	Eosinophils
CCL13/MCP-4	CCR3	Monocytes, eosinophils, T cells, basophils
CCL20/MIP-3α	CCR6	Lymphocytes
CCL22	CCR4	Monocytes, dendritic cells, activated T cells
CCL24/Eotaxin 2		Eosinophils
CCL26/Eotaxin 3	CCR3	Eosinophils
CCL28	CCR3	Resting T cells, eosinophils
β Family		
CXCL1	CXCR2	Neutrophils
CXCL8/IL-8	CXCR1, CXCR2	Neutrophils
CXCL12	CXCR4	Monocytes, T cells
CXCL13	CXCR5	B cells
γ Family		
XCL1/lymphotactin	XCR1	T cells
δ family		
CX3CL1/fractalkine	CX3CR1	T cells, monocytes

The classification of chemokines is based on the location and spacing of their cysteine (C) residues and their separation by other (X) amino acids. *L*, Ligand; *R*, receptor.

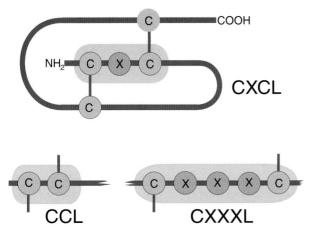

Fig. 3.6 The classification of chemokines is based on the location and spacing of their cysteine (C) residues and their separation by other (X) amino acids.

fibroblasts, keratinocytes, and endothelial cells. It attracts and activates monocytes, stimulating their respiratory burst and lysosomal enzyme release. CCL5 is produced by T cells and macrophages. It attracts monocytes, eosinophils, and some T cells. It activates eosinophils and stimulates histamine release from basophils.

Two chemokines fall outside the CC and CXC families. Lymphotactin (XCL1) is a C (only one cysteine residue) or gamma chemokine that is chemotactic for lymphocytes. Its receptor is XCR1. Fractalkine (CX3CL1) is a CXXXC (two cysteines separated by three amino acids) or delta chemokine that triggers adhesion by T cells and monocytes. Its receptor is CX3CR1.

Most chemokines are produced in infected or damaged tissues and attract other cells to sites of inflammation or microbial invasion. It is likely that the chemokine mixture produced by damaged or infected tissues regulates the precise composition of incoming inflammatory cell populations. In this way, the body can adjust the inflammatory response to optimize the destruction of different microbial invaders. Many chemokines, such as CXCL4, CCL20, and CCL5, are structurally similar to the antimicrobial proteins called defensins and, like them, have antibacterial activity (Gangur et al., 2002).

Chemokines play a major role in inflammation in domestic animals. Cattle possess chemokines not found in humans (Mestas and Hughes, 2004). For example, regakine-1 is a CC chemokine found in bovine serum that acts with CXCL8 and C5a to attract neutrophils and enhance inflammation (Widdison and Coffey, 2011). Chemokines can be detected in many bovine inflammatory diseases, including bacterial pneumonia, mastitis, arthritis, and endotoxemia. Impaired neutrophil migration is associated with certain specific CXCR2 genotypes in cattle, and this may result in their increased susceptibility to mastitis (Rambeaud and Pighetti, 2005).

Interferons

Among the most important innate defenses against viral invasion is the IFN system. IFNs are antiviral cytokines. There are three types of IFNs, type I that includes most importantly IFN-α and IFN-β, type II that includes IFN-γ, and type III that includes the IFN-λs. The IFNs are generated in response to signaling through PRMs and their associated inflammasomes. When IFNs act on cellular targets, they upregulate hundreds of IFN-stimulated genes—the interferome. The interferome is complex and most importantly, differs significantly between mammalian species. As might be expected, the antagonism between the IFNs and invading viruses results in an "arms race." Comparative studies on the type I interferome have now revealed that as expected, although the number of IFN upregulated genes varies between species, their distribution pattern is generally similar. Some such as cattle and sheep are similar as expected; however, the human and pig interferomes are also closely related.

INFLAMMATORY MEDIATORS

In addition to stimulating further cytokine production, the primary cytokine wave triggers the release of diverse inflammatory compounds from nearby tissues. These small inflammatory molecules act on blood vessels and leukocytes. In its classic form, acute inflammation is said to have five major symptoms (or cardinal signs): heat, redness, swelling, pain, and loss of function. These symptoms result from changes in small blood vessels brought about by "vasoactive" molecules (Fig. 3.7). When inflammation is first triggered by TNF-α and IL-1, the blood flow through small capillaries at the injection site decreases. This gives leukocytes an opportunity to bind to the vessel walls. Shortly thereafter, the small blood vessels in the damaged area dilate, and blood flow to the injured tissue increases greatly.

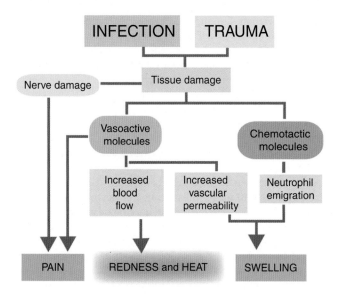

Fig. 3.7 The major signs of acute inflammation and how they are generated.

TABLE 3.2 Some Vasoactive Molecules Produced During Acute Inflammation

Mediator	Major Source	Function
Histamine	Mast cells and basophils, platelets	Increased vascular permeability, pain
Serotonin	Platelets, mast cells, Basophils	Increased vascular permeability
Kinins	Plasma kininogens and tissues	Vasodilation Increased vascular permeability, pain
Prostaglandins	Arachidonic acid	Vasodilation, increased vascular permeability
Thromboxanes	Arachidonic acid	Increased platelet aggregation
Leukotriene B_4	Arachidonic acid	Neutrophil chemotaxis Increased vascular permeability
Leukotrienes C, D, E	Arachidonic acid	Smooth muscle contraction Increased vascular permeability
Platelet-activating factor	Phagocytic cells	Platelet secretion Neutrophil secretion Increased vascular permeability
Fibrinogen breakdown products	Clotted blood	Smooth muscle Neutrophil chemotaxis Increased vascular permeability
C3a and C5a	Serum complement	Mast cell degranulation Smooth muscle contraction Neutrophil chemotaxis (C5a)

At the same time as these changes in blood flow occur, cellular responses are also taking place. Changes in nearby vascular endothelial cells permit neutrophils and monocytes to adhere to them. If the blood vessels are damaged, platelets may bind to the injured endothelium and release vasoactive and clotting molecules. Inflamed tissues swell as a result of the leakage of fluid from blood vessels. This leakage occurs in two stages. First, there is an immediate increase caused by vasoactive molecules produced by sentinel cells, damaged tissues, and nerves (Table 3.2). The second phase of leakage occurs several hours after the onset of inflammation, at a time when the leukocytes are beginning to emigrate. Endothelial and perivascular cells contract so that they pull apart and allow fluid and cells to escape through the intercellular gaps. After the invaders are eliminated, the inflammation is terminated, and blood flow returns to normal.

Vasoactive molecules come from multiple sources. Some are derived from inactive precursors in plasma. Others are derived from sentinel cells such as macrophages and mast cells; from leukocytes such as neutrophils, basophils, and platelets; or from damaged tissue cells. Stimulated sensory nerves may also produce neurotransmitters that cause vasodilation and increased permeability.

Vasoactive Amines

Two of the most important of the vasoactive molecules released by mast cells are histamine and serotonin. Histamine is a small amine of 111 kDa derived from the amino acid L-histidine by decarboxylation (Fig. 3.8). Histamine receptors are expressed on nerve cells, smooth muscle cells, endothelial cells, neutrophils, eosinophils, monocytes, dendritic cells, and T and B cells. When histamine binds to these receptors, it stimulates endothelial cells to produce nitric oxide, a potent vasodilator. At the same time, the histamine causes blood vessel leakage, leading to fluid escape and tissue edema. Histamine also upregulates TLR expression on sentinel cells (Talreja et al., 2004; Peters and Kovacic, 2009).

Serotonin (5-hydroxytryptamine, 5-HT) is a derivative of the amino acid L-tryptophan (Fig. 3.8). Serotonin is stored in blood platelets and in the mast cells of some rodents and the large domestic herbivores. Serotonin normally causes a vasoconstriction that results in a rise in blood pressure (except in cattle, in which it is a vasodilator). It has little effect on vascular permeability, except in rodents, in which it induces acute inflammation.

Vasoactive Lipids

When tissues are damaged or sentinel cells are stimulated, inflammasomes activate phospholipases that act on cell wall phospholipids to produce arachidonic acid (Von Moltke et al., 2012). The enzyme 5-lipoxygenase then converts this arachidonic acid to biologically active lipids called leukotrienes (Fig. 3.9). Another enzyme, called cyclooxygenase, converts the arachidonic acid to a second family of vasoactive lipids called prostaglandins. The collective term for all these complex lipids is eicosanoids. Both leukotrienes and prostaglandins act as local inflammatory mediators (Harizi et al., 2008).

Four leukotrienes promote leukocyte recruitment, survival, and activation. The most important of these leukotriene B_4 (LTB_4) is a neutrophil attractant and activator produced by neutrophils, macrophages, and mast cells. LTB_4 also stimulates eosinophil chemotaxis and random motility. Leukotrienes C_4, D_4, and E_4, in contrast, increase vascular permeability and cause slow, smooth muscle contraction. All three contain the amino acid cysteine conjugated to the lipid backbone, so they are called cysteinyl leukotrienes. They are produced by mast cells, eosinophils, and basophils. The cytokine IL-13 upregulates the production of LTD_4 and its receptor, whereas LTD_4 upregulates IL-13 production. This feedback loop is a major contributor to severe inflammation.

There are four groups of proinflammatory prostaglandins: PGE_2, PGF_2, the thromboxanes (TxA_2, PGA_2), and the prostacyclins (PGI_2).

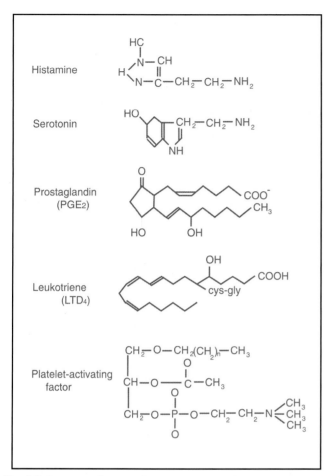

Fig. 3.8 Structure of some of the major vasoactive molecules generated during acute inflammation.

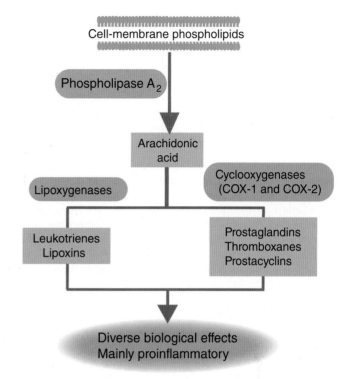

Fig. 3.9 The production of leukotrienes and prostaglandins by the actions of lipoxygenase and cyclooxygenase on arachidonic acid. Both prostaglandins and leukotrienes may have proinflammatory or antiinflammatory activity depending on their chemical structure. Note that the leukotrienes are linked to the amino acid cysteine.

Although prostaglandins can be generated by most nucleated cells, the prostacyclins are produced by vascular endothelial cells, and the thromboxanes come from platelets. The biological activities of the prostaglandins vary widely, and since many different prostaglandins are released in inflamed tissues, their net effect on inflammation may be complex (Ricciotti and Fitzgerald, 2011).

As neutrophils enter inflamed tissues, their 15-lipoxygenase generates lipoxins from arachidonic acid. These oxidized eicosanoids inhibit neutrophil migration. Thus, as inflammation proceeds, there is a gradual switch in production from proinflammatory leukotrienes to antiinflammatory lipoxins. The rise in PGE$_2$ in tissues also inhibits 5-lipoxygenase activity and eventually suppresses inflammation.

Activated neutrophils, mast cells, platelets, and eosinophils produce a phospholipid called platelet-activating factor (PAF). PAF makes endothelial cells even stickier and thus enhances neutrophil adhesion and emigration. PAF aggregates platelets, makes them release their vasoactive molecules, and synthesizes thromboxanes. It acts on neutrophils in a similar fashion. Thus it promotes neutrophil aggregation, degranulation, chemotaxis, and the release of oxidants. PAF is about 10,000 times more effective than histamine in increasing vascular permeability. It is incredibly potent, and its activity can be detected at concentrations as low as 10^{-12} M.

Vasoactive Peptides

When the complement system is activated, several small peptides are cleaved off from their peptide chains (see Chapter 5). Two of these small peptides, C3a and C5a, have significant proinflammatory activity and are called anaphylatoxins. The anaphylatoxins are potent inflammatory mediators. They mediate chemotaxis, regulate vascular dilation and permeability, and kill bacteria. They cause smooth muscle contraction, induce wheal-and-flare reactions on intradermal injection, and activate platelets. They can induce a respiratory burst in macrophages, neutrophils, and eosinophils. The anaphylatoxins bind to receptors on mast cells, promoting degranulation and the release of histamine and leukotrienes. They stimulate the release of eosinophil cationic protein and promote eosinophil migration. They modulate the release of IL-6 and TNF-α from B cells and monocytes. They are also potent attractants for monocytes, neutrophils, activated B and T cells, basophils, and mast cells (Klos et al., 2009).

Kinins

Much of the mast cell granule contents consist of the highly sulfated proteoglycan heparin. This is released when mast cells degranulate. The heparin promotes the activation of proteases called kallikreins. Once activated, the kallikreins in turn act on kininogens to release small vasoactive peptides called kinins. Kinins not only increase vascular permeability but they also stimulate smooth muscle contraction and trigger pain receptors. They may also have antimicrobial activity. The most important of these kinins is bradykinin. Bradykinin contains nine amino acids: Arg-Pro-Pro-Gly-Phe-Ser-Pro-Phe-Arg. It increases vascular permeability and vasodilation. Bradykinin also causes pain and fever. Bradykinin is involved in the activation of neutrophils, dendritic cells, and macrophages (Oschatz et al., 2011).

Neuropeptides

Many peptides produced by neurons affect both inflammation and immunity. One of the most important of these peptides is substance P (SP). SP acts both as a neurotransmitter as well as a mediator of inflammation. SP is released from sensory nerve terminals in response to stressors. It is also produced by inflammatory cells including macrophages, eosinophils, lymphocytes, and dendritic cells. SP induces degranulation and the release of histamine and serotonin by mast cells. SP activates the arachidonate pathway to trigger prostaglandin synthesis. It is a potent vasodilator and a bronchoconstrictor and plays an important role in pain and itch perception (Harrison et al., 2001).

THE COAGULATION SYSTEM

When blood vessels dilate and fluid leaks from the bloodstream into the tissues, the blood coagulation system is activated. Platelet aggregation accelerates this process. Activation of the coagulation system generates large quantities of thrombin, the main clotting enzyme. Thrombin acts on fibrinogen in tissue fluid and plasma to produce insoluble fibrin. Fibrin fibers are therefore deposited in inflamed tissues, where they form a barrier to the spread of infection. Activation of the coagulation cascade also initiates the fibrinolytic system. This leads to the activation of plasminogen activator, which in turn generates plasmin, a potent fibrinolytic enzyme. In destroying fibrin, plasmin releases peptide fragments that attract neutrophils.

REFERENCES

Baggiolini, M., 1998. Chemokines and leukocyte traffic. Nature 392, 565–568.

Baggiolini, M., 2001. Chemokines in pathology and medicine. J. Intern. Med. 250, 91–104.

Bryant, C., Fitzgerald, K.A., 2009. Molecular mechanisms involved in inflammasome activation. Trends Cell Biol. 19, 455–464.

Cui, H., Zhang, L., 2021. Key components of inflammasome and pyroptosis pathways are deficient in canines and felines, possibly affecting their responses to SARS-CoV-2 Infection. Front. Immunol. https://doi.org/10.3389/fimmu.2020.592622.

Dinarillo, C.A., 2018. Overview of the IL-1 family in innate inflammation and acquired immunity. Immunol. Revs. 281, 8–27.

Dinarello, C.A., Novick, D., Kim, S., Kaplanski, G., 2013. Interleukin-18 and IL-18 binding protein. Front. Immunol. 4 (Article 289), 1–10.

Dudeck, J., Kotrba, J., Immler, R., Hoffmann, A., et al., 2021. Directional mast cell degranulation of tumor necrosis factor into blood vessels primes neutrophil extravasation. Immunity 54, 468–483.

Gangur, V., Birmingham, N.P., Thanesvorakul, S., 2002. Chemokines in health and disease. Vet. Immunol. Immunopathol. 86, 127–136.

Harizi, H., Corcuff, J.B., Gualde, N., 2008. Arachidonic-acid-derived eicosanoids: roles in biology and immunopathology. Trends Mol. Med. 14, 461–469.

Harrison, S., Geppetti, P., 2001. Substance P. Int. J. Biochem. Cell. Biol. 33, 555–576.

Kaplanski, G., Marin, V., Montero-Julian, F., et al., 2003. IL-6: a regulator of the transition from neutrophil to monocyte recruitment during inflammation. Trends Immunol. 24, 25–30,.

Klos, A., Tenner, A.J., Johswich, K.O., Ager, R.R., Reis, E.S., Kohl, J., 2009. The role of anaphylatoxins in health and disease. Mol. Immunol. 46 (14), 2753–2766. https://doi.org/10.1016/j.molimm.2009.04.027.

Lamkanfi, M., Dixit, V.M., 2014. Mechanisms and functions of inflammasomes. Cell 157, 1013–1022.

Luster, A.D., 2019. Introduction: global positioning by chemokines and other mediators. Immunol. Revs. 289, 5–8.

Mestas, J., Hughes, C.C.W., 2004. Of mice and men: differences between mouse and human immunology. J. Immunol. 172, 2731–2738.

Oschatz, C., Maas, C., Lecher, B., et al., 2011. Mast cells increase vascular permeability by heparin-initiated bradykinin formation in vivo. Immunity 34, 258–268.

Peters, L.J., Kovacic, J.P., 2009. Histamine: metabolism, physiology, and pathophysiology with applications in veterinary medicine. J. Vet. Emerg. Crit. Care 19, 311–328.

Rambeaud, M., Pighetti, G.M., 2005. Impaired neutrophil function associated with specific bovine CXCR2 genotypes. Infect. Immun. 73, 4955–4959.

Ricciotti, E., Fitzgerald, G.A., 2011. Prostaglandins and inflammation. Arterioscler. Thromb. Vasc. Biol. 31, 986–1000.

Talreja, J., Kabir, M.K., Filla, M.B., et al., 2004. Histamine induces toll-like receptor 2 and 4 expression in endothelial cells and enhances sensitivity to gram-positive and gram-negative bacterial cell wall components. Immunology 113, 224–233.

Von Moltke, J., Trinidad, N.J., Moayeri, M., Kintzer, A.F., et al., 2012. Rapid induction of inflammatory lipid mediators by the inflammasome in vivo. Nature 490, 107–111.

Vrentas, C.E., Schaut, R.G., Boggiatto, P.M., Olsen, S.C., et al., 2018. Inflammasomes in livestock and wildlife: insights into the intersection of pathogens and natural host species. Vet. Immunol. Immunopathol. 201, 49–56.

Widdison, S., Coffey, T.J., 2011. Cattle and chemokines: evidence for species-specific evolution of the bovine chemokine system. Anim. Genet. 42, 341–353.

4

Humoral Innate Immunity: Antimicrobial Peptides

Given the essential nature of innate immunity in a world dominated by microbes, it is unsurprising that animals and plants employ their own antibiotics to provide an immediate barrier to microbial invasion. These molecules are antimicrobial peptides that are constitutively present in normal tissues, especially just under body surfaces. They do not have to be induced and are available immediately when they are needed. Antimicrobial peptides are widely distributed throughout the plant and animal kingdoms, and more than 800 different sequences have been identified to date. Different mammals employ their own specific sets of peptides that have evolved in response to microbial invasion. In general, they fall into three categories. One group typified by the enzyme lysozyme consists of enzymes that can destroy microbial structures. A second group consists of molecules that bind essential elements such as iron or zinc and hence restrict microbial growth. The third group discussed in this chapter is peptides that have the ability to disrupt microbial surface membranes. This third group consists of two major peptide families, the defensins and the cathelicidins. Although structurally diverse, the defensins and cathelicidins usually contain multiple arginine and lysine residues, making them cationic, and they have both hydrophobic and hydrophilic regions. The hydrophobic regions can bind and insert themselves into the lipid-rich membranes of bacteria, whereas the other regions can form channel-like pores or simply cover the bacterial membrane, resulting in membrane disruption and death. These antimicrobial peptides can kill both gram-positive and -negative bacteria as well as some fungi, protozoa, enveloped viruses, and tumor cells.

Antimicrobial peptide production is usually concentrated in sites where microbes are most likely to be encountered. Thus they are present in the largest amounts on and under epithelial surfaces. Epithelial cells of the skin (keratinocytes) and respiratory, alimentary, reproductive, and genitourinary tracts also synthesize many antimicrobial peptides. They are also produced by inflammatory cells and are thus found in the cytoplasmic granules of neutrophils and macrophages (see Chapter 6) as well as within secondary lymphoid organs (see Chapter 13).

The production of antimicrobial peptides by epithelial cells is regulated by cytokines. The two cytokines produced by Th17 cells, IL-17 and IL-22, are crucial regulators of antimicrobial peptide production in the intestine and lungs (see Chapter 23). Likewise, IL-1 stimulates epithelial cells to produce antimicrobial peptides. These antimicrobial peptides may regulate cytokine production and can also serve as immunomodulators. For example, some cathelicidins stimulate the production of the cytokines, IL-6, and IL-10.

These defense peptides have the ability to lyse any negatively charged cell membrane that doesn't contain cholesterol (Linde et al., 2008). Thus they can bind strongly to bacterial surface phospholipids and cause the bacterial membrane to collapse, forming pores (Fig. 4.1). As a result, they can destroy both gram-positive and -negative bacteria, fungi, intracellular parasites, and enveloped viruses. Some of these peptides may also kill some cancer cells. In addition to their killing ability, some peptides can act as chemoattractants for immature dendritic cells, thus serving to promote adaptive immunity. They can also induce CXCL8 production, attracting neutrophils to infection sites. They can also promote phagocytosis by acting as opsonins, and they enhance the cytotoxicity of natural killer (NK) cells (see Chapter 20; Linde et al., 2008).

DEFENSINS

The most important of the antimicrobial peptides are the defensins (Fig. 4.2; Sahi et al., 2005). Defensins are peptides containing 28 to 42 amino acids arranged in a β-sheet crosslinked by three or four disulfide bonds. More than 50 different mammalian defensins have been identified. They are classified as α-, β-, or θ-defensins based on their origin and on the number and position of their intrachain disulfide bonds (Bagnicka et al. 2010). The α-defensins account for about 15% of the total protein in human neutrophil granules. In cattle, at least 13 different α-defensins are produced by neutrophils alone. They are also found in the granules of Paneth cells in the small intestine of herbivores. When released into the intestine, they influence the composition of the intestinal microbiota (Fig. 23.7). α-Defensins are also present in rabbits, rodents, and primates (Lynn and Bradley, 2007).

β-Defensins are much more broadly expressed across mammalian orders. They are constitutively expressed in the epithelial cells that line the airways, skin, salivary gland, reproductive, and urinary systems (Patil et al., 2004; Sang et al., 2005a,b; Leonard et al., 2012a,b). Theta defensin is a circular peptide found only in the neutrophils of some nonhuman primates such as the rhesus macaque.

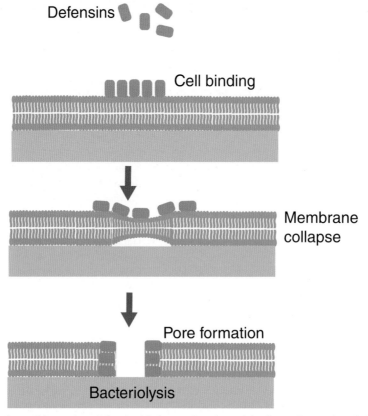

Fig. 4.1 Cationic peptides such as defensins bind strongly to bacterial cell membrane phospholipids, causing membrane collapse and pore formation. This is lethal for many bacteria.

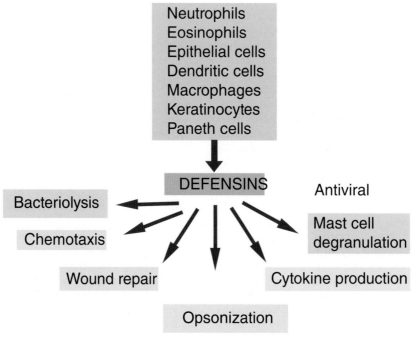

Fig. 4.2 The multiple origins and functions of the defensins.

Defensins may be produced at a constant rate (constitutively) or in response to microbial infection. Some defensins attract monocytes, immature dendritic cells, and T cells. Their production is stimulated by the inflammatory cytokines, IL-1β and TNF-α. All defensins identified so far can kill or inactivate bacteria, fungi, or enveloped viruses. Some defensins can also neutralize microbial toxins such as those from *Bacillus anthracis*, *Corynebacterium diphtheriae*, and *Staphylococcus aureus*. Although present in normal tissues, defensin concentrations increase in response to infections (Box 4.1).

Defensins are expressed in large amounts in human neutrophils where they amount to 30% to 50% of the protein content of the azurophilic granules. Mouse neutrophils, on the other hand, do not express any defensins! Conversely, Paneth cells located in the small intestine of mice express more than 20 different defensins, while human Paneth cells express only two (Mestas and Hughes, 2004).

In humans, leukocytes are attracted toward antimicrobial peptides expressed at infected sites. Thus neutrophil-derived defensins can

---

BOX 4.1   The Big Picture

The complete bovine genome has been sequenced, and unexpectedly, it was found to contain an unusually large number of genes associated with innate immunity. For example, cattle have 10 cathelicidin genes, compared with only 1 in humans and mice. They have about 106 defensin genes, compared with 30 to 50 in humans and mice. They have many more interferon genes than other species, including a hitherto undescribed family, IFN-X (see Chapter 28). It has been suggested that this duplication and divergence of genes involved in innate immunity may be a consequence of the huge load of microorganisms in the rumen and the resulting increased need to prevent microbial invasion. Alternatively, these new genes may be necessary since living within dense herds may promote infectious disease transmission between individuals and thus require a more effective immune system. Additionally, cattle show substantial differences from other mammals in the genes related to lactation. Many of these lactation-associated genes, such as those for serum amyloid A, β$_2$-microglobulin, and the cathelicidins, are also related to innate immunity. Finally, the cattle genome contains 10 lysozyme genes, largely expressed in the abomasum and gastrointestinal tract. It is speculated that they may play a role in killing bacteria entering the intestine from the rumen.

From Elsik, C.G., Tellam, R.L., Worley, K.C., et al., 2009. The genome sequence of taurine cattle: a window to ruminant biology and evolution. Science 324, 522–527.

---

attract monocytes, naïve T cells, and immature dendritic cells. There are also variations in gene copy numbers (1–12 in humans), and it is suggested that this may affect their susceptibility to some autoimmune diseases (Machado and Ottolini, 2015).

CATHELICIDINS

A second major family of antibacterial peptides found in neutrophil granules is the cathelicidins (Zhu and Gao, 2017)—otherwise called myeloid antimicrobial peptides (Fig. 4.3). They are stored in the secretory granules of neutrophils and macrophages and released only when these cells are activated. They are 12 to 100 amino acids in size with a characteristic "cathelin" domain at their C-terminus. They are stored in inactive form and activated by proteolytic cleavage when released. In addition to their antibacterial activity, they are also immunomodulatory (van Harten et al., 2018). Humans, dogs, cats, and mice have only a single cathelicidin gene, whereas pigs, cows, goats, and horses have multiple cathelicidins. Pig skin, for example, generates 11 cathelecidins. Porcine cathelicidin PR-39 has been shown to promote wound repair, angiogenesis, and neutrophil chemotaxis. They all have broad-spectrum antibacterial activity. As with other antimicrobial peptides, they interact with the negatively charged lipid membranes of microorganisms. However, because of their high cationic charge, they can also interfere with protein synthesis and DNA replication since cathelicidins efficiently bind bacterial nucleic acids. They can then deliver these nucleic acids to dendritic cells and as a result trigger a very strong IFN-α response (Baumann et al., 2014). The bovine cathelicidin BMAP-28 induces apoptosis and may serve to get rid of unwanted cells. Canine cathelicidin K9CATH has broad-spectrum activity against both gram-positive and -negative bacteria (Sang et al., 2007). Many cathelicidins have been given species specific names such as protegrins from pigs and ovispirins from sheep. Cathelicidins have a variety of immunomodulatory functions including the control of inflammation by influencing wound repair, angiogenesis, and chemotaxis (Araujo et al., 2022).

OTHER PEPTIDES

Platelet Microbicidal Proteins

In addition to their roles in the blood coagulation cascade, platelets play an important defensive role. They produce many diverse peptides that also have antimicrobial activity. For example, they produce multiple chemokines with bactericidal properties (termed kinocidins).

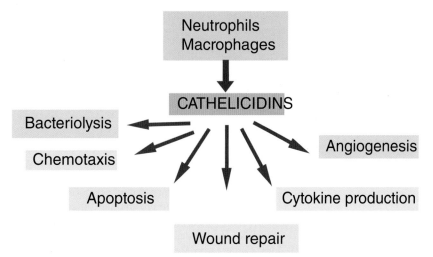

Fig. 4.3 The origins and multiple functions of cathelicidins.

Kinocidins are larger than the major cationic peptides described above and are more structurally complex. In addition to their bactericidal functions, they can also potentiate leukocyte activities. Platelets also produce several beta-defensins (thrombocidins), and in humans, they produce a bactericidal RNAse (Aquino-Dominguez et al., 2021). Equine platelet lysates have in vitro bacteriostatic effects against *S. aureus* but not *Escherichia coli* (Avellar et al., 2022).

Pentraxin 3

Pentraxin 3 (PTX3) is an octameric protein with eight pentraxin domains and a long N-terminus. PTX3 is rapidly produced in response to TNF-α, IL-1β, and some microbial components. It is produced by monocytes/macrophages, neutrophils, endothelial cells, and stromal cells. Neutrophils synthesize PTX3 during myelopoiesis and store it in their granules. They release it on exposure to microbial products (Mantovani and Garlanda, 2023). PTX3 levels rise faster than C-reactive protein in acute-phase responses (see Chapter 8) since it is stored preformed and thus rapidly released from neutrophil granules. PTX3 has been identified in the lung fluids, endothelial cells, alveolar macrophages, and neutrophils of pigs, foals, and calves. In pigs, it has antibacterial effects against *Streptococcus suis* (Xu et al., 2015). PTX3 can bind to diverse bacteria, fungi, and viruses and promote innate immunity to them. It can activate complement and play a role in the removal of apoptotic and necrotic cells (Townsend et al., 2023).

Other Peptides

Granulysins are peptides produced by cytotoxic T cells and NK cells. In addition to their antibacterial functions, granulysins attract and activate macrophages. Two other important antibacterial proteins are bactericidal permeability-increasing protein (BPI) and calprotectin. BPI is a major constituent of the primary granules of human and rabbit neutrophils. It kills gram-negative bacteria by binding to lipopolysaccharides and damaging their inner membrane. Calprotectin is found in human neutrophils, monocytes, macrophages, and epidermal cells. It forms about 60% of neutrophil cytosolic protein and is released in large amounts into the blood and tissue fluid during inflammation. Calprotectin sequesters zinc and manganese during bacterial infections and thus makes them unavailable for bacterial growth. Serprocidins are a family of antimicrobial serine proteases also found in human neutrophil granules.

Lysozyme

The enzyme lysozyme cleaves the bond between *N*-acetyl muraminic acid and *N*-acetyl glucosamine and destroys cell wall peptidoglycans in gram-positive bacteria. Lysozyme is found in all body fluids except cerebrospinal fluid and urine. It is present in large amounts in inflammatory tissue fluid. While absent from bovine neutrophils and tears, it is present in high concentrations in the tears of other mammals. Although many of the bacteria killed by lysozyme are nonpathogenic, it might reasonably be pointed out that this susceptibility could account for their lack of pathogenicity. Lysozyme is found in high concentrations in neutrophil granules and accumulates in areas of acute inflammation, including sites of bacterial invasion. Lysozyme is also a potent opsonin, binding to bacterial surfaces and facilitating phagocytosis in the absence of specific antibodies and under conditions in which its enzyme activity is ineffective (see Chapter 27).

SPECIES DIFFERENCES

Bovine

Four gene clusters encode the β-defensins in cattle and dogs. Cattle possess at least 106 β-defensin genes; the most found in any mammal so far (There are 34 in pigs, 38 in dogs, 48 in mice, and 48 in humans). Cattle do not possess any α-defensins. Their defensins play a major role in combating bacterial infections and possibly in regulating the gut microbiota. The defensins are mainly expressed in the respiratory tract, the mammary gland, small intestine, colon, and reproductive organs. *Mannheimia hemolytica* infection in bovine lungs induces increased defensin expression in airway epithelium. Calves infected with *Cryptosporidium parvum* or *Mycobacterium paratuberculosis* also show a significant increase in intestinal defensin (cryptdin) production (Cormican et al. 2008).

Milk Peptides

Antibacterial peptides such as lactoferrin and casecidin are found in bovine milk. Lactoferrin sequesters iron. Casecidin and multiple other antimicrobial peptides are derived by proteolytic chymosin digestion of milk caseins and can inhibit the growth of multiple streptococcal and staphylococcal species (Mohanty et al., 2015). A related casein-derived 23 amino acid N-terminal peptide has been called, isracidin. This has potent antibacterial activity against staphylococci. It also has antifungal activity as well as some immunostimulating activity (Lahov and Regelson, 1996). Kappacidin is a peptide derived from bovine κ-casein. Other active peptides may be derived from β-lactoglobulin.

Indolicidin is an antibacterial peptide found in bovine neutrophils. It only contains 13 amino acids and thus is one of the smallest antimicrobial peptides known. Its sequence is ILPWKWPWWPWRR-NH$_2$. Note that it contains five tryptophan(W) residues, and it can assume multiple configurations. It is a member of the cathelicidin family. It can readily insert itself into lipid bilayers. It does not appear to cause membrane disruption but interferes with protein and DNA synthesis. It is active against both gram-positive and -negative bacteria, fungi, and some viruses (Araujo et al., 2022).

Bactenecin is also a very small (12 amino acid) antibacterial peptide found in bovine neutrophils. Its sequence is RLCRIVVIRVCR-NH$_2$. The two cysteine residues form a disulfide bond thus folding the chain over. Bactenecin is especially active against gram-negative bacteria (Sun et al., 2019).

Sheep

Two β-defensins have been identified in the respiratory and gastrointestinal tracts of sheep. However, unlike cattle, these are not found in neutrophils (Linde et al., 2008). Sheep β1-defensin is upregulated in the lungs of newborn lambs infected with ovine parainfluenza virus but not with respiratory syncytial virus. There are potentially eight sheep cathelicidins but only two have been isolated.

Pigs

Multiple host defense peptides have been identified in pigs (Chen et al., 2010). They are active against a diverse spectrum of organisms both in vitro and in vivo. Among the gene families that have expanded in the porcine immunome are the cathelicidins. Thus pigs have ten cathelicidin genes compared to just one in humans and mice. They possess at least five protegrin sequences. Protegrins are elastase-activated cathelicidins with potent antibacterial properties. At least 12 different β-defensins have been reported in pigs as well (Sang et al., 2005a,b). Porcine β-defensin 1 is absent from the upper respiratory tract of newborn piglets perhaps explaining their susceptibility to pneumonia at that age. No α-defensins have been detected in pigs. There are also significant breed differences in the expression of defensins in different pig tissues. Thus their levels are much higher in Meishan pigs than in Duroc × Yorkshire × Landrace crossbreeds (Chen et al., 2010).

Horses

Horses are equipped with a diverse variety of bactericidal peptides. These include at least one lysozyme, five cathelicidins, nine defensins, one psoriasin, one hepcidin, and five equinins (Bruhn et al., 2011). Equinins are a group of closely related proteinase inhibitors found in the granules of equine neutrophils as well as in their tracheobronchial secretions. They can inhibit microbial proteinase K and subtilisin and some have antibacterial and antiviral functions. For example, they can kill *Streptococcus zooepidemicus*, *E. coli*, and *Pseudomonas aeruginosa*. They are also active against equine herpesvirus 2 (Pellegrini et al., 1998).

The horse relies to a much greater extent than other mammals on intestinal α-defensins. (They are absent from cattle, pigs, and dogs.) Transcription analysis has identified at least 38 α-defensin transcripts in the horse. Of these, at least 20 are functional (Bruhn et al. 2011).

Horse β-defensins are constitutively expressed in many different tissues including the heart, liver, lungs, pancreas, kidney, and especially the Paneth cells of the gastrointestinal tract (Fig. 23). Analysis has identified nine possible β-defensin genes. Horses also possess multiple α-defensin genes. The equine defensin DEFA1, is an enteric defensin exclusively produced in Paneth cells. It has potent activity against the major horse pathogens, especially *Prescotella (Rhodococcus) equi* and *Streptococcus equi* (Bruhn et al., 2009; Leonard et al., 2012a,b). The equine cathelicidins are stored in an inactive form in neutrophil granules.

Dogs

Analysis of the canine genome has identified 43 β-defensin genes and pseudogenes arranged in four clusters (Leonard et al., 2012a,b). The canine β-defensin genes *(CBD)* are numbered, *CBD1, CBD 102* to *CBD 142*. Two additional defensin genes are sperm associated. Defensins are expressed in many canine tissues. These include the testes, kidney, palatine tonsil, trachea, lung, gastrointestinal tract, liver spleen, mononuclear cells, bone marrow, and skin. One of these defensins CBD 103 has been widely studied. It has been shown to have antibiotic activity against *E. coli*, many species of *Staphylococci, Streptococci, Micrococcus,* and *Bacilli* as well as *P. aeruginosa, Enterococcus faecium, Lactobacillus acidophilus, Actinobacillus actinomycetemcomitans, Porphyromonas gingivalis, Burkholderia cepacia,* and *Bordetella bronchiseptica* as well as fungi such as *Candida albicans, Saccharomyces cerevisiae,* and *Malassezia pachydermatis* (Aono et al., 2019).

The single canine cathelicidin (K9CATH) is expressed in epithelial cells and leukocytes. It is present at high levels in bone marrow with lower levels in gastrointestinal tract, spleen, liver, testes, and skin. In some species, cathelicidins contain a sequence that enables them to respond to vitamin D3. This sequence is absent in canine cathelicidin. Canine cathelicidin has broad-spectrum antibacterial activity. Its targets include *S. aureus, E. coli,* and *Listeria monocytogenes*.

β-Defensins are expressed at high levels in dog skin. They not only act as endogenous antibiotics, but they also promote chemotaxis and wound healing. Canine skin and respiratory epithelium express large quantities of CBD103. As described in Box 4.2, CBD103 occurs in two forms. One allele has a 3-base pair deletion and binds to the melanocortin 1 receptor, promoting the production of black pigment and hence a black dog. There appears to be no difference in the potent bactericidal activities of the two canine alleles of CDB103 (Leonard et al., 2012a,b). Interestingly, the presence of atopic dermatitis in dogs (see Chapter 31) has no effect on skin defensin levels. This is different from humans where defensin levels are reduced in atopic skin.

Defensins have been identified in the urogenital tract of humans, and other primates as well as laboratory rodents and dogs (Defensins play a role in sperm maturation and capacitation. Sperm bind certain β-defensins on their surface. These sperm-bound defensins are important in promoting sperm migration through cervical mucus and binding to oviduct epithelial cells) (Leonard et al., 2012a,b). CBD102

BOX 4.2 Defensins and Dog Coat Color

Despite the great varieties of hair color seen in dog breeds, they are generated by a relatively simple mechanism involving just two types of pigments—Black eumelanin and yellow pheomelanin. Dogs such as Labrador Retrievers use a unique pathway to generate a black coat. Two genes control this pathway, *Agouti* and *Melanocortin 1 receptor (Mc1R)* acting through a ligand-receptor system (Fig. 4.4). A third gene influences the melanocortin pathway—a gene that encodes a β-defensin! A mutation in the canine defensin gene, *CBD103* correlates with black coat color in 38 different breeds. It has been shown that the mutated CBD103 product binds with high affinity to the Mc1R. Normally, Mc1R signals to melanocytes are blocked by the Agouti peptide so that, as a result, the cells produce pheomelanin and the dog has a yellow coat. However, if the dominant variant allele of *CBD103* binds to *Mc1R* then agouti is prevented from binding, Mc1R is activated, and signals are transmitted to the melanocyte instructing it to make eumelanin and the dog, therefore, grows a black coat.

From Candille, S.I., Kaelin, C.B., Cattanach, B.M., Yu, B., et al. 2007. A β-defensin mutation causes black coat color in domestic dogs. Science 318, 1418–1423.

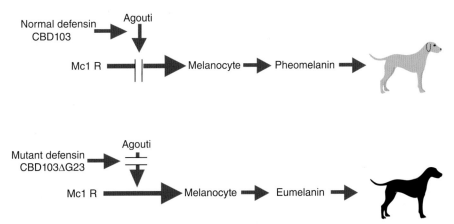

Fig. 4.4 The effect of the mutant defensin gene CBD103ΔG23, on coat color in dogs.

expression is limited to the testes. It is present in Sertoli and Leydig cells and almost certainly plays a role in the defense of the male reproductive system (Sang et al., 2005a,b).

Three defensins, CBD1, CBD103, and CBD108 are present in canine respiratory tract epithelial cells. These three are also readily expressed in skin cells. CBD 103 has antimicrobial activity against the canine pathogen *B. bronchiseptica* (Erles and Brownlie, 2010). CBD103 is expressed throughout the canine nasal cavity, especially in the nares. As well as in respiratory and olfactory epithelia. Both forms of CBD 103 caused membrane blebbing, condensation of intracellular contents, and cell wall lysis in *E. coli* and *S. aureus* (Aono et al., 2019).

Cats

Feline defensin feBD103 has been identified in cat skin (Leonard et al., 2012a,b). Feline cathelicidin is also highly expressed in the bone marrow and neutrophils. It is expressed at low levels in the skin. As in the dog, this defensin lacks a VDRE sequence suggesting that it is unresponsive to vitamin D3.

REFERENCES

Aono, S., Dennis, J.C., He, S., Wang, W., et al., 2019. Exploring pleiotropic functions of canine β-defensin 103: nasal cavity expression, antimicrobial activity, and melanocortin receptor activity. Anat. Rec. https://doi.org/10.1002/ar.24300.

Aquino-Dominguez, A.S., Romero-Tlalolini, M.A., Torres-Aguilar, H., Aguilar-Ruiz, S.R., 2021. Recent advances in the discovery and function of antimicrobial molecules in platelets. Int. J. Mol. Sci. 22, 10230. https://doi.org/10.3390/ijms221910230.

Araujo, J.B., Sastre de Souza, G., Lorenzon, E.B., 2022. Indolicidin revisited: biological activity, potential applications and perspectives of an antimicrobial peptide not yet fully explored. World J. Microbiol. Biotech. https://doi.org/10.1007/s11274-022-03227-2.

Avellar, H.K., Lutter, J.D., Ganta, C.K., Beard, W., et al., 2022. In vitro antimicrobial activity of equine platelet lysate and mesenchymal stromal cells against common clinical pathogens. Can. J. Vet. Res. 86, 59–64.

Bagnicka, E., Strzalkowska, N., Jozwik, A., Krzyzewsli, J., et al., 2010. Expression and polymorphism of defensins in farm animals. Acta Biochem. Pol. 57 (4), 487–497.

Baumann, A., Demoulins, T., Python, S., Summerfield, A., 2014. Porcine cathelicidins efficiently complex and deliver nucleic acids to plasmacytoid dendritic cells and can thereby mediate bacteria-induced IFN-alpha responses. J. Immunol. 193, 364–371.

Bruhn, O., Cauchard, J., Schlisselhuber, M., et al., 2009. Antimicrobial properties of the equine α-defensin DEFA1 against bacterial horse pathogens. Vet. Immunol. Immunopathol. 130, 102–106.

Bruhn, O., Grotzinger, J., Cascorbi, I., Jung, S., 2011. Antimicrobial proteins and peptides of the horse – insights into a well-armed organism. BMC Vet. Res. 42, 98.

Chen, J., Qi, S., Guo, R., Yu, B., et al., 2010. Different messenger RNA expression for the antimicrobial peptides, beta-defensins between Meishan and crossbred pigs. Mol. Biol. Rep. 37, 1633–1639.

Cormican, P., Meade, K.G., Cahalane, S., et al., 2008. Evolution, expression and effectiveness in a cluster of novel bovine beta-defensins. Immunogenetics 60, 147–156.

Erles, K., Brownlie, J., 2010. Expression of β-defensins in the canine respiratory tract and antimicrobial activity against *Bordetella bronchiseptica*. Vet. Immunol. Immunopathol. 135, 12–19.

Lahov, E., Regelson, W., 1996. Antibacterial and immunostimulating casein-derived substances from milk: Casecidin, Isracidin peptides. Food. Chem. Toxic 34 (1), 131–145.

Leonard, B.C., Affolter, V.K., Bevins, C.L., 2012a. Antimicrobial peptides: agents of border protection for companion animals. Vet. Dermatol. 23 (3), 177–e36.

Leonard, B.C., Marks, S.L., Outerbridge, C.A., Affolter, V.K., et al., 2012b. Activity, expression and genetic variation of canine beta-defensin 103: a multifunctional antimicrobial peptide in the skin of domestic dogs. J. Innate Immun. 4 (3), 248–259.

Linde, A., Ross, C.R., Davis, E.G., Dib, L., et al., 2008. Innate Immunity and host defense peptides in veterinary medicine. J. Vet. Intern. Med. 22, 247–265.

Lynn, D.J., Bradley, D.G., 2007. Discovery of α-defensins in basal mammals. Dev. Comp. Immunol. 31, 963–967.

Machado, L.R., Ottolini, B., 2015. An evolutionary history of defensins: a role for copy number variation in maximizing host innate and adaptive immune responses. Front. Immunol. https://doi.org/10.3389/fimmu.2015.00115.

Mantovani, A., Garlanda, C., 2023. Humoral innate immunity and acute phase proteins. N. Engl. J. Med. 388, 439–452.

Mestas, J., Hughes, C.C.W. Of mice and not men: differences between mouse and human immunology. J. Immun. 2004;172:2731–2738.

Mohanty, D., Jena, R., Choudhury, P.K., Pattnaik, R., et al., 2015. Milk derived antimicrobial bioactive peptides: a review. Int. J. Food. Prop. 19 (4), 837–846.

Patil, A., Hughes, A.L., Zhang, G., 2004. Rapid evolution and diversification of mammalian α-defensins as revealed by comparative analysis of rodent and primate genes. Physiol. Genomics 20, 1–11.

Pellegrini, A., Kalkinc, M., Hermann, M., Grünig, B., et al., 1998. Equinins in equine neutrophils: quantification in tracheobronchial secretions as an aid to the diagnosis of chronic pulmonary disease. Vet. J. 155, 257–262.

Sahi, H.-G., Pag, U., Bonness, S., et al., 2005. Mammalian defensins: structures and mechanism of antibiotic activity. J. Leukoc. Biol. 77, 466–475.

Sang, Y., Ortega, M.T., Blecha, F., et al., 2005a. Molecular cloning and characterization of three β-defensins from canine testes. Infect. Immunol. 73, 2611–2620.

Sang, Y., Ortega, M.T., Rune, K., et al., 2007. Canine cathelicidin (K9CATH): gene cloning, expression, and biochemical activity of a novel pro-myeloid antimicrobial peptide. Dev. Comp. Immunol. 31, 1278–1296.

Sang, Y., Ramanathan, B., Ross, C.R., Blecha, F., 2005b. Gene silencing and overexpression of porcine peptidoglycan recognition protein long isoforms: involvement in β-defensin-1 expression. Infect. Immun. 73, 7133–7141.

Sun, C., Gu, L., Hussain, M.A., Chen, L., et al., 2019. Characterization of the bioactivity and mechanism of bactenecin derivatives against food pathogens. Front. Microbiol. https://doi.org/10.3389/fmicb.2019.02593.

Townsend, M., Fowler, B., Aulakh, G.K., Singh, B., 2023. Expression of pentraxin 3 in equine lungs and neutrophils. Can. J. Vet. Res. 87(1), 9–16.

Van Harten, R.M., van Woudenbergh, E., Haagsman, H.P., 2018. Cathelicidins: immunomodulatory antimicrobials. Vaccines. https://doi.org/10.3390/vaccines6030063.

Xu, J., Mu, Y., Zhang, Y., Dong, W., et al., 2015. Antibacterial effect of porcine PTX3 against *Streptococcus suis* type 2 infection. Microb. Pathog. 89, 128–139.

Zhu, S., Gao, B., 2017. Positive selection in cathelicidin host defense peptides: adaptation to exogenous pathogens or endogenous receptors. Heredity 118, 453–465.

5

Humoral Innate Immunity: The Complement System

CHAPTER OUTLINE

While animals are an irresistible source of food and shelter for many microorganisms, they are not totally defenseless. Normal animal tissues are equipped with multiple antimicrobial defenses that can "automatically" kill any microbial invaders they encounter. These constitutive defenses consist of antibacterial molecules, especially peptides and enzymes that are lethal for many bacteria. The body also possesses an automatic killing system, the complement system that can destroy any microbial invaders it encounters. Thus, these defenses constitute the first line of defense against any invaders that penetrate the body's physical barriers. They make the body a hostile environment for any such invader.

THE COMPLEMENT SYSTEM

Protection from infection requires that the body responds to invaders as rapidly as possible. A critical component of this early constituent response is the complement system. This system can detect and kill invaders long before other defenses have had a chance to respond. The complement system consists of a network of interacting pattern-recognition proteins, receptors, and regulators that kill invaders fast (Fig. 5.1). The major complement proteins bind covalently (and hence irreversibly) to the surface of invading microbes and then destroy them. The complement system is activated by the presence of either microbial surface molecules or antigen-bound antibodies.

The complement system is an essential innate defense system. Although its main function is to kill pathogens immediately they enter the body, the complement system also alerts the immune system to the presence of invaders, regulates inflammation, removes damaged or altered cells, and regulates adaptive immune responses. It is also involved in the removal of antigen-antibody complexes, blood vessel formation, mobilization of stem cells, tissue regeneration, and lipid metabolism.

The first step, complement activation, is triggered by three different pathways, referred to as the alternative, the lectin, and the classical pathways (Fig. 5.2). The alternative and lectin pathways are activated by contact with microbial carbohydrates. The classical pathway, in contrast, is activated by antibodies and thus works in association with adaptive immune responses (Cagliani et al., 2016).

The mammalian complement system like other immune defenses has evolved under intense selective pressure. This selection has primarily acted on the proteins that come into direct contact with the pathogens themselves such as the binding of C3b by the alternate pathway or the recognition of polysaccharides by the lectin pathway. Thus, microbes evolve to avoid complement binding while complement components do the opposite. For example, leptospirosis is a widespread zoonosis, as well as a significant pathogen in domestic animal species. Some Leptospires produce an immunoglobulin-like protein that inactivates any complement components that bind to their surface. Some human-specific bacteria such as the two Neisserias (gonorrhea and meningitis) bind complement factor H (FH) and then inactivate it.

Complement Proteins

By convention, complement proteins are either labeled numerically with the prefix C (e.g., C1, C2, C3) or designated as "factors" by letters of the alphabet (FB, FD, FP, and so forth) (Kemper et al., 2014). Some components are found free in serum, whereas others are cell-surface receptors. Collectively, complement components account for up to 10% of the proteins in blood serum—a reflection of the critical importance of this system. Their size varies from 24 kDa for factor D (FD) to 460 kDa for C1q. Their serum concentrations in humans vary between 20 Mg/mL of C2 and 1300 Mg/mL of C3 (Table 5.1; Acierno et al., 2006). Complement proteins are synthesized at multiple sites throughout the body. Thus, C3, C6, C8, and factor B (FB) are made in the liver, whereas C2, C3, C4, C5, FB, FD, FP, and FI are made by macrophages. C1q is produced by mast cells. Neutrophil granules may store large quantities of C6 and C7. As a result, these proteins are readily available for defense at sites where neutrophils accumulate.

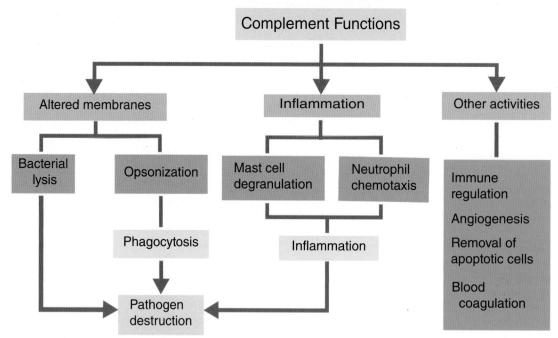

Fig. 5.1 The functions of the complement system. Complement may either alter microbial membranes or trigger inflammation. Either way, it hastens the elimination of microbial invaders and is thus a key component of the innate immune system. It has multiple other functions as well as noted here.

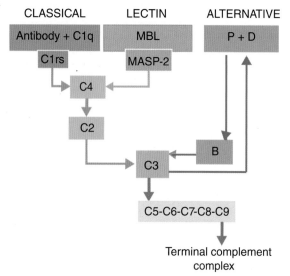

Fig. 5.2 The three pathways by which the complement system can be activated. *MASP-2*, MBL-associated serine protease; *MBL*, mannose-binding lectin.

ACTIVATION PATHWAYS

The Alternative Pathway

The alternative pathway is an evolutionary, ancient innate pathway and probably the original one. It is activated when microbial cell walls encounter complement proteins. Despite its name, the alternative complement pathway accounts for 80%–90% of all complement activation.

The most important complement protein is called C3. C3 is a disulfide-linked heterodimer of 185 kDa with α and β chains. It is synthesized by liver cells and macrophages and is the most abundant

complement component in blood serum. C3 has a reactive thioester side chain that, when activated, binds to microbes and marks them for destruction by immune cells. Activation of this thioester side chain must be carefully regulated to ensure that C3 does not bind and kill normal cells. To prevent such accidents, the thioester group in inactive C3 is hidden within the folded molecule like the blade of a pocketknife (Menger and Aston, 1985).

In healthy normal animals, C3 spontaneously breaks down into two fragments called C3a and C3b (Fig. 5.3). This breakdown exposes the reactive thioester group in C3b. The thioester then generates a carbonyl group that covalently binds the C3b to carbohydrates and proteins on nearby cell surfaces (Fig. 5.4). This breakdown of C3 also exposes binding sites for a protein called FH. When FH binds to these sites, it permits a protease called factor I (FI) to cleave the C3b, preventing further activation and breaking it into two fragments, iC3b and C3c.

The consequences of the breakdown of cell-bound C3b depend on FH binding. This binding depends in turn on the nature of the target surface. When FH interacts with normal body cells, glycoproteins rich in sialic acid (*N*-acetyl neuraminic acid) and other neutral or anionic polysaccharides enhance FH-C3b binding. As a result, FI is activated, and the C3b is promptly destroyed. In a healthy animal, therefore, there is a continuous low-level activation of C3, but FH and FI destroy the C3b as fast as it is generated.

In contrast, bacterial cell walls lack sialic acid. When C3b binds to an invading bacterium, FH cannot bind, FI is inactivated, and the C3b remains attached to the microbial surface. The bound C3b exposes a binding site for another complement protein called FB, and as a result, a complex called C3bB forms. The bound FB is then cleaved by a protease called FD, releasing a soluble fragment called Ba and leaving C3bBb attached to the bacteria. This C3bBb complex is a protease whose preferred substrate is C3. (It is therefore called the alternative C3 convertase.) FD can act only on FB after it has bound

TABLE 5.1 Complement Components

Name	MW (kDa)	Serum Concentration (mg/mL)
Classical Pathway		
C1q	460	80
C1r	83	50
C1s	83	50
C4	200	600
C2	102	20
C3	185	1300
Alternate Pathway		
FD	24	1
FB	90	210
Terminal Components		
C5	195	70
C6	120	65
C7	120	55
C8	160	55
C9	70	60
Control Proteins		
C1-INH	105	200
C4BP	550	250
FH	150	480
FI	88	35
Ana INH	310	35
FP	4 × 56	20
S	83	500

C1-INH, C1-inhibitor; *C4BP*, C4-binding protein; *FB*, factor B; *FD*, factor D; *FH*, factor H; *FI*, factor I.

to C3b but not before. This constraint is called substrate modulation and regulates several reactions in the complement pathways. It ensures that the activities of enzymes such as FD are confined to the correct molecules (Sahu and Lambris, 2001).

The alternative C3 convertase, C3bBb, cleaves bound C3 to generate more C3b. C3bBb is, however, very unstable, with a half-life of only 5 minutes. If another protein called factor P (FP or properdin) binds to the complex, it forms a stable C3bBbP complex with a half-life of 30 minutes. Since C3b generates more C3bBbP, the net effect of all this is that a positive feedback loop is established where increasing amounts of C3b are produced and irreversibly bound to the surface of the invading organism, eventually killing it (Fig. 5.5).

The Lectin Pathway

A second method of activating complement is triggered by the binding of soluble pattern-recognition molecules (lectins) to microbial carbohydrates (Matsushita and Fujita, 1992). When these lectins bind to microbes, they activate proteases that activate complement. Like the alternative pathway, this is an innate pathway triggered simply by the presence of bacterial surface carbohydrates (Fig. 5.6).

Complement-activating lectins include mannose-binding lectin (MBL) and a family of proteins called ficolins. MBL attaches to mannose or *N*-acetylglucosamine on the walls of bacteria, fungi, and protozoa. Once bound, the MBL activates a serum protease called MASP-2. (MASP stands for MBL-associated serine protease.) Activated MASP-2, in turn, acts on the complement component C4, splitting it into C4a and C4b. This exposes a thioester group on the C4b that generates a reactive carbonyl group that links the C4b to the microbial surface (Fig. 5.7). Another complement component, C2, then binds to the C4b to form a complex, C4b2. The bound C2 is then cleaved by MASP-2 to generate C4b2b (Box 5.1).

Cell-bound C4b2b is a protease that acts on C3 to generate C3a and C3b and expose the thioester group on the C3b. The activation of C3b by C4b2b is a major step because each C4b2b complex can generate as many as 200 C3b molecules. Since these reactions are confined to

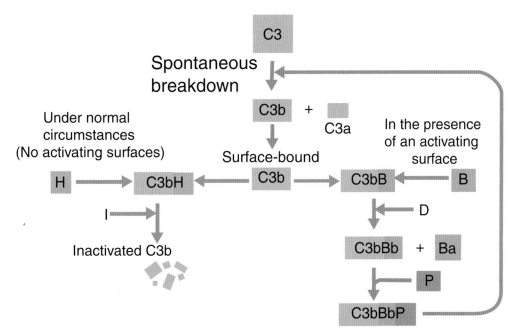

Fig. 5.3 The alternative complement pathway. Surface-bound C3b may either be destroyed, as normally happens, or activated by the presence of an activating surface such as that of an invading bacterium.

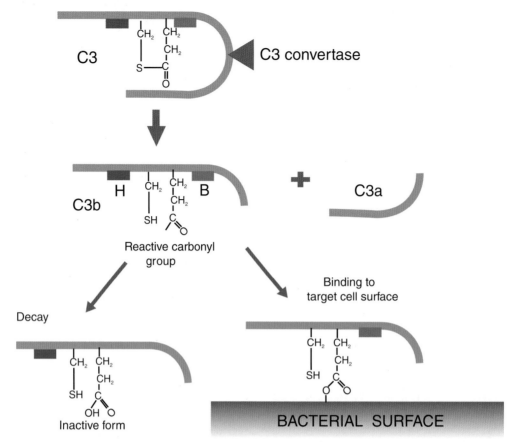

Fig. 5.4 Activation of C3 involves its cleavage by C3 convertase. This exposes a thioester bond between a cysteine and a glutamine. This bond breaks to form a reactive carbonyl group that enables the molecule to bind covalently (and hence irreversibly) to target cell surfaces. Removal of C3a also reveals the binding sites for factor H and factor B.

the microenvironment close to microbial surfaces, the newly formed C3b will bind to nearby microbes. The bound C3b can also cleave C5 to generate C5a and C5b. The complement pathway can then proceed to completion and the killing of the organism by terminal complement complexes (TCCs).

The lectin pathway is ancient, having existed for at least 300 million years (It is present in many invertebrates) (Fujita, 2002). Although in many ways it duplicates the alternative pathway, it is an example of the way the body uses redundant mechanisms to ensure protection against invasive bacteria.

The Classical Pathway

The classical complement pathway (Fig. 5.8) differs from the others since it is triggered when the complement component C1q encounters an antibody bound to an invading microorganism. Its name derives from the fact that it was the first complement pathway discovered.

Unlike the alternate and lectin pathways, the classical pathway cannot be activated until antibodies are made and immune complexes form, which may take 7–10 days after the onset of infection. When antibody molecules bind to an invader, active sites on their Fc regions are exposed. When multiple antibody molecules bind to an organism, these active sites collectively trigger the classical complement pathway.

The first component of the classical pathway is a protein complex called C1. C1 consists of three subunits (C1q, C1r, C1s) bound together by calcium. The completely assembled C1q looks like a six-stranded whip when viewed by electron microscopy (Fig. 5.9). Two molecules each of C1r and C1s form a complex located between the C1q strands. C1q is activated when its strands bind to activating sites on clustered antibody molecules. This binding triggers a conformational change in C1q that permits C1r to interact with C1s, and C1s is converted into an active protease.

Single, antigen-bound molecules of immunoglobulin M (IgM) or paired, antigen-bound molecules of IgG are required to activate C1. The polymeric IgM structure readily provides several closely spaced complement-activating sites. In contrast, two IgG molecules must be located close to each other to have the same effect. Thus IgG is much less efficient than IgM in activating the classical pathway (see Chapter 17).

Active C1s cleaves C4 into C4a and C4b. C2 then binds to C4b to form the complex C4b2. Activated C1s then splits the bound C2, generating a small peptide fragment C2a and the C4b2b complex. C1s cannot act on soluble C2; the C2 must first be bound to C4b before it can be split (another example of substrate modulation). The C4b2b complex is a potent protease whose target is C3, and it is therefore called classical C3 convertase. The newly generated C3b binds and activates C5. Subsequent reactions lead to the formation of the TCC and microbial killing.

In addition to binding immune complexes, C1 can also be activated directly by some viruses, or by bacteria such as *Escherichia coli* and *Klebsiella pneumoniae*. C1q can also bind to apoptotic and necrotic

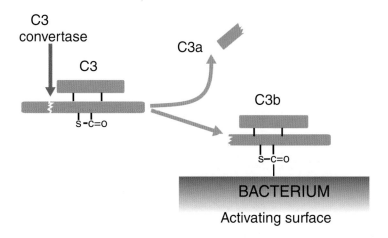

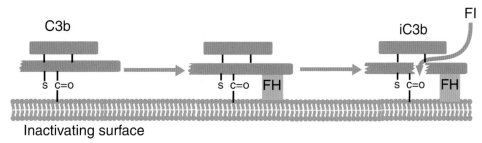

Fig. 5.5 Activated C3 binds to a cell surfaces. This C3b is normally inactivated by the actions of factor H (FH) and factor I (FI). However, FH must first be activated by binding to the surface. In the absence of FH, FI will not work. In this case, C3b persists and activates the terminal complement pathway.

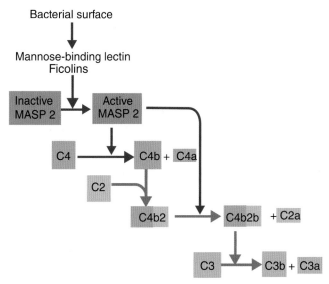

Fig. 5.6 Complement activation by the lectin pathway. *MASP-2*, Mannose-binding lectin–associated serine protease.

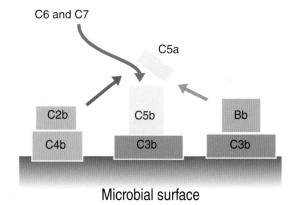

Fig. 5.7 The two C3 convertases, C4b2b and C3bBb, act on C5 when it is linked to C3b and cleave off a small peptide called C5a. In so doing they reveal a site that binds C6 and C7.

cells, extracellular matrix proteins, pentraxins such as C-reactive protein, amyloid and prion proteins, and DNA. However, all these substances with the exception of immune complexes can also bind the complement inhibitors C1-BP and FH, so that full complement activation does not occur. If these inhibitory processes are blocked, uncontrolled complement activation may lead to unwanted inflammation (Thielens et al., 2017).

BOX 5.1 The Defense Collagens

C1q and mannose-binding lectin (MBL) are members of a unique protein family called the defense collagens. Other members of this family include surfactant protein A, adiponectin, conglutinin, and ficolin. These are soluble lectins characterized as containing a conserved collagen-like region as well as a carbohydrate recognition domain. Like C1q, they commonly polymerize and serve as soluble pattern-recognition receptors. They can bind to foreign pathogens and subsequently interact with phagocytic cells or complement. Thus, MBL recognizes mannose-containing carbohydrates. On binding to their ligands, they trigger an immediate protective response such as activation of complement or promotion of phagocytosis.

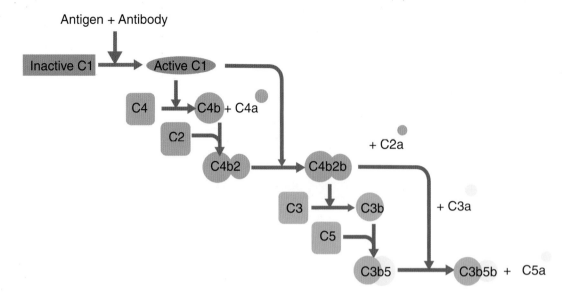

Fig. 5.8 The basic features of the classical complement pathway.

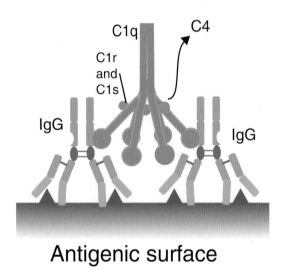

Fig. 5.9 The structure of C1 and its role in interacting with antibodies to initiate the classical complement pathway.

The Terminal Pathway

The three activating complement pathways, alternate, lectin, and classical all converge by generating C3 convertases bound to the microbial surface. These surface-bound C3 convertases, regardless of their origin, can induce the final steps in complement activation, the terminal pathway (Fig. 5.10). Once C5 binds to C3b, substrate modulation occurs, and the C5 is then cleaved by C3bBb (Fig. 5.11). The convertases break C5 (195 kDa) into a small fragment called C5a, leaving a large fragment C5b attached to the C3b. This cleavage also exposes a site on C5b that can bind two new proteins, C6 and C7, to form a multimolecular complex called C5b67 (Fig. 5.12). The C5b67 complex can then insert itself into the microbial cell wall. Once inserted in the surface of an organism, the complex first binds a molecule of C8 to form C5b678. 12–18 C9 molecules then polymerize with the C5b678 complex to form a tubular structure called the TCC, also called the membrane attack complex or C5b6789 (Muller-Eberhard, 1986). The TCC inserts into

microbial cell membranes and punches a hole in its surface (DiScipio, 1991). As a result, the invader will be killed by osmotic lysis. These TCCs can be seen by electron microscopy as ring-shaped structures on the microbial surface with a central electron-dense area surrounded by a lighter ring of poly C9 (Fig. 5.12).

Just as important as the direct TCC-mediated lysis of invaders are the potent inflammatory effects of the small peptide C5a. C5a can degranulate mast cells and stimulate platelets to release histamine and serotonin. C5a is a powerful attractant for neutrophils and macrophages. It increases vascular permeability, causes lysosomal enzyme release from neutrophils and thromboxane release from macrophages, and regulates some T-cell responses (Fig. 5.13). C5a is not bactericidal although the other small complement peptides, C3a and C4a, can kill bacteria such as *E. coli*, *Pseudomonas aeruginosa*, *Enterococcus faecalis*, and *Streptococcus pyogenes*. C3a, like other antimicrobial peptides, acts by disrupting bacterial membranes. (C3a and C5a are also called anaphylatoxins since, when injected in sufficient amounts, they can kill an animal in a manner similar to anaphylaxis [see Chapter 30; Zhang et al., 2022].)

REGULATION OF COMPLEMENT

The consequences of complement activation are so significant and potentially dangerous that each of the activation pathways must be carefully regulated by soluble and cell-bound regulatory proteins (Fig. 5.14; Hourcade et al., 1989; Ricklin et al., 2010). The most important regulator of the classical pathway is C1-inhibitor (C1-INH). C1-INH blocks active C1r and C1s. Other regulatory proteins control the activities of the C3 and C5 convertases. Some compete with the MASPs for binding sites on MBL and ficolins. CD55, or decay accelerating factor, is a glycoprotein expressed on red blood cells, neutrophils, lymphocytes, monocytes, platelets, and endothelial cells. CD55 binds to the convertases and accelerates their decay. Its function is to protect normal cells from complement attack. Other proteins that accelerate degradation of the convertases include FH and C4-binding protein (C4BP), found in plasma, and CD35 (CR1) and CD46, found on cell membranes. The terminal pathway is controlled by three glycoproteins: vitronectin, clusterin, and, most important, protectin (CD59). They all inhibit assembly of the TCC by blocking C5b678 insertion and C9 polymerization.

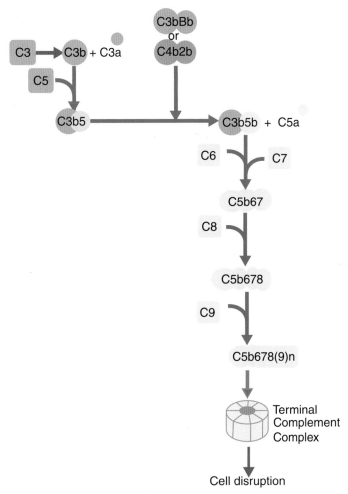

Fig. 5.10 The terminal complement pathway. The progressive aggregation of the terminal complement components eventually leads to the polymerization of C9 and the assembly of a membrane attack complex on the surface of its target.

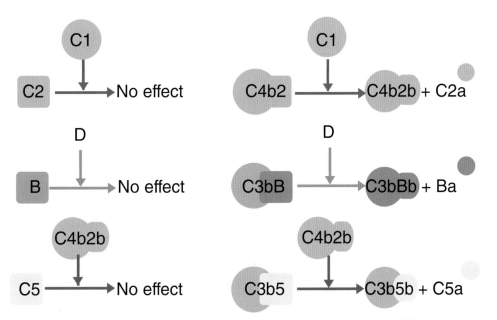

Fig. 5.11 Substrate modulation is one way in which the complement system is regulated. The target for a protease cannot be cleaved unless it is first bound to another protein. Examples of substrate modulation include the cleavage of factors C2, B, and C5 only after they have bound to C4, C3, and C3, respectively.

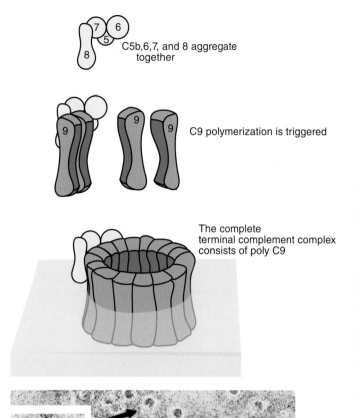

C5b,6,7, and 8 aggregate together

C9 polymerization is triggered

The complete terminal complement complex consists of poly C9

Fig. 5.12 Formation of poly C9 by the amplification pathway and an electron micrograph of poly C9-complement lesions on an erythrocyte membrane. The *insert* shows a mouse complement lesion. The *arrow* points to a possible C5b678 complex. Compare these lesions to the NK cell polyperforins in Fig. 19.8. From Podack, E.R., Dennert, G., 1983. Assembly of two types of tubules with putative cytolytic function by cloned natural killer cells. *Nature* 307, 442.

Complement Receptors

Cells express five receptors for C3 or its fragments. These are called CR1 (CD35), CR2 (CD21), CR3 (CD11a/CD18), CR4 (CD11c/CD18), and CRIg.

CR1 is found on primate red cells, neutrophils, eosinophils, monocytes, macrophages, B cells, and some T cells. It is a receptor for C3b and C4b as well as for the C3b breakdown product, iC3b. Red cell CR1 accounts for 90% of all CR1 in the blood. In primates, CR1 removes immune complexes (antigen-antibody-complement complexes) from the circulation. These immune complexes bind to CR1 on red cells, and the coated red cells are then removed in the liver and spleen (see Chapter 38). Deficiencies of complement components or their receptors may allow circulating immune complexes to accumulate in the kidney and cause damage. C3-deficient dogs develop immune complex–mediated kidney lesions for the same reason (see Chapter 33; Pringle et al., 2012).

CR2 (CD21) is the receptor for C3d found on B cells. CR2 associates with another B-cell surface protein called CD19. This CD21-CD19 complex regulates B cell responses (Fig. 16.11; Pringle et al., 2012). In order to respond optimally to foreign antigens, B cells must be stimulated by C3d acting through CR2. When C3d binds to CR2 on B cells, it reduces their activation threshold a 1000-fold. As always, mice are not always a good guide to the situation in other mammals. Bovine CR2 consists of four distinct receptors that are generated by alternative splicing. They include two variants that are homologs of mouse CR1 and CR2, and each is expressed in a short and long form (Liu et al., 2008).

CR3 (CD11a/CD18) is an integrin that binds iC3b. It is found on macrophages, neutrophils, and natural killer cells. An inherited deficiency of CR3 (leukocyte adherence deficiency, LAD) occurs in humans, cattle, and dogs. Affected individuals are killed by overwhelming infections (see Chapter 40).

CR4 (CD11c/CD18) is an integrin found on neutrophils, T cells, natural killer cells, a few platelets, and macrophages. It is also a receptor for breakdown fragments of C3.

CRIg (Complement receptor of the Ig family) is expressed on tissue macrophages. It is a receptor for the C3-dependent opsonization of blood-borne pathogens.

OTHER CONSEQUENCES

Although microbial destruction mediated by TCCs is the most obvious beneficial activity of the complement system, its protective effects go far beyond this (Reis et al., 2019).

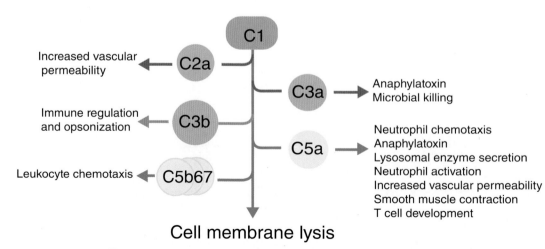

Fig. 5.13 Some of the biological consequences of complement activation.

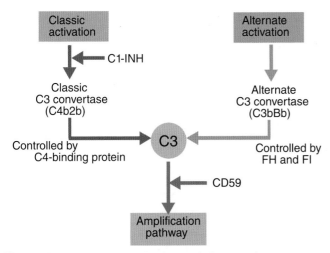

Fig. 5.14 Basic control mechanisms of the complement system. *C1-INH*, C1-inhibitor; *FH*, factor H; *FI*, factor I.

TABLE 5.2 Complement-Derived Chemotactic Factors

Factor	Target
C3a	Eosinophils
C5a	Neutrophils, eosinophils, macrophages
C567	Neutrophils, eosinophils
FBb	Neutrophils
C3e	Promotes leukocytosis

Opsonization

Bacteria normally lack complement regulators so that uncontrolled complement activation occurs on their surface. This leads to proinflammatory signaling, opsonization, phagocytosis, and in some organisms, especially Gram-negative bacteria and some parasites, TCC assembly and bacterial lysis. C3b and C4b are very effective opsonins (see Chapter 6). Phagocytic cells express CR1 and tissue macrophages also express CRIg. C3b-coated organisms will be bound to these cells and undergo type II phagocytosis. If, for some reason, these organisms cannot be ingested, neutrophils may secrete their lysosomal enzymes and oxidants into the surrounding tissue fluid. This can cause inflammation and tissue damage, a reaction classified as type III hypersensitivity (see Chapter 33). Given the long evolutionary history of the complement system, it is not surprising that many bacteria have evolved mechanisms to neutralize the effects of complement (see Chapter 27).

Removal of Apoptotic Cells

Complement contributes to recovery from inflammation by promoting the removal of dead (apoptotic) cells and immune complexes. Apoptotic cells lose their complement inhibitors CD46 and CD59. As a result, they are opsonized by C3b and C4b and removed by phagocytosis. Apoptotic cells also bind CRP that can then bind C1q, leading to classical pathway activation. Properdin (FP) also binds to apoptotic T cells, resulting in C3b-mediated opsonization and destruction (Kemper et al., 2008).

Inflammation

Just as important as direct complement-mediated lysis are the potent inflammatory effects of two small peptides C3a and C5a generated during complement activation. C3a and C5a can degranulate mast cells and stimulate platelets to release histamine and serotonin. As a result, they trigger inflammation. C5a is also a powerful attractant for neutrophils and macrophages. It increases vascular permeability, causes lysosomal enzyme release from neutrophils, and regulates some T-cell responses. As a result, complement activation within tissues plays a key role in inflammatory diseases such as systemic lupus and rheumatoid arthritis (Nordahl et al., 2004; Nemali et al., 2008).

Blood Coagulation

The complement system enhances blood coagulation and inhibits fibrinolysis. Thus C5a induces the expression of tissue factor and plasminogen activator inhibitor I. Likewise, components of the clotting system amplify the complement system. Activated clotting factor XII can cleave C1 and so activate the classical pathway. Thrombin acts on C5 to generate C5a.

Chemotaxis

Activation of the complement system generates chemotactic peptides, including C5a and C5b67 (Table 5.2). C5b67 attracts neutrophils and eosinophils, whereas C5a attracts not only neutrophils and eosinophils but also macrophages and basophils. C5a also stimulates the neutrophil respiratory burst and upregulates CR1 and integrin expression.

Immune Regulation

The complement system regulates both humoral and cell-mediated adaptive immunity (Carroll and Isenman, 2012). When an antigen molecule binds to a B cell antigen receptor, any attached C3d will also bind to CR2/CD19 complexes on the B cell and enhances B cell antigen receptor signaling (see Chapter 16). Conversely, depletion of C3 is associated with reduced B cell responses (Sorman et al., 2014). Many complement proteins also influence T-cell activation (Clarke and Tenner, 2014). Thus C3 is present within CD4+ T cells (see Chapter 15). This C3 is cleaved when T cells are activated and the C3a moves to the cell surface and drives T-cell cytokine production.

Conglutinin

Conglutinin is an oligomeric protein that can range in size from 34 to 630 kDa. The reduced conglutinin monomer is 40–44 kDa in size. It is a heat-stable beta-globulin consisting of four trimeric subunits. The trimers are stabilized by interchain disulfide bonds. On electron microscopy the conglutinin molecule is X-shaped.

Conglutinin is a member of the subfamily of C-type (Ca++-dependent) lectins called collectins. It is found in cattle and related mammals. Conglutinin can bind, and agglutinate (conglutinate) complement-coated particles and it has the ability to trigger phagocytosis. It can bind the surface polysaccharides on invading bacteria and parasites and so serve both as a complement activator and an opsonin. It has both antibacterial and antiviral properties. In addition to conglutinin, other bovine collectins include mannose-binding protein, surfactant proteins A and D, and bovine collectin 43. Conglutinin is found not only in adult bovine serum but also in colostrum, milk, and in fetal calf serum. Conglutinin is synthesized by neutrophils and macrophages as well as by hepatocytes.

INTRACELLULAR COMPLEMENT

Recent studies have also shown that the complement system is also active within cells. This "complosome" appears to play an important role in apoptosis and the destruction of intracellular pathogens (Kunz and Kemper, 2021). Thus the major complement components C3, C1q, FH, and CD59 are all present and functional within cells. As a result, they can kill intracellular invaders. Activation of

C5 and C3 within T cells is involved in maintaining immunological tolerance and promotes their differentiation into Th1 cells. They also play a role in the migration of monocytes and T cells from the bloodstream into tissues. This is also linked to cellular metabolic processes and stimulation of immune cell activity, especially IFN-γ production (Reichhardt and Meri, 2018; King and Blom, 2023).

COMPLEMENT GENES

The genes coding for the complement proteins are scattered throughout the genome. However, two major gene clusters have been identified. Thus the genes for C4, C2, and FB are located within the major histocompatibility complex class III region (see Chapter 12). Likewise, the genes for C4BP, CD55, CD35, CD21, CD46, and FH are linked within the RCA (regulation of complement activation) cluster.

Complement components, like other proteins, show multiple genetic variations and collectively these variants form an animal's "complotype" (Harris et al., 2012). These genetic variations may influence an animal's susceptibility to infectious and inflammatory diseases. The precise number of variants varies between components and species. For example, bovine FH has three alleles, equine C3 has six, and canine C3 has two. Canine C6 has seven alleles, and porcine C6 has 14 (Shibata et al., 1993). Eleven alleles of canine C7 have been identified, whereas canine C4 has at least five. There is an association among C4-4 allele expression, low serum C4 levels, and the development of autoimmune polyarthritis in dogs (Day et al., 1985). Feline and equine C4 each have at least four alleles. Pigs have multiple C6 alleles (Shibata et al., 1993).

COMPLEMENT DEFICIENCIES

Canine C3 Deficiency

Because the complement system is an essential innate defensive mechanism, any deficiency will increase susceptibility to infections. The most severe of these occurs in animals deficient in C3. For example, some Brittany spaniels may suffer from an autosomal recessive C3 deficiency (Fig. 5.15). Dogs that are homozygous for this trait have no detectable C3, whereas heterozygous animals have C3 levels that are approximately half normal. Heterozygous animals are clinically normal (Ameratunga et al., 1998). The homozygous-deficient animals have lower IgG levels than normal, and their ability to make antibodies is reduced (O'Neil et al., 1988). These dogs tend to make more IgM and less IgG. They experience recurrent sepsis, pneumonia, pyometra, and wound infections. The organisms involved include *Clostridium* species, *Pseudomonas* species, *E. coli*, and *Klebsiella* species. Some affected dogs develop amyloidosis, and many develop immune complex–mediated kidney disease (see Chapter 33). The mutation responsible for this deficiency (deletion of a single cytosine) shortens the C3 chain as a result of a frameshift that generates a premature stop codon (Fig. 5.16).

Porcine Factor H Deficiency

FH is a critical component of the alternative complement pathway. It normally inactivates C3b as soon as it is generated and so prevents excessive complement activation. If an animal fails to make FH, C3b will be generated in an uncontrolled fashion. FH deficiency has been identified as an autosomal recessive trait in Yorkshire pigs. Affected piglets are healthy at birth and develop normally for a few weeks. However, eventually they fail to thrive, stop growing, become anemic, and die of renal failure (Hogasen et al., 1995).

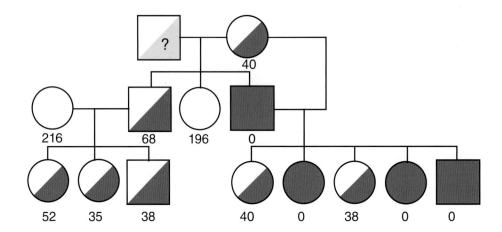

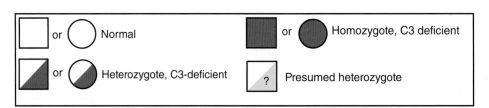

Fig. 5.15 Inheritance of a C3 deficiency in a colony of Brittany spaniels. The number below each circle or square represents the animal's C3 level as a percentage of a standard reference serum. The mean level in healthy spaniels was 126. (*Squares* denote males, *circles* denote females.) From Winkelstein, J.A., Cork, L.C., Griffin, D.E., et al., 1981. Genetically determined deficiency of the third component of complement in the dog. Science 212, 1169–1170.

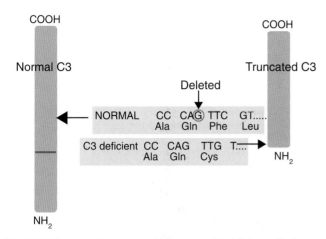

Fig. 5.16 The mutation that results in canine C3 deficiency. Deletion of a cytosine results in a frameshift and premature termination of transcription of the C3 gene.

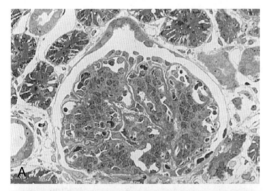

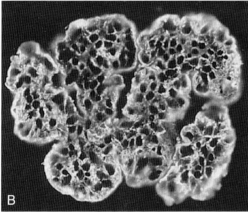

Fig. 5.17 (A) A thin section of the glomerulus of a piglet with factor H deficiency. Note the thickened basement membrane and increased numbers of mesangial cells, hence the name membranoproliferative glomerulonephritis. (B) An immunofluorescence photomicrograph of another glomerulus from a factor H–deficient piglet. This is stained with fluorescent anti-C3. The bright fluorescence indicates the presence of C3 deposited in this glomerulus. (A) Courtesy Johan, H. Jansen; (B) From Jansen, J.H., Hogasen, K., Mollnes, T.E., 1993. Extensive complement activation in hereditary porcine membranoproliferative glomerulonephritis type II (porcine dense deposit disease. Am. J. Pathol. 143, 1356–1365.

On necropsy, there are multiple petechial hemorrhages on the surface of the kidneys, accompanied by atrophy of the renal papillae. Mesangial cell proliferation and capillary basement membrane thickening occur within glomeruli (Fig. 5.17). On electron microscopy, extensive intramembranous electron-dense deposits are found

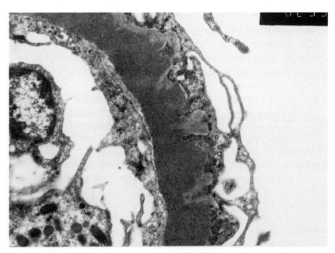

Fig. 5.18 Electron micrograph showing dense intramembranous deposits in the glomerulus of a piglet with factor H deficiency. From Jansen, J.H., 1993. Porcine membranoproliferative glomerulonephritis with intramembranous dense deposits (porcine dense deposit disease. APMIS 101, 281–289.

in the glomerular basement membranes (Fig. 5.18). This is typical of type II membranoproliferative glomerulonephritis (see Chapter 33). Indirect immunofluorescence tests demonstrate massive deposits of C3 but no immunoglobulins in the basement membranes. C3 can be found in the glomeruli before birth, but mesangial proliferation and intramembranous dense deposits develop after 5 days of age (Jansen et al., 1993, 1995).

Nephritic piglets are almost totally deficient in FH (2% of normal levels), whereas heterozygotes have half the normal levels. If FH is replaced by plasma transfusions, the progress of the disease can be slowed and piglets survive longer. Affected pigs have no plasma C3. Since heterozygotes are readily detected by measuring plasma C3, this disease can be eradicated from affected herds.

Other Complement Deficiencies

In contrast to the severe effects of a C3 deficiency, congenital deficiencies of other complement components in laboratory animals or humans are not necessarily lethal. Thus, individuals with C6 or C7 deficiencies have been described who are quite healthy. Apparently, healthy C6-deficient pigs have been described. The lack of discernible effect of these deficiencies suggests that the terminal portion of the complement pathway leading to terminal complex formation may not be biologically essential.

REFERENCES

Acierno, M.J., Labato, M.A., Stern, L.C., et al., 2006. Serum concentrations of the third component of complement in healthy dogs and dogs with protein-losing nephropathy. Am. J. Vet. Res. 67, 1105–1109.

Ameratunga, R., Winkelstein, J.A., Brody, L., et al., 1998. Molecular analysis of the third component of canine complement (C3) and identification of the mutation responsible for hereditary canine C3 deficiency. J. Immunol. 160, 2824–2830.

Cagliani, R., Forni, D., Filippi, G., Mozzi, A., et al., 2016. The mammalian complement system as an epitome of host pathogen conflicts. Mol. Ecol. 25, 1324–1339.

Carroll, M.C., Isenman, D.E., 2012. Regulation of humoral immunity by complement. Immunity 37, 199–207.

Clarke, E.V., Tenner, A.J., 2014. Complement modulation of T cell immune responses during homeostasis and disease. J. Leukoc. Biol. 96, 745–756.

Day, M.J., Kay, P.M., Clark, W.T., et al., 1985. Complement C4 allotype association with and serum C4 concentration in an autoimmune disease in a dog. Clin. Immunol. Immunopathol. 35, 85–91.

DiScipio, R., 1991. The relationship between polymerization of complement component C9 and membrane channel formation. J. Immunol. 147, 4239–4247.

Fujita, T., 2002. Evolution of the lectin-complement pathway and its role in innate immunity. Nat. Rev. Immunol. 2, 346–386,.

Harris, C.L., Heurich, M., Rodriguez De Cordoba, S., Morgan, B.P., 2012. The complotype: dictating risk for inflammation and infection. Trends Immunol. 33, 513–521.

Høgåsen, K., Jansen, J.H., Molines, T., et al., 1995. Hereditary porcine membranoproliferative glomerulonephritis type II is caused by factor H deficiency. J. Clin. Invest. 95, 1054–1061.

Hourcade, D., Holers, V.M., Atkinson, J.P., 1989. The regulators of complement activation (RCA) gene cluster. Adv. Immunol. 45, 381–416.

Jansen, J.H., Høgåsen, K., Grøndahl, A.M., 1995. Porcine membranoproliferative glomerulonephritis type II: an autosomal recessive deficiency of factor H. Vet. Rec. 137, 240–244.

Jansen, J.H., Høgåsen, K., Molines, T.E., 1993. Extensive complement activation in hereditary porcine membranoproliferative glomerulonephritis type II (porcine dense deposit disease). Am. J. Pathol. 143, 1356–1365.

Kemper, C., Mitchell, L.M., Zhang, L., Hourcade, D.E., 2008. The complement protein properdin binds apoptotic T cells and promotes complement activation and phagocytosis. Proc. Natl. Acad. Sci. U.S.A. 105, 9023–9028.

Kemper, C., Pangburn, M.K., Fishelson, Z., 2014. Complement nomenclature 2014. Mol. Immunol. 61, 56–58.

King, B.C., Blom, A.M., 2023. Intracellular complement: evidence, definitions, controversies and solutions. Immunol. Rev. 313, 104–119.

Kunz, N., Kemper, C., 2021. Complement has brains—do intracellular complement and immunometabolism cooperate in tissue homeostasis and behavior? Front. Immunol. https://doi.org/10.3389/fimmu.2021.629986

Liu, D., Zhu, J.Y., Niu, Z.X., 2008. Molecular structure and expression of anthropic, ovine, and murine forms of complement receptor type 2. Clin. Vaccine Immunol. 15, 901–910.

Matsushita, M., Fujita, T., 1992. Activation of the classical complement pathway by mannose-binding protein in association with a novel C1s-like serine protease. J. Exp. Med. 176, 1497–1502.

Menger, M., Aston, W.P., 1985. Isolation and characterization of the third component of bovine complement. Vet. Immunol. Immunopathol. 10, 317–331.

Muller-Eberhard, H.J., 1986. The membrane attack complex of complement. Annu. Rev. Immunol. 4, 503–528.

Nemali, S., Siemsen, D.W., Nelson, L.K., et al., 2008. Molecular analysis of the bovine anaphylatoxin C5a receptor. J. Leukoc. Biol. 84, 537–549.

Nordahl, E.A., Rydengard, V., Nyberg, P., et al., 2004. Activation of the complement system generates antibacterial peptides. Proc. Natl. Acad. Sci. U. S. A. 101, 16879–16884.

O'Neil, K.M., Ochs, H.D., Heller, S.R., et al., 1988. Role of C3 in humoral immunity: defective antibody formation in C3-deficient dogs. J. Immunol. 140, 1939–1945.

Pringle, E.S., Firth, M.A., Chattha, K.S., Hodgins, D.C., Shewen, P.E., 2012. Expression of complement receptors 1 (CR1/CD35) and 2 (CR2/CD21), and co-signaling molecule CD19 in cattle. Dev. Comp. Immunol. 38, 487–494.

Ricklin, D., Hajishengallis, G., Yang, K., Lambris, J.D., 2010. Complement: a key system for immune surveillance and homeostasis. Nat. Immunol. 11, 785–797.

Reichhardt, M.P., Meri, S., 2018. Intracellular complement activation – an alarm raising mechanism? Sem. Immunol. 38, 54–62.

Reis, E.S., Mastellos, D.C., Hajishengallis, G., Lambris, J.D., 2019. New insights into the immune functions of complement. Nat. Revs. Immunol. 19, 503–516.

Sahu, A., Lambris, J.D., 2001. Structure and biology of complement protein C3, a connecting link between innate and acquired immunity. Immunol. Rev. 180, 35–48.

Shibata, T., Akita, T., Abe, T., 1993. Genetic polymorphism of the sixth component of complement (C6) in the pig. Anim. Genet. 24, 97–100.

Sorman, A., Zhang, L., Ding, Z., Heyman, B., 2014. How antibodies use complement to regulate antibody responses. Mol. Immunol. 61, 79–88.

Thielens, N.M., Tedesco, F., Bohlson, S.S., Gaboriaud, C., Tenner, A.J., 2017. C1q: a fresh look at an old molecule. Mol. Immunol. 89, 73–83.

Zhang, X.-J., Zhong, Y.-Q., Ma, Z.-Y., Hu, Y.-Z., et al., 2022. Insights into the antibacterial properties of complement peptides, C3a, C4a, and C5a across vertebrates. J. Immunol. 209, 2330–2340.

6

Cellular Innate Immunity: Leukocytes

CHAPTER OUTLINE

Although physical barriers such as the skin exclude many organisms, these barriers are not impenetrable, and microbes can gain access to body tissues through wounds, by inhalation, or with food. Once sentinel cells recognize the invaders, signals are generated that activate and attract defensive cells to the sites of invasion. Depending upon the nature of the invader, these defensive cells may include dendritic cells, mast cells, eosinophils, neutrophils, macrophages, and innate lymphoid cells. The most significant and abundant of these, at least in the early stages of inflammation, are neutrophils. Huge numbers of these are attracted to sites of invasion where they kill and eat bacterial invaders. This process is called phagocytosis (Greek for "eating by cells"). One prime purpose of inflammation is to ensure that phagocytic cells can intercept and destroy invading bacteria as rapidly, and efficiently as possible.

Defensive cells circulate in the bloodstream where they are collectively called leukocytes (white blood cells) (Fig. 6.1). All leukocytes originate from bone marrow (myeloid) stem cells, and all help defend the body. Two types of leukocytes specialize in killing and eating invading microorganisms. These, called neutrophils and macrophages, originate from a common stem cell but look very different and have different, but complementary, functions. Thus, neutrophils are the first responders and eat invading organisms rapidly but are incapable of sustained phagocytic effort. Macrophages, in contrast, move more slowly but are highly effective phagocytes and are capable of repeated phagocytosis. They complete the task of eliminating the invaders. In this chapter, we review the properties of neutrophils and their role in inflammation and innate immunity (Soehnlein and Lindbom, 2010). We will look at their partners, the macrophages in Chapter 7.

LEUKOCYTE CLASSIFICATION

Examination of a stained blood smear reveals several different types of leukocytes. Those with a cytoplasm filled with granules are called granulocytes (Fig. 6.2). Granulocytes also have a characteristic lobulated, irregular nucleus, so they are described as "polymorphonuclear" (as opposed to the single-rounded nucleus of "mononuclear" cells such as

macrophages). Granulocytes are classified based on the staining properties of their granules. Cells whose granules take up basic dyes such as hematoxylin are called basophils; those that take up acidic dyes such as eosin are called eosinophils; and those that take up neither are called neutrophils. All three populations play important defensive roles. Likewise, the degree of nuclear lobulation varies among mammals. The nuclei of mice and some rodents may be U-shaped without obvious lobules. Conversely, the neutrophils of nonhuman primates tend to be hyperlobulated.

NEUTROPHILS

Polymorphonuclear neutrophil granulocytes, otherwise called neutrophils, predominate in the blood of most mammals (Fig. 6.3). As a result, about two-thirds of the hematopoietic activity of their bone marrow is devoted to neutrophil production. Neutrophils are the major phagocytic cells that participate in acute inflammation (Siwicki and Kubes, 2022). They are structurally similar among the mammals but may vary somewhat based on the size and specific staining properties of their granules (Fig. 6.4; Bertram, 1985). They have a short life cycle, respond rapidly, and are present in enormous numbers. Neutrophils are formed by stem cells in the bone marrow at a rate of about 8 million per minute in humans; they migrate to the bloodstream and about 12 hours later move into tissues such as the spleen and lungs where they continue to serve a defensive role. They live for only a few days unless activated by inflammation and must therefore be constantly replaced (Hidalgo et al., 2019). Neutrophils constitute about 60%–75% of the blood leukocytes in most carnivores, about 50% in the horse, and 20%–30% in cattle, sheep, and laboratory rodents. Normally, however, blood neutrophils account for only 1%–2% of their total population. The vast majority of neutrophils are normally sequestered in capillaries within the liver, spleen, lungs, and bone marrow. During bacterial infections, the number of circulating neutrophils may increase 10-fold as these stored cells are released from these organs (Baldridge et al., 2011). These neutrophils migrate into the bloodstream and eventually into inflamed tissues. They eventually die by apoptosis (Burn et al.,

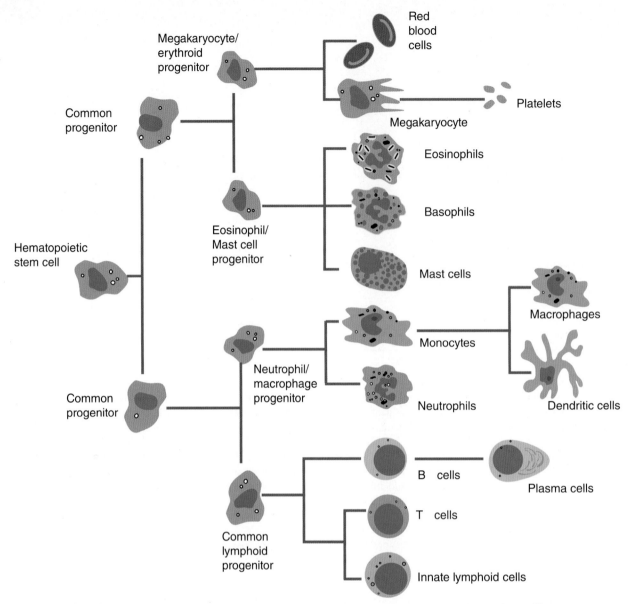

Fig. 6.1 The origin of leukocytes from the bone marrow. Note that lymphoid cells originate from different stem cells than the cells of the myeloid system. Note too that cells such as eosinophils and basophils are probably closely related despite significant morphological differences.

2021). This in turn brings their partners, the monocytes to the scene to finish the job (Siwicki and Kubes, 2022).

The production of neutrophils by stem cells is regulated by a cytokine called granulocyte colony-stimulating factor (G-CSF) (Baldridge et al., 2011). The production of G-CSF is coordinated with the rate of neutrophil apoptosis. Thus apoptotic neutrophils are removed by macrophages. These macrophages then produce interleukin-23 (IL-23) so that, as neutrophils die, IL-23 production increases. IL-23 in turn promotes IL-17 production by lymphocytes and the IL-17 in turn stimulates G-CSF production and stem cell activity. As a result, the rate of neutrophil production matches the rate of their removal (Vietinghoff and Ley, 2008). Toll-like receptors (TLRs) are also expressed on myeloid stem cells. During microbial infections, pathogen-associated molecular patterns (PAMPs) such as lipopolysaccharides bind to these TLRs and trigger the production of more neutrophils. TLRs thus provide a mechanism whereby neutrophil availability increases rapidly in response to infection. Administration of G-CSF stimulates neutrophil production.

If administered to cattle around calving time, it will increase neutrophil numbers and as a result reduce the prevalence of mastitis. A modified form of G-CSF is currently available for this purpose in dairy cattle (see Chapter 35).

Structure

Neutrophils are round cells, about 10–20 μm in diameter. They have a finely granular cytosol at the center of which is an irregular sausage-like or segmented nucleus (Fig. 6.4). Their nuclear chromatin is condensed so that neutrophils cannot divide. Electron microscopy shows three major types of enzyme-rich granules in their cytosol (Fig. 6.5). Primary (azurophil) granules contain enzymes such as myeloperoxidase, lysozyme, elastase, β-glucuronidase, and cathepsin B. Secondary (specific) granules lack myeloperoxidase but contain lysozyme and collagenase and the iron-binding protein lactoferrin. Tertiary granules contain gelatinase (Borregaard and Sorensen, 2007). Mature neutrophils have a small Golgi apparatus, some mitochondria, a few ribosomes, and a little rough endoplasmic reticulum. Although neutrophil DNA is tightly condensed and they have a very short life span, they produce many proteins. Neutrophils express a broad repertoire of PRMs and can respond dynamically to PAMPs by producing pro-inflammatory cytokines. As a result, they are major mediators of innate immunity (Rahman et al., 2008).

Rabbit neutrophils contain large cytoplasmic granules that stain dark pink with Romanowsky stains. As a result, they are called heterophils or pseudo-eosinophils. Despite this different staining pattern, rabbit heterophils are functionally the same as neutrophils in other mammals. True eosinophils have larger and more spherical granules (see Fig. 30.15) and stain with eosin-based stains (Hawkey, 1975). Guinea pigs and related rodents also possess heterophils.

EMIGRATION

Neutrophils in the bloodstream are simply carried along by the flow. In inflamed tissues, however, these fast-moving cells slow down, stop, bind to blood vessel walls, and emigrate into the tissues. This emigration is triggered by changes in the endothelial cells lining the blood vessels (Muller, 2013).

Changes in Endothelial Cells

In aggregate, the endothelial cells that line blood vessels collectively have a huge surface area (estimated at $4000\,m^2$ in humans) and thus serve as a broad sensor of microbial invasion. When PAMPs and damage-associated molecular patterns (DAMPs) such as LPS or histamine and platelet-activating factor (PAF) from damaged tissues reach blood vessels, they stimulate these endothelial cells to express a sticky glycoprotein called P-selectin (CD62P). P-selectin is stored in cytoplasmic granules but moves to the cell surface within minutes after stimulation. The P-selectin binds a protein called L-selectin (CD62L) expressed on passing neutrophils. At first, this binding is weak and transient because the neutrophils shed their L-selectin, but the neutrophils progressively

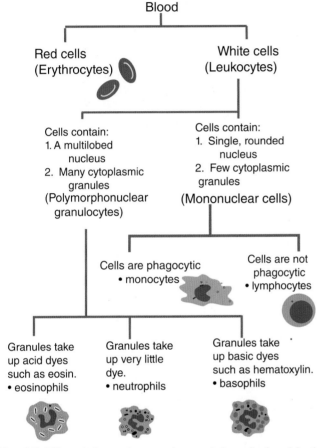

Fig. 6.2 Differentiation and nomenclature of the cells found in the blood. Leukocytes are first classified on the basis of their nuclear shape. Polymorphonuclear cells are then differentiated on the basis of their granule staining. Lymphocytes and macrophages are classified on the basis of nuclear shape and extent of cytoplasm. Note that the different subpopulations of lymphocytes cannot be distinguished on the basis of their morphology.

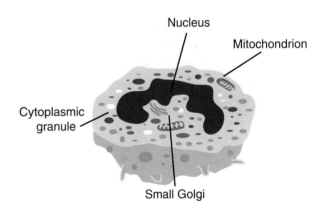

Fig. 6.3 The major structural features of a neutrophil. Note the characteristic nucleus and the plentiful cytoplasmic granules.

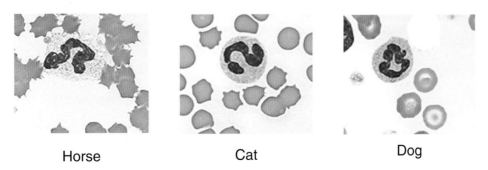

Fig. 6.4 Neutrophils in peripheral blood smears: (A) horse, (B) cat, and (C) dog. These cells are about 10 μm in diameter. Giemsa stain. Courtesy Dr. M.C. Johnson.

express more selectins so that they gradually slow, roll along the endothelial cell surface, and eventually stop (Fig. 6.6). This mainly happens in venules where the vessel wall is thin and its diameter is sufficiently small to permit the neutrophils to make firm contact with the endothelium.

Changes in Neutrophils

As neutrophils roll along the endothelial surface, PAF, chemokines, and leukotrienes from the endothelial cells act on the rolling neutrophils, causing them to express the adhesive protein, leukocyte function–associated antigen–1 (LFA-1) (Foster et al., 1992). LFA-1 is an integrin that binds to intercellular adhesion molecule-1 (ICAM-1 or CD54) on endothelial cells (Fig. 6.7). Their strong binding brings the neutrophils to a complete stop and attaches them firmly to the vessel wall, despite the shearing force of the blood flow. After several hours, endothelial cells activated by cytokines such as tumor necrosis factor–α (TNF-α) also express the strongly adhesive E-selectin (CD62E). IL-1 and IL-23 also induce endothelial cells to produce chemokines that attract more neutrophils (Vestweber, 2015).

Integrins

Many cell surface proteins bind cells together, but the most important of these are the integrins (Luscinskas and Lawler, 1994). Integrins are cell membrane proteins that bind to ligands in the extracellular matrix, to other cells, and to some soluble proteins. Each consists of paired protein chains (heterodimers) that use a unique α-chain paired with a common β-chain. For example, three β_2-integrins are found in neutrophils. Their α-chain, called CD11a, b, or c, is associated with a common β_2-chain called CD18 (Fagerholm, 2022). Therefore these three neutrophil integrins are CD11a/CD18 (LFA-1), CD11b/CD18, and CD11c/CD18. As described previously, LFA-1 on activated neutrophils binds to ICAM-1 on capillary endothelial cells. CD11b/CD18 also binds leukocytes to endothelial cells and—acts as a complement receptor (complement receptor 3) (see Chapter 5). In the case of humans, they are primarily attracted to inflammatory sites by the chemokine IL-8. Neutrophils are also attracted to infection sites by *N*-formyl peptides from gram-negative bacteria.

Emigration and Swarming

After binding to blood vessel walls, neutrophils swarm into the surrounding tissues under the influence of chemokines, lipids, and other chemoattractants (Fig. 6.8; DiStasi and Ley, 2009). Most migrating neutrophils squeeze between the endothelial cells, but about 20% actually pass through these cells and produce proteases to get through the basement membrane. They then crawl toward any invading microbes.

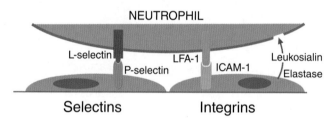

Fig. 6.7 A simplified view of the proteins and their ligands engaged in neutrophil-vascular endothelial cell binding. Selectins are carbohydrate-binding proteins that bind other glycoproteins. This selectin-mediated binding is weak and temporary. Subsequently, integrins on leukocytes, especially leukocyte function–associated antigen–1 (LFA-1), bind strongly to their ligand intercellular adhesion molecule–1 (ICAM-1) on vascular endothelial cells. Elastase secreted by endothelial cells removes leukosialin, thus permitting the neutrophil to bind strongly to the endothelial cell.

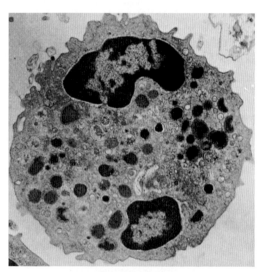

Fig. 6.5 Transmission electron micrograph of a rabbit neutrophil. Note the two lobes of the nucleus and the granule-filled cytoplasm. Courtesy Dr. S. Linthicum.

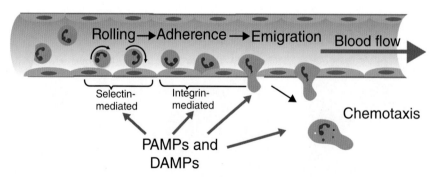

Fig. 6.6 The stages of neutrophil adhesion and emigration from blood vessels. Changes in vascular endothelial cells are triggered by tissue damage and microbial invasion. Selectins on endothelial cells tether neutrophils and stimulate them to roll. When they come to a halt, integrins bind them firmly to vascular endothelial cells and signal the neutrophils to emigrate into tissues by passing through the blood vessel walls. *DAMPs*, Damage-associated molecular patterns; *PAMPs*, pathogen-associated molecular patterns.

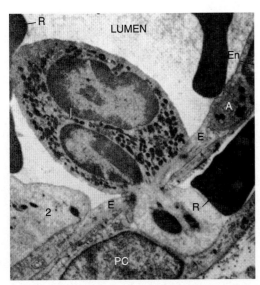

Fig. 6.8 Inflamed venule of a rat. Cell 1 is a neutrophil migrating through a capillary wall to reach the surrounding tissues. Cells 2 and 3 are also neutrophils. *E*, Endothelium; *PC*, periendothelial cell; *R*, red blood cells. From Marchesi, V.T., Florey, H.W., 1960. Electron micrographic observations on the emigration of leucocytes. Q J. Exp. Physiol. 45, 343.

Since neutrophils are the most mobile of all the blood leukocytes, (they can move at up to 12 μm/min), they are the first to arrive at damaged tissues. These first cells detect short-range chemotactic factors. Some of these neutrophils die and release even more chemoattractants. The newly arrived cells in turn synthesize leukotriene B$_4$ that is even more attractive. Within hours neutrophils gather in enormous numbers (Kameritsch and Renkawitz, 2020). Under some conditions, the number of neutrophils in these swarms may be sufficient to generate pus. This whitish-yellow liquid consists of accumulated dead neutrophils. It is produced in especially large amounts in the presence of bacteria that produce leukotoxins—toxins that kill leukocytes. Such bacteria are said to be pyogenic (see Chapter 27).

PHAGOCYTOSIS

Once they reach sites of microbial invasion, neutrophils eat and destroy the invading bacteria through phagocytosis. Although a continuous process, phagocytosis can be divided into discrete stages; activation, chemotaxis, adherence, ingestion, and destruction (Fig. 6.9; Gordon, 2016).

Activation

Neutrophils must be activated before they attack and destroy invaders. Thus, when neutrophils bind to endothelial cell integrins and are stimulated by CXCL8, or C5a, they secrete elastase, defensins, and oxidants. The elastase promotes its adhesiveness. The oxidants activate tissue proteases, which in turn release TNF-α from macrophages. The TNF-α, in turn, attracts more neutrophils, thus providing feedback amplification. PAF also activates neutrophils confirming the close functional linkage between neutrophils and blood platelets (Okabayashi et al., 2021).

Chemotaxis

Neutrophils crawl directly toward invading organisms and damaged tissues, attracted by the presence of chemotactic molecules. These chemoattractants diffuse from sites of microbial invasion and form a concentration gradient. Neutrophils crawl toward the area of highest concentration—the source of the material. The moving cells generate

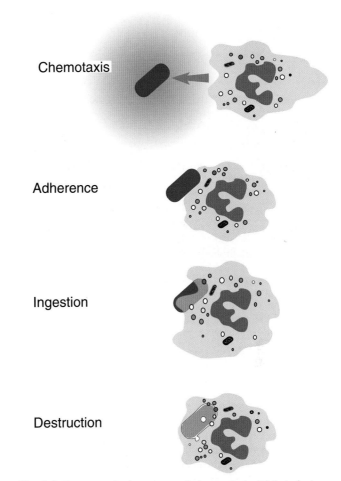

Fig. 6.9 The stages in the process of phagocytosis. While in fact a continuous process, this division into stages provides a useful method of analyzing the process.

projections (lamellipodia) at their leading edges. Chemoattractant receptors are distributed over the neutrophil surface, but the formation of lamellipodia is driven by the higher concentration of attractants at the cell's leading edge (Nourshargh and Alon, 2014).

Microbial invasion and tissue damage generate many chemoattractants. These include the complement peptide C5a (see Chapter 5); a peptide called fibrinopeptide B, derived from fibrinogen; and hydrogen peroxide. A damage-triggered gradient of H$_2$O$_2$ is established within 5 minutes of wounding, just preceding the movement of the first neutrophils toward a wound. Other attractants include chemokines cathelicidins, and lipids such as leukotriene B$_4$ (see Chapter 4; Strom and Thomsen, 1990). Invading bacteria release peptides with formylated methionine groups that are very attractive to the neutrophils of some mammals. Thus, migrating neutrophils receive a multitude of signals, causing them to swarm toward sites of invasion and tissue damage in large numbers (Durr and Peschel, 2002).

Some cattle with a specific genotype of the chemokine receptor CXCR2 have reduced neutrophil migration compared to normal cattle. Cows with this genotype also have reduced expression of the integrin chains CD18 and CD11b and as a result have decreased resistance to bacterial mastitis (Rambeaud and Pighetti, 2005).

Adherence and Opsonization

Once a neutrophil encounters a bacterium, it must "catch" it. This does not happen spontaneously because both cells and bacteria suspended

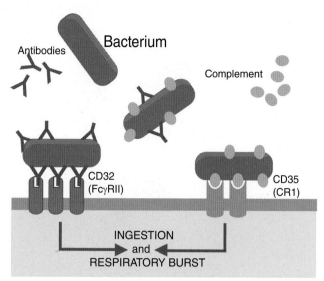

Fig. 6.10 The opsonization of a bacterium by antibodies and complement. Binding of these ligands to their receptors on neutrophils, triggers ingestion and the respiratory burst. The antibody receptor is called CD32, and the complement receptor is called CD35. Type 1 phagocytosis is mediated by antibodies through CD32. Type 2 phagocytosis is mediated by complement through CD35.

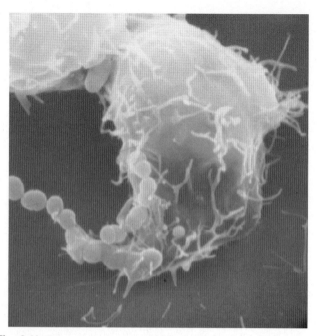

Fig. 6.11 A scanning electron micrograph of a bovine milk neutrophil ingesting *Streptococcus agalactiae*. Note how a film of neutrophil cytoplasm appears to flow over the surface of the bacterium. Original magnification ×5000.

in body fluids usually have a negative charge (zeta potential) and repel each other. The electrostatic charge on the bacteria must be neutralized by coating them with positively charged molecules. Molecules that coat bacteria in this way and promote phagocytosis are called opsonins. This word is derived from the Greek word for "sauce," implying that they make the bacterium more attractive to neutrophils. Examples of such opsonins include mannose-binding lectin, fibronectin, some complement components, and, most importantly, antibodies.

Antibodies, the major proteins produced by the adaptive immune system, are by far the most effective opsonins. They coat bacteria, link them to receptors on phagocytic cells, and trigger their ingestion. Antibody receptor-mediated phagocytosis (or type I phagocytosis) is triggered when antibody-coated bacteria attach to receptors on the neutrophil (Fig. 6.10). CD32 is an example of such an antibody receptor. It binds to the Fc region of antibody molecules (see Chapter 17). CD32 is therefore an example of an Fc receptor (FcR). (There are several different FcRs, CD32 is classified as FcγRII.) However, as pointed out in Chapter 1, antibodies are not produced until several days after the onset of an infection, and the body must rely on innate opsonins for immediate protection. CD35 (or complement receptor–1, CR1) binds the complement component C3b. C3b-coated bacteria bind to neutrophil CD35, but this may not necessarily trigger ingestion. The surface of phagocytic cells is also covered with many pattern-recognition molecules that can bind their ligands to bacteria.

Ingestion

As a neutrophil crawls toward a chemotactic source, a lamellipod advances first, followed by the main portion of the cell. The cytosol of the lamellipod contains a filamentous network of actin and myosin whose polymeric state determines the fluidity of the cytoplasm. When a neutrophil meets a bacterium, the lamellipod flows over and around the organism, and binding occurs between opsonins on the organism and receptors on the neutrophil surface (Fig. 6.11). When antibody-coated microbes are bound by neutrophil CD32, they trigger the polymerization of actin. As a result, actin-rich lamellipods extend from the cell to engulf the particle (type I phagocytosis).

In complement-mediated phagocytosis, particles sink into the neutrophil without lamellipod formation, suggesting that the ingestion process is fundamentally different from that mediated by antibodies (type II phagocytosis). The bacterium is eventually drawn into the cell, and as it is engulfed, it is enclosed in a vacuole called a phagosome. The ease of ingestion depends on the properties of the bacterial surface. Neutrophils readily flow over lipid surfaces so that hydrophobic bacteria, such as *Mycobacterium tuberculosis*, are readily ingested. In contrast, *Streptococcus pneumoniae* has a hydrophilic capsule. It is poorly phagocytosed unless made hydrophobic by opsonization. A third type of ingestion occurs with bacteria such as *Legionella pneumophila* and *Borrelia burgdorferi* where a single lamellipod may wrap itself several times around the organism. This is called coiling phagocytosis.

Destruction

Neutrophils kill ingested bacteria through two distinct processes. One involves the generation of potent oxidants by a respiratory burst. The other involves the release of lytic enzymes and antimicrobial peptides from intracellular granules (Box 6.1).

The Respiratory Burst

Within seconds after binding a bacterium, neutrophils increase their oxygen consumption nearly 100-fold by activating a cell surface enzyme complex called NADPH oxidase (NOX) (Nathan and Cunningham-Bussel, 2013). The NOX components are separate in resting cells, but when a neutrophil encounters TNF or is exposed to other inflammatory stimuli, they assemble to form a complete complex (Fig. 6.12). Activated NOX converts NADPH (the reduced form of NADP, nicotinamide adenine dinucleotide phosphate) to $NADP^+$ with the release of electrons. A molecule of oxygen accepts a donated electron, generating a superoxide anion (the dot in $\cdot O_2^-$ denotes the presence of an unpaired electron):

$$NADPH + 2O_2 \xrightarrow{NOX} NADP^+ + H^+ + 2\cdot O_2^-$$

BOX 6.1 Autophagy

Phagocytosis, as described in this chapter, involves the ingestion, killing, and digestion of extracellular particles such as invading bacteria (Behrends et al., 2010). Cells can also destroy particles within the cytosol by autophagy (Fig. 6.16). Autophagy is a form of cellular waste disposal. The structure to be destroyed, such as an intracellular microbe or a damaged cytoplasmic organelle, is first enclosed within a double membrane to form a cytosolic vesicle called an autophagosome. This then fuses with lysosomes, whose enzymes digest the contents of the autophagosome. Their macromolecules are then released back into the cytosol, where they can be recycled. Autophagy can be triggered by starvation to provide more amino acids for protein synthesis, but it can also be used to selectively remove organelles such as mitochondria, misfolded and aggregated proteins, and intracellular infectious agents. Thus TLR7 or FcγR signaling from phagosomes can initiate their targeting by the autophagy system, possibly by acting through the NOX complex. Autophagy plays important roles in the elimination of intracellular pathogens, activation of intracellular pattern recognition receptors, regulation of inflammasome activation, and intracellular antigen processing. Disorders of autophagy are associated with cancer, neurodegeneration, microbial infections, and aging (Deretic, 2016).

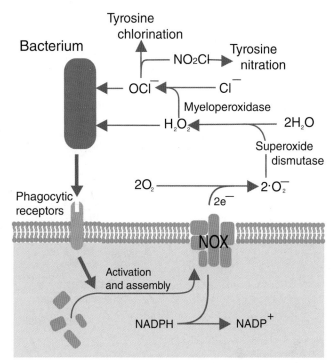

Fig. 6.12 The major features of the respiratory burst pathway in neutrophils. Binding of opsonized bacteria to phagocytic receptors such as CD32 triggers the process. It results in the assembly of the multicomponent enzyme NADPH oxidase (NOX) in the membrane of the phagosome. Once assembled, NOX catalyzes the generation of singlet oxygen. In association with other enzymes such as superoxide dismutase and myeloperoxidase, bactericidal products such as hydrogen peroxide (H_2O_2) and hypochlorite ions (Ocl⁻) are then generated.

Two superoxide anions interact spontaneously (dismutate) to generate one molecule of H_2O_2 under the influence of the enzyme superoxide dismutase:

$$2 \cdot O_2^- + 2H^+ \xrightarrow{\text{superoxide dismutase}} H_2O_2 + O_2$$

Myeloperoxidase then catalyzes the reaction between hydrogen peroxide and chloride ions to produce hypochlorite:

$$H_2O_2 + Cl^- \xrightarrow{\text{myeloperoxidase}} H_2O + OCl^-$$

Plasma Cl^- is used in most inflammatory sites except in milk and saliva, where SCN^- is also employed. Hypochlorous acid (HOCl) is the major product of neutrophil oxidative metabolism. Because of its reactivity, HOCl is rapidly consumed in multiple reactions. As long as H_2O_2 is supplied (neutrophils can generate H_2O_2 for up to 3 hours after triggering), myeloperoxidase will generate HOCl. HOCl kills bacteria by unfolding and aggregating their proteins and oxidizing their lipids, and it enhances the bactericidal activities of the lysosomal enzymes. (Remember that HOCl is the active ingredient of household bleach and is commonly used to prevent bacterial growth in swimming pools).

There are quantitative differences in neutrophil activity between the domestic species, especially in the intensity of the respiratory burst. For example, sheep neutrophils produce less superoxide than human or bovine neutrophils. Neutrophils also have safety mechanisms to detoxify oxidants and minimize collateral damage. Thus they contain large amounts of glutathione, which reduces the oxidants. Redox-active metals such as iron can be bound to lactoferrin to minimize –OH formation, and antioxidants such as ascorbate and vitamin E interrupt these reactions.

Superoxide, hydrogen peroxide, singlet oxygen, hypohalides, and organic peroxides are collectively known by the term reactive oxygen species (ROS). These molecules act at the atomic level, binding to sulfur atoms in the side chains of cysteine and methionine. They inhibit serine/threonine kinases and phosphatases, many transcription factors, signal-regulating proteins, and ion channels. They also oxidize bases in DNA and so influence transcription. ROS activate inflammasomes and promote B- and T-cell activation.

Lytic Enzymes

Once a bacterium is ingested by a neutrophil, the cell's granules (or lysosomes) migrate through the cytosol, fuse with the maturing phagosome, and release their enzymes as the pH drops. (The complete vacuole is then called a phagolysosome.) (Nordenfelt and Tapper, 2011). The rise in ionic strength within phagosomes releases elastase and cathepsin G from their sulfated proteoglycan matrix (Fig. 6.13). Other lysosomal enzymes include lysozyme, proteases, acid hydrolases, and myeloperoxidase. They also contain high concentrations of antimicrobial defensins and cathelicidins. The enzymes that accumulate in phagosomes can digest bacterial walls and kill most microorganisms, but as might be expected, variations in susceptibility are observed. Gram-positive bacteria susceptible to lysozyme are rapidly destroyed. Gram-negative bacteria such as *Escherichia coli* survive somewhat longer since their outer wall is resistant to digestion. Lactoferrin, by binding iron, may deprive bacteria of this essential nutrient and limit bacterial growth (see Chapter 4). Some organisms such as *Brucella abortus* and *Listeria monocytogenes* can interfere with phagosomal maturation in such a way that they do not come into contact with the lysosomal enzymes and can therefore grow inside phagocytic cells. Neutrophil enzymes released into tissues cleave membrane-bound TNF-α from macrophages. The TNF-α attracts and activates yet more neutrophils (Fig. 6.14).

Cytokines

Under the influence of bacterial products such as lipopolysaccharides, neutrophils can secrete many different cytokines such as IL-1,

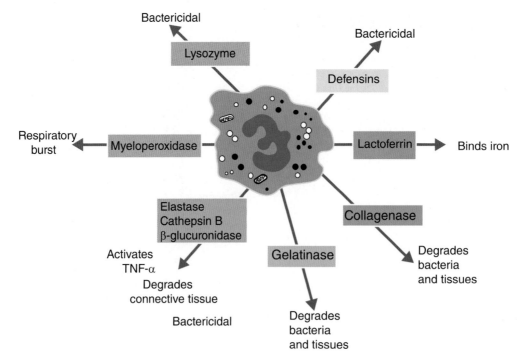

Fig. 6.13 Some of the enzymes and other antibacterial molecules found in the cytoplasmic granules of neutrophils. *TNF-α*, Tumor necrosis factor–α.

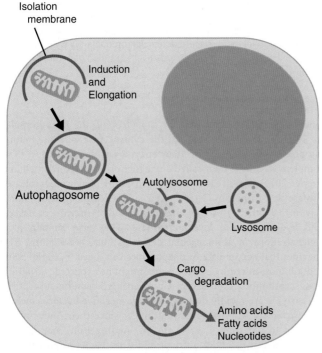

Fig. 6.14 The process of autophagy, a method of cellular waste-disposal. An autophagosome forms within the cytoplasm and encloses the organelle or microbe to be destroyed. Lysosomes fuse with the autophagosome to form an autolysosome. The contents are degraded and recycled. This is a way to get rid of old, damaged organelles as well as intracellular bacteria (Levine and Kroemer, 2008).

TNF-α, IL-6, CXCL8, IL-10, and transforming growth factor–β (TGF-β). Although individual neutrophils produce only small amounts of these cytokines, they invade inflammatory sites in enormous numbers, so their total contribution to both innate and adaptive immune responses may be significant (Rosales, 2020).

EXTRACELLULAR TRAPS

In addition to phagocytosis, neutrophils can also trap and kill extracellular bacteria. Some neutrophils undergo a form of cell death termed NETosis as an alternative to apoptosis or necroptosis (Papayannopoulos and Zychlinsky, 2009). After activation by CXCL8 or lipopolysaccharides, neutrophil oxidants release the contents of the azurophil granules. These enzymes rupture the nuclear and plasma membranes, and as a result, the cell releases long strands of sticky nuclear chromatin and its associated proteins into the extracellular fluid. The neutrophils die within 3–8 hours. The released chromatin strands form networks of decondensed DNA called neutrophil extracellular traps (NETs) (Fig. 6.15; Tan et al., 2021). On occasion, neutrophils may also release NETs in a rapid, oxidant-independent process that is not suicidal.

The NETs are coated with antimicrobial proteins, including citrullinated histones and bactericidal granule components such as elastase, myeloperoxidase, cathepsin G, lactoferrin, and gelatinase. Nets also activate the alternative complement pathway. As a result, these NETs can not only physically bind tightly to bacterial surfaces but can also kill them. It is believed that neutrophils can sense the size of their microbial targets and resort to NETosis when their targets are "too large to eat." They also use NETs to trap and kill fungi such as *Candida albicans* and protozoa such as *Leishmania amazonensis* and *Eimeria bovis* (Fig. 6.16). In cattle, NETs have also been associated with three destruction of blood parasites such as Toxoplasma tachyzoites (see Chapter 29). They have also been implicated in the pathogenesis of many bacterial infections including *Histophilus somni* infections in cattle (Xie et al., 2021) and streptococcal infections in horses (Goggs et al., 2020). NETs are abundant in sites of acute inflammation including mastitic milk. Pyometra in both dogs and cats also results in neutrophils generating NETs within the endometrium to capture the inducing bacteria (Rebordão et al., 2017).

NETs play a very important role in containing microbial invaders, by acting as physical barriers, and so preventing their spread from their initial invasion sites. However, under some circumstances, excessive neutrophil trap formation may cause tissue damage. They

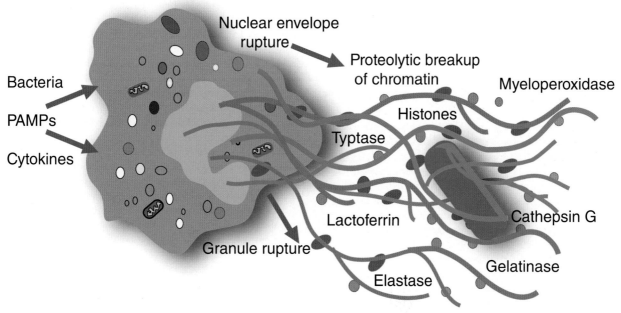

Fig. 6.15 The structure of neutrophil extracellular traps (NETs). NETs are composed of a network of DNA strands to which are attached neutrophil lysosomal enzymes such as myeloperoxidase, cathepsins, and elastases. *PAMPs*, Pathogen-associated molecular patterns.

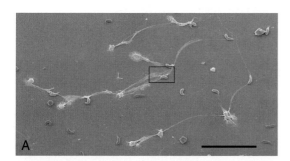

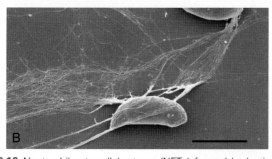

Fig. 6.16 Neutrophil extracellular traps (NETs) formed by bovine neutrophils cocultured with sporozoites of the protozoan parasite, *Eimeria bovis*. (A) Several sporozoites can be seen sticking to a network of fibers originating from dead and disrupted neutrophils (scale bar, 50 μm). (B) At higher magnification, it can be seen that the NETs consist of a meshwork of filaments, many of which are attached to a sporozoite (scale bar, 5 μm). From Behrendt, J.H., Ruiz, A., Zahner, H., et al., 2010. Neutrophil extracellular trap formation as innate immune reactions against the apicomplexan parasite *Eimeria bovis*. Vet. Immunol. Immunopathol. 133, 1–8.

can be deposited on the vessel walls to cause vasculitis and immunothrombosis. They can be deposited in the kidneys to cause glomerulonephritis (see Chapter 33). Normally, however, once their task is completed, these NETs are degraded by DNase, and normal blood flow is restored (Box 6.2).

BOX 6.2 The Role of Platelets

While platelets have been traditionally considered to play a major role in hemostasis and thrombosis, they also contribute significantly to innate immunity. Platelets express many immune receptors on their surface, and they can release a complex mixture of cytokines, bactericidal peptides, and inflammatory mediators. Platelets can readily bind to antigens and pathogens, they play a role in NET formation and inflammation.

Platelets express p-selectins and can promote lymphocyte adhesion to vascular endothelium. They express several integrins, some of which can bind the lymphocyte-activating molecule CD40L. CD40 is constitutively expressed on platelets. They can also express other cell adherence molecules such as DC-SIGN. Some TLRs are also expressed on platelets. Platelets can express many different chemokines (and their receptors), many of which are bactericidal. They are significant sources of IL-1β. They also can produce multiple cationic antimicrobial peptides known as thrombocidins. Collectively, platelets are significant players in the innate immune responses to invading pathogens.

Von Hundleshausen, P., Weber, C., 2007. Platelets as immune cells: bridging inflammation and cardiovascular disease. Circ. Res. 100, 27–40.

SURFACE RECEPTORS

Cells must interact with many molecules and other cells in their environment. To this end, they express many cell surface receptors. As described in Box 6.3, cell surface glycoproteins are classified by the cluster of differentiation (CD) system. Neutrophils carry many different CD molecules on their surface (Fig. 6.17). The most relevant of these are the receptors for opsonins and those that attach neutrophils to blood vessel walls. Other neutrophil surface molecules include receptors for inflammatory mediators such as leukotrienes, complement components such as C5a, chemokines, and cytokines (Thomas and Schroder, 2013).

FATE

Neutrophils are short-lived terminally differentiated cells that have a limited reserve of energy that cannot be replenished. They are therefore most active immediately after release from the bone marrow but are rapidly exhausted and can undertake only a limited number of phagocytic events. Most neutrophils survive for only a few days. They die as a result of apoptosis and mononuclear phagocytes remove the

cell corpses (Bratton and Henson, 2011). Most such cell death is physiological, simply removing unwanted, unused cells. As neutrophils age, they express changes in their surface that send an "eat-me" message to monocytes. For example, the phospholipid, phosphatidyl serine is normally found only on the inner side of the plasma membrane. As neutrophils age, the membrane flips, and phosphatidyl serine is exposed and recognized by macrophages that promptly eat the dying cell in a process called efferocytosis. Efferocytosis is a critical process since it initiates the healing process since the dying cells do not rupture. In its absence, dying neutrophils could release their enzymes and oxidants, and so cause further tissue damage (Bratton and Henson, 2011).

Neutrophil apoptosis also occurs in the presence of inflammatory stimuli, especially ROS. This may also involve the formation of NETs of exocytosed DNA. When dendritic cells ingest apoptotic neutrophils containing bacteria, they secrete TGF-β, IL-6, and IL-23. This IL-23 stimulates the differentiation of Th17 cells that attract even more neutrophils (see Chapter 15). Conversely, ingestion of uninfected apoptotic neutrophils triggers the secretion of IL-10 and TGF-β, promoting the production of regulatory T cells and suppressing inflammation (Lawrence et al., 2020).

Thus, neutrophils may be considered a first line of defense, converging rapidly on invading organisms and destroying them promptly, but they are incapable of sustained effort. The second line of defense is the mononuclear phagocyte system. DAMPs released by neutrophil degranulation or death, promote the recruitment and activation of both macrophages and dendritic cells, augmenting both the innate and adaptive immune responses (see Fig. 2.1).

BOX 6.3   The CD Nomenclature System

When advances in immunology made it possible to produce highly specific monoclonal antibodies against individual cell surface proteins (see Chapter 17), it was shown that mammalian cells expressed hundreds of different proteins on their surface. Initially, each protein was given a specific name and often an acronym as well. It soon became apparent, however, that such a system was unworkable. In an attempt to classify these proteins, a system has been established that assigns each protein to a numbered cluster of differentiation (CD). In many cases, a defined CD denotes a protein (or related proteins) of specific function. For example, the protein CD14 binds bacterial lipopolysaccharides and controls TLR-4 responses. As of March 2016, numbers up to CD371 have been assigned. Unfortunately, CD numbers provide no clue to a molecule's function. In practice, therefore immunologists tend to use a mixed system employing both a CD number and an abbreviation that denotes the function of a molecule. For example, CD32 is also called FcγR1. A list of selected CD molecules can be found in the Appendix.

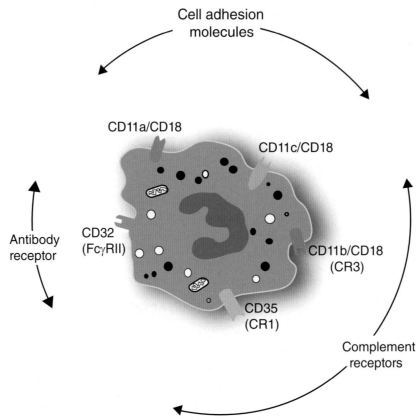

Fig. 6.17 Some of the major surface receptors on neutrophils and their functions.

REFERENCES

Baldridge, M.T., King, K.Y., Goodell, M.A., 2011. Inflammatory signals regulate hematopoietic stem cells. Trends Immunol. 32 (2), 57–65.

Behrendt, J.H., Ruiz, A., Zahner, H., Taubert, A., Hermosilla, C., 2010. Neutrophil extracellular trap formation as innate immune reactions against the apicomplexan parasite *Eimeria bovis*. Vet. Immunol. Immunopathol. 133 (1), 1–8.

Bertram, T.A., 1985. Neutrophil leukocyte structure and function in domestic animals. Adv. Vet. Sci. Comp. Med. 30, 91–129.

Borregaard, N., Sørensen, O.E., Theilgaard-Mönch, K., 2007. Neutrophil granules: a library of innate immunity proteins. Trends Immunol. 28, 340–345.

Bratton, D.L., Henson, P.M., 2011. Neutrophil clearance: when the party is over, clean-up begins. Trends Immunol. 32 (8), 350–357.

Behrends, C., Sowa, M.E., Gygi, S.P., Harper, J.W., 2010. Network organization of the human autophagy system. Nature 466, 68–76.

Burn, G.L., Foti, A., Marsman, G., Patel, D.F., Zychlinsky, A., 2021. The neutrophil. Immunity 54, 1377–1391.

Deretic, V., 2016. Autophagy in leukocytes and other cells: mechanisms, subsystem organization, selectivity, and links to innate immunity. J. Leukoc. Biol. 100 (5), 969–978.

DiStasi, M.R., Ley, K., 2009. Opening the flood-gates: how neutrophil-endothelial interactions regulate permeability. Trends Immunol. 30 (11), 547–556.

Durr, M., Peschel, A., 2002. Chemokines meet defensins: the merging concepts of chemoattractants and antimicrobial peptides in host defense. Infect. Immun. 70, 6515–6517.

Fagerholm, Sc., 2022. Integrins in health and disease. New Engl. J. Med. 387 (16), 1519–1521.

Foster, A.P., Lees, P., Cunningham, F.M., 1992. Platelet activating factor is a mediator of equine neutrophil and eosinophil migration in vitro. Res. Vet. Sci. 53, 223–229.

Goggs, R., Jeffery, U., LeVine, D.N., Li, R.H.L., 2020. Neutrophil-extracellular traps, cell-free DNA, and immunothrombosisin companion animals: a review. Vet. Pathol. 57 (1), 6–23.

Gordon, S., 2016. Phagocytosis: an immunobiologic process. Immunity 44 (3), 463–475.

Hawkey, C.M., 1975. Comparative Mammalian Hematology. Cellular Components and Blood Coagulation of Captive Wild Animals. Heinemann Medical Books, London.

Hidalgo, A., Chilvers, E.R., Summers, C., Koenderman, L., 2019. The neutrophil life cycle. Trends Immunol. 40. https://doi.org/10.1016/j.it.2019.04.013.

Kameritsch, P., Renkawitz, J., 2020. Principles of leukocyte migration strategies. Trends Cell Biol. 30 (10), 818–832.

Lawrence, S.M., Corriden, R., Nizet, V., 2020. How neutrophils meet their end. Trends Immunol. 41 (6), 531–544.

Levine, B., Kroemer, G., 2008. Autophagy in the pathogenesis of disease. Cell 132, 27–42.

Luscinskas, F.W., Lawler, J., 1994. Integrins as dynamic regulators of vascular function. FASEB J. 8, 929–938.

Muller, W.A., 2013. Getting leukocytes to the site of inflammation. Vet. Pathol. 50 (1), 7–22.

Nathan, C., Cunningham-Bussel, A., 2013. Beyond oxidative stress: an immunologist's guide to reactive oxygen species. Nat. Revs. Immunol. 13 (5), 349–361.

Nordenfelt, P., Tapper, H., 2011. Phagosome dynamics during phagocytosis by neutrophils. J. Leukoc. Biol. 90 (2), 271–284.

Nourshargh, S., Alon, R., 2014. Leukocyte migration into inflamed tissues. Immunity 41 (5), 694–707.

Okabayashi, K., Kanai, S., Katakura, F., Takeuchi, R., 2021. Activation of canine neutrophils by platelet-activating factor. Vet. Immunol. Immunopathol. https://doi.org/10.1016/j.vetimm.2021.110336

Papayannopoulos, V., Zychlinsky, A., 2009. NETs: a new strategy for using old weapons. Trends Immunol. 30, 513–521.

Rahman, M.M., Miranda-Ribera, A., Lecchi, C., et al., 2008. Alpha1-acid glycoprotein is contained in bovine neutrophil granules and released after activation. Vet. Immunol. Immunopathol. 125, 71–81.

Rambeaud, M., Pighetti, G.M., 2005. Impaired neutrophil function associated with specific bovine CXCR2 genotypes. Infect. Immun. 73, 4955–4959.

Rebordão, M.R., Alexandre-Pires, G., Carreira, M., Adriano, L., et al., 2017. Bacteria causing pyometra in bitch and queen induce neutrophil extracellular traps. Vet. Immunol. Immunopathol. 192, 8–12.

Rosales, C., 2020. Neutrophils at the crossroads of innate and adaptive immunity. J. Leukoc. Biol. 108, 377–396.

Siwicki, M., Kubes, P., 2022. Neutrophils in host defense, healing and hypersensitivity: dynamic cells within a dynamic host. J. Allergy Clin. Immunol. https://doi.org/10.1016/j.jaci.2022.12.004.

Soehnlein, O., Lindbom, L., 2010. Phagocyte partnership during the onset and resolution of inflammation. Nat. Rev. Immunol. 10, 427–439.

Strom, H., Thomsen, H.K., 1990. Effects of proinflammatory mediators on canine neutrophil chemotaxis and aggregation. Vet. Immunol. Immunopathol. 25, 209–218.

Tan, C., Aziz, M., Wang, P., 2021. The vitals of NETs. J. Leukoc. Biol. 110, 797–808.

Thomas, C.J., Schroder, K., 2013. Pattern recognition receptor function in neutrophils. Trends Immunol. 34, 317–322.

Vestweber, D., 2015. How leukocytes cross the vascular endothelium. Nat. Revs. Immunol. 15 (11), 692–704.

von Vietinghoff, S., Ley, K., 2008. Homeostatic regulation of blood neutrophil counts. J. Immunol. 181, 5183–5188.

Xie, L., Ma, Y., Opsomer, G., Pascottini, O.B., Guan, Y., 2021. Neutrophil extracellular traps in cattle health and disease. Res. Vet. Sci. 139, 4–10.

7

Cellular Innate Immunity: Macrophages and Recovery from Inflammation

Although neutrophils act as a first line of defense, mobilizing, rapidly, converging, and eating and killing invading microorganisms with enthusiasm, they cannot, by themselves, ensure that all invaders are killed. The body therefore employs a "backup" system employing multipurpose phagocytic cells collectively known as macrophages. Their name is derived from the fact that they are "large-eating" cells (Greek *macro, phage*). Macrophages differ from neutrophils in their speed of response, which is slower; in their antimicrobial abilities, which are greater; and in their ability to initiate adaptive immunity by processing antigens. They also act as sentinel cells and initiate tissue repair. Unlike neutrophils, which are specialized for a single task—the killing of invading organisms—macrophages are much more flexible. Depending on their location and environment, macrophages can respond in many different ways. The use of two phagocytic cell systems also permits cooperation between neutrophils and macrophages to enhance many aspects of innate immunity (Soehnlein and Lindbom, 2010). For example, neutrophils tend to be of greater importance in killing extracellular pathogens, whereas macrophages dominate in the fight against intracellular pathogens (Silva, 2010).

MACROPHAGES

Macrophages not only detect and kill invading microbes, but they also produce a mixture of cytokines that promote both innate and adaptive immune responses; they can control inflammation, and contribute directly to the repair of damaged tissues by removing dead, dying, and damaged cells.

Macrophages are a diverse family of cells that reside in many different tissues and, as a result, differ greatly in their transcriptional profiles and in their functions. They can change their activation status and phenotypes in response to signals, especially cytokines, from other cells and from their local environment. This adaptability and resulting diversity have given rise to a confusing nomenclature.

One population of bone marrow–derived macrophages circulates in the bloodstream, where they are called monocytes. Macrophages are found throughout the body in connective tissue, where they are called histiocytes; those found lining the sinusoids of the liver are called Kupffer cells; and those in the brain are called microglia. The macrophages in the alveoli of the lungs are called alveolar macrophages, whereas those in the capillaries of the lung are called pulmonary intravascular macrophages. Some macrophages can develop into dendritic cells. Large numbers are found in the sinusoids of the spleen, bone marrow, and lymph nodes. Irrespective of their name, origin, or location, they are all considered macrophages and collectively form the mononuclear phagocyte system (Fig. 7.1; Wynn et al., 2013).

Structure

In suspension, monocytes are round cells about 15–20 μm in diameter. They possess abundant cytoplasm, at the center of which is a single large, rounded nucleus (Fig. 7.2). Their central cytoplasm contains mitochondria, large numbers of lysosomes, some rough endoplasmic reticulum, and a Golgi apparatus, indicating that they can synthesize and secrete proteins (Figs. 7.3 and 7.4). In living cells, the peripheral cytoplasm is in continuous movement, forming and reforming veil-like ruffles. Many macrophages show variations in this basic structure. For example, blood monocytes have round nuclei, that elongate as the cells mature. Alveolar macrophages contain very little rough endoplasmic reticulum, but their cytosol is full of granules. The microglia of the central nervous system have rod-shaped nuclei and very long cytoplasmic processes (dendrites) that are lost when the cell responds to tissue damage.

Life History

Macrophages arise from multiple sources. Thus, monocytes and intestinal macrophages develop from myeloid stem cells in the bone marrow (Fig. 7.5) (Ginhoux and Jung, 2014). On the other hand, tissue macrophages such as Kupffer cells and microglia arise from the yolk sac or fetal liver stem cells. During development, the myeloid stem cells give rise in sequence to monoblasts, promonocytes, and eventually to monocytes, all under the influence of cytokines called colony-stimulating factors. Monocytes enter the bloodstream and circulate for about three days before entering tissues and developing into macrophages. They account for about 5% of the total leukocyte population in mammalian blood. Tissue macrophages either originate from monocytes or arise by mitosis of precursor stem cells within tissues. They are usually long-lived cells, replacing themselves at a rate of about 1% per day

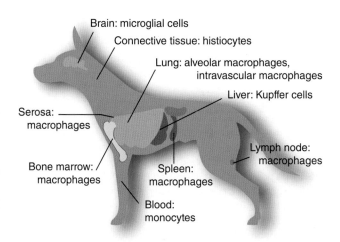

Fig. 7.1 The location of the major populations of cells of the mononuclear phagocyte system.

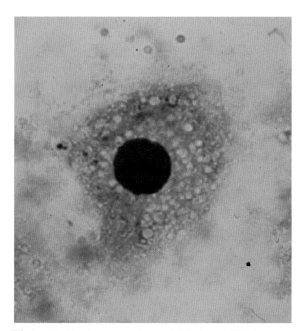

Fig. 7.2 A typical bovine macrophage. Original magnification × 500.

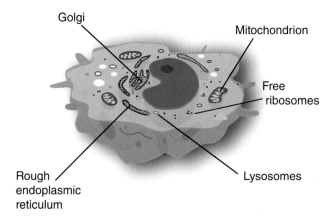

Fig. 7.3 The major structural features of a macrophage. The presence of a rough endoplasmic reticulum and Golgi apparatus demonstrates that these cells can synthesize and secrete significant amounts of proteins.

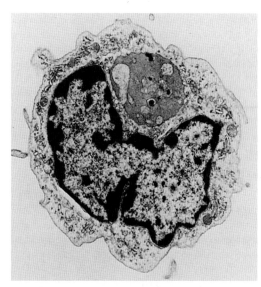

Fig. 7.4 Transmission electron micrograph of a normal rabbit macrophage. The nature of the large inclusion is unknown. Courtesy Dr. S. Linthicum.

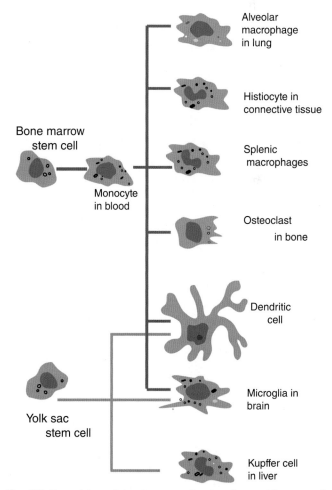

Fig. 7.5 The origin and development of macrophages. Monocytes in blood can differentiate into many different types of macrophages. They can also differentiate into dendritic cells. Some macrophage populations such as the microglia and Kupffer cells may also originate from stem cells in the fetal yolk sac.

unless activated by inflammation or tissue damage. Macrophages may live for a long time after ingesting inert particles, such as the carbon in tattoo ink, although they may fuse together to form multinucleated giant cells in response to DNA damage and mitotic defects. At least some dendritic cell populations appear to be specialized macrophages optimized for antigen processing and presentation (see Chapter 11; Guilliams et al., 2014; Box 7.1).

FUNCTIONS

Sentinel Cells

As described in Chapter 3, macrophages act as sentinel cells. They are widely distributed throughout the body and express many different pattern-recognition receptors (Scott et al., 2014). They detect and respond to invading bacteria and viruses as well as tissue damage. In addition to triggering effective phagocytosis, macrophages produce many cytokines. The most important of these are interleukin-1 (IL-1), IL-6, IL-12, IL-18, and tumor necrosis factor–α (TNF-α) (Fig. 7.6). They also produce chemokines such as CXCL8 (IL-8), that recruit and attract neutrophils.

Inflammation

Macrophages recognize tissue damage, promote the recruitment of neutrophils, and regulate the processes by which neutrophils recruit

---

monocytes. As sentinel cells, macrophages trigger neutrophil emigration from blood vessels. The release of high-mobility group box protein–1 and other damage-associated molecular patterns (DAMPs) from damaged cells stimulates macrophages to produce TNF-α and IL-6 as well as neutrophil chemotactic chemokines and reactive oxygen species.

Exosomes are small cytoplasmic vesicles, about 50–100 nm in diameter, that can transmit signals between cells. They are released by stimulated macrophages, dendritic cells, and B cells. These exosomes carry with them a mixture of immunostimulatory and proinflammatory molecules. They can spread through the extracellular fluid and interact with nearby cells. Thus, exosomes from macrophages containing ingested bacteria can express bacterial cell wall components such as glycopeptidolipids and other pathogen-associated molecular patterns (PAMPs) on their surfaces. These exosomes can bind to PRRs on nearby neutrophils and macrophages, triggering the release of TNF-α and iNOS and promoting more inflammation (O'Neill and Quah, 2008; Tan et al., 2006).

Phagocytosis

When microbial invasion occurs and inflammation develops, blood monocytes respond to PAMPs and DAMPs by binding to vascular endothelial cells in a manner similar to their partners, the neutrophils. Thus, adherence and rolling are triggered by selectin binding, and the cells are brought to a gradual halt by integrins binding to ligands on vascular endothelial cells. The monocytes bind to endothelial cell intracellular adhesion molecule 1, by using their β2-integrins and then emigrate into the tissues (and change their name to macrophages). Several hours after neutrophils have entered an inflammatory site, the macrophages arrive. Neutrophils can reach targets in damaged tissues within 3–4 hours. Macrophages require at least 12 hours. These macrophages are attracted not only by bacterial products and complement components such as C5a but also by DAMPs from damaged cells and tissues. Once neutrophils have migrated into tissues, they too attract macrophages. Thus, neutrophil granules contain macrophage chemoattractants such as azurocidin and cathelicidins. Activated neutrophils and endothelial cells also produce monocyte chemoattractant protein-1 under the influence of IL-6. Neutrophils are the martyrs of the immune system: they reach and attack foreign material first, and by undergoing apoptosis, they attract macrophages to the site of invasion. They also release defensins that augment the antimicrobial activities of macrophages (Poon et al., 2014).

BOX 7.1   Circadian Rhythm and Monocytes

There is a daily oscillation of the number of monocytes present in mouse tissues. The numbers tend to increase while an animal is resting and decrease when the animal is active. Monocytes also express an intrinsic circadian clock where their gene expression pattern varies over 24 h. The monocytes that exhibit the diurnal rhythm in tissues are "inflammatory" monocytes. At the beginning of the animal's resting time (daytime for a mouse), the circulating inflammatory monocyte numbers are low as is their tissue infiltration. At nighttime when the animal is active, the number of circulating monocytes and their tissue infiltration increase. Similar rhythms have been observed in neutrophil homing to bone marrow and in the expression of TLR9 by B cells and splenic macrophages. One practical consequence of this is that an animal's response to a vaccine may also depend on the time of day when it receives the vaccine.

From Druzd, D., Scheiermann, C., 2013. Some monocytes got rhythm. Science 341, 1462–1464.

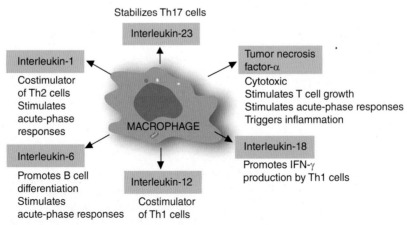

Fig. 7.6 Some of the most important cytokines produced by macrophages and their functions.

Phagocytosis by macrophages differs from the process in neutrophils in that macrophages have few cytoplasmic granules. Instead, they generate oxidants by using a respiratory burst or inducing nitric oxide (NO) synthesis. They also synthesize many new proteins including pro- and antiinflammatory cytokines, antimicrobial peptides and proteins, and enzymes as well as leukotrienes. Macrophages destroy bacteria by both oxidative and nonoxidative mechanisms. In contrast to neutrophils, however, macrophages can undertake sustained, repeated phagocytic events. In addition, macrophages produce proteases such as collagenases and elastases that destroy nearby connective tissue. They produce a plasminogen activator that generates plasmin, another potent protease. Thus, macrophages can "soften up" the local connective tissue matrix and permit more effective penetration of the damaged tissue. Macrophages phagocytose both apoptotic neutrophils and their exosomes. The contents of neutrophil granules are not always destroyed but may be carried to macrophage endosomes where they can continue to inhibit the growth of bacteria. Thus, neutrophils enhance the effectiveness of macrophages in host defense. Macrophages can also release citrullinated DNA, elastase, and histones to form macrophage extracellular traps (METs) in response to bacterial pathogens and their exotoxins (Aulik et al., 2012). Bovine monocyte-derived and alveolar macrophages exposed to *Mannheimia haemolytica* have also been shown to produce METs. These METs together with any captured bacteria are then endocytosed and destroyed by other macrophages. Like neutrophil traps, these METs have significant procoagulant activity and so trigger immunothrombosis (Granger et al., 2017).

Generation of Reactive Nitrogen Species

Major species differences emerge between macrophages in relation to the production of reactive nitrogen species (RNS), especially NO. Thus, in some mammals, especially laboratory rodents, dogs, and horses (but not in humans, pigs, cattle, sheep, goats, or rabbits), microbial PAMPs trigger macrophages to express type 2 nitric oxide synthase (NOS2) (Imrie and Williams, 2019) (The overall gene expression profile of pig macrophages is much closer to humans than to mice). NOS2 converts L-arginine and oxygen to citrulline and NO (Fig. 7.7). Nitric oxide alone is not highly toxic, but it can react with superoxide anion to produce potent RNS such as peroxynitrite and nitrogen dioxide radicals (Bogdan, 2015).

$$NO + O_2^- \rightarrow OONO^- \rightarrow HOONO \rightarrow OH + NO_2^-$$

RNS can also inactivate iron and sulfur-containing enzymes such as the heme-containing respiratory enzymes. They nitrosylate proteins, oxidize lipids, and damage DNA (Wink et al., 2011).

Macrophage Polarization

Macrophages can be divided into two functional subpopulations. One subpopulation, called M1 cells, promotes host defense through inflammation. The other subpopulation, called M2 cells, suppresses inflammation and promotes tissue repair. This polarization is not necessarily permanent. Macrophages can change their phenotype under the influence of other cytokines and microbial products. M1 and M2 cells should perhaps be considered the extremes of a spectrum of phenotypes rather than distinct subpopulations (Fairbairn et al., 2013).

M1 cells generate large amounts of iNOS, and their function is enhanced by exposure to GM-CSF, type I interferons, and especially by interferon-γ (IFN-γ) as well as by microbial pathogens and their products. The sustained production of iNOS permits M1 macrophages to kill bacteria, fungi, protozoa, and some helminths, but at the cost of some tissue damage. They also produce large amounts of TNF-α (Chow et al., 2022).

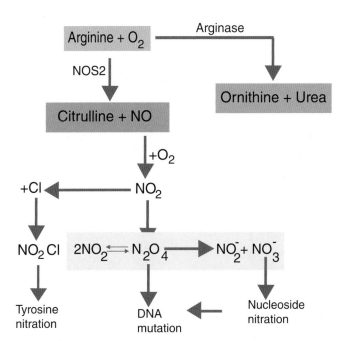

Fig. 7.7 The two pathways of arginine metabolism in macrophages. The production of nitric oxide through the use of nitric oxide synthase 2 is a major antimicrobial pathway and the key feature of M1 macrophages. The use of arginase to produce ornithine, however, reduces the antimicrobial activities of M2 cells.

M2 cells, in contrast, are generated by exposure to M-CSF, IL-4, and IL-13. M2 cells do not produce NO but instead convert arginine to ornithine using the enzyme arginase. M2 cells upregulate their production of IL-8, IL-10, and MCP1. These two macrophage populations play different roles in defending the body. M1 cells defend against microbial invaders and produce proinflammatory cytokines. M2 cells have opposite effects: they reduce inflammation and produce cytokines that suppress immune responses. M2 cells thus promote blood vessel formation, tissue remodeling, and tissue repair. M1 cells are produced early in the inflammatory process when inflammation is required. M2 cells, on the other hand, tend to appear late in the process when healing is required. M1 and M2 cells are attracted by different chemokine mixtures (Porcheray et al., 2005).

A third subset of macrophages, regulatory macrophages, are generated by exposure to the cytokine, IL-10. They have potent antiinflammatory activity and are discussed in Chapter 21.

Macrophage Activation

Although macrophages are competent phagocytes, their activities are greatly enhanced by several activating pathways. Neutrophil granule proteins enhance monocyte adherence to vascular endothelium, trigger macrophages to secrete cytokines, and activate dendritic cells, thus promoting antigen presentation. Molecules that promote M1 macrophage polarization include PAMPs such as lipopolysaccharides, CpG DNA, microbial carbohydrates, and heat-shock proteins as well as many DAMPs. Different levels of M1 activation are recognized, depending on the triggering agent, and some bacteria, such as *Mycobacterium tuberculosis*, are better able to activate macrophages than others. Thus, when monocytes first move into inflamed tissues, they produce increased amounts of lysosomal enzymes, increase phagocytic activity, increase the expression of antibody and complement receptors, and secrete more proteases (Fig. 7.8; Mosser and Edwards 2008). The cytokines produced by these macrophages, especially TNF-α and IL-12, activate a population

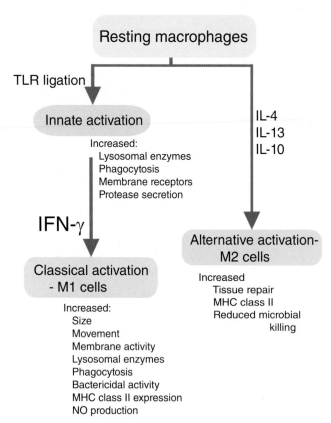

Fig. 7.8 The progressive activation of macrophages can involve three pathways. Innate activation occurs in response to TLR ligation. Additionally, macrophages can become classically activated M1 cells by exposure to microbial products and subsequent exposure to Th1 cytokines such as interferon-γ Alternatively, they may undergo "alternative activation" on exposure to Th2 cytokines and become M2 cells.

of innate lymphocytes called natural killer (NK) cells (see Chapter 19). NK cells in turn secrete IFN-γ, which activates macrophages still further. IFN-γ upregulates many different genes, especially that for NOS2. The *NOS2* gene can be upregulated 400-fold by a combination of IFN-γ and mycobacteria. This increases NO production, so that activated M1 macrophages become even more effective bacterial killers (see Chapter 19).

M2 macrophages are somewhat unique in that they can fuse with other macrophages and, as a result, differentiate into multinuclear osteoclasts in bone. Osteoclasts play a critical role in bone destruction and remodeling. They are large, bone-resorbing cells about 100 μm in diameter and contain up to 20 nuclei. Macrophages can also fuse with other macrophages to form multinucleated, giant cells in other tissues. Giant cells play important roles in chronic inflammation and the removal of foreign bodies (>45 μm) that are too large to be destroyed by single cells. Langhans giant cells are a subtype that contains a horseshoe-shaped ring of nuclei and are found in chronic granulomas. Macrophages can also fuse with somatic cells to promote tissue repair or even with tumor cells to promote cancer metastases.

Receptors

Macrophages express thousands of different receptors on their surface (Fig. 7.9). All are glycoproteins. Some are PRRs, such as the toll-like receptors (TLRs) and the mannose-binding receptor (CD206). CD206 can bind carbohydrate chains terminating in mannose, fucose, or glucose on bacteria and permits macrophages to ingest nonopsonized bacteria.

CD64 is a high-affinity antibody receptor expressed on macrophages and to a lesser extent on neutrophils. Like other antibody receptors, CD64 binds the Fc region of antibody molecules and thus is called an Fc receptor (FcγRI). Its expression is enhanced by IFN-γ-induced activation so a combination of antibody and IFN-γ are potent macrophage activators. Human macrophages also express two low-affinity antibody receptors, CD32 (FcγRII) and CD16 (FcγRIII). Cattle and sheep macrophages express a unique Fc receptor called Fcγ2 R, which can bind particles coated with a specific type of antibody called immunoglobulin G2 (see Chapter 16; Jungi et al., 1992). Macrophages also have receptors for complement components. These include CD35 (CR1) and CD11b/CD18, both of which are C3b receptors.

CD163 is a hemoglobin scavenger receptor expressed on the surface of pig macrophages. It is expressed at high levels in activated macrophages such as those responding to inflammation. By binding free hemoglobin, CD163 reduces the oxidative and proinflammatory effects of hemoglobin and hence has an antiinflammatory effect. During inflammation, it is released into the bloodstream and hence is also an acute-phase protein in the pig. CD163 is a member of the scavenger receptor, cysteine-rich, protein family and as such is closely related to another prominent pig protein, SWC1 that plays a key role in the regulation of γ/δ T cells (see Chapter 15).

Cell surface integrins bind macrophages to other cells, to connective tissue molecules such as collagen and fibronectin, and to some complement components. CD40 is used by macrophages to communicate with lymphocytes. Its ligand (CD154) is expressed on T cells. Thus T cells can activate macrophages via CD40.

FATE OF FOREIGN MATERIAL

Macrophages are located throughout the body and so can detect and capture bacteria or fungi invading by many different routes. For example, bacteria injected intravenously are rapidly removed from the blood. Their precise fate depends on the species involved. In dogs, rodents, and humans, 80%–90% are trapped and removed in the liver. The bacteria are removed by the macrophages (Kupffer cells) that line the sinusoids of the liver. The process occurs in two stages. Bacteria are first phagocytosed by blood neutrophils. These neutrophils are then ingested and destroyed by the Kupffer cells (Gregory and Wing, 2002). These processes thus resemble acute inflammation in which neutrophils are primarily responsible for the destruction of invaders, whereas the macrophages are responsible for preventing damage caused by apoptotic neutrophils (Table 7.1). In contrast, in ruminants, pigs, horses, and cats, particles are mainly removed from the bloodstream by macrophages that line the endothelium of lung capillaries (pulmonary intravascular macrophages) (Figs. 7.10 and 7.11; Brain et al., 1999).

In species where hepatic clearance is important, large viruses or bacteria may be cleared completely by a single passage through the liver (Fig. 7.12). The spleen also filters blood. It is a more effective filter than the liver, but since it is much smaller, it traps much less material. There are also differences in the type of particle removed by the liver and spleen. Splenic macrophages express antibody receptors (CD64) so that particles opsonized with antibody are preferentially removed from the spleen. In contrast, phagocytic cells in the liver express CD35, a receptor for complement C3, so that particles opsonized by C3 are preferentially removed in the liver. The clearance of particles from the blood is regulated by soluble opsonins such as fibronectin or mannose-binding lectin. Experimentally, if an animal is injected intravenously with a very large dose of particles such as colloidal carbon, these opsonins are temporarily depleted, and particles such as bacteria will not be removed from the bloodstream. In this situation, the mononuclear-phagocytic system is said to be "blockaded."

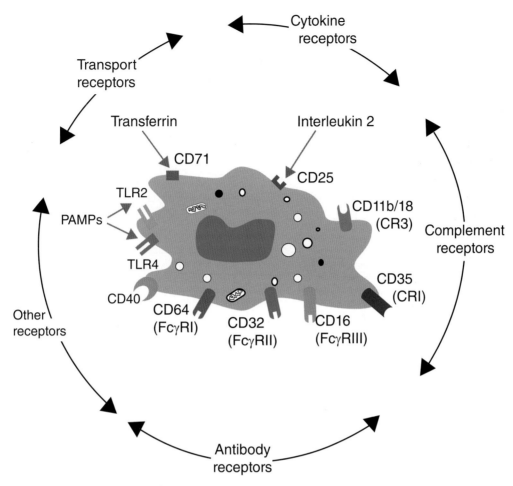

Fig. 7.9 Some of the major surface receptors expressed by macrophages.

TABLE 7.1	Sites of Clearance of Particles from the Blood in Domestic Mammals	
	LOCALIZATION (%)	
Species	**Lung**	**Liver/Spleen**
Calf	93	6
Sheep	94	6
Dog	6.5	80
Cat	86	14
Rabbit	0.6	83
Guinea pig	1.5	82
Rat	0.5	97
Mouse	1.0	94

From Winkler, G.C., 1988. Pulmonary intravascular macrophages in domestic animal species: review of structural and functional properties. Am. J. Anat. 181, 223; Chitko-McKown, C.G., Blecha, F., 1992. Pulmonary intravascular macrophages, a review of immune properties and functions. Ann. Rech. Vet. 23, 201–214.

Removal of bacteria from the bloodstream is greatly enhanced if they are opsonized by specific antibodies. If antibodies are absent or the bacteria possess an antiphagocytic polysaccharide capsule, then the rate of clearance is much slower. Some molecules, such as bacterial endotoxins, estrogens, and simple lipids, stimulate macrophage activity and therefore increase the rate of bacterial clearance. Corticosteroids and other drugs that depress macrophage activity depress the clearance rate.

Based on studies in laboratory rodents and rabbits, it was long believed that bacteria, immune complexes, and other particulate materials were removed from the bloodstream by the macrophages in the liver, spleen, and bone marrow—the mononuclear phagocytic system. However, subsequent studies revealed that in ruminants, horses, cats, and pigs, particles are mainly removed from the bloodstream by macrophages that line the endothelium of lung capillaries (pulmonary intravascular macrophages) (Fig. 15.4). These are large, mature macrophages, 20–80 μm in diameter, that are anchored to the pulmonary capillary endothelium. Intravenous inoculation of colloidal gold particles has shown that up to 60% of these particles are taken up by pulmonary intravascular macrophages in the lungs of sheep, calves, pigs, and cats.

Soluble Proteins Given Intravenously

Unless carefully treated, protein molecules in solution tend to aggregate spontaneously. If such a protein solution is injected intravenously, neutrophils, monocytes, and macrophages rapidly remove these protein aggregates. Unaggregated protein molecules remain in solution and are distributed evenly through the animal's blood. Small proteins (<60 kDa) also spread throughout the extravascular tissue fluids. Once distributed, these proteins are catabolized, resulting in a slow but progressive decline in their concentration. Within a few days, however, the animal will mount an immune response against the foreign protein. Antibodies combine with the antigen; phagocytic cells remove these

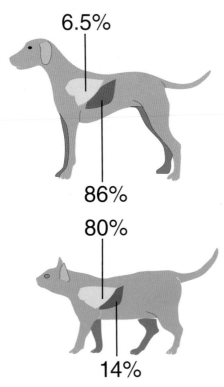

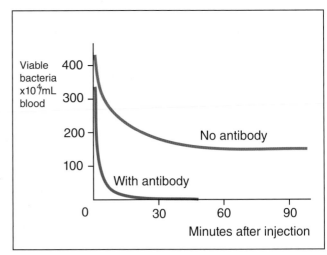

Fig. 7.12 The clearance of bacteria from the blood (in this case *Escherichia coli* from piglets). In the absence of antibodies, bacteria are slowly and incompletely removed.

Fig. 7.10 The different routes by which bacteria are cleared from the bloodstream in the dog and cat expressed as percentages of an administered dose. Dogs mainly use Kupffer cells in the liver. Cats mainly employ pulmonary intravascular macrophages.

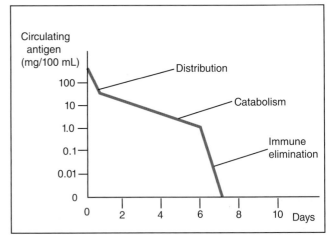

Fig. 7.13 The clearance of a soluble antigen from the bloodstream. Note the three phases of this clearance.

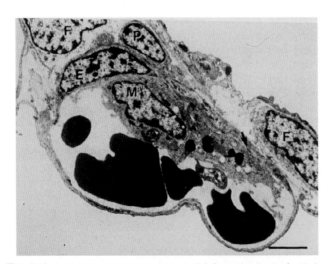

Fig. 7.11 An intravascular macrophage (*M*) from the lung of a 7-day-old pig. The cell has numerous pseudopods, electron-dense siderosomes, phagosomes, and lipid droplets. It is closely attached to the thick portion of the air-blood tissue barrier that contains fibroblasts (*F*) and a pericyte (*P*) between basal laminae of the capillary endothelium (*E*) and the alveolar epithelium. At sites of close adherence, intercellular junctions with subplasmalemmal densities are seen (*arrow*). Bar = 2 μm. Original magnification ×8000. From Winkler, G.C., Cheville, N.F., 1987. Postnatal colonization of porcine lung capillaries by intravascular macrophages: an ultrastructural morphometric analysis. Microvasc. Res. 33, 224–232.

antigen-antibody complexes from the blood; and the protein is rapidly eliminated (Fig. 7.13).

This triphasic clearance pattern of redistribution, catabolism, and immune elimination may change according to circumstances. For example, if the animal has not been previously exposed to a protein antigen, it takes between 5 and 10 days before immune elimination occurs. If, on the other hand, the animal has been primed by prior exposure to the protein, a secondary immune response will occur in 2–3 days, and the catabolic phase will be short. If antibodies are present at the time of antigen administration, immune elimination is immediate, and no catabolic phase is seen. If the injected material is not antigenic or if an immune response does not occur, catabolism will continue until all the material is eliminated.

Fate of Material Administered by Other Routes

When foreign material is injected into a tissue, some local damage and inflammation are bound to occur, and DAMPs are released. As a result, neutrophils and macrophages migrate toward the injection site and phagocytose the injected material. Some will also be captured by dendritic cells. The material captured by macrophages and the dendritic cells can be processed and used to initiate adaptive immune responses. Antibodies and complement (see Chapter 4) interact with the antigenic material, generating chemotactic factors that attract still more phagocytic cells and hastening its final elimination. In the skin, a web of antigen-trapping dendritic cells called Langerhans cells may trap foreign molecules and present them directly to lymphocytes. For this reason, intradermal injection of antigen may be most effective in stimulating an immune response.

Soluble macromolecules injected into a tissue are redistributed by the flow of tissue fluid through the lymphatic system. They eventually reach the bloodstream, so their final fate is similar to intravenously injected material. Any aggregated material present is phagocytosed by neutrophils or tissue macrophages or by the macrophages and dendritic cells of lymph nodes through which the tissue fluid flows.

Respiratory Tract

The fate of inhaled particles such as dust or aerosol droplets depends on their size. Large particles (>5 µm in diameter) stick to the mucous layer that covers the respiratory epithelium from the trachea to the terminal bronchioles. These particles are then removed by the flow of mucus toward the pharynx or by coughing. Very small particles that reach the lung alveoli are ingested by alveolar macrophages, which carry them back to the bronchoalveolar junction; from there, they are also removed by the flow of mucus. Nevertheless, some material may be absorbed from the alveoli. Small particles absorbed in this way are cleared to the draining lymph nodes, whereas soluble molecules enter the bloodstream and are distributed throughout the body. When large amounts of dust are inhaled, as occurs in animals exposed to moldy hay, the alveolar macrophage system may be "blockaded," and the lungs made more susceptible to microbial invasion.

RESOLUTION OF INFLAMMATION

It was once thought that inflammation simply went away when its cause, such as infection, was removed. This is not the case. The resolution of inflammation is an active process. Once invading organisms have been destroyed, macrophages must switch from a killing process to a repair process. Pro-resolving molecules are produced that counteract the pro-inflammatory processes. For example, as inflammation progresses, macrophages change their polarization (Fig. 7.14). The first macrophages that enter the site are activated in the classical manner by TNF-α and GM-CSF to kill invading bacteria. However, these M1 macrophages gradually convert to M2 cells and develop tissue repair and antiinflammatory properties as they receive different signals from the tissues. Thus, the same cell can act in a pro-inflammatory manner at the beginning of an infection but switch to antiinflammatory/tissue repair activities once the infection is overcome and it receives different signals. These signals come from multiple sources such as apoptotic neutrophils, tissue-specific defense collagens, and cytokines such as IL-4 and IL-13 (Bouchery and Harris, 2017). IL-4 and -13 together with efferocytosis of apoptotic cells induce the tissue repair program in macrophages.

Inflammation is also resolved by an active, coordinated process mediated by a complex mixture of lipids related to the leukotrienes. These include resolvins, protectins, maresins, and lipoxins. Produced by endothelial cells, resolving, and protectins promote phagocyte removal by reducing neutrophil emigration from the bloodstream and enhancing macrophage ingestion of apoptotic neutrophils. Maresins are produced by macrophages and enhance tissue repair while acting on nerves to reduce pain. Lipoxins enhance macrophage activity while reducing neutrophil emigration. Chemokines are destroyed by tissue metalloproteases. Apoptotic neutrophils exercise negative feedback by releasing lactoferrin that suppresses neutrophil recruitment. Dying neutrophils attract scavengers. Thus, phagocytosis of apoptotic neutrophils by macrophages promotes the production of vascular endothelial growth factor (VEGF), a cytokine that is crucial for revascularization and wound repair. Once generated, M2 cells secrete secretory leukocyte peptidase (SLP1), a serine protease inhibitor. This molecule inhibits the release of elastase and oxidants by TNF-α-stimulated neutrophils and inhibits the activity of the elastase. SLP1 also protects the antiinflammatory cytokine transforming growth factor-β (TGF-β) from breakdown, and TGF-β in turn, inhibits the release of TNF-α.

Even in normal, healthy animals, millions of cells die daily and must be promptly removed. This is the job of the macrophages. For example, dying neutrophils release the nucleotides adenosine triphosphate and uridine triphosphate. These attract macrophages that therefore move rapidly toward the apoptotic cells. Macrophages "palpate" any neutrophils that they encounter. If the neutrophil is healthy, the cells separate. If, however, the neutrophil is dead or dying, the macrophage remains in contact and eats the neutrophil. This interaction (efferocytosis) operates through CD31 (Fig. 7.15; Allen and Ruckeri, 2017). Thus CD31 on a neutrophil binds to CD31 on a macrophage. If the neutrophil is healthy, it sends a signal to the macrophage, causing it to disengage. On the other hand, if the neutrophil fails to signal, it will be eaten. It is interesting to note that this failure in CD31 signaling occurs long before a neutrophil begins to leak its enzyme contents and cause damage. Likewise, the macrophages that consume these neutrophils do not release cytokines or vasoactive lipids. Ingestion of

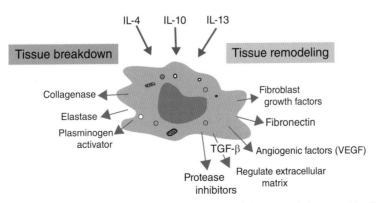

Fig. 7.14 The role of M2 macrophages in tissue breakdown and tissue repair in wound healing. In effect, damaged tissues must be removed before repair and remodeling can begin.

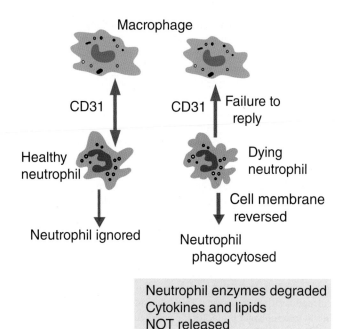

Fig. 7.15 The removal of apoptotic neutrophils. The reaction is initiated by interactions between CD31 on neutrophils and macrophages. If the neutrophil fails to reply when interrogated by a macrophage, it will be ingested and destroyed.

apoptotic neutrophils does, however, cause the macrophages to secrete more TGF-β that in turn promotes tissue repair. Efferocytosis is thus an efficient way of removing apoptotic neutrophils without causing additional tissue damage or inflammation (Martin et al., 2012).

By secreting IL-1β, macrophages also attract and activate fibroblasts. These fibroblasts enter the damaged area and produce collagen. Once sufficient collagen fibers have been deposited, their synthesis stops. This collagen is then remodeled over several weeks or months as the tissue returns to normal (Wick et al., 2010). The reduced oxygen tension in dead tissues stimulates macrophages to secrete cytokines such as VEGF that promote the growth of new blood vessels. Once the oxygen tension is restored to normal, new blood vessel formation ceases.

The final result of this healing process depends on the effectiveness of the inflammatory response. If the cause is rapidly and completely removed, healing will follow uneventfully. If tissue health is not restored, either because the invaders are not eliminated or because tissue repair is inadequate, inflammation may persist and become a damaging, chronic condition. Examples of persistent invaders include bacteria such as *M. tuberculosis*, fungi such as *Cryptococcus* species, parasites such as liver fluke, or inorganic material such as asbestos crystals. Macrophages, fibroblasts, and lymphocytes may accumulate in large numbers around the persistent material for months or years. Because they resemble epithelium in histological sections, these accumulated macrophages are called epithelioid cells. Persistent inflammation and especially prolonged TLR stimulation also cause macrophages to form various multinucleated giant cells. These develop as a result of an activated DNA damage response, repeated attempts at cell division, and defects in mitosis. In all these cases, the persistence of foreign material results in the continual influx of new M2 macrophages that continue to attract fibroblasts and stimulate the deposition of collagen. The compact aggregate of immune cells that develops around this foreign material is called a granuloma (Fig. 7.16). Granulomas consist of granulation tissue—an accumulation of macrophages, lymphocytes, fibroblasts, loose connective tissue, and new blood vessels. The term *granulation tissue* is derived from the granular appearance

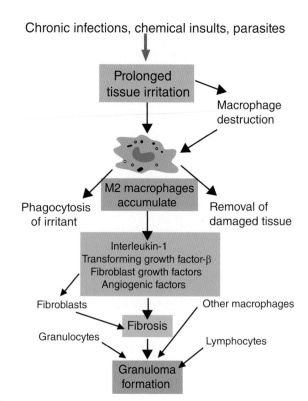

Fig. 7.16 The pathogenesis of chronic inflammation. Macrophages undergoing prolonged stimulation may switch from an M1 to an M2 phenotype. M2 cells secrete cytokine mixtures that not only promote wound healing but also promote the "walling-off" of persistent irritants by fibroblasts and extracellular matrix. Other cell types are attracted to the persistent antigen. Their precise composition will vary with the antigens involved.

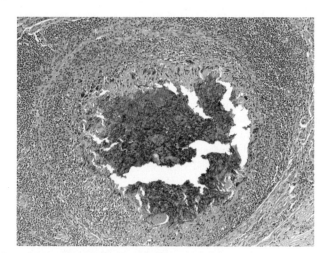

Fig. 7.17 A granulomatous inflammatory reaction around a degenerating tapeworm cyst in a bovine heart. The mass of cells around the central organism is a mixture of macrophages and fibroblasts serving to wall it off from the rest of the body. This would be classified as a type 2 granuloma. Original magnification × 250. Courtesy Dr. John Edwards.

of this tissue when cut. The "granules" are in fact new blood vessels. If the irritant is antigenic (e.g., some persistent bacteria, fungi, and parasites), the granuloma may contain many lymphocytes as well as macrophages, fibroblasts, and probably some neutrophils, eosinophils, and basophils (Fig. 7.17). The chronically activated M2 cells within these granulomas produce IL-1, which stimulates collagen deposition by fibroblasts and eventually "walls off" the lesion from the rest of the body. If the persistent foreign material is not antigenic (e.g., silica, talc, or mineral oil), few neutrophils or lymphocytes will be attracted to the lesion. Epithelioid and multinucleate giant cells, however, may continue their attempts to destroy the offending material. If the material is toxic for macrophages (as is asbestos), leaking enzymes and cytokines such as IL-6 may lead to central necrosis, chronic tissue damage, local fibrosis, and scarring (Wynn and Vanella, 2016; Fielding et al., 2014).

Chronic granulomas, whether due to immunological or foreign body reactions, may enlarge and destroy normal tissues. In liver fluke infestations, for example, death may result from the gradual replacement of normal liver cells by fibrous tissue formed as a result of the persistence of the parasites. Granulomas may be classified into type 1 granulomas as typified by tubercles. These contain macrophages and dendritic cells and are associated with significantly increased production of IFN- and IL-17 from Th1 and Th17 cells. Type 2 granulomas, as typified by those that form around parasitic worms in tissues, contain macrophages and dendritic cells, may contain eosinophils, have increased production of IL-4, -5, and -13, and have large numbers of fibroblasts (Azouz et al., 2004).

REFERENCES

Allen, J.E., Ruckeri, D., 2017. The silent undertakers: macrophages programmed for efferocytosis. Immunity. https://doi.org/10.1016/j.immune.2017.10.010

Aulik, N.A., Hellenbrand, K.M., Czuprynski, C.J., 2012. *Mannheimia haemolytica* and its leukotoxin cause macrophage extracellular trap formation by bovine macrophages. Infect. Immun. 80, 1923–1933.

Azouz, A., Razzaque, M.S., El-Hallak, M., Taguchi, T., 2004. Immunoinflammatory responses and fibrogenesis. Med. Electron. Microsc. 37, 141–148.

Bogdan, C., 2015. Nitric oxide synthase in innate and adaptive immunity: an update. Trends Immunol 36 (3), 161–178.

Bouchery, T., Harris, N.L., 2017. Specific repair by discerning macrophages. Science 356, 1014.

Brain, J.D., Molina, R.M., DeCamp, M.M., Warner, A.E., 1999. Pulmonary intravascular macrophages: their contribution to the mononuclear phagocytic system in 13 species. Am. J. Physiol. 276 (1), L145–L154.

Chow, L., Soontararak, S., Wheat, W., Ammons, D., Dow, S., 2022. Canine polarized macroiphages express distinct functional and transcriptomic profiles. Front. Vet. Sci. https://doi.org/10.3389/fvets.2022.988981.

Fairbairn, L., Kapetanovic, R., Beraldi, D., et al., 2013. Comparative analysis of monocyte subsets in the pig. J. Immunol. 190, 6389–6396.

Fielding, C.A., Jones, G.W., McLoughlin, R.M., McLeod, L., et al., 2014. Interleukin-6 signaling drives fibrosis in unresolved inflammation. Immunity 40 (1), 40–50.

Ginhoux, F., Jung, S., 2014. Monocytes and macrophages: developmental pathways and tissue homeostasis. Nat. Rev. Immunol. 14 (6), 392–404.

Granger, V., Faille, D., Marani, V., Noel, B., et al., 2017. Human blood monocytes are able to form extracellular traps. J. Leukoc. Biol. 102 (3), 775–781.

Gregory, S.H., Wing, E.J., 2002. Neutrophil-Kupffer cell interaction: a critical component of host defenses to systemic bacterial infections. J. Leukoc. Biol. 72, 239–248.

Guilliams, M., Ginhoux, F., Jakubzick, C., Naik, S.H., et al., 2014. Dendritic cells, monocytes and macrophages: a unified nomenclature based on ontogeny. Nat. Revs. Immunol. 14 (8), 571–578.

Imrie, H., Williams, D.J.L., 2019. Stimulation of bovine monocyte-derived macrophages with lipopolysaccharide, interferon−γ, interleukin-4 or interleukin-1 does not induce detectable changes in nitric oxide or arginase activity. BMC Vet. Res. https://doi.org/10.1186/s12917-019-1785-0.

Jungi, T.W., Francey, T., Brcic, M., et al., 1992. Sheep macrophages express at least two distinct receptors for IgG which have similar affinity for homologous IgG$_1$ and IgG$_2$. Vet. Immunol. Immunopathol. 33, 321–337.

Martin, C.J., Booty, M.G., Rosebrock, T.R., Nunes-Alves, C., Desjardins, D.M., Keren, I., et al., 2012. Efferocytosis is an innate antibacterial mechanism. Cell Host Microbe. 12 (3), 289–300.

Mosser, D.M., Edwards, J.P., 2008. Exploring the full spectrum of macrophage activation. Nat. Rev. Immunol. 8, 958–969.

O'Neill, H.C., Quah, B.J.C., 2008. Exosomes secreted by bacterially infected macrophages are proinflammatory. Sci. Signal 1, 1–5.

Poon, I.K., Lucas, C.D., Rossi, A.G., Ravichandran, K.S., 2014. Apoptotic cell clearance: basic biology and therapeutic potential. Nat. Revs. Immunol. 14 (3), 166–180.

Porcheray, E., Viaud, S., Rimaniol, A.-C., et al., 2005. Macrophage activation switching: an asset for the resolution of inflammation. Clin. Exp. Immunol. 142, 481–489.

Scott, C.L., Henri, S., Guilliams, M., 2014. Mononuclear phagocytes of the intestine, the skin, and the lung. Immunol. Revs. 262 (1), 9–24.

Silva, M.T., 2010. When two is better than one: macrophages and neutrophils work in concert in innate immunity as complementary and cooperative partners of a myeloid phagocytic system. J. Leukoc. Biol. 87, 93–106.

Soehnlein, O., Lindbom, L., 2010. Phagocyte partnership during the onset and resolution of inflammation. Nat. Revs. Immunol. 10 (6), 427–439.

Tan, B.H., Meinken, C.C., Bastian, M., et al., 2006. Macrophages acquire neutrophil granules for antimicrobial activity against intracellular pathogens. J. Immunol. 177, 1864–1871.

Wick, G., Backovic, A., Rabensteiner, E., et al., 2010. The immunology of fibrosis: innate and adaptive responses. Trends Immunol. 31, 110–119.

Wink, D.A., Hines, H.B., Cheng, R.Y., Switzer, C.H., Flores-Santana, W., Vitek, M.P., et al., 2011. Nitric oxide and redox mechanisms in the immune response. J. Leuko. Biol. 89 (6), 873–891.

Wynn, T.A., Chawla, A., Pollard, J.W., 2013. Macrophage biology in development, homeostasis and disease. Nature 496 (7446), 445–455.

Wynn, T.A., Vannella, K.M., 2016. Macrophages in tissue repair, regeneration, and fibrosis. Immunity 44 (3), 450–462.

8

Sickness: The Body's Innate Responses

CHAPTER OUTLINE

While inflammation often appears to be a local response, restricted to sites of tissue damage or microbial invasion, it can also have significant effects on distant parts of the body. If the local inflammation is minor, such systemic effects may not be noticed. If, however, inflammation affects multiple organ systems, or if the microbial invaders succeed in spreading throughout the body, these systemic effects become clinically significant. These include fever, changes in behavior, endocrine changes, and even cardiovascular changes. Collectively, we call them sickness. It need hardly be pointed out that in Veterinary Medicine, it is these signs of sickness that draw the attention of an owner to an animal's illness.

SICKNESS BEHAVIOR

When an animal is invaded by pathogens, inflammatory cytokines are released into the circulation and act directly on the brain and liver. The subjective feelings of sickness—malaise, lassitude, fatigue, loss of appetite, and muscle and joint pains, as well as a fever—are evidence of a systemic innate immune response. These reflect changes in the body's priorities as it fights off the invaders. Microbial PAMPs acting through the pattern-recognition molecules stimulate the production of a cytokine wave consisting of interleukin-1β (IL-1β), IL-6, and tumor necrosis factor–α (TNF-α) (Fig. 8.1). These three cytokines signal to the brain using two pathways. One pathway acts through the sensory neurons that serve damaged tissues. Stimulation by IL-1β through the vagus nerve can signal directly to the brain. (IL-1 will not trigger a fever if the vagus nerve is cut.) Lipopolysaccharide (LPS) binding to TLR4 on intestinal cells can also trigger these vagal signals. As a result, they initiate fever, nausea, and other sickness responses. Alternatively, these cytokines may diffuse directly into the brain from the bloodstream. They act on neurons and microglia to modify behavior and alter pain perception. Type 1 interferons can also enter the brain and trigger malaise, depression, and sickness behavior (Box 8.1).

High-mobility group box protein–1 (HMGB1) is a potent sickness-inducing alarmin. Although IL-1, IL-6, and TNF-α have long been known to cause septic shock and sickness behavior, it is now clear that these three molecules induce the release of HMGB1 from macrophages (Sha et al., 2008). HMGB1 has been implicated in food aversion and weight loss. It mediates endotoxin lethality, joint pain, and macrophage activation. The inflammation induced by necrotic cells is caused in part by the escape of HMGB1 from disrupted nuclei and damaged mitochondria (Yang et al., 2005).

FEVERS

The most obvious systemic response to infection is the development of a fever resulting from an increase in metabolic rate. Thus the development of a fever, 2°C above baseline body temperature, requires a 20% increase in basal metabolism. The inflammatory cytokines that can trigger this include IL-1α, IL-1β, IL-6, IFN-α, TNF-α, and TNF-β. These cytokines act on the brain where they induce cyclooxygenase-2 (COX-2) production in the preoptic nucleus of the hypothalamus as well as in the limbic system. This results in local prostaglandin-E_2 (PGE_2) production. The PGE_2 acts on warm-sensitive neurons to slow their firing rate and so alter the body's thermostatic set point. These changes in the set point result in behavioral changes. For example, affected animals conserve heat by vasoconstriction and increase their heat production by shivering, thus raising their body temperature until it reaches the new set point.

Fevers and Innate Immunity

Combating infection requires a major shift in metabolic priorities. Given that sickness consistently suppresses food intake, the body must mobilize reserves of protein and energy to support the initial innate response as well as increased thermogenesis. Fevers are protective in that they enhance many innate and adaptive immune responses (Fig. 8.2). Fever clearly modulates the outcomes of infection. Thus it

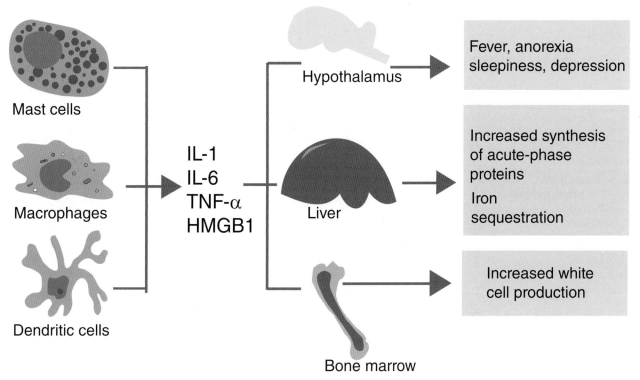

Fig. 8.1 Sickness behavior is part of the response of the body to inflammatory stimuli. Multiple systemic effects are due to the cytokines secreted by sentinel cells, mast cells, macrophages, and dendritic cells. The major sickness-inducing cytokines are interleukin (IL)-1, IL-6, tumor necrosis factor (TNF)–α, and high-mobility group band protein–1 (HMGB1) acting on the brain, liver, and bone marrow.

reduces virus replication within cells and increases the sensitivity of bacteria to complement-mediated lysis. Fever increases blood flow to infected tissues thus speeding the mobilization of effector cells (Evans et al., 2015). A high body temperature enhances many neutrophil functions. It promotes their release from the bone marrow, their trans-endothelial migration, and their chemotactic responses, increasing their accumulation within tissues. Fever-range temperatures stimulate their respiratory burst, enhancing their bacteriolytic activity.

Increased body temperatures enhance multiple macrophage functions such as phagocytosis, release of cytokines, and the expression of TLR2, TLR4, and MHC molecules. Warmed macrophages upregulate their production of TNF-α through the actions of HSP70. It also upregulates their production of nitric oxide synthase and hence NO production.

Fever enhances the phagocytic abilities of dendritic cells (DCs) as well as NK cell cytotoxicity. Fever upregulates phagocytosis by DCs and their expression of TLR2 and TLR4. It enhances DC migration to lymphoid organs. Activated DCs enhance CD4 T-cell proliferation and direct them toward Th1 responses (Walter et al., 2016).

Fevers and T-Cell Functions

High body temperatures increase the binding affinity of many immune system receptor-ligand pairs. As a result, they enhance lymphocyte, specifically T cell, behavior and effectiveness. (Fig. 8.2). Fevers enhance the passage of T cells across high endothelial venule walls, promote immunological synapse formation, and inhibit T-cell apoptosis. Fevers act on T cells through a pathway that involves heat shock protein 90 and α4 integrins (Lin et al., 2019). Thus, when mouse T cells are held at 40°C for 12 hours, they develop an increased ability to bind to integrins. As a result, these heat-treated T cells have an enhanced ability to migrate across membranes. When mice are exposed to elevated temperatures for 6 hours, their T cells show increased adherence to high endothelial venules and trafficking into lymph nodes and Peyer's patches.

Fever range temperatures enhance $CD8^+$ effector cell differentiation. Fever range temperatures also modulate cytokine production by T cells. Thus, when primed $CD4^+$ T cells are maintained at a moderate fever temperature (39°C) they tend to function as Th2 cells producing IL-4, IL-5, and IL-13 while suppressing the production of the Th1 cytokine interferon-γ (IFN-γ).

It is also clear that febrile temperatures control the differentiation and plasticity of Th17 cells. As a result, they produce greater quantities of IL-17F and IL-22. These cells and the interleukins they produce play

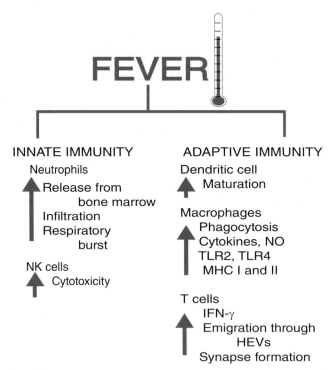

Fig. 8.2 The enhancement of both innate and adaptive immune responses as a result of a fever. *HEV,* High endothelial venule; *IFN-γ,* interferon-γ; *MHC,* major histocompatibility complex; *NK,* natural killer; *TLR,* toll-like receptor.

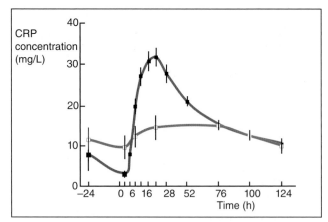

Fig. 8.3 The rise in C-reactive protein (*CRP*) levels in six dogs following anesthesia and surgery (*red line*) and in six dogs undergoing anesthesia alone (*blue line*). From Burton, S.A., Honor, D.J., Mackenzie, A.L., et al., 1994. C-reactive protein concentration in dogs with inflammatory leukograms. Am. J. Vet. Res. 55, 615.

a critical role in stimulating acute inflammation and neutrophil activation (Wang et al., 2020). Changes in body temperature also influence B cell responses but this is largely a consequence of alterations in Th cell functions.

Metabolic Changes

In addition to causing a fever, inflammatory cytokines, especially IL-1, promote the release of sleep-inducing molecules. Thus, lethargy is commonly associated with a fever. This response may reduce the energy demands of an animal and increase that available for defense and repair (Herz and Kipnis, 2016). IL-1, IL-18, and leptin (a cytokine from adipose tissue) suppress the hunger centers in the hypothalamus and so are responsible for the loss of appetite associated with infections. The benefits of this are unclear but it may oblige the animal to be more selective about its food. IL-1, IL-6, and TNF-α also act on skeletal muscle to increase protein catabolism and release free amino acids. Although this results in myalgia and muscle wastage, the newly available amino acids are available for increased antibody and cytokine synthesis. If animals are subjected to long-term, low-grade inflammation, they will be exposed to chronic, low doses of TNF-α. As a result, they lose weight, become anemic, and protein depleted. TNF-α inhibits the uptake of lipids by preadipocytes and causes mature adipocytes to lose stored lipids. TNF-α is thus responsible for the weight loss seen in animals with cancer or chronic parasitic and bacterial diseases such as Johne's disease. Weight loss is a common response to infection (and sometimes to vaccination) and is of special significance to livestock producers.

The Costs of a Fever

While on balance, the ability to develop a fever is a positive adaptive response, it does result in a temporary inability of an animal to function normally in a social context. Humans take to their beds; other mammals do not have a choice. Thus sickness behavior may result in increased vulnerability to predators. In addition, there may be social costs within animal groups. For example, febrile monkeys spend more time resting and less time feeding, just like sick humans! (McFarland et al., 2021). These febrile monkeys were targeted with twice as much aggression by their troop mates and were six times more likely to become injured. Sick elk are selectively targeted by wolves. Thus sickness behavior has significant costs for gregarious mammals and important ecological consequences. In view of these disadvantages, many mammals and birds attempt to hide their sickness, especially when a potential predator such as a human is present.

ACUTE-PHASE PROTEINS

Inflammatory cytokines also act on liver cells. Under the influence of the TNF-α, IL-1, and especially IL-6, hepatocytes are induced to synthesize many new proteins (Eckersall and Bell, 2010). Because this increase is associated with acute infections and inflammation, these newly produced proteins are called acute-phase proteins (APPs). The increase in APP levels begins about 90 minutes after injury or the onset of systemic inflammation and subsides within 48 hours (Fig. 8.3). It may also occur following prolonged stress such as road transportation or confinement. Over 30 APPs have been recognized in mammals, and many are important components of the innate immune system. They include soluble PRMs, complement components, clotting factors, protease inhibitors, and iron-binding proteins. Different species produce different APPs (Fig. 8.4; Ceron et al., 2005).

Pattern-Recognition Molecules

Pentraxins are P-type lectins that act as soluble pattern-recognition molecules (Du Clos, 2013). Two of the most important are C-reactive protein (also called PTX1) and serum amyloid P (PTX2) (see Chapter 2). C-reactive protein (CRP) is the major acute-phase protein produced in primates, rabbits, and dogs and is important in pigs in response to IL-6. Serum amyloid P (SAP) is also a pentraxin (PTX2) and the major acute-phase protein in rodents. A major function of SAP is to regulate innate immune responses. It binds to macrophage Fc receptors, reduces the binding of neutrophils to the extracellular matrix, reduces the differentiation of macrophages into fibroblasts so inhibiting fibrosis, and promotes phagocytosis of cell debris. SAP binds and stabilizes amyloid proteins (Mantovani and Garlanda, 2023).

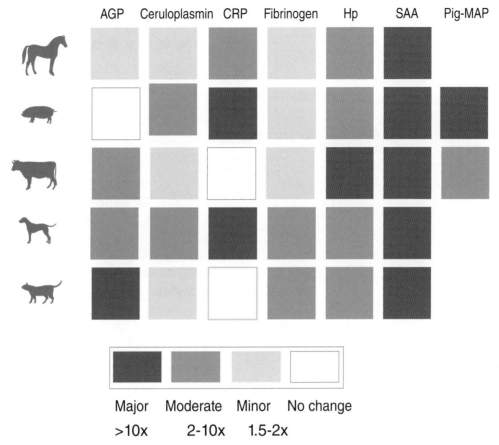

Fig. 8.4 Species differences in the major acute-phase proteins produced by the domestic mammals. *CRP,* C-reactive protein.

Pentraxin 3 (PTX3) is a large octomeric protein that is rapidly produced in response to TNF-α, IL-1β, and some microbial components. It is produced by monocytes/macrophages, neutrophils, endothelial cells, and stromal cells. PTX3 levels rise faster than CRP in acute-phase responses since it is stored preformed and rapidly released from neutrophil granules. PTX3 has been identified in the lung fluids, endothelial cells, alveolar macrophages, and neutrophils of pigs, foals, and calves (Townsend et al., 2023). In pigs, it has antibacterial effects against *Streptococcus vsuis* (Xu et al.,2015). CRP, SAP, and PTX3 can all bind to diverse bacteria, fungi, and viruses and promote their phagocytosis.

Other soluble PRMs that act as APPs include LPS-binding protein in cattle, humans, and rabbits, CD14 in humans, horses, and mice, and C-type lectins such as mannose-binding lectin and conglutinin in other mammals (Silva et al., 2013). LPS-binding protein is a type II APP that presents LPS to CD14 and TLR4 on phagocytic cells and enhances their proinflammatory activity up to 1000-fold. It can also bind lipotechoic acids on the cell wall of gram-positive bacteria and trigger inflammation through TLR2 activation (Cox et al., 2014).

Iron-Binding Molecules

One of the most important factors that determines the success or failure of bacterial invasion is the availability of iron (Fig. 8.5). Most pathogenic bacteria, such as *Staphylococcus aureus, Escherichia coli, Bacillus anthracis, Pasteurella multocida*, and *Mycobacterium tuberculosis*, require iron for growth since iron atoms form the key catalytic sites in many enzymes. Animals, however, also require iron for vital functions such as oxygen transport and energy production. As a result,

bacteria and their hosts compete for the same metal. The result of this competition may determine the outcome of an infection (Cassat and Skaar, 2013). When serum iron levels are elevated, as occurs after red cell destruction, animals become more susceptible to bacterial infections. Free iron concentrations within mammal tissues are normally very low. Mammalian blood has just 10^{-26}M free iron since almost all of the available iron is bound to proteins. These iron-binding proteins include transferrin, lactoferrin, hepcidin, siderocalin, haptoglobin, and ferritin.

Iron is usually absorbed from food through duodenal enterocytes. It binds to a cell surface iron-carrier called ferroportin and is transported to the bloodstream where it is transferred to transferrin. Most of this iron is incorporated into hemoglobin in red cells. Less than 10% of our daily needs are, however, met by importing dietary iron. Mostare derived by recycling aged or damaged red cells. Aged red cells give up their iron when ingested by splenic macrophages. The macrophages phagocytose these cells and catabolize the hemoglobin using hemoxygenase. They release the iron obtained from hemoglobin into the circulation via ferroportin. The exported iron binds to transferrin and is carried to erythroblasts for use in new red cell production (Ganz and Nemeth 2015).

Despite the low availability of free iron, bacteria such as *M. tuberculosis, B. anthracis*, and *E. coli*, can successfully invade an animal because they produce their own iron-binding proteins called siderophores. Mycobacteria use their siderophore (called carboxymycobactin) to strip iron from mammalian ferritin. *S. aureus* uses staphyloferrins to lyse red cells and access the iron in hemoglobin.

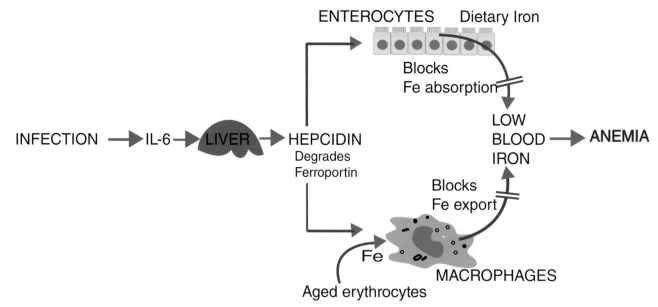

Fig. 8.5 The role of hepcidin in regulating iron availability. This protein prevents iron efflux from enterocytes and macrophages by binding to ferroportin and triggering its degradation. The net effect is to retain iron within these cells, making it unavailable for hemoglobin synthesis and leading to the development of anemia. *IL-6,* Interleukin-6.

Enterobactin is a very potent iron chelator produced and secreted by many enteric bacteria. In response, the body responds to microbial invasion by producing two additional APPs, hepcidin and haptoglobin. Hepcidin is produced by hepatocytes under the influence of IL-1 and IL-6. It binds to ferroportin and triggers its internalization and degradation. Hepcidin also suppresses intestinal iron absorption by downregulating ferroportin expression in enterocytes (Johnson et al., 2010). In healthy individuals, hepcidin production is regulated by systemic iron availability or by erythropoietic signals and hypoxia. In inflammation, however, IL-6 and IL-1 stimulate the hepcidin promoter. As a result, hepcidin increases, ferroportin decreases, iron absorption by enterocytes is blocked, and macrophages can no longer export their iron (Drakesmith and Prentice 2012). Iron availability for red blood cell production drops, and hypoferremia develops. Chronically infected animals become anemic—the anemia of infection. This is usually a mild normocytic, normochromic, nonregenerative anemia (Chikazawa and Dunning, 2016).

Haptoglobin is a major acute-phase protein in ruminants, horses, and cats. It can rise from virtually undetectable levels in normal calves to as high as 1 mg/mL in calves with acute respiratory disease. Haptoglobin also binds iron and makes it unavailable to invading bacteria.

Mammals may also capture iron by stealing bacterial siderophores. Thus, during bacterial infections, the liver, spleen, and macrophages synthesize a protein called lipocalin 2. Lipocalin 2 (also called siderocalin) binds the bacterial siderophore enterochelin with very high affinity. Lipocalin 2 is essential for limiting the growth of enterochelin-producing bacteria such as *E. coli* but does not affect bacteria that employ other methods to acquire iron.

Other iron-binding APPs include transferrin (important in birds) and hemopexin. Activation of macrophages by IFN-γ leads to downregulation of macrophage iron import through transferrin receptors and so deprives intracellular bacteria of needed iron. A similar situation occurs in the mammary gland when, in response to bacterial invasion, milk neutrophils release stored lactoferrin. The lactoferrin binds iron and makes it unavailable to the bacteria.

Serum Amyloid A

Serum amyloid A (SAA), a lipoprotein of 15 kDa, is the major acute-phase protein in cattle, cats, pigs, and horses and is also important in humans and dogs. Thus equine SAA concentrations rise several 100-fold during noninfectious arthritis, whereas canine SAA concentrations increase up to 20-fold in bacterial disease. The functions of SAA are unclear, but it binds to TLR2 and may also be an endogenous TLR4 agonist (Cheng et al., 2008). This leads to NF-kB activation and the production of multiple inflammatory cytokines. SAA recruits lymphocytes to inflammatory sites and activates enzymes that degrade the extracellular matrix. It increases significantly in mastitic milk (Nielsen et al., 2004). SAA is a chemoattractant for neutrophils, monocytes, and T cells. It regulates the intensity of inflammation by inhibiting myeloperoxidase release and inhibiting lymphocyte proliferation.

Other Acute-Phase Proteins

Alpha-1-acid glycoprotein (AGP) is a minor acute-phase protein in cattle but important in cats. Neutrophils exposed to activating agents such as phorbol myristate acetate rapidly release their stores of α_1-acid glycoprotein. This protein inhibits the respiratory burst and may reduce the damage caused by excessive inflammation. Alpha-1-acid glycoprotein has antiinflammatory and immunomodulatory effects. It inhibits complement activities and promotes the release of IL-IRA from macrophages.

Some serum protease inhibitors such as α_1-antitrypsin, α_1-antichymotrypsin, and α_2-macroglobulin are also APPs. They inhibit neutrophil proteases in sites of acute inflammation and thus reduce tissue damage. Major acute-phase protein (MAP), a 120 kDa plasma glycoprotein, is a significant protease inhibitor in pigs and a moderate one in cattle. MAP shares homology with inter-α-trypsin inhibitor heavy chain 4, a moderate acute-phase protein in dogs. Other APPs include ceruloplasmin (a copper-binding protein), haptoglobin, and fibrinogen in sheep and CRP, haptoglobin, sialic acid, apolipoprotein A, and ceruloplasmin in pigs.

Some protein levels fall during acute inflammation. These are called "negative" APPs. Two of the most important are albumin and transferrin. The albumin serves as a source of amino acids that can be used on demand, such as during infections and inflammation. Recent studies have also identified a serum enzyme associated with lipid oxygenation, paraoxonase 1, as a potentially useful negative acute phase protein for diagnostic purposes. Thus, in dogs, it is significantly reduced in cases of acute pancreatitis, leishmaniasis, and sepsis. In cats, it is significantly reduced in cases of feline infectious peritonitis (Meazzi et al., 2021).

Acute-Phase Proteins as "Biomarkers" of Disease

It is possible to identify animals with severe infections or inflammation by measuring acute-phase protein levels in the blood. This may be helpful, for example, in antemortem meat inspections by identifying animals that are suffering from inapparent inflammation or infection and hence are unfit to eat. Numerous studies have examined the specificity and sensitivity of these assays by determining their ROC curves (see Chapter 43). Different APPs increase in different inflammatory states, and different APPs may predominate at different stages of a disease. In cattle, haptoglobin increases in chronic infections such as mastitis, enteritis, respiratory disease, traumatic pericarditis, and endometritis. SAA and lipopolysaccharide-binding protein are sensitive markers of respiratory infection in calves. In calves with umbilical abscesses, fibrinogen is elevated, followed by haptoglobin and SAA. A mammary-associated isoform of SAA (M-SAA3) is elevated in mastitis. The acute-phase response in sheep is similar to that in cattle.

In horses, very high SAA levels accompanied by low iron concentrations probably reflect the presence of widespread systemic infection. Fibrinogen is a less sensitive indicator in this species. Vaccination elicits a prominent acute-phase response in horses (Andersen et al., 2012).

Pigs with tail lesions and carcass abscesses due to biting have elevated levels of CRP, SAA, and haptoglobin compared to control pigs. These tail lesions were associated with increased carcass condemnation. In experimental *Actinobacillus pleuropneumoniae* infections, CRP and SAA are significantly increased (Heinonen et al., 2010).

In dogs, CRP is the major acute-phase protein, increasing 100-fold in infectious diseases such as pyometra-associated sepsis, babesiosis, leishmaniasis, parvovirus infection, and colibacillosis. APP levels increase moderately in canine inflammatory bowel disease. CRP, haptoglobin, and SAA are significantly elevated in the cerebrospinal fluid and serum of dogs with canine steroid-responsive arteritis-meningitis (see Chapter 38). In pregnant dogs, haptoglobin, ceruloplasmin, and fibrinogen levels increase midway through gestation. SAA also increases in pyometra.

The acute-phase response to systemic infections in cats appears to differ in several respects from other mammals (Paltrinieri, 2008). For example, CRP is not a major acute-phase reactant in cats. The three major APPs in cats are SAA, alpha-1-acid glycoprotein, and haptoglobin. In feline infectious peritonitis (FIP) caused by a coronavirus, blood SAA levels increase 10- to 50-fold. They are also elevated in diabetes mellitus, other infectious diseases, traumatic injury, and cancer. α_1-Acid glycoprotein also increases in FIP and other feline virus infections.

SYSTEMIC INFLAMMATORY RESPONSE SYNDROME

While inflammation is an essential component of the innate immune response, it can, on occasion, get out of control and cause lethal damage. When animals die from infectious diseases or malignancies, death is not always attributable to a direct effect of the pathogen or its toxins but may be a result of a systemic inflammatory response syndrome (SIRS). After massive tissue damage, large amounts of cellular components including

---

BOX 8.2 Immune Reconstitution Inflammatory Syndrome!

When bats hibernate, their body temperature drops, and they may become immunosuppressed. This permits the causal agent of white-nose syndrome, a filamentous fungus called *Pseudogymnoascus destructans*, to colonize and erode the skin of their wings, ears, and muzzle. About a week after infected bats emerge from hibernation, they develop an intense inflammatory response that leads to their death. It has been suggested that the sudden reversal of immune suppression that occurs when their body temperature rises, results in the development of immune reconstitution inflammatory syndrome (IRIS). This syndrome was first reported in AIDS patients following the onset of effective antiretroviral therapy. It is believed that the recovery of T-cell function drives an exaggerated immune response against the underlying infection. Thus, in white-nose syndrome, cold-loving *P. destructans* is present in infected tissues. When body temperature returns to normal, T-cell function is rapidly restored, leading to a massive neutrophil influx that results in tissue destruction.

From Meteyer, C.U., Barber, D., Mandl, J.N., 2012. Pathology in euthermic bats with white nose syndrome suggests a natural manifestation of immune reconstitution inflammatory syndrome. Virulence 3, 10–16; Blehert, D.S., Hicks, A.C., Behr, M., Meteyer, C.U., et al., 2009. Bat white nose syndrome: an emerging fungal pathogen? Science 323, 227.

HMGB1, mitochondria, and oxidants may escape into the bloodstream and trigger hyperinflammation. These DAMPs activate sentinel cells, and as a result, large quantities of inflammatory mediators such as TNF-α, IL-1β, IL-18, IFN-γ, CXCL8, and IL-6 are released (Lee and Cron, 2023). Large amounts of the complement fragment, C5a, are also produced. These cytokines and C5a trigger the activation of yet more T cells and the release of yet more cytokines, leading to even greater cell destruction. As a result, affected animals develop high fevers, tachycardia, tachypnea, leukopenias, and coagulopathies. This "cytokine storm" can result in multiple organ failures and death. SIRS is often triggered by massive bacterial infections, tissue trauma, or burns. However, viruses such as influenza, COVID-19, and dengue, can also trigger excessive cytokine release and death (Box 8.2; Babyak and Sharp, 2016).

Severe traumatic tissue injury may also result in the development of a SIRS. This serves to limit further damage and initiate healing. However, it can also result in complications. Thus, additional tissue damage may occur as a result of the release of oxidants from activated phagocytic cells (Hietbrink et al. 2006; Huber-Lang et al., 2018).

Bacterial Septic Shock

Septic shock (or sepsis) is the name given to an SIRS caused by severe bacterial infections and complicated by reduced blood pressure and unresponsiveness to fluid therapy. It accounts for about 9% of human deaths in the United States and is a correspondingly important cause of animal deaths. Severe infections can cause excessive triggering of TLRs, leading to a massive and uncontrolled release of HMGB1. Other cytokines involved are TNF-α and IL-1β, with IFN-γ, IL-6, IL-3, and CXCL8 in supporting roles. These cytokines, in turn, stimulate nitric oxide synthase 2, leading to an increase in serum nitric oxide and COX-2, and resulting in massive prostaglandin and leukotriene synthesis. This excessive mediator release causes severe acidosis, fever, an uncontrollable drop in blood pressure, elevation of plasma catecholamines, and eventually renal, hepatic, and lung failure. Tissue damage, inflammation, and the release of damaged cell fragments all act to raise blood levels of TF, a key initiator of coagulation. The cytokines activate vascular endothelial cells so that their procoagulant activity is enhanced, leading to excessive blood clotting. The nitric oxide causes vasodilation and a drop in blood

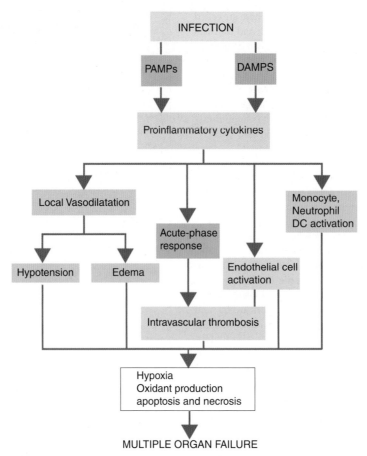

Fig. 8.6 The pathogenesis of the systemic inflammatory response syndrome. In effect, the syndrome results from massive overproduction of multiple cytokines as a result of a severe infection or massive tissue damage. This "cytokine storm" triggers a series of events that result in widespread cell death and multiple organ failure. *DAMPs,* Damage-associated molecular patterns; *DC,* dendritic cells; *PAMPs,* pathogen-associated molecular patterns.

pressure. The prostaglandins and leukotrienes also increase vascular permeability. This combination of effects may result in disseminated intravascular coagulation (Fig. 8.6; Lewis et al., 2012).

Disseminated Intravascular Coagulation

Disseminated intravascular coagulation (DIC) is a severe clinical syndrome characterized by an imbalance between the clotting and fibrinolytic systems (Fig. 8.7; Berthelsen et al., 2011). It is triggered by overwhelming infections, immune-mediated cell destruction, and some cancers. It occurs in two phases. First, there is a hypercoagulable phase as the clotting cascade is activated by damaged vascular endothelial cells. This damage results in the excessive production of a transmembrane glycoprotein called "tissue factor" (TF) (CD142). TF does not trigger blood clotting in healthy tissues. However, TF is released on exposure to cytokines, especially IL-1 and TNF-α. It is also released by massive tissue damage or by exposure to bacteria and bacterial endotoxins. The TF transforms prothrombin to thrombin to form fibrin thrombi. Simultaneous downregulation of anticoagulant systems results from reduced antithrombin synthesis (it is a "negative" acute-phase protein). Activation of the clotting cascade also leads to the formation of neutrophil NETs and platelet microthrombi in small blood vessels throughout the body. These thrombi can cause intravascular thrombosis leading to ischemia, impaired organ perfusion, and widespread damage (Wada, 2004). In addition, the newly formed thrombi consume clotting factors and platelets.

The hypercoagulable phase is followed by a hemorrhagic phase. Thus the excess thrombin activates plasminogen to generate plasmin, which causes fibrinolysis. When the microthrombi break down they release anticoagulant fibrin breakdown products such as D-dimer that therefore promote hemorrhage and uncontrolled bleeding. Plasmin also activates the complement and kinin systems and these too promote, inflammation, hypotension, and increased vascular permeability. The occurrence of DIC carries with it a poor prognosis.

Multiple-Organ Dysfunction Syndrome

Multiple-organ dysfunction syndrome (MODS) is defined as altered organ function in an acutely ill animal such that homeostasis cannot be maintained without intervention (Osterbur et al., 2014). It is usually a sequel to severe sepsis or septic shock but can also develop as a result of major trauma or anything else that will induce a SIRS (Fig. 8.8). It is characterized by hypotension, insufficient tissue perfusion, uncontrollable bleeding, and organ failure caused by hypoxia, tissue acidosis, mitochondrial dysfunction and cytopathic hypoxia, tissue necrosis, and severe local metabolic disturbances. The reported incidence of MODS in dogs is about 4% in trauma and 50% in sepsis cases. MODS results from immune system dysregulation and subsequent mitochondrial dysfunction. The immune system dysregulation may be due to overregulation of the inflammatory response and the excessive release of neutrophil reactive oxygen species (ROS), leading to lethal tissue damage. MODS can affect the liver, respiratory system, brain, adrenal, the heart, and the kidneys. It permits bacterial translocation in the gastrointestinal tract and disseminated intravascular coagulation.

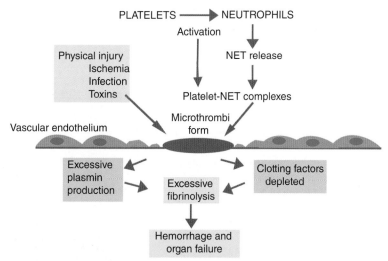

Fig. 8.7 The pathways of disseminated intravascular coagulation. Initially, the coagulation pathway is activated as a result of widespread injury to vascular endothelium, together with platelet activation and NETosis. The neutrophil extracellular trap (NET)-platelet complexes form microthrombi. The interaction of these NETs together with platelets and components of the coagulation pathway results in intravascular thrombus formation (immunothrombosis). However, in DIC, this excessive thrombosis eventually depletes the animal of clotting factors. In addition, plasmin is generated in large amounts and dissolves these thrombi through fibrinolysis. As a consequence, uncontrolled hemorrhage may result. *DIC,* Disseminated intravascular coagulation.

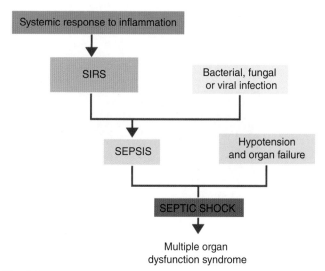

Fig. 8.8 The relationships of systemic inflammatory response syndrome (SIRS), sepsis, septic shock, and multiple organ dysfunction syndrome.

The sensitivity of mammals to septic shock varies greatly. Species with pulmonary intravascular macrophages (cats, horses, sheep, and pigs) tend to be more susceptible than dogs and rodents, which lack these cells and are relatively insusceptible to lung injury (DeClue et al., 2011).

Bacterial Toxic Shock

Some strains of *S. aureus* produce toxins that stimulate T-cell functions (Fig. 8.9). These toxins may activate up to 20% of an animal's T cells, causing them to secrete enormous quantities of IL-2 and IFN-γ. These in turn stimulate the overproduction of TNF-α and IL-1β. This leads to the development of a fever, hypotension, collapse, skin lesions, and damage to the liver, kidney, and intestines with multiple-organ dysfunctions called toxic shock syndrome. A similar syndrome has also

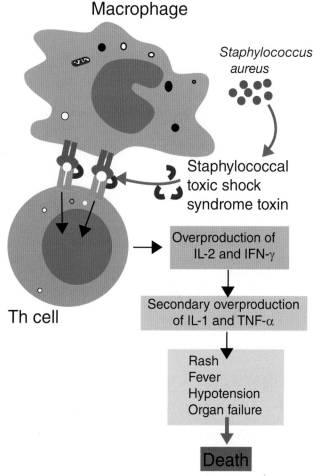

Fig. 8.9 The pathogenesis of Staphylococcal toxic shock syndrome. The toxic shock syndrome toxin is a potent superantigen that acts as a powerful stimulant of interleukin (IL)-1 and tumor necrosis factor–α (TNF-α) production. *IFN-γ,* Interferon-γ.

been observed in some streptococcal infections. In these cases, streptococcal M-protein binds to fibrinogen. The M-protein-fibrinogen complexes bind to endothelial cell integrins and trigger a respiratory burst. This causes an increase in vascular permeability and hypercoagulability, leading to toxic shock characterized by hypotension and DIC.

Systemic Inflammatory Response Syndrome–Associated Laminitis

Acute laminitis is a common debilitating disease in horses and ponies. While traditionally considered a single entity, laminitis is now recognized as a syndrome resulting from several different mechanisms: These include endocrinopathic disease caused by prolonged hyperinsulinemia, support-limb laminitis caused by prolonged weight-bearing on one hoof, and inflammation-related laminitis. Experimentally, inflammation sufficient to trigger laminitis can be triggered by carbohydrate (starch and oligofructose) overload, black walnut poisoning, or by sepsis. All of these forms of laminitis may have a final common pathway (Katz and Bailey, 2012).

In most mammals with sepsis, as described above, internal organs such as liver or lung are damaged as a result of a cytokine storm, and this results in organ failure. In the horse, in contrast, the epidermal laminae within the hoof are the vulnerable organs. (The laminar tissue is formed by the interdigitations between the dermis and epidermis formed by the basement membrane.) Infections that trigger laminitis may therefore include pleuropneumonia, endometritis, and gastrointestinal injury. In the latter case, this may be due to enterocolitis and severe colic, especially when associated with dysbiosis of the colonic microbiota as a result of carbohydrate overload. Massive death of gram-negative bacteria releases large amounts of lipopolysaccharide resulting in destruction of the epithelial barrier, gram-negative sepsis, and endotoxemia. While endotoxin alone cannot induce laminitis, other molecules escaping from the damaged gut probably play a role. The complex mixture of PAMPs and DAMPs escaping from the colon, presumably acting through PRMs, triggers acute laminar inflammation. Endothelial cells, epidermal cells, and macrophages release COX-2 and ROS, as well as IL-1β and IL-6 and many different chemokines. They also trigger leukocyte infiltration and activation. The resulting acute inflammation within the lamina upregulates the matrix and secretes metalloproteases within the hoof. These degrade the proteoglycans in the basement membrane of the lamellae as well as collagen in the intercellular matrix. This leads to basement membrane disruption and the separation of the epidermal and dermal laminar tissue. The separation may also be due to downregulation of epithelial cell adherence proteins such as integrins and to a loss of hemidesmosomes, oxidative injury, and excessive apoptosis.

Treatment includes prolonged cooling of the foot to reduce blood flow and exudation, pain management, and mechanical support for the damaged hoof. If lamellar damage is not controlled the disease may become chronic leading to rotation of the third phalanx, coffin bone remodeling, dropped sole and development of a lamellar wedge.

PROTEIN MISFOLDING DISEASES

Amyloidosis is the name given to the deposition of large quantities of insoluble protein fibrils in body organs. These deposits appear as amorphous, eosinophilic, hyaline proteins in cells and tissues (Fig. 8.10). Amyloid proteins are produced as a result of errors in the folding of newly formed protein chains. These misfolded chains eventually aggregate to form insoluble fibrils. Electron microscopy shows that amyloid proteins consist of protein fibrils, formed by peptide chains cross-linked to form β-pleated sheets (Fig. 8.11). This molecular conformation makes amyloid proteins extremely insoluble and almost totally

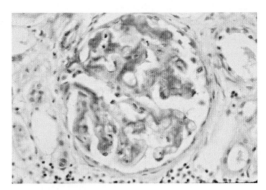

Fig. 8.10 Secondary amyloid deposited in a glomerulus. The red dye (Congo red) specifically binds to amyloid fibrils. Original magnification ×400.

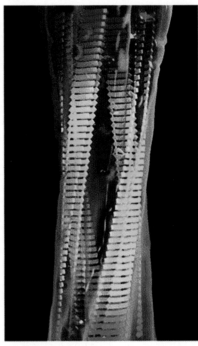

Fig. 8.11 Molecular model of an amyloid fibril. From Dobson, C.M., 1999. Protein misfolding, evolution and disease. Trends Biochem. Sci. 24, 329–332.

resistant to digestion by proteases. Consequently, once deposited in cells or tissues, amyloid is almost impossible to remove. Amyloid accumulation eventually leads to gradual cell loss, tissue destruction, and death. Amyloidosis may be systemic when it involves multiple organs, or it may be localized, involving only a single organ (Herczenik and Gebbink, 2008).

Many different proteins have been shown to misfold and form amyloid (Fig. 8.12). The most important of these proteins is the acute-phase protein, SAA. As a result of its chronic overproduction, amyloidosis develops in response to long-term, persistent inflammation. Fragments of SAA can misfold, aggregate, and then be deposited extracellularly in organs such as the liver, kidney, and spleen. This material, the most common form in domestic animals, is called reactive amyloid or AA amyloid. AA amyloidosis is associated with chronic inflammation in mastitis, osteomyelitis, abscesses, traumatic pericarditis, metritis, gangrenous pneumonia, equine recurrent uveitis, and tuberculosis. AA amyloidosis is a major cause of death in horses repeatedly immunized for commercial antiserum production.

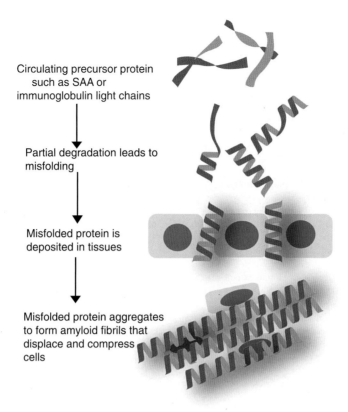

Circulating precursor protein
such as SAA or
immunoglobulin light chains

↓

Partial degradation leads to
misfolding

↓

Misfolded protein is
deposited in tissues

↓

Misfolded protein aggregates
to form amyloid fibrils that
displace and compress
cells

Fig. 8.12 The pathogenesis of reactive amyloid fibril deposition. Misfolded proteins aggregate to form insoluble fibrils that are deposited in many tissues. *SAA,* Serum amyloid A.

Multiple myelomas are plasma cell tumors that secrete huge quantities of antibody light chains (see Chapter 17). These light chains and their misfolded fragments are then deposited to form immunogenic (AL) amyloid in multiple organs. AL amyloid is the most common form of amyloid in humans but is very rare in domestic animals (Kim et al., 2005).

Several other forms of localized amyloidosis are recognized in domestic animals; for example, old dogs may suffer from vascular amyloidosis, in which amyloid is deposited in the media of leptomeningeal and cortical arteries. In humans, amyloid fibrils are deposited in the neurons of patients with Alzheimer's disease. An inherited form of amyloid has been described in Abyssinian cats and Shar Pei dogs where it is deposited in the liver. Familial amyloidosis of Shar Peis consists of AA amyloid generated as a result of chronic recurrent inflammation (Shar Pei fever). Tumor-like amyloid nodules and subcutaneous amyloid have been reported in horses, but in general, amyloid deposits are found in the liver, spleen, and kidneys, particularly within renal glomeruli. As a result, animals with amyloidosis commonly die as a result of renal failure.

Misfolded proteins may be transmissible. They form the prion proteins that cause spongiform encephalopathies such as bovine spongiform encephalopathy (BSE) and scrapie. Prions are protease-resistant forms of cellular proteins. In the case of BSE, the prion is a misfolded and aggregated form of a cellular protein PrP^c that is important for normal macrophage functions. These proteins normally play a role in resistance to intracellular bacteria such as *Brucella*. It is also of interest to note that even reactive amyloidosis is somewhat "transmissible," since inoculation of AA proteins into a laboratory mouse will hasten the development of amyloidosis. In such cases, amyloid proteins likely act by providing a substrate on which other misfolded proteins can be deposited. There is evidence that foie gras prepared from duck or goose liver can transmit AA amyloidosis when fed to mice. Similarly, silk fibers (a very stable protein composed of β-sheets) may promote amyloidosis when inserted into mice!

REFERENCES

Andersen, S.A., Petersen, H.H., Ersboll, A.K., Falk-Ronne, J., Jacobsen, S., 2012. Vaccination elicits a prominent acute phase response in horses. Vet. J. 191, 199–202.

Babyak, J.M., Sharp, C.R., 2016. Epidemiology of systemic inflammatory response syndrome and sepsis in cats hospitalized in a veterinary teaching hospital. J. Am. Vet. Med. Assn. 249 (1), 65–71.

Berthelsen, L.O., Kristensen, A.T., Tranholm, M., 2011. Animal models of DIC and their relevance to human DIC: a systematic review. Thromb. Res. 128 (2), 103–116.

Cassat, J.E., Skaar, E.P., 2013. Iron in infection and immunity. Cell Host Microbe. 13 (5), 509–519.

Ceron, J.J., Eckersall, P.D., Martinez-Subiela, S., 2005. Acute phase proteins in dogs and cats: current knowledge and future perspectives. Vet. Clin. Pathol. 34, 85–99.

Cheng, N., He, R., Tian, J., et al., 2008. Cutting edge: TLR2 is a functional receptor for acute-phase serum amyloid A. J. Immunol. 181, 22–26.

Chikazawa, S., Dunning, M.D., 2016. A review of anaemia of inflammatory disease in dogs and cats. J. Small Anim. Pract. 57 (7), 348–353.

Cox, N., Pilling, D., Gomer, R.H., 2014. Serum amyloid P: a systemic regulator of the innate immune response. J. Leukoc. Biol. 96 (5), 739–743.

De Clue, A.E., Delgado, C., Chang, C.-H., Sharp, C.R., 2011. Clinical and immunologic assessment of sepsis and the systemic inflammatory response syndrome in cats. J. Am. Vet. Med. Assn. 238, 890–897.

Drakesmith, H., Prentice, A.M., 2012. Hepcidin and the iron-infection axis. Science 338 (6108), 768–772.

Du Clos, T.W., 2013. Pentraxins: structure, function, and role in inflammation. ISRN Inflamm. 379040. 2013

Eckersall, P.D., Bell, R., 2010. Acute phase proteins: biomarkers of infection and inflammation in veterinary medicine. Vet. J. 185, 23–27.

Evans, S.S., Repasky, E.A., Fisher, D.T., 2015. Fever and the thermal regulation of immunity: the immune system feels the heat. Nat. Rev. Immunol. 15 (6), 335–349.

Ganz, T., Nemeth, E., 2015. Iron homeostasis in host defence and inflammation. Nat. Rev. Immunol. 15 (8), 500–510.

Heinonen, M., Orro, T., Kokkonen, T., et al., 2010. Tail biting induces a strong acute phase response and tail-end inflammation in finishing pigs. Vet. J. 184, 303–307.

Herczenik, E., Gebbink, M.F.B.G., 2008. Molecular and cellular aspects of protein misfolding and disease. FASEB J. 22, 2115–2133.

Hietbrink, F., Koenderman, L., Leenen, L.P.H., 2006. Trauma: the role of the innate immune system. World J. Emerg. Surg. 1, 15. https://doi.org/10.1186/1749-7922-1-15.

Herz, J., Kipnis, J., 2016. Bugs and brain: how infection makes you feel blue. Immunity 44 (4), 718–720.

Huber-Lang, M., Lambris, J.D., Ward, P.A., 2018. Innate immune responses to trauma. Nat. Immunol. 19, 327–341.

Johnson, E.E., Sandgren, A., Cherayil, B.J., et al., 2010. Role of ferroportin in macrophage-mediated immunity. Inf. Immun. 78, 5099–5106.

Katz, L.M., Bailey, S.R., 2012. A review of recent advances and current hypotheses on the pathogenesis of acute laminitis. Equine Vet. J. 44 (6), 752–761.

Kim, D.Y., Taylor, H.W., Eades, S.C., Cho, D.-Y., 2005. Systemic AL amyloidosis associated with multiple myeloma in a horse. Vet. Pathol. 42, 81–84.

Lee, P.Y., Cron, R.Q., 2023. The multifaceted immunology of cytokine storm syndrome. J. Immunol. 210, 1015–1024.

Lewis, D.H., Chan, D.L., Pinheiro, D., Armitage-Chan, E., Garden, O.A., 2012. The immunopathology of sepsis: pathogen recognition, systemic inflammation, the compensatory anti-inflammatory response, and regulatory T cells. J. Vet. Int. Med. 26 (3), 457–482.

Lin, C., Zhang, Y., Zhang, K., et al., 2019. Fever promotes T lymphocyte trafficking via a thermal sensory pathway involving heat shock protein 90 and α4 -integrins. Immunity 50, 137–151.

Mantovani, A., Garlanda, C., 2023. Humoral innate Immunity and acute phase proteins. N. Engl. J. Med. 388, 439–452.

McFarland, R., Henzi, S.P., Parrett, L., Bonnell, T., et al., 2021. Fevers and the social costs of acute infection in wild vervet monkeys. Proc. Natl. Acad. Sci. U.S.A. 118 (44) e207881118.

Meazzi S, Paltrinieri S, Lauzi S, Stranieri A, et al. Role of paraononase-1 as adiagnostic marker for feline infectious peritonitis. Vet J, 2021; https://doi:10.1016/j.tvjl.2021.105661.

Nielsen, B.H., Jacobsen, S., Andersen, P.H., et al., 2004. Acute phase protein concentrations in serum and milk from healthy cows, cows with clinical mastitis, and cows with extramammary inflammatory conditions. Vet. Rec. 154, 361–365.

Osterbur, K., Mann, F.A., Kuroki, K., DeClue, A., 2014. Multiple organ dysfunction syndrome in humans and animals. J. Vet. Intern. Med. 28, 1141–1151.

Paltrinieri, S., 2008. The feline acute-phase reaction. Vet. J. 177, 26–35.

Sha, T., Zmijewski, J., Xu, Z., Abraham, E., 2008. HMGB1 develops enhanced proinflammatory activity by binding to cytokines. J. Immunol. 180, 2531–2537.

Silva, A., Wagner, B., McKenzie, H.C., et al., 2013. An investigation of the role of soluble CD14 in hospitalized, sick horses. Vet. Immunol. Immunopathol. 155, 264–269.

Townsend, M., Fowler, B., Aulakh, G.K., Singh, B., 2023. Expression of pentraxin 3 in equine lungs and neutrophils. Can. J. Vet. Res. 87 (1), 9–16.

Wada, H., 2004. Disseminated intravascular coagulation. Clin. Chim. Acta. 344 (1–2), 13–21.

Walter, E.J., Hanna-Jumma, S., Carreretto, M., Forni, L., 2016. The pathophysiological basis and consequences of fever. Crit. Care. https://doi.org/10.1186/s13054-016-1375-5.

Wang, X., Ni, L., Wan, S., Zhao, X., et al., 2020. Febrile temperature critically controls the differentiation and pathogenicity of T helper 17 cells. Immunity 52, 328–341.

Xu, J., Mu, Y., Zhang, Y., Dong, W., et al., 2015. Antibacterial effect of porcine PTX3 against Streptococcus suis type 2 infection. Microb. Pathog. 89, 128–139.

Yang, H., Wang, H., Czura, C., Tracey, K.J., 2005. The cytokine activity of HMGB-1. J. Leukoc. Biol. 78, 1–8.

9

How Immune Cells Communicate: Cytokines and Their Receptors

CHAPTER OUTLINE

The immune systems consist of complex networks involving many different cell populations, each sending and receiving multiple messages from many sources. Target cells can be directed to behave in a specific manner by signaling through appropriate receptors. They may be told to divide or stop dividing; they may be stimulated to synthesize and secrete other signaling molecules or express new receptors; they may be told to commit suicide. Each cell may be exposed to hundreds of signals at any one time. The target cell must integrate these signals and respond appropriately. In this chapter, we review the signaling molecules produced by immune cells, the receptors that receive these signals, and the way in which these incoming signals are interpreted by a cell.

The cells of the immune system produce hundreds of proteins that control the behavior of cells in immune responses. These proteins are called cytokines (Box 9.1; Myers and Murtaugh, 1995). Cytokines differ from conventional hormones in several important respects. Unlike hormones, which tend to affect a single target cell type, cytokines can affect many cell types. Second, immune system cells rarely produce a single cytokine at a time. For instance, macrophages secrete at least four interleukins (IL-1, IL-6, IL-12, and IL-18) as well as tumor necrosis factor–α (TNF-α). Third, cytokines are "redundant" in their biological activities in that many cytokines have similar effects. For example, IL-1, TNF-α, TNF-β, IL-6, and high mobility group box protein-1, all act on the brain to cause a fever. Finally, cytokine-mediated signals are transient, and the messages delivered vary over time as the cytokine environment changes.

CYTOKINE NOMENCLATURE

The nomenclature and classification of the cytokines are not based on any systematic relationship among these proteins. Many were originally named after their cell of origin, or the bioassay used to identify them. The interleukins, for example, are cytokines that signal between lymphocytes and other leukocytes. They are numbered sequentially in the order of their discovery. Because their definition is so broad, the interleukins are a heterogeneous mixture of proteins with little in common except their name. As of 2023, 41 numbered interleukins have been described. As might be expected, we know a lot about some of these molecules and very little about others. Likewise, some are clearly critical to a successful immune response, whereas others appear to be less essential (Catalan-Dibene et al., 2018).

The interferons are cytokines produced in response to virus infection or immune stimulation. Their name is derived from the fact that they interfere with viral RNA and protein synthesis and so have antiviral activity (see Chapter 28). There are three major types of interferon. Type I interferons are a diverse mixture, the most important of which are interferon-α (IFN-α) and interferon-β (IFN-β). There is a single type II interferon, called IFN-γ. Three type III interferons (IFN-λ) have been identified. Type I interferons are primarily antiviral with a secondary immunoregulatory role. For type II and type III interferons such as IFN-γ and IFN-λ, the reverse is the case. Some type I interferons also play an important role in the maintenance of pregnancy (see Chapter 35).

The TNFs are cytokines produced by macrophages and T cells. As their name suggests, they can kill tumor cells, although this is not their primary function. Thus, TNF-α is a key mediator of acute inflammation. The TNFs belong to a family of related cytokines, the TNF superfamily, which is involved in the coordination of host defenses, cell survival, immune regulation, and inflammation. It consists of at least 50 cytokines and their receptors. Important members of the TNF superfamily include CD178 (also called CD95L or Fas ligand) (see Chapter 19) and CD154 (CD40 ligand) (see Chapter 36).

Many cytokines act as growth factors (or colony-stimulating factors) and so control cell production by regulating stem cell activities. They thereby ensure that the body is supplied with sufficient cells to defend itself. Examples include the colony-stimulating factors for leukocyte precursors such as granulocytes and macrophages. Interleukin-34 also belongs to this group (Baghdadi et al., 2018).

Chemokines are a family of at least 50 small proteins that play a role in leukocyte chemotaxis, circulation, migration, and activation, especially in inflammation. Their task is to ensure that a cell is in the right place at the right time. A typical example of a chemokine is CXCL8 (also known as IL-8). Chemokines were described in detail in Chapter 3.

CYTOKINE FUNCTIONS

Cytokines are produced in response to many stimuli. Examples of these stimuli include antigens acting through the T- or B-cell antigen receptors (TCRs or BCRs); antigen-antibody complexes acting through antibody receptors (FcR); pathogen-associated molecular patterns (PAMPs) such as lipopolysaccharides acting through pattern-recognition receptors (PRRs); and other cytokines acting through specific cytokine receptors (Fig. 9.1; Dawson et al., 2020).

Cytokines act on their targets through cell-surface receptors. Some, like IL-1α, will only act when two adjacent cells are in direct contact; this is called juxtacrine signaling. Others may bind to receptors on the cell that produced them and thus have an autocrine effect. Alternatively, they may bind only to receptors on nearby cells; this is called a paracrine effect. Some cytokines may spread throughout the body, affecting target cells in distant locations, and thus have an endocrine effect (Fig. 9.2).

BOX 9.1   **Properties of Cytokines**

- Short-lived proteins
- Highly diverse structures and receptors
- Can act locally and/or systemically
- Pleiotropic: affects many different cells
- Redundant: exhibit biologically overlapping functions
- Carefully regulated
- Toxic in high doses

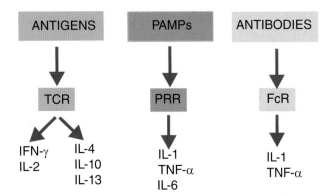

Fig. 9.1 Three of the most important pathways that trigger cytokine release are the binding of antigens to their receptors on T and B cells, the binding of pathogen-associated molecular patterns (PAMPs) to pattern-recognition receptors on sentinel cells, and the binding of antibodies to Fc receptors on phagocytic cells. *IFN-γ*, Interferon-γ; *IL*, interleukin; *PRRs*, pattern-recognition receptors; *TCRs*, T-cell antigen receptor; *TNF-α*, tumor necrosis factor–α.

When cytokines bind to their receptors, they affect cell behavior. They may induce the target cell to divide or differentiate, or they may stimulate the production of new proteins. Alternatively, they may inhibit these effects—preventing division, differentiation, or new protein synthesis. Most cytokines act on many target cell types, perhaps inducing different responses in each one, a feature that is called pleiotropy. Conversely, many cytokines may act on a single target cell, a feature known as redundancy. For example, IL-3, IL-4, IL-5, and IL-6 all affect B-cell function. Some cytokines work best when paired with other cytokines in a process called synergy. For example, the combination of IL-4 and IL-5 stimulates B cells to make immunoglobulin E (IgE) and hence promotes allergic responses. Synergy can also occur in sequence when, for example, one cytokine induces the target cell to express the receptor for another cytokine. Finally, some cytokines have opposing effects and may antagonize the effects of others. The best example of this is the mutual antagonism of IL-4 and IFN-γ. Finally, cytokines may have a cascade effect since they can stimulate the production of other cytokines or their receptors. This may result in a "cytokine storm" described in the previous chapter.

CYTOKINE STRUCTURE

Cytokines can be classified based either on their structures or on their functions (Table. 9.1). Structurally, many fall into four major families.

The group I cytokines (or hematopoietins), consist of four peptide chains forming α helices bundled together. This group can be subdivided into three families. The interferon family, the IL-2 family, and the IL-10 family (Fickenscher et al., 2002). All facilitate communication between lymphocytes and epithelial cells. Group II cytokines consist of long-chain β-sheet structures. They include the TNF family and the IL-1 family. The IL-1 family includes eight agonist cytokines, three receptor antagonists, and one antiinflammatory cytokine (Sims and Smith, 2010). IL-1 family members are first synthesized as precursor proteins that require proteolytic cleavage by enzymes such as caspases to become activated (Dinarello et al., 2010). Group III cytokines include the chemokines and related molecules. These are small proteins containing both α helices and β sheets. Group IV cytokines are heterodimers that use mixtures of domains and structural motifs. They include the IL-12 family and the IL-17 family. Many cytokines, such as IL-14, IL-16, and IL-32 are structurally unique and do not belong to any of these major families.

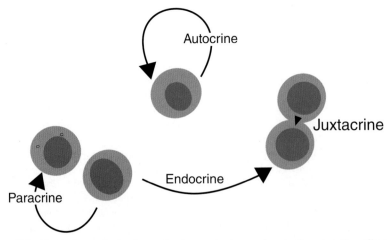

Fig. 9.2 The distinction between juxtacrine, autocrine, paracrine, and endocrine signaling effects. Cytokines differ from hormones in that most of their effects are autocrine or paracrine, whereas hormones usually act on distant cells in an endocrine fashion.

TABLE 9.1 Molecular Classification of Selected Cytokines		
Structural Families	**Structure**	**Examples**
Group 1	Four α helix bundle	IL-2, -3, -4, -5, -6, -7, -9, -11, -13, -15, -21; GM-CSF, erythropoietin, G-CSF, prolactin, leptin, TSLP
	IFN family	IFN-α/β, IFN-γ, IFN-λ
	IL-10 family	IL-10, -19, -20, -22, -24, -26, -28, -29
Group 2	β Sheets	TGF-β
	IL-1 family	IL-1α, -1, -18, -33, -36, -37, -38
	TNF family	TNFs, BAFF
Group 3	α Helices and β sheets	Chemokines
Group 4	Mixed motifs	
	IL-12 family	IL-12, -23, -27, -30, -35, -39
	IL-17 family	IL-17A-F. IL-17F is also called IL-25
Ungrouped	Unique structures	IL-14, -16, -32

BAFF, B cell–activating factor; G-CSF, granulocyte colony stimulating factor; GM-CSF, granulocyte-macrophage colony-stimulating factor; IFN-α, interferon-α; IFN-γ, interferon-γ; IL, interleukin; TGF, transforming growth factor; TNF, tumor necrosis factor; TSLP, thymic stromal lymphopoietin.

Patterns may also be seen in their biological functions. Thus, group I cytokines tend to be involved in immune cell or stem cell regulation. Group II cytokines are mainly involved in the growth and regulation of cells, cell death, and inflammation. Group III cytokines are involved in inflammation. The activities of the group IV cytokines depend on their subcomponents. For example, IL-12 is formed by a combination of a group I structure with a stem cell receptor, but it acts like a group I cytokine (Tait Wojno et al., 2019).

A more practical cytokine classification is based on their roles in adaptive immunity. Put simply, type 1 cytokines mediate cell-mediated or type 1 immune responses, while type 2 cytokines mainly mediate antibody or type 2 immune responses (see Box 1.1). The major type 1 cytokines are IL-1 and IFN-γ. The major type 2 cytokines are IL-4 and IL-13 (Wynn, 2015).

CYTOKINE RECEPTORS

Cytokines act through cell-surface receptors. These receptors usually consist of at least two functional units, one for ligand binding and one for signal transduction (Fig. 9.3). These units may or may not be on the same protein (Parham et al., 2002). Cytokine receptors can also be classified into classes based on their structure. Some also circulate in soluble form (Heaney and Golde, 1996).

One class of receptors is channel linked. These act as transmitter-gated ion channels. Thus the receptor itself is an ion channel, and the binding of its ligand opens that channel, allowing ions to pass through it. Channel-linked receptors are found in inflammatory and immune cells, but their roles are unclear. They do not serve as cytokine receptors.

A second class of receptors consists of proteins that also act as tyrosine kinases (TKs) (Fig. 9.4). These are typically growth factor and cytokine receptors. The ligand-binding site, the membrane-spanning region, and the tyrosine kinase are separate domains of a single protein.

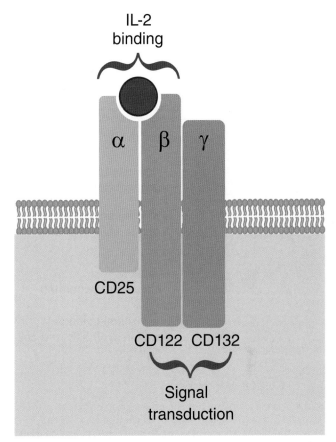

Fig. 9.3 The structure of a cytokine receptor, in this case, the interleukin-2 (IL-2) receptor complex. The alpha and beta chains contain the high-affinity IL-2-binding site, whereas the beta and gamma chains serve as signal transducers.

Binding of the ligand to two adjacent receptors draws them together to form an active dimer. Thus, when the ligand binds to the extracellular domains, the two receptor chains come together so that the two TKs can activate each other. These kinases phosphorylate tyrosine residues on other proteins or even the receptor itself (auto-phosphorylation). Since many of these other proteins are also TKs, phosphorylation also activates them. In this way, a cascade of phosphorylation develops within a cell (Fig. 9.5). Phosphorylation causes changes in cellular activities (see later). Many cytokines operate through this type of receptor, especially through TKs of the src family.

A related class of receptors consists of proteins that are not themselves TKs but activate linked TKs. This type of receptor is also widely employed in the cells of the immune system. Examples of TK-linked receptors include the TCR and the BCR. Some of these TKs may transfer their phosphate groups to transcription factors within the nucleus and activate them. Others act indirectly through the production of second messenger molecules.

A large class of receptors is coupled to membrane-bound guanosine triphosphate (GTP)-binding proteins, called G-proteins. G-proteins act as chemical switches and so control many cellular processes. When the receptor is inactive, it binds guanosine diphosphate (GDP). When activated by ligand-binding, it adds another phosphate group to form GTP (Fig. 9.6). The activated G-protein then activates other substrates, resulting in a biological response. The GTP is rapidly hydrolyzed to GDP, so that the G-protein is then turned off. The targets of G-proteins include ion channels, enzymes such as adenylate cyclase, phospholipase C, and some protein kinases.

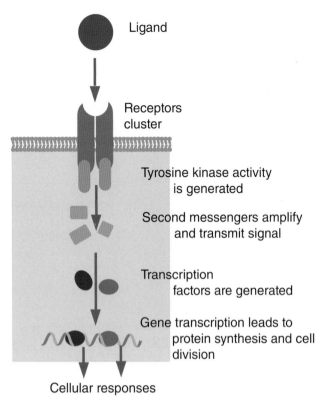

Fig. 9.4 A generic view of signal transduction involving the activation of tyrosine kinases. Although receptor signaling varies in its details and intricacy, the overall process of signal transduction has some consistent features as shown here.

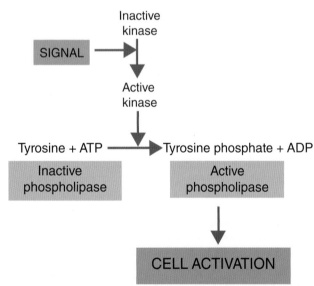

Fig. 9.5 The key to signal transduction and cellular activation is the phosphorylation of the amino acid tyrosine by the actions of a tyrosine kinase. For example, phosphorylation of tyrosine by a protein kinase can result in phospholipase activation that leads eventually to cell activation. Phosphorylation can have many other effects on protein functions and fate. *ADP,* Adenosine diphosphate; *ATP,* adenosine triphosphate.

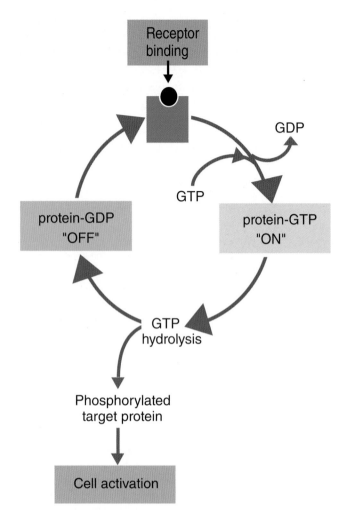

Fig. 9.6 Guanosine triphosphate (GTP)-binding proteins (G-proteins) can act as signaling switches to turn cell functions on and off. They are often activated in the initial stages of signal transduction. *GDP,* Guanosine diphosphate.

from internal stores and increases the concentration of intracellular Ca^{2+}. These calcium ions can activate many proteins. The diacylglycerol remains in the plasma membrane and along with calcium activates an enzyme called protein kinase C. Immunological receptors that employ G-proteins include the receptors for C5a, chemokine receptors, leukotriene receptors, and the platelet-activating factor receptor. In neutrophils, G-proteins control responses to chemoattractants.

A fourth class of cytokine receptors acts in a totally different manner. It activates a sphingomyelinase that then hydrolyzes the cell membrane phospholipid, sphingomyelin to form ceramide. The ceramide then activates a serine-threonine protein kinase that phosphorylates cellular proteins. This mechanism of signal transduction is used by the receptors for IL-1 and IFN-α.

Receptor Families

In general, most cytokines use receptors that act through TKs. However, within this class, one can identify subfamilies that share subunits and functions. For example, members of the IL-1/toll-like receptor (TLR) family participate in host responses to injury and infection. The family can be split into the molecules that are IL-1R-like (IL-1R1, IL-18R) and the molecules that are TLR. Ligation of these receptors triggers activation of the transcription factor nuclear factor kappa B (NF-κB) (Fig. 9.8) and generates inflammasomes.

When activated by a G-protein, phospholipase C splits the membrane-bound lipid, phosphatidylinositol 4,5-bisphosphate (PIP_2), into two molecules, inositol trisphosphate and diacylglycerol (Fig. 9.7). Inositol trisphosphate binds to intracellular receptors releasing Ca^{2+}

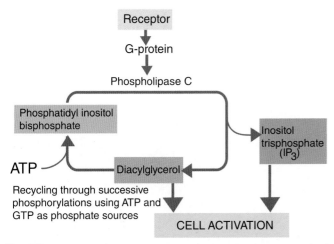

Fig. 9.7 Activation of cell membrane phospholipase C generates both inositol triphosphate and diacylglycerol. These two molecules are messengers that initiate cell activation. The signaling molecules can then be recycled by phosphorylation. *ATP*, Adenosine triphosphate; *GTP*, guanosine triphosphate.

Another cytokine receptor family shares a common beta (β_c) chain. The β_c family includes among its members the receptors for granulocyte-macrophage colony-stimulating factor (GM-CSF), IL-3, and IL-5 (Fig. 9.9; Pant et al., 2023). These regulate inflammatory responses and hematopoiesis (Dougan et al., 2019). In yet another receptor family, a common gamma chain (γ_c) is shared by the receptors for IL-2, IL-4, IL-7, IL-9, IL-15, and IL-21 (Leonard et al., 2019). These receptor chains dimerize in the presence of the ligand and form complexes with a group of kinases called Janus kinases (JAKs). JAKs in turn phosphorylate a cytosolic protein called STAT (signal transducers and activators of transcription). The STAT then dimerizes to form an active transcription factor. Depending on the specific JAKs and STATs used these may enhance or suppress cytokine signaling. This is called the JAK-STAT pathway.

The members of the IL-6 receptor family share a common signal transducer (gp130) in their receptor complex. IL-6 signals to target cells through a heterodimeric receptor with a cytokine-binding chain (IL-6Ra) and its signal-transducing component, gp130. This can be done in two ways. In its classic signaling pathway, the IL-6 can bind directly to target cells such as leukocytes and hepatocytes. In its trans-signaling pathway, soluble IL-6Ra can bind and form complexes with IL-6. These circulating cytokine-receptor complexes can then act on any target cells that express gp130. (gp130 is ubiquitous so many cell types can respond to IL-6). IL-6 is released by skeletal muscle cells in response to exercise where it exerts an antiinflammatory role (Wolf et al., 2014).

The IL-6 receptor family also includes the receptors for IL-11, IL-27, IL-35, and IL-39 (Murakami et al., 2019).

The members of the group II cytokine receptor family have a very different structure. They bind interferons (α, β, γ, and λ) and are members of the IL-10 cytokine family (IL-19, -20, -22, -24, -26). These receptors also form heterodimers in the presence of the ligand and signal through the JAK-STAT pathway (Ouyang and O'Garra, 2019).

CYTOKINE REGULATION

Cytokine signaling is regulated in three ways: by changes in receptor expression, by the presence of specific binding proteins, and

Growth factor receptor

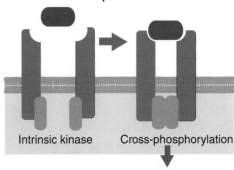

Group I cytokine receptor

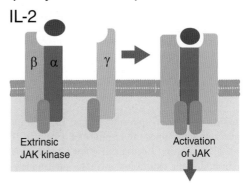

Group II cytokine receptor

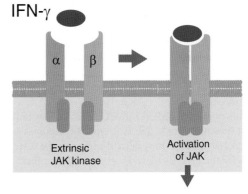

Fig. 9.8 The major types of cytokine receptors. In all cases, protein kinases are activated by ligand binding. For example, growth factor receptors associate in the presence of their ligand to form a dimer. This brings the two tyrosine kinases on the cytoplasmic domains close together. The enzymes then activated each other by cross-phosphorylation. Group I cytokine receptors, so-called because they bind the type 1 cytokines, associate in the presence of the ligand to form oligomers and form complexes with JAK kinases. When brought together, the JAK kinases are activated and in turn activate STAT proteins. The activated STAT proteins then dissociate and activate transcription factors. Group II cytokines such as the interferons and IL-10 bind receptors that have a similar mode of action to type I receptors. They differ, however, in their conserved sequences. *IFN-γ*, interferon-γ; *IL-2*, interleukin-2; *JAK*, Janus kinase.

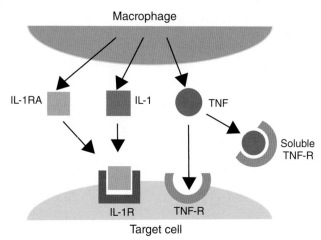

Fig. 9.9 The control of cytokine activities as exemplified by interleukin-1 (IL-1) and tumor necrosis factor (TNF)-α. IL-1 activity is regulated by the presence of interleukin-1 receptor antagonist (IL-1RA), an inert form of IL-1 that binds and blocks the IL-1 receptor, preventing signal transduction. Soluble tumor necrosis factor receptor (TNF-αR), in contrast, competes for TNF-α with the cell membrane receptor but also serves to inhibit cytokine signaling. *IL-1R*, Interleukin-1 receptor.

by cytokines that exert opposing effects. For example, IL-2 receptor expression determines the response of T cells to IL-2 (Mitra and Leonard, 2018). Resting T cells express few receptors for IL-2 but when once activated, their expression increases enormously (Boyman and Sprent, 2012). In contrast, IL-1 is regulated by a receptor antagonist called IL-1RA. IL-1RA is a form of IL-1 that binds to the IL-1 receptor but does not stimulate signal transduction. It therefore blocks active IL-1 (Fig. 9.10). Other cytokines may bind to soluble receptors in body fluids. Examples include the soluble receptors for IL-1, IL-2, IL-4, IL-5, IL-6, IL-7, IL-9, TNF-α, IL-18-binding protein, and macrophage colony-stimulating factor (Dinarello et al., 2013). In most cases, these soluble receptors compete for cytokine binding with the cell-surface receptors and hence inhibit cytokine activity. Cytokines such as IL-1, IL-12, and TGF-β may bind to connective tissue glycosaminoglycans such as heparin or CD44 that then serve as a reservoir of readily available molecules.

Some cytokine receptors can act as decoys. They bind cytokines but do not transmit signals. The IL-1 type II receptor is such a receptor. Other decoy receptors have been identified for the IL-1/IL-18 family as well as for the TNF, IL-10, and IL-13 receptor families.

The most important mechanism of cytokine regulation is through the opposing effects of different cytokines. For example, the type 2 cytokine IL-4 stimulates IgE production, whereas the type 1 cytokine, IFN-γ suppresses IgE production (see Chapter 30). Likewise, IL-10 and IL-37 inhibit the activities of many other cytokines (see Fig. 20.12). Suppressors of cytokine signaling proteins play an important role in the control of the inflammatory response. These act on both the NF-κB and the JAK-STAT pathways and so regulate inflammation. It is also important to bear in mind that at any given time, a single cell may receive signals from multiple cytokine receptors. It must somehow integrate these multiple signals to produce a coherent response.

SIGNAL TRANSDUCTION

When a cytokine binds its receptor, the receptor transmits a signal to the cell to modify its behavior. This conversion of an extracellular signal into a series of intracellular events is called signal transduction. The key components of signal transduction include binding of an agonist

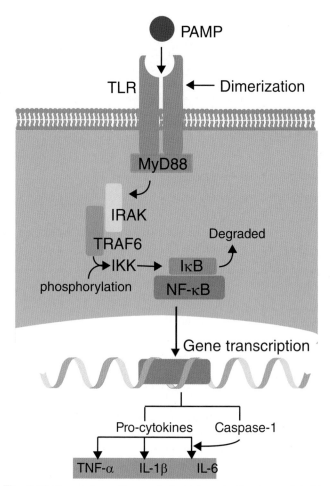

Fig. 9.10 One major pathway of signal transduction is mediated by the transcription factor nuclear factor kappa-B (NF-κB). This is widely employed in immunologic signaling such as the response to sentinel cells to activation of their toll-like receptors (TLRs) by pathogen-associated molecular patterns (PAMPs). *IL*, Interleukin; *TNF-α*, tumor necrosis factor–α.

such as a cytokine to its receptor, possibly clustering of receptor chains, activation of kinases by the receptor, activation of second messengers, generation of new transcription factors, and gene activation leading to altered protein synthesis and cell behavior (Fig. 9.4). Because cell signaling must be fast and precise, this is best accomplished by enzyme cascades. Since enzymes can produce or modify a large number of molecules in a short time, a pathway that involves the use of several enzymes in sequence can amplify cell responses very rapidly.

Protein Phosphorylation

Central to most cell signaling is the reversible modification of proteins by the addition of a phosphate group to selected amino acids. Signal transduction systems use a high-energy phosphate-rich compound such as adenosine triphosphate to modify proteins and hence send a signal to a cell. Cell growth, cell division, and other critical processes are all regulated by protein phosphorylation. The enzymes that do this, called protein kinases, enzymatically phosphorylate the amino acids serine, threonine, or tyrosine.

$$\text{Protein} + \text{ATP} \xrightarrow{\text{Protein kinase}} \text{protein-P} + \text{ADP}$$

In some proteins, only one amino acid is phosphorylated; in others, multiple amino acids may be phosphorylated. Phosphorylated and nonphosphorylated proteins have different functional properties. For example, the phosphorylation of serine or threonine activates some enzymes, whereas dephosphorylation has the opposite effect. In most cells, about 90% of the phosphate groups are linked to serine and about 10% to threonine. Only about 1/2000 of the phosphate is linked to tyrosine. Thus, tyrosine phosphorylation is a rare event. Nevertheless, it is a key mechanism in almost all the signal transduction pathways described in this book.

Transduction Pathways

Three signal transduction pathways play key roles in the immune system. These involve the generation of transcription factors belonging to three families: NF-κB, nuclear factor of activated T cells (NF-AT), and STAT.

The NF-κB Pathway

The NF-κB pathway is the most significant signal transduction pathway in the immune system. It is the pathway that is activated when antigens bind to the TCR and BCR; when PAMPs bind to the PRRs, such as the TLRs and NODs; and when TNF-α binds to its receptor. Thus NF-κB plays a critical role in both innate and adaptive immunity (Wietek and O'Neill, 2007). The term NF-κB refers to a family of five transcription factors. These factors can form many heterodimers that activate different genes. More than 150 unique stimuli can activate NF-κB, and more than 150 genes are expressed after NF-κB activation. In a resting cell, NF-κB is found in the cytosol in an inactive form bound to a protein called IκB. IκB inhibits NF-κB activity by masking its nuclear binding site. Thus, in resting cells, NF-κB cannot move to the nucleus or activate genes (Hayden and Ghosh, 2008).

The major NF-κB activation pathway is triggered by the inflammatory cytokines IL-1 and TNF-α, by TLRs, and by antigen receptors and is essential for innate immunity. The signals induced by these stimuli converge on a regulator of NF-κB, the IKK (IκB kinase) complex. This complex consists of multiple subunits with kinase activity. When activated, IKK phosphorylates IκB. As a result, the IκB dissociates from the NF-κB and is destroyed. This releases the NF-κB so that it can enter the nucleus and activate selected genes including those encoding IL-1, IL-6, IL-18, IL-33, TNF-α, GM-CSF, and IL-4. Activated NF-κB also turns on the genes coding for inflammasomes, chemokines, angiogenic factors, adhesion molecules, antiapoptotic proteins, inducible enzymes such as iNOS and cyclooxygenase-2, as well as IκB. This newly synthesized IκB will eventually bind and suppress NF-κB activation. Molecules or organisms that block the destruction of IκB have antiinflammatory and immunosuppressive effects. For example, corticosteroids stimulate the production of excess IκB, whereas some bacteria can block its degradation. Either way, the activation of cells and the development of inflammation and immune responses can be blocked.

An example of the importance of the NF-κB pathway is seen when macrophage TLRs bind their ligands (Fig. 9.8). This immediately causes the receptor to dimerize. As a result, it binds several adaptor molecules, of which one, MyD88 (myeloid differentiation primary response gene 88) is the most important. When MyD88 binds to the TLR, it also binds two kinases called IRAK-1 and IRAK-4 (Fig. 2.5). IRAK-4 activates IRAK-1, and these in turn recruit TRAF6. TRAF6 and other proteins then activate the IKK complex. Activation of IKK phosphorylates IκB, causing its destruction and the release of active NF-κB. The NF-κB in turn enters the nucleus and activates the genes that encode precursors of TNF-α, IL-1, and caspase-1. Caspase-1 activates these newly produced cytokines that then trigger inflammation.

Binding of antigen to T cell receptors also activates NF-κB. Thus, binding to the TCR activates a protein kinase C to form a protein complex that degrades IKK. Another pathway involves stabilization of

NF-κB–inducing kinase. This activates IKKα, that then promotes the destruction of IkB by proteasomes. All NF-κB members affect antigen-induced T-cell proliferation. Antigen dose and oscillations in calcium concentrations are also important because they modulate the movement of transcription factors between the nucleus and cytoplasm.

The NF-AT Pathway

The NF-AT pathway is used in many immune cells. When an antigen binds to its receptor on a T cell, the signal is first transmitted from the antigen-binding receptor (TCR) to a signal-transducing complex called CD3, where it causes the CD3 chains to cluster together in lipid rafts (Fig. 9.11). Each CD3 protein has short amino acid sequences in its cytoplasmic domains called immunoreceptor tyrosine-based, activation motifs (ITAMs). When the CD3 chains cluster, their ITAMs collectively activate several TKs. These TKs are members of the src-kinase family. They include lck and fyn in T cells and NK cells, and lyn and fyn in B cells and mast cells. In T cells, the first TK activated, called lck, phosphorylates the ITAMs. As a result, these sites then bind a second TK, called zeta-associated protein-70 (ZAP-70). The bound ZAP-70 is phosphorylated and after binding

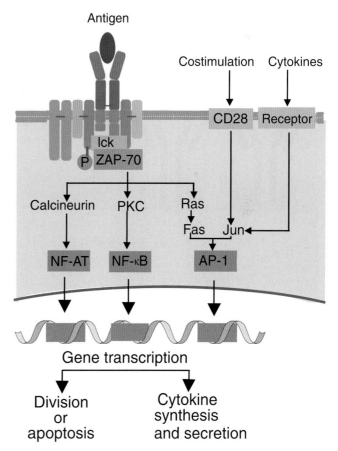

Fig. 9.11 Signal transduction mediated through T-cell antigen receptors (TCRs) generates three transcription factors: nuclear factor of activated T cells (NF-AT), nuclear factor kappa-B (NF-κB), and activator protein–1 (AP-1). When TCRs cluster, they activate several protein kinases. The most important of these is called ZAP-70. This in turn triggers three signaling pathways and, with appropriate costimulation, generates multiple transduction factors. The jun-fos heterodimer (AP-1) is required to stimulate the genes for cytokines and their receptors. The final results of the stimulus include cell division or apoptosis as well as cytokine production. *ZAP-70*, Zeta-associated protein–70.

many other proteins forms a multimolecular proximal signaling complex (PSC). Signals generated by the PSC then activate at least three families of transcription factors. One pathway generates the second messengers, diacylglycerol and inositol trisphosphate. The inositol trisphosphate releases calcium ions from intracellular organelles and opens transmembrane channels, allowing Ca²⁺ to enter the cell and raising intracellular calcium. This in turn activates a phosphatase called calcineurin. Calcineurin removes a phosphate from NF-AT. Dephosphorylated NF-AT enters the nucleus and with the help of another transcription factor called activator protein-1 (AP-1), binds to the promoters of at least 100 genes. The potent immunosuppressive drugs tacrolimus and cyclosporine bind to calcineurin and so block T cell-mediated responses (see Fig. 42-4). If the T cell receives suppressive signals, such as those provided by IL-10 or TGF-β, NF-AT will associate with a transcription factor called Foxp3. Foxp3 activates a very different set of genes and converts the cell into a regulatory T cell (Treg) that suppresses immune responses (see Chapter 15).

In B cells, the paired adaptor molecules Ig-α and Ig-β also have ITAMs. When aggregated by antigen and costimulated by CD19, they activate the src kinases, lyn and fyn. These in turn activate phospholipase C and eventually generate both NF-κB and NF-AT (Fig. 9.12).

AP-1 belongs to a family of transcription factors consisting of fos and jun heterodimers. Production of AP-1 is also triggered by the PSC. The PSC activates a protein kinase C, which in turn leads to activation of ras-mitogen protein kinase (MAPK) and increased production of c-fos. The c-fos moves to the nucleus, where it combines with

preexisting jun proteins to form AP-1. AP-1 binds to NF-AT proteins integrating the calcium signaling with the ras-MAPK pathway. Collectively they activate the genes coding for IL-2, IFN-γ, GM-CSF, TNF-α, IL-3, IL-4, IL-13, IL-5, FasL, and CD25.

The JAK-STAT Pathway

The JAK-STAT pathway provides a method of rapidly signaling from the cell surface to the nucleus. It also mediates many different aspects of the immune system. Almost 40 cytokines have been shown to use the JAK-STAT pathway, including IL-4, IL-7, IL-11, IL-12, IL-13, and IL-31, leptin, GM-CSF, and IFN-γ. These ligands use group I cytokine receptors that consist of paired identical transmembrane proteins. When a cytokine binds to its receptor the two proteins come together. This dimerization leads in turn to phosphorylation of two tightly associated JAK proteins. These activated JAK molecules then phosphorylate STAT proteins. The phosphorylated STAT proteins dimerize, dissociate from JAK, and move to the nucleus, where they act as transcription factors and induce the expression of target genes. There are four JAK and seven STAT family members currently recognized. A specific JAK-STAT combination is paired with each cytokine receptor. For example, hematopoietic growth factor receptors usually use JAK2. The cytokine receptors that employ the common γ chain preferentially use JAK1 and JAK3. The IFN-γ receptor uses JAK1 and JAK2. The IL-4R uses JAK1 and JAK3. Presumably, the genes turned on by this signaling depend on these specific combinations of JAK and STAT as well as the cell type involved (Box 9.2). The synthetic JAK inhibitor, oclacitinib maleate (Apoquel) blocks signal transduction by the cell receptor kinases, JAK1 and JAK3. These are components of the receptors for IL-2, IL-4, IL-6, IL-13, and IL-31 (Villarino et al., 2017).

Although the pathways described above are of greatest importance in cells of the immune system, many other transcription factors can trigger cell differentiation. This is especially important in the T cell system, where the cells are plastic and can readily transform from one phenotype to another. These transcription factors include T-bet, which controls transcription of IFN-γ in Th1 cells; GATA3, which controls cytokine transcription in Th2 cells; ROR γT, which acts in Th17 cells; and FoxP3, which acts within Treg cells.

GENE TRANSCRIPTION

The activity of each gene in a cell is carefully regulated. Central to gene control, however, are the transcription factors. Activation of genes depends on the presence of an appropriate mixture of transcription

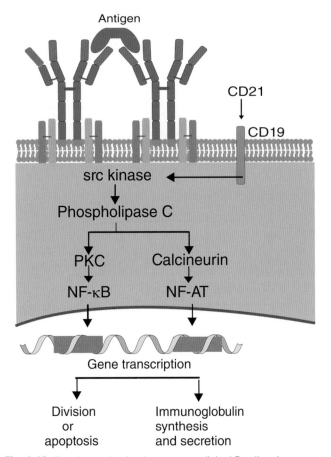

Fig. 9.12 Signal transduction by two cross-linked B-cell antigen receptors (BCRs) activates B cells, triggering cell division, differentiation, and immunoglobulin synthesis. Both nuclear factor kappa-B (NF-κB) and nuclear factor of activated T cells (NF-AT) are involved in B-cell signal transduction.

BOX 9.2 Inhibition of JAK-STAT Signaling

Inhibition of JAK-STAT signaling can have immunosuppressive and antiinflammatory effects. This may be useful in suppressing unwanted immune responses or inflammation. Drugs directed against specific JAK proteins can have profound antiinflammatory responses. For example, oclacitinib (Apoquel) is a synthetic selective inhibitor of JAK1 and JAK3. As a result, it blocks signal transduction and hence inhibits the itching caused by IL-31 (see Chapter 31). It has been approved for the treatment of dermatitis in dogs. Specifically, it is used for the treatment of severe itch (pruritus) in dogs with allergic dermatitis including flea and food allergies, atopic dermatitis, and contact dermatitis (see Chapters 31 and 34). It is administered daily for up to 15 days, and then once daily for maintenance therapy. It appears to be highly effective in most but not all animals. Presumably, this reflects the heterogeneity of the conditions classified as allergic dermatitis. Given the protective role of inflammation it is unsurprising that oclacitinib may increase susceptibility to the skin mite Demodex, bacterial skin infections, and some skin cancers.

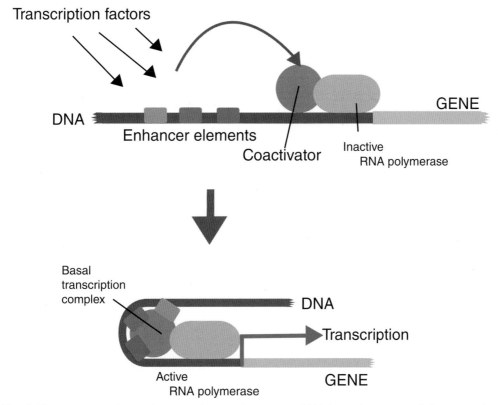

Fig. 9.13 Transcription factors bind to enhancer elements on DNA located upstream of the genes they activate. Gene transcription is turned on by a carefully regulated RNA polymerase. However, the polymerase can only be turned on when transcription factors form a basal transcription complex and activate the basic transcriptional machinery.

BOX 9.3 No Interleukin 26 in Horses

Interleukin-26 (IL-26) is a member of the IL-10 family. Its gene is located in a cluster with the interferon-gamma gene on one side and the IL-22 gene on the other. As a result of a one-base pair frame-shift mutation, the IL-26 gene is inactivated in horses and related equids such as zebras and donkeys. Since IL-26 is a stimulator of T cells and may promote inflammation and autoimmunity, this inactivation may explain, in part, why some aspects of acute inflammation differ between horses and other mammals (Shakhsi-Niaei et al., 2013).

---

factors. As described earlier, these transcription factors are only generated when a cell receives an appropriate signal. The transcription factors then collectively activate the appropriate RNA polymerase, and gene transcription begins.

Transcription factors have two binding sites. One site binds DNA; the other binds regulatory proteins. When a transcription factor is generated, it enters the nucleus and binds to specific DNA control elements located between 50 and 200 bases upstream from the start site of the gene (Fig. 9.13). Transcription factors may also bind to enhancer elements located thousands of bases upstream. These bound transcription factors then use their other binding site to bind either directly to basal transcription complexes or to coactivator molecules. This leads to the assembly of a basal transcription complex. The basal transcription complex, together with its attached coactivator molecules, then binds to the RNA polymerase and activates it. It is believed that the conformation of the polymerase changes once activated. The polymerase then begins the process of transcribing the selected genes leading eventually to the production of the required proteins (Box 9.3).

REFERENCES

Baghdadi, M., Umeyama, Y., Hama, N., Kobayashi, T., et al., 2018. Interleukin 34, a comprehensive review. J. Leukoc. Biol. 104, 931–951.

Boyman, O., Sprent, J., 2012. The role of interleukin-2 during homeostasis and activation of the immune system. Nat. Revs. Immunol. 12 (3), 180–190.

Catalan-Dibene, J., McIntyre, L.L., Zlotnik, A., 2018. Interleukin 30 to interleukin 40. J. Interferon Cytokine Res. 38 (10), 423–439.

Dawson, H.D., Sang, Y., Lunney, J.K., 2020. Porcine cytokines, chemokines and growth factors: 2019 update. Res. Vet. Sci. 131, 266–399.

Dinarello, C., Arend, W., Sims, J., et al., 2010. IL-1 family nomenclature. Nat. Immunol. 11, 973.

Dinarello, C.A., Novick, D., Kim, S., Kaplanski, G., 2013. Interleukin-18 and IL-18 binding protein. Front. Immunol. 4 Article 289, 1-10.

Dougan, M., Dranoff, G., Dougan, S.K., 2019. GM-CSF, IL-3, and IL-5 family of cytokines: Regulators of inflammation. Immunity 50, 796–811.

Fickenscher, H., Hor, S., Kupers, H., et al., 2002. The interleukin-10 family of cytokines. Trends Immunol. 23, 89–96.

Hayden, M.S., Ghosh, S., 2008. Shared principles in NF-kB signaling. Cell 132, 344–362.

Heaney, M.L., Golde, D.W., 1996. Soluble cytokine receptors. Blood 87, 847–857.

Leonard, W.J., Lin, J.-X., O'Shea, J.J., 2019. The γ_c family of cytokines, basic biology and therapeutic ramifications. Immunity 50, 832–850.

Mitra, S., Leonard, W.J., 2018. Biology of IL-2 and its therapeutic modulation: mechanisms and strategies. J. Leukoc. Biol. 103, 643–655.

Myers, M.J., Murtaugh, M.P. (Eds.), 1995. Cytokines in Animal Health and Disease. Marcel Dekker, New York.

Murakami, M., Kamimura, D., Hirano, T., 2019. Pleiotropy and specificity: insights from the interleukin 6 family of cytokines. Immunity 50, 812–831.

Ouyang, W., O'Garra, A., 2019. IL-10 family cytokines, IL-10 and IL-22. From basic science to clinical translation. Immunity 50, 871–891.

Pant, H., Hercus, T.R., Tumes, D.J., Yip, K.H., et al., 2023. Translating the biology of β common receptor-engaging cytokines into clinical medicine. J. Allergy Clin. Immunol. 151, 324–344.

Parham, C., Chirica, M., Timans, J., et al., 2002. A receptor for the heterodimeric cytokine IL-23 is composed of IL-12γ1 and a novel cytokine receptor subunit, IL-23R. J. Immunol. 168, 5699–5708.

Shakhsi-Niaei, M., Drogemuller, M., Jagannathan, V., Gerber, V., Leeb, T., 2013. IL26 gene inactivation in Equidae. Anim. Genet. 44 (6), 770–772.

Sims, J.E., Smith, D.E., 2010. The IL-1 family: regulators of immunity. Nat. Rev. Immunol. 10, 89–102.

Tait Wojno, E.D., Hunter, C.A., Sturnhofer, J.S., 2019. The immunobiology of the interleukin 12 family: room for discovery. Immunity 50, 851–870.

Villarino, A.V., Kanno, Y., O'Shea, J.J., 2017. Mechanisms and consequences of Jak-STAT signaling in the immune system. Nat. Immunol. 18 (4), 374–384.

Wietek, C., O'Neill, L.A.J., 2007. Diversity and regulation in the NF-κB system. Trends Biochem. Sci. 32, 301–309.

Wolf, J., Rose-John, S., Garbers, C., 2014. Interleukin-6 and its receptors: a highly regulated and dynamic system. Cytokine 70, 11–20.

Wynn, T.A., 2015. Type 2 cytokines: mechanisms and therapeutic strategies. Nat. Revs. Immunol. 15 (5), 271–282.

Antigens: Triggers of Adaptive Immunity

Up to now, we have considered only the body's innate reactions to microbial invasion. Innate responses are triggered by recognition of a limited number of conserved microbial pathogen-associated molecular patterns such as microbial nucleic acids or lipopolysaccharides. The triggering of inflammation and the mobilization of phagocytic cells such as neutrophils and macrophages by these molecules contribute to the rapid destruction of microbial invaders. Although effective in the short term, innate immunity cannot be guaranteed to provide complete resistance to infection. Nor does the body learn from the experience. Thus a more potent immune response should ideally recognize all the foreign molecules in rapidly evolving microbes. In addition, such a response should be able to learn from this experience and, given time, evolve more efficient procedures to combat subsequent invasions. This new and improved response is the function of the adaptive immune system.

Since the function of the adaptive immune system is to defend the body against invading microorganisms, it is essential that these organisms be recognized immediately after they invade the body. The body must be able to recognize that these are foreign (and dangerous) if they are to stimulate an immune response. To this end, the adaptive immune system uses cells with receptors that can bind and respond to almost all the foreign macromolecules present in an invading microorganism. These foreign macromolecules are called antigens.

During an adaptive immune response, molecules from invading organisms are captured, processed, and presented to the cells of the immune system. These immune cells have surface receptors that can bind appropriately presented foreign molecules. These bound molecules then trigger a powerful response by cells called lymphocytes that ultimately destroys the invaders and ensures an animal's survival. In addition, the immune system generates memory cells that "remember" these antigens, makes some improvements, and, by adapting, ensures that an animal will respond even more effectively when it encounters these organisms again (Borek, 1972).

MICROBIAL ANTIGENS

Bacterial Antigens

Bacteria are single-celled prokaryotic organisms consisting of a cytoplasm containing the essential elements of cell structure, surrounded by a lipid-rich cytoplasmic membrane (Fig. 10.1). Outside the cytoplasmic membrane is a thick, carbohydrate-rich cell wall. The major components of the bacterial surface thus include the cell wall and its associated protein structures, the capsule, the pili, and the flagella. The cell wall of Gram-positive organisms is largely composed of peptidoglycan (chains of alternating *N*-acetyl glucosamine and *N*-acetyl muramic acid cross-linked by short peptide side chains) (see Fig. 2.2). Gram-positive cell walls also contain lipoteichoic acids that are involved in the transport of ions across the cell wall. The cell wall in gram-negative organisms, in contrast, consists of a thin layer of peptidoglycans covered by an outer layer consisting of lipopolysaccharides. Most of the antigenicity of gram-negative bacteria is associated with these lipopolysaccharides. Each consists of an oligosaccharide attached to a lipid (lipid A) and to a series of repeating trisaccharides. The structure of these trisaccharides determines the antigenicity of the organism. Many bacteria are classified according to this antigenic structure. For example, the genus *Salmonella* contains a major species, *Salmonella enterica*, that is classified into more than 2300 serovars based on their antigenicity. These polysaccharide antigens are called O-antigens. The outer cell wall lipopolysaccharides of Gram-negative bacteria bind to toll-like receptors (TLRs) and other pattern-recognition receptors and induce the production of inflammatory cytokines when an animal is infected. These cytokines cause fever and sickness, so bacterial lipopolysaccharides are also called endotoxins.

Bacterial capsules consist mainly of polysaccharides that are usually good antigens. The capsules protect bacteria against phagocytosis and intracellular destruction, whereas anticapsular antibodies can overcome the benefits of the capsule and protect an infected animal. Capsular antigens are collectively called K-antigens.

Pili and fimbriae are short projections that cover the surfaces of some gram-negative bacteria; they are classified as F- or K-antigens. Pili bind bacteria together and play a role in bacterial conjugation and movement. Fimbriae bind bacteria to cell surfaces. Antibodies to fimbrial proteins may be protective since they can prevent bacteria from sticking to body surfaces. Bacterial flagella are long filaments used for bacterial movement. They consist of a single protein called flagellin. Flagellar antigens are collectively called H antigens.

Other significant bacterial antigens include the porins, the heat-shock proteins, and the exotoxins. The porins are proteins that form pores on the surface of gram-negative organisms. Heat-shock proteins

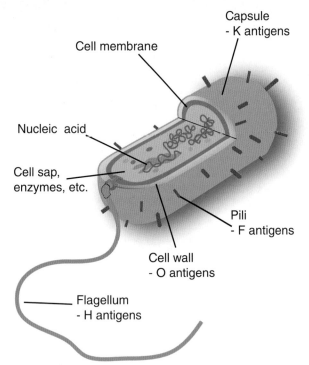

Fig. 10.1 The structure of a typical bacterium and the location of its most important antigens.

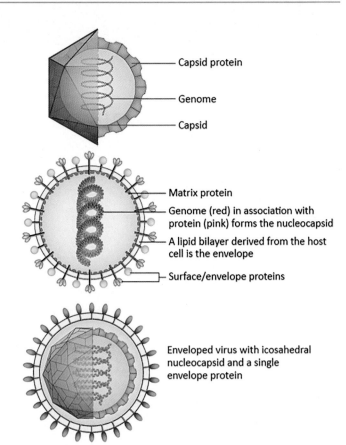

Fig. 10.2 The structure of a typical virus. The antigenic proteins include the capsids and envelope proteins. Courtesy Dr. S. Payne.

are produced in large amounts in stressed bacteria. The exotoxins are toxic proteins secreted by bacteria or released into the surrounding environment when they die. Exotoxins are highly effective antigens and stimulate the production of antibodies called antitoxins. Many exotoxins, when treated with a mild protein-denaturing agent such as formaldehyde, lose their toxicity but retain their antigenicity. Toxins modified in this way are called toxoids. Toxoids may be used as vaccines to prevent disease caused by toxigenic bacteria such as *Clostridium tetani*. Bacterial nucleic acids rich in unmethylated CpG sequences serve both as effective antigens for the adaptive immune system and as potent stimulators of innate immunity acting through TLRs. The presence of the enormous and diverse intestinal microbiota provides a source of many different microbial antigens. These too can stimulate adaptive immune responses.

Viral Antigens

Viruses are very small molecular constructs that grow only inside living cells. They are thus "obligate," intracellular parasites. Viruses usually consist of a nucleic acid core covered by a protein layer (Fig. 10.2). This protein layer is termed the capsid and consists of multiple subunits called capsomeres. Capsid proteins are good antigens, well capable of stimulating antibody responses. Some viruses may also be surrounded by an envelope containing lipoproteins and glycoproteins. A complete viral particle is called a virion. When a virus infects an animal, its proteins are processed, recognized, and trigger adaptive immune responses. Viruses, however, are not always found free in circulation but live within cells, where they are protected from the unwelcome attentions of antibodies. Indeed, viral nucleic acids may be integrated into a cell's genome. In this situation, the integrated viral genes encode new proteins, some of which are expressed on the surface of infected cells. These viral proteins, although they are synthesized inside an animal's own cells, can still bind to antigen receptors and provoke adaptive immunity. These newly synthesized foreign proteins are called

endogenous antigens to distinguish them from the foreign antigens that enter from the outside and are called exogenous antigens (Green et al., 1982).

Other Microbial Antigens

In addition to bacteria and viruses, animals may be invaded by fungi, protozoan parasites, parasitic arthropods, and even parasitic worms. Each of these organisms consists of many complex structures composed of proteins, carbohydrates, lipids, and nucleic acids. Many of these molecules can serve as antigens and trigger adaptive immunity. However, their degree of antigenicity does vary, and the adaptive responses triggered by these organisms are not always successful in protecting an animal or eliminating the invader.

NONMICROBIAL ANTIGENS

Invading microorganisms are not the only source of foreign material entering the body. Food contains many foreign molecules, especially proteins, that under some circumstances may trigger immune responses and cause allergic reactions. Likewise, inhaled dust can contain antigenic particles such as pollen grains or mold spores, and these may enter the body through the respiratory system. Foreign molecules may be injected directly into the body through a snake or mosquito bite, or by a veterinarian. Furthermore, foreign proteins may be injected into animals for experimental or therapeutic purposes.

Cell Surface Antigens

Organ grafts are an effective way of delivering large amounts of foreign antigens to an animal. The surface of mammalian cells consists of a fluid lipid bilayer with a complex mixture of protein molecules embedded in it. These proteins can act as antigens if they are injected into another species or even into a different individual of the same species. For example, glycoproteins known as blood-group antigens are found on the surface of red blood cells. Early attempts to transfuse blood between unrelated humans usually met with disaster because the transfused cells were rapidly destroyed. Investigation revealed that the problem was due to the presence of naturally occurring antibodies against these foreign red cell glycoproteins.

Nucleated cells, such as leukocytes, possess hundreds of different protein molecules on their surface. Many of these proteins are good antigens and readily provoke an immune response when injected experimentally into a different species. These surface molecules are classified by the CD system (Box 6.3). Other cell surface proteins may provoke an immune response (such as graft rejection) if transferred to a genetically different individual of the same species. The cell surface proteins that trigger graft rejection are called histocompatibility antigens. Histocompatibility antigens are of such importance in immunology that they warrant a complete chapter of their own (see Chapter 12; Katz et al. 1982).

Autoantigens

In some situations (and not always abnormal ones), an animal may mount immune responses against normal body components. These are called autoimmune responses. Antigens that induce autoimmunity are called autoantigens. They can include hormones, such as thyroglobulin; structural components such as basement membranes; complex lipids, such as myelin; intracellular components such as the mitochondrial proteins, nucleic acids, or nucleoproteins; and cell surface proteins such as hormone receptors. The production of autoantibodies and the consequences of this are discussed in detail in Chapter 37.

WHAT MAKES A GOOD ANTIGEN?

Molecules vary in their ability to act as antigens (their antigenicity) (Fig. 10.3). In general, foreign proteins make the best antigens, especially if they are big (greater than 1000 Da is best). Many of the major microbial antigens such as the clostridial toxins, bacterial flagella, virus capsids, and protozoan cell membranes are large proteins. Other important antigenic proteins include components of snake venoms, serum proteins, cell surface proteins, milk and food proteins, hormones, and even foreign antibody molecules.

Simple polysaccharides, such as starch or glycogen, are not antigenic because they are rapidly degraded before the immune system has time to respond to them. More complex carbohydrates may be effective antigens, especially if bound to proteins. These include the major cell wall antigens of gram-negative bacteria and the blood-group glycoproteins of red blood cells. Many of the so-called natural antibodies found in the serum of unimmunized animals are directed against polysaccharides and probably arise as a result of exposure to glycoproteins or carbohydrates derived from the intestinal microbiota or from food. To this extent, they can also be considered part of the innate immune system.

Lipids tend to be poor antigens because of their wide distribution, relative simplicity, structural instability, and rapid metabolism. Nevertheless, when linked to proteins or polysaccharides, lipoproteins, glycolipids, and lipopolysaccharides can trigger immune responses. Some lymphocytes possess specific receptors, called CD1 molecules, that can bind lipid, lipoprotein, and glycolipid antigens and present them to antigen-sensitive cells (see Chapter 20; DeLibero et al., 2009).

Mammalian nucleic acids are very poor antigens because of their relative simplicity and flexibility and because they are very rapidly degraded. Microbial nucleic acids, on the other hand, have a structure very different from that found in eukaryotes with many unmethylated CpG sequences. As a result, they can stimulate potent immune responses. It is perhaps for this reason that autoantibodies to nucleic acids are produced in some important autoimmune diseases (see Chapter 39).

Proteins are the most effective antigens because they have properties that best trigger an immune response. (More correctly, the adaptive immune system has evolved to trap, process, and then recognize foreign proteins.) Thus large molecules are better antigens than small molecules, and proteins can be very large indeed (Fig. 10.4).

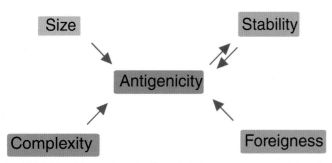

Fig. 10.3 The factors that significantly influence the antigenicity of a molecule. Of these, either excessive or insufficient stability will reduce antigenicity. The best antigens are large, complex, and foreign. However, their ability to stimulate an immune response is also determined by their route of administration, by the amount of antigen administered, and by the genetic makeup of the immunized animal.

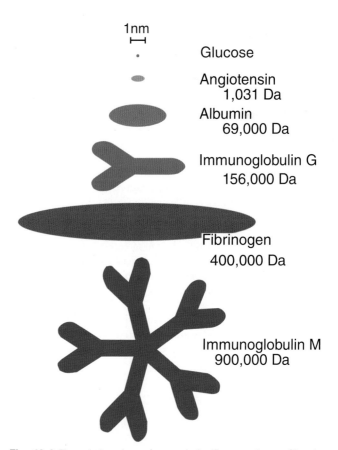

Fig. 10.4 The relative sizes of several significant antigens. Size does matter! Big molecules are generally much more antigenic than small molecules. Molecules as small as angiotensin are poor antigens.

For example, hemocyanin, a very large protein from invertebrate blood (670 kDa), is a potent antigen. Serum albumin from other mammals (69 kDa) is a fairly good antigen but may also provoke tolerance. The small peptide hormone angiotensin (1031 Da) is a poor antigen.

Similarly, the more complex an antigen is, the better. For example, simple repeating polymers are poor antigens, but complex bacterial lipopolysaccharides are good. Complex proteins containing many different amino acids, especially aromatic ones, are better antigens than large, repeating polymers, such as lipids, carbohydrates, and nucleic acids (Wilson et al., 1984; Atassi, 1978).

Structural stability is an important feature of good antigens, especially those that trigger antibody responses. To bind to specific foreign molecules, the cell surface receptors of the adaptive immune system must recognize their shape. Consequently, highly flexible molecules that have no fixed shape are poor antigens. For example, gelatin, a protein well known for its structural instability (which is why it can wobble), is a poor antigen unless it is stabilized by the incorporation of tyrosine or tryptophan molecules, which cross-link the peptide chains. Similarly, flagellin, the major protein of bacterial flagella, is a flexible, weak antigen. Its rigidity, and thus its antigenicity, is greatly enhanced by polymerization. Remember too that the route of antigen administration, its dose, and the genetics of the recipient animal also influence antigenicity (Marx 1984).

Not all foreign molecules can stimulate an immune response. Stainless steel bone pins and plastic heart valves are commonly implanted in animals without triggering an immune response. The lack of antigenicity of metals or large organic polymers, such as plastics, is due not only to their molecular uniformity but also to their inertness. These polymers cannot be degraded and processed by cells into a form suitable for triggering an adaptive response. Conversely, since immune responses are antigen driven, foreign molecules that are unstable and destroyed very rapidly may not persist for a sufficient time to stimulate an immune response (Tizard, 1982).

Foreignness

The cells that respond to foreign antigens consist of lymphocytes that have been selected so that their receptors do not bind to molecules originating within an animal (self-antigens). Cells that bind self-antigens are eliminated but that still leaves lymphocytes with a huge variety of receptors that can bind foreign molecules. These are sufficient to protect animals against almost all potential pathogens. They will bind and respond to a huge variety of foreign molecules that differ, even in minor respects, from those normally found within the body.

The immunogenicity of a molecule also depends on its degree of foreignness. The greater the difference in molecular structure between a foreign antigen and an animal's own antigens, the greater will be the intensity of the immune response. For example, a kidney graft from an identical twin will be readily accepted because its proteins are identical to those on the recipient's own kidney. A kidney graft from an unrelated animal of the same species will be rejected in about 10 days unless prevented by drugs. A kidney graft between different species such as from a pig to a dog will be rejected within a few hours despite the use of immunosuppressive drugs.

EPITOPES

Foreign particles, such as invading bacteria, transplanted nucleated cells, and transfused red blood cells, consist of an enormously complex mixture of proteins, glycoproteins, polysaccharides, lipopolysaccharides, lipids, and nucleoproteins (Sercarz, 1989). The adaptive immune response against such foreign invaders or cells is therefore a mixture

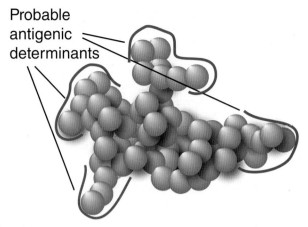

Fig. 10.5 A hypothetical antigen. Note that the cells of the immune system preferentially recognize the prominent structures on the surface of the molecule as a result of their characteristic shapes.

of many simultaneous immune responses directed against each of the foreign molecules in the mixture (Atassi, 1978).

A large complex molecule such as a protein can be recognized by many different lymphocytes and thus stimulate multiple immune responses. Large molecules have regions on their surface that are recognized by lymphocyte antigen receptors and against which immune responses are therefore directed. These regions, usually on the surface of the molecule, are called epitopes, or antigenic determinants (Fig. 10.5). In a large, complex protein molecule, many different epitopes may be recognized by lymphocytes, but some are much more immunogenic than others. Thus, animals may respond to a few favored epitopes, and the remainder of the molecule may be ignored. Such favored epitopes are said to be immunodominant. In general, the number of epitopes on a molecule is directly related to its size, and there is usually about one epitope for every 5 kDa of a protein (Sela 1969). When we describe a molecule as "foreign," therefore, we are implying that it contains epitopes that are absent from self-antigens. The cells of the immune system bind and respond to these foreign epitopes. A good example of a well-defined epitope is the peptide proline-glutamic acid-proline-lysine, which binds to antibodies against the bacterium *Streptococcus equi*. Presumably, the shape of this peptide is identical to the major antigenic determinant on *S. equi*.

Haptens

Small molecules, such as drugs or hormones of less than 1000 Da, are far too small to be appropriately processed and presented to the immune system. As a result, they are not immunogenic. If, however, these small molecules are chemically bound to a large protein molecule, they will form new epitopes on the surface of the larger molecule (Fig. 10.6). If this complex molecule is injected into an animal, immune responses will be triggered against all its epitopes. Some of the antibodies made in response to the complex will be directed against new epitopes formed by the small molecules. Small molecules that can function as epitopes only when bound to other larger molecules are called haptens (in Greek, *haptein* means "to grasp or fasten"). The antigenic molecule to which the haptens are attached is called the carrier. Many drug allergies occur because the drug molecules, although small, bind covalently to normal body proteins and so act as haptens (Landsteiner, 1945).

By using haptens of known chemical structure, it is possible to study the interaction between antibodies and epitopes in great detail. For example, antibodies raised against one hapten can be tested for their ability to bind to other, structurally related molecules. Simple tests have shown that any alteration in the shape, size, or charge of a hapten alters its ability to bind to antibodies. Even minor modifications to the shape of a hapten may influence its ability to bind an antigen receptor or an antibody. Since there exist an enormous number of potential haptens, and since each hapten can provoke its own specific antibodies, it follows that animals must be able to generate an incredibly large variety of

antigen receptors and specific antibody molecules. It is this enormous diversity that enables animals to successfully fight the multitude of rapidly evolving pathogenic microbes encountered throughout life (Eisen and Chakraborty, 2010).

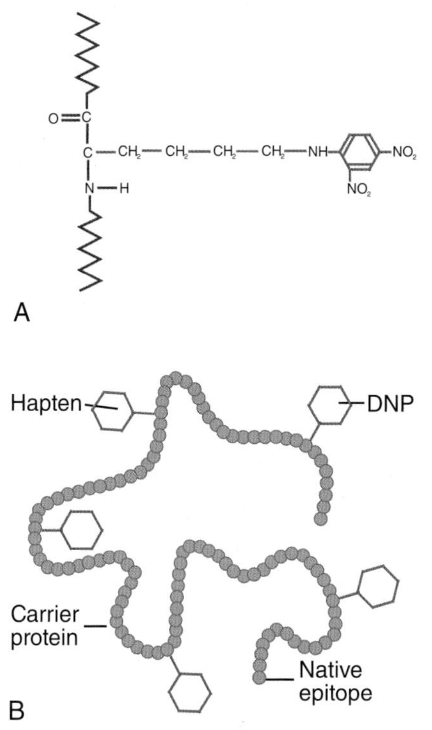

Some Examples of Haptens

Although the concept of haptens and carrier molecules provides the basis for much of our knowledge concerning the specificity of the antibody response, haptens may also be of clinical importance. For example, the antibiotic penicillin is a small, nonimmunogenic molecule. Once degraded within the body, however, it forms a reactive "penicilloyl" group, which can bind to serum proteins such as albumin to form penicilloyl-albumin complexes (Fig. 10.7). The penicilloyl hapten is recognized as a foreign epitope by some individuals and so provokes an immune response, resulting in penicillin allergy.

A second example of a naturally occurring reactive chemical that binds spontaneously to normal proteins and so acts as a hapten is the toxic component of the poison ivy plant (*Rhus radicans*). The resin of this plant, called urushiol, will react with any protein with which it comes into contact, including the skin proteins of a person who rubs against the plant. These modified skin proteins are then regarded as foreign and attacked by lymphocytes in a manner similar to the rejection of a skin graft. The result is an uncomfortable skin rash called allergic contact dermatitis (see Chapter 34).

CROSS-REACTIONS

Identical or similar epitopes may sometimes be found on apparently unrelated molecules. As a result, antibodies directed against one antigen may bind unexpectedly to an unrelated antigen. In another situation, the epitopes on a protein may differ in only minor respects from those on the same protein obtained from an animal of a related species. Consequently, antibodies directed against a protein in one species may also react in a detectable manner with the homologous or similar protein in another species. Both phenomena are called cross-reactions.

An example of a cross-reaction of the first type is seen when blood typing. Many bacteria possess cell wall glycoproteins with carbohydrate

Fig. 10.6 (A) A typical hapten, in this case, dinitrophenol attached to a lysine side chain. (B) When several haptens are attached to a peptide chain, they serve as new epitopes and will stimulate immune responses.

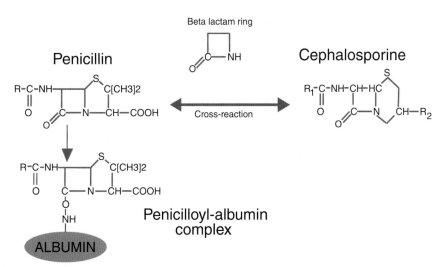

Fig. 10.7 Penicillin as a hapten. Penicillin can break down in vivo by several different pathways. The most important derivative is an acid that combines with amino groups in a protein such as serum albumin to form a penicilloyl-protein complex. This complex may provoke an immune response and result in a penicillin allergy. Cephalosporins also contain a beta-lactam ring. As a result of a cross-reaction, penicillin-allergic individuals may also be allergic to cephalosporins.

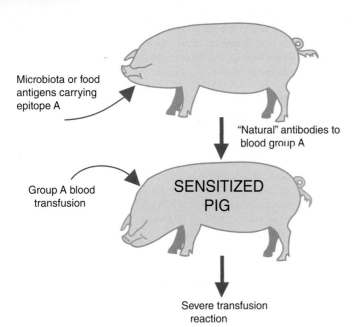

Microbiota or food antigens carrying epitope A

"Natural" antibodies to blood group A

Group A blood transfusion

SENSITIZED PIG

Severe transfusion reaction

Fig. 10.8 Food or bacterial antigens encountered in the diet carry epitopes that cross-react with blood group glycoprotein A. As a result, pigs of blood group O make antibodies to the A epitope despite never having received group A red cells. Should these animals be inadvertently transfused with group A blood, they will suffer an immediate and severe transfusion reaction.

side chains that are identical to those found on mammalian red blood cell glycoproteins. For example, some of the intestinal microbiota possess glycoproteins with A or B side chains on their cell walls (see Chapter 32). These glycoproteins are absorbed through the intestinal wall and trigger an antibody response. For example, blood-group glycoprotein side chain A is foreign to a pig of blood group O (Fig. 10.8). Pigs of blood group O therefore develop antibodies that react with red cells from pigs of blood group A. These antibodies arise not as a response to previous immunization with group A red cells but following exposure to glycoproteins from the intestinal microbiota. Another example of cross-reactivity occurs between *Brucella abortus* and some strains of *Yersinia enterocolitica*. *Y. enterocolitica*, a relatively unimportant organism, may provoke cattle to make antibodies that cross-react with *B. abortus*. Since *Brucella*-infected

animals are detected by testing for the presence of serum antibodies, a *Yersinia*-infected animal may be wrongly thought to carry *B. abortus* and so be killed. In another example, cross-reactivity occurs between the coronavirus of feline infectious peritonitis (FIP) and the virus of pig transmissible gastroenteritis (TGE). It is difficult to grow the FIP virus in the laboratory. TGE virus, on the other hand, is readily propagated. By detecting antibodies to TGE in cats, it is possible to diagnose FIP without having to culture the FIP virus.

The second type of cross-reactivity, which occurs between related proteins, may be demonstrated in many different biological systems. One example is a method used to determine relationships between mammalian species. Thus antisera to bovine serum albumin cross-react strongly with sheep and goat serum albumin but weakly with serum albumin from other mammals. Presumably, this reflects the degree of structural similarity between the epitopes on serum proteins and is thus a useful tool in determining evolutionary relationships.

REFERENCES

Atassi, M.Z., 1978. Precise determination of the entire antigenic structure of lysozyme. Immunochemistry 15, 909–936.

Borek, F., 1972. Immunogenicity, Frontiers of Biology Series. Elsevier North-Holland, Amsterdam.

De Libero, G., Collmann, A., Mori, L., 2009. The cellular and biochemical rules of lipid antigen presentation. Eur. J. Immunol. 39, 2648–2656.

Eisen, H.N., Chakraborty, A.K., 2010. Evolving concepts of specificity in immune reactions. Proc. Natl. Acad. Sci. U.S.A. 107, 22373–22380.

Green, N., Alexander, H., Olsen, A., et al., 1982. Immunogenic structure of the influenza virus hemagglutinin. Cell 28, 477–487.

Katz, M.E., Maizels, R.M., Wicker, L., et al., 1982. Immunological focusing by the mouse major histocompatibility complex: mouse strains confronted with distantly related lysozymes confine their attention to very few epitopes. Eur. J. Immunol. 12, 535–540.

Landsteiner, K., 1945. The Specificity of Serological Reactions. Harvard University Press, Cambridge.

Marx, J.L., 1984. Do antibodies prefer moving targets? Science 226, 819–821.

Sela, M., 1969. Antigenicity: some molecular aspects. Science 166, 1365–1374.

Sercarz, E. (Ed.), 1989. Antigenic determinants and immune regulation. In: Chemical Immunology, vol. 46, Karger, Basel.

Tizard, I., 1982. Antigen structure and immunogenicity. JAVMA 181, 978–982.

Wilson, I.A., Niman, H.L., Houghten, R.A., et al., 1984. The structure of an antigenic determinant in a protein. Cell 37, 767–778.

Dendritic Cells, Antigen Processing, and Presentation

Innate immune defenses have evolved to destroy microbes as soon as they enter the body. Most invaders, especially if they are of low virulence, are rapidly eliminated. However, in addition to being uncomfortable and damaging, inflammation is not a foolproof process. If the body is to be defended effectively, an animal must have defenses that detect and eliminate all microbial invaders without the damage and discomfort associated with inflammation. This is the task of the adaptive immune system.

Adaptive immune responses proceed in four major steps. These are: Step 1: Antigen capture, processing, and presentation. Step 2: Helper T-cell activation. Step 3: B cell and/or cytotoxic T cell–mediated responses that eliminate the invaders. And finally, Step 4: The generation of large populations of memory cells. It is these persistent memory cells that provide a vaccinated animal with the ability to respond rapidly and effectively to subsequent microbial infections.

Step 1: Antigen Capture, Processing, and Presentation

To trigger adaptive immunity, a sample of foreign material must first be captured, processed, and then presented in the correct fashion to cells that can recognize it. The induction of adaptive immune responses requires the activation of antigen-presenting cells. Their activation is mediated by cytokines generated during the initial innate response. Three different cell types are considered to function as "professional" antigen-presenting cells. These are dendritic cells, B cells, and macrophages. (Fig. 11.1) Of these, dendritic cells are the most important and effective. They present processed antigens to helper T cells.

DENDRITIC CELLS

Dendritic cells (DCs) perform three major functions. First, they serve as sentinel cells and activate innate defenses when they first encounter invaders. Second, they process exogenous antigens and thus initiate adaptive immune responses. Third, they regulate adaptive immunity by determining whether an antigen will trigger an antibody-mediated or a cell-mediated response or even prevent an immune response from occurring (a condition called tolerance). DCs are at least 100 times more effective antigen-presenting cells than are macrophages or B cells. DCs can take up many different antigens, including dead microorganisms, soluble foreign antigens in tissue fluids, and antigens released by dying cells, and present them to helper T cells. DCs are the only antigen-presenting cells that can activate helper T cells that have never previously encountered an antigen (naïve cells) and therefore are essential for initiating primary immune responses.

Origin

DCs are derived from hematopoietic stem cells in the bone marrow. Immature DCs migrate through the body and form networks in virtually every tissue. Monocytes may also develop into DCs when exposed to appropriate cytokines. DCs are found in all organs except the brain, parts of the eye, and the testes. They are especially prominent in lymph nodes, skin, and under mucosal surfaces, sites where invading microbes are most likely to be encountered. The number of dendritic cells varies among tissues. Thus, DCs are present in large numbers within the dermis. As a result, intradermally administered antigens are readily captured. Likewise, circulating DCs are common in well-vascularized muscles, the preferred site of injection for many vaccines. (There are fewer DCs in the subcutis and adipose tissue, thus explaining why these are usually less effective routes of vaccine administration) (Geissmann et al., 2010).

Structure

The shape of a DC depends on its state of activation. Typically, however, they are characterized by having a small, round cell body with many long cytoplasmic processes known as dendrites extending from it (Fig. 11.2). These dendrites increase the efficiency of antigen trapping and maximize contact between DCs and other cell types.

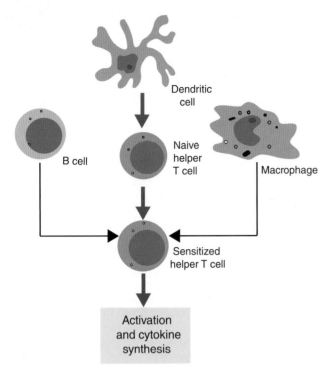

Fig. 11.1 The three major populations of antigen-presenting cells: B cells, Dendritic cells (DCs), and macrophages. Of these, only DCs can activate naïve T cells and trigger a primary immune response.

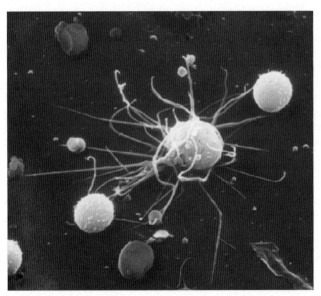

Fig. 11.2 A scanning electron micrograph of a dendritic cell from a guinea pig lymph node. Note the relatively small cell body and the numerous long dendrites. Original magnification ×4000.

Subpopulations

Like other immune cell populations, DCs consist of multiple subpopulations. The two most prominent of these are classical/conventional (cDC) and plasmacytoid DCs (pDC) (Fig. 11.3). These subpopulations differ in their origins, morphology, surface antigens, and functions, although they share adhesion molecules, costimulatory molecules, and activation markers. Other important dendritic cell subpopulations are found in the skin (Langerhans cells) and in lymphoid organs (follicular DCs). Each DC subpopulation expresses different cell surface

receptors, signaling receptors such as TLRs and FcRs, and each produces a diverse and complex mixture of cytokines and chemokines. As with other cells described in this text, many of the details of DC function have been worked out in humans and mice. It must not be assumed that the structure and functions of DCs in domestic mammals are identical.

As pointed out in Chapter 1, the adaptive immune system mounts two types of response: the antibody-mediated (type two) and cell-mediated (type one) responses. The type of response mounted is determined by the type of helper T (Th) cells activated when an antigen is encountered. Thus there are multiple types of helper cells (see Fig. 14.12). One major type, T-helper 1 cells (Th1 cells), stimulates cell-mediated immune responses that protect animals against intracellular organisms. The other major type, T-helper 2 cells (Th2 cells), stimulates antibody-mediated immune responses optimized to protect animals against extracellular invaders. Which of these helper cell populations is activated is determined by antigen-presenting DCs (Kushwah and Hu, 2011).

Classical Dendritic Cells

The relationships between macrophages and dendritic cells are complex and may differ between species (Sallusto and Lanzavecchia, 2010). Blood monocytes are the immediate precursors of some tissue macrophages and some cDCs. Which cell type is produced depends on the mixture of cytokines and cells encountered by the monocyte as it differentiates. Each type can convert to the other until late in the differentiation process. cDCs can therefore be considered part of the mononuclear phagocytic system being derived from a common stem cell, respond to the same growth factors, express the same surface markers, and in effect are in no specific way uniquely different from other macrophages. Their main function is antigen presentation and induction of T-cell responses.

Plasmacytoid Dendritic Cells

Plasmacytoid DCs (pDCs) are long-lived sentinel cells found in blood, bone marrow, and lymphoid organs. They lack myeloid antigens but retain some lymphoid characteristics. pDCs serve as an early warning system for viral infections since they are rapidly activated by viral nucleic acids acting through TLRs7 and 9. They respond to viruses by synthesizing massive amounts of the type I interferons (IFN-α and IFN-β). (Ten- to 100-fold more than other cell types.) They are also major producers of type III interferons (IFN-λ) (see Chapter 9). Their numbers increase during infection. pDCs have a unique ability to link innate and adaptive immunity. After producing large amounts of type I interferon, they are still able to differentiate into mature DCs that can stimulate naïve T cells. Because pDCs secrete large amounts of IFN-α, they can also activate natural killer (NK) cells (Reizis, 2019). As discussed in Chapter 20, pDCs may actually be a type of innate lymphoid cell.

Langerhans Cells

Langerhans cells are specialized, long-lived dendritic cells found in the skin. Their cytoplasm contains characteristic rod- or racquet-shaped granules called Birbeck granules whose function is unclear. Their long dendrites form an extensive network that is ideally situated to trap foreign antigens (Fig. 11.4). These antigens include not only invading microbes but also topically applied antigens, such as the resins of poison ivy, or intradermally injected antigens, such as those in mosquito saliva. Langerhans cells influence the development of skin inflammatory responses, such as delayed hypersensitivity and allergic contact dermatitis (see Chapter 34). They express multiple pattern-recognition receptors, including the C-type lectins langerin and DC-SIGN that can

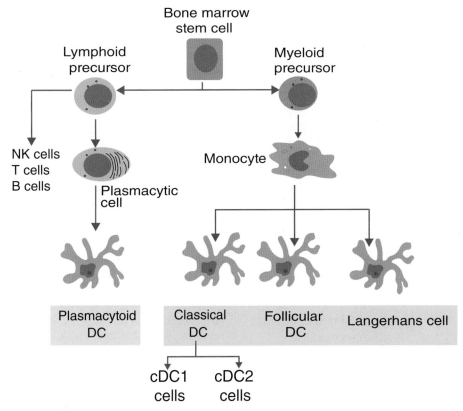

Fig. 11.3 The origins of dendritic cells (DCs). One population, the plasmacytoid DCs, originates from lymphoid precursors. The second major population arises from myeloid precursors and is closely related to monocytes. These, together with follicular DCs and Langerhans cells, constitute the conventional dendritic cells (cDC1) type. *NK*, Natural killer.

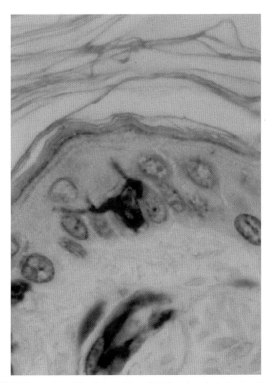

Fig. 11.4 The red cell in the epidermis of a dog is a Langerhans cell stained for the protein vimentin. Note that its dendrites extend between the epidermal cells so that it can effectively trap antigens. Courtesy Dr. K.M. Credille.

bind bacteria, fungi, and some viruses. Once they have captured antigens, the Langerhans cells migrate to draining lymph nodes, where they present the antigen to T cells. Some immunologists regard Langerhans cells simply as specialized macrophages (de Jong and Geijtenbeek, 2010; Palucka and Banchereau, 2006).

Follicular Dendritic Cells

Another population of specialized DCs called follicular DCs (fDCs) are found in the germinal centers of the spleen, lymph nodes, and Peyer's patches (see Chapter 13). They are also found around localized infection sites and chronic inflammatory lesions. Follicular DCs are essential for antibody production and the development of B cell memory (DeShane and Chaplin, 2010). In an animal that has not previously been exposed to the antigen, antigen presentation is a passive process. The fDCs simply provide a surface on which antigen can be presented to B cells. In contrast, in animals that have previously been exposed to an antigen and possess antibodies, the antigen and antibody combine to form antibody-antigen complexes (also called immune complexes). Follicular DCs take up these immune complexes on their surface and then shed them in extracellular membrane vesicles called exosomes. These exosomes express both antigen-MHC complexes as well as costimulatory molecules and so can also present antigen to T and B cells. Likewise, B cells can also take up these exosomes, and after processing the antigen, present its fragments to antigen-sensitive T cells (Hodge et al., 2022). Follicular DCs can retain antigens on their surface receptors for more than three months. They also integrate signals from toll-like receptors (TLRs) and other sources to support effective germinal center responses (see Chapter 13; Heesters et al., 2014).

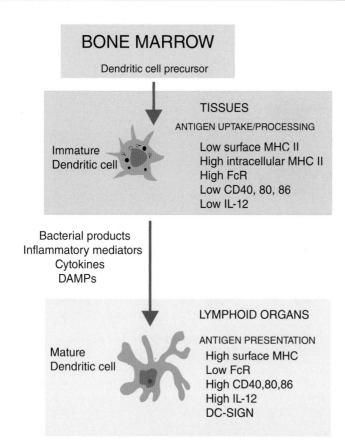

Fig. 11.5 As dendritic cells (DCs) mature, they change their function. Immature DCs are specialized antigen-trapping and processing cells. Mature DCs, on the other hand, are specialized antigen-presenting cells. *DAMPs,* Damage-associated molecular patterns; *IL-12,* interleukin-12; *MHC,* major histocompatibility complex.

Dendritic Cell Maturation

Although multiple DC subpopulations have been characterized, their most important properties are determined by their state of maturity (Fig. 11.5). Thus immature DCs are specialized, efficient antigen-trapping cells. As they mature, DCs undergo cellular reorganization and become specialized, efficient antigen-presenting cells.

Immature Dendritic Cells—Antigen-Trapping Cells

Newly generated DCs migrate from the bone marrow to lymph nodes or other tissues. Here they act as sentinels whose role is to capture invading microbes. With their short life span, they can be regarded as disposable antigen-trapping cells. If they do not encounter antigens, they die in a few days. If, however, they encounter antigens and are stimulated by tissue damage or inflammation, they become activated and mature rapidly. Immature DCs have receptors that help them carry out their functions. These include the receptors for interleukin-1 (IL-1R) and tumor necrosis factor, chemokine receptors, C-type lectins, Fc receptors (FcγR and FcεR), mannose receptors (CD206), and heat-shock protein receptors, as well as TLRs.

Although the most important functions of DCs are to trap, process, and present antigen to helper T cells of the immune system, they must also be able to kill any pathogens they encounter. Thus DCs can kill invaders by mounting a respiratory burst. Activation of their TLRs by pathogen-associated molecular patterns (PAMPs) enhances their production of superoxide.

DCs mature in response to interleukin-1 (IL-1) and tumor necrosis factor-α (TNF-α) as well as to PAMPs and damage-associated

molecular patterns (DAMPs). Injured and inflamed tissues release large amounts of soluble heparan sulfate that binds to TLR4 and activates DCs. Breakdown of nucleic acids generates uric acid, another potent dendritic cell activator. One of the most important activators of immature DCs is high mobility group box protein-1 (HMGB1) (see Chapter 3). Immature DCs are attracted to areas of inflammation by chemokines, defensins, and HMGB1.

Immature DCs can capture antigens and cell fragments by phagocytosis, by pinocytosis (the uptake of fluid droplets—cell drinking), and by binding to cell surface receptors. If they ingest bacteria, they can usually kill them. They can distinguish between normal tissue debris and foreign organisms by selectively sampling their environment. This differentiation depends on the ability of the foreign material to bind to TLRs. Activation of TLRs by PAMPs ensures that ingested material is processed in such a way that it triggers antigen presentation. Material that does not activate TLRs is not processed and will not trigger an adaptive response.

The pH in the phagosomes of conventional phagocytic cells such as neutrophils and macrophages is highly acidic and hence optimized for proteolytic destruction of foreign material. The pH within dendritic cell and B cell phagosomes is, in contrast, relatively alkaline since these phagosomes do not fuse with lysosomes. Cysteine and aspartyl proteases are inhibited at these high pH levels, and as a result, ingested antigens are not completely degraded but rather are preserved for presentation by MHC class I molecules.

Mature Dendritic Cells—Antigen-Presenting Cells

Once they have captured and processed antigens, immature DCs carry these antigens to sites where they can be recognized by T cells. The activated DCs are attracted to lymphoid organs by chemokines. Infection or tissue damage also promotes the migration of antigen-bearing DCs to lymph nodes or the spleen. Once they enter a lymphoid organ, the cells mature rapidly.

Mature DCs first secrete chemokines that attract T cells, that accumulate in clusters around the dendritic cell (Fig. 11.6). The DCs embrace the T cells in a net of dendrites as they interact. During this time, the T cells examine the mature DCs for the presence of antigen fragments. If their antigen receptors can bind these presented fragments, the T cells will be triggered to respond.

As DCs mature, their MHC molecules move from intracellular endosomes and lysosomes to the cell surface. Cell surface expression of their costimulatory molecules also increases. As a result, MHC molecules and MHC-peptide complexes are found at levels 100 times higher on mature DCs than on other cell types such as B cells or macrophages. Their expression of costimulatory molecules such as CD86 may also rise 100-fold.

Mature DCs are the only cells that can trigger a primary T-cell response. One reason for this is that mature DCs can assemble complete T-cell activation complexes (antigen-loaded MHC plus costimulatory molecules) within the cell before they are carried to the cell surface. Mature DCs also express DC-SIGN (CD209), a C-type lectin that binds a ligand called intercellular adhesion molecule-3 (ICAM-3 or CD50) on naïve T cells. DC-SIGN permits transient binding between DCs and T cells. It allows a single dendritic cell to rapidly screen thousands of T cells to find the few that are expressing compatible antigen receptors. Thus one dendritic cell may activate as many as 3000 T cells (Yamakawa et al., 2008).

Tolerance Induction

Under steady-state conditions, in the absence of inflammation or infection, some immature DCs spontaneously mature and migrate to lymphoid tissues carrying processed normal tissue antigens on their

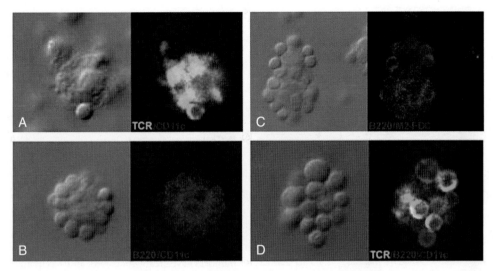

Fig. 11.6 When dendritic cells (DCs) and T cells interact, they form visible clusters as the cells converse among themselves. Thus, in these figures, DCs are stained with a blue fluorescent dye (anti-CD11c), T cells are stained with a green dye (anti-CD3), and B cells are stained with a red dye (anti-B220). (A) T cells are interacting with a dendritic cell. (B) B cells are binding to a dendritic cell. (C) B cells are binding to a follicular dendritic cell. (D) There is a mixed B and T-cell cluster. Note that some B cells appear to be attached to T cells. From Hommel, M., Kyewski, B., 2003. Dynamic changes during the immune response in T cell-antigen-presenting cell clusters isolated from lymph nodes. J. Exp. Med. 197, 269–280.

MHC molecules. If a T cell recognizes this "normal" antigen, the T cell will undergo apoptosis and die. Alternatively, these DCs may trigger the production of IL-10, a suppressive cytokine that generates regulatory T cells. As a result, the processing of normal tissue antigens or even harmless environmental antigens by these DCs can lead to T-cell deletion and immunological tolerance (see Chapter 21). In humans, a subset of DCs express the immunosuppressive molecule indoleamine 2,3-dioxygenase. This subset has a regulatory function and may be able to promote tolerance. The decision to induce either a tolerogenic response or a defensive immune response likely depends upon the presence of microbial PAMPs or tissue DAMPs. A good example of this is the tolerance expressed in the intestine to food antigens and commensal bacteria. DCs that sample these antigens are potent inducers of retinoic acid and TGF-β (see Chapter 22). This retinoic acid promotes the differentiation of regulatory T cells and thus prevents the development of inappropriate immune responses to commensals and food. It has also been shown that under inflammatory conditions, TNF-α can kill these tolerogenic DCs and thus free other cells to respond actively to invaders (Bourque and Hawiger, 2023).

cDC1, cDC2, and DC3 Cells

When cDCs stimulate helper T cells, they deliver three signals. The first signal is delivered when T-cell antigen receptors bind antigen fragments presented on MHC molecules. The second signal provides the cells with additional critical costimulation through cell surface molecules such as CD40 and CD80/86. The third signal determines the direction in which naïve helper T cells will develop and is provided by secreted cytokines. For example, some microbial antigens trigger cDCs to secrete IL-12 (Fig. 11.7). These are called cDC1 cells since this IL-12 activates Th1 cells and triggers cell-mediated type 1 immune responses. Because they promote cytotoxic T-cell functions cDC1 cells play an important role in cancer immunotherapy.

Other microbial antigens induce cDCs to secrete IL-1 and IL-6. These cytokines stimulate Th2 differentiation and are produced by cDC2 cells. They stimulate antibody-mediated type 2 responses. Other antigens may induce cDC2s to secrete IL-23 and so provoke the development of Th17 cells and type 3 responses.

A third cDC population designated DC3 forms a distinctly separate lineage. Their phenotype is CD88⁻, CD14⁺, CD2⁺, and CD163⁺. They originate from hematopoietic stem cells and appear to activate CD8⁺ T cells, but their specific functions remain unclear (Villar and Segura, 2020).

Different PAMPs and DAMPs acting through different TLRs influence the development of these dendritic cell subpopulations and thus the nature of immune responses induced. The stimuli that promote cDC1 production include double-stranded RNA acting through TLR3, lipopolysaccharide acting through TLR4, flagellin acting through TLR5, and nucleic acids acting through TLR7 and TLR9. On the other hand, inflammatory mediators, such as IL-10, transforming growth factor–α (TGF-α), prostaglandin E_2 (PGE₂), histamine, extracts of parasitic worms, or the toxin of *Vibrio cholerae*, promote cDC2 production. cDC2 responses may also be triggered by bacterial lipopolysaccharides and proteoglycans acting through TLR2, TLR6, or TLR1. Ligands of TLR2 promote the production of IL-23 and hence promote Th17 cell responses. As pointed out previously, a similar functional subdivision occurs among macrophages. Thus, M1 and M2 macrophages, when acting as antigen-presenting cells, also promote different helper cell responses.

It may also be that the same dendritic cell can promote a type 1, type 2, or type 3 response, depending on the dose and type of antigen it encounters. The response may also depend on its location. For example, DCs from the intestine or airways seem to preferentially secrete IL-10 and IL-4 and thus promote type 2 responses. In such cases, the intestinal microbiota may provide the cDC2-polarizing signals.

pDCs increase dramatically during inflammation and infection. They are relatively inefficient in promoting helper cell proliferation but produce large quantities of IFN-γ and IL-17. They thus promote Th1 polarization and type 1 responses.

Interleukin-12

IL-12 is a key cytokine produced by macrophages, DCs, B cells, and neutrophils. Its targets are T cells and NK cells. IL-12 primarily

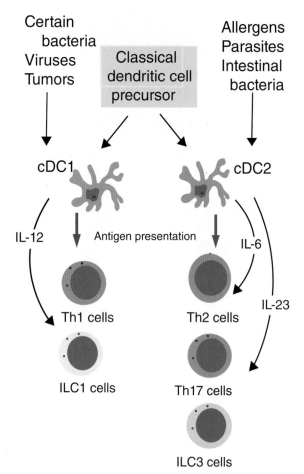

Fig. 11.7 Two populations of conventional dendritic cells (cDCs) can activate helper T-cell subpopulations. cDC1 cells promote type 1 responses by producing IL-12 and activating Th1 cells. Whereas cDC2 cells promote type 2 responses by producing interleukin-6 (IL-6) and IL-23 and so activating Th2 cells and Th17 cells. The helper cell population that is activated depends on the cytokine mixture produced by these dendritic cell subpopulations. These specific dendritic cell subpopulations depend upon the nature of the inducing antigens. Dendritic cells also activate innate lymphoid cells (ILCs). CDC1s activate ILC1s and cDC2s activate ILC3s (see Chapter 20).

determines Th1/Th2 polarization. Th1 cells develop when it is present. Th2 cells develop when it is absent. IL-12 is a member of a family of related proteins that also includes IL-23, IL-27, IL-35, and IL-39. These are all heterodimeric proteins. For example, IL-12 is formed by two chains, p35 and p40. Some of these chains are shared with other family members. All the members of the family regulate T-cell function. Thus IL-12 and IL-27 generate Th1 cells, whereas IL-23 generates Th17 cells (Wojno et al., 2019).

OTHER ANTIGEN-PROCESSING CELLS

Naïve T cells require prolonged close interaction with DCs before they can respond to antigens. Once primed, however, these T cells may be further activated by relatively brief interactions with two other major cell types: antigen-presenting macrophages and B cells.

Macrophages

Macrophages are the most accessible and best understood of the antigen-processing cells. Their properties are described in Chapter 7. Once

antigens are taken up by macrophages, a portion is processed, bound to MHC molecules, and presented to sensitized T cells. Macrophages, however, are unable to engage in prolonged interactions with T cells. As a result, they cannot activate naïve T cells. In addition, antigen processing by macrophages is inefficient since much of the ingested antigen is destroyed by lysosomal proteases and oxidants. Indeed, macrophages and B cells can be considered cells with other priorities (some call them "semiprofessional" antigen-processing cells) (Hume, 2008).

B Cells

B cells, like macrophages, cannot undertake prolonged interactions with T cells. They do, however, have antigen receptors that enable them to bind and process large amounts of specific antigen. They ingest and process antigens before presenting them, in association with MHC class II molecules, to sensitized T cells (see Fig. 16.7). B cells probably play a minor role in antigen processing in a primary immune response but a much more significant one in a secondary response when their numbers have greatly increased, and T cells are easier to stimulate.

Other Cells

T cells may also be activated by many different "amateur" antigen-presenting cells. These include neutrophils, eosinophils, basophils, T cells, mast cells, endothelial cells, fibroblasts, NK cells, smooth muscle cells, astrocytes, microglial cells, platelets, and some epithelial cells such as thymic epithelial cells and corneal cells. Their effectiveness may depend on the local environment and collaboration with other "professional" antigen-presenting cells. Thus fibroblasts may be very effective antigen-processing cells when located within granulomas. Presumably, costimulation can come from other nearby cells in this cytokine-rich environment. Vascular endothelial cells can also take up antigens, synthesize IL-1, and under the influence of IFN-γ, express MHC class II molecules. Even skin keratinocytes can secrete cytokines similar to IL-1, express MHC class II molecules, and present antigen to T cells. In pigs, a subpopulation of circulating γ/δ T cells may also act as professional antigen-processing cells (Schuijs et al., 2019).

ANTIGEN PROCESSING

One type of foreign antigen is typified by the invading bacteria that grow in the tissues and extracellular fluid. These live outside cells and so are called "exogenous antigens." Exogenous antigens must first be captured, processed, and presented in the correct fashion to helper T cells if they are to trigger a defensive response. This is the responsibility of dendritic cells using the MHC class II pathway (Pishesha et al., 2022).

Major Histocompatibility Complex Class II Pathway

The presentation of exogenous antigens is regulated by MHC class II molecules. These are cell surface receptors that bind processed peptide fragments. Although many cells can phagocytose foreign antigens, only those that can express antigen fragments bound to MHC class II molecules will trigger an immune response. As described previously, the most efficient antigen-processing cells are thus mature MHC class II+ cDCs. Unlike macrophages, DC lysosomes have limited proteolytic activity and degrade internalized antigens slowly. As a result, antigen fragments may persist within these cells for a long time. MHC class II molecules can bind these fragments of ingested antigens and present them to helper cells (Fig. 11.8). T-helper cells recognize and respond to antigen fragments only when they are bound to MHC class II molecules. If an antigen is presented to T cells in the absence of MHC class II, the T cells will be turned off or die, and tolerance may result (see Chapter 21).

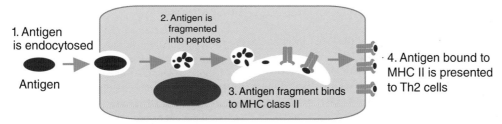

Fig. 11.8 The processing of exogenous antigen by an antigen-presenting cell. Ingested antigens are taken into phagosomes where they are fragmented by proteases. Peptides are then carried to the endosomal compartments where the antigenic peptides are placed in the binding grooves of major histocompatibility complex (MHC) class II molecules. The antigen-MHC complexes are then carried to the cell surface where they are presented to helper T cells.

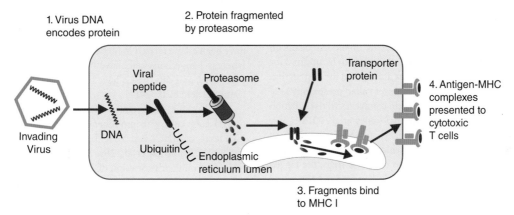

Fig. 11.9 The processing of endogenous antigen. Samples of newly synthesized proteins are ubiquinated before being chopped into peptides by a proteasome. The peptides attach to a transporter protein located in the membrane of the endoplasmic reticulum. They are then carried into the lumen of the endoplasmic reticulum, where they are placed in the antigen-binding groove of major histocompatibility complex (MHC) class I molecules. The MHC class I–peptide complexes are carried to the cell surface, where they encounter cytotoxic T cells.

Exogenous antigen processing involves multiple steps. First, the antigen must be endocytosed and taken into phagosomes. These phagosomes then fuse with lysosomes. The ingested proteins are broken up by the lysosomal proteases into peptide fragments of varying length. The endosomes containing these peptide fragments then fuse with other endosomes carrying newly synthesized MHC class II molecules to generate the lysosome-MHC class II compartment (MIIC). Endogenous antigens may also enter the MIIC through autophagy (see Chapter 6).

Newly synthesized MHC class II chains are translocated to the endosomes, where, together with a peptide called the invariant chain (Ii), they form a protein complex. The invariant chain occupies the MHC antigen-binding site. This complex travels to the MIIC, where the invariant chain is digested, leaving a small peptide called the class II-associated Ii peptide (CLIP), filling the MHC antigen-binding groove. When antigen-containing phagosomes fuse with the MHC-containing endosomes, the foreign peptide fragments are exchanged for the CLIP chain. An MHC class II antigen-binding groove can hold a peptide of 12–24 amino acids as a straight, extended chain that projects out of both ends of the binding groove. Side chains from the peptide fit into pockets on the walls of the binding groove.

The presence of the CLIP chain prevents endosomes containing MHC class II molecules from being prematurely transported to the cell surface. Thus, unlike most new transmembrane proteins that are expressed minutes after assembly, MHC class II molecules are retained

inside the cell for several hours until they are needed. Once an antigen peptide binds to an MHC molecule, the MIIC vesicle moves toward the cell surface. When it reaches the surface, the vesicle fuses with the cell membrane and the MHC-peptide complex is exposed and available for inspection by any passing T cell.

It has been calculated that an antigen-processing DC contains about 2×10^5 MHC class II molecules that can present peptide fragments to T cells. If costimulation is provided, a single T cell can be activated by exposure to as few as 200–300 of these peptide-MHC complexes. It is therefore possible for a single antigen-processing cell to present many different antigens to different T cells simultaneously.

Since T-helper cells must recognize MHC-antigen complexes in order to respond to an antigen, the MHC class II molecules effectively determine whether or not an animal will mount an adaptive immune response to any antigen. Class II molecules can bind some, but not all, peptides created during antigen processing, and in effect, they select those antigen fragments that are to be presented to T cells. (Further coverage of MHC molecules is provided in Chapter 12.)

Major Histocompatibility Complex Class I Pathway

One function of T cell–mediated immune responses is the identification and destruction of cells producing abnormal or foreign proteins. The best examples of such cells are those infected by viruses. Viruses take over the protein-synthesizing machinery of infected cells and use it to make new viral proteins (Fig. 11.9). To control virus infections, cytotoxic T cells must be able to recognize any viral proteins expressed on the surface of infected cells. T cells can indeed recognize and respond to these endogenous antigens but only if they are processed and bound to MHC class I molecules (see Chapter 12).

The MHC class I molecule is a cell surface receptor folded in such a way that a large antigen-binding groove is formed (see Fig. 12.5). This binding groove, however, differs from that on MHC class II molecules in that it is closed at each end. Overall, however, the antigen-binding sites on class II and class I molecules function in a similar manner. The processing of endogenous peptides differs from the processing of exogenous peptides.

Living cells continually break up and recycle the proteins they produce. As a result, abnormal proteins are removed, regulatory peptides do not accumulate, and amino acids are recycled. As a first step, the unwanted protein must be tagged. To do this, ubiquitin, a small protein found in all eukaryote cells, attaches to lysine residues in target proteins. Additional ubiquitin molecules then attach to the protein-bound ubiquitin so that multiple ubiquitin molecules are linked like beads on a string. A chain of four ubiquitin molecules appears to be optimal for processing. These polyubiquinated proteins are marked for destruction since they are recognized by enzyme complexes called proteasomes.

Proteasomes are large multisubunit protein complexes whose function is to degrade unwanted intracellular proteins (Finley et al., 2016). They are tubular structures with an inner channel that contains the protease activity and two outer rings that regulate which proteins can enter and be destroyed. Ubiquitinated proteins bind to the outer rings, the tagged protein is unfolded, and the ubiquitin is released and reused (Bhoj and Chen, 2009). The unfolded protein is inserted into the inner channel of the proteasome, where it is chopped up into 8- to 15-amino acid long peptides (like a meat grinder). Most of these peptide fragments are recycled into new proteins. For about 1 in a million molecules, however, the peptides are rescued from further breakup by attachment to transporter proteins. Two transporter proteins are used: TAP-1 and TAP-2 (TAP stands for transporter for antigen processing). TAP-1 and TAP-2 form a heterodimer that binds peptide fragments and transports them into endosomes. Ideally, an 8- to 10-amino acid peptide precisely fits the binding site on the heterodimer. In this case, the peptide is loaded into the TAP dimer, carried to a newly formed MHC, and if it fits the MHC antigen-binding site it is transferred. Once loaded on the MHC, the MHC-peptide complex is carried to the cell surface by its normal secretory pathway where it is displayed for many hours.

A cell can express about 10^6 MHC-peptide complexes at any one time. A minimum of about 200 MHC class I molecules loaded with the same viral peptide is required to activate a cytotoxic T cell. Thus the MHC-peptide complexes can provide passing T cells with fairly complete information on virtually all the proteins being made by a cell. Analyses of peptide binding indicate that the binding groove of a class I protein can bind over a million different peptides with significant affinity. The number is not unlimited because each MHC type usually shows preferences for peptides with certain structures. In fact, out of the great number of peptides generated from the proteome of a pathogen, only a few "immunodominant" peptides are recognized by most of the host's T cells. Thus cytotoxic T cells can screen these peptides to determine whether any are "foreign" and bind to their TCRs.

Normally the two ends of the MHC class I peptide binding groove are closed. This is in contrast to the MHC class II binding groove where the ends are open and long antigenic peptides can extend out of the groove at either end. An interesting feature of pig MHC class I peptide binding is the fact that they can also recognize long antigenic peptides whose N-terminus can extend out beyond the MHC binding groove. This novel form of antigen presentation has also been observed in some human MHC class I molecules (Wei et al., 2022).

Cross-Priming

It must not be assumed that the two antigen-processing pathways function in isolation. In fact, the pathways interact extensively. For example, under some circumstances, exogenous antigens may enter the cytoplasm, join the endogenous antigen pathway, and be presented on MHC class I molecules. Thus, in antigen-presenting cells such as macrophages and DCs, endocytosed viral antigen may not be degraded in lysosomes but by proteasomes and so is processed as an endogenous antigen. This antigen thus binds to MHC class I molecules and is recognized by cytotoxic T cells. This may be important in promoting immunity to viruses since it ensures that the antigens from dead virions may still be able to trigger a response by cytotoxic T cells (see Chapter 19).

DENDRITIC CELLS IN DOMESTIC ANIMALS

DCs are found in all the major domestic mammals and do not appear to differ in any significant respect from DCs in humans and mice. cDCs have been characterized in horses, ruminants, pigs, dogs, and chickens, whereas Langerhans cells have been described in horses, ruminants, pigs, dogs, and cats. pDCs have been characterized in pigs and horses (Summerfield et al., 2014).

Equine DCs have typical dendritic cell morphology—irregularly shaped large cells with prominent cytoplasmic processes. They express high levels of MHC1 and MHC II, in addition to CD11, EqWC1, LFA1, and EqWC2 (Siedek et al., 1997). Different subsets have been identified based on their expression of MHC class II and other markers. Thus, dendritic cells from lymph nodes are CD1b positive but blood DCs are not. Equine pDCs have been characterized and shown to produce large amounts of IFN-α on stimulation with TLR9 agonists (Ziegler et al., 2016).

Bovine DCs express MHC II, CD80, CD86, and CD40 (Fig. 11.10). Cattle possess two dendritic cell subpopulations that differ in their ability to stimulate CD4 and CD8 T cells (Seo et al., 2009). One population synthesizes more IL-12, whereas the other population produces more IL-1 and IL-10. These may well represent cDC1 and cDC2 subpopulations. Cattle also possess some DCs that produce large amounts of type I interferons and are therefore likely functional equivalents of pDCs (González-Cano et al., 2014). DCs derived from sheep peripheral blood monocytes express MHC class II, CD11c, and are CD14-negative. pDC, cDC1, and cDC2 cells have been identified in this species (Chan et al., 2002).

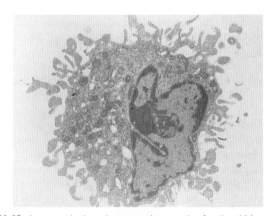

Fig. 11.10 A transmission electron micrograph of a dendritic cell from bovine afferent lymph. It has been stained with a monoclonal antibody specific for bovine CD1b. (The antibody is linked to colloidal gold particles, which are visible as small, electron dense dots around the outside of the cell.) Courtesy Dr. C.J. Howard and Dr. P. Bland, Institute for Animal Health, Compton, United Kingdom.

Pigs have both conventional cDCs and plasmacytic pDCs (Facci et al., 2010). Pig cDCs are CD172a+, CD11R1+, CD1+/−, and CD80/86+/−, whereas their pDCs are CD172a+, CD4+, CD1+/−, and CD80/86+/−. Both types secrete IL-10 and IL-12. Porcine DCs also express FcγRII and FcγRIII on their surface and thus can be activated by immune complexes. They express TLRs and are responsive to stimulation by bacterial LPS and CpG DNA. Pig blood pDCs are the major source of TNF-α, IL-12p40, and IFN-α in addition to some complement components (Calzada-nova et al., 2010). Neonatal pig dendritic cells are also activated by ligands of TLR4 or TLR9. TLR7 and TLR9 are restricted to pDCs and not expressed on cDCs as in mice (Johansson et al., 2003).

Pig pDCs are also unique in that they express functional NKp46 receptors (Mair et al., 2022). In other mammals these are considered to be strictly NK cell markers. However, pig DCs do not express perforins so they are not cytotoxic but these may be activating receptors. It is also of interest to note that pig pDCs produce IFN-α in response to several common viruses, including transmissible gastroenteritis, pseudorabies, and swine flu, but not porcine reproductive and respiratory syndrome virus (PRRSV). This virus impairs antigen presentation by cDCs and enhances their IL-10 production. It is not surprising therefore that PRRSV causes persistent infection and stimulates only a weak immune response (Auray et al., 2010, 2016).

Canine dendritic cells are potent T-cell stimulators. They can be generated from blood monocytes by treatment with IL-4 and GM-CSF. They can also be derived from CD34+ progenitors stimulated by GM-CSF and TNF-α in the bone marrow. As in other species, their state of maturity makes a big difference to their functionality. Dog dendritic cells possess a unique ultrastructure since there are multiple, variable-sized, electron-dense granules with a wasp's nest-like appearance in their cytoplasm.

Dog DCs can be stimulated to differentiate by many different cytokine mixtures but the most widely employed is GM-CSF plus interleukin 4. There are two main populations of canine DCs (Qeska et al., 2013). One is MHC class II+, CD11c+, CD34+, and CD14−; the other is MHC class II+, CD34+, and CD14+. CD40 is expressed on canine DCs but not on monocytes. Canine DCs produce a diverse array of cytokines. The precise mixture produced depends on the stimulus employed, but in general, it resembles those produced by DCs in humans and mice. One unusual feature is, however, the production of large amounts of IL-10, IL-12, IL-13, and IFN-α by LPS-stimulated canine DCs. Canine DCs also express functional CD1 molecules that can bind and present lipid antigens to lymphocytes. They also express low levels of CD4 and CD8. As in other species, depending on whether they are DC1 or DC2 cells, they can secrete polarizing cytokines (Ricklin Gutzwiller et al., 2010).

As in other species, cat DCs are readily activated by exposure to GM-CSF and IL-4. Feline Langerhans cells are CD18+, MHC class II+, CD1a+, and CD4+. DCs from feline blood mononuclear cells are CD1+, CD14+, and MHC class I and II+ (Fig. 11.11).

HISTIOCYTOSIS AND HISTIOCYTOMAS

Domestic animals suffer from several diseases in which macrophages or DCs proliferate excessively. These are called histiocytomas or histiocytosis. The most common of these, canine cutaneous histiocytosis, is a benign epidermal neoplasm of Langerhans cell origin that usually regresses spontaneously. However, it may metastasize in some animals. Langerhans cell histiocytosis is a nonneoplastic reactive lesion whose trigger is unknown but may be an infectious agent. This condition is not premalignant, and it may occur in cutaneous or systemic forms. Both forms of Langerhans cell histiocytosis present with a lesion or lesions in the skin or subcutis, but systemic histiocytosis also involves other tissues. Cutaneous histiocytosis shows no breed predilection,

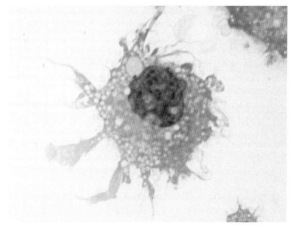

Fig. 11.11 A feline dendritic cell cultured in the presence of recombinant human interleukin-4 and granulocyte-macrophage colony-stimulating factor. Note the extensive dendrites so characteristic of these cells. Bright-field illumination ×100. From Sprague, W.S., Pope, M., Hoover, E.A., 2005. Culture and comparison of feline myeloid DCs vs macrophages. J. Comp. Pathol. 133, 139.

occurs in adult dogs between 3 and 9 years old, and is characterized by the development of nonpainful solitary or multiple nodules in the skin or subcutis. These lesions tend to occur on the head, neck, extremities, perineum, and scrotum. In contrast, systemic histiocytosis tends to occur in large breeds such as Bernese Mountain dogs, Rottweilers, Golden Retrievers, and Labradors. The age of onset is between 4 and 7 years. The lesions develop in the skin, mucous membranes, eyes, nasal cavity, spleen, lung, liver, bone marrow, and spinal cord. Histologically, these lesions are characterized as containing a mixture of cells. The cells express CD1, CD11c, MHC class II, CD4, and CD90, a phenotype typical of Langerhans cells (Kaim et al., 2006). The lesions also contain T cells and neutrophils and may be successfully treated with corticosteroids, cyclosporine, or leflunomide (see Chapter 42). As many as 30% of cutaneous cases and 10% of systemic cases spontaneously regress following infiltration by CD4+ T cells and the production of Th1 cytokines such as IL-2, TNF-α, and IFN-γ, as well as NOS2, and subsequent recruitment of antitumor effector cells.

Feline progressive histiocytosis is a skin disease presenting as solitary or multiple nonpruritic nodules on the feet, legs, and face. These histiocytes express CD1a, CD1c, CD18, and MHC class II molecules. About 10% of cases express E-cadherin, a characteristic of Langerhans cells. This is a slowly progressive disease that may involve internal organs in terminal cases (Faller et al., 2016).

REFERENCES

Auray, G., Facci, M.R., van Kessel, J., et al., 2010. Differential activation and maturation of two porcine DC populations following TLR ligand stimulation. Mol. Immunol. 47, 2103–2111.

Auray, G., Keller, I., Python, S., Gerber, M., et al., 2016. Characterization and transcriptomic analysis of porcine blood conventional and plasmacytoid dendritic cells reveals striking species-specific differences. J. Immunol. 197 (12), 4791–4806.

Bhoj, V.G., Chen, Z.J., 2009. Ubiquitylation in innate and adaptive immunity. Nature 458, 430–437.

Bourque, J., Hawiger, D., 2023. Life and death of tolerogenic dendritic cells. Trends Immunol. 44 (2), 110–118.

Calzada-Nova, G., Schnitzlein, W., Husmann, R., Zuckermann, F.A., 2010. Characterization of the cytokine and maturation responses of pure populations of porcine plasmacytoid DCs to porcine viruses and toll-like receptor agonists. Vet. Immunol. Immunopathol. 135, 20–33.

Chan, S.S., McConnell, I., Blacklaws, B.A., 2002. Generation and characterization of ovine DCs derived from peripheral blood monocytes. Immunology 107, 366–372.

de Jong, M.A., Geijtenbeek, T.B., 2010. Langerhans cells in innate defense against pathogens. Trends Immunol. 31 (12), 452–459.

Deshane, J., Chaplin, D.D., 2010. Follicular dendritic cell makes environmental sense. Immunity 33, 2–4.

Facci, M.R., Auray, G., Buchanan, R., et al., 2010. A comparison between isolated blood DCs and monocyte-derived DCs in pigs. Immunology 129, 396–405.

Faller, M., Lamm, C., Affolter, V.K., Valerius, K., Schwartz, S., Moore, P.F., 2016. Retrospective characterisation of solitary cutaneous histiocytoma with lymph node metastasis in eight dogs. J. Small Anim. Pract. 57 (10), 548–552.

Finley, D., Chen, X., Walters, K.J., 2016. Gates, channels, and switches: elements of the proteasome machine. Trends Biochem. Sci. 41 (1), 77–93.

Geissmann, F., Manz, M.G., Jung, S., et al., 2010. Development of monocytes, macrophages and DCs. Science 337, 656–661.

González-Cano, P., Arsic, N., Popowych, Y.I., Griebel, P.J., 2014. Two functionally distinct myeloid dendritic cell subpopulations are present in bovine blood. Dev. Comp. Immunol. 44, 378–388.

Heesters, B.A., Myers, R.C., Carroll, M.C., 2014. Follicular dendritic cells: dynamic antigen libraries. Nat. Rev. Immunol. 14 (7), 495–504.

Hodge, A.L., Baxter, A.A., Poon, I.K.H., 2022. Gift bags within the sentinel cells of the immune system: the diverse role of dendritic cell-derived extracellular vesicles. J. Leukoc. Biol. 111, 903–920.

Hume, D.A., 2008. Macrophages as APC and the dendritic cell myth. J. Immunol. 181, 5829–5835.

Johansson, E., Domeika, K., Berg, M., et al., 2003. Characterization of porcine monocyte-derived dendritic cells according to their cytokine profile. Vet. Immunol. Immunopathol. 91, 183–197.

Kaim, U., Moritz, A., Failing, K., Baumgärtner, W., 2006. The regression of a canine Langerhans cell tumour is associated with increased expression of IL-2, TNF-α, IFN-γ and iNOS mRNA. Immunology 118, 472–482.

Kushwah, R., Hu, J., 2011. Complexity of dendritic cell subsets and their function in the host immune system. Immunology 133 (4), 409–419.

Mair, K.H., Stadler, M., Saalmueller, A., Gerner, W., 2022. Porcine plasmacytoid dendritic cells are unique in their expression of a functional NKp46 receptor. Front. Immunol. https://doi.org/10.3389/fimmu.2022.822258.

Palucka, A.K., Banchereau, J., 2006. Langerhans cells: daughters of monocytes. Nat. Immunol. 7, 223–224.

Pishesha, N., Harmand, T.J., Ploegh, H.L., 2022. A guide to antigen processing and presentation. Nat. Rev. Immunol. 22, 751–764.

Qeska, V., Baumgartner, W., Beineke, A., 2013. Species-specific properties and translational aspects of canine DCs. Vet. Immunol. Immunopathol. 151, 181–192.

Reizis, B., 2019. Plasmacytoid dendritic cells: development, regulation and function. Immunity 50, 37–50.

Ricklin Gutzwiller, M.E., Moulin, H.R., Zurbriggen, A., et al., 2010. Comparative analysis of canine monocyte- and bone marrow-derived DCs. Vet. Res. 41, 40.

Sallusto, F., Lanzavecchia, A., 2010. Monocytes join the dendritic cell family. Cell 143 (3), 339–340.

Schuijs, M.J., Hammad, H., Lambrecht, B.N., 2019. Professional and "amateur" antigen-presenting cells in type 2 immunity. Trends Immunol. 40 (1), 22–34.

Seo, K.S., Park, J.Y., Davis, W.C., et al., 2009. Superantigen-mediated differentiation of bovine monocytes into DCs. J. Leuko. Biol. 85, 606–616.

Siedek, E., Little, S., Mayall, S., Edington, N., Hamblin, A., 1997. Isolation and characterization of equine dendritic cells. Vet. Immunol. Immunopathol. 60, 15–31.

Summerfield, A., Auray, G., Ricklin, M., 2014. Comparative dendritic cell biology of veterinary mammals. Ann. Rev. Anim. Biosci. https://doi.org/10.1146/annurev-animal-022114-111009.

Villar, J., Segura, E., 2020. The more, the merrier: DC3s join the human dendritic cell family. Immunity. https://doi.org/10.1016/j.immuni.2020.07.014.

Wei, X., Wang, S., Wang, S., Xie, X., et al., 2022. Structure and peptidomes of swine MHC class I with long peptides reveal the cross-species characteristics of the novel N-terminal extension presentation mode. J. Immunol. 208, 480–491.

Wojno, E.D.T., Hunter, C.A., Stumhofer, J.S., 2019. The immunobiology of the interleukin-12 family: room for discovery. Immunity 50, 851–870.

Yamakawa, Y., Pennelegion, C., Willcocks, S., et al., 2008. Identification and functional characterization of a bovine orthologue to DC-SIGN. J. Leuko. Biol. 83, 1396–1403.

Ziegler, A., Marti, E., Summerfield, A., Baumann, A., 2016. Identification and characterization of equine blood plasmacytoid dendritic cells. Dev. Comp. Immunol. 65, 352–357.

The Major Histocompatibility Complex

Resistance to infectious diseases is one of the most strongly inherited disease traits. After all, a lethal infection effectively removes susceptible individuals from the gene pool. "Survival of the fittest" applies most strongly to individuals who successfully defend themselves against infectious diseases. As a result, many genes influence resistance to infection. The most important of these genes are those encoding the cell-surface glycoproteins that constitute the major histocompatibility complex (MHC).

In order to trigger an adaptive immune response, antigen molecules must first be processed. They are broken up inside cells, and the resulting fragments are bound to appropriate antigen-presenting receptors (Fig. 12.1). These receptors are cell-surface glycoproteins encoded by genes clustered together to form the MHC. The receptors are therefore called MHC molecules. Antigens can only trigger an adaptive immune response after binding to MHC molecules. These MHC molecules present their attached antigens to T-cell antigen receptors, and if they are recognized, they trigger a response. Since MHC molecules act as antigen-presenting receptors, the genes encoding them effectively determine which antigens can be bound and so trigger adaptive immunity. Thus the MHC can be considered a cluster of those genes that control antigen presentation and so determine resistance or susceptibility to infectious diseases. The ability of pathogens to evade, escape, or subvert immune defenses has placed strong selection pressures on MHC genes and has resulted in their rapid evolution (Nei et al., 1997).

MAJOR HISTOCOMPATIBILITY COMPLEX

All mammals possess an MHC. Each MHC contains about 200 expressed genes divided into three regions (I, II, and III) (Fig. 12.2). The class I region contains genes coding for MHC molecules expressed on most nucleated cells. Class I genes can be subdivided into those that are highly polymorphic (class Ia genes) and those that show very little polymorphism (class Ib, Ic, or Id genes). (Polymorphism refers to structural variations between proteins.) Class Id genes are located outside the MHC on a different chromosome. The genes in MHC class II regions encode polymorphic MHC molecules, usually restricted to the professional antigen-presenting cells (dendritic cells, macrophages, and B cells) (Table 12.1). Genes within the MHC class III region encode diverse proteins, many of which are important in innate immunity

such as complement components. Although each MHC contains all three gene regions, their gene content and arrangement vary among species (Kumanovics et al., 2003).

The collective name given to the proteins encoded by MHC genes depends on the species. In humans, these molecules are called human leukocyte antigens (HLA); in dogs, they are called DLA; in rabbits, RLA; in cattle (bovines), BoLA; in horses, ELA; in swine, SLA; and so forth. In some species, MHC molecules were identified as transplantation antigens before their true function was recognized and their nomenclature is anomalous. Thus, in the mouse, the MHC is called H-2, and in chickens, it is called B. The complete set of alleles found within an individual animal's MHC is called its MHC haplotype.

While the human and mouse MHC class I genes exhibit extreme allelic polymorphism, this is not the case in all mammals. In other species, MHC diversity is generated by variations in the number of MHC class I genes expressed. If some MHC genes are expressed in some MHC haplotypes but not in others, the effect will be to generate even more diversity than alternative combinations of alleles of a fixed gene. Gene content variation and allelic polymorphism can therefore be considered as two alternative strategies to diversify MHC haplotypes. Nonhuman primates, rodents, horses, pigs, and ruminants all rely on variations in MHC gene content. In contrast, humans, mice, dogs, and cats have relatively few functional MHC class I genes and rely on allelic polymorphism.

MAJOR HISTOCOMPATIBILITY COMPLEX CLASS I MOLECULES

Class I molecules are expressed on most nucleated cells. In pigs, for example, class I molecules have been detected on lymphocytes, platelets, granulocytes, hepatocytes, kidney cells, and sperm. They are not usually found on mammalian red cells, gametes, neurons, or trophoblast cells. Some cells, such as myocardium and skeletal muscle, may express very few class Ia molecules. The function of these molecules is to present endogenous antigens, such as viral antigens, to T cells.

Structure

Class I molecules consist of paired glycoprotein chains. An α-chain (45 kDa) is associated with a much smaller chain called

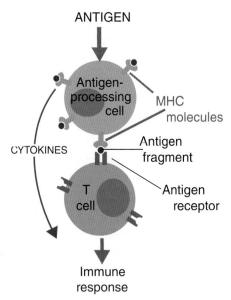

Fig. 12.1 The key initial step in any immune response is the presentation of antigens by antigen-processing cells to antigen-sensitive cells. This step is mediated by major histocompatibility complex (MHC) molecules located on the surface of antigen-processing cells. The complex is recognized by the T-cell antigen receptors.

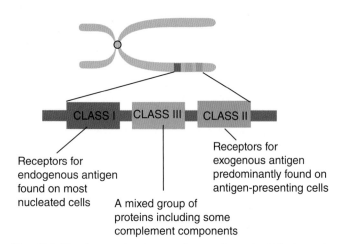

Fig. 12.2 The three major classes of genes located within the major histocompatibility complex are grouped together into three regions: their cell distribution and functions differ.

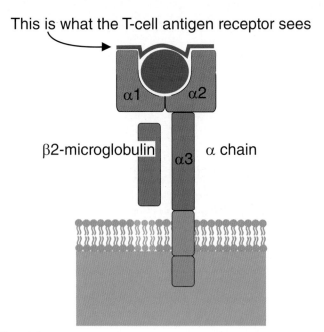

Fig. 12.3 The structure of a class Ia major histocompatibility complex. molecule on a cell membrane. Its antigen-binding site is formed by the folding of both its α_1 and α_2 domains. The β_2M serves to stabilize the structure.

ß$_2$-microglobulin (ß$_2$M) (12 kDa) (Fig. 12.3). The α-chain is inserted in the cell membrane. It consists of five domains: three extracellular domains called α_1, α_2, and α_3, each about 100 amino acids long; a transmembrane domain; and a cytoplasmic domain. The antigen-binding site is formed by the α_1 and α_2 domains. The β_2M chain consists of a single domain and serves to stabilize the structure.

Gene Arrangement

The size of the MHC class I gene region varies. Humans and rodents have the largest, and pigs have the smallest. Each MHC class I region has a common framework of non-MHC genes, and size differences are mainly due to variations in these framework genes. The number of class Ia genes also varies between mammals, ranging from rats with more than 60 to pigs with 11 and seven in dogs. Not all these genes are functional. In mice, only two or three class I genes are expressed. The remainder are pseudogenes (defective genes that cannot be expressed). In humans, the three functional polymorphic genes are called *A*, *B*, and *C*. In mice, they are called *K* and *D* (and, in some strains, *L*). In other mammals, they are usually numbered (Fig. 12.4).

Polymorphism

In mice and humans, the class Ia genes show extreme diversity. As a result, there are many variations in the amino acid sequences in the α_1 and α_2 domains of their encoded proteins. The most extreme polymorphism is restricted to three to four small regions within the α_1 and α_2 domains. In these "hypervariable" regions, two or three alternative amino acids can occur at each position. The other domains of MHC class Ia molecules have a constant structure with little sequence variation.

The α_1 and α_2 domains of MHC class I molecules fold together to form an open-ended groove. A flat ß sheet forms the floor of this groove, and its walls are formed by two α helices (Fig. 12.5). This groove can contain antigenic peptides that are 8–10 amino acids long. The variable sequences located along the walls of this groove determine its shape. The shape of the groove in turn determines which peptides can be bound and used to trigger immune responses (Hulpke and Tampe, 2013).

TABLE 12.1	**Comparison of Major Histocompatibility Complex Class I and Class I Structure**	
	Class I	Class II
Loci include	Typically A, B, and C	DP, DQ, and DR
Distribution	Most nucleated cells	B cells, macrophages, and dendritic cells
Function	Present antigen to cytotoxic T cells	Present antigen to T helper cells
Result	T cell–mediated toxicity	T cell–mediated help

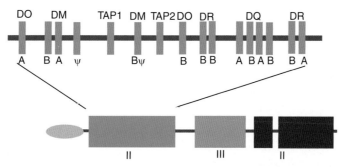

Fig. 12.4 Arrangement of the major loci within the major histocompatibility complex (MHC) of the horse—a typical mammalian MHC. The ELA class II region is provided in more detail. ψ denotes a pseudogene. A and B denote genes encoding α and β chains, respectively.

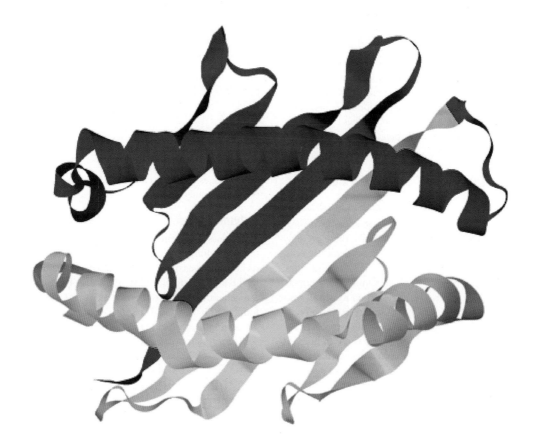

Fig. 12.5 A view (from above) of the antigen-binding groove on a major histocompatibility complex class I molecule. The floor of the groove is formed by an extensive β-pleated sheet. The walls of the groove are formed by two parallel α helices. This structure is formed by the folding of the α_1 (blue) and α_2 (yellow) domains of the α chain. Courtesy Dr. B. Breaux.

The amino acid polymorphism in the α_1 and α_2 domains results from variations in the nucleotide sequences between MHC alleles. These sequence variations result from point mutations, reciprocal recombination, and gene conversion. Point mutations are simply changes in individual nucleotides. Reciprocal recombination involves crossing over between two chromosomes. In gene conversion, small blocks of DNA are exchanged between different class I genes in a non-reciprocal fashion. The donated DNA blocks may come from nearby nonpolymorphic class I genes, from nonfunctional pseudogenes, or from other polymorphic class I genes. As a result of all this, class I

MHC genes have the highest mutation rate of any germline genes yet studied, 10^{-3} mutations per gene per generation in mice. This high mutation rate implies that there must be significant advantages to be gained by having very polymorphic MHC genes and diverse MHC antigen receptors.

Nonpolymorphic Major Histocompatibility Complex Class I Molecules

Mammalian cells also express many nonpolymorphic class I molecules. Some are encoded by genes found within the MHC class I region, others by genes located on other chromosomes. They are classified according to their evolutionary origin.

Class Ib molecules show reduced expression and tissue distribution compared to class Ia molecules but are part of the MHC complex. They have limited polymorphism, and they probably originated from class Ia precursors by duplication. For example, the class Ib genes in mice are found in three loci called *Q*, *T*, and *M*. They code for proteins on the surface of regulatory and immature lymphocytes and on hematopoietic cells. These also consist of a membrane-bound α-chain associated with β_2-microglobulin, so their overall shape and antigen-binding groove are similar to those in MHC class Ia molecules. Since they are not polymorphic, however, MHC class Ib molecules bind only a limited range of ligands. They act as pattern-recognition receptors for commonly encountered, microbial PAMPs (Birch et al., 2008a,b).

Class Ic genes also have limited polymorphism and are found within the MHC. Their products include MICA and MICB, specialized proteins that are involved in signaling to natural killer (NK) cells but do not bind antigenic peptides (see Chapter 20).

Class Id genes are nonpolymorphic class I-related genes not located on the MHC chromosome. Many of their products contribute to innate immunity since they bind PAMPs. For example, CD1 molecules are antigen-presenting receptors that bind lipid antigens (see Chapter 20). FcRn is a class Id MHC molecule that acts as an antibody (Fc) receptor on epithelial cells. It is expressed on the mammary gland epithelium and on the enterocytes of newborns (see Chapter 24).

MAJOR HISTOCOMPATIBILITY COMPLEX CLASS II MOLECULES

MHC class II molecules play a key role in the presentation of processed exogenous antigens to T cells. Thus, in rodents, these are only expressed on the professional antigen-presenting cells (dendritic cells, macrophages, and B cells) but can be induced on T cells, keratinocytes, and vascular endothelial cells. In pigs, dogs, cats, mink, and horses, MHC class II molecules are constitutively expressed on nearly all resting adult T cells. In cattle, MHC class II molecules are expressed only on B cells and activated T cells. In pigs, resting T cells express MHC class II molecules at about the same level as macrophages. In humans and pigs, MHC class II molecules are expressed on renal vascular endothelium and glomeruli—a fact of significance in kidney graft rejection. The expression of class II molecules is enhanced in rapidly dividing cells and in cells treated with IFN-γ (see Chapter 19).

Structure

MHC class II molecules consist of paired peptide chains called α and β. Each chain has two extracellular domains (one constant and one variable), a connecting peptide, a transmembrane domain, and a cytoplasmic domain (Fig. 12.6). A third chain, called the Ii or γ-chain, is associated with the assembly of class II molecules within cells and was discussed in Chapter 11.

Gene Arrangement

A "complete" MHC class II region contains three paired loci. In primates, these are called DPA and DPB, DQA and DQB, and DRA and DRB. (The genes for the α-chains are designated A, and the genes for the β-chains are called B.) Some of these genes are polymorphic. There may also be additional nonpolymorphic loci present such as DM and DO in humans. The DM and DO gene products regulate the loading of antigen fragments into the MHC groove. Not all mammals possess a complete set of class II genes since nonprimates lack DPA and DPB. Not all loci contain genes for both chains, and some contain many

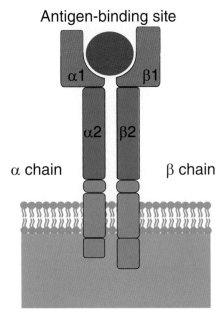

Fig. 12.6 Diagram showing the structure of a major histocompatibility complex class II antigen located on a cell surface. Note that the antigen-binding site is formed by the variable domains from both peptide chains.

pseudogenes. These pseudogenes can serve as DNA donors that may be used to generate class II polymorphism by gene conversion.

Polymorphism

MHC class II proteins have an antigen-binding groove formed by their α_1 and β_1 domains. Its walls are formed by two parallel α-helices, and its floor consists of a β-sheet. Gene polymorphism results in variations in the amino acids forming the walls of the groove. These variations are generated in the same way as in class Ia molecules. Other genes found within the class II region code for molecules involved in antigen processing. These include the transporter proteins TAP1 and TAP2 and some proteasome components.

MAJOR HISTOCOMPATIBILITY COMPLEX CLASS III MOLECULES

Most of the remaining genes located within the MHC are found in the class III region. This is usually located centrally between the class I and II regions.

The MHC class III is the most gene-dense region within the human genome with 62 genes containing more than 500 exons over 706 kb and one gene per 11387 bp. These genes code for proteins with diverse functions. Some are important in the defense of the body such as the genes encoding the complement components C4, factor B (*FB*), and C2 (Fig. 12.7). They also include genes that encode tumor necrosis factor–α (TNF-α), several lymphotoxins, and some NK cell receptors. Thus, one subregion contains several cytokine genes, such as lymphotoxin-beta LTB and TNF-α, as well as regulatory genes, such as IFN-β. This subregion has been referred to as the Class IV region or the "Inflammatory region." This cluster is highly conserved between species. Comparative analysis suggests that the genes in this cluster have remained together for over 450 million years and predate the emergence of mammals (Deakin et al., 2006). The class III genes are unrelated to either MHC class I or II or even often to each other.

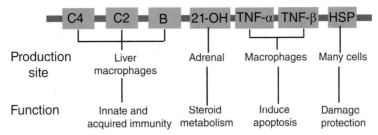

Fig. 12.7 The arrangement of selected genes within the major histocompatibility complex class III region. These genes all play a role in innate and adaptive immunity. There are many other genes within this region that have no apparent role in immunity. *TNF*, Tumor necrosis factor.

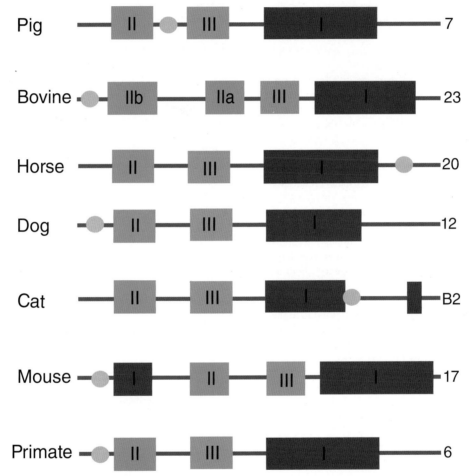

Fig. 12.8 The arrangement of gene regions within the major histocompatibility complex in different domestic mammal species. The yellow circle denotes the location of the centromere. The number denotes the chromosome location.

MAJOR HISTOCOMPATIBILITY COMPLEX OF DOMESTIC ANIMALS

Every mammalian MHC contains class I, class II, and class III regions. When the MHCs of different mammals are compared, some regions such as class III are conserved, whereas others are highly diverse. Likewise, the precise arrangement and number of loci vary among species (Fig. 12.8). In general, genes within the class II and class III regions possess obvious orthologs in all species. That is, they are clearly derived from a single ancestor and have not been subjected to major rearrangements during evolution. Class I genes, in contrast, have evolved so

frequently and been reorganized so many different times by deletion and duplication that their amino acid sequences differ widely, and it is very difficult to compare class I genes between different species. They are said to be paralogous.

Equine: The equine MHC, designated ELA, is located on chromosome 20. Fifteen different MHC class I genes have been identified in the horse class I region. Of these, seven appear to be functional (Janova et al., 2009). The equine class II region is about 1.2 mb in size. It contains 35 gene loci (Barbis et al., 1994).

Bovine: The bovine MHC has been mapped to autosome 23 and is collectively termed the BoLA (Bovine leukocyte antigen) system (Birch et al., 2008a,b). The MHC class 1 molecules are expressed on all nucleated cells. MHC class II molecules are also heterodimers with an alpha chain of 33 kDa linked to a beta chain of 28 kDa. In general, class II MHC molecules are only expressed on professional antigen-presenting cells in this species. MHC class III molecules, as in other mammals, are a diverse mixture of molecules connected in some way with adaptive or innate immune functions (Amills et al., 1998). The MHC of the sheep (OLA) has also been well characterized (Deverson et al., 1991; Dukkipati et al., 2006)

The ruminant MHC class II region is unique in that it is split into two subregions (IIa and IIb) from *DOB* in the class IIb region to *DQB* in the class IIa region. They are separated by a spacer sequence of 15 cM. This splitting of the class II region probably resulted from a chromosomal inversion early in ruminant evolution. The class IIb region is close to the centromere, while the class I region is telomeric to the class IIa genes. This class II inversion is found not only in cattle but also in the MHC of other ruminants such as sheep, goats, antelope, and deer (Ballingall et al., 2008; Gao et al., 2010).

Pigs: The MHC of the pig (SLA) spans about 2.4 mb on chromosome 7. At least 150 MHC genes have been characterized (Ho et al., 2009, 2010). It differs from other mammals in that its class II region is separated from the class I and class III regions by the presence of the centromere (Lunney et al., 2009). Thus the class II region is located on the q arm, while the telomeric class I and the centromeric class III regions are located on the p arm of the chromosome. This is an unusual example of the loss of the tight linkage that is usually present between MHC regions (Charon et al., 1999).

Dogs: The canine MHC is classified as the DLA—Dog Leukocyte Antigen complex. The entire canine MHC spans 3.9 mb compared to 4.6 in humans and 3.3 mb in cats. As in other mammals it is arranged in the order, class II-class III-class I in the pericentromeric region of chromosome 12. However, a small number of MHC genes (about 500 bp) are also located on chromosome 35. A similar situation is seen in cats where most of their MHC is located on the long arm of chromosome B2, but a small fragment has been inverted and so is found in the subtelomeric region of the short arm of the same chromosome. The break has occurred in the same location in cats and dogs, between *TRIM 39* and *TRIM 26*. Two additional class I genes are also located on canine chromosomes 7 and 18 (Wagner et al., 2002; Kennedy et al., 2002).

Cats: The feline MHC complex (FLA) is similar to that of other mammals and the three gene classes are arranged in the usual order I, III, II on chromosome B2 (Holmes et al., 2013).

MAJOR HISTOCOMPATIBILITY COMPLEX MOLECULES AND DISEASE

Since the function of MHC molecules is to present antigens to the cells of the immune system, MHC genes regulate immune responses. A foreign molecule that cannot be bound to at least one MHC molecule cannot trigger an adaptive immune response (Fig. 12.9). Thus, the expression of specific MHC alleles determines resistance to many infectious and autoimmune diseases. Because class Ia and class II MHC molecules are structurally diverse, each MHC allele can bind and present a different set of antigenic peptides. The more diversity within an animal's MHC, the more antigens it can respond to. Thus, an MHC-heterozygous animal will express many more alleles and can respond to a greater diversity of antigens than a homozygous animal (Fig. 12.10; Radwan et al., 2020).

MHC polymorphism is maintained in populations by a process called overdominant selection or heterozygote advantage. Simply put, MHC heterozygotes have a survival advantage because they can respond to a greater diversity of microbial antigens and so are best fitted to resist

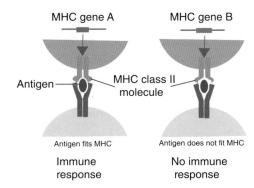

Fig. 12.9 Major histocompatibility complex (MHC) molecules regulate the immune response. Only antigen fragments that can bind in the groove of an MHC molecule will trigger an immune response. This is called MHC restriction. Thus the genes that code for these MHC molecules will also determine immune responsiveness.

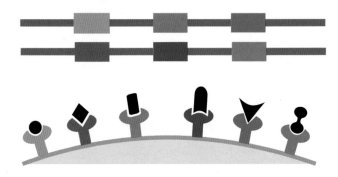

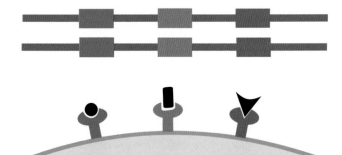

Fig. 12.10 Heterozygous animals with two different major histocompatibility complex (MHC) alleles coded for at each locus express six different antigen-presenting molecules on the cell surface. Therefore they generate more diverse and effective immune responses than homozygous animals with only one MHC a single allele coded for at each locus. An example of heterozygote advantage.

infectious diseases. The antigen-binding sites of MHC class Ia or II molecules are also very nonspecific, and it has been estimated that an average MHC molecule can bind about 2500 different peptides. This is because the MHC groove binds to the peptide backbone rather than to its amino acid side chains. Nevertheless, structural constraints limit the efficiency of binding of each allele. As a result, it is likely that only one or two peptides from an average antigenic protein can bind to any given MHC molecule. The ability of MHC molecules to bind antigens is therefore a limiting factor in generating adaptive immunity and resistance to infectious agents. Increasing the diversity of MHC molecules increases the diversity of antigens that can be bound and so increases resistance to infectious diseases. Because most individuals are MHC heterozygotes, each individual normally expresses, at most, six different class Ia molecules (in humans, for example, two each are coded for by the HLA-A, -B, and C loci). The number of expressed MHC molecules is not greater because that would increase the risk that the MHC molecules could bind and present more self-antigens. This would require the elimination of many more self-reactive T cells during development (see Chapter 21). Thus the presence of six different MHC class Ia molecules appears to be a reasonable compromise between maximizing the recognition of foreign antigens while at the same time minimizing the chances of recognizing self-antigens, at least in humans (Fig. 12.11).

MHC class Ia loci can encode very polymorphic genes. For example, the H-2K locus in the mouse codes for more than 100 alleles. Since there can never be more than two alleles per locus in any individual animal, it appears that this number of alleles has evolved to maximize polymorphism in the mouse population. This may protect the population as a whole from complete destruction. Because of MHC polymorphism, most individuals in a population carry a unique set of class Ia alleles, and each individual can therefore respond to a unique mixture of antigens. When a new infectious disease strikes a population, it is likely that at least some individuals will possess MHC molecules that can bind the new antigens and trigger immunity. Those that can respond will mount an immune response and live. Those that lack these molecules cannot respond and will die.

When large populations of humans or mice are examined, no single MHC haplotype predominates. In other words, no single MHC haplotype confers major survival advantages on individual animals. This reflects the futility of the host attempting to bind all the antigens in a population of invading microorganisms. Microbes will always be able to mutate and evade the immune response faster than we mammals can develop resistance. Any changes in an MHC allele may increase resistance to one organism but at the same time decrease resistance to another. It is therefore more advantageous for the members of a population to possess many highly diverse MHC alleles so that any pathogen spreading through a population will have to adapt anew to each individual.

Highly adaptable social animals, such as humans or mice, with large populations through which disease can spread rapidly, usually show extensive MHC polymorphism (Fig. 12.12). In contrast, low-density solitary species such as marine mammals (whales and elephant seals), moose, or Tasmanian devils have much less polymorphism. It is also of interest to note the case of the cheetah, where some wild populations have reduced MHC class II polymorphism as a result of recent population bottlenecks. Because of this low MHC diversity, some cheetahs will accept allografts from other, unrelated cheetahs. Likewise, an infectious disease such as feline infectious peritonitis causes 60% mortality in captive cheetahs compared with 1%–2% mortality in domestic cats. However, there is little evidence to suggest that wild cheetah populations have reduced immune competence (Castro-Prieto et al., 2011).

There are many examples of links between MHC haplotype and resistance to infectious disease (Berry et al., 2011). For example, in cattle there is an association between possession of certain BoLA alleles and resistance to bovine leukosis, squamous cell eye carcinoma, trypanosomiasis; responsiveness to foot-and-mouth disease virus; and susceptibility to the tick *Rhipicephalus microplus* (Baxter et al., 2009). In sheep, there is an association of the class I allele SY1 with resistance to *Trichostrongylus colubriformis*. Resistance to scrapie and caseous lymphadenitis is also associated with certain MHC class I alleles. In goats, the class I allele Be7 is associated with resistance, and Be1 and Be14 are associated with susceptibility, to caprine arthritis-encephalitis. In horses, an allergic response to the bites of *Culicoides* midges is linked to ELA-Aw7. In pigs, the SLA complex also affects major reproduction parameters such as ovulation rate, litter size, and piglet viability.

Selection for specific MHC haplotypes has potential for use in developing disease-resistant strains of domestic animals. However, it must be pointed out that by selecting for a specific gene locus, one may also inadvertently select for susceptibility at closely linked loci. This may outweigh the benefits of a resistant allele at one locus. An animal cannot be resistant to all possible infectious diseases (Rastislav et al., 1997).

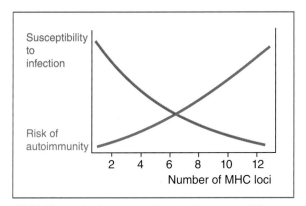

Fig. 12.11 The optimal number of major histocompatibility complex (MHC) loci is a balance between the need to respond to as many different microbial antigens as possible and the need to avoid autoimmune responses. Computer modeling suggests that the optimal number of MHC loci in humans is six.

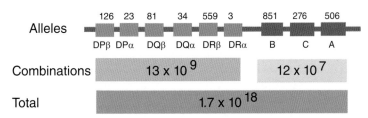

Fig. 12.12 An example of how major histocompatibility complex (MHC) polymorphism can generate an enormous number of different MHC haplotypes. The numbers above each locus are the number of identified alleles in the human MHC. The number of different combinations can be determined by multiplying all of them together. Thus there are 13×10^9 class II combinations, 12×10^7 class I combinations, and 1.7×10^{18} total possible combinations; more than sufficient to give every human a unique haplotype.

Berry, D.P., Bermingham, M.L., Good, M., More, S.J., 2011. Genetics of animal health and disease in cattle. Irish Vet. J. 64 (1), 5.

Birch, J., Codner, G., Guzman, E., Ellis, S.A., 2008a. Genomic location and characterization of nonclassical MHC class I genes in cattle. Immunogenetics 60, 267–273.

Birch, J., Sanjuan, C.D.J., Guzman, E., Ellis, S.A., 2008b. Genomic localization and characterization of MIC genes in cattle. Immunogenetics 60, 477–483.

Castro-Prieto, A., Wachter, B., Sommer, S., 2011. Cheetah paradigm revisited: MHC diversity in the world's largest free-ranging population. Mol. Biol. Evol. 28 (4), 1455–1468.

Charon, P., Renard, C., Vaiman, M., 1999. The major histocompatibility complex in swine. Immunol. Rev. 167, 179–192.

Deakin, J.E., Papenfuss, A.T., Belov, K., Cross, J.C.R., et al., 2006. Evolution and comparative analysis of the MHC class III inflammatory region. BMC Genomics. https://doi.org/10.1186/1471-2164/7/281.

Deverson, E.V., Wright, H., Watson, S., et al., 1991. Class II major histocompatibility complex genes of the sheep. Anim. Genet. 22, 211–225.

Dukkipati, V.S.R., Blair, H.T., Garrick, D.J., Murray, A., 2006. "Ovar-MHC"—ovine major histocompatibility complex: structure and gene polymorphisms. Gen. Mol. Res. 5, 581–608.

Fan, W., Liu, Y.C., Parimoo, S., Weissman, S.M., 1995. Olfactory receptor-like genes are located in the human major histocompatibility complex. Genomics 27 (1), 119–123.

Gao, J., Liu, K., Blair, H.T., Li, G., et al., 2010. A complete DNA sequence map of the ovine Major Histocompatibility Complex. BMC Genomics 11, 466.

Ho, C.S., Lunney, J.K., Franzo-Romain, M.H., et al., 2009. Molecular characterization of swine leucocyte antigen class I genes in outbred pig populations. Anim. Genet. 4, 468–478.

Ho, C.S., Lunney, J.K., Lee, J.H., et al., 2010. Molecular characterization of swine leucocyte antigen class II genes in outbred pig populations. Anim. Genet. 41, 428–432.

Holmes, J.C., Holmer, S.G., Ross, P., et al., 2013. Polymorphisms and tissue expression of the feline leukocyte antigen class I loci FLAI-E, FLAI-H, and FLAI-K. Immunogenetics 65, 675–689.

Hulpke, S., Tampe, R., 2013. The MHC I loading complex: a multitasking machinery in adaptive immunity. Trends Biochem. Sci. 38 (8), 412–420.

Janova, E., Matiasovic, J., Vahala, J., et al., 2009. Polymorphism and selection in the major histocompatibility complex DRA and DQA genes in the family Equidae. Immunogenetics 61, 513–527.

Kennedy, L.J., Barnes, A., Happ, G.M., et al., 2002. Extensive interbreed, but minimal intrabreed, variation of DLA class II alleles and haplotypes in dogs. Tissue Antigens 59, 194–199.

Kumanovics, A., Takada, T., Fischer Lindahl, K., 2003. Genomic organization of the mammalian MHC. Annu. Rev. Immunol. 21, 629–657.

Leinders-Zufall, T., Brennan, P., Widmayer, P., et al., 2004. MHC class I peptides as chemosensory signals in the vomeronasal organ. Science 306, 1033–1037.

Lunney, J.K., Ho, C.-S., Wysocki, M., Smith, D.M., 2009. Molecular genetics of the swine major histocompatibility complex, the SLA complex. Dev. Comp. Immunol. 33, 362–374.

Nei, M., Gu, X., Sitnikova, T., 1997. Evolution by the birth-and-death process in multigene families of the vertebrate immune system. Proc. Natl. Acad. Sci. U.S.A. 94, 7799–7806.

Radwan, J., Babik, W., Kaufman, J., Lenz, T.L., Winternitz, J., 2020. Advances in the evolutionary understanding of MHC polymorphism. Trends Genet. 36, 298–311.

Rastislav, M., Mangesh, B., 1997. BoLA-DRB3 exon 2 mutations associated with paratuberculosis in cattle. Vet. J. 192 (3), 517–519. 2012.

Santos, P.S.C., Mezger, M., Kolar, M., Michler, F.-U., Sommer, S., 2018. The best smellers make the best choosers: mate choice is affected by female chemosensory receptor gene diversity in a mammal. Proc. Roy. Soc. B. https://doi.org/10.1098/rspb.2018.2426.

Tizard, I.R., Skow, L., 2021. The olfactory system: the remote sensing arm of the immune system. Anim. Hlth. Res. Revs. https://doi.org/10.1017/s1466252320000262.

Wagner, J.L., Sarmiento, U.M., Storb, R., 2002. Cellular, serological, and molecular polymorphism of the class I and class II loci of the canine major histocompatibility complex. Tissue Antigens 59, 205–210.

> ## BOX 12.1   Major Histocompatibility Complex (MHC) and Sperm Counts in Horses
>
> The MHC haplotype is closely linked to body odors. Mate choice appears to be determined in some species by odor. For example, twelve stallions were exposed to an MHC-similar mare and then to an MHC-dissimilar mare or vice versa for four weeks. Blood testosterone levels were determined weekly. Ejaculates were collected at the end of the experiment. Testosterone levels were higher in the stallions exposed to the MHC-dissimilar mare than to the MHC-similar mare. Sperm numbers were correlated with mean testosterone levels and were higher if MHC-dissimilar mares were presented last than if MHC-similar mares were presented last. Thus MHC-linked olfactory signals influence testosterone levels and sperm counts.
>
> From Burger, D., Dolivo, G., Marti, E., Sieme, H., Wedekind, C., 2015. Female major histocompatibility complex type affects male testosterone levels and sperm number in the horse (*Equus caballus*). Proc. R Soc. B. 282, 20150407.

MAJOR HISTOCOMPATIBILITY COMPLEX AND BODY ODORS

Mammals use odors to detect information about another individual's gender, status, and health (Tizard and Skow, 2021). The molecules that carry this information are small, volatile peptides found in urine. These peptides can bind to the antigen-binding grooves of MHC class I molecules. Thus, peptides known to bind to two mouse MHC class I molecules of different haplotypes have been shown to induce responses (field potentials) in mouse vomeronasal organs. The responses were not haplotype-specific, but different peptides induced different activation patterns. This finding may well explain how mammals such as mice can recognize the MHC of other mice by smell (Leinders-Zufall et al., 2004).

The class I region of humans, mice, cattle, and pigs contains numerous genes coding for pheromone olfactory receptors (Fan et al., 1995). As a result, the MHC haplotype affects the recognition of peptide ligands, causing individual odors in an allele-specific fashion, and thus influences the mating preferences of mammals. Thus, under controlled conditions, mice prefer to mate with MHC-incompatible individuals. Such matings preferentially generate heterozygote advantage, resulting in optimized disease resistance (Box 12.1). However, this type of mating could also prevent genome-wide inbreeding. Inbreeding avoidance may be the most important function of MHC-based mating preferences and therefore the fundamental selective force diversifying MHC genes in species with such mating patterns. Despite not having a vomeronasal organ, humans also have the ability to sense MHC peptides in body odor, and this may influence human mate choice (Santos et al., 2018).

REFERENCES

Amills, M., Ramiya, V., Norimine, J., Lewin, H.A., 1998. The major histocompatibility complex of ruminants. Rev. Sci. Tech. Off. Int. Epiz. 17, 108–120.

Ballingall, K.T., Miltiadou, D., Chai, Z.W., et al., 2008. Genetic and proteomic analysis of the MHC class I repertoire from four ovine haplotypes. Immunogenetics 60, 177–184.

Barbis, D.P., Bainbridge, D., Crump, A.L., Zhang, C.H., et al., 1994. Variation in expression of MHC class II antigens on horse lymphocytes determined by MHC haplotype. Vet. Immunol. Immunopathol. 42 (1), 103–114.

Baxter, R., Craigmile, S.C., Haley, C., et al., 2009. BoLA-DR peptide binding pockets are fundamental for foot-and-mouth disease virus vaccine design in cattle. Vaccine 28, 28–37.

Lymphoid Organs: Their Structure and Functions

Although antigens are trapped and processed by dendritic cells, macrophages, and B cells, adaptive immune responses are actually mounted by cells called lymphocytes. Lymphocytes are the small, unspectacular round cells that predominate in organs such as the spleen, lymph nodes, and thymus (Fig. 13.1). These are called lymphoid organs. Lymphocytes have antigen receptors on their surface and so can recognize and respond to foreign antigens. Lymphocytes are eventually responsible for the production of antibodies and for cell-mediated immune responses. The lymphoid organs must therefore provide an environment for efficient interaction among lymphocytes, antigen-presenting cells, and foreign antigens as well as sites where lymphocytes can respond optimally to processed antigens.

Immune responses must be carefully controlled. Lymphocytes must be selected so that their receptors will only bind foreign antigens, and the response of each lymphocyte must be regulated so that it is sufficient but not excessive for the body's requirements. The lymphoid organs may therefore be classified on the basis of their roles in generating lymphocytes, regulating the production of lymphocytes, and providing an environment for trapping foreign antigens, processing them, and maximizing the opportunity for lymphocytes to encounter and interact with these foreign antigens (Fig. 13.2).

SOURCES OF LYMPHOCYTES

Lymphoid stem cells first appear in the fetal omentum, liver, and yolk sac. In older fetuses and adults, these stem cells move to the bone marrow. The bone marrow has multiple functions in adult mammals. It is a hematopoietic organ containing the precursors of all blood cells, including lymphocytes. In some mammals, such as primates, it is also a primary lymphoid organ (a site where newly produced lymphocytes can mature). Like the spleen, liver, and lymph nodes, the bone marrow is also a secondary lymphoid organ. It contains many dendritic cells and macrophages and thus removes foreign material from the blood. It contains large numbers of antibody-producing cells and is therefore a major source of antibodies. Because of these multiple functions, the bone marrow is divided into hematopoietic and vascular compartments. These compartments alternate, in wedge-shaped areas within long bones. The hematopoietic compartments contain stem cells for all the blood cells as well as macrophages, dendritic cells, and lymphocytes and are enclosed by a layer of adventitial cells. In older animals, these adventitial cells may become so loaded with fat that the marrow may have a fatty yellow appearance. The vascular compartments, where antigens are mainly trapped, consist of blood sinuses lined by endothelial cells and crossed by a network of reticular cells and macrophages.

PRIMARY LYMPHOID ORGANS

The organs where lymphocytes first develop are called the primary lymphoid organs. Lymphocytes fall into two major populations called T cells and B cells, based on the primary organ in which they mature. Thus, all T cells mature in the thymus, but B cells, in contrast, mature within different organs depending on species. These include the bursa of Fabricius in birds, the bone marrow in primates and rodents, and the intestinal lymphoid tissues in rabbits, ruminants, and pigs. These primary lymphoid organs all develop early in fetal life. As animals develop, newly produced, immature lymphocytes migrate from the bone marrow to the primary lymphoid organs where they complete their development (Table 13.1).

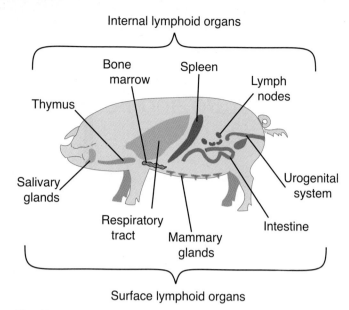

Fig. 13.1 The major lymphoid tissues of the pig, a typical mammal.

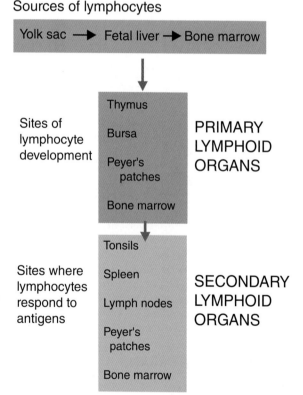

Fig. 13.2 The lymphoid organs can conveniently be divided into three groups based on their role in the origin, development, and functioning of lymphocyte populations.

TABLE 13.1 Comparison of Primary and Secondary Lymphoid Organs

	Primary	Secondary
Origin	Ectoendodermal junction or endoderm	Mesoderm
Time of development	Early in embryonic life	Late in fetal life
Persistence	Involutes after puberty	Persists in adults
Effect of removal	Loss of lymphocytes	No or minor effects
Response to antigen	Unresponsive	Fully reactive
Examples	Thymus, bursa, some Peyer's patches	Spleen, lymph nodes

thyroid gland. The thymus in pigs is also located in the thorax above the pericardium, but it too extends to the thoracic inlet. The two lobes, however, extend into the cervical region along the carotid artery to the pharynx—a cervical thymus (Sisson and Grossman, 1953). The size of the thymus varies, its relative size being greatest in the newborn animal and its absolute size being greatest before puberty. It may be very small and difficult to find in adult animals.

Structure

The thymus consists of lobules of loosely packed epithelial cells, each covered by a connective tissue capsule. The outer part of each lobule, the cortex, is densely infiltrated with lymphocytes (or thymocytes), but the inner medulla contains fewer lymphocytes, and the epithelial cells are clearly visible (Fig. 13.3). Within the medulla are also found round, layered bodies called Hassall's corpuscles (Fig. 13.4). These contain keratin, and the remains of a small blood vessel may be found at their center. In cattle these corpuscles may also contain immunoglobulin A (see Chapter 17). An abnormally thick basement membrane and a continuous layer of epithelial cells surround the capillaries that supply the thymic cortex. This barrier prevents circulating foreign antigens from entering the cortex. No lymphatic vessels leave the thymus. As an animal ages, the thymus shrinks and is gradually replaced by fat. However, the aged thymus still contains small amounts of lymphoid tissue and remains functionally active (Pierce, 2006).

Function

The functions of the thymus are best demonstrated by studying the effects of its removal in rodents of different ages. For example, thymectomized neonatal mice become susceptible to infections and fail to grow. These animals have very few circulating lymphocytes and cannot reject foreign organ grafts because they lose the ability to mount cell-mediated immune responses (Table 13.2). In contrast, thymectomy has no immediate obvious effect on adult mice. But if thymectomized adult mice are monitored for several months, their blood lymphocyte numbers and their ability to mount cell-mediated immune responses gradually decline. This suggests that the thymus remains functional in adults, but there is a reservoir of long-lived thymus-derived cells that must be exhausted before the effects of adult thymectomy become apparent (Cunningham et al., 2001).

The results of thymectomy indicate that the neonatal thymus is the source of most blood lymphocytes and that these lymphocytes are mainly responsible for mounting cell-mediated immune responses. They are called thymus-derived lymphocytes or T cells. T-cell precursors originate in the bone marrow but then enter the thymus. Once

Thymus

The thymus is located within the thoracic cavity in front of and below the heart. Large mammals such as humans, other primates, and dogs have a bilobed thymus located within the anterior thoracic cavity. In smaller mammals such as rats, there may be an extension of one or both lobes out of the thoracic cavity into the cervical region. In horses, cattle, sheep, pigs, and chickens, it also extends up the neck as far as the

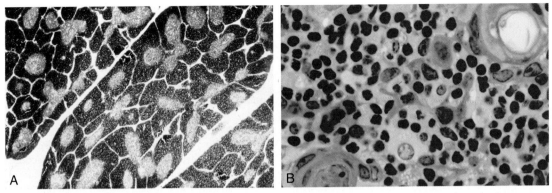

Fig. 13.3 (A) A section of a monkey thymus. Each lobule is divided into a cortex rich in lymphocytes, hence staining darkly, and a paler medulla consisting mainly of epithelial cells. Original magnification ×10. (B) A high-power view of the medulla of a monkey thymus showing several pale-staining epithelial cells with cytoplasmic processes and many dark-staining, round lymphocytes. Original magnification ×1000.

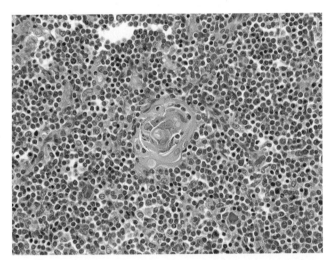

Fig. 13.4 A Hassall's corpuscle in the thymus of a 2-month-old puppy. Original magnification ×40. Courtesy Dr. Brian Porter.

TABLE 13.2 Effects of Neonatal Thymectomy and Bursectomy

Function	Thymectomy	Bursectomy
Numbers of circulating lymphocytes	Disappear	No effect
Presence of lymphocytes in T-dependent areas	Disappear	No effect
Graft rejection	Suppressed	No effect
Presence of lymphocytes in T-independent areas	Minor depletion	Disappear
Plasma cells in lymphoid tissues	Minor drop	Disappear
Serum immunoglobulins	Minor drop	Major drop
Antibody formation	Minor effects	Major drop

within the thymus, the cells (called thymocytes) divide rapidly. Of the new cells produced, most die by apoptosis, whereas the survivors (about 5% of the total in rodents and about 25% in calves) remain in the thymus for 4–5 days before leaving and colonizing the secondary lymphoid organs.

T cells that enter the thymus have two conflicting tasks. They must recognize foreign antigens but at the same time must not respond strongly to normal body constituents (self-antigens). A two-stage selection process in the thymic medulla accomplishes this feat. Thus, thymocytes with receptors that bind self-antigens strongly and that could therefore cause autoimmunity are killed by apoptosis. Thymocytes with receptors that cannot bind any major histocompatibility complex (MHC) class II molecules and thus cannot react to any processed antigen are also killed.

On the other hand, those thymocytes that survive this "negative selection" process but can still recognize specific MHC class II-antigen complexes with moderate affinity are stimulated to grow—a process called positive selection. These surviving cells eventually leave the thymus as mature T cells, circulate, and colonize the secondary lymphoid organs.

Thymic epithelial cells are unusual since they express more than 1900 antigens normally expressed in other tissues. In addition, these cells have a very high level of autophagy. As a result, their intracellular antigens are bound to MHC class II molecules and expressed in large amounts on the epithelial cell surfaces. This "promiscuous" antigen presentation ensures that developing thymocytes encounter a diverse array of normal tissue antigens. Since T cells with receptors that bind and respond to these antigens are killed, the system ensures that those T cells leaving the thymus lack receptors for most self-antigens and, as a result, cannot respond to normal body components.

Thymic Hormones

Within the thymus, cells are regulated by a complex mixture of cytokines and small peptides collectively known as thymic hormones. These include peptides variously called thymosins, thymopoietins, thymic humoral factor, thymulin, and the thymostimulins. Thymulin is especially interesting because it is a zinc-containing peptide secreted by the thymic epithelial cells, and it can partially restore T-cell function in thymectomized animals. Zinc is an essential mineral for the development of T cells. Consequently, zinc-deficient animals have defective cell-mediated immune responses (see Chapter 41). Hassall's corpuscles play a functional role in regulating thymic activity since they produce a growth factor called thymic stromal lymphopoietin (TSLP) (see Chapter 30). TSLP activates thymic dendritic cells that can stimulate regulatory T cells and so control the positive selection process (Wang et al., 2018).

Thymic Involution

The thymus shrinks with age. While thymic involution is associated with increasing age, it is not really a form of immunosenescence. Thus, in many mammals including dogs and humans involution may commence by one year. During the neonatal period, however, the thymus increases in absolute size as it supplies the developing animal with a fresh, carefully selected, supply of new T cells. In humans, the thymus epithelial space starts decreasing from the first year of life at a rate of 3% annually until around age 40. Thereafter, it decreases by about 1% annually until death (Steinmann et al., 1985). The thymus of humans over 40 cannot rebuild a new T-cell compartment. As a result of this involution, naive T-cell output drops steadily, and by around age 65. there is a marked drop in T-cell diversity. Acute involution can also be induced in animals by stresses including malnutrition and infectious diseases. Involution during pregnancy is associated with progesterone-mediated downregulation of chemokine production (Laan et al., 2016). The thymus also decreases in size in hibernating mammals.

The aging of the thymus is readily observed in larger mammals. By age 30 the human thymus mainly consists of adipose and connective tissues. The functional thymic tissue shrinks to be replaced by adipocytes, stromal cells, epithelial cords, and tubules, especially in the medulla. In most species, this involution becomes most apparent at the onset of sexual maturity and is presumably driven at this stage by hormonal influences. As the thymic lymphocytes undergo apoptosis, phagocytic cells remove the cell debris, and increased numbers of macrophages invade the structure (Haley, 2017). There are some species differences in this process so that, in dogs there is a great diversity of thymic sizes and weights. Likewise, nonhuman primates vary greatly depending on if they are wild-caught (stressed) or bred in captivity. Other age-related changes include cystic dilation of Hassall's corpuscles and the accumulation of cellular debris. The process is progressive and inexorable (Haley, 2017).

Bursa of Fabricius

The bursa of Fabricius is found only in birds. It is a round sac located just above the cloaca (Fig. 13.5). Like the thymus, the bursa reaches its greatest size in the chick about 1–2 weeks after hatching and then shrinks as the bird ages. It is difficult to identify in older birds.

Structure

Like the thymus, the bursa consists of lymphocytes embedded in epithelial tissue. The epithelial tissue lines a hollow sac connected to the cloaca by a duct. Inside the sac, folds of epithelium extend into the lumen, and scattered through the folds are round lymphoid follicles (Fig. 13.6). Each follicle is divided into a cortex and a medulla. The cortex contains lymphocytes, plasma cells, and macrophages. At the corticomedullary junction, there is a basement membrane and capillary network on the inside of which are epithelial cells. These medullary epithelial cells are replaced by lymphoblasts and lymphocytes in the center of the follicle. Specialized neuroendocrine dendritic cells of unknown function surround each follicle.

Function

The bursa may be removed either surgically or by infecting newborn chicks with a virus that destroys the bursa (infectious bursal disease virus). Since the bursa shrinks when chicks become sexually mature, bursal atrophy can also be provoked by administration of testosterone. Bursectomized birds have very low levels of antibodies in their blood, and antibody-producing cells disappear from lymphoid organs. However, they still possess circulating T cells and can reject foreign skin grafts. Thus bursectomy has little effect on the cell-mediated immune response. Bursectomized birds are more susceptible than normal to leptospirosis and salmonellosis but not to intracellular bacteria such as *Mycobacterium avium* (Ekino et al., 1985).

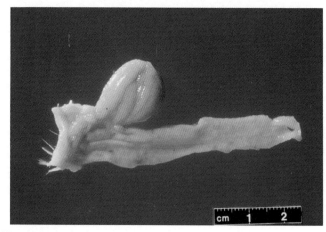

Fig. 13.5 The Bursa of Fabricius and cloaca obtained from a 1-week-old chicken. The bursa has been cut open to reveal the folds inside.

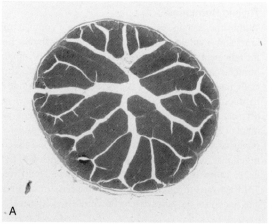
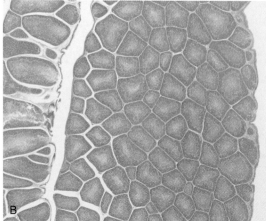

Fig. 13.6 Photomicrographs showing the structure of the Bursa of Fabricius. (A) Low-power micrograph showing the bursa of a 13-day-old chick. Original magnification ×5. (B) A high-power view. Original magnification ×360. From a specimen provided by Drs. N.H. McArthur and L.C. Abbott.

Thus the bursa is a primary lymphoid organ that functions as a maturation and differentiation site for the cells of the antibody-forming system. Lymphocytes originating in the bursa are therefore called B cells. The bursa acts like the thymus insofar as immature cells produced in the bone marrow migrate to the bursa. These cells then proliferate rapidly, but 90%–95% of them eventually die by apoptosis, the negative selection of self-reactive B cells (Motyka and Reynolds, 1991). Once their maturation is complete, the surviving B cells emigrate to secondary lymphoid organs.

A close examination shows that the bursa is not a pure primary lymphoid organ because it can also trap antigens and undertake some antibody synthesis. It also contains a small focus of T cells just above the bursal duct opening. Several different hormones have been extracted from the bursa. The most important of these is a tripeptide (Lys-His-glycylamide) called bursin that activates B cells but not T cells (Audhya et al., 1986).

Peyer's Patches

Structure

Peyer's patches (PPs) are lymphoid organs located in the walls of the small intestine. Their structure and functions vary among species. Thus mammals can be divided into two distinct groups based on the functions of their PPs (Liebler-Tenorio and Pabst, 2006).

Group I mammals. In ruminants, pigs, horses, dogs, and humans (Group I), most PPs are primary lymphoid organs that serve as a source of B cells (Yasuda et al., 2006). In these species, up to 90% of the PPs are found in the ileum, where they form a single continuous structure that extends forward from the ileocecal junction. In young ruminants and pigs, the ileal PP may be as long as 2 m. Ileal PPs consist of densely packed lymphoid follicles, each separated by a connective tissue sheath, and contain only B cells (Fig. 13.7). They export these B cells to all the other secondary lymphoid organs (Reynolds and Morris, 1983).

In Group I species, the ileal PPs reach maximal size and maturity before birth at a time when they are shielded from foreign antigens. They collectively form the largest lymphoid tissue in 6-week-old lambs. (They constitute about 1% of total body weight, like the thymus.) They disappear by 15 months of age and cannot be detected in adult sheep. Dogs also have two types of PPs, including a single ileal PP that involutes early and contains predominantly immature B cells.

The Group I species also have a second type of PP that consists of multiple discrete accumulations of follicles in the jejunum. These jejunal PPs persist for the life of the animal. They consist of pear-shaped follicles

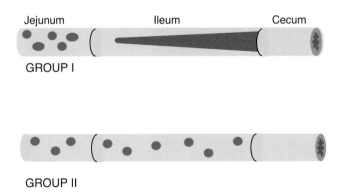

GROUP I

GROUP II

Fig. 13.7 Schematic diagram showing the differences between the arrangement of Peyer's patches in group I and group II mammals. The large ileal Peyer's patch in group I mammals (*red*) is a primary lymphoid organ that regresses at about a year of age. The small jejunal Peyer's patches (*blue*) are secondary lymphoid organs involved in the defense of the intestinal tract and control of the microbiota.

separated by extensive interfollicular tissue and contain mainly B cells with up to 30% T cells. These function like secondary lymphoid organs.

The pig is a Group I species. Pigs have about 30 jejunal PPs of conventional structure and a single, large ileal PP. Their ileal PP lacks T cells and has a structure similar to that seen in sheep. It regresses within the first year of life, but unlike the other Group I species, it does not appear to be a primary lymphoid organ since it is not required for B-cell development. It appears to be a secondary lymphoid organ that plays a role in the immune response to the intestinal microbiota (Sinkora et al., 2011).

Group II mammals. Nonhuman primates, rabbits, and rodents belong to Group II. In these mammals, the PPs are located at random intervals along the ileum and jejunum. Their PPs do not develop until 2–4 weeks after birth and persist into old age. The development of the PPs in some Group II mammals appears to depend entirely on stimulation by the normal intestinal microbiota since they remain small and poorly developed in germ-free animals. Thus, they are secondary lymphoid organs.

The rabbit's small intestine contains oval PPs located on the antimesenteric border of the intestine. They increase progressively in size and number from the duodenum to the ileum. There are no obvious patches in newborn rabbits, but they become apparent around day 15. The number of patches in adult rabbits varies from two to ten and averages about four. The covering epithelium contains multiple M cells. (Microfold [M] cells are specialized antigen-sampling epithelial cells.) There are also two large lymphoid patches located at the beginning of the large intestine. Each patch has the usual structure with multiple lymphoid follicles and a specialized overlying epithelium containing M cells (see Fig. 23.8). Rabbits possess two other sites containing organized lymphoid tissues. The sacculus rotundus is located at the ileocecal junction in a location consistent with the terminal ileal Peyer's patch in other species. It is, however, much larger than any Peyer's patch and contains large numbers of lymphoid follicles as well as M cells in the follicle-associated epithelium. Rabbits also possess a prominent appendix at the distal end of the cecum that is also packed with lymphoid follicles (Smith et al., 2009).

Functions

The ileal PPs of some Group I species such as sheep and cattle, function in a manner similar to the avian bursa. Thus ileal PPs are sites of rapid B-cell proliferation, although most cells then undergo apoptosis, and the survivors are released into the circulation (Reynolds, 1986; Motyka and Reynolds, 1991). If their ileal PPs are surgically removed, lambs become B cell deficient and fail to produce antibodies. The bone marrow of lambs contains many fewer lymphocytes than the bone marrow of laboratory rodents, and the ileal PPs are therefore their most significant source of B cells (Raynaud et al., 1991).

The intestinal lymphoid tissues in conventional animals are in intimate contact with the billions of bacteria that make up the gut microbiota. As a result, developing B cells are exposed to a diverse universe of products generated by these commensal organisms. It is believed that this complex mixture promotes B-cell diversification and furthers the development of the preimmune repertoire. It is clear that products derived from the microbiota are required for proper development not only of the gut-associated lymphoid tissue (GALT) but also of the antibody system itself. Products from the intestinal bacteria, possibly acting through pattern recognition receptors, activate the developing B cells and promote gene diversification (Chen et al., 2020). This diversification may also depend on the presence of selected bacterial species such as *Bacillus subtilis*, *Bacteroides fragilis*, or certain Clostridia. Bacterial structural proteins such as lipoarabinomannans, lipopolysaccharides, some superantigens such as Staphylococcal protein A, or even metabolites such as fatty acids and retinoic acid may also influence the B-cell diversification process. Likewise, endogenous stimulatory molecules from helper cells such as IL-4, IL-13, or IL-33 may also be required. Two very obvious cytokines that promote B-cell development are BAFF (B cell–activating factor) and APRIL (a proliferation-inducing ligand), which are upregulated by bacterial products and promote B-cell proliferation in an autocrine fashion (see Chapter 15).

Lymphoglandular Complexes

Lymphoglandular complexes are present in the walls of the large intestine and cecum in horses, ruminants, dogs, and pigs. They consist of submucosal masses of lymphoid tissue penetrated by radially branching extensions of mucosal glands. These glands penetrate both the submucosa and the lymphoid nodules. They are lined by intestinal columnar epithelium containing goblet cells, intraepithelial lymphocytes, and M cells (see Chapter 23). Their function is unknown, but they contain many plasma cells, suggesting that they are sites of antibody production.

Bone Marrow

The specialized ileal PP is the primary lymphoid organ for B cells only in group I mammals such as ruminants. In group II mammals, the bone marrow probably serves this function. There is no exclusive B-cell development site in the bone marrow, although it is suggested that precursor B cells develop at the outer edge of the marrow and migrate to the center as they mature and multiply. Negative selection occurs within the bone marrow so that, as in other primary lymphoid organs, most preB cells generated are destroyed. Not all bones contain active bone marrow, especially in adults. For example, the major sites of proliferative bone marrow in adult dogs are the vertebral column, the ossa coxarum, the proximal femur, and the sternum (Rowe et al., 2019).

SECONDARY LYMPHOID ORGANS

The cells of the immune system must be able to respond to the huge diversity of pathogens that an animal may encounter. It is especially important that antigen-specific lymphocytes can readily encounter their target antigens. To maximize the probability of such encounters, the body employs secondary lymphoid organs. In contrast to the primary lymphoid organs, the secondary lymphoid organs arise late in fetal life and persist in adults. Unlike primary lymphoid organs, they enlarge in response to antigenic stimulation. Surgical removal of one of them does not significantly reduce immune capability. Examples of secondary lymphoid organs include the spleen, the lymph nodes, the tonsils, and other lymphoid tissues in the intestinal, respiratory, and urogenital tracts. These organs contain dendritic cells that trap and process antigens and then present them to lymphocytes that mediate the immune responses. The overall anatomical structure of these organs therefore facilitates antigen trapping and provides an optimal environment for the initiation of immune responses. Secondary lymphoid organs are connected to both the blood and lymphoid systems, thus allowing them to continuously sample and respond to circulating antigens.

Lymph Nodes
Structure

Humans possess about 500 lymph nodes located throughout the body (Willard-Mack, 2006). These are round or bean-shaped filters strategically placed on lymphatic vessels in such a way that they can sample antigens carried in the lymph (Fig. 13.8). Lymph nodes consist of a capsule beneath which is a reticular network filled with lymphocytes,

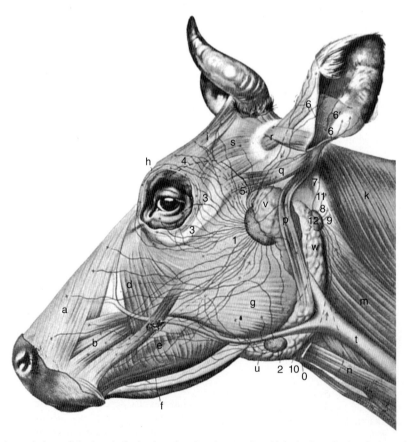

Fig. 13.8 Lateral view of the head of a bovine showing the way in which the lymphatics drain to the parotid lymph node. From Sisson S [revised by Grossman JD]., 1953. Anatomy of the Domestic Animals, fourth ed. Saunders, Philadelphia.

macrophages, and dendritic cells and through which lymphatic sinuses penetrate (Fig. 13.9). The lymph node thus acts as a filter for lymph fluid. A subcapsular sinus is located immediately under the connective tissue capsule. Other sinuses pass through the body of the node but are most prominent in the medulla. Afferent lymphatics enter the node around its circumference, and efferent lymphatics leave from a depression or hilus on one side. The blood vessels supplying a lymph node also enter and leave through the hilus.

The interior of lymph nodes is divided into three regions: a peripheral cortex, a central medulla, and an ill-defined region in between, called the paracortex (Fig. 13.10). B cells predominate in the cortex, where they are arranged in aggregates called follicles. In lymph nodes that are responding to antigen, some of these follicles form specialized structures called germinal centers (Fig. 13.11).

Germinal centers are sites where B cells grow, mutate, and mature. They are round, ovoid clusters of cells divided into light and dark zones. The germinal center originates when a few antigen-specific B cells enter a follicle and then divide rapidly to become the centroblasts that form the dark zone. This is the site where B cells proliferate and undergo a process called somatic mutation. The centroblasts eventually produce nondividing centrocytes that migrate to the light zone. The light zone is the site where immunoglobulin class switching and memory B-cell formation occur (see Chapter 16). Light zones are rich in antigen-trapping follicular dendritic cells (fDCs) and CD4+ helper T cells (Fig. 13.12; Allen et al., 2007).

T cells and dendritic cells predominate in the lymph node paracortex. These cells are arranged in cords between the lymphatic sinuses. At the center of each paracortical cord is a high endothelial venule (HEV). These vessels are lined with tall, rounded endothelial cells, quite unlike the flattened endothelium found in other blood vessels (Fig. 13.13). HEVs are surrounded by concentric layers of fibroblastic reticular cells and a narrow space called the perivenular channel.

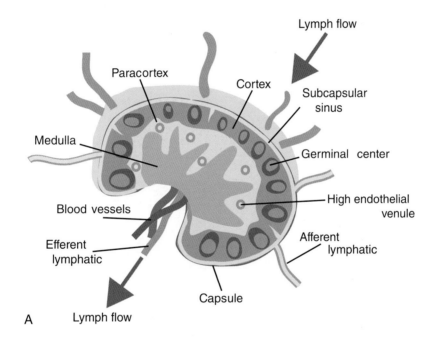

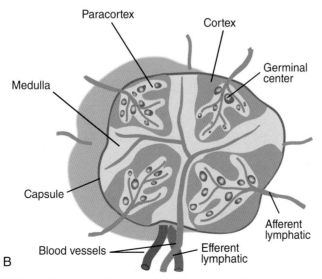

Fig. 13.9 (A) The major structural features of a typical mammalian lymph node. (B) Structure of a pig lymph node. The pig node is effectively inverted so that the medulla is exterior, and the cortex is interior. This has implications for the flow of lymphocytes through the node.

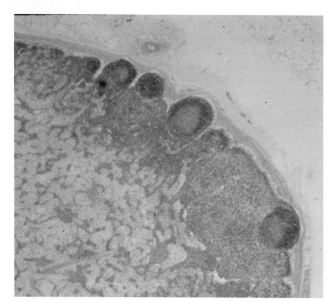

Fig. 13.10 A section of bovine lymph node. Original magnification × 12. From a specimen provided by Dr. W.E. Haensly.

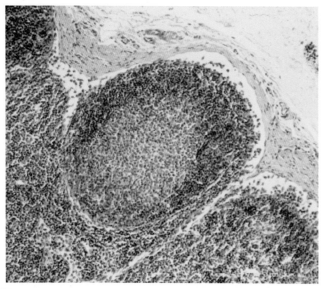

Fig. 13.11 A germinal center in the cortex of a cat's lymph node. Note the obvious light zone in the center of the germinal center. Original magnification × 120. From a specimen provided by Dr. W.E. Haensly.

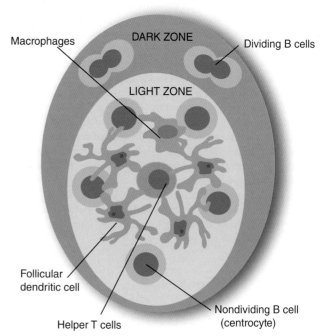

Fig. 13.12 A schematic diagram showing the structure of a germinal center. The outer dark zone contains dividing B cells. The central pale zone is a location where antigen-presenting dendritic cells, helper T cells, and B cells interact.

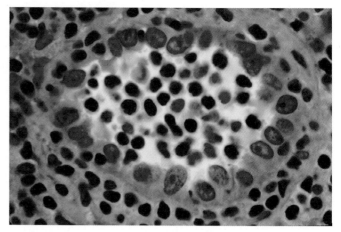

Fig. 13.13 A section of human tonsil showing a high endothelial venule with its characteristic high, rounded endothelial cells. Note the lymphocytes emigrating between the endothelial cells.

The lymph node medulla contains lymph-draining sinuses separated by medullary cords containing many plasma cells, macrophages, and memory T cells.

Lymph nodes are very busy places with cells coming and going in response to a multitude of signals. These signals are delivered through the reticular fibers that provide the structural scaffolding of the lymph node. These fibers are hollow and serve as conduits for the rapid transmission of signaling molecules and antigens (Fig. 13.14; Roozendaal et al., 2009). The conduits consist of bundles of collagen fibers ensheathed by fibroreticular cells. The fibroreticular cell wall is not continuous, so that follicular B cells and dendritic cells can insert their processes through tiny gaps and sample the antigens within the lymphatic fluid (Fig. 13.15). A similar network of conduits occurs within the T-cell zones where antigens are sampled by dendritic cells. The conduits provide for the rapid delivery of soluble antigens from the afferent

lymph to the lumen of HEVs and enable these antigens to reach deep into a node (Harwood and Batista, 2009).

Function

The principal function of lymph nodes is to capture circulating antigens and facilitate the subsequent interactions between antigen-presenting cells and antigen-sensitive T and B cells. Each cell must be guided to its appropriate contacts with great precision. A complex mixture of chemokines directs these cells. Thus, chemokines drive the emigration of lymphocytes from HEVs into the lymph node. Once they enter the lymph node, the T and B cells are guided to their respective regions by chemokines secreted by stromal cells and fDCs. Immature dendritic cells, once they encounter antigen, are also guided into lymph nodes

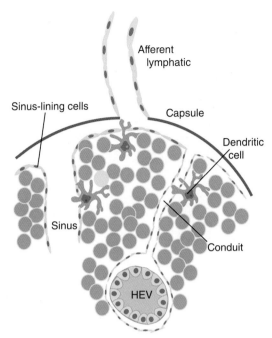

Fig. 13.14 Conduits connect the subcapsular sinus directly to the perivenular space around high endothelial venules. As soluble antigens flow through these conduits, they can be sampled by dendritic cells. *HEV,* High endothelial venule.

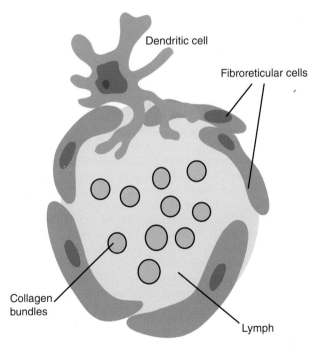

Fig. 13.15 Conduits consist of loosely attached fibroreticular cells surrounding collagen bundles. Dendritic cell processes can reach into the conduits to sample their antigen content.

by chemokines. For example, dendritic cells are attracted to the paracortex, where they present their antigen to T cells. Once this is accomplished, the dendritic cells change their chemokine receptors and can then leave the node.

Lymph nodes also contain innate lymphoid cells that are located close to sentinel macrophages lining the lymphatic sinuses. They are thus exposed to cytokines such as IL-18 released when the macrophages encounter invaders. The innate lymphocytes in turn rapidly

increase their IFN-γ secretion that activates the macrophages still further and enhances their antimicrobial activities.

An important feature of secondary lymphoid organs is the fact that both B and T cells are highly active and motile. The T cells in the paracortex and B cells in the cortex are guided by fDCs. Chemokines control the relocation and recirculation of lymphocytes and ensure that they end up in the right place. For example, T cells are attracted to the perifollicular area of the cortex. B cells, on the other hand, are attracted to the interior of germinal centers. When T cells are activated, they too may enter germinal centers where they "help" B cells respond to antigens. Other secondary lymphoid organs employ different homing receptors. For example, MAdCAM-1 is a homing receptor found in blood vessels in PPs. Lymphocytes that recirculate to the intestine express high levels of the MAdCAM-1 ligand.

Soluble antigens entering the node through its afferent lymphatics first pass into the subcapsular sinus. From there, they enter the conduit network and are carried into the cortex. Larger antigens such as viruses are captured by macrophages within the subcapsular sinus. These macrophages carry the viral particles through the sinus floor and present them directly to B cells in the underlying follicles. The B cells then migrate to the T cell-B cell boundary, where they receive specific T-cell help. B cells can also enter the paracortex directly from HEVs. There is a specialized population of fDCs clustered around these blood vessels so that immigrating B cells can interact with any antigens they may be carrying. This is also a perfect location to receive T-cell help.

When bacteria invade tissues, the resident dendritic cells are activated and migrate to the draining lymph node where they accumulate in the paracortex and cortex. These dendritic cells form a web through which antigens must pass. Captured antigens are presented by the dendritic cells to T cells. T cells are initially activated in the paracortex, whereas the B cells remain randomly dispersed in the primary follicles. Both cell populations then migrate to the edges of the follicles where they interact. Once antibody production is stimulated, the progeny of these B cells move to the medulla and begin to secrete antibodies. Some of these antibody-producing cells may escape into the efferent lymph and colonize downstream lymph nodes. Several days after antibody production is first observed in the medulla, germinal centers appear in the cortex.

In the presence of antigen, T cells and dendritic cells form stable complexes lasting for many hours. However, before selecting, its partner a dendritic cell might sample as many as 500 different T cells/hour and can interact with up to 10 simultaneously.

Adherence to fDCs is the predominant means of antigen trapping once an animal has been sensitized by previous exposure to an antigen. In a secondary response, the germinal centers become less obvious as activated memory cells emigrate in the efferent lymph. Once this stage is completed, the germinal centers redevelop.

Antigen-stimulated lymph nodes also trap lymphocytes. Interactions between infectious agents and mast cells result in the production of tumor necrosis factor–α (TNF-α). The TNF-α blocks the passage of lymphocytes through these organs, the lymphocytes accumulate, and the lymph nodes swell. This trapping concentrates lymphocytes close to sites of antigen accumulation. After about 24 hours, the lymph nodes release their trapped cells, and their cellular output is increased for several days after.

Lymphocyte Circulation

In adult animals, most cell types reside in stable tissues and do not move a lot. The cells of the immune system are, in contrast, highly mobile. Cells move from the bone marrow to the thymus and secondary lymphoid organs; cells migrate around the body looking for invaders and also move from lymphoid organs to sites of microbial

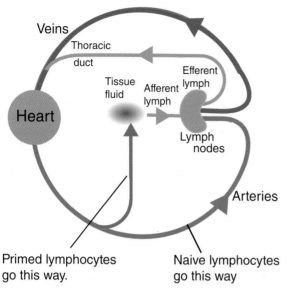

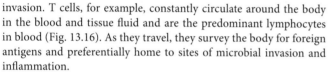

Fig. 13.16 The circulation of lymphocytes. T cells circulate in both the bloodstream and the lymphatic fluid. Their precise route through a lymph node depends on whether they are naïve or primed. Thus, naïve lymphocytes enter lymph nodes through the bloodstream and the high endothelial venules. Primed lymphocytes, in contrast, migrate through the tissues and enter through afferent lymphatics. They all leave through efferent lymphatics.

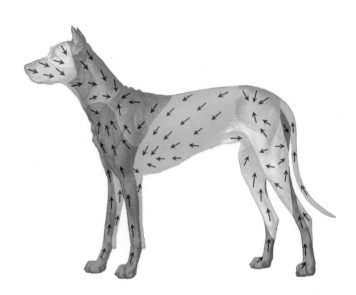

Fig. 13.17 Color coded diagram of 10 superficial lymphosomes in the dog with arrows showing the direction of lymph flow. From Suami, H., Yamashita, S., Soto-Miranda, M.A., Chang, D.W., 2013. Lymphatic territories (lymphosomes) in a canine: an animal model for investigation of postoperative lymphatic alterations. PLoS ONE 8(7), e69222.

invasion. T cells, for example, constantly circulate around the body in the blood and tissue fluid and are the predominant lymphocytes in blood (Fig. 13.16). As they travel, they survey the body for foreign antigens and preferentially home to sites of microbial invasion and inflammation.

Circulating T cells leave the bloodstream by two routes. T cells that have not previously encountered antigens ("naïve" T cells) bind to HEV in lymph nodes. The high endothelial cells in these vessels are not joined by tight junctions but are linked by discontinuous "spot-welded" junctions. This means that lymphocytes can pass easily between the high endothelial cells. Circulating lymphocytes can adhere to these high endothelial cells and then migrate into the lymph node paracortex (Harp et al., 1990). The immigration of lymphocytes from HEVs resembles that of neutrophils in inflamed blood vessels. Thus, the cells first roll along the endothelial surface, binding to selectins. As they roll, they become activated and express integrins. This results in their complete arrest and emigration. The number and length of HEVs are variable and controlled by local activity. Thus, stimulation of a lymph node by the presence of antigens results in a rapid increase in the length of its HEVs. If, however, a lymph node is protected from antigens, its HEVs shorten. Recognizable HEVs are not normally found in ruminant lymph nodes, but paracortical venules serve the same function (von Andrian and Mempel, 2003).

In contrast to naïve T cells, memory T cells leave the bloodstream through conventional blood vessels in tissues and are then carried to lymph nodes through afferent lymphatics. They leave the lymph nodes through the efferent lymphatics. Typically, afferent lymph in sheep contains 85% T cells, 5% B cells, and 10% dendritic cells. Efferent lymph contains more than 98% lymphocytes, of which 75% are T cells and 25% are B cells. The efferent lymphatics eventually join together to form large lymph vessels. The largest of these lymph vessels is the thoracic duct, which drains the lymph from the lower body and intestine and empties it into the anterior vena.

Lymphosomes

It is possible to map the body regions (lymphosomes) drained by each lymph node based on the tracing of injected colored dyes. Ten lymphosomes have been identified in the dog (Fig. 13.17).

Species Differences

Domestic pigs and related swine are different. Their lymph nodes consist of several lymphoid "nodules" oriented so that the cortex of each nodule is located toward the center of the node, whereas the medulla is at the periphery (Fig. 13.9; Binns and Pabst, 1994). Each nodule is served by a single afferent lymphatic that enters the central cortex as a lymph sinus. Thus, afferent lymph is carried deep into the node. A cortex surrounds the lymph sinus. Outside this region are a paracortex and a medulla. This medulla may be shared by adjacent nodules (Fig. 13.18). Lymph passes from the cortex at the center of the node to the medulla at the periphery before leaving through the efferent vessels that drain the region between nodules (Dubreil et al., 2022). The cortex and paracortex have a similar structure to that seen in other mammals. The medulla has very few sinuses but consists of a dense mass of cells that is relatively impermeable to cells in the lymph. As a result, few cells migrate through the medulla. T cells in these species enter the lymph node in the conventional way through HEVs. However, they do not leave the lymph node through the lymphatics but migrate directly back to the bloodstream through the HEVs of the paracortex (Fig. 13.19). Very few lymphocytes are found in pig lymph.

Hemolymph Nodes

Hemal nodes (technically hemolymph nodes) are structures similar to lymph nodes found in association with some blood vessels of cattle, deer, and related mammals (Sakita et al., 1997). Because of their dark red or black color and their size (mm to pea-sized), they are very obvious on necropsy. They are found in adipose and connective tissue in the neck, around the kidneys, and around large blood vessels. Their

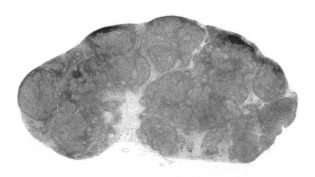

Fig. 13.18 A section of a pig lymph node. Note how the germinal centers are located in the interior of the node. Compare this to Figure 12.8. Original magnification × 12. From a specimen provided by Dr. Brian Porter.

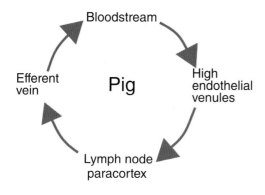

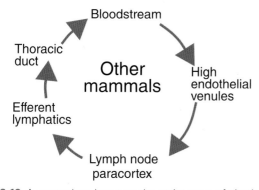

Fig. 13.19 A comparison between the major route of circulation of T cells in the pig compared to other mammals. Note that pig lymphocytes are largely confined to the bloodstream.

numbers and prominence vary greatly between individual animals. Their function is unclear and somewhat controversial. The general arrangement of their lymphoid tissue is similar to that in conventional lymph nodes. However, they differ from conventional lymph nodes in that their sinuses contain numerous red cells, and, in some respects, they resemble small spleens. They have a cortex containing germinal centers and B cells. T cells predominate at the medulla in association with lymphatic sinuses. They are surrounded by blood-filled sinuses. These cells differ, however, from those found in conventional lymph nodes by containing more γ/δ+, WC1+ T cells, and fewer CD8+ T cells (Thorp et al., 1991). Intravenously injected carbon particles are trapped in the sinusoids of hemal nodes, suggesting that they may combine features of both the spleen and lymph nodes. As a result, they can both trap antigen and trigger cellular and humoral immune responses.

Spleen

Just as lymph nodes filter antigens from lymph, so the spleen filters blood-borne pathogens and antigens. The filtering process removes antigenic particles such as microorganisms, cellular debris, and aged blood cells. This filtering function, together with highly organized lymphoid tissue, makes the spleen an important component of the immune system. In addition to its immune functions, the spleen also stores red cells and platelets, recycles iron, and in some species, undertakes fetal red cell production. As a result, the spleen consists of two forms of tissue. One is used predominantly for blood filtering and for red cell storage, called the red pulp. It contains large numbers of antigen-presenting cells, lymphocytes, and plasma cells (Odroiu, 2017). Macrophages in the red pulp specialize in removing aged red blood cells and so regulate iron recycling. The other tissue is rich in both B and T cells. This is where immune responses occur and is called the white pulp. The white pulp is separated from the red pulp by a region called the marginal zone. This zone contains numerous macrophages and dendritic cells as well as a large population of B cells. The spleen is not supplied with lymphatic fluid, although it does possess efferent lymphatics.

Structure of White Pulp

Arteries entering the spleen pass through muscular trabeculae before entering the white pulp and branching into arterioles. Immediately after leaving the trabeculae, each arteriole is surrounded by a layer of lymphoid tissue called a periarteriolar lymphoid sheath (Fig. 13.20). The arteriole eventually leaves this sheath and branches into penicillary arterioles. In some mammals, these penicillary arterioles are surrounded by periarteriolar macrophage sheaths (ellipsoids). These arterioles then open, either directly or indirectly, into venous sinuses that drain into the splenic venules. Ellipsoids are relatively large and prominent in pigs, mink, dogs, and cats; are small and indistinct in horses and cattle; and are absent in laboratory animals such as mice, rats, guinea pigs, and rabbits. The function of ellipsoids is to trap circulating particulate material (Sorby et al., 2005). In species that lack ellipsoids, particles are trapped primarily in the marginal zone of the white pulp (Onkar and Govardhan, 2013).

The white pulp contains both B and T cells, which accumulate in specific zones under the influence of chemokines. The periarteriolar lymphoid sheaths consist largely of T cells. Within these, the T cells interact with dendritic cells and passing B cells. The B-cell areas, in contrast, consist of round primary follicles scattered through the sheaths. These follicles are sites where germinal center formation, clonal expansion, isotype switching, and somatic hypermutation occur.

The white pulp is separated from the red pulp by a marginal sinus, a reticulum sheath, and a marginal zone of cells. This marginal zone is an important transit area for white cells moving between the blood and the white pulp. It is rich in macrophages, dendritic cells, and B cells. Most of the blood that enters the spleen flows into the marginal sinus and through the marginal zone before returning to circulation through venous sinuses. This flow pattern ensures that these antigen-presenting cells can capture any blood-borne antigens and deliver them to the B cells in the marginal zone. The white pulp is involved in adaptive immune responses, whereas cells of the marginal zone can participate in both innate and adaptive responses. Splenic white pulp does not contain HEVs. Instead, lymphocytes enter the white pulp through the marginal zone, although the route by which they leave is unclear.

Function

Intravenously administered antigens are trapped in the spleen. Depending on the species, they are taken up by dendritic cells in the marginal zone or in the periarteriolar macrophage sheaths. These

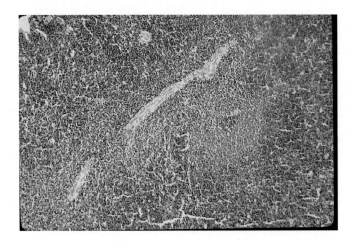

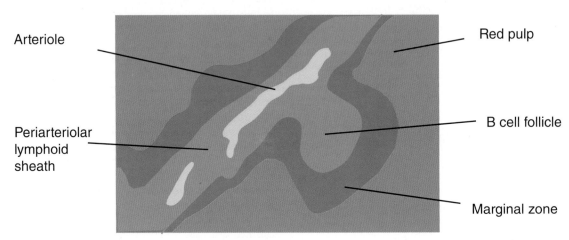

Fig. 13.20 Histological section and diagram showing the structure of the bovine spleen. Original magnification ×50. From a specimen provided by Dr. J.R. Duncan.

dendritic cells and macrophages carry the antigen to the primary follicles of the white pulp, from which, after a few days, antibody-producing cells migrate. These antibody-producing cells (plasma cells and plasmablasts) colonize the marginal zone and move into the red pulp. Antibodies produced by these cells diffuse rapidly into the bloodstream. The germinal center formation also occurs in the primary follicles. In an animal possessing circulating antibodies, trapping by dendritic cells within the follicles becomes significant. As in primary immune response, the antibody-producing cells migrate from these follicles into the red pulp and the marginal zone where antibody production occurs.

Tonsils

The tonsils are located within the pharynx and serve to capture and process ingested antigens. Some organisms, however, can overcome the defenses of the tonsils and use them as a portal of entry into the body. For example, pathogens such as bovine herpesvirus-1, *Mannheimia hemolytica*, *Streptococcus suis*, and *Mycobacterium tuberculosis* can persist indefinitely within the tonsils.

There are two types of tonsils: those with crypts and those without. A tonsillar crypt is a blind invagination of the surface epithelium surrounded by a mass of lymphoid tissue. A single crypt together with its associated lymphoid tissue constitutes a tonsillar follicle. They have no afferent lymphatics. Tonsils with crypts and follicles include the palatine tonsils of humans, horses, ruminants, and pigs. Tonsils without crypts are formed by a single layer of lymphatic tissue that may bulge outward. These include the tonsils of carnivores, the pharyngeal tonsils, and the tubal tonsils of ruminants. In general, tonsils are larger in young animals (Velinova et al., 2001).

The Genital Lymphoid Ring

Lymphoid tissues consisting of organized lymphoid follicles as well as diffuse lymphocytic infiltrates are found in the lamina propria of the vaginal vestibule of cows where they form a ring of lymphoid tissue. These lymphoid follicles may contain germinal centers. They also contain both lymphocytes and macrophages and HEV. The lymphocytes are predominantly B cells. The epithelial covering of these follicles is infiltrated with lymphocytes as well. It is suggested that this genital lymphoid ring serves a similar function as the tonsils in the pharynx (Chuluunbaatar et al., 2022).

Other Secondary Lymphoid Organs

Secondary lymphoid organs include not only the spleen and lymph nodes but also the bone marrow and lymphoid tissues scattered throughout the body, most notably in the mucosa of the digestive, respiratory, and urogenital tracts (Meek et al., 2022). The lymphoid tissues of the intestinal tract constitute the largest pool of lymphocytes in the body, but the bone marrow also contains very large numbers of lymphocytes. If antigen is given intravenously, much will be trapped not only in the liver and spleen but also in the bone marrow. During a primary immune response, antibodies are mainly produced in the spleen and lymph nodes (Fig. 13.21). Toward the end of that response,

memory cells leave the spleen and colonize the bone marrow. When a second dose of an antigen is given, the bone marrow produces very large quantities of antibodies and is the major source of antibodies in adult rodents. Up to 70% of the antibody to some antigens may be produced by cells in the bone marrow (Fig. 13.22). Fat-associated lymphoid clusters are small secondary lymphoid nodules within adipose tissues underlying serosal membranes such as the mesentery.

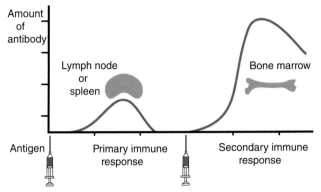

Fig. 13.21 Although the primary immune response to intravenously injected antigen takes place in lymph nodes or spleen, the antibodies produced in a secondary response are largely produced in the bone marrow.

TERTIARY LYMPHOID ORGANS

Within the body are found lymphoid structures that are structurally similar to secondary lymphoid organs but develop in response to microbial colonization and chronic immune stimulation. These are organized masses of lymphocytes with clearly discrete T- and B-cell regions that contain germinal centers and other lymphoid tissue components (Neyt et al., 2012). These can be called tertiary lymphoid organs. Good examples of these develop in the intestinal wall in response to the intestinal microbiota. Other examples include the lymphoid nodules that develop in rheumatoid arthritis joints and in atherosclerotic plaques. The initial trigger for their development probably comes from stimulated fibroblasts that produce appropriate chemokines attracting and accumulating T cells, B cells, and dendritic cells (Pabst et al., 2005).

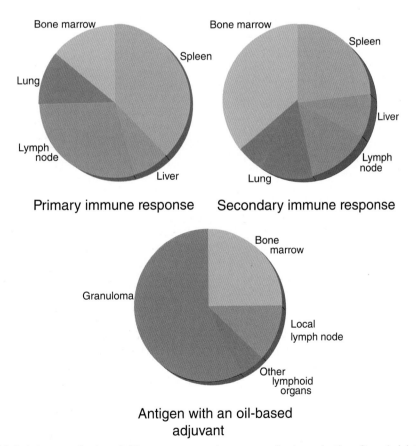

Fig. 13.22 Relative contribution of different organs or tissues to antibody production after administration of antigen either intravenously or intramuscularly with Freund's complete adjuvant. The adjuvant (see Chapter 25) causes the accumulation of lymphocytes and antigen-processing cells. It thus forms a lymphoid nodule where antibodies are produced.

REFERENCES

Allen, C.D., Okada, T., Cyster, J.G., 2007. Germinal-center organization and cellular dynamics. Immunity 27, 190–202.

Audhya, T., Kroon, D., Heavner, G., et al., 1986. Tripeptide structure of bursin, a selective B cell differentiating hormone of the bursa of Fabricius. Science 231, 997–999.

Binns, R.M., Pabst, R., 1994. Lymphoid tissue structure and lymphocyte trafficking in the pig. Vet. Immunol. Immunopathol. 43, 79–87.

Chen, H., Zhang, Y., Ye, A.Y., Du, Z., et al., 2020. BCR selection and affinity maturation in Peyer's patch germinal centers. Nature 582, 421–425.

Chuluunbaatar, I., Ichii, O., Masum, M.A., Namba, T., et al., 2022. Genital organ-associated lymphoid tissues arranged in a ring in the mucosa of cow vaginal vestibule. Res. Vet. Sci. 145, 147–158.

Cunningham, C.P., Kimpton, W.G., Holder, J.E., Cahill, R.N., 2001. Thymic export in aged sheep: a continuous role for the thymus throughout pre- and postnatal life. Eur. J. Immunol. 31, 802–811.

Dubreil, L., Ledevin, M., Hervet, C., Menard, D., Philippe, C., et al., 2022. The internal conduit system of the swine inverted lymph node. Front. Immunol. 13, 869384.

Ekino, S., Suginohara, K., Urano, T., et al., 1985. The bursa of Fabricius: a trapping site for environmental antigens. Immunology 55, 405–410.

Haley, P.J., 2017. The lymphoid system: a review of species differences. J. Toxicol. Pathol. 30, 111–123.

Harp, J.A., Pesch, B.A., Runnels, P.L., 1990. Extravasation of lymphocytes via paracortical venules in sheep lymph nodes: visualization using an intracellular fluorescent label. Vet. Immunol. Immunopathol. 24, 159–168.

Harwood, N.E., Batista, F.D., 2009. The antigen expressway: follicular conduits carry antigen to B cells. Immunity 30, 177–179.

Laan, M., Haljasorg, U., Kisand, K., Salumets, A., Peterson, P., 2016. Pregnancy-induced thymic involution is associated with suppression of chemokines essential for T-lymphocyte progenitor homing. Eur. J. Immunol. 46, 2008–2017.

Liebler-Tenorio, E.M., Pabst, R., 2006. MALT structure and function in farm animals. Vet. Res. 37, 257–280.

Meek, H.C., Stenfeldt, C., Arzt, J., 2022. Morphological and phenotypic characterization of the bovine nasopharyngeal mucosa and associated lymphoid tissue. J. Comp. Path. 198, 62–79.

Motyka, B., Reynolds, J.D., 1991. Apoptosis is associated with the extensive B cell death in the sheep ileal Peyer's patch and the chicken bursa of Fabricius: a possible role in B cell selection. Eur. J. Immunol. 21, 1951–1958.

Neyt, K., Perros, F., Corine, H., van Kessel, G., Hammad, H., Lambrecht, B.N., 2012. Tertiary lymphoid organs in infection and autoimmunity. Trends Immunol. 33, 297–305.

Onkar, D.P., Govardhan, S.A., 2013. Comparative histology of human and dog spleen. J. Morphol. Sci. 30 (1), 16–20.

Pabst, O., Herbrand, H., Worbs, T., Feiedrichsen, M., et al., 2005. Cryptopatches and isolated lymphoid follicles. Dynamic lymphoid tissues dispensable for the generation of intraepithelial lymphocytes. Eur. J. Immunol. 35, 98–107.

Pearse, G., 2006. Normal structure, function and histology of the thymus. Toxicol. Pathol. 34, 504–514.

Reynaud, C.-A., Mackay, C.R., Müller, R.G., Weill, J.-C., 1991. Somatic generation of diversity in a mammalian primary lymphoid organ: the sheep ileal Peyer's patches. Cell 64, 995–1005.

Reynolds, J.D., 1986. Evidence of extensive lymphocyte death in sheep Peyer's patches. I. A comparison of lymphocyte production and export. J. Immunol. 136, 2005–2010.

Reynolds, J.D., Morris, B., 1983. The evolution and involution of Peyer's patches in fetal and postnatal sheep. Eur. J. Immunol. 73, 627–635.

Roozendaal, R., Mempel, T.R., Pitcher, L.A., et al., 2009. Conduits mediate transport of low molecular weight antigen to lymph node follicles. Immunity 30, 264–276.

Rowe, J.A., Morandi, F., Osborne, D.R., Wall, J.S., et al., 2019. Relative skeletal distribution of proliferating marrow in the adult dog determined by using 3'-deoxy-3'-[^{18}F]fluorothymidine. Anat. Histol. Embryol. 48, 46–52.

Sakita, K., Fujino, M., Koshikawa, T., Ohmiya, N., et al., 1997. The structure and function of the hemolymph node in rats. Nagoya J. Med. Sci. 60, 129–137.

Sinkora, M., Stepanova, K., Butler, J.E., Francis, D., et al., 2011. Ileal Peyer's patches are not necessary for systemic B cell development and maintenance and do not contribute significantly to the overall B cell pool in swine. J. Immunol. 187, 5150–5161.

Sisson, S., Grossman, J.D., 1953. The Anatomy of the Domestic Animals, fourth ed. Saunders, Philadelphia.

Smith, H.F., Fisher, R.E., Everett, M.L., Thomas, A.D., et al., 2009. Comparative anatomy and phylogenetic distribution of the mammalian cecal appendix. J. Evol. Biol. 22, 1984–1999.

Sørby, R., Wein, T.N., Husby, G., Espenes, A., Landsverk, T., 2005. Filter function and immune complex trapping in splenic ellipsoids. J. Comp. Pathol. 132, 313–321.

Steinmann, G.G., Klaus, B., Muller-Hermelin, H.K., et al., 1985. The aging of the human thymic epithelium is independent of puberty. A morphometric study. Scand. J. Immunol. 22 (5), 563–575.

Thorp, B.H., Seneque, S., Staute, K., Kimpton, W.G., 1991. Characterization and distribution of lymphocyte subsets in sheep hemal nodes. Dev. Comp. Immunol. 15, 393–400.

Udroiu, I., 2017. Storage of blood in the mammalian spleen: an evolutionary perspective. J. Mammal. Evol. 24, 243–260.

Velinova, M., Theilen, C., Melot, F., et al., 2001. New histochemical and ultrastructural observations on normal bovine tonsils. Vet. Rec. 149, 613–617.

von Andrian, U.H., Mempel, T.R., 2003. Homing and cellular traffic in lymph nodes. Nat. Rev. Immunol. 3, 867–878.

Wang, J., Sekai, M., Matsui, T., Fujii, Y., et al., 2018. Hassall's corpuscles with cellular senescence features maintain IFNα production through neutrophils and pDC activation in the thymus. Int. Immunol. 31 (3), 127–139.

Willard-Mack, C.K., 2006. Normal structure, function, and histology of lymph nodes. Tox. Pathol. 34, 409–424.

Yasuda, M., Jenne, C.N., Kennedy, L.J., Reynolds, J.D., 2006. The sheep and cattle Peyer's patch as a site of B cell development. Vet. Res. 37, 401–415.

Lymphocytes

Lymphocytes are the cells responsible for adaptive immunity and the defense of the body. There are three major types of lymphocytes. These are innate lymphoid cells that play a role in innate immunity; T cells that regulate adaptive immunity and are responsible for cell-mediated immune responses; and B cells that are responsible for antibody production. Within these three major types are many subpopulations, each with different characteristics and functions. This chapter reviews the structure and properties of T and B lymphocytes and some of their important subpopulations.

LYMPHOCYTE STRUCTURE

Lymphocytes are small, round (spherical) cells, 7 to 15 μm in diameter. Each contains a single large, round nucleus that stains intensely and evenly with hematoxylin (Fig. 14.1). Their nucleus is surrounded by a thin rim of cytoplasm containing some mitochondria, free ribosomes, and a small Golgi apparatus (Fig. 14.2). Scanning electron microscopy shows that some lymphocytes are smooth surfaced, whereas others are covered by many small projections (Fig. 14.3). Innate lymphoid cells are often larger than T or B cells and may contain obvious cytoplasmic granules. With this exception, lymphocyte structure provides no clue as to their function or complexity (Fig. 14.4).

LYMPHOCYTE POPULATIONS

Lymphocytes are found throughout the body in lymphoid organs, in the bloodstream, and scattered under body surfaces. Despite their uniform appearance, they are a diverse mixture of distinct cell populations. Although these populations cannot be identified by structural differences, they can be identified by their characteristic cell surface molecules and by their behavior (Table 14.1). The pattern of cell surface molecules expressed on a cell is called its phenotype. By analyzing cell phenotypes, it is possible to identify and classify many lymphocyte populations.

The loss of cell-mediated immunity as a result of neonatal thymectomy first demonstrated the existence of T cells (Fig. 14.5). After T cells leave the thymus, they accumulate in the paracortex of lymph nodes, the periarteriolar lymphoid sheaths of the spleen, and the interfollicular areas of the Peyer patches. T cells also account for 60% to 80% of the lymphocytes circulating in the bloodstream (Table 14.2).

Similar experiments involving bursectomy in chickens pointed to the existence of B cells. In mammals, B cells originate in the bone marrow but mature within Peyer patches or the bone marrow before migrating to the secondary lymphoid organs. B cells predominate in the cortex of lymph nodes, in follicles within the Peyer patches and spleen, and in the marginal zone of the white pulp of the spleen. B cells account for 10% to 40% of blood lymphocytes (see Table 14.2).

Natural killer cells, a population of innate lymphoid cells, were identified as a result of the detection of cytotoxic lymphocytes in unsensitized animals. NK cells probably originate from the same stem cells as T cells but do not undergo thymic processing. They are widely distributed throughout the lymphoid organs. They account for 5% to 10% of blood lymphocytes. Other innate lymphoid cell populations are also found in tissues, especially in the intestine, respiratory tract, and skin (see Chapter 20).

LYMPHOCYTE SURFACE MOLECULES

All cells express thousands of different protein molecules on their surface. Hundreds of these surface molecules have been characterized, especially in human and mouse lymphocytes (Box 14.1). As each molecule is characterized, it is usually given a functional or chemical name. It is also usually given a cluster of differentiation (CD) designation as well (Figs. 14.6 and 14.7). Currently, the CD system assigns sequential numbers to each molecule: CD1, CD2, CD3, and so on, up to CD371. Since arbitrary numbers are difficult to remember, the basic principle used in this text is that if the molecule's common name is well accepted or describes its function, that name will be used. Examples include the

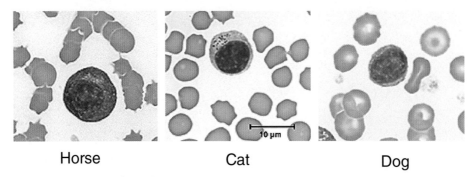

Fig. 14.1 Photomicrographs showing lymphocytes in stained blood smears from horse, cat, and dog. Giemsa stain. Courtesy Dr. M.C. Johnson.

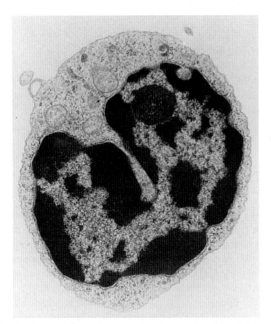

Fig. 14.2 Transmission electron micrograph of a blood lymphocyte from a rabbit. Courtesy Dr. S. Linthicum.

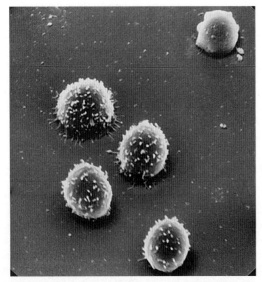

Fig. 14.3 Scanning electron micrograph of lymphocytes from a mouse lymph node. Recent studies have indicated that antigen-binding receptors are concentrated on the tips of the small projections (called microvilli). Original magnification ×1500.

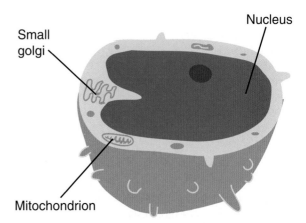

Fig. 14.4 Essential structural features of a lymphocyte. There are actually very few characteristic structural features.

IgA receptor, FcαR (CD89), the interleukin-6 receptor (CD126), and L-selectin (CD62L). CD nomenclature is also used for molecules for which the designation is well accepted, such as CD8 and CD4. A list of the most relevant CD molecules and their functions can be found in Appendix 1.

CD molecules expressed on the cells of domestic mammals fall into two categories. Most are also expressed on human and mouse cells (homologs) and thus have the same CD number. There are, however, several cell surface molecules in domestic mammals that have no recognized homolog in humans or mice. These unattributable molecules are given a species abbreviation and the prefix WC (Workshop Cluster); for example, BoWC1 and BoWC2 are expressed on cattle lymphocytes. Some of these WC molecules have subsequently been shown to be homologous to previously recognized CD molecules, while others are species-specific. The phenotypes of cells as expressed by their cell surface molecules are characterized through the use of an instrument called a flow cytometer. How this works is described in Chapter 43.

Antigen Receptors

While lymphocytes express thousands of proteins on their surface, from an immunological viewpoint, the most important structures are the receptors they use to recognize antigens. These are abbreviated TCR (T-cell antigen receptor) or BCR (B-cell antigen receptor). Both the TCR and BCR are complex structures assembled from many different protein chains. Some of these protein chains bind the antigen, whereas others are used for signal transduction. Additional complexity occurs within lymphocyte subpopulations. For example, there are two different T-cell populations differentiated by their antigen-binding receptors.

TABLE 14.1 Identifying Features of T and B Cells

Property	B Cells	T Cells
Develop within	Bone marrow, bursa, Peyer patches	Thymus
Distribution	Lymph node cortex	Lymph node paracortex
	Splenic follicles	Spleen periarteriolar sheath
Circulate	No	Yes
Antigen receptors	BCR—immunoglobulin	TCR—protein heterodimer
		Associated with CD3, CD4, or CD8
Important surface antigens	Immunoglobulins	CD2, CD3, CD4, or CD8
Mitogens	Pokeweed, lipopolysaccharide	Phytohemagglutinin, concanavalin A, BCG vaccine, pokeweed
Antigens recognized	Free foreign proteins	Processed foreign proteins in MHC antigens
Tolerance induction	Difficult	Easy
Progeny cells	Plasma cells, memory cells	Effector T cells, memory T cells
Secreted products	Immunoglobulins	Cytokines

BCR, B-cell antigen receptor; TCR, T-cell antigen receptor.

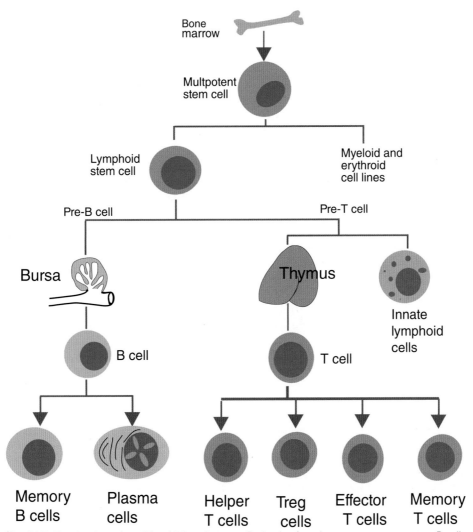

Fig. 14.5 The development of T and B lymphocytes. Both arise from bone marrow precursors. B cells develop in the bursa, Peyer patches, or bone marrow. T cells develop in the thymus. Innate lymphoid cells are a third population of lymphocytes that are distinct from T and B cells.

TABLE 14.2   Major Peripheral Blood Lymphocyte Populations in Mammals as Percentages of the Total Population

	T Cells	B Cells	CD4$^+$	CD8$^+$	CD4/CD8
Horses	38–66	17–38[a]	56[b]	20–37[a]	4.75[b]
Bovine	45–53[c]	16–21[c]	8–31	10–30	1.53[c]
Sheep	56–64[d]	11–50[e]	8–22[e]	4–22[e]	1.55[d]
Pigs	45–57[f]	13–38[g]	23–43	17–39	1.4[h]
Dogs	46–72	7–30	27–33[i]	17–18[i]	1.7[i]
Cats	31–89[j]	6–50[j]	19–49[j]	6–39[j]	1.9[j]
Humans	70–75	10–15	43–48[k]	22–24[k]	1.9–2.4[k]

[a]From McGorum, B.C., Dixon, P.M., Halliwell, R.E., 1993. Phenotypic analysis of peripheral blood and bronchoalveolar lavage fluid lymphocytes in control and chronic obstructive pulmonary disease affected horses, before and after "natural (hay and straw) challenges". Vet. Immunol. Immunopathol. 36, 207–222.

[b]From Grunig, G., Barbis, D.P., Zhang, C.H., et al., 1994. Correlation between monoclonal antibody reactivity and expression of CD4 and CD8 alpha genes in the horse. Vet. Immunol. Immunopathol. 42, 61–69.

[c]From Park, Y.H., Fox, L.K., Hamilton, M.J., Davis, W.C., 1992. Bovine mononuclear leukocyte subpopulations in peripheral blood and mammary gland secretions during lactation. J. Dairy Sci. 75, 998–1006.

[d]From Thorp, B.H., Seneque, S., Staute, K, Kimpton, W.G., 1991. Characterization and distribution of lymphocyte subsets in sheep hemal nodes. Dev. Comp. Immunol. 15, 393–400.

[e]From Smith, H.E., Jacobs, R.M., Smith, C., 1994. Flow cytometric analysis of ovine peripheral blood lymphocytes. Can. J. Vet. Res. 58, 152–155.

[f]From Pescovitz, M.D., Sakopoulos, A.B., Gaddy, J.A., et al., 1994. Porcine peripheral blood CD4$^+$/CD8$^+$ dual expressing T-cells. Vet. Immunol. Immunopathol. 43, 53–62.

[g]From Saalmüller, A., Bryant, J., 1994. Characteristics of porcine T lymphocytes and T-cell lines, Vet. Immunol. Immunopathol. 43, 45–52.

[h]From Joling, P., Bianchi, A.T., Kappe, A.L., Zwart, R.J., 1994. Distribution of lymphocyte subpopulations in thymus, spleen, and peripheral blood of specific pathogen free pigs from 1 to 40 weeks of age, Vet. Immunol. Immunopathol. 40, 105–118.

[i]From Rivas, A.L., Kimball, E.S., Quimby, F.W., Gebhard, D. 1995. Functional and phenotypic analysis of in vitro stimulated canine peripheral blood mononuclear cells. Vet. Immunol. Immunopathol. 45, 55–71.

[j]From Walker, R., Malik, R., Canfield, P.J., 1995. Analysis of leucocytes and lymphocyte subsets in cats with naturally-occurring cryptococcosis but differing feline immunodeficiency virus status. Aust. Vet. J. 72, 93–97.

[k]From Bleavins, M.R., Brott D.A., Alvey J.D., 1993. de la Iglesia FA: flow cytometric characterization of lymphocyte subpopulations in the cynomolgus monkey (Macaca fascicularis). Vet. Immunol. Immunopathol. 37, 1–13.

BOX 14.1   A Note on Cell Phenotypes

All the cells of the body arise from a single precursor cell, the fertilized ovum. As the embryo develops and grows, cells differentiate both structurally and biochemically. They do this by activating required genes while turning off unneeded ones. One obvious result is that cells acquire a characteristic morphology. Histologic examination shows these structural differences and has provided much useful guidance regarding a cell's function. Structural differences are limited, however, in what they can tell us. For example, T and B cells look identical but differ significantly in their biochemistry and function. As a result, biochemical differences must be determined to identify functional cell types. One of the best ways to do this is to examine the proteins expressed on the cell surface. Cells express hundreds of different proteins on their surface, and their identification provides a powerful tool to characterize cells. The CD system of identifying cell surface proteins is an organized attempt to catalog these cell surface proteins.

Two otherwise identical cell populations may be distinguished by the set of cell surface molecules they express. By identifying cells in this way, it is possible not only to identify cell subpopulations but also to follow cell development and differentiation as different genes are turned on and off depending on changes in the cell's function.

In many cases, it has proven possible to identify cell subpopulations or changes in a cell's phenotype without determining the cell's functional significance. Different phenotypes occur in different domestic animal species. Students will therefore find much of the literature in this area confusing, especially if large numbers of CD molecules are reported for a specific cell phenotype.

innate cells will kill target cells that fail to express MHC molecules (see Chapter 20).

CD3 is the collective designation given to the complex of six signal-transducing proteins within the TCR. CD3 is therefore found on all T cells. Another protein, CD4, is found only on helper T cells. CD4 molecules can bind to major histocompatibility complex (MHC) class II molecules on antigen-presenting cells, and so they are found on helper T cells. A third protein, CD8, is, in contrast, only expressed on T cells that attack and kill abnormal cells, the cytotoxic T cells. CD8 molecules bind to MHC class I molecules. Most human and mouse T cells express either CD4 or CD8, but rarely both. For example, about 65% of human T cells are CD4$^+$, CD8$^-$, and 30% are CD4$^-$, CD8$^+$. The remaining T cells express neither (CD4$^-$, CD8$^-$) and are said to be double negative. The ratio of CD4$^+$ to CD8$^+$ cells in the blood may be used to estimate lymphocyte function. An elevated CD4 count implies increased lymphocyte reactivity because helper T cells predominate, whereas a high CD8 count implies depressed reactivity. The relative proportions of CD4 and CD8 cells differ between humans and other mammals (Table 14.3). Neither CD4 nor CD8 are expressed by B cells or NK cells.

CD45 is the name of a large family of TCR-linked tyrosine phosphatases that are also required for T-cell responses to antigens. They are expressed in large amounts in all T-cell populations. For example, about 10% of the T-cell surface is covered by CD45 molecules. Different forms of CD45 have been identified. For example, naïve T cells express one form of CD45, whereas stimulated and memory T cells express another.

The signal-transducing components of the B-cell antigen receptor complex are protein heterodimers formed by pairing CD79a (Ig-α) with CD79b (Ig-β). These are discussed in detail in Chapter 16.

Molecules That Regulate Lymphocyte Function

Proteins on cell surfaces serve physiological functions. Some are enzymes, some are transport proteins, and many are receptors. All cells

One uses paired α and β peptide chains (TCR α/β), and the other uses paired γ and δ chains (TCR γ/δ) (see Chapter 15). Subpopulations of B cells may use one of five different heavy chains (γ, μ, α, ε, or δ) in their BCRs. BCRs also differ from TCRs in that they are shed from the B cell in large amounts into the tissue fluid and blood, where they are called antibodies. Thus, antibodies are simply soluble BCRs.

Innate lymphoid cells do not have variable antigen receptors. Instead, they have germline-encoded receptors that can bind to molecules such as MHC molecules expressed on healthy normal cells but not on diseased, abnormal cells. Innate cells are "turned off" when they bind to these target molecules on normal cells. On the other hand,

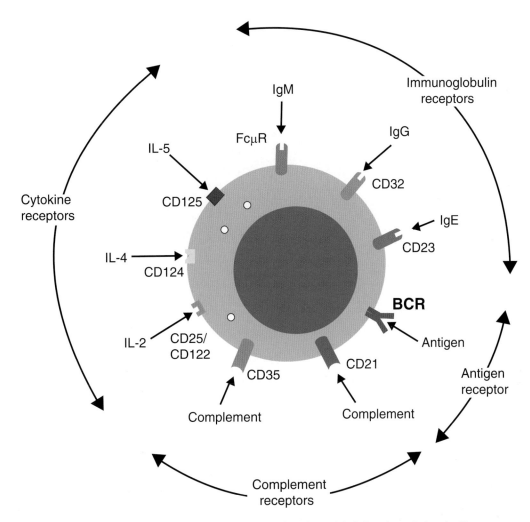

Fig. 14.6 Major surface receptors of B cells, their ligands, and their functions. *IL*, Interleukin.

Cytokine Receptors

Lymphocytes express many different cytokine receptors. Examples include CD25, a part of the interleukin-2 (IL-2) receptor; CD118, an interferon (IFN) receptor; CD120, the tumor necrosis factor (TNF) receptor; and CD210, the IL-10 receptor. (These are discussed in Chapter 21.)

Antibody Receptors

Lymphocytes receive signals from and hence must have receptors for antibodies. Since these receptors bind to the Fc regions of antibody molecules, they are called Fc receptors (FcRs). (The meaning of the term Fc can be found in Chapter 16.) The FcRs for immunoglobulin G (IgG) are designated FcγR since they bind the γ chain of IgG. Likewise, those for IgA are designated FcαR, and those for IgE are FcεR. Receptors for IgM have been identified on both B and T cells but are not well characterized.

Four different IgG receptors have been described on mouse leukocytes (Table 14.4). They are called FcγRI (CD64), FcγRII (CD32), FcγRIII (CD16), and FcγRIV. All are multichain glycoproteins. One chain usually binds the antibody, whereas the other chains are used for signal transduction. CD64 (FcγRI) is found on dendritic cells,

monocytes, and macrophages and, to a much lesser extent, on neutrophils. (It is not found on lymphocytes but is mentioned here for the sake of completeness.) CD64 binds IgG with high affinity.

CD32 (FcγRII) is found on B cells, dendritic cells, and myeloid cells. It has a moderate affinity for IgG and will therefore only bind immune complexes (antibody molecules attached to an antigen). There are three subtypes of CD32 called a, b, and c. CD32a is expressed on macrophages and neutrophils, where it is an activating receptor. It promotes phagocytosis and stimulates the release of cytokines. CD32b is found on B cells, where it is an inhibitory receptor and regulates antibody production. The function of CD32c is unclear. All three subtypes are expressed on dendritic cells and stimulate dendritic cell maturation and antigen presentation.

CD16 (FcγRIII) binds IgG with low affinity and will therefore only bind immune complexes. It is found on granulocytes, NK cells, and macrophages, but not on B cells. Signaling through CD16 can trigger NK cell activation.

Mice have an additional receptor for IgG called FcγRIV, and related proteins are found in humans, chimpanzees, rats, dogs, cats, pigs, and cattle. This receptor binds IgG2 antibodies with moderate affinity, but it does not bind IgG1 or IgG3. It is expressed exclusively on neutrophils, macrophages, and dendritic cells. (Nimmerjahn et al., 2005)

Cattle and sheep also have a unique FcR called Fcγ2R. It is not related to other mammalian FcγRs but belongs to a novel gene family that includes the IgA receptor, FcαRI (CD89), and the KIRs (see

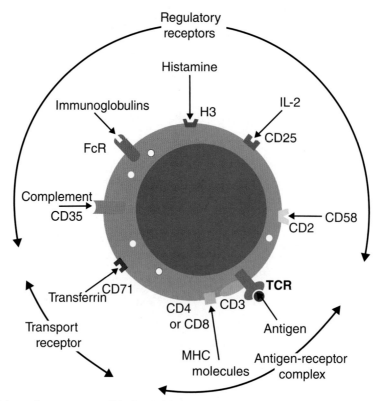

Fig. 14.7 Major surface receptors of T cells, their ligands, and their functions. *IL-2*, Interleukin-2; *MHC*, major histocompatibility complex; *TCRs*, T-cell antigen receptor.

TABLE 14.3 Surface Molecules on Peripheral Blood T Cells

Marker	Cell Percentage			
	Mouse	Bovine	Swine	Sheep
TCRα/β	85–95	5–30	14–34	5–30
TCRγ/δ	5–15	45–50	31–66	22–68
CD2	95	41–60	58–72	10–36
CD4	24	8–28	23–43	8–22
CD8	11	10–30	17–39	4–22
WC1	–	5–44	40	15–70

CD, Cluster of differentiation; *TCR*, T-cell antigen receptor; *WC1*, workshop cluster 1.

TABLE 14.4 Receptors for Immunoglobulin G (FcγR)

Property	FcγRI	FcγRII	FcγRIII	FcγRIV
CD designation	CD64	CD32	CD16	
Molecular weight (kDa)	75	39–48	50–65	
Cells	Monocytes, macrophages	B cells, macrophages granulocytes eosinophils	NK cells, granulocytes, macrophages	Neutrophils, macrophages, dendritic cells
Affinity	High	Moderate	Low	Intermediate/high
Function	Phagocytosis	B cells: inhibition Macrophages: phagocytosis	NK cells: ADCC Granulocytes: phagocytosis	Proinflammatory

CD, Cluster of differentiation; *NK*, natural killer.

Chapter 20). It is expressed on myeloid cells and binds only IgG2. It is important in promoting phagocytosis of antibody-opsonized bacteria in these species (Qiao et al., 2009).

FcαRI (CD89) is expressed on neutrophils, eosinophils, monocyte-macrophages, and dendritic cells. It binds IgA and mediates its endocytosis and recycling. FcεRI is a high-affinity IgE receptor found on mast cells and discussed in Chapter 30. It plays an important role in allergies. CD23, or FcεRII, in contrast, is a low-affinity IgE receptor expressed on activated B cells, platelets, eosinophils, macrophages, NK cells, dendritic cells, and possibly even T cells. Activated B cells can secrete soluble CD23, which then regulates allergic responses.

The polymeric Ig receptor (PIgR) and the neonatal Ig receptor (FcRn) are FcRs involved in immunoglobulin transport across epithelial surfaces such as the intestinal epithelium. They are described in Chapters 23 and 24.

Complement Receptors

There are four major complement receptors on lymphocytes (CR1 to CR4). B cells and activated T cells express CR1 (CD35), which binds C3b and C4b, and CR2 (CD21), which binds C3d and C3bi. CR2 is closely associated with the BCR and regulates B-cell responses to antigen. NK cells express CR3 and CR4.

Adherence Molecules

As discussed in Chapter 6, some cell surface molecules serve to bind cells together. They regulate signal network transmission between the cells of the immune system and control the movement of leukocytes in tissues. The cell adhesion molecules found on lymphocytes include integrins, selectins, and members of the immunoglobulin superfamily (IgSF) (Elangbam et al., 1997).

Integrins

Integrins are heterodimeric proteins formed by paired α and β chains. The β_1-integrins consist of a β_1 chain (CD29) paired with one of several different α chains (CD49). They bind cells to extracellular matrix proteins such as fibronectin, laminin, and collagen. The β_2-integrins consist of a β_2 chain (CD18) paired with one of several α chains (CD11). They control the binding of leukocytes to the vascular endothelium and bind T cells to antigen-presenting cells. For example, LFA-1 (CD11a/CD18) on a T-cell binds to its ligand, intercellular adhesion molecule-1 (ICAM-1), on the antigen-presenting cell. By prolonging and stabilizing cell interactions, this binding permits successful antigen recognition (Fig. 14.8).

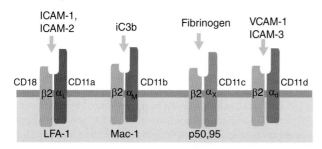

Fig. 14.8 The β_2-integrins act as cell surface adhesion molecules to link cells together so that they can communicate privately. The integrins consist of families of paired peptide chains (heterodimers). These families are based on pairing many different α chains with a limited number of β chains.

Selectins

The emigration of lymphocytes from the bloodstream into tissues is regulated by P-selectin (CD62P), L-selectin (CD62L), and E-selectin (CD62E). P- and E-selectins are found on vascular endothelial cells. When these cells are activated by inflammation, they express selectins that bind neutrophils, activated T cells, and monocytes. L-selectin binds lymphocytes to high endothelial venules in lymphoid organs (see Chapter 13).

Immunoglobulin Superfamily

Some members of the IgSF act as lymphocyte adhesion molecules. For example, ICAM-1 (CD54) binds to the integrin, CD11a/CD18 (see Fig. 14.8). ICAM-1 is normally expressed on dendritic cells and B cells. Inflammation induces ICAM-1 expression on the vascular endothelium and permits phagocytic cells to bind and move into inflamed tissues. ICAM-1 is also responsible for the migration of T cells into areas of inflammation (so-called delayed hypersensitivity reactions; see Chapter 34). Another IgSF family member is vascular cell adhesion molecule-1 (VCAM-1) or CD106. VCAM-1 is expressed on inflamed vascular endothelial cells. It binds the β_1-integrin, CD49d/CD29, on lymphocytes and monocytes.

CD58 and CD2

CD58 is the ligand for CD2. CD2 is found only on T cells, whereas CD58 is widely distributed on many cell types. When cytotoxic T cells encounter their target cells, the T-cell binds them through CD2 and CD58. CD58 facilitates T-cell attachment to any cell undergoing surveillance (see Chapter 19). CD58 is found on antigen-presenting cells such as dendritic cells and macrophages. When it binds to T cell CD2, CD58 enhances the recognition of antigen by the T cell and at the same time stimulates the antigen-presenting cell to secrete cytokines.

Changes in Phenotype

Lymphocytes do not express the same phenotype at all stages in their life cycle. A cell's phenotype depends on its maturity and activation status. For example, immature human T cells carry both CD9 and CD10. As the T cells mature within the thymus, CD9 is lost, and the cells gain CD4 and CD8. Mature thymocytes can then split into two subpopulations; one population becomes CD4+, the other becomes CD8+. The phenotype of lymphocytes also changes after exposure to antigen. For example, naïve T cells express high levels of CD45R and L-selectin and low levels of CD44. Memory T cells show the reverse of this: low levels of CD45R and L-selectin and high levels of CD44.

SPECIES DIFFERENCES

Lymphocytes of the major domestic mammals express several cell surface proteins not found in either humans or mice. The best-defined of these belong to the bovine WC1 family. WC1 are single-chain type 1 glycoproteins of 220 kDa belonging to the "scavenger receptor cysteine-rich" (SRCR) protein superfamily. These are expressed exclusively on a subpopulation of γ/δ T cells. Homologs of WC1 have been identified in pigs, camels, llamas, deer, elk, and chicken.

Horses

Horse lymphocytes express two species-specific proteins. EqWC1 is found on 70% of equine T cells, 30% of B cells, and 50% of granulocytes and may be a homolog of CD90. EqWC2 is found on granulocytes and most T cells (Antczak and Kidd, 1994).

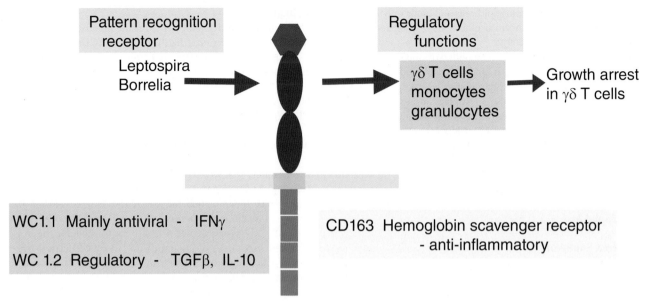

Fig. 14.9 The WC1 proteins are transmembrane glycoproteins belonging to the scavenger receptor cysteine-rich (SRCR) family. They are expressed in camels, pigs, cattle, and sheep. They are formed by multiple extracellular repeats of the SRCR class B domain. *IFNγ*, Interferonγ; *IL-10*, interleukin-10; *TGF-β*, transforming growth factor–β; *WC1*, workshop cluster 1.

Bovine

Bovine lymphocytes express several cell major surface proteins not found in either humans or mice. The best-defined of these belong to the Workshop cluster 1 (WC1) family (Hsu et al., 2015) (Fig. 14.9). Cattle possess a multigene family of 13 WC1 genes. They are expressed exclusively on γ/δ T cells. Between 50% and 99% of ruminant blood γ/δ T cells express WC1 family proteins on their surface (Telfer et al., 2015).

WC1$^+$ T cells are found in high numbers in the skin and mucus membranes as well as in the hemal nodes and the thymus. (WC1$^-$ γ/δ T cells predominate in the gut, mammary gland, and uterus). About 13 *WC1* gene family members occur in cattle, whereas 50 to 100 are found in sheep (Wijngaard et al., 1992). Bovine WC1 molecules show extensive polymorphism, and there are differences in their expression between *B.t. taurus* and *B.t. indicus*. A gene encoding WCI has been detected in the genome of the extinct aurochs (Loonie et al., 2021).

WC1 Functions

WC1 proteins serve multiple roles. Thus they function as pattern recognition receptors and can bind to surface components of some bacterial pathogens (Hsu et al., 2015). When the binding specificities of the different WC1 proteins are examined, it is clear that like other PRRs they bind to selected bacterial ligands. There is an active, antigen-binding site on one of their SRCR domains (Hsu et al., 2015). In addition, bovine WC1 proteins can serve as signaling coreceptors with the γ/δ TCRs. Individual WC1 receptors generate antigen specificity through colligation with the γ/δ TCR.

WC1+ γ/δ T cells

Cattle possess two WC1$^+$ T-cell subpopulations, WC1.1$^+$ and WC1.2$^+$. These two subpopulations differ in their ability to respond to specific pathogens. For example, WC1.1$^+$ cells can recognize and bind Leptospiral antigens as well as the Bacille Calmette-Guérin (BCG) vaccine strain of *Mycobacterium bovis*. WC1.2$^+$ cells in contrast can bind *Anaplasma marginale* and virulent strains of *M. bovis* (Yirsaw et al., 2022). WC1.1 binds Leptospiral antigens through multiple

SRCR domains. Thus, Leptospira, WC1, and γ/δTCR interact directly on the T-cell surface (Gillespie et al., 2021; Wang et al., 2011). As a result of this binding to WC1, TCR-induced activation is significantly enhanced, so that the cells respond through proliferation and IFN-γ production.

WC1$^+$ γ/δ T are also found in granulomas surrounding schistosomes and Mycobacteria. In these cases, the initial T-cell infiltration is dominated by γ/δ T cells, and this is followed by a wave of α/β T cells. A second wave of γ/δ T cells may terminate the response. These WC1$^+$ cells secrete IL-12 and IFN-γ and may promote a Th1 bias in the immune response (Baldwin et al., 2021).

In resting T cells, the WC1 and γ/δ TCR molecules exist as separate entities on the T-cell surface. However, once these cells bind antigen, the receptors come together. These cells can then be activated by stimuli acting through their TCR or through their WC1. In response, they produce TNF-α, IL-1, IL-12, and IFN-γ. This mixture suggests that they contribute to both inflammation and a Th1 bias in the bovine immune response and thus link the innate and adaptive immune systems. WC1.2$^+$ γ/δ T cells can act as Tγ/δ17 cells and produce IL-17 (Damani-Yokota et al., 2022).

WC1$^-$ γ/δ T Cells

Not all bovine γ/δ T cells express WC1. WC1$^+$ and WC1$^-$ cells have a different tissue distribution. In the spleen and uterus, the majority of T cells are WC1$^-$. In the blood, up to 50% of the γ/δ T cells can be WC1$^-$. This WC1$^-$ cell population increases with age, while WC1$^+$ cell numbers decrease.

WC1$^+$ cells can be considered to be more engaged in innate immunity, while WC1$^-$ cells are more adaptive. The WC1$^-$ γ/δ T cells appear to be more myeloid in character, whereas the positive cells are associated with the production of IFN-γ (Baldwin et al., 2015). In the absence of WC1$^+$ cells, cattle preferentially make IgG1, whereas in their presence, they make IgG2. These subpopulations also respond differently to type I IFNs. WC1$^-$ cells proliferate in response to IFN-τ, whereas WC1$^+$ cells are suppressed by IFN-τ and IFN-α. WC1-negative γ/δ cells may act as regulatory cells.

CD4 is expressed on 20% to 30% of blood lymphocytes in adult ruminants. Double-negative T cells constitute 15% to 30% of the blood T cells in young ruminants, but this may reach 80% in newborn calves. Most of these double-negative cells are γ/δ+ and WC1+.

Sheep

Sheep T cells express OvWC1 (also called T19). The isoform of this molecule expressed on α/β T cells differs from that on γ/δ T cells. In newborn lambs, γ/δ T cells account for 60% of blood T cells, but this drops to 30% by 1 year and to 5% by 5 years. The genes encoding these γ/δ T cells show much less diversity than the genes encoding their α/β T cells (O'Keeffe et al., 1999).

Pigs

Pig leukocytes express nine unique surface proteins (SWC1 to SWC9). SWC1 is expressed on resting T cells, monocytes, and granulocytes but not on B cells. It is homologous to CD52. SWC2 is homologous to CD 27 and is found on T and NK cells. SWC3 is found on monocytes and macrophages. SWC9 is expressed only by mature macrophages. Pigs are a γ/δ-high species. In young pigs, up to 66% of blood T cells are γ/δ positive, but this drops to 25% to 50% in adults. Pigs have two subpopulations of γ/δ T cells (Gerner et al., 2015). One is CD2+ and the other is CD2−, which have not been identified in other species (Binns, 1994). Some pig γ/δ T cells can function as antigen-presenting cells using MHC class II molecules. Up to 60% of T cells in pig blood are double positive (CD4+, CD8+) (Piriou-Guzylack and Salmon, 2008). The rest are predominantly double negative (CD4−, CD8−). Some CD4+ T cells also express CD8α/α homodimers and are cytotoxic (Yang and Parkhouse, 1996).

Dogs and Cats

In dogs, CD4 is expressed on neutrophils and macrophages but not on monocytes, whereas in cats, CD4 is found on only a subset of T cells and their precursors.

LYMPHOCYTE MITOGENS

In addition to their surface proteins, lymphocytes can be characterized by the stimulants that make them divide in vitro. The most important of these are the lectins that bind to cell surface glycoproteins and trigger cell division (Box 14.2). These lectins are commonly obtained from plants. Examples include phytohemagglutinin (PHA) obtained from the red kidney bean (*Phaseolus vulgaris*), concanavalin A (Con A) obtained from the jack bean (*Canavalis ensiformis*), and pokeweed mitogen (PWM) obtained from the pokeweed plant (*Phytolacca americana*). Lectins bind sugar residues on glycoprotein side chains. For example, PHA binds *N*-acetylgalactosamine, and Con A binds α-mannose and α-glucose. Not all lymphocytes respond equally well to all lectins. Thus, PHA primarily stimulates T cells, although it has a slight effect on B cells. Con A is also a T-cell mitogen, whereas PWM acts on both T and B cells.

Although the plant lectins are the most efficient lymphocyte mitogens, mitogens may also be found in other unexpected sources. For example, an extract from the snail *Helix pomata* stimulates T cells, whereas lipopolysaccharide from Gram-negative bacteria stimulates B cells. Other important B-cell mitogens include proteases, such as trypsin, and Fc fragments of immunoglobulins. BCG vaccine, an avirulent strain of *M. bovis* that is used as a vaccine against tuberculosis, is a T-cell mitogen. These mitogens can assist in the differentiation of T and B cells and, by measuring the response provoked, provide an estimate of lymphocyte responsiveness (Becker and Misfeldt, 1993).

BOX 14.2 How to Measure Mitogenicity

To measure the effect of mitogens, lymphocytes are grown in tissue culture. Lymphocytes can be obtained directly from blood. The lymphocytes are cultured for at least 24 hours before the mitogen is added. Once this is done, they begin to divide, synthesize new DNA, and take up any available nucleotides from the medium. It is usual to incorporate a small quantity of thymidine labeled with the radioactive isotope of hydrogen, tritium (^{3}H), in the tissue culture fluid. The thymidine is only incorporated into the DNA of cells that are dividing. After about 24 hours, the cultured cells are separated from the tissue culture fluid, either by centrifugation or filtration, and their radioactivity is counted. The amount of radioactivity in the mitogen-treated cells may be compared with that in an untreated lymphocyte culture. This ratio is called the stimulation index (see Fig. 34.8). As an alternative to the use of tritiated thymidine, a radiolabeled amino acid such as ^{14}C-leucine can be used. Uptake of this compound indicates increased protein synthesis by the cells.

REFERENCES

Antczak, D.F., Kydd, J., 1994. Equine leukocyte antigens. Vet. Immunol. Immunopathol. 42, 1–116.

Baldwin, C.L., Damani-Yokota, P., Kirsaw, A., Loonie, K., et al., 2021. Special features of γδ T cells in ruminants. Mol. Immunol. 134, 161–169.

Baldwin, C.L., Telfer, J.C., 2015. The bovine model for elucidating the role of γδ T cells in controlling infectious diseases of importance to cattle and humans. Mol. Immunol. 66, 35–47.

Becker, B.A., Misfeldt, M.L., 1993. Evaluation of the mitogen-induced proliferation and cell surface differentiation antigens of lymphocytes from pigs 1 to 30 days of age. J. Anim. Sci. 71, 2073–2078.

Binns, R.M., 1994. The null/γδ+ T cell family in the pig. Vet. Immunol. Immunopathol. 43, 69–77.

Damani-Yokota, P., Zhang, F., Gillespie, A., Park, H., et al., 2022. Transcriptional programing and gene regulation in WC1+ γδ T cell populations. Mol. Immunol. 142, 50–62.

Elangbam, C.S., Qualls Jr, C.W., Dahlgren, R.R., 1997. Cell adhesion molecules: update. Vet. Pathol. 34, 61–73.

Gerner, W., Talker, S.C., Koinig, H.C., Sedlak, C., Mair, K.H., Saalmuller, A., 2015. Phenotypic and functional differentiation of porcine alpha/beta T cells: current knowledge and available tools. Mol. Immunol. 66 (1), 3–13.

Gillespie, A., Gervasi, M.G., Sathiyaseelan, T., Connelley, T., et al., 2021. Gamma delta TCR and the WC1 coreceptor interactions in response to Leptospira using imaging flow cytometry and STORM. Front. Immunol. https://doi.org/10.3389/fimmu.2021.712123.

Hsu, H., Chen, C., Nenninger, A., Holz, L., Baldwin, C.L., Telfer, J.C., 2015. WC1 is a hybrid gammadelta TCR coreceptor and pattern recognition receptor for pathogenic bacteria. J. Immunol. 194 (5), 2280–2288.

Loonie, K., Gillespie, A., Baldwin, C., 2021. The WC1 γδ T cell pathogen receptor of ruminants is preserved in the genome of the ancient extinct auroch. Immunogenetics. https://doi.org/10.1007/s00251-021-01211-y.

Nimmerjahn, F., Bruhns, P., Horluchi, K., Ravetch, J.V., 2005. FcγRIV: a novel FcR with distinct IgG subclass specificity. Immunity 23, 41–51.

O'Keeffe, M.A., Metcalfe, S.A., Cunningham, C.P., Walker, I.D., 1999. Sheep CD4+ αβ T cells express novel members of the T19 multigene family. Immunogenetics 49, 45–55.

Piriou-Guzylack, L., Salmon, H., 2008. Membrane markers of the immune cells in swine: an update. Vet. Res. 39, 54.

Qiao, S., Yang, Y., Liu, Y., Zhang, G., Xi, J., 2009. Characterization and ligand specificity of sheep IgG2 receptor. Immunogenetics 61, 597–601.

Telfer, J.C., Baldwin, C.L., 2015. Bovine gamma delta T cells and the function of gamma delta T cell specific WC1 co-receptors. Cell Immunol. 296 (1), 76–86.

Wang, F., Herzig, C.T., Chen, C., Hsu, H., Baldwin, C.L., Telfer, J.C., 2011. Scavenger receptor WC1 contributes to the gammadelta T cell response to Leptospira. Mol. Immunol. 48 (6-7), 801–809.

Wijngaard, P.L.J., Metzelaar, M.J., MacHugh, N.D., et al., 1992. Molecular characterization of the WC1 antigen expressed specifically on bovine CD4⁻CD8⁻ γ/δ T lymphocytes. J. Immunol. 149, 3273–3277.

Yang, H., Parkhouse, R.M.E., 1996. Phenotypic classification of porcine lymphocyte subpopulations in blood and lymphoid tissues. Immunology 89, 76–83.

Yirsaw, A.W., Gillespie, A., Zhang, F., Smith, T.P.L., et al., 2022. Defining the caprine γδ T cell WC1 multigenic array and evaluation of its expressed sequences and gene structure among goat breeds and relative to cattle. Immunogenetics. https://doi.org/10.1007/s00251-022-01254-9.

Helper T Cells: Diverse Responses to Antigens

CHAPTER OUTLINE

When T cells emerge from the thymus they migrate to lymphoid and nonlymphoid tissues where they remain quiescent until they encounter an antigen that binds to their antigen receptors. It is estimated that there are about 2×10^{11} naive T cells in a human body with 10^{10} different antigen receptors (TCRs) (Chopp et al., 2023). When they encounter the appropriate antigen, these T cells differentiate into subpopulations based on the antigen, the microenvironment, and other signals. There are four major populations of lymphocytes with antigen-binding receptors. These include helper and regulatory T cells that regulate immune responses; effector or cytotoxic T cells that destroy abnormal cells; and B cells that produce antibodies. Each of these cell types responds to antigens that bind to their receptors. This chapter describes the first of these major lymphocyte populations, the helper T cells.

The cells of the adaptive immune system must respond appropriately to diverse microbial pathogens. They must be able to assume different functional configurations depending on the nature of the microbial challenge. This is largely achieved by employing differentiated T-cell subpopulations. For example, mammals can mount a cell-mediated, type 1 immune response by activating Th1 cells, generating cytotoxic T cells, destroying virus-infected cells, and hence effectively combatting viral invasion. Alternatively, they can turn on an antibody-mediated immune response by activating Th2 cells and B cells and so combat extracellular bacteria. In other situations, Th17 cells may be activated and promote local inflammation or generate antiviral interferons. If required, they can also act as regulatory (Treg) cells and control inappropriate responses. T cells can also change their phenotype rapidly if the situation demands it. This flexibility results from the use of multiple polymorphic gene families that are selected based on the nature of the invader, fine-tuned to identify specific invaders, activate the appropriate defenses, and so maximize an animal's chances of survival. Thus the emergence of multiple T-cell subsets, when correctly selected, will yield the best results, namely, survival. The selection process involves the use of pattern recognition receptors, antigen-binding by major histocompatibility complex (MHC) encoded receptors, and the use of very specific antigen receptors by T and B cells. The responding immune system makes a choice between different T-cell subsets. These subsets are triggered by different stimuli depending upon the nature of the invaders and their routes of invasion. The responding T cells employ different transcription factors to generate different cytokine mixtures. These cytokines, in turn, trigger different forms of immune defense, ideally optimized to rapidly eliminate invaders with a minimum of damage to the defender.

When DCs present their processed antigen to helper T cells, they generate three signals. The first signal is delivered when T-cell antigen receptors bind antigen fragments attached to MHC class II molecules. The second signal provides the T cells with additional costimulation through other cell surface receptors such as adhesion molecules. The third signal determines the direction in which naïve helper T cells will develop and is generated by cytokines (Walsh and Mills, 2013). For example, some microbial antigens trigger DCs to secrete IL-12. These are called DC1 cells since their IL-12 activates Th1 cells and so triggers type 1 responses. Other microbial antigens can cause DCs to secrete IL-4 and IL-6. These cytokines stimulate Th2 differentiation and are produced by DC2 cells. They stimulate type 2 responses. It may also be that the same dendritic cell can promote a type 1 or type 2 response, depending on the dose and type of antigen encountered. The response may also depend on its location. For example, DCs in the intestine or airways preferentially secrete IL-4 and thus promote type 2 IgA–mediated antibody responses.

Because MHC molecules can bind many different antigenic peptides, any individual peptide will only be displayed in small amounts. T cells must be able to recognize these few specific peptide-MHC complexes among a vast excess of MHC molecules carrying irrelevant peptides. The number of MHC-peptide complexes signaling to the T cell is also important since the stimulus required to trigger a T-cell response can vary greatly depending upon circumstances.

THE IMMUNOGLOBULIN SUPERFAMILY

Peptide chains spontaneously fold into structures called domains. Complete protein molecules are then constructed by linking multiple domains together. Each domain usually has a specialized function. For example, in proteins located on cell surfaces, the membrane-binding domain contains hydrophobic amino acids that can penetrate the cell membrane lipid bilayer. Other domains may be responsible for the structural stability of a protein or its biological activities. In antibody (immunoglobulin) molecules, one domain is used to bind antigen, and other domains are responsible for cell binding. The presence of similar domains in diverse proteins suggests that they have a common origin, and proteins may be classified into families or superfamilies based on their domain structure.

Proteins belonging to the immunoglobulin superfamily play key roles in immunity. The members of this superfamily all contain at least one immunoglobulin domain. In a typical immunoglobulin domain, the peptide chains weave back and forth to form a pleated sheet that folds into a taco-like structure. Immunoglobulin domains were first

identified in antibody molecules (immunoglobulins). They have since been found in many other proteins. Important proteins with multiple immunoglobulin domains include the B-cell antigen receptors (BCRs), the T-cell antigen receptors (TCRs), and the MHC class I and II molecules (Fig. 15.1). All of the members of this superfamily are receptors; most are found on cell surfaces; and none has enzymatic activity. Many responses in the immune system are triggered by interactions between cells bearing two different members of the superfamily, for example, between TCR and MHC molecules.

T-CELL ANTIGEN RECEPTORS

Unlike innate immune responses that are triggered by a limited number of molecular patterns from pathogenic microbes, the lymphocytes of the adaptive immune system are able to recognize and respond to "everything," or at least to a large number of very diverse foreign antigens. They can do this because they have receptors that bind these antigens and, under the right conditions, respond by mounting cell-mediated or antibody-mediated immune responses.

Antigen-Binding Component

Foreign antigens are captured by antigen-processing cells and then presented to helper T cells. Each T cell is covered by about 30,000 identical antigen receptors (TCRs). If these receptors bind sufficient antigen in the correct manner, the helper T cell will respond and initiate an immune response. It does this by secreting multiple cytokines, dividing, and differentiating. As you will learn later, the other antigen-responsive cell populations, B cells and cytotoxic T cells, cannot respond to antigens unless they too are stimulated by helper T cells.

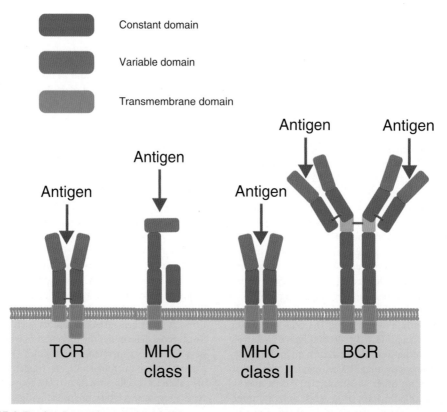

Fig. 15.1 The four key antigen receptors of the immune system—T-cell antigen receptor (TCR), major histocompatibility complex (MHC) class I, MHC class II, B-cell antigen receptor (BCR)—are each constructed using immunoglobulin domains as building blocks. Each binds antigen through the use of variable domains. All are members of the immunoglobulin superfamily.

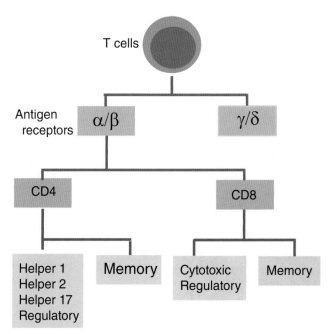

Fig. 15.2 T cells can be divided into subpopulations based on the antigen receptors they employ, on the accessory molecules that support their activity, and ultimately on their functions.

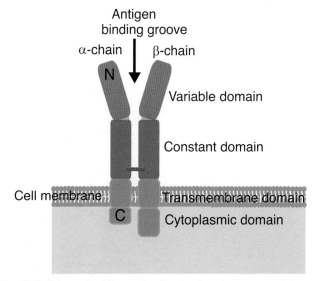

Fig. 15.3 Schematic diagram showing the domain structure of the two peptide chains that make up the antigen-binding component of an α/β T-cell antigen receptor.

Each TCR is constructed from multiple glycoprotein chains. Two of these chains are paired to form the antigen-binding site; the remaining chains in the complex form a cluster that transmits the signal generated by antigen binding to the cell. Two major types of TCR have been identified based on their use of antigen-binding chains (Fig. 15.2). One type employs chains designated γ and δ (γ/δ) chains. The other employs α and β (α/β) chains. In humans, carnivores, and rodents, 90%–99% of T cells use α/β chains. In calves, lambs, and piglets up to 66% of T cells use γ/δ chains (Morath and Schamel, 2020).

The four antigen-binding chains (α, β, γ, and δ) are similar in structure, although they differ in size as a result of variations in glycosylation. Thus, the α chain is 43–49 kDa, the β chain is 38–44 kDa, the γ chain is 36–46 kDa, and the δ chain is 40 kDa. Each chain is constructed from four domains (Fig. 15.3). The N-terminal domain contains about 100 amino acids, and its sequence varies greatly among T cells. This is therefore called the variable (V) domain. The second domain contains about 150 amino acids. Its amino acid sequence does not vary, so it is called the constant (C) domain. A third, very small domain consisting of 20 hydrophobic amino acids passes through the T-cell membrane. The C-terminal domain within the cytoplasm of the T cell is only 5–15 amino acids long. The paired chains are linked by a disulfide bond between their constant domains to form a stable heterodimer (Fig. 15.4). As a result, a groove is formed between the two V domains that function as the antigen-binding site. The precise shape of this antigen-binding groove varies among different TCRs because of variations in the V domain amino acid sequences. The specificity of the binding between a TCR and an antigen is determined by the shape of this groove.

Within each V domain are smaller regions where the amino acid sequence is very highly variable. These are the regions that actually come into contact with the antigen. For this reason, they are called the hypervariable or complementarity-determining regions (CDR). The antigen-binding site of the TCR is formed by the CDRs from each chain that lines the groove. The rest of the V domain outside the CDRs has a constant sequence and is called the framework region.

Signal Transduction Component

CD3 Complex

The ability of the immune system to mount a rapid and appropriate response to a specific invader centers on the responses of the responding T cells. It is they that make the decision that will result in survival or death. Much of this decision-making depends upon the signals sent to the T cell by bound antigen together with multiple costimulatory signals. A key part of this pathway is the signal-transducing component of the TCR. When antigen binds to its TCR a signal is generated that triggers the T-cell response. The paired antigen-binding chains of each TCR are associated with a cluster of signal-transducing proteins called the CD3 complex (Fig. 15.5). The CD3 complex consists of six chains (γ, ε, ζ, and δ) arranged as three dimers γ-ε, δ-ε, and ζ-ζ. The TCR β chain is linked to the γ-ε dimer and the TCR α chain is linked to the δ-ε dimer (Box 8.1).

CD4 and CD8

Two additional proteins closely associated with the TCR, are called CD4 and CD8. CD4 is a single-chain molecule of 55 kDa, while CD8 is a dimer of 68 kDa (one chain of CD8 is called α, the other is β. In humans, pigs, mice, and cats, CD8 is an α-β heterodimer or, less commonly, an α-α homodimer). CD4 and CD8 determine the class of antigen-presenting MHC molecule that can be recognized by the T cell (Fig. 15.6). For example, CD4, found only on helper T cells, cross-links to MHC class II molecules on antigen-presenting cells. CD8, in contrast, is found only on cytotoxic T cells, and it binds MHC class a molecules expressed on virus-infected or other abnormal cells. Both CD4 and CD8 enhance TCR signal transduction by tightly binding the T cell to the antigen-presenting cell through the MHC.

COSTIMULATORS

The binding of a T-cell antigen receptor to an antigen-MHC complex is not sufficient by itself to trigger a helper T-cell response. Additional signals are needed if the T cell is to respond fully. For example, adhesion molecules must bind the T cells and antigen-presenting cells firmly together and so permit prolonged, strong signaling between the cells. TCR-antigen binding then triggers the initial signaling steps.

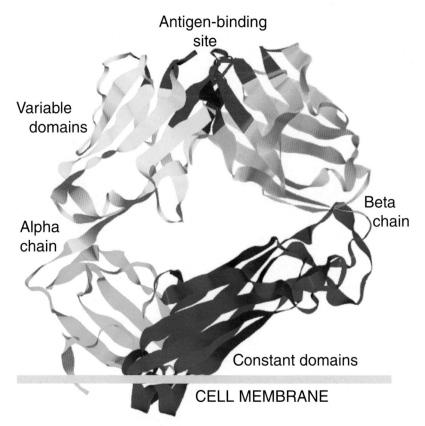

Fig. 15.4 A "Ribbon diagram" showing the three-dimensional structure of a T-cell antigen receptor α/β dimer. Courtesy Dr. B. Breaux.

Receptors on antigen-presenting cells also bind to their ligands on T cells and amplify these signals. The helper T cells must also be stimulated by cytokines secreted by the antigen-presenting cells. These cytokines determine the way in which a T cell responds to antigen, turning on some pathways and turning off others. Multiple cellular receptor pairs must be stimulated in order to fully activate T cells and determine how they will respond. This is called costimulation.

CD40-CD154 Signaling

CD40 is a receptor expressed on antigen-presenting cells. Its ligand is CD154, expressed on helper T cells (Fig. 15.7). When CD154 and CD40 bind, signals are sent in both directions. The signal from the antigen-presenting cell to the T cell causes it to express a receptor called CD28. The signal from the T cell to the antigen-presenting cell stimulates it to express either CD80 or CD86. CD40-CD154 signaling also stimulates the antigen-presenting cell to secrete multiple cytokines, including interleukin-1 (IL-1), IL-6, IL-8, IL-12, CCL3, and tumor necrosis factor–α (TNF-α) (Clarke, 2000).

CD28-CD80/CD86 Signaling

CD28, a receptor induced by CD40-CD154 signaling on T cells, has two alternative ligands: either CD80 on dendritic cells, macrophages, and activated B cells or CD86 on B cells. When CD80 or CD86 binds to CD28, signals are generated that cause the T cell, in turn, to express yet another receptor, CTLA-4. CTLA-4 may bind to either CD80 or CD86. The binding of CD28 to its ligands amplifies the stimulus to the T cell eightfold. CD28 stimulation enhances the production of IL-2 and other cytokines, upregulates cell survival genes, promotes energy

metabolism, and facilitates T-cell division. On the other hand, when CTLA-4 binds to CD80 or 86, T-cell activation is suppressed. The balance between these opposing signals delivered to T cells through these two receptors, CD28 and CTLA-4, regulates the intensity of T-cell responses. (Inhibitors of CTLA-4 enhance T-cell cytotoxicity and have proven to be highly effective anticancer treatments [see Chapter 36].)

Resting antigen-presenting cells express neither CD80 nor CD86. It takes 48–72 hours after T cell CD154 binds to CD40 before the antigen-presenting cells begin to express CD80/86 and the T cells express CTLA-4. CD80 and CD86 can bind to either CD28 or CTLA-4. However, because CTLA-4 binds these molecules with a higher affinity than does CD28, the inhibitory effect of CTLA-4 gradually predominates. When CTLA-4 binds to CD80 on antigen-presenting cells, it induces the production of indoleamine dioxygenase, an enzyme that destroys tryptophan. In the absence of this amino acid, T cells cannot respond to antigen, and so the T-cell response is terminated (see Chapter 21).

Costimulatory Cytokines

Cytokines, as described in Chapter 9, are proteins that regulate immune cell functions. Antigen-presenting cells are major sources of these cytokines. Antigen-presenting cells are triggered to produce cytokines by many different stimuli. These include microbial PAMPs binding to TLRs, as well as T cells signaling through CD40 and CD154. As described in Chapter 11, different dendritic cell populations secrete different cytokine mixtures. These mixtures in turn determine the nature of the helper T-cell response. For example, IL-12 from cDC1 cells promotes the differentiation of Th1 cells. Further differentiation is promoted by IFN-γ and IL-18. In the absence of IL-12, T cells differentiate into Th2 cells, and their further differentiation is promoted by IL-4, -13, -25, -33, and TSLP. cDC2 dendritic cells and macrophages stimulated through TLR2 secrete IL-23. This cytokine, together with

IL-6 and transforming growth factor–β (TGF-β), results in the development of Th17 cells (Fig. 15.8).

Adhesion Molecules

In addition to the dialog mediated by costimulatory molecules, T cells, and antigen-presenting cells stimulate each other most effectively if they are bound together by adhesion molecules such as the integrins. For example, CD2 and CD11a/CD18 on T cells bind to their

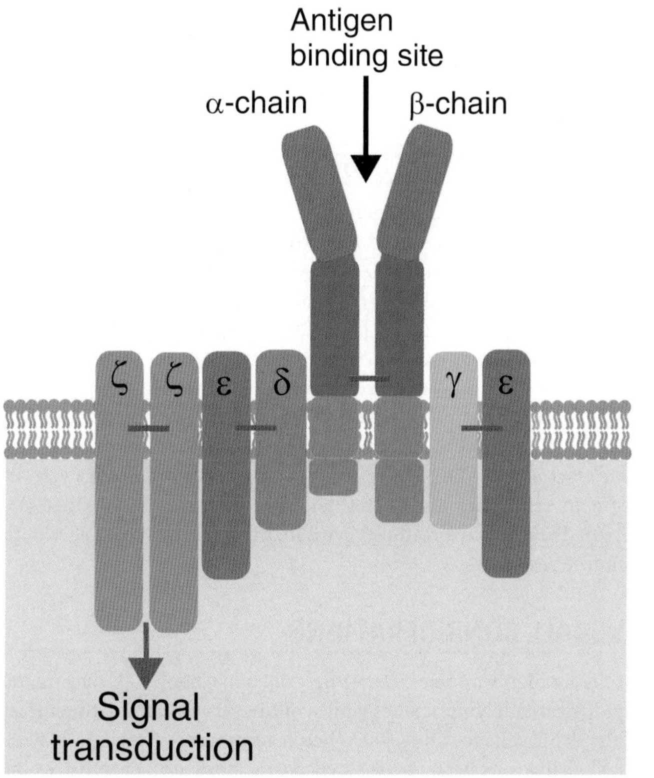

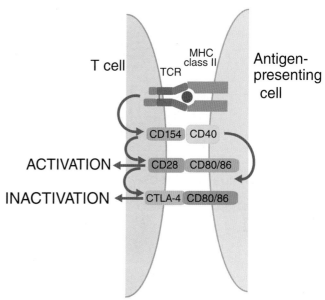

Fig. 15.7 Antigen-presenting cells and helper T cells engage in a dialog. Thus binding of antigen to the T-cell antigen receptor (TCR) causes the T cell to express CD40 ligand (CD154). This engages CD40 on the antigen-presenting cell. As a result, CD28 and CD152 are expressed on the T cell, and CD80 or CD86 is expressed on the antigen-presenting cell. Depending on which receptors are engaged, the T cell may be stimulated or suppressed. *MHC,* Major histocompatibility complex.

Fig. 15.5 Overall structure of the T-cell antigen receptor (TCRs)/CD3 complex. The signal transduction proteins are collectively classified as CD3. About 80% of α/β TCRs use ζ-ζ dimers. The remaining 20% use δ-ε heterodimers. Most γ/δ TCRs probably use a completely different signal transduction complex.

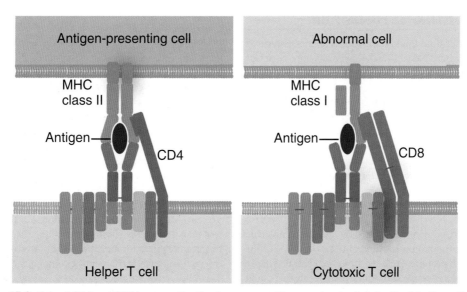

Fig. 15.6 Role of CD4 and CD8 in promoting T-cell responses. These molecules link the T cell to the antigen-presenting cell, binding the two cells together and ensuring that an effective signal is transmitted between them. CD4 binds to major histocompatibility complex (MHC) class I molecules. This interaction is seen in Fig. 10.6A.

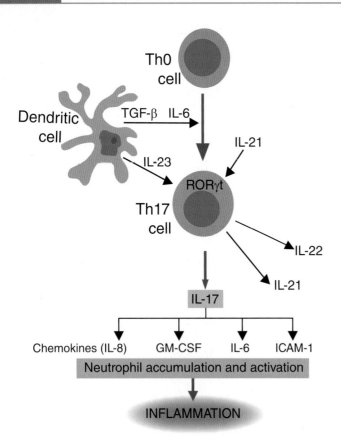

Fig. 15.8 The induction of Th17 cells by exposure to a cytokine mixture containing transforming growth factor–β (TGF-β) and interleukin (IL)-6. Differentiation is promoted by IL-21 and maintained by IL-23. Th17 cells promote neutrophil accumulation and acute inflammation. *GM-CSF,* Granulocyte-macrophage colony-stimulating factor.

ligands CD58 and CD54 on antigen-presenting cells and bind the cells together. Once tightly bound, an immunological synapse forms where the cells come into contact (Zhang and Wang, 2012).

IMMUNOLOGICAL SYNAPSE FORMATION

Cell membranes consist of fluid lipid bilayers that contain segregated areas called lipid rafts, where patches in the membrane are enriched in sphingolipids, cholesterol, and proteins. Small rafts are distributed evenly over the surface of resting T cells. When a T cell and an antigen-presenting cell come into contact, their cell membrane rafts aggregate so that the TCR-peptide-MHC complexes and the costimulatory receptors cluster together in the area of contact to form an immunological synapse (Fig. 15.9; Janes et al., 2000). This synapse consists of concentric rings of molecular complexes called supramolecular activation clusters (SMACs). They form a characteristic "bull's eye structure" consisting of a central (c) SMAC surrounded by a peripheral (p) SMAC and an outer ring (Dustin, 2014). The cSMAC of Th1 cells contains the MHC and TCR molecules as well as CD4, CD3, CD2, CD28, CD80/86, and CD40/154. The pSMAC contains CD45, the adhesion molecule ICAM-1, and leukocyte function-associated antigen–1 (LFA-1). The third, outer ring contains proteins excluded from the central synapse such as CD43. (CD43 is a very large anti-adhesive molecule that could interfere with the functioning of the synapse) (Nel, 2002).

Th2 cells, in contrast, do not form a "bull's eye" synapse with APCs. They form multifocal immunological synapses at high antigen concentrations (Thauland et al., 2008). Whereas the immunological synapse

is on the cell surface, mitochondria in the cytosol cluster beneath the synapse and reduce the local concentration of calcium ions. This activates Ca channels in the plasma membrane, resulting in a sustained Ca influx and activation of transcription factors such as NF-AT.

It is important to note that T cells may initially form synapses with multiple antigen-presenting cells but then polarize toward the cell providing the strongest stimulus. Thus, in effect, the T cell selects the cell presenting an antigen that binds most strongly to its TCR. Once signaling is complete, the synapse is endocytosed and degraded, terminating cell interactions (Padhan and Varma, 2010).

SIGNAL TRANSDUCTION

Once a TCR binds to antigen on a presenting cell and an immunological synapse forms, the receptor signals to the T cell (Nel and Slaughter, 2002). Several TCRs cluster so that the immunoreceptor tyrosine-based activation motifs on the CD3 chains can activate their tyrosine kinases (see Chapter 9). These form a signaling complex that acts through calcineurin to activate NF-AT. It also activates the Ras-mitogen-activated protein kinase pathway that triggers AP-1 production and a protein kinase C–dependent pathway that activates NF-κB. These three transcription factors activate multiple cytokine genes (see Fig. 9.11). As a result, the T cells enter the cell cycle and begin to synthesize and secrete another mixture of cytokines (Fig. 15.10). These newly produced cytokines trigger the next stages of the immune responses.

OVERALL CONSIDERATIONS

T cells are highly mobile cells. As described in Chapter 11, they migrate rapidly through lymph nodes while continuously scanning the surfaces of dendritic cells for antigens. When it recognizes a foreign antigen, a T cell changes its behavior. It slows down, stops, and eventually binds strongly to the antigen-presenting cell and forms a synapse. Whether or not a T cell stops depends on how strongly it binds to the target antigen. It will not stop for weakly binding antigens.

Once the synapse forms, TCRs and costimulatory molecules signal to the T cell. However, the TCR does not function simply as an on/off switch. Instead, differences in the strength of binding, in the amount of costimulation, and in the duration of the cell interaction determine the nature of a T-cell response.

Because MHC molecules can bind many different antigenic peptides, any individual peptide will only be displayed in small amounts. T cells must be able to recognize these few specific peptide-MHC complexes among a vast excess of MHC molecules carrying irrelevant peptides on the cell surface. The number of MHC-peptide complexes signaling to the T cell is also important since the stimulus needed to trigger a T-cell response varies. For example, only a single MHC-peptide complex is needed to trigger a cytotoxic CD8+ T-cell response. On the other hand, at least 8000 TCRs must bind antigen for a helper CD4+ T cell to become activated in the absence of CD28, but only about 1000 TCRs need to be engaged if CD28 is present (Fig. 15.11).

The duration of signaling also determines a T cell's response. In the presence of appropriate costimulation, T cells need to bind DCs for less than 15 seconds (Brodovitch et al., 2013). Sustained signaling is, however, required for maximal T-cell activation. During prolonged cell interactions, each MHC-peptide complex may trigger up to 200 TCRs. This serial triggering depends on the kinetics of TCR-ligand interaction. CD28, for example, reduces the time needed to trigger a T cell and lowers the threshold for TCR triggering. Adhesion molecules stabilize the binding of T cells to antigen-processing cells and allow the signal to be sustained for hours.

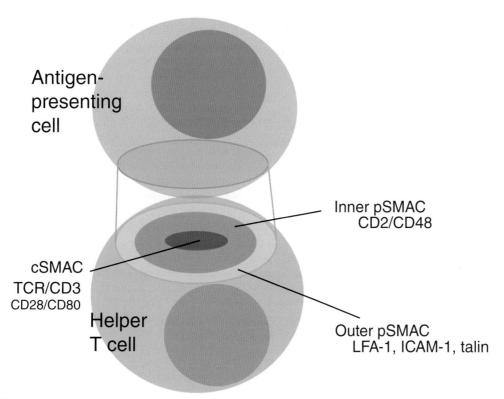

Fig. 15.9 Interaction between a T cell and an antigen-presenting cell generates the supramolecular structure called an immunological synapse. Thus a series of concentric rings supramolecular activation clusters (SMACs) form around the interacting T-cell antigen receptor–major histocompatibility complex (TCR-MHC) complex. These rings contain different costimulating molecules depending upon whether they are central or peripheral.

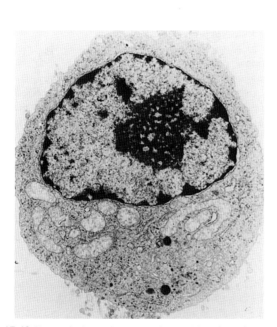

Fig. 15.10 Transmission electron micrograph of a lymphoblast. Compare this with an unstimulated lymphocyte in Fig. 14.2. Note the extensive cytoplasm, ribosomes, and large mitochondria. Courtesy Dr. S. Linthicum.

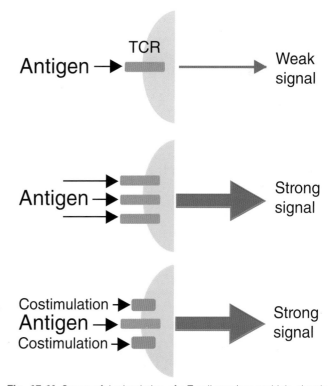

Fig. 15.11 Successful stimulation of a T cell requires multiple signals. Depending on the antigen, the T cell may be activated by signals from multiple T-cell antigen receptors (TCRs) or by appropriate costimulation.

Naïve T cells have strict requirements for activation. They must receive a sustained signal for at least 10 hours in the presence of costimulation or for up to 30 hours in its absence. This level of costimulation can only be provided by dendritic cells, which supply high levels of costimulatory and adhesion molecules. In contrast, other antigen-presenting cells act only transiently. Although macrophages and B cells can briefly trigger a TCR, they are unable to complete the process and thus fail to activate naïve T cells. Once primed, however, T cells require about an hour to reach commitment. Only then can they be activated by macrophages and B cells. In the absence of effective costimulation, T cells undergo abortive activation. They do not divide or produce cytokines but either become unresponsive to antigen (anergic) or undergo apoptosis.

SUPERANTIGENS

Fewer than 1 in 10,000 T cells can bind and respond to any specific foreign epitope. However, some microbial molecules called superantigens are unique in that they may stimulate as many as one in five T cells. These molecules are not simply nonspecific mitogens. Superantigens only activate T cells with specific TCR Vβ domains. Unlike conventional antigens that must bind within the grooves of both an MHC molecule and a TCR, superantigens directly link the TCR Vβ domain to the MHC class II molecule on the antigen-presenting cell. All superantigens come from microbial sources such as streptococci, staphylococci, and mycoplasma and from viruses such as rabies. The immune responses to superantigens are not MHC restricted (i.e., they do not depend on specific MHC haplotypes), but the presence of MHC antigens is required for an effective response since superantigens do not bind to the antigen-binding groove of the MHC class II molecule but attach elsewhere on its surface (Fig. 15.12). Because of this strong binding, superantigens trigger a powerful T-cell response. Some superantigens may stimulate the secretion of so many cytokines that they trigger a toxic shock syndrome (see Chapter 8).

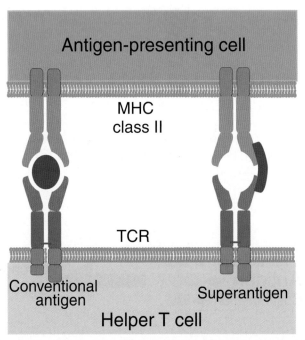

Fig. 15.12 Differences in binding to a T-cell antigen receptor (TCR) between a conventional antigenic peptide that fills the groove between the α and β chains as opposed to a superantigen that binds only to the β chain. *MHC,* Major histocompatibility complex.

HELPER T-CELL SUBPOPULATIONS

As pointed out at the beginning of this chapter, the immune system has to be flexible if it is to respond to a multitude of diverse invaders. Much of this flexibility comes from T cells. As naïve CD4+ T cells develop and differentiate, four major subpopulations emerge. They are classified into helper 1 (Th1), helper 2 (Th2), helper 17 (Th17), and regulatory (Treg) cells, and each is distinguished by the mixture of cytokines that they secrete (Fig. 15.13). As always, many of the details of their function have been investigated in mice and humans, and it must not be assumed that they function in a completely identical manner in other domestic mammals. Immune responses mediated through Th1 cells are classified as type 1 immune responses. Likewise, those mediated by Th2 cells are classified as type 2 responses. Type 3 immune responses are mediated by Th17 cells (Annunziato and Romagnani, 2015).

Th1 Cells

The production of Th1 cells is driven by IL-12 from antigen-presenting dendritic cells (cDC1), macrophages (M1), and B cells plus costimulation by CD80. Complete Th1-cell activation, proliferation, and IFN-γ production are achieved by additional stimulation from IL-18. IL-18 and IFN-γ thus reinforce each other's activities. These cytokines activate the transcription factor T-bet. T-bet is the master regulator of Th1-cell differentiation. Once activated, Th1 cells produce IL-2, IFN-γ, TNF-α, and lymphotoxin (TNF-β) (Fig. 15.14). Th1 cells promote cell-mediated immune responses such as macrophage activation and are strongly protective. They thus generate immunity to intracellular organisms such as mycobacteria and viruses (Fig. 15.15). The "type 1"-associated cytokines may also inhibit type 2 immune responses (see later).

Interferon-γ

Interferon-γ has some antiviral activity, but its major function is the mediation of Th1-cell responses (Fig. 15.16). IFN-γ is mainly produced by Th1 cells, CD8+ cytotoxic T cells, and natural killer (NK) cells, with lesser amounts from antigen-presenting cells, B cells, and natural killer (NKT) T cells (see Chapter 20). It activates cells through the JAK-STAT pathway. It promotes macrophage activation, suppresses Th2 cells, and enhances NK cell activities (Box 15.1).

Interleukin-2

IL-2 is produced by activated CD4+ Th1 cells. Some are also produced by CD8+ cells, NKT cells (see Chapter 20), dendritic cells, and mast cells. Its targets are T, B, and NK cells and macrophages. IL-2 is a potent stimulator of T-cell proliferation, IFN-γ production, and antibody production by B cells. It enhances the cytotoxicity of CD8+ and NK cells (Fig. 15.17). It promotes T-cell differentiation into Th1 and Th2 subsets while also inhibiting Th17 differentiation. IL-2 is essential for the survival of regulatory T cells as well as for activation-induced cell death. Thus, it has a broad range of essential functions.

Th2 Cells

Th2 cells are responsible for protective type 2 immune responses including resistance to parasitic helminths and tissue repair. They are regulated in turn by dendritic cells. Classical type 2 dendritic cells (cDC2) preferentially promote Th2 cell differentiation. The major Th2 stimulators are IL-33, IL-25, and TSLP. These Th2 cells respond optimally to antigen presented by cDC2 and macrophages, and less well to antigen presented by B cells. The cDC2 cells provide additional costimulation through CD86. Th2 cells may also require costimulation by IL-1 from macrophages or dendritic cells (Walker and McKenzie 2018).

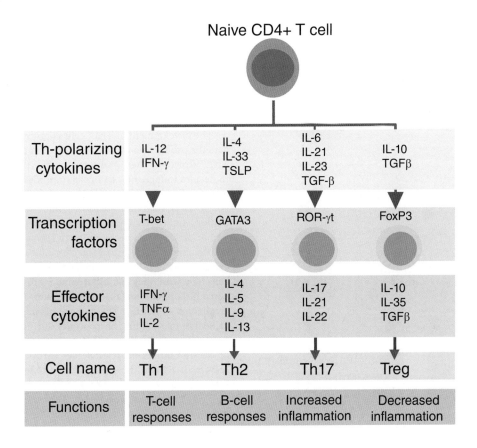

Fig. 15.13 The major populations of helper T cells. Note that their differentiation is induced by different mixtures of polarizing cytokines. These induce specific transcription factors in each population. Once polarized, the T cells synthesize and secrete different mixtures of effector cytokines. *IFN*, Interferon; *IL*, interleukin; *TGF-β*, transforming growth factor–β; *TNF-α*, tumor necrosis factor–α.

Activated Th2 cells secrete IL-4, IL-5, IL-9, and IL-13 and so mediate "type 2" immune responses (Fig. 15.18). These cytokines stimulate B-cell proliferation and immunoglobulin secretion but tend to suppress cell-mediated responses. The cytokines from Th2 cells enhance B-cell production of immunoglobulin G (IgG) and IgA up to 20-fold and production of IgE up to 1000-fold. Type 2 responses are associated with enhanced immunity to parasitic worms but decreased resistance to mycobacteria and other intracellular organisms. They suppress some autoimmune diseases; they neutralize toxins and regulate wound and tissue repair following infection and injury. If not carefully regulated, type 2 responses may trigger damaging allergic responses.

Interleukin-4

IL-4 is a glycoprotein produced by Th2 cells and mast cells. Its targets are T cells, B cells, and macrophages. IL-4 activates the Th2-specific transcription factor GATA3. GATA3 is the master regulator of Th2 differentiation. IL-4 promotes IgG and IgE production and inhibits IFN-γ expression and Th17 cell production. In humans and rodents, IL-4 is essential for antibody production because it stimulates B-cell activity (Fig. 15.19). In pigs, however, IL-4 blocks antibody and IL-6 production and suppresses antigen-induced B-cell proliferation. Thus IL-4 may play a very different role in pigs than it does in mice or humans (Murtaugh et al., 2009). IL-4 shares overlapping intracellular signaling pathways and biological functions with IL-13.

Some helper T cells secrete a mixture of Th1 and Th2 cytokines. These cells may be precursors of Th1 and Th2, or of cells that are in transition between the two populations. Some IL-2-secreting T cells may switch to become IL-4-secreting cells after exposure to antigen, implying a change in phenotype from Th1 to Th2. The principal molecules that control this switch are IL-4 and IL-12. When cultured in the presence of IL-4, undifferentiated helper cells become Th2 cells. When cultured in the presence of IL-12, they become Th1 cells. Mixed cell populations are most obvious early after the initiation of an immune response, whereas Th1 and Th2 subsets are more obvious in chronic diseases where the antigens are persistent.

Interleukin-9

Interleukin-9 is a glycoprotein of about 40 kDa produced by T lymphocytes. A subset of Th2 cells that can be stimulated by a combination of IL-4 and TGF-β to produce large quantities of IL-9 have been called Th9 cells. These Th9 cells are generated by a combination of IL-4 and TGF-β. IL-25 and TSLP treatment of these cells also induces IL-9 release and so enhances allergic responses. Other cells that can produce IL-9 include ILC2 cells and a subset of mucosal mast cells.

IL-9 affects Th2 and ILC2 cells by promoting their differentiation; Th1 cells in which it reduces differentiation; mast cells where it promotes mediator release; and eosinophils where it promotes their development and survival. The main function of the IL-9-producing cells is probably to defend against parasitic helminths. They are, however, present in the blood of allergic patients where they appear to enhance inflammation by promoting mast cell activation. Th9 cells play important roles in the development of atopic dermatitis, allergic contact dermatitis, and food allergies.

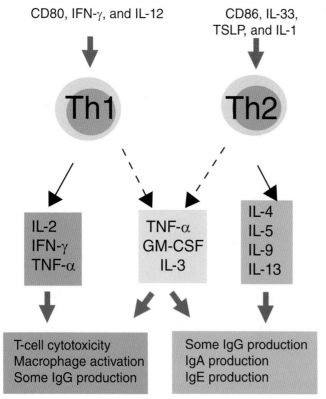

Fig. 15.14 Major differences between Th1 and Th2 populations. Note that the costimuli that trigger them are different as are the set of effector cytokines they secrete. *IFN-γ*, Interferon-γ; *IL*, interleukin; *TNF-α*, tumor necrosis factor–α; *GM-CSF*, granulocyte-macrophage colony-stimulating factor.

Th17 Cells

The third major population of CD4+ T cells produces IL-17 and are therefore called Th17 cells (Fig. 15.20; Crome et al., 2010). Th17 cells are conventional small lymphocytes that are abundant in mucosal surfaces. Their presence in these surface tissues is regulated by the gut microbiota (Bettelli et al., 2008). They mediate type 3 immune responses (Schnell et al., 2023).

The development of Th17 cells is promoted by IL-23. IL-23 triggers the production of a unique transcription factor called ROR-γt. Th17 growth is then promoted by IL-1β, IL-6, and IL-21. These molecules induce the Th17 cells to produce a mixture of cytokines, namely, IL-17A, IL-17F, IL-21, and IL-22 (Parrish-Novak et al., 2002). Th17 cells have two major functions: they mediate inflammation, and they are potent B-cell helpers. Cytokines of the IL-17 family play a key role in protective type 1 responses to extracellular bacteria and assist in the clearance of fungi. Under some circumstances, Th17 cells may convert into IFN-γ-producing Th1 cells. Likewise, they can differentiate into regulatory T cells (Tregs) when inflammation is resolved (Annunziato and Romagnani, 2010; Gagliani et al., 2015). The balance between Th17 and Treg cells is critical to maintaining homeostasis during immune and inflammatory responses. Excessive Th17 activity can lead to the development of chronic inflammatory diseases (Mills, 2023). Many γ/δ T cells secrete IL-17, and these may also be found in significant numbers under mucosal surfaces (Box 15.2).

Type 3 responses mediated by Th17 cells play a key role in immunity to extracellular bacteria and fungi since they recruit neutrophils through their actions on stem cells. IL-17 stimulates the production of GM-CSF leading to a neutrophilia (see Chapter 19). It promotes the recruitment and survival of macrophages, and it stimulates the production of pro-inflammatory cytokines and antibacterial peptides

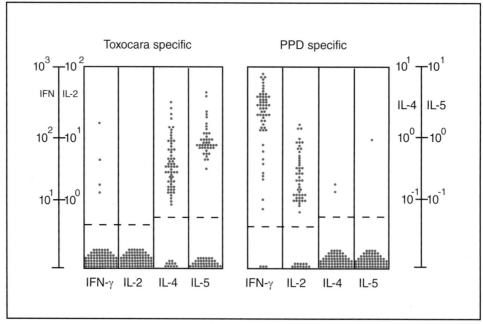

Fig. 15.15 Different antigens can trigger distinctly different Th-cell subpopulations. For example, T cells exposed to a parasite antigen from the roundworm *Toxocara canis* mount a type 2 response and secrete interleukin (IL)-4 and IL-5. In contrast, T cells exposed to PPD, an antigen from *Mycobacterium tuberculosis*, mount a type 1 response characterized by secretion of interferon-γ (IFN-γ) and IL-2. *PPD*, Tuberculin, purified protein derivative. From Del Prete, G., De Carli, G., Mastromauro, C., 1991. Purified protein derivative of *Mycobacterium tuberculosis* and excretory-secretory antigen(s) of *Toxocara canis* expand in vitro human T cells with stable and opposite (type 1 T helper or type 2 T helper) profile of cytokine production. J. Clin. Invest. 88, 346–350.

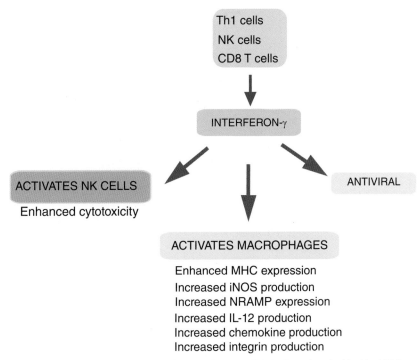

Fig. 15.16 The origins and some properties of interferon-γ (IFN-γ). *IL-12*, Interleukin-12; *MHC*, major histocompatibility complex; *NK cells*, natural killer cells.

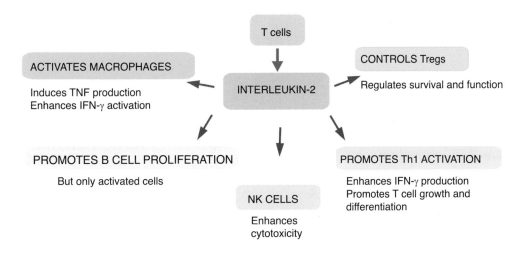

Fig. 15.17 The origins and some properties of interleukin-2. *IFN-γ*, Interferon-γ; *NK cells*, natural killer cells; *TNF*, tumor necrosis factor.

BOX 15.1   Type 1 and type 2 Immunity

There is a growing tendency among immunologists to classify protective immune responses into two types. Type 1 immunity encompasses the use of Th1 cells. However, it also involves the use of Th17 cells, cytotoxic T cells, group 1 and 3 innate lymphoid cells, and M1 macrophages as well as immunoglobulins G, M, and A. Type 1 responses are responsible for immunity to bacteria, viruses, protozoa, and fungi. It employs the cytokines, IFNγ, IL-12, -17, and -18. Type 2 immunity, in contrast, encompasses the use of Th2 cells. In addition, it includes group 2 innate lymphoid cells, basophils, mast cells, eosinophils, M2 macrophages, and immunoglobulin E. It also employs the cytokines, IL-4, -5, -9, -13, -25, -33, and TSLP. Type 2 responses are responsible for immunity to parasitic helminths and arthropods as well as for allergic responses.

from many cell types. It attracts neutrophils and macrophages (but not eosinophils) to inflammatory sites. Th17 cell numbers are normally controlled by Treg cells as well as by the suppressive cytokines, IL-10, TGF-β and IL-35. Dysregulated IL-17 production contributes significantly to inflammatory diseases such as asthma, systemic lupus, and rheumatoid arthritis (Mills, 2023; McGeachy et al., 2019).

Interleukin -17

Six related cytokines belong to the IL-17 family (IL-17A through IL-17F), but the two most important members are IL-17A and IL-17F. IL-17A is involved in the development of autoimmunity, inflammation, and some tumors. IL-17F is mainly involved in mucosal defense. IL-17E (also known as IL-25) promotes Th2 responses. The functions of the others are unclear. IL-17A is a homodimer of 35 kDa produced

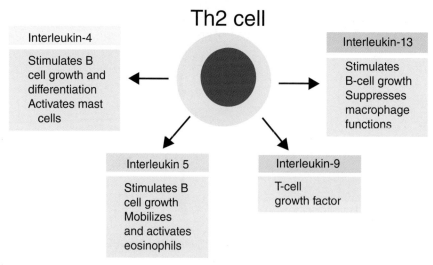

Fig. 15.18 The cytokines produced by Th2 cells and their major properties.

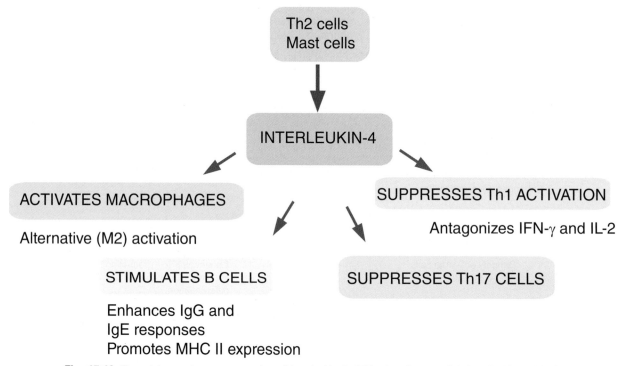

Fig. 15.19 The origins and some properties of interleukin-4. *IFN-γ*, interferon-γ; *IL-2*, Interleukin-2; *MHC*, major histocompatibility complex.

by Th17 cells. IL-17 binds to a family of cell surface receptors (IL-17RA through RE) that signal through NF-κB. Endothelial cells and macrophages are the main targets of these cytokines since IL-17 plus TNF-α can stimulate them to produce chemokines, G-CSF, GM-CSF, IL-1, and IL-6, inflammatory mediators such as acute-phase and complement proteins, and antibacterial defensins (Fig. 15.21).

IL-17 is crucial for coordinating host defenses against many bacteria and fungi. For example, Th17 cells play a key role in defense against pathogens such as *Klebsiella pneumoniae, Salmonella enterica, Mycobacterium tuberculosis,* and *Candida albicans.* It is believed that they do so by triggering the recruitment of inflammatory cells leading to rapid pathogen eradication. Engagement of dectin-1 and -2 drives Th17 responses in fungal infections (McGeachy et al., 2019).

Th22 Cells

Th22 cells, as their name implies, secrete the cytokine IL-22 (Eyerich et al., 2009). They promote mucosal immunity. They are induced by IL-1, IL-18, and IL-23. They are also induced by signals from the microbiota acting through the aryl hydrocarbon receptor (Chopp et al., 2023).

Regulatory T Cells

Regulatory T cells (Tregs) are typical lymphocytes that express CD4 and CD25 (the α-chain of the IL-2 receptor). (They are discussed in

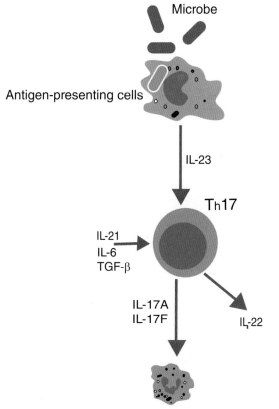

Fig. 15.20 The production of Th17 cells. The original differentiation signal comes from transforming growth factor–β (TGF-β) and interleukin (IL)-6. This signal is amplified by IL-21 and then the cell phenotype is stabilized by IL-23.

detail in Chapter 19.) Their most characteristic feature, however, is their use of the transcription factor, Foxp3. Treg cells act through several pathways. They can directly contact other cells to deliver suppressive molecules such as TGF-β, or cytotoxic granzymes and perforins. They also produce suppressive cytokines such as IL-10, and IL-35. They also express a pair of ectoenzymes, CD39 and CD73 that convert extracellular ATP into adenosine which has potent antiinflammatory effects (Dikiy and Rudensky, 2023). As a result, Treg cells suppress the responses of both Th1 and Th2 cells and prevent inappropriate T-cell activation in the absence of antigens. The balance between Treg cells and Th2 cells regulates many inflammatory and allergic diseases. Treg cell function is modulated through the checkpoint molecules, CTLA-4 and PD-1.

BOX 15.2   Interleukin-23

Interleukin (IL)-23 is closely related to IL-12. Both are heterodimers consisting of an identical p40 subunit and a second smaller subunit, IL-23p19 or IL-12p35, respectively. Both cytokines are produced by macrophages and dendritic cells in response to LPS, and both enhance T-cell proliferation and the production of IFN-γ. Whereas IL-12 drives a pathway leading to Th1-cell production, IL-23 drives a pathway leading to the stabilization of IL-17-producing CD4+ T cells. IL-23 recruits diverse inflammatory cells in addition to Th17 cells and is thus involved in the pathogenesis of several immune-mediated diseases. The production of IL-23 is increased in some tumors, where it promotes inflammation and enhances angiogenesis (see Chapter 36).

From Gaffen, S.L., Jain, R., Garg, A.V., Cua, D.J., 2014. The IL-23-IL-17 immune axis: from mechanisms to therapeutic testing. Nat. Rev. Immunol. 14 (9), 585–600.

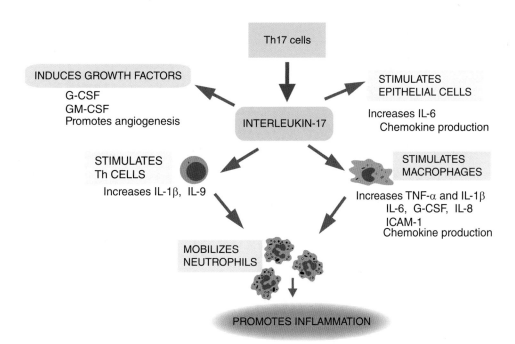

Fig. 15.21 The origins and properties of interleukin (IL)-17. GM-CSF, Granulocyte-macrophage colony-stimulating factor; TNF-α, tumor necrosis factor–α.

Follicular Helper T Cells

Follicular helper T cells (Tfh cells) are a type of CD4+ cell that is specialized for providing help to B cells within germinal centers. Their production is tightly regulated to ensure a sufficient supply of functional B cells (Belanger and Crotty, 2016). Unlike the other T cells that are defined by the cytokines they produce, Tfh cells express the cytokine receptor CXCR5. As a result, they localize in the B cell-rich areas of follicles and germinal centers. Tfh cells must be activated twice. They are initially activated by dendritic cells and subsequently activated by B cells. They promote B-cell survival, proliferation, and differentiation. They drive B-cell affinity maturation through IL-21 and CD40L. Several different Tfh subsets have been identified.

SPECIES DIFFERENCES

The proportion of T cells with γ/δTCRs differs greatly between the domestic mammals. In species such as humans and mice, fewer than 5% have γ/δ TCRs and so are classified as γ/-low. In others, such as piglets and calves, 60%–80% of T cells express γ/δ TCRs (γ/δ-high) (Fig. 15.22; Holderness et al., 2013).

γ/δ-High Species
Bovine

T cells expressing γ/δ receptors may comprise up to 66% of the circulating T cells in young calves. They decrease steadily with age, but their numbers still remain relatively high until adulthood. Thus 8%–18% of adult bovine peripheral blood T cells are γ/δ+. CD4 is expressed on 20%–30% of blood lymphocytes in adult ruminants. Double-negative T cells constitute 15%–30% of the blood T cells in young ruminants, but this may reach 80% in newborn calves. Most of these double-negative cells are γ/δ+ and WC1+. Thus the major circulating T cells in ruminants (γ/δ+, WC1+, CD4−, CD8−) differ from the predominant

T cells in humans and mice (α/β+, WC1−, CD4+, CD8−) (Baldwin and Telfer, 2015).

Most bovine γ/δ T cells also express the coreceptor called WC1 (see Chapter 14). As a result, these cells can be activated either through their TCR or through WC1. In response, they produce TNF-α, IL-1, IL-12, and IFN-γ. This mixture suggests that they contribute to both inflammation and a Th1 bias in the bovine immune response and thus link the innate and adaptive immune systems (Baldwin et al., 2021).

Bovine γ/δ T cells colonize the skin, mammary gland, reproductive organs, tonsils, and the intestinal mucosa. They fall into two major subsets, innate cells, and regulatory cells (Telfer and Baldwin, 2015). Between 50% and 99% of bovine γ/δ T cells are major contributors to innate immunity especially since many of them have non-polymorphic TCRs. They recognize antigenic glycolipids presented by CD1-positive antigen-presenting cells and release cytokines and lyse target cells just like conventional α/β NKT cells (Chapter 20). Some WC-bovine γ/δ T cells serve a regulatory function (Guzman et al., 2004). They spontaneously secrete IL-10 and can inhibit antigen-specific and nonspecific CD4+ and CD8+ T-cell proliferation in vitro (Baldwin et al., 2021).

WC1 T Cells

Bovine WC1+ and WC1− T cells have a different tissue distribution. WC1− cells predominate in the spleen and uterus. WC1+ γ/δ T cells are found in granulomas surrounding Schistosomes and Mycobacteria (Chen et al., 2009). In these cases, the initial T-cell infiltration is dominated by γ/δ T cells, and this is followed by α/β T cells. A second wave of γ/δ T cells may terminate the response. These WC1+ cells may secrete IL-12, IL-17, and IFN-γ and so promote a Th1 bias in the immune response. IFN-γ-producing bovine γ/δ WC1+ cells are the major population involved in recall immune responses to Leptospira (Baldwin et al., 2014).

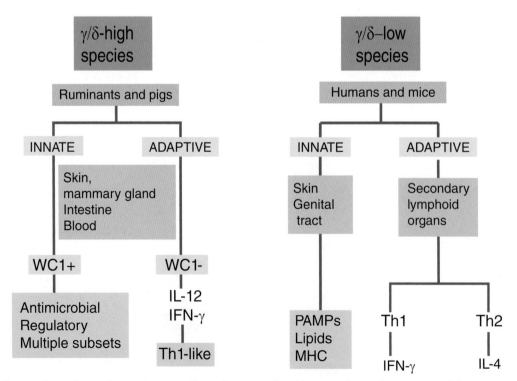

Fig. 15.22 γ/T cells may, depending on the species, act as innate immune cells with an invariant antigen receptor. Others may act as classic helper T cells with diverse T-cell antigen receptors (TCRs) of polyclonal origin. *IFN-γ*, Interferon-γ; *IL-12*, interleukin-12; *WC1*, Workshop Cluster1.

Sheep

Two-thirds of the circulating T cells in young lambs are γ/δ positive. They recognize a very wide diversity of antigens and mount adaptive rather than innate responses. Vaccine-induced γ/δ T-cell responses have been reported in pigs and lambs.

Pigs

As many as 85% of T cells in neonatal piglets express γ/δ TCRs. It drops to around 30% in adult pigs. Like cattle and sheep, pig γ/δ T cells can also be distinguished by their expression of WC1 (see Chapter 14). Pig γ/δ cells accumulate in large numbers in epithelial tissues and at inflammatory sites. Pigs also have multiple subpopulations of γ/δ T cells. Some may produce IFN-γ alone, TNF-α alone, or both. Other subpopulations can produce IL-17 (Charerntantanakul and Roth, 2007).

Up to 60% of γ/δ T cells in pig blood are double positive (CD4$^+$, CD8$^+$). The rest are predominantly double negative (CD4$^-$, CD8$^-$). Pigs also have two subpopulations of circulating γ/δ T cells based on their expression of the adhesion molecule CD2. Thus CD2$^-$ and CD2$^+$ may reflect two different cell lineages (Stepanova and Sinkora, 2013). Some pig γ/δ T cells can function as antigen-presenting cells using MHC class II molecules (Thome et al., 1994).

Pig α/β T cells can be subdivided into three populations based on their expression of CD4 and CD8. These are CD8αβ$^+$CD4$^-$, CD8$^-$CD4$^+$ and CD8αα$^+$CD4^{++}. Pig T cells also constitutively express MHC class II molecules which is also a unique feature of this species.

γ/δ Low Species

γ/δ-low mammals are those that have less than 10% γ/δ T cells in their blood. These species include humans and mice with 0.5%–10%; rats, 1%–5%; dogs 2.5%; and guinea pigs with 8.6%. Thus γ/δ T cells constitute a very small portion of their entire T-cell population.

In these γ/δ-low species, there are two subsets of γ/δ cells. One subset has limited γ/δ receptor diversity, is mainly found in the skin and genital tract, and is engaged in innate immunity. The second subset is engaged in adaptive immunity, has extensive receptor diversity, and is found in secondary lymphoid organs and the digestive tract (see Chapter 20). These innate γ/δ T cells respond to lipid antigens presented by CD1 molecules (Porcelli and Modlin, 1999). When stimulated, they secrete IL-17 and IFN-γ. Like Th17 cells, human innate γ/δ T cells are activated by IL-23.

Dogs

In dogs, α/β T cells far outnumber γ/δ T cells in peripheral blood and lymphoid organs. On average, newborn puppies have about 2% γ/δ T cells and this does not change for many years. The numbers of γ/δ cells eventually drop in old dogs, 10–13 years of age, to around 0.5% (10 ± 3 cells/μL).

MEMORY T CELLS

When naïve T cells encounter antigens with appropriate costimulation, they differentiate into multiple effector T-cell populations. These effector cells are usually short-lived. However, some resist apoptosis and develop into long-lived memory cells. These can be thought of as "antigen-experienced" stem cells. Memory T cells can be the most abundant T-cell population in the body, especially in older animals since they accumulate throughout life. Compared to naïve T cells, memory cells are easier to activate, live longer, and have enhanced effector activity. As a result, they mount a strong rapid cytokine response the next time they encounter the antigen and can provide life-long protection against pathogens. The differences in behavior between naïve and memory

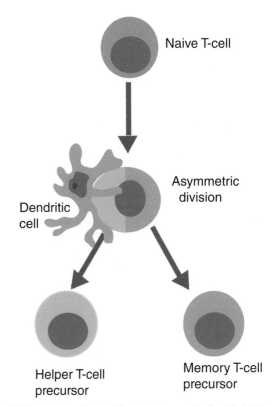

Fig. 15.23 Following T cell-DC interactions, the T cell divides asymmetrically. The cell at the pole in contact with the antigen-presenting dendritic cell synapse becomes a helper T cell. The cell at the opposite pole receives different signals and so becomes a memory T cell.

T cells likely result from epigenetic modifications that alter gene transcription (mainly histone methylation, see Chapter 21) and hence cell functions (Schenkel and Masopust, 2014).

The development of effector and memory T-cell populations results from asymmetrical T-cell division (Fig. 15.23; Barnett et al., 2012). As described earlier, naïve T cells interact with antigen-presenting cells for several hours through an immunological synapse. Once they have received sufficient stimulation the T cells begin to divide even before they have separated from their antigen-presenting cells. The dividing T cells are polarized since one pole of the cell contains the immunological synapse and associated structures. The other pole contains molecules excluded from the synapse. Thus, when these cells divide, they form two distinctly different populations of daughter cells. The daughter cells adjacent to the synapse are the precursors of the effector T cells. The daughter cells formed at the opposite pole are the precursors of the memory T cells (Ciocca et al., 2012).

Three types of memory T cells have been characterized. These are central memory T cells, tissue-resident memory T cells, and effector memory T cells. Central memory T cells circulate through secondary lymphoid tissues, such as lymph nodes, awaiting the arrival of invaders. They lack immediate effector function but have very rapid recall responses. Effector memory T cells, in contrast, have receptors enabling them to home to inflamed tissues, where they immediately attack invaders without the need to differentiate further. Tissue-resident memory T cells occupy tissues and provide a first response to pathogens invading through body surfaces. They rapidly produce cytokines after infection. They do not circulate in peripheral blood. All memory T-cell populations express either CD4 or CD8 and persist in the absence of antigen. CD8$^+$ memory cells tend to accumulate under epithelial surfaces while CD4$^+$ memory cells are scattered through the tissues in memory lymphocyte clusters. These cells slowly divide and replenish their numbers. IL-7 and IL-15 are both required for the survival of memory CD8$^+$ T cells, whereas only IL-7 is needed for the survival of CD4$^+$ T cells. These cytokines maintain the cells in a state of slow proliferation. In humans, memory CD4$^+$ T cells have a half-life of 8–12 years, whereas memory CD8$^+$ T cells have a half-life of 8–15 years. The size of the immune system is fixed somewhat, but the effector memory CD8$^+$ T-cell pool can double without loss of preexisting memory cells (Vezys et al., 2009).

REFERENCES

Annunziato, F., Romagnani, S., 2010. The transient nature of the Th17 phenotype. Eur. J. Immunol. 40, 3312–3316.

Annunziato, F., Romagnani, S., 2015. The 3 major types of innate and adaptive cell-mediated effector immunity. J. Allergy Clin. Immunol. 135, 626–635.

Baldwin, C.L., Hsu, H., Chen, C., Palmer, M., et al., 2014. The role of bovine γδ T cells and their WC1 co-receptor in response to bacterial pathogens and promoting vaccine efficacy: A model for cattle and humans. Vet. Immunol. Immunopathol. 159, 144–155.

Baldwin, C.L., Damani-Yokota, P., Yirsaw, A., Loonie, K., et al., 2021. Special features of γ T cells in ruminants. Mol. Immunol. 134, 161–169.

Baldwin, C.L., Telfer, J.C., 2015. The bovine model for elucidating the role of gammadelta T cells in controlling infectious diseases of importance to cattle and humans. Mol. Immunol. 66 (1), 35–47.

Barnett, B.E., Ciocca, M.L., Goenka, R., Barnett, L.G., Wu, J., Laufer, T.M., et al., 2012. Asymmetric B cell division in the germinal center reaction. Science 335 (6066), 342–344.

Belanger, S., Crotty, S., 2016. Dances with cytokines, featuring Tfh cells, IL-21, IL-4 and B cells. Nat. Immunol. 17 (10), 1135–1136.

Bettelli, E., Korn, T., Oukka, M., Kuchroo, V.K., 2008. Induction and effector functions of T(H)17 cells. Nature 453, 1051–1057.

Brodovitch, A., Bongrand, P., Pierres, A., 2013. T lymphocytes sense antigens within seconds and make a decision within one minute. J. Immunol. 191, 2064–2071.

Charerntantanakul, W., Roth, J.A., 2007. Biology of porcine T lymphocytes. Anim. Health Res. Rev. 8, 1–16.

Chen, C., Herzig, C.T., Telfer, J.C., Baldwin, C.L., 2009. Antigenic basis of diversity in the gamma/delta T cell co-receptor WC1 family. Mol. Immunol. 46, 2565–2575.

Chopp, L., Redmond, C., O'Shea, J.J., Schwartz, D.M., 2023. From thymus to tissues and tumors: a review of T-cell biology. J. Allergy Clin. Immunol. 151, 81–97.

Ciocca, M.L., Barnett, B.E., Burkhardt, J.K., Chang, J.T., Reiner, S.L., 2012. Cutting edge: asymmetric memory T cell division in response to rechallenge. J. Immunol. 188 (9), 4145–4148.

Clarke, S.R.M., 2000. The critical role of CD40/CD40L in the CD4-dependent generation of CD8$^+$ T cell immunity. J. Leukoc Biol. 67, 607–613.

Crome, S.Q., Wang, A.Y., Levings, M.K., 2010. Translational mini-review series on Th17 cells: function and regulation of human T helper 17 cells in health and disease. Clin. Exp. Immunol. 159, 109–119.

Dikiy, S., Rudensky, A.Y., 2023. Principles of regulatory T cell function. Immunity 56, 240–255.

Dustin, M.L., 2014. What counts in the immunological synapse? Mol. Cell 54 (2), 255–262.

Eyerich, S., Eyerich, K., Pennino, D., et al., 2009. Th22 cells represent a distinct human T cell subset involved in epidermal immunity and remodeling. J. Clin. Invest. 119, 3573–3585.

Gagliani, N., Amezcua Vesely, M.C., Iseppon, A., Brockmann, L., Xu, H., Palm, N.W., et al., 2015. Th17 cells transdifferentiate into regulatory T cells during resolution of inflammation. Nature. 523 (7559), 221–225.

Guzman, E., Hope, J., Taylor, G., Smith, A.L., et al., 2004. Bovine γδ T cells are a major regulatory T cell subset. J. Immunol. 193, 208–222.

Holderness, J., Hedges, J.F., Ramstead, A., Jutila, M.A., 2013. Comparative biology of γ T cell function in humans, mice and domestic animals. Ann. Rev. Anim. Biosci. 1, 99–124.

Janes, P.W., Ley, S.C., Magee, A.I., Kabouridis, P.S., 2000. The role of lipid rafts in T cell antigen receptor (TCR) signaling. Immunology 12, 23–34.

McGeachy, M.S., Cua, D.J., Gaffen, S.L., 2019. The IL-17 family of cytokines in health and disease. Immunity 50, 892–906.

Mills, K.H.G., 2023. IL-17 and IL-17 producing cells in protection versus pathology. Nat. Rev. Immunol 23, 38–54.

Morath, A., Schamel, W.W., 2020. αβ and g T cell receptors: similar but different. J. Leukoc. Biol. https://doi.org/10.1002/JLB.2MR1219-233R.

Murtaugh, M.P., Johnson, C.R., Xiao, Z., et al., 2009. Species specialization in cytokine biology: is interleukin-4 central to the Th1-Th2 paradigm in swine? Dev. Comp. Immunol. 33, 344–352.

Nel, A.E., 2002a. T-cell activation through the antigen receptor. 1: Signaling components, signaling pathways, and signal integration at the T-cell antigen receptor synapse. J. Allergy Clin. Immunol. 109, 758–770.

Nel, A.E., Slaughter, N., 2002b. T-cell activation through the antigen receptor. 2: role of signaling cascades in T-cell differentiation, anergy, immune senescence, and development of immunotherapy. J. Allergy Clin. Immunol. 109, 901–915.

Padhan, K., Varma, R., 2010. Immunological synapse: a multi-protein signaling cellular apparatus for controlling gene expression. Immunology 129, 322–328.

Parrish-Novak, J., Foster, D.C., Holly, R.D., Clegg, C.H., 2002. Interleukin-21 and the IL-21 receptor: novel effectors of NK and T cell responses. J. Leukoc. Biol. 72, 856–863.

Porcelli, S.A., Modlin, R.L., 1999. The CD1 system: antigen-presenting molecules for T cell recognition of lipids and glycolipids. Annu. Rev. Immunol. 17, 297–329.

Schenkel, J.M., Masopust, D., 2014. Tissue-resident memory T cells. Immunity 41 (6), 886–897.

Schnell, A., Littmann, D.R., Kuchroo, V.K., 2023. T$_H$17 cell heterogeneity and its role in tissue inflammation. Nat. Immunol 24, 19–29.

Stepanova, K., Sinkora, M., 2013. Porcine γδ T lymphocytes can be categorized into two functionally and developmentally distinct subsets according to expression of CD2 and level of TCR. J. Immunol. 190, 2111–2120.

Telfer, J.C., Baldwin, C.L., 2015. Bovine gamma delta T cells and the function of gamma delta T cell specific WC1 co-receptors. Cell Immunol. 296 (1), 76–86.

Thauland, T.J., Koguchi, Y., Wetzel, S., et al., 2008. Th1 and Th2 cells form morphologically distinct immunological synapses. J. Immunol. 181, 393–399.

Thome, M., Hirt, W., Pfaff, E., et al., 1994. Porcine T-cell receptors: molecular and biochemical characterization. Vet. Immunol. Immunopathol. 43, 13–18.

Vezys, V., Yates, A., Casey, K.A., et al., 2009. Memory CD8 T-cell compartment grows in size with immunological experience. Nature 457, 196–200.

Walker, J.A., McKenzie, N.J., 2018. T$_H$2 cell development and function. Nat. Rev. Immunol. 18, 121–134.

Walsh, K.P., Mills, K.H., 2013. Dendritic cells and other innate determinants of T helper cell polarisation. Trends Immunol. 34 (11), 521–530.

Zhang, Y., Wang, H., 2012. Integrin signalling and function in immune cells. Immunology 135 (4), 268–275.

B Cells and Their Response to Antigens

The division of the adaptive immune system into two major components is based on the need to recognize two distinctly different forms of foreign invaders. Some invaders such as most bacteria enter the body and grow in extracellular fluids. These "exogenous" invaders are destroyed by antibodies. Other invaders such as viruses, replicate inside cells where antibodies cannot reach. They are destroyed by T cell–mediated responses. Antibodies are produced by the lymphocytes called B cells. This chapter describes B cells and their response to antigens.

B cells are found in the cortex of lymph nodes, in the marginal zone in the spleen, in the bone marrow, throughout the intestine, and in Peyer's patches. A few B cells circulate in the blood. Like T cells, B cells have a large number of identical antigen-binding receptors on their surface. Each B cell, therefore, will only bind and respond to a single antigen. These antigen receptors are generated at random during B-cell development in a process described in Chapter 18. If a B cell encounters an antigen that binds its receptors, it will, with appropriate costimulation, respond by secreting these receptors into body fluids, where they are called antibodies.

B-CELL ANTIGEN RECEPTORS

Each B cell is covered with about 200,000–500,000 identical antigen receptors (BCRs); many more than the 30,000 antigen receptors (TCRs) expressed on each T cell. Each BCR is constructed from multiple peptide chains, and, like the TCR, they can be divided into antigen-binding and signaling components. Unlike the TCR, however, the BCR can also bind antigens when in solution. Antibodies are simply soluble BCRs released into body fluids; they all belong to the family of proteins called immunoglobulins (see Chapter 17).

Antigen-Binding Component

The antigen-binding component of the BCR (or immunoglobulin) is a glycoprotein of 160–180 kDa consisting of four linked peptide chains. These chains consist of two identical pairs: two heavy chains, each

60 kDa in size, and two light chains, about 25 kDa each (Fig. 16.1). The light chains are linked by disulfide bonds to the heavy chains, so that the complete molecule forms the letter Y. The tail of the Y (called the Fc region) is formed from paired heavy chains and attaches to the B-cell surface. The arms of the Y (called the Fab regions) are formed by paired light and heavy chains, and they bind antigens (Fig. 16.2). The antigen-binding sites are formed by the grooves between the light and heavy chains. Thus each BCR has two identical antigen-binding sites.

Light Chains

Light chains are constructed from two domains, each containing about 110 amino acids. The amino acid sequences in the C-terminal domains in the BCRs from different B cells are identical and are called constant domains (C_L). In contrast, the sequences in the N-terminal domains differ in each B cell and so form variable domains (V_L). Mammals also make two types of light chains, called κ (kappa) and λ (lambda). Although their amino acid sequences are different, they are functionally identical. The ratio of κ to λ chains in BCRs varies among mammals, ranging from mice and rats, which have more than 95% κ chains, to cattle and horses, which have 95% λ chains. Primates such as the rhesus monkey and the baboon have 50% of each, whereas humans have 70% κ chains. Carnivores such as cats and dogs have 90% λ chains (Tizard, 2023).

Heavy Chains

Immunoglobulin heavy chains are constructed from four or five domains each of about 110 amino acids. The N-terminal domain is the variable (V_H) domain. The remaining three or four domains show few sequence differences and thus are constant (C_H) domains.

Mammalian B cells make five different classes of heavy chains that differ in their sequence and domain structure. As a result, each class has a different biological activity. The five different immunoglobulin heavy chains are called α, γ, δ, ε, and μ. These heavy chains determine the immunoglobulin class (or isotype). Thus immunoglobulin molecules

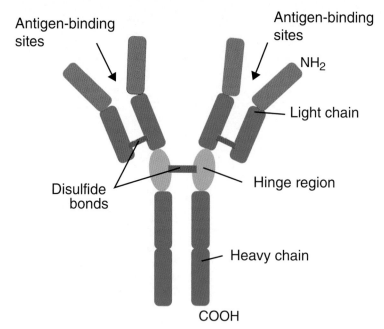

Fig. 16.1 The overall structure of an immunoglobulin molecule. When expressed on B-cell surfaces, these molecules act as antigen receptors (BCR). When released by the B cell and free in circulation, they function as antibodies. Note that, unlike a T-cell antigen receptor, BCRs have two antigen-binding sites.

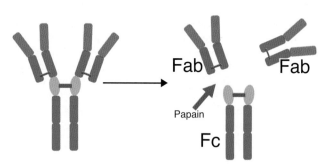

Fig. 16.2 Fragmentation of an immunoglobulin molecule using the proteolytic enzyme papain. The names of these fragments denote the nomenclature of different regions of an immunoglobulin molecule. *Fab*, Fragment-antibody binding; *Fc*, fragment crystalizable.

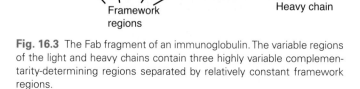

Fig. 16.3 The Fab fragment of an immunoglobulin. The variable regions of the light and heavy chains contain three highly variable complementarity-determining regions separated by relatively constant framework regions.

that use α heavy chains are called immunoglobulin A (IgA), and those that use γ chains are called IgG; μ chains are used in IgM, δ chains in IgD, and ε chains in IgE.

Variable Regions

When the sequences of the V domains from light and heavy chains are examined in detail, two features become apparent. First, their sequence variation is largely confined to three regions, each containing 6–10 amino acids, within the variable domain (Fig. 16.3). These regions are said to be hypervariable. Between the three hypervariable regions are relatively constant regions called framework regions. The hypervariable regions on paired light and heavy chains determine the shape of the antigen-binding site and thus the specificity of antigen binding. Since the shape of the antibody-binding site is complementary to the conformation of the antigenic determinant, the hypervariable sequences are also called complementarity-determining regions (CDRs). Each V-domain is folded in such a way that its three CDRs come into close contact with the bound antigen (Fig. 16.4).

Constant Regions

Mammals employ different antibody molecules for different tasks. These differences are determined by the shape, size, and functionality of their heavy chains. For example, the number of constant domains differs between immunoglobulin heavy chain classes. There are three constant domains in a γ heavy chain; they are labeled, from the N-terminal end, as C_H1, C_H2, and C_H3. Three constant domains are also found in α and most δ chains, whereas μ and ε chains have a fourth constant domain called C_H4.

Since heavy chains are paired, the domains in each chain come together to form structures by which antibody molecules can exert their biological functions. Thus, V_H and V_L together form the antigen-binding site, and C_H1 and C_L together stabilize the antigen-binding site. The paired C_H2 domains of IgG contain a site that activates the classical complement pathway (see Chapter 5) and a site that binds to Fc receptors on phagocytic cells (Fig. 16.5). The heavy chain also regulates the transfer of IgG into colostrum (see Chapter 24) and antibody-mediated cellular cytotoxicity (see Chapter 19). When immunoglobulin molecules act as BCRs, their Fc region is embedded in the B-cell

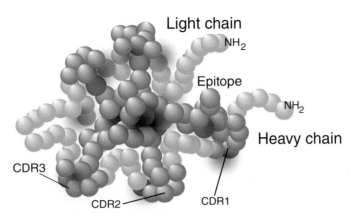

Fig. 16.4 A schematic diagram showing the way in which the complementarity-determining regions of both light and heavy chains are folded to form an antigen-binding site on an immunoglobulin molecule. A similar folding occurs in the peptide chains of the T-cell antigen receptor.

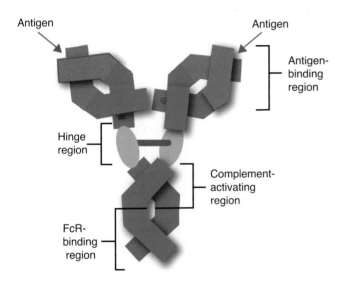

Fig. 16.5 The structure of an immunoglobulin G molecule, showing how the light and heavy chains intertwine to form clearly defined regions within the molecule. Each region has defined biological functions.

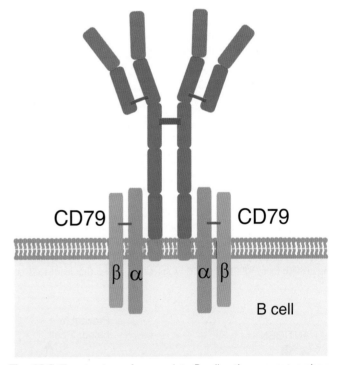

Fig. 16.6 The structure of a complete B-cell antigen receptor, showing both the antigen-binding component (immunoglobulin) and the signal transducing components (CD79). Note the small transmembrane domain at the end of each heavy chain.

surface membrane. These cell-bound immunoglobulins differ from the secreted form in that they have a small transmembrane domain attached to their C-terminus. This contains the hydrophobic amino acids that associate with the cell-membrane lipids.

Hinge Region

One important feature of the immunoglobulins is that their Fab regions can swing freely around the center of the molecule as if hinged. This hinge consists of a short domain of about 12 amino acids located between the C_H1 and C_H2 domains. The hinge region contains many hydrophilic and proline residues that cause the peptide chain to unfold and make this region readily accessible to proteases (Fig. 16.5). This region also contains the interchain disulfide bonds that bind the four peptide chains together. Proline, because of its configuration, produces a 90-degree bend when inserted in a polypeptide chain. Because amino acids can rotate around peptide bonds, the effect of closely spaced proline residues is to produce a universal joint around which the immunoglobulin chains can swing freely. The μ chains of IgM do not possess a hinge region.

Signal Transducing Component

BCR immunoglobulins cannot signal directly to their B cells since their cytoplasmic domains contain only three amino acids. However, their C_H4 and transmembrane domains associate with two glycoprotein heterodimers formed by pairing CD79a (Ig-α) with CD79b (Ig-β). These CD79β heterodimers act as the signal transducers (Fig. 16.6). The CD79β chains are identical in all BCRs. The CD79α chains differ depending on their associated heavy chains and employ different signaling pathways (Clark et al., 1992).

Antigen-BCR binding and cross-linking of two receptors expose activating sites (ITAMs) on CD79α and CD79β. Phosphorylation of these ITAMs by src kinases leads to phosphorylation of a phospholipase

C and a G-protein (see Fig. 9.12). Subsequent hydrolysis of phosphatidylinositol and calcium mobilization generates a protein kinase C and calcineurin and activates the transcription factors NF-κB and NF-AT (Tedder et al., 1994). This eventually results in cell division and immunoglobulin production—providing the B cell also receives appropriate costimulatory signals from other sources (Gold, 2002).

ANTIGEN PRESENTATION BY B CELLS

In addition to their role as antibody producers, B cells are also effective antigen-presenting cells. Following antigen binding, the BCR is internalized and either degraded or transported to an intracellular compartment, where major histocompatibility (MHC) class II molecules and antigen fragments combine (Finkelman et al., 1992). These antigen-MHC class II complexes are then carried to the B-cell surface and presented to helper T cells (Fig. 16.7). Since all the antigen receptors on a single B cell are identical, each B cell can bind only a single antigen. This makes them much more efficient antigen-presenting cells than macrophages that must present any foreign material that comes their way. This is especially true in primed animals, in which large numbers of B cells can bind and present a specific antigen. As a result, B cells can activate Th cells with 1/1000 of the dose of antigen required by activating macrophages (Batista and Harwood, 2009).

COSTIMULATION

Although the binding of antigen to a BCR is an essential first step, this alone is insufficient to activate B cells. Complete activation of a B cell requires multiple signals from other sources. Thus it requires costimulation by helper T cells and cytokines, by complement, and by toll-like receptors (TLRs) (Fig. 16.8).

T Cell Help

When helper T cells "help" B cells they signal through multiple pathways to promote B-cell functions. These signals result in increased B-cell expression of BCRs and MHC class II molecules, as well as receptors for IL-4, IL-5, IL-6, tumor necrosis factor–α and transforming growth factor–β (TGF-β). They start the process that leads to B-cell

division and differentiation into antibody-secreting cells. The helper T cells provide B cells with signals from secreted cytokines as well as through interacting receptor pairs. T-cell signals also trigger somatic mutation and immunoglobulin class switching within germinal centers and thus increase antibody-binding affinity.

To provide these signals, however, the helper T cells must themselves be stimulated by the antigen. This antigen can be presented by one of the professional antigen-presenting cells, such as dendritic cells, macrophages, or even by B cells. Thus a B cell can capture and process antigen, present it to a T cell, and then receive costimulation from the same T cell.

Cytokine Stimulation

Type 2 helper T (Th2) cells produce multiple cytokines that activate B cells. The most important of these are interleukin-4 (IL-4), IL-5, IL-6, IL-13, and IL-21. IL-4 stimulates the growth and differentiation of B cells and enhances their expression of MHC class II and Fc receptors. It also induces immunoglobulin class switching and thus stimulates IgA and IgE production (Table 16.1). The actions of IL-4 are neutralized by IFN-γ, which inhibits both IgA and IgE synthesis as well as B-cell proliferation. IL-5 promotes the differentiation of activated B cells into plasma cells. It stimulates IgG and IgM production and

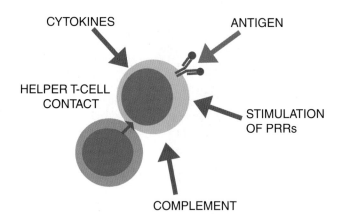

Fig. 16.8 Not only must B cells be stimulated by antigen, but they must also receive costimulation from helper T cells and their cytokines as well as complement and PRRs if they are to respond optimally. *PRRs*, Pattern-recognition receptors.

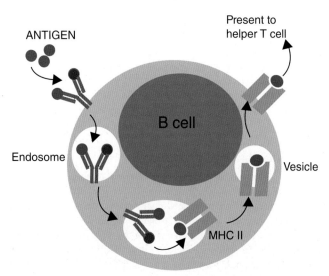

Fig. 16.7 The processing and presentation of antigens by B cells. This is a very efficient process since the B-cell antigen receptors can capture large amounts of identical antigen molecules. *MHC*, Major histocompatibility complex.

TABLE 16.1   **Immunoglobulins Produced by Mouse B Cells in the Presence of Th1 and Th2 Antigen-Specific helper T Cell Clones.**

Class	Th1 Cells (ng/mL)	Th2 Cells (ng/mL)
IgG1	<8	21,600
IgG2a	14	39
IgG2b	<8	189
IgG3	<8	354
IgM	248	98,000
IgA	<1	484
IgE	<1	187

Adapted from Coffmann, R.L., Seymour, B.W., Lebman, D.A., et al., 1988. The role of helper T cell products in mouse B cell differentiation and isotype regulation. Immunol. Rev. 102, 5.

enhances IL-4-induced IgE production. IL-5 selectively stimulates IgA production in mucosal B cells. IL-6 is needed for the final differentiation of activated B cells into plasma cells. It acts together with IL-5 to promote IgA production and with IL-1 to promote IgM production. IL-13 has biological activities similar to those of IL-4. This stimulates B-cell proliferation and increases immunoglobulin secretion. IL-13 is required for optimal induction of IgE, especially if IL-4 is low or absent.

IL-21 is produced by several helper cell populations including both Tfh cells and Th17 cells. It induces the differentiation of B cells into plasma cells and memory B cells. It stimulates IgG production in conjunction with IL-4. IL-21 also promotes the IgM to IgG class switch, while IL-4 induces the switch to IgE.

Cell-Cell Signaling

Cytokines alone cannot fully activate B cells. Complete activation also requires juxtacrine signaling between Th cells and B cells through receptor pairs such as CD40 and CD154 (Durie et al., 1994). CD154 is expressed on activated helper T cells, while its receptor CD40 is expressed on resting B cells. CD40 must receive a signal from CD154 for the B cell to begin its cell cycle and upregulate its IL-4 and IL-5 receptors (Figs. 16.9 and 16.10). The signals from CD154 synergize with those from IL-4 and IL-5 receptors to drive B-cell activation, memory cell development, and immunoglobulin class switching. CD28, also found on helper T cells, must also provide costimulation by signaling through CD86 on activated B cells.

Complement Help

Effective costimulation of B cells also requires signals from the complement system transmitted through CD21/CD19 on the B-cell surface. CD21 is a receptor (CR2) whose ligand is C3d. CD19 is its accompanying signaling component. If an antigen with C3d attached binds to CD21, a signal is transmitted through CD19 to the B cell (Fig. 16.11).

Stimulation of a BCR plus CD19/CD21 lowers the threshold for B-cell activation 100-fold. The importance of complement in stimulating B cells is emphasized by the observation that dogs deficient in C3 have very low immunoglobulin levels (see Chapter 5).

The B-cell Fc receptor, FcγRIIb, is a negative regulator of B-cell function. When an IgG molecule binds and links this receptor to a BCR

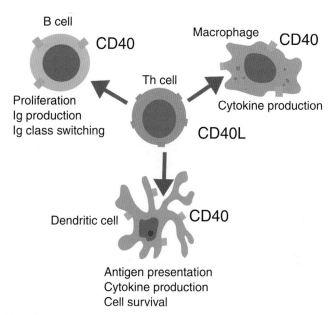

Fig. 16.10 CD40 and CD154 participate in a dialog between T cells and the three populations of antigen-presenting cells. In each case, both cell types are stimulated. In the case of B cells, T-cell stimulation permits B-cell proliferation and immunoglobulin production. *Ig*, Immunoglobulin.

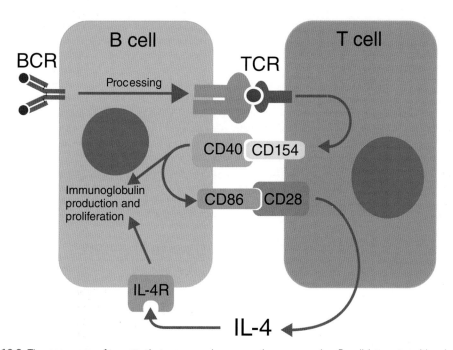

Fig. 16.9 The sequence of events that occurs when an antigen-processing B cell interacts with a helper T cell. During a primary immune response, antigen is processed by a dendritic cell and presented to the helper T cell. During a secondary immune response, the B cell itself can act as an antigen-presenting cell. Costimulators, such as CD154 and CD28, engage serially to trigger interleukin-4 (IL-4) secretion by the T cell and IL-4 receptor (IL-4R) expression by the B cell. *BCR*, B-cell antigen receptor; *TCR*, T-cell antigen receptor.

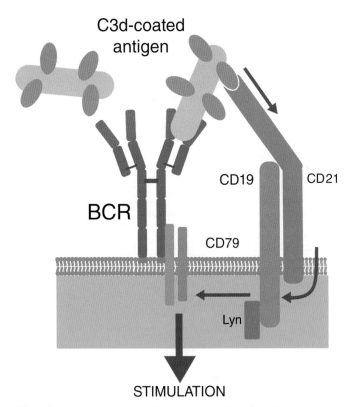

Fig. 16.11 The stimulation of B cells by antigen-bound complement through the CD21/CD19 complex. CD21 binds to C3d on the antigen. Signaling through CD19, the C3d generates a potent costimulatory signal that enhances B-cell responses. *BCR*, B-cell antigen receptor.

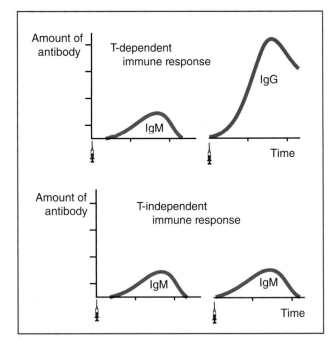

Fig. 16.12 The differences in the nature of T-dependent and -independent antibody responses. T-independent antigens cannot induce an immunoglobulin switch or immunological memory. As a result, they cannot trigger a secondary antibody response.

through antigen, it inhibits antibody formation. This has important practical consequences when vaccinating young animals (Chapter 26).

Toll-like Receptor Help

Although BCR-antigen-binding plus T-cell costimulation trigger initial B-cell division, they cannot induce a prolonged, self-sustaining B-cell response. Complete activation of B cells also requires coordinated signals from their TLRs (Hayashi et al., 2005). The B cell–stimulating ligands include flagellins, lipopolysaccharides, and CpG DNA. Signaling through TLR4 enhances B-cell antigen presentation, promotes germinal center formation, and is required for optimal antibody production against T-dependent antigens. TLR signaling to memory B cells increases antibody production, but it does not appear to be required for IgA and IgE production. Thus TLR signaling can substitute in part for T cell help and explains why antibody production still occurs in AIDS patients despite their lack of T cells (Pasare and Medzhitov, 2005).

B-CELL RESPONSES

Once it receives stimuli from the multiple sources described above, the B cell is ready to respond.

Differential Signaling

Like the TCR, the BCR probably produces a tunable signal. That is, it generates signals that depend on the properties of the antigen and the amount of costimulation received. The affinity of a BCR for its antigen influences B-cell proliferation and antibody secretion. On the other hand, receptor occupancy influences MHC class II expression and signal transduction. The direction of the immunoglobulin class switch also depends on signals received from Th1 or Th2 cytokines.

Certain antigens can provoke antibody formation in the absence of helper T cells. These so-called T-independent antigens are usually simple repeating polymers such as *Escherichia coli* lipopolysaccharide, polymerized salmonella flagellin, and pneumococcal polysaccharide. These T-independent antigens can bind directly to B-cell TLRs and cross-link several BCRs, providing a sufficient signal for B-cell proliferation. Characteristically, T-independent antigens only trigger IgM responses and fail to generate memory cells (Fig. 16.12).

It is appropriate to emphasize at this stage that the BCR has the same antigen-binding ability as antibody molecules. Thus, antibodies can bind free intact antigens in solution. This is very different from the α/β TCR that can only bind processed antigen fragments bound to an MHC molecule (Fig. 16.13). This difference in the antigen-binding ability of B and T cells is significant in that B cells can respond to a greater variety of antigens than T cells. Likewise, antibodies are directed, not against breakdown products of antigens, but against intact antigen molecules. As a result, antigen-antibody interactions usually depend on maintenance of the conformation of an antigen. A good example of this is seen with tetanus toxoid. Antibodies raised against the intact molecule will bind only to the intact molecule and may be unable to bind proteolytic fragments such as those produced by macrophage processing.

CELLULAR RESPONSES

The term clonotype is used to describe a clone of B cells expressing a BCR capable of responding to a single epitope. A newborn animal with few B cells has only a limited variety of clonotypes available, but their diversity increases with age as a result of increased use of alternative sets of V genes and of somatic mutation (see Chapter 18). This diversity is also increased by signals from the intestinal microbiota (see Chapter 22). In an adult animal, the number of B cells within a given clonotype depends on their exposure to different antigens over the animal's lifetime. Thus, the most used clonotypes will increase greatly in number, and there may be as many as 10^4 responsive B cells per clonotype (Box 16.1).

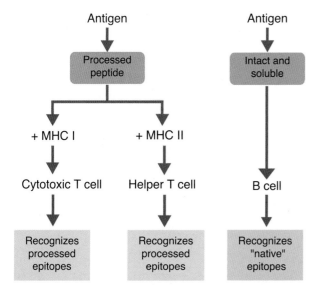

Fig. 16.13 T-cell antigen receptors (TCRs) and B-cell antigen receptors (BCRs) recognize antigen in a very different fashion. Thus BCRs can bind and respond to free, soluble antigens. TCRs, in contrast, can recognize only processed antigenic peptides presented on a major histocompatibility complex (MHC) molecule. This means that B-cell antigen receptors may readily bind to normal body components. But in the absence of a helper T-cell response, this will normally fail to lead to an antibody response or autoimmunity.

BOX 16.1   Cell Membrane Exchange

It has generally been assumed that individual cells conserve their major structural components and do not share them with other cells. In recent years, however, it has become abundantly clear that cells may exchange cell surface membranes and their associated receptors. Thus macrophages may accept fragments of neutrophil membranes. Activated B cells can also donate their antigen receptors to nearby bystander cells. This process is mediated by membrane transfer between adjacent B cells and is amplified by the interaction of the BCR with specific antigen. The net effect is to permit a dramatic expansion of the number of antigen-binding B cells in vivo. The B cells with their newly acquired receptors can act as antigen-presenting cells for CD4+ T cells. This is yet another example of the remarkable efficiency of the adaptive immune system in responding to a specific antigen once an animal is primed.

From Quah, B.J., Barlow, V.P., McPhun, V., et al., 2008. Bystander B cells rapidly acquire antigen receptors from activated B cells by membrane transfer. Proc. Natl. Acad. Sci. U.S.A. 105, 4259–4264; Davis, D.M., 2007. Intercellular transfer of cell-surface proteins is common and can affect many stages of an immune response. Nat. Rev. Immunol. 7, 238–243.

Conversely, a completely novel antigen may have as few as 10 responsive B cells in their spleen or bone marrow.

In most newborn mammals, each B cell initially expresses both IgM and IgD BCRs on its surface with about 10 times as many IgD molecules as IgM. These unstimulated B cells may secrete small amounts of monomeric IgM.

When appropriately stimulated and costimulated, B cells undergo repeated division. The B-cell division that results from this is asymmetric, so that one daughter cell gets a lot of antigen while the other daughter cell gets very little or none. The cell that gets lots of antigen then differentiates into a plasma cell. The cell that gets very little antigen continues the cycle of dividing and mutating and eventually becomes a memory cell. The cells destined to become plasma cells develop a rough endoplasmic

BOX 16.2   BAFF/APRIL System

B cell–activating factor (BAFF) (CD257) and "a proliferation-inducing ligand" (APRIL) (CD256) are two related cytokines. BAFF is produced by monocytes, dendritic cells, T cells, and neutrophils. APRIL is produced by monocytes, dendritic cells, T cells, and intestinal epithelial cells. They bind to the same or related receptors on B cells. BAFF is expressed on the cell membranes of producing cells but can be cleaved off as a soluble cytokine. It functions in both situations. APRIL only functions as a soluble cytokine. They both promote B-cell division and inhibit their apoptosis. Both BAFF and APRIL are crucial survival factors for B cells and essential for their production and differentiation. Overexpression of BAFF results in severe autoimmune disease.

From Ng, L.G., Mackay, C.R., Mackay, F., 2005. The BAFF/APRIL system: life beyond B lymphocytes. Mol. Immunol. 42, 763–772; He, B., Xu, W., Santini, P.A., Polydorides, A.D., et al., 2007. Intestinal bacteria trigger T cell-independent immunoglobulin A(2) class switching by inducing epithelial-cell secretion of the cytokine. Immunity 26, 812–826.

---

reticulum, increase their rate of protein synthesis, and secrete large quantities of immunoglobulins. Within a few days, these responding cells switch from making IgM to making another immunoglobulin class. This switch occurs within the germinal center and leads to the production of IgG, IgA, or IgE. This class switch results from the deletion of unwanted heavy chain genes and the joining of variable-region genes to the next available heavy chain genes (see Chapter 17). The specificity of the antibody produced remains unchanged.

Class switching is controlled by IL-4, IFN-γ, and TGF-β (Cerutti et al., 2005). Thus IL-4 from Th2 cells directs mouse B cells to produce IgG1 and IgE, whereas it directs human B cells to produce IgG4 and IgE (see Table 16.1). IL-4 alone is insufficient for class switching, and additional signals are required from CD40 and CD154. IFN-γ from Th1 cells stimulates a switch to IgG2a and IgG3 in mouse B cells and effectively suppresses the effects of IL-4. IFN-γ acts by promoting the production of the B cell–stimulating cytokines BAFF and APRIL (Box 16.2). TGF-β promotes the switch to IgA production on body surfaces. As described previously, signals from IL-5 and IL-6 also contribute to class switching.

PLASMA CELLS

Antigen-stimulated B cells develop into plasma cells (Fig. 16.14). These are mainly located in the secondary lymphoid organs. Early plasma cells (plasmablasts) can be identified in the lymph node cortex and paracortex and in the marginal zone in the spleen. As the B cells differentiate, the plasma cells emigrate from these areas to the spleen, the medulla of lymph nodes, and especially to the bone marrow where they may persist for years. During this time, many continue to produce specific antibodies. The bone marrow provides a cytokine environment where plasma cells can survive for long periods. This is probably due to the stimulating cytokines, BAFF, and APRIL. Plasma cells are ovoid cells, 8 to 9 μm in diameter (Fig. 16.15). They have a round, eccentrically placed nucleus with unevenly distributed chromatin. As a result, the nucleus may resemble a clock face or cartwheel. Plasma cells have an extensive cytoplasm that is rich in rough endoplasmic reticulum and so stains strongly with basic dyes and pyronin. They have a large, pale-staining Golgi apparatus (Figs. 16.16 and 16.17). Plasma cells can secrete up to 10,000 molecules of immunoglobulin per second. The immunoglobulin produced by a plasma cell is of identical binding specificity to the BCRs on its parent B cell. Plasma cells with cytoplasmic globules (Russell bodies) are called Mott cells. Plasma cells with a pink fringe of cytoplasm are called "flame cells."

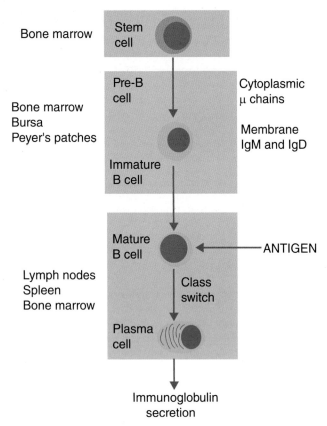

Bone marrow

Stem cell

Bone marrow
Bursa
Peyer's patches

Pre-B cell

Cytoplasmic µ chains

Immature B cell

Membrane IgM and IgD

Lymph nodes
Spleen
Bone marrow

Mature B cell

ANTIGEN

Class switch

Plasma cell

Immunoglobulin secretion

Fig. 16.14 B cells originate in the bone marrow and proceed through a series of differentiation developmental stages before becoming able to respond to antigen. When B cells respond to antigen, they respond by division and differentiation of their progeny into plasma cells. *Ig,* Immunoglobulin.

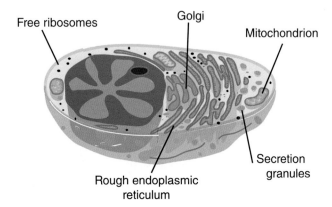

Free ribosomes

Golgi

Mitochondrion

Secretion granules

Rough endoplasmic reticulum

Fig. 16.15 The structure of a typical plasma cell. The possession of an extensive rough endoplasmic reticulum is typical of a cell dedicated to the rapid production of large amounts of protein such as immunoglobulin.

MEMORY B CELLS

One reason that the primary immune response ends is that the responding B cells and plasma cells undergo apoptosis. If all these cells died, however, immunological memory could not develop. Clearly, some B cells must survive as memory cells. B cells are activated by antigen and helper T cells in the paracortex of lymph nodes. Most of these B cells differentiate into plasma cells and migrate to the bone marrow, spleen, and other organs, but some memory precursors remain in the

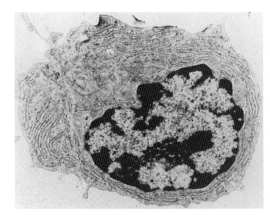

Fig. 16.16 A transmission electron micrograph of a plasma cell from a rabbit. Courtesy Dr. S. Linthicum.

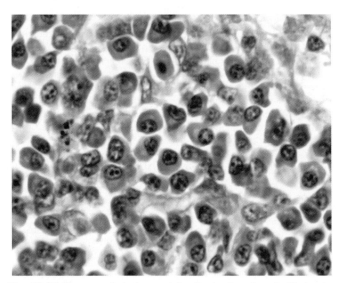

Fig. 16.17 Plasma cells in the medulla of a dog lymph node. Their cytoplasm is rich in ribosomes and so stains intensely with pyronin, giving a dark red appearance. Original magnification ×450. From a specimen kindly provided by Drs. N. McArthur and L.C. Abbott.

cortex, proliferate, and form germinal centers. (Asymmetric division as described earlier likely accounts for these two different fates) (Barnett et al., 2012). These cells persist under the influence of programming and rescue signals. Thus, memory cells are first screened for their ability to bind antigen. This induces CD154 on nearby T cells, which in turn promotes the expression of *bcl*-2. *Bcl*-2 protects them against apoptosis and allows the B cells to survive and differentiate into memory cells.

Memory cells form a reserve of long-lived antigen-sensitive cells to be called upon following subsequent exposure to an antigen. There are several populations of memory B cells distinguishable by their immunoglobulin class, their location, and their passage through germinal centers. For example, one population consists of small, long-lived resting cells with IgG BCR. These cells, unlike plasma cells, look like generic lymphocytes. Their survival does not depend on antigen contact. On exposure to antigen, they proliferate and differentiate into plasma cells without undergoing further mutation. It has been calculated that in a secondary immune response, the clonal expansion of memory B cells results in 8- to 10-fold more plasma cells than does a primary immune response.

A second memory B-cell population consists of large, dividing cells with IgM BCRs. These cells persist in germinal centers, where their

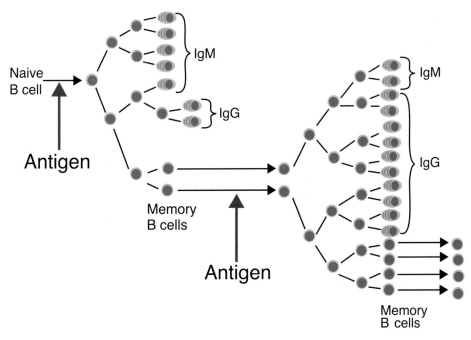

Fig. 16.18 The time course of a B-cell response and the cellular events that accompany it. Note that some IgG is made in the primary immune response, whereas a small amount of IgM is also made in a secondary immune response.

continued survival depends on exposure to antigen by follicular dendritic cells. There are two distinct populations of plasma cells: a short-lived population that lives for 1–2 weeks and produces large amounts of antibodies shortly after antigen exposure, and a long-lived population that can survive for months or years. (In humans, these plasma cells have a half-life of 8–15 years.) These antibodies provide immediate immunity to microbial pathogens. The short-lived cells are found in the spleen and lymph nodes soon after immunization. The long-lived plasma cells, in contrast, accumulate in the bone marrow. These long-lived plasma cells probably develop from a population of self-renewing, slowly dividing memory B cells (Ahuja et al., 2007). These memory B cells require a functional BCR to survive, suggesting that constant low-affinity antigen binding keeps them alive. Thus, cats immunized with killed panleukopenia virus will continue to produce antibodies at low levels for many years. The source of these antibodies is believed to be the long-lived plasma cells stimulated to secrete antibodies by exposure to PAMPs and T cell help.

If a second dose of antigen is given to a primed animal, it will encounter large numbers of memory B cells that respond in the manner described previously for antigen-sensitive B cells (Fig. 16.18). As a result, a secondary immune response is much greater than a primary immune response. The lag period is shorter since more antibodies are produced, and they can be detected earlier. IgG is also produced in preference to the IgM characteristic of the primary response.

GERMINAL CENTERS

A key feature of the humoral immune response is the progressive increase in antigen-binding affinity over time. This process takes place within germinal centers (Fig. 16.19). Thus germinal centers are sites where antigen-driven B-cell proliferation, somatic mutation, and positive- and negative- selection of B-cell populations occur (Berek, 1992). Germinal centers are divided into two zones based on staining patterns, a light zone containing dendritic cells, some B cells and Tfh cells, and a dark zone that mainly consists of

dividing B cells. In the early stages of the reaction, B cells stimulated by antigen and Tfh cells migrate to the dark zone. There they proliferate and as they do so, they mutate their antibody V genes. B cells divide every 6–8 hours so that within just a few days a single B cell develops into a clone of several thousand cells. During this phase of rapid B-cell division, the BCR V region genes mutate randomly, once per division (Dale et al., 2019). This repeated mutation generates B cells whose BCRs differ from the parent cell. Once these cells have been clonally expanded, a process that takes 10–20 days, they migrate to the light zone where they are presented with antigen by the dendritic cells. Because of their altered V regions, some of these B cells bind the antigen with greater affinity, while others bind it less strongly. A process of selection thus occurs. If a mutation has resulted in greater binding affinity, this stimulates more B-cell proliferation. Thus cycles of rapid somatic mutation and selection lead to a rapid improvement in antigen binding—a process called affinity maturation. These antigen-selected B cells eventually leave the germinal center to form either plasma cells or memory B cells. In contrast, those B cells with BCRs that have reduced antigen binding undergo apoptosis. Thus the B-cell population that emerges from a germinal center is very different from the population of cells that entered it. In addition to somatic mutation of BCR V genes, BCRs also undergo class switching within germinal centers. Germinal centers eventually dissipate after the B-cell response has peaked (Elsner and Shlomchik, 2020).

B-Cell Subpopulations

In mice, there are two subpopulations of B cells that develop from different precursor stem cells. These are called B1 and B2 cells. B2 cells are conventional B cells that are central to the adaptive antibody responses and are discussed in this chapter and throughout the book. B2 cells appear late in neonatal life, are the predominant population in adult bone marrow, and produce most of the body's IgG.

Mouse B1 cells originate from stem cells in the fetal liver or omentum rather than the bone marrow. They are innate-like cells that share

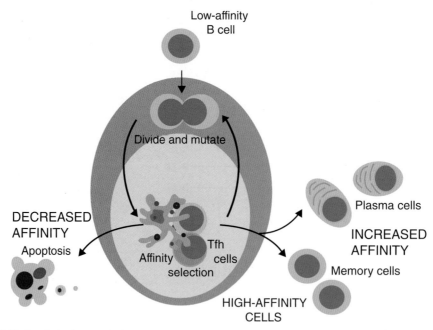

Fig. 16.19 B cells in the germinal center undergo somatic mutation as they respond to antigen presented by dendritic cells. If the mutation enables them to bind antigen with increased affinity, they will be stimulated to continue dividing. If, on the other hand, the mutation reduces their antigen-binding affinity, they will undergo apoptosis.

some features with macrophages. They are, for example, phagocytic and microbicidal (they produce ROS) and can present antigen to CD4⁺ T cells. There are two subpopulations of B1 cells, termed B1a and B1b. B1a cells develop exclusively in the neonate, are self-replenishing, and are responsible for most "natural" IgM in serum. They thus participate in innate immunity. B1a cells express CD5, an adhesion and receptor molecule. (CD5 is the receptor for CD72.) They recognize common bacterial molecules such as phosphoryl-choline as well as molecules such as immunoglobulins and DNA. They produce antibodies in a T-independent manner. B1a cells also differ from conventional B2 cells in that they are found in the peritoneal and pleural cavities and can renew themselves. B1b cells are distinguished from B1a cells by lacking CD5. They are, however, required for protection against several parasites and bacteria. B1b cells are produced throughout adult life. Many of the IgA-producing cells in the intestine originate from B1 cells. B1 cells have been identified in humans, mice, rabbits, guinea pigs, pigs, sheep, and cattle. It is unclear, however, whether the B1-B2 classification applies to all these species (Appleyard and Wilkie, 1998; Wilson and Wilkie, 2007).

MYELOMAS

If a B cell turns cancerous, it may develop into a clone of immunoglobulin-producing tumor cells. These cells are usually recognizable as plasma cells (Fig. 16.20). Plasma cell tumors are called myelomas or plasmacytomas. Because myelomas arise from a single precursor cell or clone, they secrete a homogeneous immunoglobulin called a myeloma protein. On serum electrophoresis, this homogeneous myeloma protein will appear as a sharp, well-defined peak. This is called a monoclonal gammopathy (Fig. 16.21).

Myeloma proteins may belong to any immunoglobulin class. For example, IgG, IgA, and IgM myelomas have been reported in dogs. In humans, in addition to myelomas of the major immunoglobulin classes, rare cases of IgD and IgE myelomas have also been described.

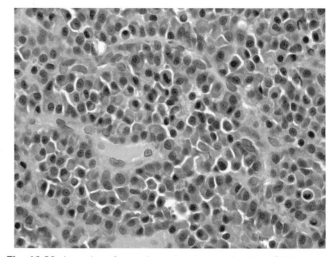

Fig. 16.20 A section of a myeloma tumor mass in a dog. Original magnification ×600. These cells are clearly plasma cells. Courtesy Dr. Brian Porter.

The prevalence of myelomas expressing the various immunoglobulin classes in myeloma proteins correlates with their quantities in normal serum. Light chain disease is caused by a myeloma in which light chains alone are produced, or the production of light chains is greatly in excess of the production of heavy chains. Similarly, there is a very rare form of myeloma in which Fc fragments alone are produced. This condition is erroneously termed heavy chain disease.

Myelomas have been described in humans, mice, dogs, cats, horses, cows, pigs, ferrets, and rabbits. They account for less than 1% of all canine tumors, and they are considerably rarer in the other domestic species. The clinical presentations of myelomas include bleeding disorders, hyperviscosity, renal failure, and hypercalcemia. Other signs include lethargy, recurrent infections, anemia, lameness, bone

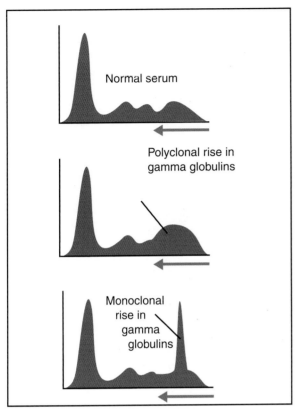

Fig. 16.21 Serum electrophoretic patterns showing the normal pattern and the characteristic features of monoclonal and polyclonal gammopathies. The monoclonal antibody spike reflects the production of large amounts of homogenous immunoglobulins. Monoclonal gammopathies commonly result from the presence of a myeloma. The arrow denotes the direction of protein migration.

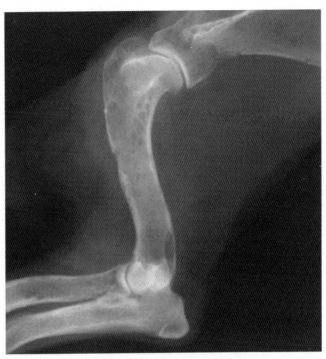

Fig. 16.22 A radiograph of a dog, showing the round, radiolucent areas where bone has been eroded by the presence of a myeloma. Courtesy Dr. Claudia Barton.

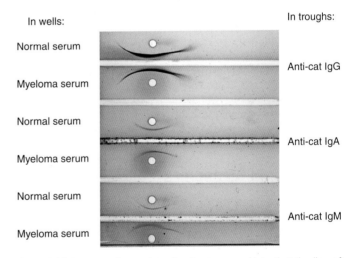

Fig. 16.23 Immunoelectrophoresis of cat serum. Note that the line of precipitate formed by the reaction between anti-cat immunoglobulin M (IgM) and the myeloma serum is distorted (*bottom well*). The line is much thicker than the control, and it forms two distinct joined arcs as a result of the presence of a monoclonal IgM myeloma protein. (Details of this technique can be found in Chapter 43.). Courtesy Dr. G. Elissalde.

fractures, and neurological signs, including dementia and peripheral neuropathy. The most common clinical manifestation in dogs is excessive bleeding as a result of a thrombocytopenia and a loss of clotting components as they bind to myeloma proteins. The presence in serum of abnormally large quantities of immunoglobulins results in a hyperviscosity syndrome, which is especially severe in animals with IgM myelomas (macroglobulinemia). As a result of the increase in blood viscosity, the heart must work harder, and congestive heart failure, retinopathy, and neurological signs may result. Because myeloma cells stimulate osteoclast activity, the presence of tumors in bone marrow may lead to severe bone destruction. Multiple radiolucent osteolytic lesions and diffuse osteoporosis develop and are readily seen by radiography (Fig. 16.22). These lesions result in pathological fractures. Light chains, being relatively small, are excreted in the urine. Unfortunately, they are toxic for renal tubular cells and, as a result, may cause renal failure. The light chains may be detected by electrophoresis of concentrated urine or, in some cases, by heating the urine. Light chains precipitate when heated to 60°C but redissolve as the temperature is raised to 80°C. Proteins possessing this curious property are called Bence-Jones proteins, and their presence in urine suggests a myeloma (Fig. 16.23). They occur in about 40% of canine cases. Nonsecretory myelomas are occasionally diagnosed in dogs.

Because of the overwhelming commitment of the body's immune resources to the production of neoplastic plasma cells, as well as the replacement of normal marrow tissue by tumor cells and the negative feedback induced by elevated serum immunoglobulins, animals with myelomas are immunosuppressed and anemic. In humans, renal failure and overwhelming infection are the most common causes of death in myeloma patients.

Affected animals should receive supportive therapy. Antibiotics can be used to control secondary infections, and fluid therapy should be administered to combat dehydration resulting from renal failure. Steroids and diuretics may assist in promoting calcium excretion. The serum hyperviscosity may be reduced by plasmapheresis to remove the myeloma protein. The tumor itself can be treated with specific chemotherapy. The drug of choice is melphalan, an alkylating agent. Prednisone may be used in association with melphalan. In unresponsive cases, cyclophosphamide or thalidomide may be employed. In humans, major improvements in survival have resulted from the use of monoclonal antibodies against malignant B-cell antigens (see Chapter 36).

Sometimes, in clinically normal humans, dogs, and horses, a monoclonal gammopathy may develop that is not due to a myeloma. These monoclonal antibodies are usually an accidental finding on serum electrophoresis, and their origin is unclear. They may disappear spontaneously within a short period, or they may persist for many years. Affected animals may show abnormally large numbers of plasma cells in their internal organs on necropsy.

Polyclonal Gammopathies

In contrast to monoclonal gammopathies, which are usually produced by a myeloma, polyclonal gammopathies are observed in many different diseases. Polyclonal gammopathies are characterized by an increase in all immunoglobulins as a result of excessive activity of many different clones of plasma cells. The condition that most resembles a myeloma is Aleutian disease in mink (see Chapter 28). Animals infected by the Aleutian disease parvovirus show marked plasmacytosis and lymphocyte infiltration of many organs and tissues, as well as a polyclonal (occasionally monoclonal) gammopathy. As a result of the elevated immunoglobulin levels, affected mink experience a hyperviscosity syndrome and are severely immunosuppressed.

Other causes of polyclonal gammopathy include autoimmune diseases such as systemic lupus erythematosus, rheumatoid arthritis, and myasthenia gravis (see Chapter 39), as well as infections such as tropical pancytopenia in dogs due to *Ehrlichia canis*, African trypanosomiasis, and chronic bacterial infections such as pyometra and pyoderma. In horses heavily parasitized with *Strongylus vulgaris*, polyclonal IgG3 levels rise significantly. Polyclonal gammopathy also occurs in virus diseases such as feline infectious peritonitis and African swine fever and in diseases in which there is extensive liver damage.

IgG4-related diseases are a group of inflammatory disorders characterized by excessive IgG4 production. Affected dogs develop abnormalities in innate immunity including activation of macrophages, mast cells, basophils, and dendritic cells. The IgG4 antibodies can activate macrophages that then cause extensive tissue fibrosis.

MONOCLONAL ANTIBODIES

The plasma cells in myelomas become neoplastic in an entirely random manner, so the immunoglobulins that they secrete are not usually directed against any antigen of practical importance. Nevertheless, myeloma cells can be grown in tissue culture, where they survive indefinitely. This has provided an opportunity to obtain large quantities of pure, specific immunoglobulins directed against an antigen of interest. This can be done by fusing normal plasma cells, making the antibody of interest with myeloma cells that can grow in tissue culture. The resulting mixed cell is called a hybridoma.

The first stage in making a hybridoma is to generate antibody-producing plasma cells (Fig. 16.24). This is done by immunizing a mouse against the antigen of interest and repeating the process several times to ensure that a good antibody response is mounted. 2–4 days after the antigen is administered, the spleen is removed and broken up to form a cell suspension. The spleen B cells are suspended in culture medium, together with cultured mouse myeloma cells. Generally, myeloma cells that do not secrete immunoglobulins are used since this simplifies purification later on. Polyethylene glycol is added to the mixture. This compound induces many of the cells to fuse (although it takes about 200,000 spleen cells on average to form a

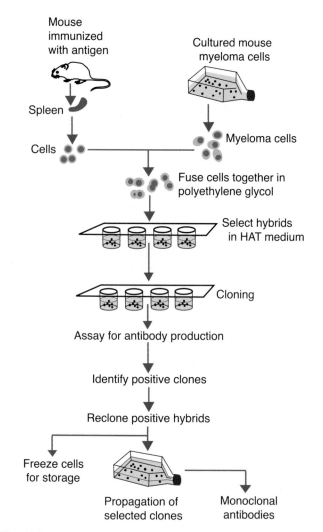

Fig. 16.24 A schematic diagram showing the method of production of monoclonal antibodies. Antibody-producing plasma cells are fused with myeloma cells. The resulting hybridoma cells are then cultured, cloned, and selected so that the selected cells only produce antibodies against the antigen of interest. (For details see text.) *HAT*, Hypoxanthine, aminopterin, and thymidine.

viable hybrid with one myeloma cell). If the fused cell mixture is cultured for several days, any unfused spleen cells will die. The myeloma cells would normally survive, but they are eliminated by blocking their nucleic acid synthesis.

There are three pathways by which cells can synthesize nucleotides and therefore nucleic acids. The myeloma cells are selected so that they lack two enzymes: hypoxanthine phosphoribosyl transferase and thymidine kinase. As a result, they cannot use either thymidine or hypoxanthine and are obliged to use an alternative biosynthetic pathway to convert uridine to nucleotides. The fused cell mixture is therefore grown in a culture containing three compounds: hypoxanthine, aminopterin, and thymidine (known as HAT medium). Aminopterin is a drug that prevents cells from making their own nucleotides from uridine. Since the myeloma cells cannot use hypoxanthine or thymidine and the aminopterin stops them from using the alternative synthetic pathway, they cannot make nucleic acids and soon die. Hybrid cells made from a myeloma and a normal cell are able to survive and grow since they possess the critical enzymes. The hybridomas divide rapidly in the HAT medium, doubling their numbers every 24–48 hours.

On average, about 300–500 different hybrids can be isolated from a mouse spleen, although not all will make antibodies of interest.

If a mixture of cells from a fusion experiment is cultured in wells on a plate with about 50,000 myeloma cells per well, it is usual to obtain about one hybrid in every three wells. After culturing for 2–4 weeks, the growing cells can be seen, and the supernatant fluid can be screened for the presence of antibodies. It is essential to use a sensitive assay at this time. Radioimmunoassays or enzyme-linked immunosorbent assays are preferred (see Chapter 43). Clones that produce the desired antibody are grown in mass tissue culture and recloned to eliminate non–antibody-producing hybrids. The monoclonal antibodies produced are then purified using antigen affinity purification.

The classical methods of making hybridomas produce only mouse immunoglobulins and these are of limited usefulness in other mammals. Mouse antibodies are regarded as foreign in these species and are rapidly removed by the recipient's immune response. Two strategies have been used to prevent or minimize this. One involves the genetic manipulation of hybridomas so that they produce antibodies of reduced antigenicity. Thus, we can use only purified Fab'2 fragments—this eliminates the immunogenic Fc region but reduces their biological activities. It is possible however to join this fragment to the Fc region of the target species using molecular biological approaches to produce a chimeric molecule. For example, mouse myeloma variable regions can be attached to dog constant regions to make a canine monoclonal antibody for use in that species. By subsequently modifying the sequence in the V region framework regions, the monoclonal antibody may be fully "caninized." For example, a caninized monoclonal antibody directed against interleukin-31 is used to prevent itch in dogs with atopic dermatitis (see Chapter 31). Alternatively, it is possible to produce monoclonal antibodies of the desired species using "display technologies" such as phage displays. In these cases, huge libraries of antibody fragments are generated from the species of interest and then screened for their antigen-binding abilities.

Monoclonal antibodies are the preferred source of antibodies for much immunological research and new medical treatments. They are absolutely specific for single epitopes and are available in large amounts. Because of their purity, they are used in clinical diagnostic tests in which large quantities of antibodies of consistent quality are required. Although mouse cells have been the preferred source, studies have shown that cattle and goats can be genetically engineered to produce monoclonal antibodies in their milk. It has even proved possible to incorporate antibody genes into plants such as soy, corn, and tobacco. These "plantibodies" are produced in very large quantities and appear to be functional. "Humanized" monoclonal antibodies are being employed to treat cancers as well as inflammatory and autoimmune diseases. Similar species-modified monoclonal antibodies are being increasingly employed in veterinary medicine (see Chapter 42).

REFERENCES

Ahuja, A., Anderson, S.M., Khalil, A., Siomchik, M.J., 2007. Maintenance of the plasma cell pool is independent of memory B cells. Proc. Natl. Acad. Sci. 105, 4802–4807.

Appleyard, G.D., Wilkie, B.N., 1998. Characterization of porcine CD5 and CD5+ B cells. Clin. Exp. Immunol. 111, 225–230.

Barnett, B.E., Ciocca, M.L., Goenka, R., Barnett, L.G., Wu, J., Laufer, T.M., et al., 2012. Asymmetric B cell division in the germinal center reaction. Science 335 (6066), 342–344.

Batista, F.D., Harwood, N.E., 2009. The who, how and where of antigen presentation to B cells. Nat. Rev. Immunol. 9, 15–27.

Berek, C., 1992. The development of B cells and the B-cell repertoire in the microenvironment of the germinal center. Immunol. Rev. 126, 5–19.

Cerutti, A., Qiao, X., He, B., 2005. Plasmacytoid dendritic cells and the regulation of immunoglobulin heavy chain class switching. Immunol. Cell Biol. 83, 554–562.

Clark, M.R., Campbell, K.S., Kazlauskas, A., et al., 1992. The B cell antigen receptor complex: association of Ig-α and Ig-β with distinct cytoplasmic effectors. Science 258, 123–125.

Dale, G.A., Wilkins, D.J., Bohannon, C.D., Dilernia, D., et al., 2019. Clustered mutations at the murine and human IgH locus exhibit significant linkage consistent with templated mutagenesis. J. Immunol. 203, 1252–1264.

Durie, F.H., Foy, T.M., Masters, S.R., et al., 1994. The role of CD40 in the regulation of humoral and cell-mediated immunity. Immunol. Today 15, 406–411.

Elsner, R.A., Shlomchik, M.J., 2020. Germinal center and extrafollicular B cell responses in vaccination, immunity and autoimmunity. Immunity. https://doi.org/10.1016/j.mmuni.2020.11.006.

Finkelman, F.D., Lees, A., Morris, S.C., 1992. Antigen presentation by B lymphocytes to CD4+ T lymphocytes in vivo: importance for B lymphocyte and T lymphocyte activation. Semin. Immunol. 4, 247–255.

Gold, M.R., 2002. To make antibodies or not: signaling by the B-cell antigen receptor. Trends Pharm. Sci. 23, 316–324.

Hayashi, E.A., Akira, S., Nobrega, A., 2005. Role of TLR in B cell development: signaling through TLR4 promotes B cell maturation and is inhibited by TLR2. J. Immunol. 174, 6639–6647.

Pasare, C., Medzhitov, R., 2005. Control of B-cell responses by Toll-like receptors. Nature 438, 364–368.

Tedder, T.F., Zhou, L.-J., Engel, P., 1994. The CD19/CD21 signal transduction complex of B lymphocytes. Immunol. Today 15, 437–442.

Tizard, I.R., 2023. The Comparative Immunology of the Mammals. Acadmic Press, San Diego, CA.

Wilson, S.M., Wilkie, B.N., 2007. B-1 and B-2 B-cells in the pig cannot be differentiated by expression of CD5. Vet. Immunol. Immunopathol. 115, 10–16.

17

Antibodies: Soluble Antigen Receptors

CHAPTER OUTLINE

The properties of B-cell antigen receptors (BCRs) were discussed in the previous chapter. These receptors are, however, not restricted to the B-cell surface. Once a B-cell response is triggered, it becomes a plasma cell and its antigen receptors are produced in huge amounts and shed into the surrounding fluid, where they act as antibodies. These antibodies bind to foreign antigens and mark them for destruction or elimination. Antibodies are found in many body fluids but are present in the highest concentrations and are most easily obtained from blood serum. Antibodies defend an animal against many different microbes, including bacteria, viruses, helminths, and protozoa. They also act in several different environments, for example, in blood and milk or on body surfaces. It is not surprising, therefore, that multiple immunoglobulin classes exist. Each class is optimized for action in a specific environment; for example, IgA protects body surfaces. Immunoglobulins may also be optimized for activity against a specific group of pathogens. For example, IgE is important in the defense against parasitic worms.

IMMUNOGLOBULINS

Antibody molecules are glycoproteins called immunoglobulins. There are five structural classes (or isotypes) of immunoglobulins. The class found in the highest concentrations in serum is called immunoglobulin G (abbreviated to IgG). The class with the second highest serum concentration (in most mammals) is immunoglobulin M (IgM). The third-highest concentration in most mammals is immunoglobulin A (IgA). IgA is, however, the predominant immunoglobulin in secretions such as saliva, milk, and intestinal fluid. Immunoglobulin D (IgD) is primarily a BCR and is rarely encountered in body fluids. Immunoglobulin E (IgE) is found in very low concentrations in serum and mediates allergic reactions. The characteristics of each of these classes are shown in Table 17.1.

When serum is subjected to electrophoresis, its protein mixture separates into four major fractions (Fig. 17.1). The most negatively charged fraction consists of a single homogeneous protein called serum albumin. The other three fractions contain proteins classified as α, β, and γ globulins, according to their electrophoretic mobility (Fig. 17.2). Most immunoglobulins migrate in the γ globulins. Immunoglobulin molecules consist of four linked peptide chains. Together they form a bilaterally symmetrical Y-shaped molecule with two identical Fab regions linked to a stem consisting of an Fc region. The Fab regions bind antigens, and the Fc region binds to cells and activates complement.

IMMUNOGLOBULIN CLASSES

Immunoglobulin G

IgG is produced by plasma cells in the spleen, lymph nodes, and bone marrow. It is the immunoglobulin found in the highest concentration in the blood and plays a major role in antibody-mediated defenses. It has a molecular weight of about 180 kDa and a typical BCR structure with two identical light chains and two identical γ heavy chains (Fig. 17.3). Its light chains may be of the κ or λ type. Because it is the smallest of the immunoglobulin molecules, IgG can escape from blood vessels more easily than the others. This is especially important in inflammation, where increased vascular permeability allows IgG to participate in the defense of tissues and body surfaces. IgG binds to specific antigens such as those found on bacteria. The binding of these antibody molecules to bacteria can cause clumping (agglutination) and opsonization. IgG antibodies activate the classical complement pathway only when sufficient molecules have clustered on the antigenic surface (see Chapter 5).

It has generally been assumed that once an antibody molecule has formed, its structure remains unchanged until it is destroyed by catabolic processes. That assumption is incorrect. The IgG4 subclass in humans can exchange regions with other antibody molecules to generate a hybrid antibody with two different Fab arms. As a result, this

	IMMUNOGLOBULIN CLASS				
TABLE 17.1 Major Immunoglobulin Classes in the Domestic Mammals					
Property	**IgM**	**IgG**	**IgA**	**IgE**	**IgD**
Molecular weight	900,000	180,000	360,000	200,000	180,000
Subunits	5	1	2	1	1
Heavy chain	μ	γ	α	ε	δ
Largely synthesized in	Spleen and lymph nodes	Spleen and lymph nodes	Intestinal and respiratory tracts	Intestinal and respiratory tracts	Spleen and lymph nodes

Ig, Immunoglobulin.

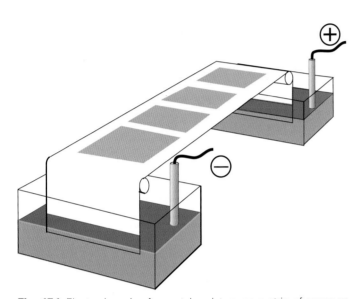

Fig. 17.1 Electrophoresis of a protein mixture on a strip of paper or gel. The support bridges two buffer baths, and an electrical potential is applied across them. It provides a convenient way to analyze serum proteins based on their charge.

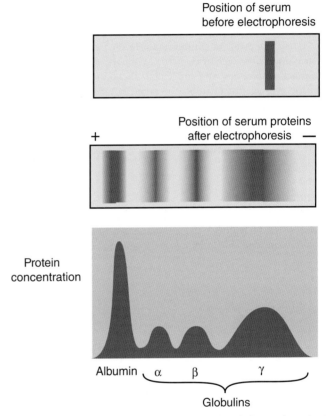

Fig. 17.2 Schematic diagram showing the results of electrophoresis of whole serum. It consistently separates serum proteins into four major bands: one albumin and three globulin bands.

antibody can cross-link two different antigens. IgG4 is the least abundant human IgG subclass. This exchange of Fab arms between IgG4 molecules is dynamic. Thus, a homogeneous IgG4 antibody, when administered to a human, will rapidly begin to swap arms. It is not known whether this Fab-arm exchange occurs in domestic mammals.

Immunoglobulin M

IgM is produced by plasma cells in the secondary lymphoid organs. It has the second highest concentration after IgG in most mammalian sera. When still attached to the B cell and acting as a BCR, IgM is a 180 kDa monomer. However, the secreted form of IgM consists of five (occasionally six) 180 kDa units linked by disulfide bonds in a circular fashion. Its total molecular weight is then 900 kDa (Fig. 17.4). A small polypeptide called the J chain (15 kDa) joins two of the units to complete the circle. Each IgM monomer is of conventional immunoglobulin

structure and consists of two κ or λ light chains and two μ heavy chains; μ chains differ from γ chains in that they have an additional, fourth constant domain (C_H4), as well as an additional 20-amino acid segment on their C-terminus, but they have no hinge region. The complement activation site on IgM is located on its C_H4 domains.

IgM is the major immunoglobulin produced during primary immune responses (Fig. 17.5). Smaller quantities are also produced in secondary responses. Although produced in small amounts, IgM is more efficient (on a molar basis) than IgG at complement activation, opsonization, neutralization of viruses, and agglutination. Because of their very large size, IgM molecules rarely enter tissue fluids even at sites of acute inflammation.

Immunoglobulin A

IgA is mainly produced by plasma cells located under body surfaces. Thus it is made in the walls of the intestine, respiratory tract, urinary system, skin, and mammary gland. Although produced in large amounts, most goes into the intestine, bronchi, or milk. As a result, its serum concentration in most mammals is usually lower than that of IgM. IgA monomers have a molecular weight of 150 kDa, but they are normally secreted as dimers. Each IgA monomer consists of two light chains and two α heavy chains containing three constant domains. In dimeric IgA, the two monomers are joined by a J chain (Fig. 17.6). Higher polymers of IgA are occasionally found in serum.

IgA produced in body surfaces is transported through epithelial cells into external secretions bound to the polymeric immunoglobulin receptor (also called secretory component) (see Fig. 23.13). Secretory component is a peptide that binds to IgA dimers to form secretory IgA (SIgA). It protects the IgA from digestion by microbial and intestinal proteases.

SIgA is the major immunoglobulin in the external secretions of nonruminants. As such, it is of critical importance in protecting the intestinal, respiratory, and urogenital tracts, the mammary gland, and the eyes against microbial invasion. IgA does not activate the classical complement pathway, nor can it act as an opsonin. It can, however, agglutinate particulate antigens and neutralize viruses. IgA mainly acts by preventing the adherence of invading microbes to body surfaces. Because of its importance, IgA is examined in more detail in Chapter 23.

Immunoglobulin E

IgE, like IgA, is mainly made by plasma cells located beneath body surfaces. It is a typical Y-shaped, four-chain immunoglobulin with four constant domains in its ε heavy chains and a molecular weight of 190 kDa (Fig. 17.7). Most IgE is bound to tissue mast cells and thus occurs in extremely low concentrations in serum.

IgE does not act simply by binding and coating antigens, as do the other immunoglobulins. IgE acts as a signal-transducing molecule on the surface of mast cells. When two mast cell-bound IgE molecules are cross-linked by an allergen, they trigger FcεR1 receptor activation, leading to the release of inflammatory molecules.

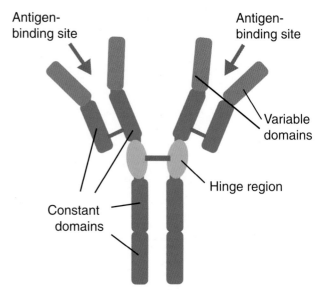

Fig. 17.3 The structure of immunoglobulin G, a typical immunoglobulin molecule.

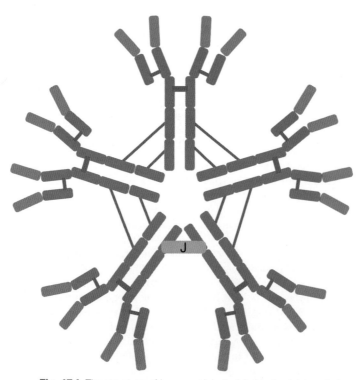

Fig. 17.4 The structure of immunoglobulin M. J is the joining chain.

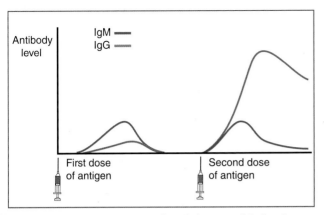

Fig. 17.5 The relative amounts of each immunoglobulin class produced during the primary and secondary immune responses. Note that immunoglobulin (Ig) M predominates in a primary immune response, whereas IgG predominates in later responses.

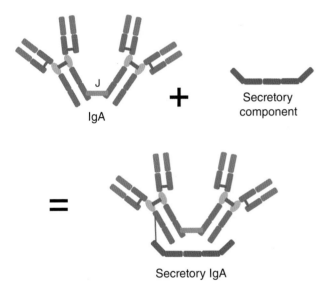

Fig. 17.6 The structure of dimeric immunoglobulin A (IgA) and secretory IgA (SIgA). Secretory component consists of five linked immunoglobulin domains. It is found on the surface of certain epithelial cells, where it acts as a receptor for polymeric immunoglobulins (pIgR). It can also bind to IgM.

IgE is found in exquisitely small quantities in serum, especially in humans but its concentration varies greatly within species (see Table 30.4). In domestic, and especially wild, mammals, IgE levels are greatly influenced by the presence of parasites. IgE also has a very short half-life of 2–3 days in humans and about 12 hours in mice. As a result, it has to be produced continuously in order to maintain its serum levels. Most of the body's IgE is firmly bound to high-affinity FcεRI receptors on the surface of tissue mast cells. As a result, the IgE serum concentration does not reflect its total amount in the body. The function of IgE is to trigger an acute inflammatory process that serves to eliminate parasites, especially helminth parasites, from the tissues and the gastrointestinal tract. IgE is readily

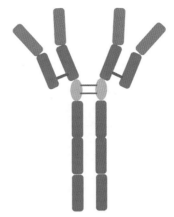

Fig. 17.7 The structure of immunoglobulin E. Note the presence of four constant domains in addition to a hinge in the heavy chain.

destroyed by mild heat treatment. It does not activate complement and its ability to cross the placenta in primates is limited. It is, however, found in colostrum.

Immunoglobulin D

IgD is present in horses, cattle, sheep, pigs, dogs, rodents, and primates but has not yet been detected in rabbits or cats (Wan et al., 2021). It is present in many bony fish and many birds, but not in chickens. IgD mainly remains attached to B cells, and very little is released into the bloodstream. IgD molecules consist of two δ heavy chains and two light chains. In contrast to the other immunoglobulin classes, IgD is evolutionarily labile and shows many structural variations (Rogers et al., 2006). For example, mouse IgD lacks a Cδ2 domain and thus has only two constant domains in its heavy chains. It has a molecular weight of about 170 kDa (Fig. 17.8). Horse, cow, sheep, dog, monkey, and human IgD, in contrast, have three heavy-chain constant domains and a very long hinge domain coded for by two exons (Fig. 17.9). Pig IgD has a short hinge coded for by a single exon. In cattle, sheep, and pigs, but not horses or dogs, the Cδ1 domain is almost identical to the Cμ1 domain of IgM, whereas the other constant domains are distinctly different (Zhao et al., 2002). In mice, the two constant region domains (Cδ1 and Cδ3) are separated by a very long exposed hinge region. Because of this long hinge region and the fact that it has no interchain disulfide bonds, mouse IgD is unusually susceptible to destruction by proteases and cannot be detected in serum, although it may be detected in plasma. Like IgE, IgD is destroyed by mild heat treatment.

The role of IgD has so far defied explanation, but it probably regulates B-cell responses. IgM to IgD class switching has been described in the upper respiratory mucosa of humans. This generates IgD-producing plasma cells whose products bind bacteria. The circulating IgD also binds to basophils through galectin 9 and induces them to produce cathelicidins, as well as the Th2 cytokines, IL-1, IL-4, and B cell-activating factor (see Chapter 15; Shan et al., 2018). Thus, in humans, IgD orchestrates a defense system at the interface between innate and adaptive immunity.

Recent studies on the role of IgD have determined that B-cell class switching from IgM to IgD in mice is initiated by the intestinal microbiota! In mice, much IgD is produced by the B cells of the intestinal mucosa-associated lymphoid tissues. However, it is not produced in germ-free mice (Choi et al., 2017).

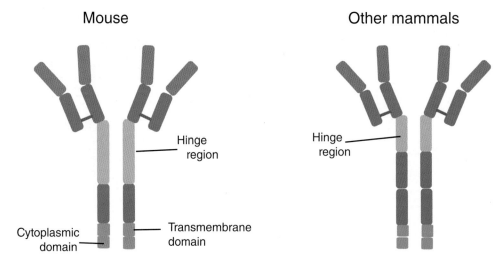

Fig. 17.8 The structure of immunoglobulin D (IgD) in mice and other mammals. Note the long, exposed hinge region in mouse IgD that makes this molecule very unstable.

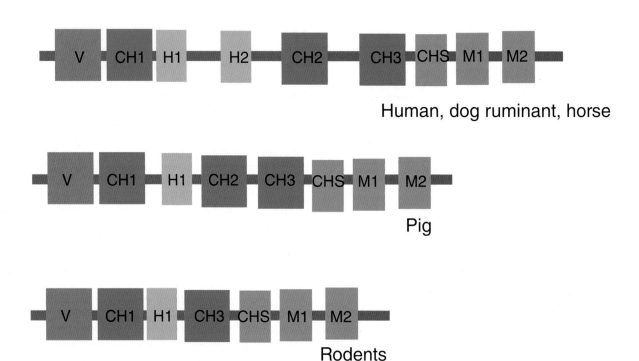

Fig. 17.9 The gene structure of Immunoglobulin D (IgD) differs greatly among mammals. This diagram shows the exon structure of IgD heavy chains in different species. No other immunoglobulin class shows such variation, and its significance is unknown.

THREE-DIMENSIONAL STRUCTURE OF IMMUNOGLOBULINS

Immunoglobulin peptide chains fold in such a way that an IgG molecule consists of three globular regions (two Fab regions and one Fc region) linked by flexible hinges (Fig. 17.10). Each globular region is made up of paired domains. Thus, the Fab regions each consist of two paired domains (V_H-V_L and C_H1-C_L), whereas the Fc region contains either two or three paired domains, depending on the immunoglobulin class (i.e., C_H2-C_H2, C_H3-C_H3, and in IgE or IgM, C_H4-C_H4). The peptide chains within each domain are closely intertwined. In the Fab regions, a groove is formed between the two variable domains, V_H and V_L. The amino acids of the complementarity-determining regions (CDRs) line this groove, and as a result, the surface of the groove has a highly variable shape. This groove forms the antigen-binding site. The CDRs from both light and heavy chains contribute to the binding of an antigen, although the heavy chain contributes most to the process. Because immunoglobulins are bilaterally identical, the CDRs on each of the Fab regions are also identical. Since the antigen-binding sites on each Fab region are identical, immunoglobulins are able to cross-link two identical epitopes at the same time. The presence of a hinge region in the middle of their heavy chains makes immunoglobulins such as IgG very flexible.

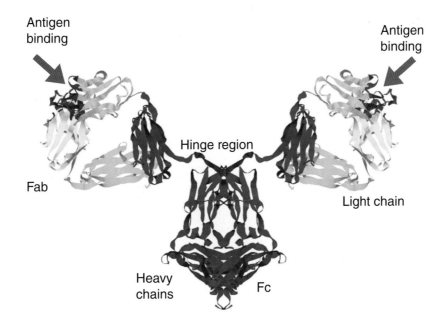

Fig. 17.10 A ribbon diagram showing the folding of the peptide chains in bovine immunoglobulin G (IgG). Compare this with the very schematic diagrams of IgG structure seen elsewhere in the text. The globular domain structure is very obvious. It is also clear that the peptide chains in the hinge region are very exposed to breakage by proteases. Blue denotes constant domains, orange/yellow denotes variable domains while red denotes hypervariable regions. Courtesy Dr. B. Breaux.

IMMUNOGLOBULIN VARIANTS

Subclasses

All immunoglobulin molecules are made of two heavy and two light chains. Several different heavy chains are employed in making these molecules. Thus, when γ chains are used, the resulting immunoglobulin is IgG. IgM contains μ chains, IgA contains α chains, and so on. However, closer examination shows that even these immunoglobulin classes consist of mixtures of molecules using structurally different heavy chains known as subclasses.

Immunoglobulin subclasses have arisen as a result of gene duplication. During the course of evolution, heavy-chain (*IGH*) genes have been duplicated, and the new gene is then gradually changed through mutation. The amino acid sequences coded by these new genes may differ from the original in only minor respects. For example, bovine IgG is a mixture of three subclasses, IgG1, IgG2, and IgG3, coded for by three heavy-chain genes *IGHG1*, *IGHG2*, and *IGHG3*, respectively. They differ in amino acid sequence and in physical properties such as electrophoretic mobility. These immunoglobulin subclasses also have very different biological activities; for example, bovine IgG2 agglutinates antigenic particles, whereas IgG1 does not. The four canine IgG subclasses differ in their ability to bind Fc receptors and thus have different functional abilities. The number and properties of immunoglobulin subclasses vary among species. For example, most mammals have only one or two IgA subclasses, but rabbits have 15. These species differences are probably not of major biological significance; they simply reflect the number of immunoglobulin heavy-chain gene duplications a species has undergone.

Allotypes

In addition to subclass differences, individual animals have inherited variations in immunoglobulin amino acid sequences. Thus, the immunoglobulins of one individual may differ from those of another individual of the same species (Fig. 17.11). These allelic sequence variations in heavy-chain genes are reflected in structural differences called allotypes.

Idiotypes

The third group of structural variants found in immunoglobulins results from the variations in the amino acid sequences within the variable domains on light and heavy chains. These variants are called idiotopes. The collection of idiotopes on an immunoglobulin is called its idiotype. Most idiotopes are located within the antigen-binding site.

PRODUCTION OF IMMUNOGLOBULIN HEAVY CHAINS

Two genes code for each immunoglobulin heavy chain. One gene codes for the variable domain (and thus the antigen-binding site), whereas a separate gene encodes the constant domains. The way in which genes code for the variable domains is discussed in Chapter 17. The genes that code for the constant regions of the immunoglobulin heavy chain (*IGH* genes) each consist of multiple expressed sequences or exons. One exon codes for each constant domain, and one codes for the hinge region (Fig. 17.12). A complete IgM constant region gene (*IGHM*) therefore consists of five exons, whereas an IgA constant region gene (*IGHA*) contains four exons. The heavy-chain constant region genes are clustered on a single chromosome. They are generally arranged in the order 5′-*IGHM*-*IGHD*-*IGHG*-*IGHE*-*IGHA*-3′. Thus, the gene for the μ chain is followed by the gene for the δ chain, and these are followed by the γ chain genes, and so on.

As they mature, B cells undergo two DNA recombination events. The first, called V(D)J recombination, creates the V domain with the complete antigen-binding site of the BCR. This happens while the B cells are developing within the bone marrow. Once antigens have activated the B cells, a second DNA recombination event occurs. This second event results in a switch in the class of BCR and thus antibodies produced by a B cell. This class switch recombination does not affect the antigen-binding site, just the constant domains.

All cattle possess a
complete set of classes
and subclasses (ISOTYPES)

Within a population
individual cattle possess
different ALLOTYPES.
For example, some possess
IgG2(A1), others possess
IgG2(A2)

Each individual animal
has a very large number
of different IDIOTYPES

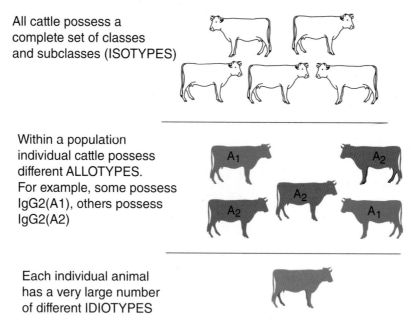

Fig. 17.11 A schematic diagram showing the differences among the inheritance of the major immunoglobulin variants.

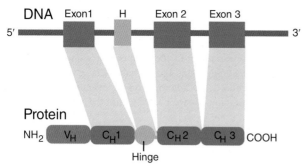

Fig. 17.12 A peptide chain such as an immunoglobulin heavy chain is coded for by a series of expressed sequences (exons) separated by intervening sequences or introns. Usually, each exon codes for a single domain. When transcription occurs, the introns are spliced out and the exon sequences joined together in mRNA before translation into peptide chains.

Class Switch Recombination

During the course of a B-cell response, the class of immunoglobulin produced by a cell changes. This "class switch" can be explained by the way in which heavy-chain genes are assembled.

During an antibody response, the immunoglobulins are synthesized in a standard sequence. Thus a responding B cell first uses the *IGHM* gene to make IgM BCRs. The remaining genes located 3′ to *IGHM* are ignored. In species that make IgD, the B cell may also transcribe the *IGHD* gene and then express both IgM and IgD. As the immune response progresses, responding B cells switch to using *IGHG*, *IGHA*, or *IGHE* genes and become committed to synthesizing IgG, IgA, or IgE. The unwanted, unused *IGH* genes are excised as a DNA circle and are lost from the cell, so that the required *IGH* constant gene can be spliced directly to the *IGHV* gene.

For example, if IgM is to be synthesized, an *IGHV* gene is spliced directly into the *IGHM* gene (Fig. 17.13). On the other hand, if IgA is to be synthesized, the genes coding for Cμ to Cε inclusive are deleted, and

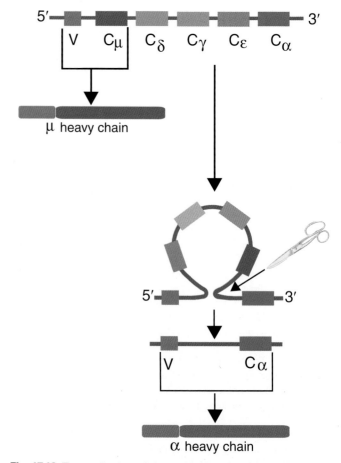

Fig. 17.13 The mechanism of class switching. In this example, a switch is made from immunoglobulin M production to immunoglobulin A production by deleting intervening heavy-chain genes and joining the V genes to the appropriate heavy-chain gene.

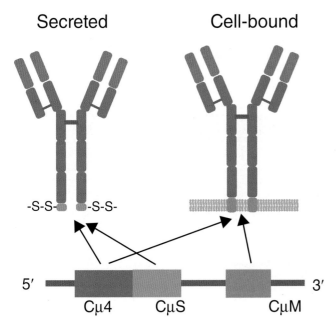

Secreted   Cell-bound

Cμ4   CμS   CμM

Fig. 17.14 IgM immunoglobulins serving as B-cell antigen receptors have a choice as to which C-terminal domain they will use. The membrane-bound form uses a hydrophobic transmembrane domain (CμM). In contrast, the secreted form deletes this sequence and uses the CμS gene. The difference between the two forms is determined by RNA splicing following transcription.

TABLE 17.2 **Serum Immunoglobulin (Ig) Levels in the Domestic Animals and Humans**				
	Ig LEVELS (MG/DL)			
Species	**IgG**	**IgM**	**IgA**	**IgE**
Horses	1000–1500	100–200	60–350	4–106
Cattle[a]	1700–2700	250–400	10–50	
Sheep	1700–2000	150–250	10–50	
Pigs	1700–2900	100–500	50–500	
Dogs	1000–2000	70–270	20–150	2.3–4.2
Cats[b]	400–2000	30–150	30–150	
Chickens	300–700	120–250	30–60	
Humans	800–1600	50–200	150–400	0.002–0.05

[a]Cattle show significant seasonal differences in serum immunoglobulin levels.
[b]Immunoglobulin levels in pathogen-free cats are about half those in pet cats.

the *IGHV* gene is then spliced directly to the *IGHA* gene. There are several ways by which these intervening genes can be excised. The simplest is called looping out-deletion. In this case, the V region and C genes come together by looping out and then excising the intervening DNA using an enzyme called a recombinase. Two signals are needed to initiate class switching in a B cell. First, the B cell must receive an activation signal generated when CD40 on the B cell binds to CD154 on a helper T cell. Second, the specific class switch is determined by signals from cytokines, especially by IL-4, TGF-β, and IFN-γ. Signals from CD40 and the antigen activate the recombinase in the B cell while signals from the cytokine receptors, by activating specific promoter regions, target the recombinase to a specific heavy-chain gene.

B-Cell Antigen Receptors and Soluble Immunoglobulins

Immunoglobulins are first produced as cell-bound BCRs and are subsequently secreted as antibodies. The heavy chains of BCRs have a hydrophobic transmembrane C-terminal domain that attaches them to a B-cell surface. This domain is absent from the secreted antibody. The switch between the two forms results from the differential splicing of exons. For example, the *IGHM* gene contains two short exons: called CμS and CμM located 3′ to Cμ4 (Fig. 17.14). CμS codes for the C-terminal domain of the secreted form, whereas CμM codes for the hydrophobic domain of the membrane-bound form. When IgM is made, all the Cμ exons are first transcribed to messenger RNA (mRNA). To produce membrane-bound IgM, the mRNA for the CμS exon is deleted, and the Cμ4 exon is spliced directly to the CμM exon. To produce secreted IgM, the exon coding for the CμM domain is deleted, and translation is stopped after Cμ4 and CμS are read.

IMMUNOGLOBULINS OF DOMESTIC MAMMALS

All mammals examined possess genes for and express four or five major immunoglobulin classes (IgG, IgM, IgA, IgE, and IgD) (Table 17.2).

The basic characteristics of each of these classes are as described previously. However, during the course of evolution, as pointed out earlier, the immunoglobulin heavy-chain (*IGH*) genes have duplicated, sometimes several times (Fig. 17.15). Over time, these duplicated genes mutate so that animals may produce multiple subclasses of a specific immunoglobulin. If a duplicated gene mutates in such a way that it is no longer functional, it becomes a pseudogene. The number of duplications, and hence the number of immunoglobulin subclasses and pseudogenes, varies among species (Table 17.3).

Horses

The horse heavy-chain gene locus is located on chromosome 24. The locus contains 11 *IGHC* genes of which seven are expressed (Walther et al., 2015). Thus there are seven IgG subclasses: IgG1 thru IgG7. (The previous nomenclature for IgG1 thru IgG4 was IgGa, IgGc, IgG[T], and IgGb. IgG6 was previously called IgG[B]). The order of the Ig heavy-chain genes in the horse is:

5′-M-D-G1-G2-G3-G7-G4-G6-G5-E-A-3′.

IgG7 is closely related to IgG4 and likely resulted from a recent duplication of the *IGHG4* gene. IgG1, IgG4, and IgG7 are produced in response to intracellular infections while IgG3 and IgG5 are mainly produced in response to extracellular invaders (Overesch et al., 1998). Horses also express IgM, IgD, IgA, and IgE (Wagner et al., 2004). The horse *IGHD* gene is located downstream from *IGHM*. It appears to be expressed at least at the mRNA level. Horses have two IgG4 alleles (IgG4[a] and IgG4[b]) and four IgE alleles (IgE[1-4]) (De Camargo et al., 2009; Wagner, 2009).

Cattle

Cattle are unusual in that they are the only mammals known to possess two functional heavy-chain loci. Most of these *IGH* genes are located on chromosome 21 but a truncated μCH2 exon is present on chromosome 11. The genes on chromosome 21 are organized thus: (*n* denotes a variable number of these genes, and *p* denotes a pseudogene).

5′-Vn-Dn-Jn-M1- (D1p-V3-D1n)$_3$-Jn-M2-D-G3-G1-G2-E-A-3′.

Thus, there are internal duplications of D_H, J_H, and C region genes in the bovine IGH locus (Ma et al., 2016). Both IgM genes can be expressed independently or sequentially by class switching. Cattle have three *IGHG* genes corresponding to their three subclasses: IgG1, IgG2,

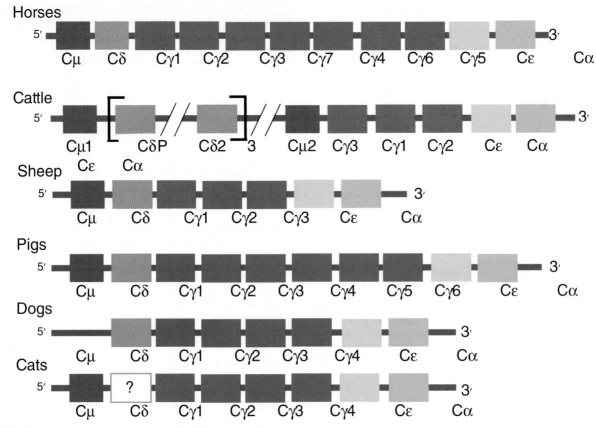

Fig. 17.15 The arrangement of the immunoglobulin heavy-chain genes of the major domestic mammals.

TABLE 17.3 Immunoglobulin (Ig) Classes and Subclasses in Selected Mammals

Species	IG CLASSES				
	IgG	IgA	IgM	IgE	IgD
Horses	G1, G2, G3, G4, G5, G6, G7	A	M	E	D
Cattle	G1, G2, G3	A	M1, M2	E	D
Sheep	G1, G2, G3	A1–A13	M	E	D
Pigs	G1, G2a, G2b, G3, G4	A	M	E	D
Dogs	G1, G2, G3, G4	A	M	E1, E2	D
Cats	G1, G2?	A1, A2?	M	E	-
Humans	G1, G2, G3, G4	A1, A2	M1, M2	E	D

cattle. Cattle IgD may be expressed on B cells. About 95% of bovine Ig have λ light chains.

Ultralong V$_H$ CR3

A unique feature of bovine IgG molecules is the presence of a subset (<10%), with an unusually long third complementary determining region (CDR3) in their variable domains. As a result, they have significantly different antigen-binding properties(Fig. 17.16) (Stanfield et al., 2016; Wang et al., 2013).

Mammals such as humans and mice have IgG heavy-chain variable domains with CDR3 regions that average about 10–13 amino acids in length. Cattle are different. About 10% of bovine IgG molecules have V domains with CDR3s that may contain over 60 amino acids (Oyola et al., 2021).

This extreme length is due to the use of a very long germline *D* gene segment that encodes four cysteines that form interchain bonds with each other, together with repeated glycine, serine, and tyrosine residues. (Koti et al., 2010). The 23 gene segments that constitute the bovine *D* gene cluster can be divided into nine subfamilies, *D1* to *D9*. Most contain only 14–30 nucleotides. However, *D8* contains 149 nucleotides. The extreme length of the CDR3 in some antibodies is due to the use of *D8* (Deiss et al., 2019).

In addition, CDR3 may also use an unusually long IGHV gene (*IGHV1-7*) in association with the *D8* segment. This generates a stalk structure within the ultralong CDR3 (Fig. 17.17; Deiss et al., 2019). (The CDR1 and CDR2 regions of this V gene segment show limited sequence variability and are of normal length) (Ma et al., 2016).

These ultralong heavy-chain CDR3s fold into a long beta-stranded stalk supporting a "knob" domain located far from the rest of the molecule. The ultralong CDRs may also show significant structural diversity

and IgG3. IgG1 constitutes about 50% of the serum IgG and is the predominant immunoglobulin in cows' milk rather than IgA. IgG2 levels are highly heritable, and its concentrations vary greatly among cattle. Cattle possess a unique Fc receptor on their macrophages and neutrophils that binds only IgG2. Since bovine IgG2 has a very small hinge region, this receptor might represent a special adaptation to the structure of this immunoglobulin. Cattle also possess IgE (Gershwin, 2009).

Two heavy-chain allotypes (a and b) have been identified in all three bovine IgG classes. Allotype B1 is found on light chains of some cattle but is relatively uncommon. IgA, IgM, and IgE also occur in

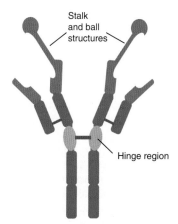

Fig. 17.16 The unusual variable regions of the bovine immunoglobulin M with a stem and knob structure.

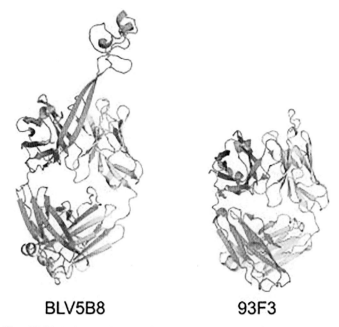

Fig. 17.17 A ribbon diagram showing the structure of a bovine Fab (BLV5B8) as compared to a "normal" Fab (93F3) showing the superlong β-stranded stalk protruding from the VH immunoglobulin domain. From Wang et al., 2013. Reshaping antibody diversity. Cell 153, 1379–1393.

as a result of somatic mutation and combinations of somatically generated disulfide bonds. The knob can fold into multiple mini-domains and can bind diverse antigens. The benefits of this unusual structure are unclear, but it almost certainly enables the CDR3 region of these molecules to bind otherwise inaccessible antigenic determinants on some viruses.

Sheep

The three IgG subclasses of sheep are IgG1, IgG2, and IgG3. Some sheep have an IgG1a allotype. An *IGHD* gene has been detected in sheep. Three IgA heavy-chain allotypes have been identified, as have three IgE allotypes. The sheep CDR3 region is much shorter than in cattle (average

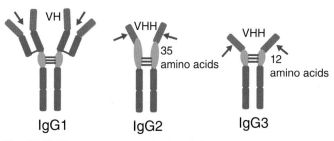

Fig. 17.18 The structural organization of dromedary immunoglobulins is unique. They possess a conventional immunoglobulin, IgG1, and two different heavy chains only, immunoglobulins, IgG2 and IgG3. The two different IgG2 isotypes differ in the size of their hinge region. The red arrows denote their antigen-binding sites.

length, 16 amino acids) so they do not make the knob and ball structure. They primarily use lambda chain alleles (Park et al., 2023).

Goats

As expected, there is a broad similarity between the antibody loci in cattle, sheep, and those in the domestic goat. The goat heavy-chain locus is found on chromosome 21q24. Goats possess seven heavy-chain constant region genes, *IGHM, IGHD,* three *IGHG* genes, *IGHE,* and *IGHA.* The *IGHG* genes differ in their hinge regions and share ancestry with cattle and sheep (Schwartz et al., 2017). Their products are predicted to be functionally equivalent to those in cattle (Du et al., 2018).

Camels

Members of the camel family from both the Old and New Worlds (dromedaries and llamas) have three IgG subclasses: IgG1, IgG2, and IgG3. IgG1 has a conventional four-chain structure and, therefore, has a molecular weight of 170 kDa. In contrast, IgG2 and IgG3, which together account for 75% of camel Ig, are 100 kDa heavy-chain dimers that have no light chains! (Conrath et al., 2003). In addition, camel IgG2 heavy chains lack a C_H1 domain but compensate for this by having a very long hinge region (Fig. 17.18). Despite lacking light chains, these antibodies can still bind to many antigens. For example, camel antibodies bind effectively to the substrate pockets of enzymes. The antigen-binding site on these heavy chains is very convex. This enables it to fit snugly into the concave active site on an enzyme. Thus, these single-chain antibodies may have a structural advantage over conventional immunoglobulins in neutralizing antigenic enzyme activity (Brooks et al., 2018; Griffin et al., 2014).

Pigs

The pig IGH region is about 190 kb in size. The first genomic studies performed on the European breeds such as Landrace and Duroc identified single *IGHM, IGHD, IGHE,* and *IGHA* genes in addition to six *IGHG* subclass genes (Fig. 17.15; Kacsovics et al., 1994; Eguchi-Ogawa et al., 2012). Eleven pig IGHG gene sequences have since been described. These encode the six IgG subclasses, named IgG1 through IgG6. There are two allelic forms of each of these subclasses except for IgG3 (Butler et al., 2009). The IGHG genes form a cluster located between IGHD and IGHE. They encode the six subclasses as well as their alleles. They are arranged in order:

$5'$-G3-G5^a-G5^b-G6^a-G6^b-G4^a-G4^b-G2^b-G2^a-G1^a-G1^b-$3'$

The differences between the alleles may be minor. For example, IgG2^a and IgG2^b differ by only three amino acids. IgG3 has an extended hinge, is structurally unique, and appears to be the most evolutionarily conserved porcine IgG. IgG5[b] differs most from its allele, and its C$_H$1 domain shares sequence homology with the C$_H$1 domain of IgG3. Some pigs may have two *IGHG5* and two *IGHG6* genes but no *IGHG2* or *IGHG4*. Other pigs may lack IgG4 or IgG6.

These IGH sequences were initially derived from the genome of a single Landrace pig with a haplotype designated Lan-1. Subsequent genomic studies have shown that other breeds of pigs have different numbers of IGHG genes (Butler and Wertz, 2014). It is believed that all of these IgG genes were present in the ancestral wild boar, but some have been lost following domestication. Only IGHG1, IGHG3, and IGHG4 are present in all pig breeds. Presumably, these three IgG genes are ancestral. IGHG3 appears to be the most ancient and is found at the upstream (5') end of the cluster (Paudyal et al., 2022).

IgG is the predominant serum immunoglobulin in pigs, accounting for about 85% of the total. IgM accounts for about 12% and dimeric IgA for about 3% of serum Ig. Pigs have a single *IGHA* gene with two alleles. IgA[b] differs from IgA[a] by a 12-nucleotide deletion in the hinge region owing to a mutation in its splice acceptor site. The consequences of this are unclear. An *IGHD* gene has been identified in pigs. Its first constant domain may be coded by either a C$_H$1 δ gene or by a C$_H$1 μ gene! Thus, pig IgD heavy-chain transcripts may contain either *VDJ-CH1μ-CH2δ-CH3δ* or *VDJ-CH1δ-CH2δ-CH3δ*. This pattern has not been reported in other mammals. These two genes, however, show almost 99% similarity, so the biological consequences are probably not great. IgD has not been identified and may not be expressed in pigs. Pig IgE has been identified (Roe et al., 1993). One IgM allotype has been reported.

Dogs and Cats

Dogs have four *IGHG* genes and hence four IgG subclasses, named IgG1, IgG2, IgG3, and IgG4 in order of abundance (Bergeron et al., 2014). In addition, dogs have IgA, IgM, IgD, and IgE. Four alleles have been identified in the dog *IGHA* gene. All are restricted to the hinge region. An IgM allotype has been described in the dog. Dogs also make a small quantity of IgD (Yang et al., 1995).

Biochemical and genetic studies on polyclonal canine IgE have identified two biochemically, physically, and biologically distinct IgE subclasses, IgE1, and IgE2 (Peng et al., 1997). These can be distinguished by their reactivity with monoclonal IgE antiglobulins and by binding to protein A (a staphylococcal immunoglobulin-binding protein). While sharing the major characteristics of IgE such as heat lability, molecular weight, mast cell binding, and reactivity with polyclonal anti-IgE, they differ in their reactivity with monoclonal antibodies and their isoelectric point. These differences are not due to altered glycosylation. They also appear to have different biological properties in that IgE2 levels are highly variable when compared to IgE1 in ragweed-sensitized dogs. Examination of the canine IgE heavy-chain gene locus confirms the existence of two functional IgE heavy-chain genes, IGEH1 and IGEH2. The biological significance of this gene duplication remains unclear. Perhaps the existence of two IgE subclasses may account in part, for the relatively high levels of IgE in dogs when compared to other mammals (see Table 30.4).

Cats have two *IGHG* genes (IgG1 and IgG2), one IgM gene, possibly two IgA genes (IgA1 and IgA2), and one IgE gene (Baldwin and Denham, 1994). The IgG1 gene consists of two allotypes designated IgG1a and IgG1b. Together IgG1 accounts for about 98% of serum IgG. About 2% of cat serum IgG belongs to the IgG2 subclass (Strietzel et al., 2014).

Primates

Humans have four *IGHG* genes coding for IgG1 to IgG4. Chimpanzees and rhesus macaques possess three *IGHG* genes coding for IgG1, IgG2, and IgG3. The chimpanzee IgG2 molecule contains epitopes also found on both human IgG2 and IgG4, suggesting that the *IGHG2* and *IGHG4* genes split after humans separated from chimpanzees. Baboons have four *IGHG* genes, but they differ significantly from human IgG in their hinge region. Rhesus macaques may have two IgM subclasses. All the great apes, with the exception of the orangutan, have two IgA subclasses.

Other Mammals

Rats and mice have four or five functional *IGHG* genes. In contrast, rabbits have only one *IGHG* gene despite having 15 *IGHA* genes, at least 12 of which are functional! They appear to lack IgD. The expression of these rabbit IgA subclasses varies among tissues. It is believed that these IgA subclasses differ in their susceptibility to bacterial proteolytic cleavage. Given the importance of the gut microbiota in rabbits, it is entirely possible that the microbiota have played a role in the evolution and persistence of the multiple IgA isotypes. Alternatively, the expansion of the rabbit IgA subclasses may be a mechanism to compensate for the lack of diversity among their IgG subclasses.

REFERENCES

Baldwin, C.I., Denham, D.A., 1994. Isolation and characterization of three subpopulations of IgG in the common cat (*Felis catus*). Immunology 81, 155–160.

Bergeron, L.M., McCandless, E.E., Dunham, D., Dunkle, B., et al., 2014. Comparative functional characterization of canine IgG subclasses. Vet Immunol. Immunopathol. 157, 31–41.

Brooks, C.L., Rossotti, M.A., Henry, K.A., 2018. Immunological functions and evolutionary emergence of heavy chain antibodies. Trends Immunol. 39 (12), 956–960.

Butler, J.E., Wertz, N., 2014. The immunoglobulin genes of domestic swine. In: Kaushik, A.K., Passman, Y. (Eds.), Comparative Immunoglobulin Genetics. Apple Academic Press, Toronto.

Butler, J.E., Wertz, N., Deschacht, N., Kacsovics, I., 2009. Porcine IgG: structure, genetics, and evolution. Immunogenetics 61, 209–230.

Choi, J.H., Wang, K.-W., Zhang, D., Zhan, X., et al., 2017. IgD class switching is initiated by microbiota and limited to mucosa-associated lymphoid tissue in mice. Proc. Natl. Acad. Sci. 114, E1196–E1204.

Conrath, K.E., Wernery, U., Muyldermans, S., Nguyen, V.K., 2003. Emergence and evolution of functional heavy chain antibodies in *Camelidae*. Dev. Comp. Immunol. 27, 87–103.

De Camargo, M.M., Kuribayashi, J.S., Bombardieri, C.R., Hoge, A., 2009. Normal distribution of immunoglobulin isotypes in adult horses. Vet. J. 182, 359–361.

Deiss, T.C., Vadnais, M., Wang, F., Chen, P.L., et al., 2019. Immunogenetic factors driving formation of ultralong VH CDR3 in *Bos taurus* antibodies. Cell Mol. Immunol. 16, 53–64.

Du, L., Wang, S., Zhu, Y., Zhao, H., et al., 2018. Immunoglobulin heavy chain variable region analysis in dairy goats. Immunobiology 223, 599–607.

Eguchi-Ogawa, T., Toki, D., Wertz, N., Butler, J.E., Uenishi, H., 2012. Structure of the genomic sequence comprising the immunoglobulin heavy constant (IGHC) genes in *Sus scrofa*. Mol. Immunol. 52, 97–107.

Gershwin, L.J., 2009. Bovine immunoglobulin E. Vet. Immunol. Immunopathol. 132, 2–6.

Griffin, L.M., Snowden, J.R., Lawson, A.D.G., Wernery, U., et al., 2014. Analysis of heavy and light chain sequences of conventional camelid antibodies from *Camelus dromedarius* and *Camelus bactrianus* species. J. Immunol. Meth. 405, 35–46.

Kacsovics, I., Sun, J., Butler, J.E., 1994. Five putative subclasses of swine IgG identified from the cDNA sequence of a single animal. J. Immunol. 153, 3565–3574.

Koti, M., Kataeva, G., Kaushik, A.K., 2010. Novel atypical nucleotide insertions specifically at VH-DH junction generate exceptionally long CDR3H in cattle antibodies. Mol. Immunol. 47, 2119–2128.

Ma, L., Qin, T., Chu, D., Cheng, X., et al., 2016. Internal duplications of DH, JH and C region genes create an unusual IgH gene locus in cattle. J. Immunol. 196, 4358–4366.

Overesch, G., Wagner, B., Radbruch, A., Leibold, W., 1998. Organization of the equine immunoglobulin constant heavy chain genes II: equine Cγ genes. Vet. Immunol. Immunopathol. 66, 273–287.

Oyola, S.O., Henson, S.P., Nzau, B., Kibwana, E., Nene, V., 2021. Access to ultra-long IgG CSRH3 bovine antibody sequences using short read sequencing technology. Mol. Immunol. 139, 97–105.

Park, M., Nunez de Diaz, T., Lange, V., Wu, L., et al., 2023. Exploring the sheep (*Ovis aires*) immunoglobulin repertoire by next generation sequencing. Mol. Immunol. 156, 20–30.

Paudyal, B., Mwangi, W., Rijal, P., Schwartz, J.C., et al., 2022. Fc-mediated functions of porcine IgG subclasses. Front. Immunol. https://doi.org/10.3389/fimmu.2022.903755.

Peng, Z., Arthur, G., Rector, E.S., Kierek-Jaszczul, D., et al., 1997. Heterogeneity of polyclonal IgE characterized by differential charge, affinity to protein A, and antigenicity. J. Allergy Clin. Immunol. 100, 87–95.

Roe, J.M., Patel, D., Morgan, K.L., 1993. Isolation of porcine IgE and preparation of polyclonal antisera. Vet. Immunol. Immunopathol. 37, 83–97.

Rogers, K.A., Richardson, J.P., Scinicariello, F., Attanasio, R., 2006. Molecular characterization of immunoglobulin D in mammals: immunoglobulin heavy constant delta genes in dogs, chimpanzees and four old world monkey species. Immunology 118, 88–100.

Schwartz, J.C., Philp, R.L., Bickhart, D.M., Smith, T.P.L., Hammond, J.A., 2017. The antibody loci of the domestic goat (*Capra hircus*). Immunogenetics. https://doi.org/10.1007/s00251-017-1033-3

Shan, M., Carillo, J., Yeste, A., Gutzeit, C., et al., 2018. Secreted IgD amplifies humoral T helper 2 cell responses by binding basophils via galectin-9 and CD44. Immunity 49, 709–724.

Stanfield, R.L., Wilson, I.A., Smider, V.V., 2016. Conservation and diversity in the ultralong third heavy-chain complementarity-determining region of bovine antibodies. Science Immunol. 1, 1–12. aaf7962.

Strietzel, C.J., Bergeron, L.M., Oliphant, T., Mutchler, V.T., Choromanski, L.J., Bainbridge, G., 2014. In vitro functional characterization of feline IgGs. Vet. Immunol. Immunopathol. 158 (3-4), 214–223.

Wagner, B., 2009. IgE in horses: occurrence in health and disease. Vet. Immunol. Immunopathol. 132, 21–30.

Wagner, B., Miller, D.C., Lear, T.L., Antczak, D.F., 2004. The complete map of the Ig heavy chain constant gene region reveals evidence for seven IgG isotypes and for IgD in the horse. J. Immunol. 173, 3230–3242.

Walther, S., Rusitzka, T.V., Diesterbeck, U.S., Czerny, C.-P., 2015. Equine immunoglobulins and organization of immunoglobulin genes. Dev. Comp. Immunol. 53, 303–319.

Wan, Z., Zhao, Y., Sun, Y., 2021. Immunoglobulin D and its encoding genes: an updated review. Dev. Comp. Immunol., 124. https://doi.org/10.1016/j.dci.2021.104198

Wang, F., Ekiert, D.C., Ahmad, I., et al., 2013. Reshaping antibody diversity. Cell 157, 1379–1393.

Yang, M., Becker, A.B., Simons, E.R., Peng, Z., 1995. Identification of a dog IgD-like molecule by a monoclonal antibody. Vet. Immunol. Immunopathol. 47, 215–224.

Zhao, Y., Kacskovics, I., Pan, Q., et al., 2002. Artiodactyl IgD: the missing link. J. Immunol. 169, 4408–4416.

18

How Antigen-Binding Receptors Are Made

Because bacteria and viruses have such a short generation time, they have the ability to mutate and change rapidly. As a result, the immune system must be able to respond not only to existing organisms but also, within reason, to newly evolved organisms. The ability of the adaptive immune responses to respond specifically to an enormous number of foreign antigens implies the existence of an enormous number of lymphocytes, each with its own specific antigen receptors. This then raises the question; how do lymphocytes generate such an enormous diversity of antigen receptors?

The ability of a receptor to bind an antigen is determined by the shape of its binding site. This shape depends on the folding of its peptide chains, which is governed, in turn, by their amino acid sequences. Each amino acid in a peptide chain exerts an influence on its neighboring amino acids, which determines their relative configuration. The shape of a peptide chain, therefore, represents the contributions of all amino acids in the chain as the peptide assumes its most energetically favorable conformation. The folding of a protein is determined by its amino acid sequence, and that sequence is determined by the sequence of bases in the DNA encoding that protein. The diversity of antigen receptors implies either a corresponding diversity in the genes coding for these receptors or a mechanism that generates diversity from a limited pool of receptor genes. This second mechanism is now known to be the method used by the adaptive immune system.

RECEPTOR-ANTIGEN BINDING

When an antigen and its receptor bind, they interact through the chemical side chains on the antigen and the complementarity-determining regions (CDRs) of the receptor. In classic chemical reactions, molecules are assembled through the establishment of firm, covalent bonds. These bonds can be broken only by the input of a large amount of energy, that is not readily available. In contrast, the formation of noncovalent bonds provides a rapid and reversible way of forming complexes and permits the reuse of molecules in a way that covalent bonding does not allow. However, noncovalent bonds act over short intermolecular distances and, as a result, form only when two molecules approach each other very closely. The binding of an antigen to a BCR or TCR is exclusively noncovalent, so the strongest binding occurs when the shape of the antigen and the shape of the receptor perfectly match. This requirement for a close conformational fit has been likened to the specificity of a key for its lock.

The major bonds formed between an antigen and its receptor are hydrophobic (Fig. 18.1). When antigen and antibody molecules come together, they exclude water molecules from the area of contact. This frees some water molecules from constraints imposed by the proteins and is therefore energetically stable. (The bond can be likened to two wet glass microscope slides stuck together. Anyone who has tried to separate two wet glass slides can confirm the effectiveness of this type of bonding.)

A second type of binding between an antigen and its receptor is through hydrogen bonds. When a hydrogen atom bound to an electronegative atom, for example, an –OH group, approaches another electronegative atom such as an O=C– group, the hydrogen is shared between the two electronegative atoms. This situation is energetically favorable and is called a hydrogen bond. The major hydrogen bonds formed in antigen-receptor interaction are O–H–O, N–H–N, and O–H–N.

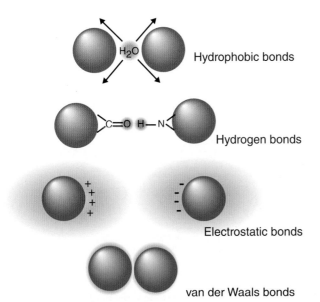

Fig. 18.1 Noncovalent bonds that link an antigen with its receptor arranged in order of relative importance. All these bonds are effective only over a very short distance. It is, therefore, essential that the shape of the antigen and its receptor site interact closely if strong binding is to be achieved.

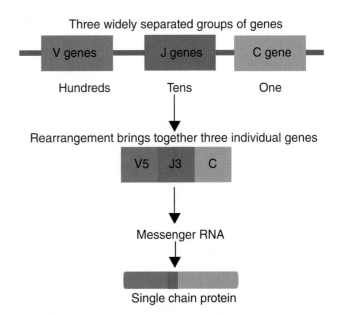

Fig. 18.2 Antigen receptor chains are coded for by genes originating in three distinct clusters. The genes for a complete receptor chain are assembled by joining one gene selected from each cluster.

Hydrogen bonds are already present between proteins and water molecules in an aqueous solution, so the binding of an antigen to its receptor by hydrogen bonds requires relatively little net energy change.

Electrostatic bonds formed between oppositely charged amino acids may contribute to antigen-receptor binding, but the charge on many protein groups is commonly neutralized by electrolytes in solution. As a result, the importance of electrostatic bonding is unclear.

When two atoms approach very closely, a nonspecific attractive force, called a van der Waals force, becomes operative. It occurs as a result of a minor asymmetry in the charge of an atom because of the position of its electrons. This force, although very weak, may become collectively important when two large molecules come into contact. It can, therefore, contribute to antigen-receptor binding.

The binding of a receptor to its antigen is, therefore, mediated by multiple noncovalent bonds. Each bond is relatively weak in itself, but collectively they may have a significant binding strength. All these bonds act only across short distances and weaken rapidly as that distance increases. Electrostatic bond and hydrogen bond strengths are inversely proportional to the square of the distance between the interacting molecules; the van der Waals forces and hydrophobic bonds are inversely proportional to the seventh power of that distance. Thus, the strongest binding between an antigen and its receptors occurs when their shapes match perfectly and multiple noncovalent bonds form. Antigens can bind to receptors when they fit less than perfectly, although their binding affinity will be much reduced.

ANTIGEN RECEPTOR GENES

The information needed to make all proteins, including antigen receptors, is stored in an animal's genome. All that is required for the production of these molecules is that the necessary genes be turned on. Once the appropriate genes are activated, they can be transcribed into RNA and translated into the appropriate receptor protein on B or T cells. It has been estimated that mammals can produce up to 10^{15} different antigen receptors to be expressed on B and T cells. To produce this enormous receptor diversity, they use fewer than 500 genes!

Multiple genes code for each receptor peptide chain. Several genes code for each variable domain, whereas only one code for each constant domain. As a result, the single constant-region gene can be joined to any one of several variable-region genes to make a complete receptor chain (Fig. 18.2). Instead of having genes for all possible receptor chains, it is only necessary to have genes for all the variable regions and to join these to an appropriate constant-region gene as required. In addition, antigen-receptor chains may be paired in different combinations to yield even greater diversity, a process called combinatorial association.

IMMUNOGLOBULIN DIVERSITY

To make as many different antibodies as possible, it is necessary to diversify the amino acid sequences of the variable domains in both light and heavy chains. Since these amino acid sequences are determined by the nucleotide sequences, mechanisms must exist for generating this nucleotide sequence diversity. In practice, gene diversity is generated through three mechanisms: gene recombination, somatic mutation, and gene conversion. The relative importance of each of these mechanisms differs among species, and the diversity-generating mechanisms that operate in humans and mice are not the same as those that operate in domestic mammals. The assembly of these diverse antigen receptors is carefully controlled during lymphocyte development by such factors as DNA methylation, chromatin structure, and location within the nucleus.

GENE RECOMBINATION

Three gene loci code for immunoglobulin peptide chains, and each is found on a different chromosome (Fig. 18.3). One locus, called *IGL*, uses three gene segments to code for λ light chains; one, called *IGK*, uses three gene segments to code for κ light chains; and one, called *IGH*, uses four gene segments to encode heavy chains. Gene recombination results within each locus from the random selection of one gene segment from the variable cluster, followed by combining these selected genes to generate a complete sequence. This is well seen in the genes that code for immunoglobulins (Table 18.1).

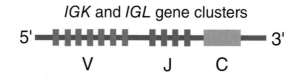

IGK and *IGL* gene clusters

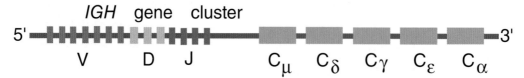

IGH gene cluster

Fig. 18.3 Genes coding for immunoglobulin light chains and heavy chains. Note that there are two distinct light chain loci, one coding for kappa chains (IGK) and one coding for lambda chains (IGL). These are located on different chromosomes. The precise number of V, D, and J gene segments varies among species.

TABLE 18.1	Examples of Immunoglobulin Gene Segment Numbers Used in Mammals						
Species	**IGKV**	**IGKJ**	**IGLV**	**IGLJ**	**IGHV**	**IGHJ**	**IGHD**
Horses	60	5	144	7	52	8	40
Bovine	22	3	25	4	36	6	14
Sheep	10	3	>100	1	7	6	>1
Pigs	14	5	23	4	20	1	2
Mice	169	9	14	3	161	7	18
Humans	48	9	69	8	215	27	30
Rats	163	7	3	2	174	5	21

The Heavy-Chain (IGH) Locus

Four different gene segments, IGHV, IGHD, IGHJ, and IGHC, are required to form a complete gene encoding an immunoglobulin heavy chain. The IGH locus contains multiple (~100) IGHV segments as well as multiple IGHJ segments. The J segments are situated 3′ to the IGHV genes. In addition, several short segments, called IGHD (D for diversity), are positioned between the IGHV and IGHJ regions. The IGHC genes consist of a series of constant-region genes, one for each heavy-chain class and subclass, usually arranged in the order 5′-M-D-G-E-A-3′ along the chromosome. There is great variation in the number of heavy-chain V genes among the mammals. These range from 7 in sheep to 215 in humans (Table 18.1). Likewise, the number of heavy-chain IGHG genes varies between species, ranging from one in the rabbit to seven in the horse. Each of these constant genes consists of multiple exons encoding the sequences for each heavy-chain domain including one or two for the hinge region, as well as exons encoding the transmembrane and intracellular domains in cell-bound immunoglobulins (see Fig. 17.9).

The Lambda Light Chain (IGL) Locus

Each λ light chain is encoded by three gene segments: IGLV, IGLJ, and IGLC. Mammals may also possess multiple IGLC genes. For example, dogs have nine and pigs have two. The IGLV segment codes for the variable domain from the N-terminus to position 95. The IGLC segment codes for the constant domain starting at position 110. The amino acids between 95 and 110 are encoded by IGLJ segments. The number of each of the IGLV segments varies among domestic species. However, not all of these are functional—many are pseudogenes.

The Kappa Light Chain (IGK) Locus

Kappa light chains are also encoded by three segments, IGKV, IGKJ, and IGKC. In general, mammals possess only a single IGKC gene segment. In the rabbit, there are two IGKC segments as a result of lineage-specific duplication. In rodents, IGKV segments are much more abundant than IGLV segments. In humans, they are present in similar numbers.

GENERATION OF JUNCTIONAL DIVERSITY

Gene Segment Rearrangement

The most obvious way to generate V-region diversity is to select one V gene segment at random from the available pool and join it to one randomly selected J segment, a process called recombination. Since many V and J segments are available, the number of possible combinations can be very large. For example, if there are 100 V segments and 10 J segments, then $100 \times 10 = 1000$ different V region genes can be constructed simply by random selection.

Light chain assembly requires the combination of one V, one J, and one C segment. During B-cell development, the intervening segments must first be removed and discarded. The first step in this process is to identify the sites where the DNA has to be cut. Thus V and J segments have sites called switch regions at each end that guide the process (Fig. 18.4). Cutting is the function of an "activation-induced" cytidine deaminase (AID). When a B cell receives the appropriate signals telling it to eliminate unwanted genes, AID deaminates the cytidines in the specific switch regions involved (Fig. 18.5). As a result, these cytidines

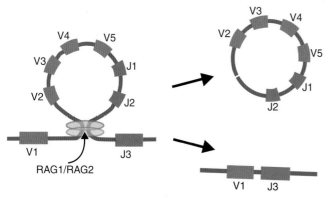

Fig. 18.4 One of the most important mechanisms of deleting unwanted genes is by "looping out." In this case, unwanted V and J gene segments form a loop that is then cut off by an enzyme complex consisting of RAG1 and RAG2 and the cut ends then joined together by a DNA ligase. As a result, the desired V segment is linked directly to a J segment. The excised loop is destroyed.

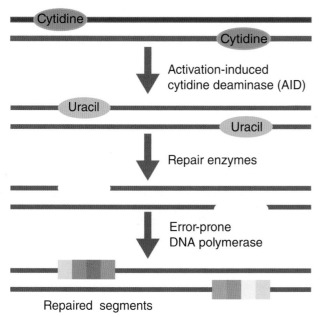

Fig. 18.5 The mechanism of somatic mutation. An "activation-induced" cytidine deaminase (AID) converts the cytidines in specific switch regions to uracils. Both strands of the DNA are cut by an endonuclease at these points. The free ends of the DNA are "rejoined" but the gaps are filled by randomly selected nucleotides.

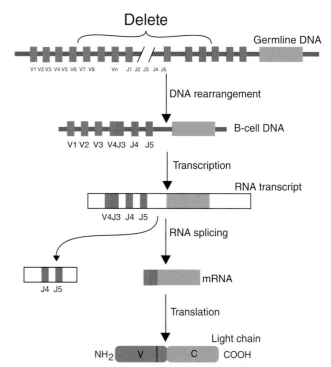

Fig. 18.6 Construction of an immunoglobulin light chain. Selected V and J gene segments are first joined as the intervening segments are deleted. The VJ and C segments remain separated until RNA splicing occurs. At that time the intervening RNA segments are deleted leaving the V, J, and C segments linked together in the messenger RNA. DNA rearrangement occurs during early B-cell development so that each individual B cell is committed to making a single form of light chain for its antigen receptor.

are converted to uracils. This conversion results in DNA "damage," and as a result, both strands of the DNA are cut by enzymes called recombinases at these specific points. There are two recombinases, RAG1 and RAG2, that act as components of a multiprotein structure that chop off the looped DNA, a "hairpin" structure. The free ends of the DNA are "rejoined" by a DNA ligase so that the V and J segments form a continuous sequence. Two sets of enzymes are used in this process; RAG endonucleases cut the DNA at two points, thus excising unwanted genes. Following this, DNA ligases join the free ends to form a continuous sequence.

Light chain gene recombination occurs in two steps. Randomly selected V and J segments are first joined to form a complete V-region gene. The joined V-J genes remain separated from the C gene until

messenger RNA (mRNA) is generated. At that time, the unwanted J segments are excised, and the complete V-J-C mRNA is then translated to form a light chain (Fig. 18.6).

When a heavy-chain V region is assembled, its construction requires the splicing together of *IGHV*, *IGHD*, and *IGHJ* segments (Fig. 18.7). This use of three randomly selected gene segments enormously increases the amount of possible variability. For example, if a pool of 100 V, 10 J, and 10 D segments are combined, then $100 \times 10 \times 10 = 10{,}000$ different V regions can be constructed. The recombination of these segments also occurs in a specific order. Thus *IGHD* is first joined to *IGHJ*, and then *IGHV* is attached to make a complete V-region gene. After transcription, any unwanted J gene segments are deleted, the *IGHC* gene mRNA is attached, and the assembled V-D-J-C mRNA is then translated to form a heavy chain.

Base Deletion

Although random recombination of two or three gene segments generates much V-region diversity, additional mechanisms can increase this diversity still further. For example, endonucleases can remove nucleotides randomly from the cut ends of the genes. As a result, the precise nucleotide at which V and J segments join varies, leading to changes in the nucleotide sequence at the splice site and variations in the amino acid sequence in the V region.

Base Insertion

In immunoglobulin heavy-chain gene processing, additional nucleotides may also be inserted at the V-D and D-J splice sites. Some of these nucleotides (N-nucleotides) are added randomly by an enzyme called

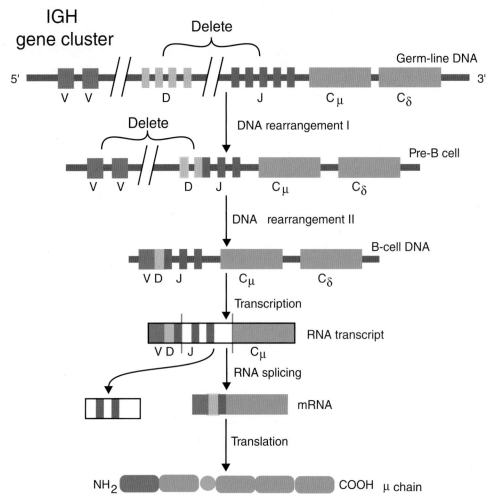

Fig. 18.7 Construction of a complete immunoglobulin heavy-chain gene. Two DNA rearrangement events are required to link V, D, and J genes together. The first event joins selected D and J gene segments; the second event adds a selected V segment. Finally, unwanted J segments are excised and VDJ joined to C in the messenger RNA.

terminal deoxynucleotidyltransferase (TdT). Up to 10 N-nucleotides may be inserted between V and D and between D and J.

Although the random selection of gene segments from two or three pools generates a huge number of combinations, not all of these combinations encode usable antibodies. Some combinations may generate sequences that cannot be translated into proteins. These are called nonproductive rearrangements. For example, nucleotides are read as triplets called codons, each of which codes for a specific amino acid. If the codons are to be read correctly, then the sequence must be in the correct reading frame. If nucleotides are inserted or deleted so that the codon reading frame is changed, the resulting gene may code for a totally different amino acid sequence. If this "frameshift" results in inappropriate splicing, the translation is prematurely terminated.

It is probable that nonproductive rearrangements are produced in two out of three attempts during B-cell development. When this happens, the B cell has several additional opportunities to produce a functional antibody. For example, immature B cells initially rearrange one of the *IGK* genes (Fig. 18.8). If this fails to produce a functional light chain, they switch to the other *IGK* allele for a second attempt. If this does not work, the B cell will use one of the *IGL* alleles, and if this fails, the second *IGL* allele represents the last resort. If all four efforts fail to produce a functional light chain, the B cell cannot make a functional

immunoglobulin. It will then undergo apoptosis without participating in an immune response.

The sequence of events described above has been worked out in mice and humans; the details differ in domestic mammals. One obvious difference lies in the use of κ and λ light chains. In mice, rabbits, pigs, and humans, κ chains are preferentially used. In the other domestic species, λ light chains predominate. The reasons for these differences are unknown.

It should also be pointed out that immunoglobulin gene rearrangement is, in fact, not entirely random. For example, in rabbits, mice, and humans, the most 3′ *IGHV* gene segments tend to be used most often. This preferential use of certain segments results from a combination of factors, including the recombination signal sequences, the accessibility of the genes to the recombinase enzyme, sequences at the splicing sites, and the way in which DNA folds.

Receptor Editing

Although each new B cell expresses a specific antigen receptor, developing B cells may continue to rearrange their V, D, and J genes and alter their receptor structure even after exposure to antigen. Thus, a B cell expressing a specific κ chain may restart V gene rearrangement by switching to the other *IGKV* genes or even switching

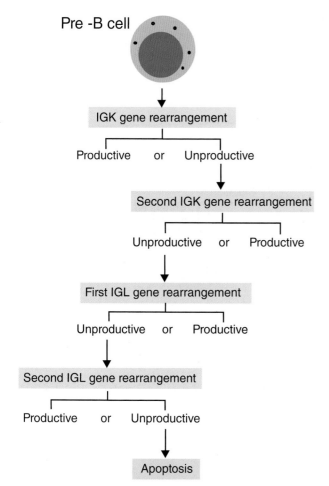

Fig. **18.8** During its development, each B cell has four attempts to make a productive gene rearrangement coding for a functional immunoglobulin. If it fails in all four attempts, the cell undergoes apoptosis.

to either of the *IGLV* genes. The cell can continue to rearrange upstream non-rearranged V genes or downstream non-rearranged J genes. This receptor editing, which occurs within germinal centers, may be a method of eliminating receptors that bind to self-antigens (see Chapter 37).

SOMATIC MUTATION

Recombination cannot account for all the sequence variability seen in immunoglobulin V regions. For example, there are three hypervariable regions (CDRs) located within each V region (Fig. 18.9). One of these, CDR3, is located around position 96 and is generated by recombination between V and J gene segments. However, the other two, CDR1 and CDR2 are located far from any V-J or V-D-J splice sites. Other mechanisms of generating antibody variability must therefore exist. In fact, gene segment recombination is only the first step in generating antibody diversity. It is followed by somatic mutation that generates even more DNA diversity and results in the production of antibodies that bind much more strongly and specifically to antigens (Papavasiliou and Schatz, 2002).

Following initial exposure to an antigen, B cells proliferate and undergo antigen-driven selection in the dark zones of germinal centers (see Chapter 16). The mutations in immunoglobulin V genes are generated by the same enzymes used for class switch recombination. They are triggered by antigen cross-linking of two BCRs, by the binding of CD40 to CD154, and by the binding of CD80 to CD28. These signals activate cytidine deaminase (AID) which deaminates the cytidines in V gene DNA and converts them to uracils. These uracils are recognized as errors (after all, uracil is not normally found in DNA), and their appearance, therefore, triggers repair processes. Other enzymes delete the uracils and leave a gap that is repaired by DNA polymerases using short sequences of randomly selected nucleotides. As a result of this "repair," V gene sequences change progressively as the B cells respond to antigens. On average, one amino acid changes each time a B cell divides (Faili et al., 2002).

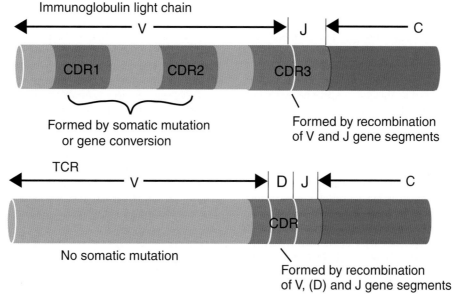

Fig. **18.9** The major difference between the variable regions of the T-cell antigen receptor (TCR) and immunoglobulins is in the formation of CDRs. Immunoglobulins have three CDRs. CDR1 and CDR2 are generated by somatic mutation. CDR3 is generated by gene conversion. This option is not available to the TCR, in which somatic mutation is stringently avoided to prevent self-reactivity.

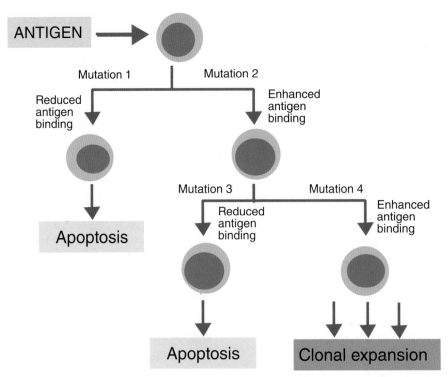

Fig. 18.10 The selection of somatic mutants. Spontaneous mutation during the expansion of a B-cell clone results in the development of cells with antigen receptors that differ in their affinity for antigen. Cells that bind antigen strongly will be more intensely stimulated than cells that bind it weakly. As a result of this selection pressure, the B-cell population gradually increases its binding affinity during the course of an antibody response.

The degree to which a B cell responds to an antigen is directly related to the strength (affinity) with which its receptors bind that antigen. The better the fit between antigen and receptor, the greater will be the stimulus received by the B cell. If a BCR cannot bind an antigen, the B cell will not be stimulated and will die. In contrast, those B cells whose receptors bind antigen with a high affinity survive and proliferate (Fig. 18.10). Thus, as B cells respond to an antigen, successive cycles of mutation and selection of the highest affinity receptors eventually generate populations of B cells producing very-high-affinity antibodies.

Somatic mutation does not begin until after B cells have switched from making immunoglobulin M (IgM) to making either IgG or IgA. This suggests that the mutation mechanism is not activated until after a responding B cell had committed to utilizing a specific heavy-chain V gene. As a result, the affinity of IgM antibodies does not increase during an immune response, whereas the affinity of IgG antibodies does.

GENE CONVERSION

Mammals other than the human and mouse may have relatively few V gene segments and gene recombination cannot explain their immunoglobulin diversification. In these species, V region diversity is generated by gene conversion (Fig. 18.11). Species that employ gene conversion must have available a supply of multiple V segments or pseudogenes. (Pseudogenes are segments of DNA that are defective and so cannot be transcribed.) During gene conversion, B-cell cytidine deaminase inserts a uracil, which is then removed, leaving a gap in the nearest V gene. This gap is then filled by randomly selected short segments of DNA obtained from an upstream V-region segment or pseudogene. The "repaired" V gene will, therefore, have a different sequence than its precursor. Some of these gene conversion events may

not generate a functional V region. In these cases, these defective B cells are eliminated.

RECEPTOR ASSEMBLY

When B-cell antigen receptors are generated, in most mammals (except pigs), the first chain to be assembled is the heavy chain. This chain is capable of generating much more junctional and combinatorial diversity than the light chain and is the major contributor to antigen binding. This heavy chain is linked to signal transduction molecules, and a surrogate partner chain is provided so that the preB cell can respond in a limited way to antigens. As a result, a small clone of B cells expressing only the heavy chain is formed. Signaling through this prereceptor triggers limited proliferation. This is followed by the assembly of a light chain. The light chain uses only V and J segments and thus contributes much less diversity to the antigen receptor although it tends to "fine-tune" its antigen-binding abilities. Once a complete first chain is formed using V, D, and J segments, further recombination and rearrangement are stopped, thus preventing assembly of the second heavy-chain allele. As pointed out elsewhere, pigs assemble their immunoglobulins in reverse order from other mammals (Sinkora et al., 2022).

POTENTIAL IMMUNOGLOBULIN DIVERSITY

Gene segment rearrangement generates enormous V-region diversity and antigenic specificity in several ways. In humans, for example, only 1 of a possible 80 *IGKV* segments is selected for transcription, as is only 1 of the 5 *IGKJ* segments. Random joining of these will generate 400 (80×5) different light chain V regions. With 300 *IGHV*, 5 *IGHD*, and 2 *IGHJ* gene segments available, as many as 3000 (300×5×2) different

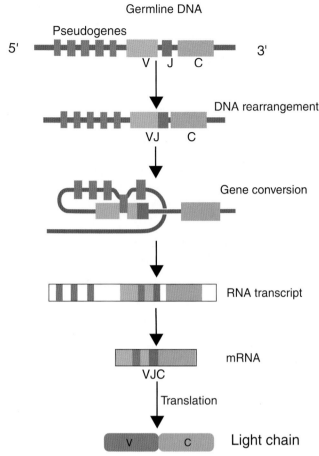

Fig. 18.11 The process of gene conversion. In this process, segments of upstream genes or pseudogenes are inserted into a single V region to generate sequence diversity.

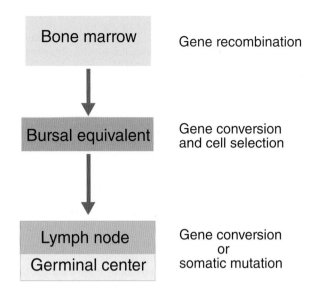

Fig. 18.12 The lymphoid organs where gene recombination, gene conversion, and somatic mutation occur.

heavy-chain V regions can be generated. Since paired heavy and light chains are used to form the antigen-binding site, the total number of possible combinations is 1.2 million (400 × 3000). In addition, the presence of two splice sites multiplies the potential for diversity generated as a result of base deletion and insertion. However, as pointed out previously, many of the gene combinations so formed may be of little functional use.

Taking all possible mechanisms into account, the number of antigen-binding sites and hence binding specificities generated in humans is about 1.8×10^{16} without accounting for somatic mutation (This figure may be compared with the estimated 1×10^7 antigens that the immune system may recognize).

SPECIES DIFFERENCES

Antigen receptor diversity is generated in different ways depending on the species. Some mammals rely on gene segment recombination followed by somatic mutation. In these species, immunoglobulin diversity is continuously generated from B-cell precursors throughout an animal's life. Other mammals, in contrast, use gene conversion for a short period early in life. After initial B-cell diversity is generated, this pool of B cells expands by a self-renewing mechanism with little somatic mutation (Fig. 18.12).

Horses

The equine IGH locus contains 40 D segments, 8 J segments, and 52 V segments as well as 11 C genes of which seven are expressed. The IGK locus contains a single C segment, 5 J segments, and 60 V segments (Sun et al., 2010). The IGL locus contains 7 C segments, each preceded by a single J segment and 144 V segments located downstream of the J-C cluster. Horses, therefore, predominantly employ gene recombination with extensive junctional diversity. More than 45% of their antibody clones have 10 or more inserted nucleotides (Navas et al., 2022). Lambda light chains constitute 92% of the antibody repertoire in horses (Walther et al., 2015).

Cattle

Cattle likely employ recombination for their immunoglobulin light chains and a combination of recombination and conversion for their heavy chains. Initial diversification occurs in lymphoid organs followed by somatic mutation in ileal Peyer patches (Liljavirta et al., 2014). They have at least 42 IGHV segments divided into 3 subgroups. Subgroup IGHV1 contains at least 11 and perhaps as many as 20 functional genes. Subgroups IGHV2 and IGHV3 consist entirely of pseudogenes (Table 18.1). Heavy-chain diversity in older cattle is generated primarily by somatic mutation. IGHJ contains 6 segments of which 2 are functional. IGHD contains 23 long and short segments. As a result, their heavy-chain CDR3 regions range from 31 to 154 nucleotides in length. In addition, conserved short nucleotide sequences of 13 to 18 nucleotides may be inserted at V-D junctions encoding IgM, so that the CDR3 loop is exceptionally long and may contain more than 60 amino acids. As pointed out in the previous chapter, this leads to the generation of a stem and knob structure where the knob shows significant structural heterogeneity as a result of somatic mutation. This knob can fold into multiple mini-domains and can bind diverse antigens (Butler, 1998).

The bovine IGL locus contains 25 V segments, of which 17 are functional, organized in three subclusters 5′ to four J-C segments. The predominantly expressed IGLV1 segments are found in two 5′ subclusters, whereas the rarely expressed *IGLV*2 and *IGLV*3 segments are proximal to the J-C genes (Pasman et al., 2010). Cattle have more than one *IGLJ* segment, but only one is expressed. Many of the pseudogenes are fused to *IGLJ* in the germline. Cattle also have four *IGLC* genes. Two of these (*IGLC2* and *IGLC3*) are functional, whereas the other two (*IGLC1* and *IGLC4*) are pseudogenes. *IGLC3* is preferentially expressed. Over 90% of bovine antibodies use lambda light chains (Chen et al., 2008).

Sheep

Fetal and neonatal lambs initially use both recombination and gene conversion to generate most of their immunoglobulin diversity (Jenne et al., 2003). However, as sheep age, their immunoglobulin diversity progressively increases probably as a result of increased use of somatic mutation. Immature B cells first diversify their V (D) and J segments in central lymphoid tissues such as the spleen or bone marrow. The immature cells then migrate to follicles in the ileal Peyer patches where further diversification occurs . Sheep have only seven functional IGHV segments and probably, therefore, use gene conversion to diversify their heavy chains. They have six IGHJ segments, two of which are pseudogenes. One of the active segments, IGHJ1, is used in 90% of expressed heavy chains, suggesting that recombination is minimal. More than 98% of all rearrangement events are in-frame, and there are few N-nucleotides inserted. Among the light chain segments, five Vλ segments account for >70% of the repertoire (Jenne et al., 2003). The sheep lambda locus contains more than 90 IGLV segments and a single IGLJ segment, so these are diversified by recombination. Unlike rabbits, humans, or mice, stimulation by the intestinal microbiota is not absolutely necessary for V gene diversification in sheep. In lambs, new rearrangements continue to occur for several months after birth (Gontier et al., 2005).

Goats

Thirty-four IGHV segments have been identified in goats but only three of these appear to be functional. Goats also possess four D gene segments (three functional) and six IGHJ gene segments (two functional) and D_H-D_H fusion is not infrequent. Neither sheep nor goats express the ultralong heavy-chain D gene segments that are present in cattle. The goat IGL locus spans 460 kb and is located on chromosome 17. The 63 IGLV segments are separated into two clusters as in cattle and sheep. Of these 25 appear to be functional. It contains two Jλ-Cλ cassettes. The goat IGK locus is located on chromosome 11. It contains only 15 IGKV segments and four IGKJ segments. Light chain usage is more balanced in the goat with kappa chains constituting 20%–35% of the B-cell antigen receptors compared to only 5% in cattle.

Pigs

Pigs have about 30 IGHV segments, 5 IGHD segments, and 5 IGHJ segments (Zhao et al., 2003). Early in fetal life, the pig uses only four or five IGHV segments, and their early repertoire consists of only 8–10 combinations. Later in fetal life, this restricted repertoire is compensated for by early TdT activity and extensive, in frame, N-region addition leading to significant junctional diversity. V_H use is independent of gene position, but three IGHV segments account for 40% of the preimmune repertoire and six segments for 70%. The neonatal piglet has very little diversity available at birth (Butler et al., 2000).

Pigs produce kappa and lambda light chains in approximately equal amounts. They have 23 IGLV segments of which 10 are functional. The constant loci consist of three tandem IGLJ-IGLC cassettes plus a fourth downstream IGLJ segment. The kappa locus contains at least 14 IGKV segments of which 9 are functional, five IGKJ segments and one IGKC segment (Guo et al., 2016; Schwartz et al., 2012a, 2012b).

Dogs and Cats

Over 5500 alleles across 550 genes in the three immunoglobulin loci and the four TCR loci have been identified across 19 dog breeds. Dogs have 89 IGHV, 6 IGHD, 6 IDHJ gene segments and 22 IGHC segments in their IGH locus. Presumably not all are functional (Martin et al., 2018; Bao et al., 2010).

Cats possess 64 IGHV segments with 42 functional sequences and 22 pseudogenes. They have seven IGHD genes and six IGHJ genes. Their expressed IGHV segments map to chromosomes B3 and D1 (Weiss et al., 2008). As in the dog, the feline repertoire is dominated by IGHV3 (Steiniger et al., 2017).

Humans and Mice

Humans and mice use recombination to generate most of their antibody diversity (Table 18.2). Additional diversity is generated by base deletion and insertion and by somatic mutation. In these species, B cells with diverse antigen receptors are produced throughout life.

Intestinal Bacteria and Expansion of the B Cell Repertoire

The generation of B-cell diversity is driven in part by the commensal microbiota. The importance of this is demonstrated by the failure of germ-free pigs to develop significant B-cell diversity. Intestinal bacteria play an especially critical role in this process. For example, in rabbits, normal intestinal lymphoid tissue development can take place in the presence of both *Bacteroides fragilis* and *Bacillus subtilis* but not with either alone. Other bacterial combinations are also effective, suggesting that some form of bacterial interaction is needed for optimal effect.

TABLE 18.2   Immunoglobulin Diversity Among Mammals

Species	CH GENE PRODUCTS					C_L GENES		V_H AND V_L FAMILIES		
	IgM	IgD	IgG	IgE	IgA	λ	κ	H	λ	κ
Horses	1	1	7	1	1	7	1	7	1	?
Bovine	2	1	3	1	1	4	1	1	2	?
Sheep	1	1	3	1	2	>1	1	1	6	3
Pigs	1	1	8–12	1	1	1?	1	1	?	?
Dogs	1	1	4	2?	1	5	4			
Rabbits	1	0	1	1	13	8	2	1	?	?
Mice	1	1	4	1	1	3	1	14	3	4
Humans	1	1	4	1	2	7	1	7	7	7

From Butler, J.E., 1997. Immunoglobulin gene organization and the mechanism of repertoire development. Scand J. *Immunol.* 45: 455–462.

Analysis of the expansion of intestinal B cells driven by commensal bacteria also shows that it tends to affect B cells with specific V_H domains. Thus this expansion is not simply due to a immune response to microbial antigens but rather a polyclonal, non–antigen-specific response. It may be triggered through toll-like receptors or be a result of microbial superantigens binding to the BCRs, or some combination thereof.

Mammals can be divided into two groups based on the manner in which their B-cell receptor repertoire develops (see Chapter 13). Thus pigs, rodents, and primates provide the immune system with a constant supply of new B cells simply by generating them in the bone marrow throughout life. Other mammals, including the large domestic herbivores, develop their B-cell antibody repertoire in two stages. The first diversification stage involves rearrangements of a small number of V, D, and J gene segments within the bone marrow. These early B cells then migrate to the intestinal lymphoid tissues such as Peyer's patches, where they greatly increase their numbers of B cells as well as the diversity of their B-cell repertoire. This second phase of B-cell diversification generally takes place in intestinal lymphoid organs in direct contact with products from the intestinal microbiota. In addition, antigens derived from the microbiota trigger these B cells to produce large quantities of IgA. This "innate" IgA, in turn, permits controlled bacterial entrance into Peyer's patches and initiates a positive feedback loop for IgA production. This IgA thus directly influences microbial diversification.

T-CELL RECEPTOR DIVERSITY

T-cell antigen receptor and immunoglobulin gene rearrangements are specific in that immunoglobulin genes are not rearranged in T cells and TCR genes are not rearranged in B cells. Like immunoglobulins, the four peptide chains, α, β, γ, and δ, that make up the two types of TCR can bind many specific antigens. They are able to do this because each consists of a variable region attached to a constant region. The diversity of TCR V regions is generated exclusively by gene recombination. This is significantly different from the diverse mechanisms employed by B cells.

T-Cell Receptor Gene Structure

The four TCR peptide chains are coded for by three gene loci. The TRA/D locus codes for both α and δ chains since the *TRD* genes are embedded within the TRA locus. The TRB locus codes only for β chains, and the TRG locus codes only for γ chains. All three TCR loci contain V, J, and C gene segments, and the TRB and TRD loci also contain D segments (Fig. 18.13).

Each of the three TCR loci contains two or more C genes. In the TRA/D locus one C gene codes for *TRAC* and the other for *TRDC*. The TRB and TRG loci, in contrast, may contain multiple C genes. For example, there are eight *TRGC* genes in dogs.

Cells with α/β TCRs rearrange and express *TRA* and *TRB* V segments whereas γ/δ T cells express *TRG* and *TRD* segments. α/β T cells and γ/δ T cells arise from a common precursor and the TCR class switch is mediated by signals within the thymus. Developing T cells committed to the α/β TCR lineage delete their *TRD* genes by looping-out and switch to using their *TRA* genes. Some of the V segments in the TRA/D locus may be used by either α or δ TCR chains.

TRA/D Chain

The TRA and TRD genes are joined in a single chromosomal region with TRD embedded within the TRA locus—the TRA/D locus. Despite this, each locus is independently controlled. There is great variability in the numbers and arrangement of both TRAV and TRDV gene

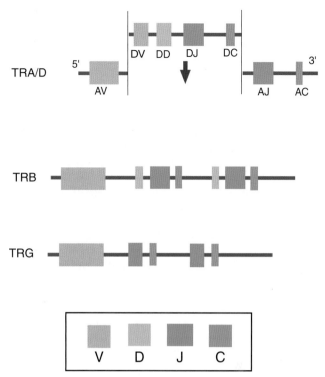

Fig. 18.13 The basic structure of the three gene loci that code for the four T-cell antigen receptor (TCR) chains. The genes encoding the TCR δ chains are embedded within the TCR α-chain genes to form a single TRA/D locus.

segments across the mammalian spectrum. The number of TRAV gene segments ranges from 5 (so far) in the horse, to 51 in the dog, and 48 in the pig, to 183 in cattle and 66 in sheep. Likewise, TRAJ gene segment numbers range from 5 in the horse to 61 in mouse, and human. Only one TRAC gene is present in the mammals investigated so far (Reinink and Van Rhijn, 2009).

The TRD locus contains between 5 and 55 V gene segments depending on species, 2 to 10 J segments, 2 to 7 D segments, and a single C gene in all mammals examined. As mentioned previously, D segment use is optional. Pigs have at least six TRDD gene segments compared to three and two in the human and mouse, respectively. These pig segments may form transcripts in a chain that encodes up to four connected TRDD domains.

TRB Chain

The TRB locus contains a cluster of V gene segments located upstream of two D-J-C cassettes, each containing several functional J segments. The D segments are all similar in sequence and length and their use is optional. Any of the TRBV segments may be joined to either of the two D-J-C cassettes, and a V segment may be linked to either a D or a J segment. A single TRBV segment in an inverted configuration is usually located at the 3' end of the gene cluster. In most mammals including humans, mouse, chimpanzee, rhesus macaque, dog, rabbit, ferret, and cat, there are two TRBD-J-C clusters, whereas in artiodactyls, there has been a duplication event, so they have a third TRBD-J-C cluster thus permitting more somatic rearrangements (Connelly et al., 2009; Conrad et al., 2002; Eguchi-Ogawa et al., 2009).

Dogs have about 38 TRBV segments, but about one-third of these are used to make up 90% of the beta chain repertoire. TRBV segment use may, in fact, be restricted to a single V gene family in the dog. In the pig, 43 TRBV segments and three D-J-C cassettes have been identified. Other mammals may have very diversified TRBV segments, ranging from 16 in the horse to 134 in cattle (Di Tommaso et al., 2010).

TRG Chain

In contrast to the TRB and TRA/D loci, the TRG locus is structurally highly variable (Antonacci et al., 2020). It generally consists of 15 TRGV segments linked to 5 TRGJ and 2 TRGC segments arranged in J-C clusters. The typical human TRGV locus contains about 160 kb, but its orientation is reversed. it consists of 12–15 TRGV segments upstream of two J-C clusters. The first containing three J segments and a single TRGC1 gene. The second cluster contains two TRGJ segments and the TRGC2 gene (Vaccarelli et al., 2008). Horses have 47 variable (TRGV) genes, 25 TRGJ genes, and 17 TRGC genes arranged in 17 V-J-(J)-C cassettes.

In the dog, the TRG locus is organized into eight cassettes, each containing a basic V-J-J-C unit, except for a J-J-C cassette at the 3′end (Massari et al., 2009). It contains a total of 40 gene segments (16 V, 16 J, and 8 C). Eight of the 16 canine TRGV segments, seven of 16 TRGJ segments, and six of eight TRGC segments are functional. The existence of these multiple TRGC segments suggests that the TCRs they generate may have diverse biological properties. Variations in gamma chain sequence length and amino acid residues have been reported in many other mammals (Conrad et al., 2007). A similar structure is seen in cats (Weiss et al., 2008).

GENERATION OF T-CELL RECEPTOR DIVERSITY

There are three hypervariable regions (CDRs) in each TCR V region. The first two, located within the V segments, have probably arisen through selection. The third is by far the most variable and is located in the region where V, D, and J segments recombine (Table 18.3). Neither somatic mutation nor gene conversion occurs in TCR genes. The genes that are separate in the germline are brought together by DNA rearrangement and are then modified by base insertion or deletion as the T cells differentiate (Fig. 18.14).

Gene Rearrangement

TCR α and γ chains are constructed using only V, J, and C segments. TCR β and δ chains use V, D, J, and C segments and can use multiple D segments. As a result, V-D-D-J or longer constructs can be formed. This amount of recombination also means that the reading frame of the D segments may change and can yield productive rearrangements. Looping-out and deletion account for more than 75% of TCR rearrangements. The rest of the rearrangements are due to either unequal sister chromatid exchange or inversion. That is, moving an inverted segment of gene into a position beside a segment in the opposite orientation.

Base Insertion and Deletion

Although in general, TCRs are constructed from a smaller V-, D-, and J-gene pool than immunoglobulins, their diversity is greater as a result of junctional diversity. Random N-nucleotides may be inserted at the V, D, and J junctions using TdT. Up to five nucleotides may be added between V and D and four between D and J segments. Likewise, random nucleotides may be removed by nucleases. This insertion of N-nucleotides and base deletion is probably the most significant component of TCR junctional diversity.

Somatic Mutation

Somatic mutation does not occur in TCR V genes, with the notable exception of the camels and llamas (Ciccarese et al., 2014). As pointed out earlier, T cells can only recognize a foreign antigenic peptide in association with a presenting MHC molecule. If random somatic mutation were to occur, it would carry the unacceptable risk of preventing MHC binding and rendering the foreign antigen unrecognizable. It might also lead to the production of TCRs able to bind self-antigens and thus trigger autoimmunity. The reasons why camels and llamas are different is unknown.

Where Does This Happen?

TCR segments are rearranged and expressed in developing T cells within the thymus. Immature thymocytes begin to rearrange *TRB*, *TRG*, and *TRD*. If *TRB* is productively rearranged, *TRG* is silenced, and *TRD* is deleted, so that the cell commits to using *TRA* and expressing α/β TCR. Because of the geometry of the TRA/D locus, joining a *TRAV* segment to *TRAJ* inevitably deletes the *TRD* segments on that allele. Thus α-chain rearrangements eliminate any possibility of δ-chain expression. Alternatively, the cell may successfully rearrange *TRG* and *TRD* and so express γ/δ TCR.

TABLE 18.3 TCR Gene Segment Diversity Among Mammal Germlines[a]

Species	TRA			TRD				TRB				TRG		
	V	J	C	V	J	D	C	V	D	J	C	V	J	C
Horses	5	5	1	8	3		1	16	1	14	2	45	7	117
Bovine	183	60	1	55	4	5	1	134	3	21	3	17	8	6
Sheep	66	61	1	25	4	7	1	120	3	18	3	13	13	5
Pigs	48	61	1	31	10	6	1	43	3	21	3			6
Dogs	51	59	1	5	4	2	1	38	2	12	2	16	16	8
Cats	62	64	1	11	5	2	1	33	2	12	2	12	12	6
Mice	100	61	1	10	2	2	1	52	2	13	2	7	4	4
Humans	54	61	1	8	4	3	1	68	2	14	2	15	5	8

[a]The numbers in this table have been drawn from multiple references. They represent the number of germline genes reported at each locus. Not all these genes will be expressed, and many are pseudogenes. When sources differ, I have chosen the highest number of genes reported since as genetic analysis proceeds, more and more genes are being identified, and these numbers may be expected to rise.

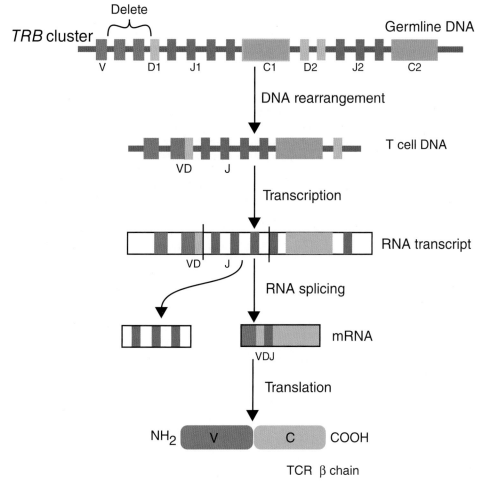

Fig. 18.14 The production of a complete T-cell antigen receptor peptide chain. Note the similarities between this and Fig. 18.7.

T-CELL DIVERSITY

In the human TRA locus, there are at least 61 *TRAJ* segments and 54 *TRAV* segments, giving more than 3000 possible combinations. N-region addition and base deletion also occur resulting in great junctional diversity. After correction for codon redundancy and correct reading frame, the number of potentially different TCR α chains is about 10^6. In the human TRB locus, there are at least 88 *TRBV* segments, 2 *TRBD* segments, and 14 *TRBJ* segments giving $88 \times 2 \times 14 = 2464$ possible combinations. In addition, there is junctional diversity and the use of many *TRBD* combinations. After corrections, there are about 5×10^9 possible *VDJ* ß sequences. Thus the number of possible TCR α/β combinations is about 5×10^{15}.

EPIGENETICS

While every cell in an animal body contains a complete copy of the genome, they only employ the genes needed for their specific function. Thus, a hepatocyte, for example, only uses those genes required for liver cell function. How do they do that? Processes that collectively control gene expression determine which genes are transcribed in each cell. This is called epigenetic regulation and has been likened to the software in a computer. Like software, a cell selects the most appropriate components (genes) for the task at hand. The importance of

epigenetic regulation is well seen in the regulation of immunoglobulin production. Consider, for example, how somatic hypermutation and class switch recombination are regulated.

There are three major mechanisms of epigenetic regulation: DNA methylation is one. By adding a methyl group to the 5-position in certain cytosines within a gene, a gene can be turned off. Conversely, demethylation results in gene activation (Li et al., 2013).

A second epigenetic mechanism involves histone modification. DNA in the nucleus is closely bound to the nuclear proteins called histones. These histones can be subjected to many chemical modifications such as methylation, phosphorylation, or acetylation. These histone modifications are introduced or removed by histone-modifying enzymes. The modifications influence the interactions between the histones and DNA and, as a result, may activate or inhibit gene transcription.

The third major epigenetic mechanism involves the production of microRNAs (miRNAs). These are small, noncoding RNAs that regulate gene expression by binding to mRNAs and influencing their functions. Collectively, these three epigenetic mechanisms determine which genes are active and which are inactive in any given cell type.

Thus B-cell activation and differentiation are associated with genome-wide hypomethylation, an increase in histone acetylation, and the appearance of a specific set of miRNAs. In the case of immunoglobulin synthesis, class switch recombination and somatic hypermutation are regulated by all three of these epigenetic processes. In effect, the production of the appropriate recombinases, polymerases, AID, TdT, and repair enzymes is turned on by activating histone modifications and DNA hypomethylation triggered by exposure to antigen and the presence of appropriate cytokines. These epigenetic pathways regulate immunoglobulin somatic hypermutation, class switch DNA recombination as well as the differentiation of B cells into plasma cells, and long-lived memory B cells. Histone modifications affect the class switch and possibly somatic hypermutation. DNA methylation and miRNAs also influence the activities of cytidine deaminase as well as plasma cell differentiation. These epigenetic pathways influence the normal immune response and, if dysregulated, also influence the development of abnormal B-cell responses and autoimmunity.

REFERENCES

Antonacci, R., Massari, S., Linguiti, G., Jambrenghi, A.C., et al., 2020. Evolution of the T-cell receptor (TR) loci in the adaptive immune response: the tale of the TRG locus in mammals. Genes 11, 624. https://doi.org/10.3390/genes11060624

Bao, Y., Guo, Y., Xiao, S., Zhao, Z., 2010. Molecular characterization of the V$_H$ repertoire in Canis familiaris. Vet. Immunol. Immunopathol. 137, 64–75.

Butler, J.E., 1998. Immunoglobulin diversity, B-cell and antibody repertoire development in large farm animals. Rev. Sci. Tech. 17, 43–70.

Butler, J.E., Sun, J., Weber, P., et al., 2000. Antibody repertoire development in fetal and newborn piglets, III. Colonization of the gastrointestinal tract selectively diversifies the preimmune repertoire in mucosal lymphoid tissues. Immunology 100, 119–130.

Chen, L., Li, M., Yang, X.Y., et al., 2008. Characterization of the bovine immunoglobulin lambda light chain constant IGLC genes. Vet. Immunol. Immunopathol. 124, 284–294.

Ciccarese, S., Vaccarelli, G., Lefranc, M.P., Tasco, G., et al., 2014. Characteristics of the somatic hypermutation in the Camelus dromedarius T cell receptor gamma (TRG) and delta (TRD) variable domains. Dev. Comp. Immunol. 46, 300–313.

Connelly, T., Aerts, J., Law, A., Morrison, W.I., 2009. Genomic analysis reveals extensive gene duplication within the bovine TRB locus. BMC Genomics 10, 192–200.

Conrad, M.L., Mawer, M.A., Lefranc, M.-P., et al., 2007. The genomic sequence of the bovine T cell receptor gamma TRG loci and localization of the TRGC cassette. Vet. Immunol. Immunopathol. 115, 346–356.

Conrad, M.L., Pettman, R., Whitehead, J., et al., 2002. Genomic sequencing of the bovine T cell receptor beta locus. Vet. Immunol. Immunopathol. 87, 439–441.

Di Tommaso, S., Antonacci, R., Ciccarese, S., Massari, S., 2010. Extensive analysis of D-J-C arrangements allows the identification of different mechanisms enhancing the diversity in sheep T cell receptor β-chain repertoire. BMC Genomics 11, 3–9.

Eguchi-Ogawa, T., Toki, D., Uenishi, H., 2009. Genomic structure of the whole D-J-C clusters and the upstream region coding V segments of the TRB locus in pig. Dev. Comp. Immunol. 33, 1111–1119.

Faili, A., Aoufouchi, S., Flatter, E., et al., 2002. Induction of somatic hypermutation in immunoglobulin genes is dependent on DNA polymerase iota. Nature 419, 944–946.

Gontier, E., Ayrault, O., Godet, I., Nau, F., Ladeveze, V., 2005. Developmental progression of immunoglobulin heavy chain diversity in sheep. Vet. Immunol. Immunopathol. 103, 31–51.

Guo, X., Schwartz, J.C., Murtaugh, M.P., 2016. Genomic variation in the porcine immunoglobulin lambda variable region. Immunogenetics 68 (4), 285–293.

Jenne, C.N., Kennedy, L.J., McCullagh, P., Reynolds, J.D., 2003. A new model of sheep Ig diversification: shifting the emphasis toward combinatorial mechanisms and away from hypermutation. J. Immunol. 170, 3739–3750.

Li, G., Zan, H., Xu, Z., Casali, P., 2013. Epigenetics of the antibody response. Trends Immunol. 34, 460–469.

Liljavirta, J., Niku, M., Pessa-Morikawa, T., Ekman, A., Iivanainen, A., 2014. Expansion of the preimmune antibody repertoire by junctional diversity in Bos Taurus. PLoS ONE 9 (6), e99808. https://doi.org/10.1371/journal.pone.0099808

Martin, J., Ponsting, H., Lefranc, M.-P., Archer, J., et al., 2018. Comprehensive annotation and evolutionary insights into the canine (Canis lupus familiaris) antigen receptor loci. Immunogenetics 70, 223–236.

Massari, S., Bellahcene, F., Vaccarelli, G., et al., 2009. The deduced structure of the T cell receptor gamma locus in Canis lupus familiaris. Mol. Immunol. 46, 2728–2736.

Navas, C., Manso, T., Martins, F., Minto, L., et al., 2022. The major role of junctional diversity in the horse antibody repertoire. Mol. Immunol. 151, 231–241.

Papavasiliou, F.N., Schatz, D.G., 2002. Somatic hypermutation of immunoglobulin genes: merging mechanisms for genetic diversity. Cell 109, S35–S44.

Pasman, Y., Saini, S.S., Smith, E., Kaushik, A.K., 2010. Organization and genomic complexity of bovine λ-light chain gene locus. Vet. Immunol. Immunopathol. 135, 306–313.

Reinink, P., Van Rhijn, I., 2009. The bovine T cell receptor alpha/delta locus contains over 400 V genes and encodes V genes without CDR2. Immunogenetics 61, 541–549.

Schwartz, J.C., Lefranc, M.P., Murtaugh, M.P., 2012a. Organization, complexity and allelic diversity of the porcine (Sus scrofa domestica) immunoglobulin lambda locus. Immunogenetics 64 (5), 399–407.

Schwartz, J.C., Lefranc, M.P., Murtaugh, M.P., 2012b. Evolution of the porcine (Sus scrofa domestica) immunoglobulin kappa locus through germline gene conversion. Immunogenetics 64 (4), 303–311.

Sinkora, M., Stepanova, K., Butler, J.E., Sinkore, M., et al., 2022. Comparative aspects of immunoglobulin gene rearrangement assays in different species. Front. Immunol. 13. https://doi.org/10.3389/fimmu.2022.823145

Steiniger, S.C., Glanville, J., Harris, D.W., Wilson, T.L., et al., 2017. Comparative analysis of the feline immunoglobulin repertoire. Biologicals 46, 81–87.

Sun, Y., Wang, C., Wang, Y., et al., 2010. A comprehensive analysis of germline and expressed immunoglobulin repertoire in the horse. Dev. Comp. Immunol. 34, 1009–1020.

Vaccarelli, G., Miccoli, M.C., Antonacci, R., et al., 2008. Genomic organization and recombinational unit duplication-driven evolution of ovine and bovine T cell receptor gamma loci. BMC Genomics 9, 81.

Walther, S., Rusitzka, T.V., Diesterbeck, U.S., Czerny, C.P., 2015. Equine immunoglobulins and organization of immunoglobulin genes. Dev. Comp. Immunol. 53 (2), 303–319.

Weiss, A.T.A., Hecht, W., Henrich, M., Reinacher, M., 2008. Characterization of C-, J-, and V-region genes of the feline T-cell receptor γ. Vet. Immunol. Immunopathol. 124, 63–74.

Zhao, Y., Pan-Hammarstrom, Q., Kacskovics, I., Hammarstrom, L., 2003. The porcine Ig delta gene: unique chimeric splicing of the first constant region domain in its heavy chain transcripts. J. Immunol. 171, 1312–1318.

19

T Cells and the Destruction of Intracellular Invaders

Antibodies bind to invading organisms in blood or tissue fluids, hastening their destruction by complement and phagocytosis. However, not all foreign organisms are found outside cells. All viruses and some bacteria grow inside cells at sites inaccessible to antibodies. Antibodies are therefore of limited use in defending the body against such invaders. Viruses and other intracellular organisms must be eliminated by other mechanisms. For this, the body uses two different cell-mediated processes. Either infected cells are killed rapidly by T cells so that the invader has no time to grow, or alternatively, infected macrophages develop the ability to destroy the intracellular organisms. In general, organisms such as viruses that enter the cell cytosol or nucleus are killed by cytotoxicity, whereas organisms such as bacteria or parasites that reside within endosomes are destroyed by macrophage activation. T cells mediate both processes. The antigens that trigger these immune responses are generated within infected cells and are thus called endogenous antigens.

ENDOGENOUS ANTIGENS

As described in Chapter 12, every time a cell makes a protein, a sample is processed, and peptides are carried to the cell surface bound to major histocompatibility complex (MHC) class I molecules (Fig. 19.1). If these peptides are not recognized by T cells, no response is triggered. If, however, the peptide-MHC complex triggers T-cell's antigen receptors (TCR), then that T cell will respond. For example, when a virus infects a cell, T cells can recognize the viral peptides presented on the cell surface. The T cells that respond to these endogenous antigens are CD8+. They use their CD8 to bind to MHC class I molecules on the infected cells, thus promoting intercellular signaling and eventually the killing of the infected cells.

APOPTOSIS

Cells can kill themselves. Old, surplus, damaged, or abnormal cells that would otherwise interfere with normal tissue functions can be persuaded to die as necessary. This cell suicide is called apoptosis. Apoptosis is carefully regulated and must only be triggered when a cell must die. Structurally, apoptosis is characterized by membrane blebbing, nuclear fragmentation, and cell death without lysis. These dying cells and fragments are readily phagocytosed by macrophages (Hotchkiss et al., 2009).

There are two major pathways of apoptosis. The extrinsic or death receptor pathway and the intrinsic or mitochondrial pathway. The extrinsic pathway is triggered by cytokines such as tumor necrosis factor-α (TNF-α) acting through specific death receptors. Death receptors are a family of cell surface receptors that when activated trigger apoptosis. They all possess an 80-amino acid cytoplasmic sequence called a death domain. The most important of these death receptors are Fas (CD95) and the receptors for tumor necrosis factor–α (TNFR). Death receptors are activated by ligands expressed on cytotoxic cells. The ligands bind to the receptors and cause the target cells to assemble multiple adaptor proteins into a signaling complex. This complex then activates initiator caspases-8 and -10 (Fig. 19.2).

The mitochondrial pathway, in contrast, is triggered by noxious stimuli that cause mitochondrial injury. The damaging stimuli (e.g., oxidants, radiation) activate pro-apoptotic bcl-2 proteins, which then release cytochrome C from mitochondria (Fig. 19.3). The cytochrome C triggers the formation of a large multiprotein complex called an apoptosome. The apoptosome then activates initiator caspase 9 (Pinkoski et al., 2001).

The initiator caspases activated by either pathway activate a cascade of "effector caspases" (caspases-3, -6, and-7) that degrade cell proteins, activate endonucleases, and break down organelles, resulting in cell death and disassembly. The DNA of apoptotic cells is broken into many low-molecular-weight fragments. This fragmentation may be responsible for the characteristic way in which the nuclear chromatin condenses against the nuclear membrane (Fig. 19.4). Affected cells shrink and detach from the surrounding cells. Eventually, nuclear breakup and cytoplasmic budding form cell fragments called apoptotic bodies (Fig. 19.5).

As cells undergo apoptosis, their cell membrane "flips" so that the lipid phosphatidylserine is exposed on their surface. This lipid binds to receptors on macrophages and dendritic cells and triggers phagocytosis of the dying cells. It also triggers the release of antiinflammatory cytokines such as TGF-β while minimizing the release of proinflammatory cytokines such as TNF-α (Box 19.1).

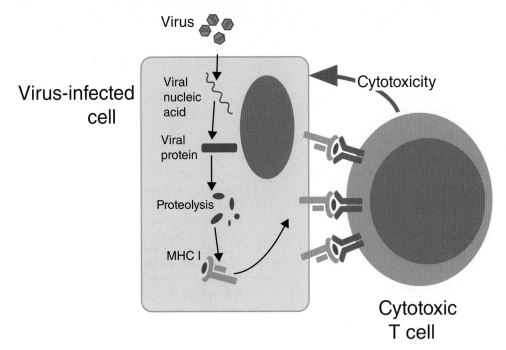

Fig. 19.1 A simplified view of the processing of endogenous antigens. Endogenous antigens are first broken down into small peptides and inserted into the antigen-binding groove of major histocompatibility complex (MHC) class I molecules. When presented on a cell surface, antigenic peptides bound to the MHC class I molecules trigger a cytotoxic T-cell response.

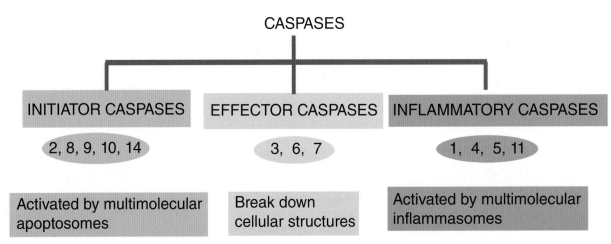

Fig. 19.2 The role of the three different types of caspase in inflammation and apoptosis. The inflammatory caspases are described in Chapter 3.

CELL COOPERATION

During a primary immune response, CD8⁺ cytotoxic T cells cannot respond to all infected cells. There are about 10^{13} nucleated cells in a human-sized body and possibly several hundred naïve T cells with receptors for each individual viral antigen. Clearly, it would be almost impossible for these T cells to find and kill all the virus-infected cells without help. In practice, dendritic cells link processed antigens to MHC class I molecules and carry them to lymphoid organs where they are presented to CD8⁺ T cells. To respond fully, the CD8⁺ cells must also be costimulated by CD4⁺ helper cells. Costimulation is only effective when both the CD8⁺ and CD4⁺ T cells recognize antigen on the same antigen-presenting cell. Thus, a helper T cell first interacts with

an antigen-presenting dendritic cell through CD40 and CD154. The helper T cells activate the dendritic cells, upregulate their expression of MHC class I, and stimulate their production of interleukin-12 (IL-12). Once activated, dendritic cell MHC class I–linked peptides bind to CD8⁺ T cells. For complete activation, the cytotoxic T cells require three signals. The first is IL-12 from activated dendritic cells. The second is an antigen-specific signal from the antigen–MHC class I complex on their target cell. The third signal comes from IL-2 and IFN-γ produced by the Th1 cells. Only after all three signals are received, can the CD8 T cells fully respond.

Different levels of stimulation trigger different activation responses in CD8⁺ T cells. As with helper cells, the duration of the stimulus is important. Although activated cytotoxic T cells can be triggered by

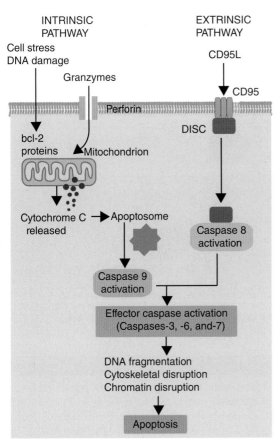

Fig. 19.3 The two pathways by which apoptosis may be triggered. Both lead to caspase activation, DNA fragmentation, and cell death. The extrinsic pathway is activated by activation of death receptors such as CD95 and formation of the death-inducing signaling complex (DISC). The intrinsic pathway is initiated by multiple damage signals, leading to the escape of cytochrome C from mitochondria, the formation of an apoptosome, and activation of caspase 9.

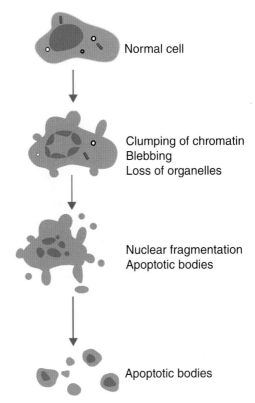

Fig. 19.4 Major morphological features of cell death by apoptosis.

brief exposure to antigen, naïve T cells must be stimulated for several hours before responding. The required stimulation time may be shortened by increasing TCR occupancy or by providing additional costimulation. Once activated, naïve CD8⁺ T cells begin to divide. They undergo multiple rounds of division to generate large numbers of cytotoxic effector cells. Some calculations have suggested that they undergo as many as 19 cell divisions in the week following antigen exposure, and they probably divide every 4–6 hours (Nolz et al., 2016). All this is regulated by extracellular signals from the TCR, costimulatory molecules, and cytokines such as IL-2, -12, -21, and -27. These activated T cells migrate to peripheral sites and differentiate into effector and memory cells. Short-lived effector cells form the bulk of the population, and these will mostly die once infections are cleared. Other cells that may have received less stimulation survive and become long-lived memory cells.

CYTOTOXIC T-CELL RESPONSES

Once fully activated, CD8⁺ T cells leave lymphoid organs and seek out infected cells by themselves. When they recognize an antigen expressed on another cell, the T cells will bind, induce apoptosis, and kill their target (Fig. 19.6).

The density of peptide-MHC complexes on a target cell required to stimulate T-cell cytotoxicity is much lower than that needed to

stimulate cytokine production. Thus T cell binding to a single peptide-MHC complex may be sufficient to trigger killing, whereas binding to 100–1000 complexes is required to stimulate cytokine production and clonal expansion. Presumably cytotoxic T cells need to be highly sensitive to viral peptides, so that they can kill infected cells as effectively as possible.

These differences in signal thresholds are probably related to the structure of the immunological synapse formed when a cytotoxic T-cell encounters a target (Fig. 19.7). (de la Roche et al., 2016). This synapse has two "centers." One of these contains clustered TCR-CD8 complexes. The other "center" attracts secretory lysosomes that release their contents into the synaptic space and so destroy the target cell. Both are surrounded by a pSMAC rich in adhesion molecules that form a "gasket," preventing the accidental escape of cytotoxic molecules into tissues (Stinchcombe et al., 2001). Once the synapse forms, cytotoxic T-cell killing is efficient. Within seconds after contacting a T cell, the organelles and the nucleus of the target show apoptotic changes, and the target is dead in less than 10 minutes. Cytotoxic T cells can disengage and move on to kill other targets within 5–6 minutes. In addition, several cytotoxic cells can join in killing a single target (Dieckmann et al., 2016).

Cytotoxic T cells kill their targets through two pathways. The perforin pathway involves the secretion of perforins and granzymes from secretory lysosomes (Fig. 19.8). These kill cells through intrinsic apoptotic mechanisms. The other pathway kills cells by signaling through the CD95 death receptor. The perforin pathway is used to destroy virus-infected cells, whereas the CD95 pathway is mainly used to kill unwanted surplus T cells (Carter and Dutton, 1995).

Perforin Pathway

The killing process mediated by T-cell perforins can be divided into three phases: adhesion, lethal hit, and cell death (see Fig. 19.8).

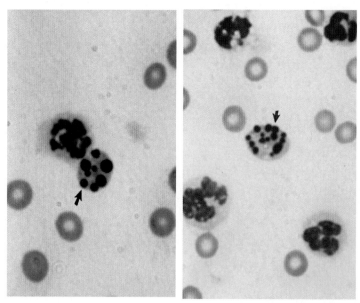

Fig. 19.5 Two rat neutrophils showing nuclear condensation and fragmentation characteristic of apoptosis. Courtesy Ms. K. Kennon.

BOX 19.1   Immunologic Cell Death

Mammalian cells respond to environmental changes by adjusting cellular pathways in an effort to maintain homeostasis. If, however, these changes exceed the ability of the cell to respond, it may have to be eliminated. Cellular death is a feature of many innate and adaptive immune responses. The body has to get rid of 200 billion cells daily. Cells can die in several different ways. Thus, irreparable damage to an essential pathway will kill a cell in an uncontrolled manner. However, there are several different ways in which a cell can participate in its own death. These forms of programmed cell death can benefit the body by stopping microbial infections, sparing uninfected nearby cells, and by not generating alarmins and inflammatory mediators. These are essentially "cell suicide" (Green and Victor 2012).

The commonest way many cells are killed is through phagocytosis (phagoptosis). Thus the removal of aged erythrocytes and blood leukocytes is mediated by phagocytic macrophages. Likewise, some cancer cells can be phagocytosed and killed by macrophages. Some neurologic diseases result from phagocytosis of stressed neurons. However, there are several other common pathways that cause death by suicide (Fig. 19.9).

Apoptosis

This is the "normal" way unwanted healthy cells are eliminated. It occurs through two pathways. An extrinsic pathway where the cell receives signals from extracellular molecules that bind to cell surface "death" receptors. This generates a cascade of activated caspases that cause mitochondrial permeability. The intrinsic pathway is activated by internal cellular events such as DNA damage or microbial infection and also leads to mitochondrial permeabilization, the release of cytochrome C into the cytoplasm, the formation of an apoptosome, and the activation of lethal caspase 9. Apoptotic cells are characterized by distinctive morphological changes. They form apoptotic bodies. These cell fragments are destroyed by other phagocytes before their plasma membranes rupture and, as a result, apoptosis does not trigger inflammation. These dying cells do, however, release nucleotides such as ATP and UTP that function as signals that attract professional scavenger cells such as macrophages and monocytes, so that the dying cells are promptly engulfed and digested (Fig. 19.9).

Pyroptosis

Pyroptosis is a form of programed cell death characterized by the formation of pores in the cell membrane, the release of IL-1 and IL-18, and DNA fragmentation. Cell swelling is followed by a breakdown in membrane integrity and the escape of cell contents. This is normally a defensive process that prevents the replication of intracellular microbial invaders. Pyroptosis is triggered by the formation of a specific type of inflammasome that activates caspase 1. The caspase, in turn, cleaves a pore-forming effector protein called gasdermin D to generate an active fragment. The activated gasdermin fragment binds to cell membrane lipids and forms oligomeric pores in the plasma membrane. These pores permit the escape of cell contents and some cytokines into the tissues. The dying cells eventually rupture as a result of increased osmotic pressure, thus releasing the rest of their contents into the tissues.

The pyroptosis pores permit the escape of inflammatory mediators such as IL-1β, HMGB-1, and ATP that act as alarmins and activate local immune cells. They also release both nuclear and mitochondrial DNA. When first released, cellular DNA is largely intact and consists of very long strands. However, it is rapidly fragmented into much smaller pieces of about 166 base pairs—about the length of a strand of DNA wrapped around a single nucleosome. Mitochondrial DNA is released at the same time. It is a potent proinflammatory DAMP since its nucleotide composition reflects its microbial origins. Thus, gasdermins also promote NETosis (Yu et al., 2021) (Fig. 19.9). Interestingly, carnivores, including dogs and cats, have inflammasomes that lack certain key components and so do not mediate normal pyroptosis.

Necroptosis

Necroptosis is a form of programed necrosis triggered by death receptors such as TNFR, nucleic acid sensors, or by TLR-signaling. They activate receptor-activating threonine kinases and form molecular complexes called necrosomes. Together with proteases and kinases, they generate a pore-forming protein, which inserts itself into the cell wall and allows the escape of cellular contents. Mitochondria are not involved in necroptosis. Like pyroptosis, necroptosis causes inflammation because of the escape of intracellular DAMPs such as HMGB-1 and interleukin 33 (IL-33) into the surrounding tissues. Dogs do not mount a normal necroptosis response (Fig. 19.9).

Panoptosis

The programmed cell death pathways described above talk to each other. A unique inflammatory programed cell death is called panoptosis. It works by integrating the other programmed cell death pathways described earlier.

From Green, D.R., Victor, B. 2012. The pantheon of the fallen: why are there so many forms of cell death? Trends Cell Biol. 22, 555–556.

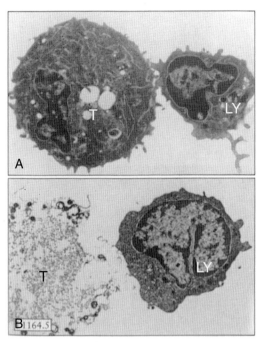

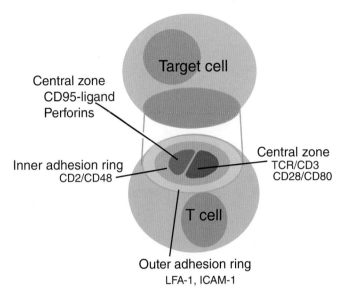

Fig. 19.6 Destruction of target cells by cytotoxic T cells. (A) Conjugation between a peritoneal exudate lymphocyte (the small cell on the right) and a target cell. Note the lysosome-like bodies *(LY)* and the nuclear fragmentation of the target cell *(T)*. (B) A lymphocyte with the remains of a lysed target cell. From Zagury, D., Bernard, J., Thierness, N., Feldman, M., Berke, G. 1995. Isolation and characterization of individual functionally reactive cytotoxic T lymphocytes, conjugation, killing and recycling at the single cell level. Eur. J. Immunol. 5, 881–822.

Fig. 19.7 Structure of the immunological synapse that forms between a cytotoxic T cell and its target. The outer ring of adhesive proteins forms an effective "gasket" that prevents leakage of cytotoxic molecules into tissue fluid. There are, however, two central supramolecular activation complexes (SMACs). The central one is dedicated to signaling and contains the T-cell antigen receptor (TCR) together with accessory molecules and costimulators. The other is dedicated to cytotoxic mechanisms. It is through this cSMAC that perforins, granzymes, and the Fas-FasL signals are transmitted.

Adhesion Phase

When TCRs on cytotoxic T cells bind to antigen-MHC complexes on the target cell, an immunological synapse rapidly forms around the area of contact. The TCRs and other signaling molecules cluster at one of the centers of the complex. The CD8 molecules bind target cell MHC class I and strengthen T cell—target binding. If the TCR has a very high affinity for the target antigen, costimulation through CD8 may not be necessary.

In addition to receiving signals from antigen-MHC-CD8 complexes, cytotoxic T cells need costimulation. As with CD4+ helper T cells, CD8+ cytotoxic cells require signals from CD28 bound to CD86 on the target cell. Additional adhesion between cytotoxic T cells and their targets is mediated by T-cell CD2 binding to target cell CD58 (in nonrodents) or CD48 (in rodents) and T-cell CD11a/CD18 (LFA-1) binding to target cell CD54 (ICAM-1).

Lethal Hit

Within a few minutes of binding to a target, the T cells orientate their microtubule organizing center, their Golgi complex, and their granules toward the target cell. Their cytoplasmic granules migrate to the center of the synapse. Here they fuse with the T-cell membrane in such a way that the toxic granule contents are injected into the target. Cytotoxic T-cell granules contain several lethal molecules, of which the most important are perforins, granzymes, and granulysin (Brodovitch et al., 2013).

Perforins are pore-forming glycoproteins produced by cytotoxic T cells and natural killer (NK) cells. Perforins insert themselves into the target cell membrane and oligomerize to form tubular transmembrane channels (Fig. 19.10) (Law et al., 2010). Between 19 and 24 perforin monomers aggregate to form a circular membrane attack complex that forms large (130–200 Å) pores in target cell membranes. These perforins are related to and act in a similar manner to C9, the molecule that forms the terminal complement complex (Chapter 5). Although the size of the central pore of the polyperforin permits granzyme

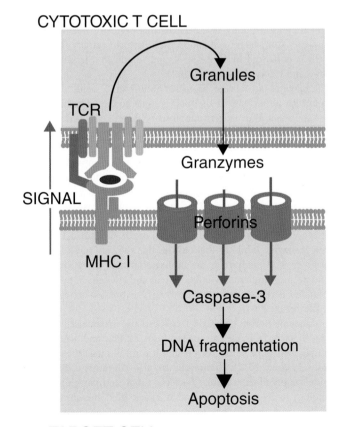

Fig. 19.8 The perforin pathway by which T cells kill targets. *MHC,* Major histocompatibility complex; *TCRs,* T-cell antigen receptor.

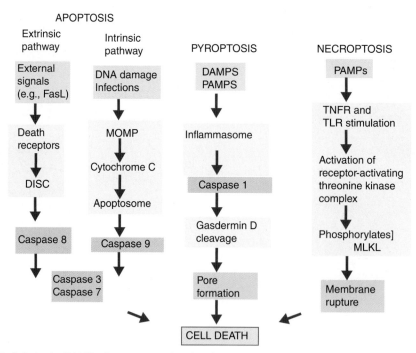

Fig. 19.9 Cell death. *DAMPs*, Damage-associated molecular patterns; *DISC*, death-inducing signaling complex; *PAMPs*, pathogen-associated molecular patterns; *TLR*, toll-like receptors; *TNFR*, tumor necrosis factor receptors.

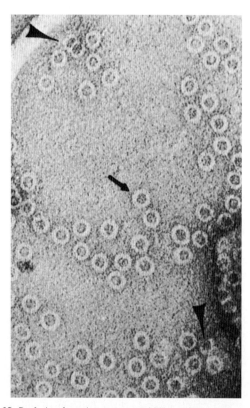

Fig. 19.10 Perforins from human natural killer cells on the surface of a rabbit erythrocyte target. The arrowheads point to incomplete rings and double rings. From Podack, E.R., Dennert G., Assembly of two types of tubules with putative cytolytic function by cloned natural killer cells. Nature 301, 442–445.

monomers and dimers to enter target cells, killing also occurs at low perforin concentrations. It is believed that perforins may also release granzymes from target cell endosomes. Perforin activity in cytotoxic T cells is enhanced by IL-2, -3, -4, and -6 and to a lesser degree by TNF-α and IFN-γ (Lowin et al., 1994).

Granzymes are serine proteases found in T cells, where they account for about 90% of the total granule contents. Granzyme A is most abundant and triggers apoptosis of target cells. It destroys histones and releases a nuclear DNase. It is this enzyme that causes the DNA damage. Granzyme B enters the target cell, either by injection through the central pore of the perforin complex or by endocytosis. It activates pro-apoptotic bcl-2 proteins, triggering the release of mitochondrial cytochrome C. As described previously, the cytochrome C generates an apoptosome that in turn activates caspase 9 and the effector caspase cascade. The effector caspases activate endonucleases that cause DNA fragmentation and cell death. Cytotoxic T cells possess a granzyme inhibitor that ensures that they are not killed during this process. Granulysin is an antibacterial lipid-disrupting peptide found in the granules of cytotoxic T cells and NK cells in primates and ruminants. A related molecule (Bo-lysin) is expressed in bovine T cells (Endsley et al., 2004).

Granzyme B from cytotoxic T cells can also activate cell death programs in bacteria. It disrupts the synthesis, folding, and degradation of multiple critical proteins. As a result, it can kill intracellular bacteria (Dotiwala et al., 2017). Granulysin can also kill target cells as well as a wide variety of extracellular bacteria, fungi, and parasites. It shares homology with other proteins that attack lipid membranes called saposins. Saposins do not form pores but activate lipid-degrading enzymes such as sphingomyelinases. An increase in saposins therefore increases ceramide content, and ceramide can induce apoptosis. For example, cytotoxic T cells can control *Listeria monocytogenes* and

Mycobacterium tuberculosis infections simply by killing infected cells. It is possible that living bacteria released from these killed cells might infect healthy cells. To avoid this, the T cell–derived granulysin kills not only infected macrophages but also any bacteria that happen to be inside them.

CD95 Pathway

The second pathway of T cell–mediated cytotoxicity involves the binding of a T-cell surface protein called CD95L (Fas ligand or CD178) to a target cell death receptor called CD95 (Fas) (Fig. 19.11; Guicciardi and Gores, 2009). CD95L is expressed on activated CD8+ T cells and NK cells. It binds to CD95 on target cells. When the cells come into contact, CD95L binds to CD95, and the CD95 trimerizes. This leads to the formation of a death-inducing signaling complex that activates initiator caspases-8 and -10. These, in turn, activate caspase-3 and trigger the apoptosis cascade. The CD95L-CD95 system regulates T-cell survival. Unwanted surplus or self-reactive T cells are conveniently eliminated once they have served their functions. For example, when activated T cells have completed their task of killing their targets, they themselves undergo CD95-mediated apoptosis (Krammer, 2000).

In mice, *lpr* (lymphoproliferation) and *gld* (generalized lymphoproliferative disease) are loss-of-function mutations in the genes encoding CD95 and CD95L, respectively. Both mutations permit activated T cells to accumulate and accelerate autoimmune diseases. For example, *lpr* mice do not express CD95 on their thymocytes. As a result, their thymocytes do not undergo apoptosis (negative selection), and they escape into the secondary lymphoid organs. Here they proliferate, resulting in a gross increase in the size of their lymphoid organs

(lymphadenopathy). Many of these cells respond to self-antigens and *lpr* mice develop an autoimmune disease similar to systemic lupus erythematosus (Chapter 39).

Feline autoimmune lymphoproliferative syndrome is an inherited disease of cats resulting from a *gld* mutation in the gene encoding CD95L. Affected kittens develop a generalized, rapidly progressive, lymphadenopathy accompanied by splenomegaly and hepatomegaly. All their lymph nodes are enlarged as a result of the accumulation of T cells. They may develop autoimmune diseases. Affected kittens die within a few months.

TNF-β (also called lymphotoxin-α [LT-α]) is secreted by some cytotoxic T cells and has a similar mode of action to CD95L. Structural changes are seen by 2–3 hours, and by 16 hours more than 90% of target cells exposed to TNF-β are dead.

CYTOTOXIC T-CELL SUBSETS

Subsets of CD8+ T cells have been identified in mice, where they are called Tc1 and Tc2 cells. Tc1 cells secrete IL-2 and IFN-γ, whereas Tc2 cells secrete IL-4 and IL-5. A third subset, Tc0, has an unrestricted cytokine profile. Unlike helper cells that can differentiate readily into Th1 or Th2 cells, CD8+ T cells show a strong preference for the Tc1 phenotype. Differentiation into Tc2 requires exposure to large amounts of IL-4. All three subsets are cytotoxic (Chopp et al., 2023).

As described in Chapter 15, T-cell interactions with their targets are regulated by positive costimulation from CD28 and negative signals from CTLA-4. In some human cancers where T-cell cytotoxicity is insufficient to kill the cancer cells, blockage of CTLA-4 by monoclonal antibodies, enhances T-cell cytotoxicity, and induces long-term tumor remission.

Another molecule that limits T-cell cytotoxicity is called programmed cell death-1 (PD-1, CD279). This is a T-cell receptor that binds to ligands (PD-L1 and PD-L2) on target cells and then inhibits signaling from the TCR. Upregulation of PD-1 is a normal consequence of T-cell activation and is required to terminate an immune response. Persistent viral infections and some cancers induce strong stable expression of PD-1 on activated T cells. This leads to T-cell exhaustion, failure of activation, and a loss of T-cell function. When PD-L1 is expressed on tumor cells, it protects them from attack by cytotoxic T cells. Conversely, inhibition of PD-1 signaling will enhance T cell–mediated destruction of certain cancers. Both CTLA-4 and PD-1 are regarded as immune checkpoint molecules and their inhibition by monoclonal antibodies has resulted in successful cancer treatments in humans. You can read more about these checkpoint inhibitors in Chapter 36.

OTHER MECHANISMS OF CELLULAR CYTOTOXICITY

T cell–mediated cytotoxicity is not the only way by which the immune system can destroy abnormal cells (Table 19.1 and Fig. 19.12). For example, cells that possess the antibody receptors FcγRI or FcγRII may bind to target cells or bacteria through specific antibodies and then kill them. These cytotoxic cells may include monocytes, eosinophils, neutrophils, B cells, and NK cells (Chapter 20). The mechanism of this antibody-dependent, cell-mediated cytotoxicity (ADCC) is unclear. However, neutrophils and eosinophils probably release lethal oxidants and toxic granule contents. ADCC is slower and less efficient than direct T cell–mediated cytotoxicity, taking 6–18 hours to occur.

Whether a macrophage participates in ADCC depends on its Fc receptors and its degree of activation. Macrophage-activating cytokines

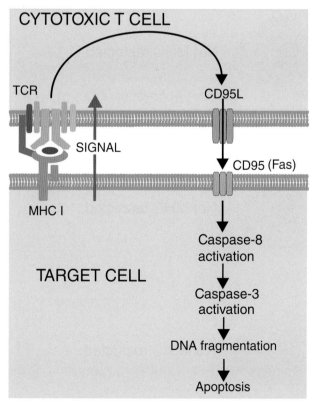

Fig. 19.11 The CD95 pathway of T cell–mediated cytotoxicity. *MHC*, Major histocompatibility complex; *TCR*, T-cell antigen receptor.

TABLE 19.1   Comparison of the Three Major Mechanisms of Cell-Mediated Cytotoxicity

Cytotoxic Cells	Time	Mechanism	MHC Restricted	Antigen Specific
NK cells	24 h	NK-mediated cytotoxicity	No	No
Normal lymphocytes or macrophages with FcγRIII with specific antibody	6 h	ADCC activity	No	Yes
Primed T cells	10 min	T cell–mediated cytotoxicity	Yes	Yes

ADCC, Antibody-dependent, cell-mediated cytotoxicity; *NK*, natural killer.

such as IFN-γ or granulocyte-macrophage colony-stimulating factor promote ADCC. Macrophages may also destroy target cells in an antibody-independent process. For example, when they ingest bacteria or parasites, macrophages release nitric oxide, proteases, and TNF-α. The nitric oxide will kill nearby bacteria and cells, whereas the TNF-α is cytotoxic for some tumor cells.

MACROPHAGE ACTIVATION

When macrophages attack and ingest invading bacteria, they produce enzymes and oxidants that normally kill and digest the invaders. These enzymes and oxidants, however, may be insufficient to kill some invaders. For example, bacteria such as *L. monocytogenes*, *M. tuberculosis*, and *Brucella abortus*, and protozoa such as *Leishmania* and *Toxoplasma*, can survive and multiply inside normal macrophages. Once inside a cell, antibodies are ineffective against these organisms, so protection against this type of infection requires that macrophages must be activated (Fig. 19.13). Activated macrophages are functionally polarized (see Chapter 7). Classically activated or

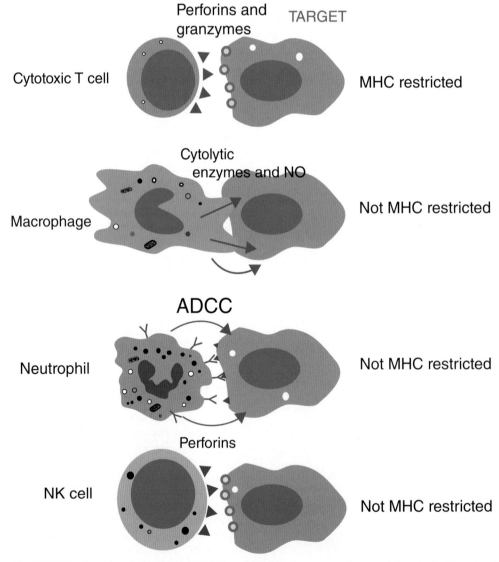

Fig. 19.12 The four major pathways by which the cells of the immune system can kill nucleated target cells. These targets would normally be tumor cells or virus-infected cells. T cells and NK cells are directly cytotoxic. Macrophages secrete nitric oxide synthase and enzymes that kill nearby cells. Cells with Fc receptors act through ADCC mechanisms. *ADCC*, Antibody-dependent, cell-mediated cytotoxicity; *MHC*, major histocompatibility complex; *NK cell*, natural killer cell; *NO*, nitric oxide.

M1 macrophages serve as proinflammatory effector cells that are key to the body's defenses against intracellular invaders. Alternatively activated or M2 macrophages have antiinflammatory properties and play a role in tolerance induction, in resolving inflammation and in wound healing.

Classical Macrophage Activation

M1 macrophages become fully activated in stages. Initial activation of sentinel cells is triggered through PRRs by exposure to PAMPs and DAMPs from invading bacteria and damaged tissues as described previously (Figs. 19.14 and 19.15). Thus, when naïve macrophages encounter bacteria or viruses that activate their TLRs, signals are generated via their inflammasome to produce cytokines. Two of these, TNF-α and IL-12, act on NK cells, causing them to produce large amounts of IFN-γ. Some TLR ligands can also activate pathways that result in IFN-β production. This endogenous IFN-β also promotes M1 cell polarization.

Macrophages also present antigen to Th1 cells as described in Chapter 15. In return, the Th1 cells can cause the macrophages to become even more activated. For example, stimulation of Th1 cells by IL-12 will trigger their IFN-γ production. These "armed" Th1 cells also produce IL-2, which further promotes M1 polarization and complete cell activation. Th1-macrophage interactions through CD40-CD40L also promote M1 activation.

M1 macrophages are polarized by IFN-γ acting through the JAK/STAT pathway. The interferon induces a rapid switch to aerobic glycolysis in M1 macrophages. This change permits increased ROS and nitric oxide production (Wang et al., 2018). IFN-γ exposure alters the expression of more than 1000 macrophage genes as a result of the activities of microRNAs. These activated macrophages secrete proteases, that can activate complement. They increase their expression of CD40 and TNF-α receptors. They secrete interferons as well as thromboplastin, prostaglandins, fibronectins, plasminogen activator, and the complement components C2 and FB. They increase their expression of MHC class II, delay production of phagosomal proteases and promote antigen loading onto MHC molecules, so enhancing antigen presentation. M1 macrophages are enlarged and show increased membrane activity (especially ruffling), increased formation of pseudopodia, and increased pinocytosis (uptake of fluid droplets) (Fig. 19.16). They move faster in response to chemotactic stimuli. They produce

more lysosomal enzymes and respiratory burst metabolites, and they are more avidly phagocytic than resting macrophages. These M1 cells produce greatly increased amounts of nitric oxide synthase 2 (NOS2). As a result, they can kill intracellular organisms or tumor cells by generating high levels of nitric oxide (Fig. 19.17). IFN-γ-activated M1 macrophages can also inhibit the growth of intracellular bacteria by down-regulating their transferrin receptors (CD71), degrading ferroportin, and by reducing the concentration of intracellular ferritin, their major iron storage protein (see Chapter 8; Trost et al., 2009).

Alternative Macrophage Activation

Macrophages have an alternative choice of phenotype. When they are activated under the influence of Th2 cytokines such as IL-4 and IL-13 they become M2 cells. M2 cells differ from M1 cells in receptor expression, cytotoxic function, cytokine production and their overall functions (Fig. 19.18) (Gordon and Martinez, 2010). M2 cells are both regulatory and antiinflammatory, and they promote the resolution of inflammation and wound repair. They are protective in some parasitic diseases by walling off parasites such as schistosomes. Instead of producing nitric oxide, M2 cells use arginase to produce ornithine. They secrete large quantities of IL-10 and IL-1RA (Anderson and Mosser, 2002).

TGF-β from M2 cells stimulates extracellular matrix (ECM) production by fibroblasts. M2 cells also secrete the matrix component fibronectin. They secrete transglutaminase, which promotes ECM cross-linking, and osteopontin, which promotes cell-binding to the ECM. Arginase is involved in proline and polyamine synthesis. Proline is required for ECM construction, whereas polyamines are required for cell proliferation. M2 cells secrete platelet-derived growth factor, insulin-like growth factor, and TGF-β, all of which promote cell proliferation. They secrete fibroblast-like growth factor–β (FGF-β), TGF-α, and vascular endothelial growth factor, which promote angiogenesis. Thus, the cytokines secreted by M2 cells promote resolution of inflammation and wound repair and have antiinflammatory, fibrotic, proliferative, and angiogenic properties. (M2 macrophages may be further subdivided into M2a cells whose primary role is promotion of wound healing, and M2b cells that are primarily antiinflammatory).

The importance of macrophage activation can be seen in diseases such as tuberculosis. Thus mycobacteria that enter the lungs

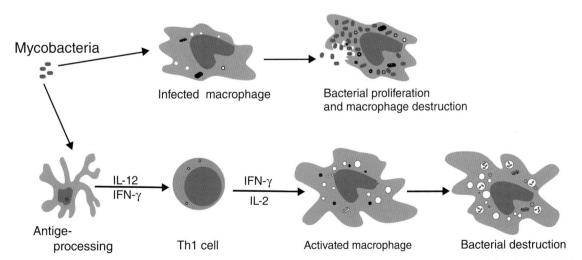

Fig. 19.13 Normal macrophages are killed by growing intracellular bacteria. Interferon-γ (IFN-γ) and interleukin-2 (IL-2) released by Th1 cells can activate macrophages and enable them to kill otherwise resistant intracellular bacteria.

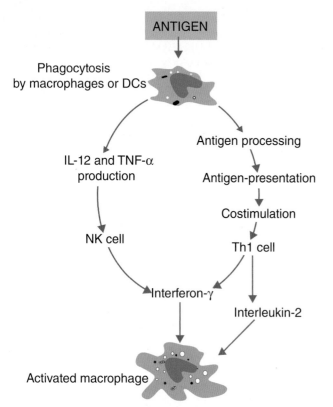

Fig. 19.14 The two pathways by which M1 macrophages can be activated. One involves interferon-γ (IFN-γ) production by natural killer cells and is thus an innate pathway. The other is mediated by IFN-γ from Th1 cells and is an adaptive response. *DCs*, Dendritic cells; *IL-12*, interleukin-12; *NK*, natural killer; *TNFα*, tumor necrosis factor–α.

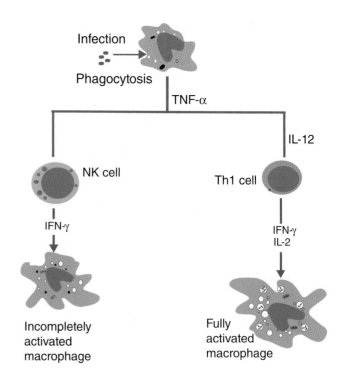

Fig. 19.15 M1 macrophage activation probably develops in stages. Thus interferon-γ (IFN-γ) produced by natural killer (NK) cells probably activates macrophages in the early stages of an immune response. If this is insufficient, then Th1 cells are activated, and the combination of IFN-γ and interleukin-2 (IL-2) that they produce causes maximal M1 activation and polarization. *IL-12*, Interleukin-12; *TNFα*, tumor necrosis factor–α.

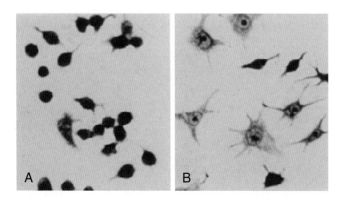

Fig. 19.16 Stained cultures of mouse macrophages grown under identical conditions: (A) normal unstimulated macrophages. (B) Macrophages activated by exposure to interferon-γ and acemannan. Note the cytoplasmic spreading of the activated cells. These cells secrete large quantities of cytokines and nitric oxide. Original magnification ×400. (Courtesy Dr. L. Zhang).

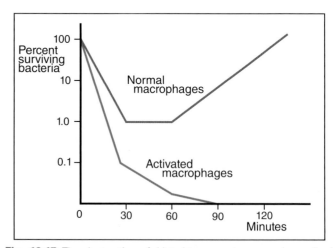

Fig. 19.17 The destruction of *Listeria monocytogenes* when mixed in vitro with cultures of normal macrophages and "activated" macrophages from *Listeria*-infected mice.

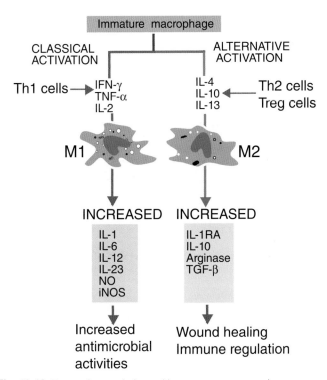

Fig. 19.18 Depending on their cytokine exposure, macrophages may be classically activated (M1 cells) or become alternatively activated (M2 cells). M2 cells have a major regulatory role and are critical to granuloma formation and wound healing. They produce very different cytokine mixtures. *IFN-γ*, Interferon-γ; *IL-2*, interleukin-2; *NO*, nitric oxide; *TGF-β*, transforming growth factor-β; *TNF-α*, tumor necrosis factor-α.

TABLE 19.2 Effects of Cytokines on Macrophage Function

Cytokine	Major Source	Effect
IL-2	Th1 cell	Activates
IFN-γ	Th1 cell, NK cell	Activates
IFN-α/β	Macrophages, T cells	Activates
TNF-α	Macrophages, Th1 cells	Activates
TNF-β	Th1 cells	Activates
GM-CSF	Many cell types	Activates
IL-4	Th2 cells	Suppresses
IL-10	Th2 cells, macrophages	Suppresses
IL-13	Th2 cells	Suppresses
TGF-β	T cells	Suppresses

GM-CSF, Granulocyte-macrophage colony-stimulating factor; *IFN-γ*, interferon-γ; *IL-2*, interleukin-2; *TGF-β*, transforming growth factor-β; *TNF-α*, tumor necrosis factor–α.

are readily phagocytosed by alveolar macrophages that then mount a respiratory burst and secrete proinflammatory cytokines. These cytokines act on NK cells, triggering IFN-γ production and limited macrophage activation. This rapid response can slow mycobacterial growth significantly. Nevertheless, these macrophages cannot destroy the bacteria by these mechanisms alone. After several days, however, recruitment of Th1 cells occurs. The Th1 cells are stimulated by mycobacteria-infected dendritic cells secreting IL-12, TNF-α, and IFN-α. In response, the Th1 cells secrete more IFN-γ and fully activate the macrophages (Table 19.2). In most individuals, this activation to the M1 level is sufficient to control the infection (Harris et al., 2009).

Cytotoxic T cells generated in cattle infected with *M. bovis* will kill infected macrophages. This cytotoxicity is mediated by both WC1+ γ/δ and CD8+ T cells. Presumably any *Mycobacteria* released are killed by granulysin (Stenger et al., 1998).

Delayed Hypersensitivity Reactions

When certain antigens are injected into the skin of a sensitized animal, an inflammatory response, taking many hours to develop, may occur at the injection site. This is a T cell–mediated response called delayed hypersensitivity. Delayed hypersensitivity reactions are classified as type IV hypersensitivity reactions (see Chapter 34). An important example of a delayed hypersensitivity reaction is the tuberculin response, the skin reaction that follows an intradermal injection of tuberculin in an infected animal.

EFFECTOR T-CELL MEMORY

In contrast to the prolonged antibody response, the effector phase of T-cell responses is relatively brief. Indeed, cytotoxicity is seen only in the presence of antigen. This is logical. Sustained and unnecessary T-cell cytotoxic activities or overproduction of cytokines could result in severe tissue damage (Dooms and Abbas, 2002).

Naïve CD8+T cells are long-lived resting cells that continuously recirculate between the bloodstream and lymphoid organs. Once they encounter antigen, they multiply rapidly in an effort to keep pace with the growth of invading pathogens. The number of responding cells may increase more than 1000-fold within a few days. They reach a peak 5–7 days after infection when pathogen-specific, cytotoxic T cells can make up 50%–70% of the total CD8+ T cells. As with other lymphocytes, asymmetric division results in two daughter cells with different fates. In the case of CD8+ cells it results in the generation of effector and memory effector T cells. The effector cells are derived from the daughter cell closest to the antigen-presenting cell. The memory T cells are derived from the daughter distal to the APC. The proximal cell has increased glycolytic activity and increased expression of effector molecules. The distal cell has increased lipid metabolism, increased expression of antiapoptotic molecules and lives very much longer (Ciocca et al., 2012). Once the infection has cleared, most of the effector cells are superfluous. Therefore, up to 95% of them undergo apoptosis 1–2 weeks after infection. Elimination of these excess T cells is a tightly controlled process involving the CD95 pathway.

The number of surviving memory cells is directly related to the intensity of the primary response. In general, only 5%–10% of the peak number of cytotoxic T cells survive as memory T cells. Survival may be a function of duration of exposure to antigen. Cells exposed to antigen for prolonged periods may die, whereas cells exposed only briefly may live. The observation that chronic viral infections can exhaust T cells and impair both cytotoxicity and memory is consistent with this idea.

Memory T cells can be distinguished from naïve T cells by their phenotype, by secreting a different mixture of cytokines, and by their behavior (Weng et al., 2012). For example, memory T cells are CD44+ and express high levels of IL-2Rβ, a receptor that binds both IL-2 and

IL-15. They express increased amounts of adhesion molecules, so they can bind more efficiently to antigen-presenting cells. They produce more IL-4 and IFN-γ and respond more strongly to stimulation of their TCR. They continue to divide very slowly, in the absence of antigen. This division requires cell-bound IL-15 and is inhibited by soluble IL-2. IL-15 is a unique cytokine that persists for very long periods attached to its receptor on T cells. It thus acts as a persistent stimulus for the memory cell microenvironment and stimulates nearby cells by cell-cell contact. The balance between IL-15 and IL-2 regulates the persistence of memory T cells. In the absence of IL-15, memory cells undergo apoptosis. In humans the CD8+ memory T-cell half-life is 8–15 years. Memory T cells persist in numerous tissues such as secondary lymphoid organs, barrier tissues such as the lung, skin and intestine as well as white adipose tissue where they constitute a readily available reservoir when needed (Han et al., 2017; Schenkel and Masopust, 2014) (Fig. 19.9).

Over an animal's lifetime, immunological memories accumulate. Older animals have more memory cells than young animals and are thus much better prepared to respond to antigens than younger animals. Repeated vaccination generates new memory cells. However, the size of the memory cell compartment expands to accommodate them. Previously generated memory cells are not removed to make space for the newcomers (Vezys et al., 2009).

REFERENCES

Anderson, C.F., Mosser, D.M., 2002. A novel phenotype for an activated macrophage: the type 2 activated macrophage. J. Leukocyte. Biol. 72, 101–106.

Brodovitch, A., Bongrand, P., Pierres, A., 2013. T lymphocytes sense antigens within seconds and make a decision within one minute. J. Immunol. 191, 2064–2071.

Carter, L.L., Dutton, R.W., 1995. Relative perforin- and Fas-mediated lysis in T1 and T2 CD8 effector populations. J. Immunol. 155, 1028–1031.

Chopp, L., Redmond, C., O'Shea, J.J., Schwartz, D.M., 2023. From the thymus to tissues and tumors: A review of T cell biology. J. Allergy Clin. Immunol. 151, 81–97.

Ciocca, M.L., Barnett, B.E., Burkhardt, J.K., Chang, J.T., Reiner, S.L., 2012. Cutting edge: asymmetric memory T cell division in response to rechallenge. J. Immunol. 188 (9), 4145–4148.

de la Roche, M., Asano, Y., Griffiths, G.M., 2016. Origins of the cytolytic synapse. Nat. Rev. Immunol. 16 (7), 421–432.

Dieckmann, N.M., Frazer, G.L., Asano, Y., Stinchcombe, J.C., Griffiths, G.M., 2016. The cytotoxic T lymphocyte immune synapse at a glance. J. Cell Sci. 129 (15), 2881–2886.

Dooms, H., Abbas, A.K., 2002. Life and death in effector T cells. Nat. Immunol. 9, 797–798.

Dotiwala, F., Santara, S.S., Binker-Cosen, A., Li, B., et al., 2017. Granzyme B disruots central metabolism and protein synthesis in bacteria to promote an immune cell death program. Cell 171, 1–13.

Endsley, J.J., Furrer, J.L., Endsley, M.A., et al., 2004. Characterization of bovine homologues of granulysin and NK-lysin. J. Immunol. 173, 2607–2614.

Gordon, S., Martinez, F.O., 2010. Alternative activation of macrophages: mechanism and functions. Immunity 32, 593–604.

Green, D.R., Victor, B., 2012. The pantheon of the fallen: why are there so many forms of cell death? Trends Cell Biol. 22, 555–556.

Guicciardi, M.E., Gores, G.J., 2009. Life and death by death receptors. FASEB J. 23, 1625–1637.

Han, S.-J., Zaretsky, A.G., Andrade-Oliveira, V., Collins, N., et al., 2017. White adipose tissue is a reservoir for memory T cells and promotes protective memory responses to infection. Immunity 47, 1–15.

Harris, J., Master, S.S., De Haro, S.A., et al., 2009. Th1-Th2 polarisation and autophagy in the control of intracellular mycobacteria by macrophages. Vet. Immunol. Immunopathol. 128, 37–43.

Hotchkiss, R.S., Strasser, A., McDunn, J.E., Swanson, P.E., 2009. Cell death. N. Engl. J. Med. 361, 1570–1583.

Krammer, P.H., 2000. CD95's deadly mission in the immune system. Nature 407, 789–795.

Law, R.H., Lukoyanova, N., Voskoboinik, I., et al., 2010. The structural basis for membrane binding and pore formation by lymphocyte perforin. Nature 468, 447–451.

Lowin, B., Hahne, M., Mattmann, C., Tschopp, J., 1994. Cytolytic T-cell cytotoxicity is mediated through perforin and Fas lytic pathways. Nature 370, 650–652.

Nolz, J.C., Hill, A.B., 2016. Strength in numbers: visualizing CTL-mediated killing in vivo. Immunity 44 (2), 207–208.

Pinkoski, M.J., Waterhouse, N.J., Heibein, J.A., et al., 2001. Granzyme B-mediated apoptosis proceeds predominantly through Bcl-2-inhibitable mitochondrial pathway. J. Biol. Chem. 276, 12060–12067.

Schenkel, J.M., Masopust, D., 2014. Tissue-resident memory T cells. Immunity 41 (6), 886–897.

Stenger, S., Hanson, D.A., Teitelbaum, R., et al., 1998. An antimicrobial activity of cytolytic T cells mediated by granulysin. Science 282, 121–125.

Stinchcombe, J.C., Bossi, G., Booth, S., Griffiths, G.M., 2001. The immunological synapse of CTL contains a secretory domain and membrane bridges. Immunity 15, 751–761.

Trost, M., English, L., Lemieux, S., et al., 2009. The phagosomal proteome in interferon-gamma-activated macrophages. Immunity 30, 143–154.

Vezys, V., Yates, A., Casey, K.A., et al., 2009. Memory CD8 T-cell compartment grows in size with immunological experience. Nature 457, 196–200.

Wang, F., Zhang, S., Jeon, R., Vuckovic, I., et al., 2018. Interferon gamma induces reversible metabolic reprogramming of M1 macrophages to sustain cell viability and pro-inflammatory activity. EbioMedicine 30, 303–316.

Weng, N.P., Araki, Y., Subedi, K., 2012. The molecular basis of the memory T cell response: differential gene expression and its epigenetic regulation. Nat. Rev. Immunol. 12 (4), 306–315.

Yu, P., Zhang, X., Liu, N., Tang, L., et al., 2021. Pyroptosis: mechanisms and diseases. Signal Transduction and Targeted Therapy. https://doi.org/10.1038/s41392-021-00507-5

Innate Lymphoid Cells

The structure of lymphocytes reveals few clues as to their functions. The two major cell types involved in adaptive immunity, the T and B cells, as described in previous chapters, employ millions of highly diverse, randomly generated, antigen receptors. T and B cells, however, require time to develop in sufficient numbers to affect the outcome of an infection. They also undergo selection to ensure that cells with self-reactive receptors are eliminated before they can cause damage.

Some lymphocytes, however, have a different role. They serve as environmental sensors and defenders of body surfaces. As such they interact with the microbiota and are able to respond to foreign antigens or abnormal cells immediately they are produced. These innate lymphoid cells (ILCs) are critical components of the body's defenses. ILCs fall into two functional groups (Fig. 20.1). One group serves primarily as helper cells. They regulate immune responses to the intestinal microbiota and play important roles in allergic diseases, autoimmunity, and obesity. The second group consists of cytotoxic cells. They serve as a first line of defense against viruses, some intracellular bacteria, fungi, and parasitic worms. They eliminate stressed or damaged cells. Some also play a major role in defense against tumors.

INNATE HELPER CELLS

Innate helper cells perform functions that were once thought to be performed only by helper T cells. Thus, there are innate counterparts of Th2 cells, Th22 cells, and Th17 cells. Each innate cell population is characterized by their cell-surface antigens, by the signals that trigger their production, by their transcription factors as well as by their products and their functions. ILCs play an important role in the very early stages of antimicrobial immune responses. They also contribute to tissue repair and defense and the maintenance of epithelial integrity (Colonna, 2018). ILCs are classified into three groups: Group 1 that defends against viruses, intracellular bacteria, and parasites; Group 2 that defends against helminths; and Group 3 that promotes immunity to intracellular bacteria (Artis and Spits, 2015).

Group 1 Innate Lymphoid Cells

Group 1 ILCs are located under body surfaces such as the intestinal mucosa where they are scattered through the lamina propria. They develop from lymphoid stem cells through the use of the transcription factor T-bet. Group 1 ILCs produce large amounts of Th1-associated cytokines such as interferon-γ (IFN-γ) and tumor necrosis factor–α (TNF-α) in response to activation by IL-12, -15, and -18 from dendritic cells (cDC1 cells) (Fig. 20.2). As a result, they can activate macrophages. They differ from NK cells in that they do not produce perforins and so are not cytotoxic. ILC1 cells play an essential role in the defense against viruses, intracellular bacteria and protozoa, and some cancers through their production of IFN-γ and TNF-α. As a result, they also antagonize type 2 responses.

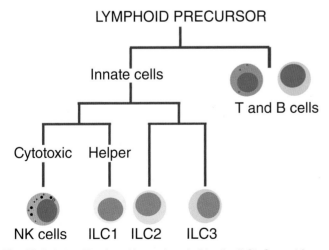

Fig. 20.1 A classification of innate lymphoid cells. *ILC1,* Group 1 innate lymphoid cells; *NK cell,* natural killer cell.

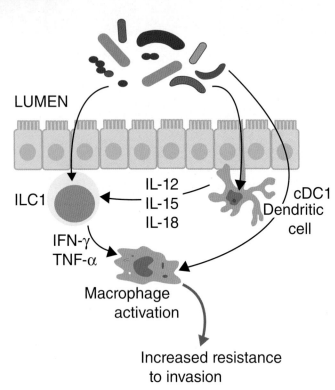

Fig. 20.2 The role of group 1 innate lymphoid cells (ILC1). Located in the intestine, they are activated by interleukin-12 (IL-12) generated by dendritic cells. They respond by producing type 1 cytokines and activating macrophages. They can be considered the functional partners of Th1 cells. *cDC1*, Classical type 1 dendritic cells; *DCs*, dendritic cells; *IFN-γ*, interferon-γ; *TNF-α*, tumor necrosis factor–α.

ILC1 cells can be converted into ILC3 cells by exposure to IL-23, IL-1β, and retinoic acid. Conversely, ILC3 cells may turn into ILC1 cells under the influence of IL-12, IL-15, and IL-18. NK cells are closely related to group 1 ILCs since they too produce IFN-γ and rely on T-bet for gene transcription. NK cells can be converted to ILC1 cells by exposure to TGF-β.

Group 2 Innate Lymphoid Cells

Group 2 ILCs are a diverse cell type found in the lung, skin, bone marrow, liver, mesenteric fat, and the small intestine (Splits and Mjosberg, 2022). They arise from lymphoid stem cells through the use of two unique transcription factors, GATA-binding protein-3 and retinoic acid receptor-related orphan receptor-α (ROR-α). ILC2s produce large amounts of the Th2-associated cytokines IL-5 and IL-13 and smaller amounts of IL-4 and IL-9 in response to thymic stromal lymphopoietin (TSLP), IL-25, and IL-33 produced by epithelial cells (Fig. 20.3). ILC2 cells are required for the development of early innate immunity to parasitic helminths (ILC2s are the major source of IL-13 during helminth infections) as well as regulating some type 2 inflammatory responses such as asthma and allergic diseases (see Chapter 30). They maintain the commensal stability of the parasitic mite, *Demodex folliculorum* within the skin and their loss may result in the development of demodectic mange (Box 20.1). ILC2s play a key role in regulating type 2 immunity by acting on macrophages, mast cells, and eosinophils. Thus, they control eosinophil production and so can induce an eosinophila. They also induce mucus production by goblet cells, alternative activation of macrophages, and promote tissue repair (Jarick et al., 2022). ILC2s can be readily converted into ILC1s by IL-12, and this can be reversed by IL-4 (Belz, 2016).

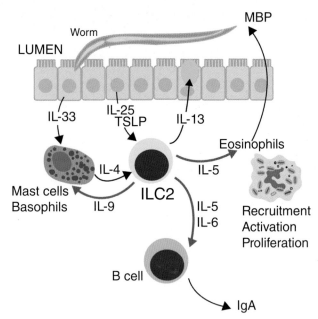

Fig. 20.3 The role of group 2 innate lymphoid cells. Activated by the presence of intestinal helminths, and mast cell products, they generate type 2 cytokines and hence stimulate both eosinophil and Immunoglobin A (IgA) production. They can be considered functional partners of Th2 cells. *IL-6*, Interleukin-6; *TSLP*, thymic stromal lymphopoietin.

BOX 20.1   Group 2 Innate Lymphoid Cells (ILC2) Cells and Demodex Mites

Demodex mites (*D. folliculorum*) are common commensal ectoparasites that live within mammalian hair follicles. Their presence is normally asymptomatic, but occasionally, they cause demodectic mange as a consequence of immunodeficiency, malnutrition, or aging. It appears that ILC2 cells are essential for the control of Demodex populations and the maintenance of stable commensalism. In the absence of ILC2 cells, the mites can trigger aberrant inflammation characterized by increased epithelial proliferation, decreased repair processes resulting in a loss of skin barrier function, increased transepidermal water loss, and hair follicle exhaustion. This control is normally mediated through the production of IL-13 by the ILC2 cells. IL-13 from ILC2s is coupled to the hair cycle and so restrains both stem cell proliferation and hair follicle regrowth. In its absence, manage results.

Ricardo-Gonzalez, R.R., Kotas, M.E., O'Leary, C.E., Singh, K., et al., 2022. Innate type 2 immunity controls hair follicle commensalism by *Demodex* mites. Immunity 55, 1–18.

Group 3 Innate Lymphoid Cells

Group 3 ILCs are primarily involved in the defense of body surfaces. They are found in the mucosa of the gastrointestinal tract (lamina propria, tonsils, Peyer's patches, and appendix) as well as in the lungs and skin. They use RORγt as their transcription factor and their maintenance and function depend on signals from the aryl hydrocarbon receptor (Box 22.1).

ILC3s produce IL-17 and IL-22 in response to stimulation by TSLP and IL-23 and thus resemble Th17 cells in their cytokine profile (Fig. 20.4). They play a central role in immunity on mucosal surfaces by resisting extracellular bacteria and fungi. They do this by producing IL-22. On exposure to IL-22, enterocytes produce antimicrobial

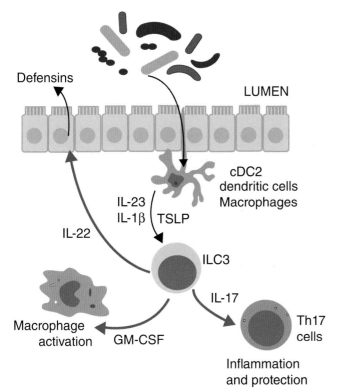

Fig. 20.4 The functions of group 3 innate lymphoid cells. Microbial products stimulate classical type 2 dendritic cells (cDC2) cells to produce interleukin (IL)-23 and IL-1β. Activated by these cytokines they release IL-23, IL-17, and granulocyte-macrophage colony-stimulating factor (GM-CSF). This causes inflammation, macrophage activation, and the production of defensins. *TSLP,* Thymic stromal lymphopoietin.

BOX 20.2 Are Plasmacytoid Dendritic Cells Really Innate Lymphocytes?

As described in Chapter 11, plasmacytoid dendritic cells have a lymphoid origin in contrast to conventional DCs that have a myeloid origin. They also have very different properties from conventional DCs. They are potent interferon producers so it has been suggested that should be categorized as a subfamily of ILCs.

From Zeigler-Heitbrock, L., Ohteki, T., Ginhoux, F. et al., 2023. Reclassifying plasmacytoid dendritic cells as innate lymphocytes. Nat. Rev. Immunol. 23, 1–2.

---

peptides that protect the intestinal epithelium. ILC3-derived IL-22 also inhibits T cell-mediated intestinal inflammation by suppressing those cells that respond to antigens from commensal bacteria. This IL-22 from ILC3s also inhibits the growth of segmented filamentous bacteria (see Chapter 22; Valle-Noguera et al., 2021).

Because they are required for the development of lymph nodes, Peyer's patches, and isolated lymphoid follicles, ILC3s are also called lymphoid tissue inducer cells. In this role, they regulate the differentiation of B cells. They activate dendritic cells (cDC2 cells) and so influence IgA class switching on surfaces. In the spleen, ILC3s express the B-cell growth factors BAFF, APRIL, and CD40L and stimulate IgM production (Lane et al., 2009; Withers, 2011).

There is also evidence for the presence of a population of innate regulatory cells in the intestines that control inflammatory responses through the release of IL-10 (Wang et al., 2017) (Box 20.2).

INNATE CYTOTOXIC CELLS

Natural Killer Cells

The first ILCs identified were called natural killer (NK) cells because they were able to kill foreign, virus-infected, and tumor cells without requiring prior activation. They are thus important defenders of the animal body. NK cells can be considered to be rapidly responding, cytotoxic ILC1s. In most mammals, NK cells are large, granular lymphocytes. In cattle, NK cells are large cells, but may not contain large cytoplasmic granules (Fig. 20.5). There is debate about NK cell morphology in the pig. Some investigators claim that they are large granular lymphocytes, whereas others believe that they are small lymphocytes without obvious cytoplasmic granules.

Origins and Location

NK cells are produced by stem cells located in the bone marrow and are found in peripheral blood, lymph nodes, spleen, lung, liver, and bone marrow but not in the thymus. They range from 2% of the lymphocytes in mouse spleen to 15% of the lymphocytes in human blood. Their characteristic cell surface phenotype is CD3$^-$, CD56$^+$, and NKp46$^+$. However, because they express many different combinations of inhibitory and activating receptors and reside in many different tissues, the NK cell population is highly diverse, and it has been estimated that there may be as many as 30,000 distinct NK cell phenotypes in any given individual (Freud et al., 2017). Much of this diversity is a result of the random expression of different MHC receptors.

Target Cell Recognition

NK cells do not make the enormous diversity of antigen receptors employed by T and B cells. Instead, they use two types of receptors to distinguish normal from abnormal cells. One type monitors the expression of MHC class I antigens by target cells; the other detects "stress" molecules on unhealthy cells such as tumors or infected cells.

NK cells thus recognize abnormal cells using two different strategies. One is a "missing-self" strategy by which NK receptors bind MHC class I molecules expressed on healthy cells, and as a result, this inhibits NK cell killing (Fig. 20.6). If, however, a cell fails to express MHC class I, then inhibitory signals are not generated, and the cell will be killed. This occurs, for example, when a virus suppresses cellular MHC class I

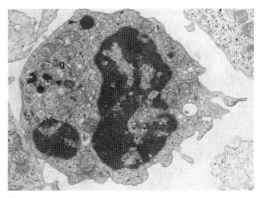

Fig. 20.5 A transmission electron micrograph of a human natural killer cell. The nucleus is indented and rich in chromatic. The cytoplasm is abundant and contains many granules. Numerous mitochondria, centrioles, and a Golgi are visible. Original magnification ×17,000. From Carpen, O., Virtanen, I., Saksela, E., 1982. Ultrastructure of human natural killer cells: nature of the cytolytic contacts in relation to cellular secretion. J. Immunol. 128, 2691.

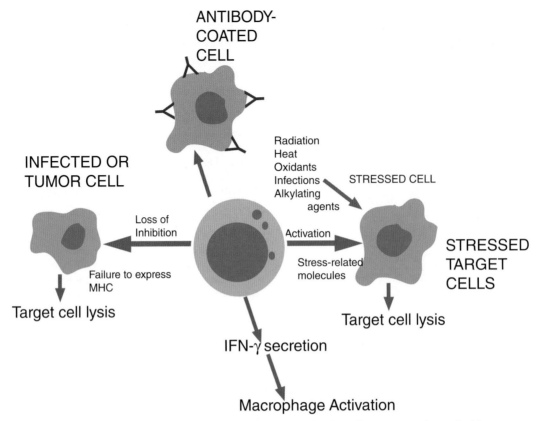

Fig. 20.6 The activities of natural killer cells. They kill stressed cells, cells not expressing major histocompatibility complex class I, and antibody-coated targets. By releasing interferon-γ (IFN-γ) they also activate macrophages. *MHC,* Major histocompatibility complex.

expression to avoid destruction by cytotoxic T cells. Likewise, tumor cells that fail to express MHC class I are also killed by NK cells.

The second NK cell strategy employs receptors that recognize stress-induced proteins on cells. When the NK cells detect these stress proteins, an activating signal is generated, and the NK cells kill the stressed cells (Fig. 20.7). Cells infected by viruses and intracellular bacteria, as well as some cancer cells express these stress proteins (Vivier et al., 2008).

MHC-Binding Receptors

The NK cell receptors for MHC class I proteins on target cells differ between species. Thus killer cell immunoglobulin (Ig)-like receptor (KIR) family members are expressed by NK cells in most mammals including humans and cattle. The second NK receptor family consists of C-type lectins, employed by rodents and horses only. The third type of receptor family, called NKG2D, is expressed on NK cells in dogs, rodents, and primates and recognizes proteins expressed by stressed cells. All three receptor families contain many members and include both inhibitory and activating receptors (Fig. 20.8). Other important NK cell receptors include CD2, CD16 (FcγRIII), CD178 (CD95L or Fas ligand), CD40L (CD154), toll-like receptors (TLR3 and TLR9), and leukocyte function–associated antigen-1 (Fig. 20.9). NK cells do not express conventional antigen receptors such as BCRs or TCRs, nor do they express a CD3 complex (see Chapter 13).

The Killer Immunoglobulin-Like Receptor Family

On the NK cells of primates, and cattle, the MHC receptors belong to a family of proteins called killer immunoglobulin-like receptors (KIR or CD158). These receptors, unlike T or B cell receptors, recognize conserved

amino acids located outside the MHC antigen-binding pocket. KIRs may be either inhibitory or stimulatory but inhibitory receptors predominate. As a result, when these inhibitory KIRs bind to MHC class I molecules on a target cell, cytotoxicity is inhibited, and healthy cells are not destroyed. On the other hand, if the target cell fails to express MHC and the inhibitory KIRs are not activated, then the target cell will be killed. Other members of the KIR family may stimulate NK cell cytotoxicity, but these receptors tend to have low binding affinities compared to the inhibitory receptors, so this contributes to the dominance of inhibition.

The human *KIR* gene locus is extremely polymorphic. Indeed, allelic polymorphism is so extensive in this locus that it is difficult to find unrelated individuals with identical *KIR* haplotypes. *KIR* gene polymorphism affects the MHC class I binding sites of these receptors. As a result, it determines their binding specificity. *KIR* gene expression patterns also vary clonally, so that individual NK cells can express random combinations of KIR receptors. This extreme diversity at the primate KIR locus results from selection pressure analogous to that seen in MHC loci. In other words, resistance to specific infections conferred by the KIR locus will depend on an animal's haplotype.

Although primate KIR genes vary in their number and diversity, four are present in virtually all haplotypes and are called framework loci. The total number of *KIR* genes expressed by a single individual ranges between 7 and 12, depending on the presence or absence of activating KIR loci. Other members of the KIR family include the leukocyte Ig-like receptors (LILRs) and NCR1 (NKp46, CD335). NCR1 (natural cytotoxicity triggering receptor 1) is only expressed on NK cells, while the LILRs are expressed on other leukocytes.

NORMAL CELL

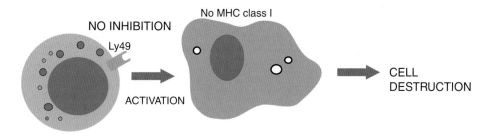

ABNORMAL CELL

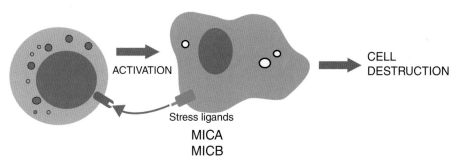

STRESSED CELL

Fig. 20.7 The activation of natural killer (NK) cells is triggered by two situations. Target cells may fail to express major histocompatibility complex (MHC) class I molecules. As a result, NK cells lose their inhibitions about attacking such cells. Alternatively, NK cells may be activated by the expression of stress-related proteins on target cells. *MICA*, Major histocompatibility complex, class I chain-related A; *MICB*, major histocompatibility complex, class I chain-related B.

C-Type Lectin Receptors

In rodents and horses, in contrast to humans and cattle, the predominant NK cell MHC-binding receptors are C-type lectins that belong to the Ly49 family of glycoproteins. They have the same function as KIR receptors in that they bind MHC class I molecules and are exceptionally polymorphic. There are at least 23 members (Ly49A to Ly49W) in this family of mice. All are homodimeric type II transmembrane C-type lectins. Ly49 haplotypes also contain variable numbers of inhibitory and activating receptors, some of which can recognize MHC class I molecules. Horses and donkeys have at least five highly conserved Ly49 genes. Unlike mice and horses, humans, pigs, dogs, cats, and cattle possess only a single Ly49-like gene. This is a pseudogene in humans but may be functional in cattle.

NKG2 Receptors

The third family of MHC-binding receptors on NK cells consists of C-type lectins that belong to the NKG2 receptor system. They are linked to CD94 to form heterodimers. NKG2D receptors bind to nonclassical MHC class I proteins produced by stressed cells. The most important of their ligands are two polymorphic MHC class I-like molecules called MIC-A (*m*ajor histocompatibility complex, class *I* chain-related *A*) and MIC-B coded for by MHC class I genes (see Chapter 12). Unlike conventional class I molecules, these do not bind antigenic peptides. While minimally expressed on normal, healthy cells MIC-A and MIC-B are expressed in large amounts by stressed cells. These stresses may include DNA damage due to ionizing radiation or alkylating agents, heat shock, and oxidative stress. MIC-A and MIC-B are overexpressed in tumor cells and virus-infected cells. When these ligands bind to NKG2D, they override the inhibitory effects of conventional MHC class I molecules and trigger NK cytotoxicity. NKG2D is also expressed on activated γ/δ and α/β T cells, suggesting that they too have a role in innate immunity. It may be that the combination of γ/δ T cells and NK cells kills tumors on body surfaces, whereas a combination of α/β T cells and NK cells is most effective within the body (Govaerts and Goddeeris, 2001).

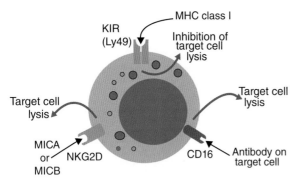

Fig. 20.8 The three major receptor types found on natural killer (NK) cells. Killer immunoglobulin-like receptors (KIRs) in most mammals and Ly49 in mice and horses recognize major histocompatibility complex (MHC) class I molecules and suppress NK cytotoxicity. NKG2D is a receptor for molecules such as major histocompatibility complex, class I chain-related A (MICA) and major histocompatibility complex, class I chain-related B (MICB). These molecules are commonly expressed on stressed, virus-infected, or tumor cells. CD16 binds immunoglobulins and triggers target cell death by antibody-dependent cellular cytotoxicity.

Fc Receptors

NK cells can also recognize and kill target cells using an antibody-dependent pathway employing the Ig receptor, CD16 (FcγRIII). CD16 is a 38 kDa transmembrane protein linked to either the γ chain of FcγRI (in macrophages) or to the zeta chain of CD3 (in NK cells). When antibodies bind to target cells, the bound antibody links to NK cell CD16, triggers cytotoxicity, and the target cells are killed. NK cells can spontaneously release their CD16 so that the NK cell can detach from an antibody-coated target after it has delivered its lethal hit.

Effector Mechanisms

In addition to be potently cytotoxic, NK cells are major producers of cytokines, especially IFN-γ and TNF-α (Mace, 2023). NK cell activities are also regulated by cytokines. For example, IL-2 and IL-4 enhance their cytotoxicity, whereas IL-3 promotes NK survival. Although NK cells are active in nonimmune animals, virus infections or interferon inducers enhance their activity (Fig. 20.10). When macrophages phagocytose invading organisms and produce TNF-α and IL-12, these cytokines then induce IFN-γ production by NK cells. The IFN-γ enhances NK activity further by promoting the rapid differentiation of pre-NK cells.

NK cells can act as "serial killers," and a single NK cell can thus kill multiple targets. Once activated, NK cells kill target cells through either the perforin/granulysin/NK-lysin pathway or through contact-dependent death receptors. These include Fas-Fas ligand (CD95L), and TRAIL-R1/R2 on target cells (Chen et al., 2015). Fully functional NK cell granules are stored in resting NK cells (in contrast to cytotoxic T cells, which only produce theirs on demand). Once an NK cell encounters a target cell, a synapse forms at the contact site. Activating KIRs

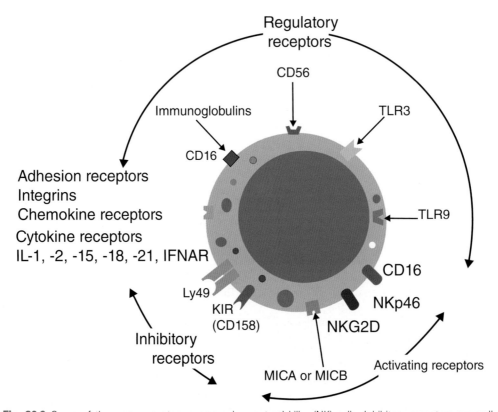

Fig. 20.9 Some of the many receptors expressed on natural killer (NK) cells. Inhibitory receptors generally predominate in healthy situations. Stimulatory receptors are activated by cancer cells and virus-infected cells. *IL-1*, Interleukin-1; *KIR*, killer inhibitory receptors; *MICA*, major histocompatibility complex, class I chain-related A; *MICB*, major histocompatibility complex, class I chain-related B; *TLR3*, toll-like receptor 3.

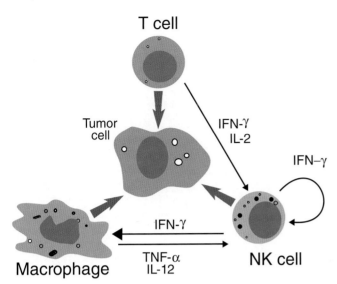

Fig. 20.10 The interactions between natural killer (NK) cells, macrophages, T cells, and abnormal cells. Interferon-γ (IFN-γ) is a potent stimulant of both NK cells and macrophages. Macrophages stimulate NK cell activities with tumor necrosis factor–α (TNF-α) and interleukin-12 (IL-12).

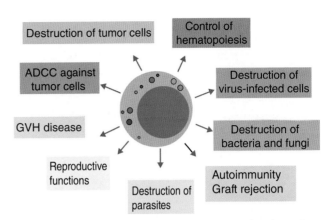

Fig. 20.11 A schematic diagram showing the many functions of natural killer cells. *ADCC*, Antibody-dependent cellular cytotoxicity; *GVH*, graft-versus-host.

induce MHC molecules to form a ring around a cluster of adhesion molecules. At the center of the synapse, there is a cSMAC through which the NK cell granule contents can pass. Receptors and signaling molecules also segregate in the cSMAC, whereas integrins and talin accumulate in the pSMAC. Inhibitory KIRs, in contrast, prevent the localization of lipid rafts to the immune synapse (Orange, 2008).

Perforins, granulysin, and NK-lysin are found in NK cell granules, and their expression is increased by exposure to IL-2 and IL-12. NK cell perforin is a protein of 70–72 kDa (slightly larger than that produced by T cells). It produces small (5–7 nm dia) channels in target cell surfaces. Presumably, granzymes are injected into the target cells through the perforin channels.

Functions

Unlike T and B cells that circulate as resting cells and so require several days to become fully activated, NK cells are "on call" and can be rapidly activated by IFNs released from virus-infected cells or by IL-12 from stimulated macrophages. As a result, NK cells promptly attack tumors and virus-infected cells. They participate in innate defenses long before antigen-specific primary adaptive responses can be generated (Box 19.2). Because they produce numerous cytokines and chemokines, they also modulate other aspects of the immune system.

NK cells kill some tumor cells, foreign cells, and virus-infected cells (Fig. 20.11). Thus they are active against herpesviruses, influenza, and poxviruses. Some Ly49 molecules on mouse NK cells can also recognize viruses directly so that, for example, they can kill cytomegalovirus-infected cells.

NK cells can also destroy some cultured tumor cells, and there is a positive correlation between this activity in vitro and resistance to tumor cells in vivo. Experimentally, it is possible to increase resistance to tumor growth in vivo by passive transfer of NK cells from a resistant animal. NK cells destroy human leukemia, myeloma, and some sarcoma and carcinoma cells in vitro, and this activity is enhanced by IFN-γ. NK cells can also invade small primary mouse tumors. Some carcinogenic agents and low doses of radiation inhibit NK activity. Stressors such as surgery may also depress NK activity and so promote

tumor growth. NK cells also play an important role in the maintenance of pregnancy (Chapter 35).

NK cells can kill bacteria, fungi, and parasites in addition to the abnormal cells described above. Thus, NK cells are cytotoxic for fungi such as Cryptococcus or Aspergillus. This is mediated by secreted perforins. It appears that NK cells bind bacteria through cell surface receptors such as NKp46 and NKG2D. Their perforins and granzymes can kill bacteria such as *Mycobacterium tuberculosis, Pseudomonas aeruginosa, E. coli, Staph aureus*, and *Listeria monocytogenes* (Mody et al., 2019). The protease granzyme B can activate a cell death program in many bacteria by cleaving vital conserved biosynthetic and metabolic enzymes. As a result, it disrupts bacterial protein synthesis, folding, and degradation. Because it destroys so many proteins, bacteria are unlikely to develop resistance to NK cell attack (Dotiwala et al., 2017).

Trained Natural Killer Cells

NK cells increase in numbers in response to stimulation and are removed once invaders have been eliminated. Some may, however, persist, develop a "memory" and mount a form of secondary response to some antigens (Netea et al., 2016). For example, mouse NK cells bearing a KIR specific for cytomegalovirus can expand their numbers in response to viral antigen. These cells can persist in both lymphoid and nonlymphoid tissues for several months. They can also be reactivated on reexposure to the viral antigen. Adoptive transfer of these reactivated NK cells leads to a rapid expansion of their numbers and protective immunity to cytomegalovirus. NK cells, in contrast to T and B cells, employ multiple activating receptors with different specificities (Moorlag et al., 2018). Thus an NK cell initially activated through one receptor may be reactivated through a different receptor. For example, NK cells initially activated through Ly49 may be reactivated through NKG2D. This NK "memory" response could be more accurately described as training rather than memory (Hu et al., 2022). There is also some evidence that this trained immunity may be vertically transmitted (Katzmarski et al., 2021).

Innate immune memory is not restricted to NK cells. It has also been demonstrated in monocytes. In vivo, treatment with BCG or beta-glucans can act on hematopoietic stem cells through GM-CSF to induce persistent myelopoiesis following a secondary challenge through lipopolysaccharide or infection. In vitro, monocytes can be treated with a stimulant such as BCG vaccine. After several days of rest, they can be restimulated, and their production of cytokines and reactive oxygen species can be measured. Cells primed in this way showed enhanced stimulation after exposure to unrelated stimuli, as shown by

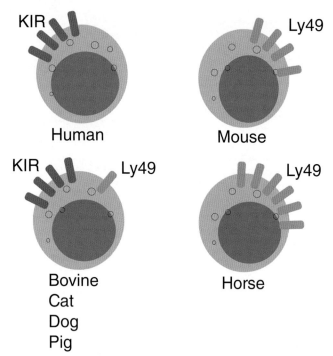

Fig. 20.12 The species difference between the major histocompatibility complex (MHC) class I receptors on natural killer cells. Humans possess a single, nonfunctional *Ly49* gene. Thus, they rely totally on killer inhibitory receptors (KIR) molecules, whereas mice rely totally on Ly49 molecules for the recognition of their MHC ligands. Most domestic species resemble humans except for the horse that resembles the mouse in its receptor usage.

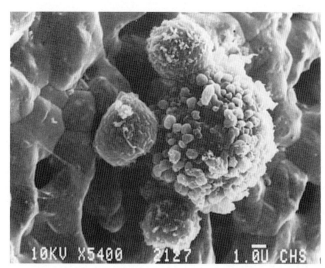

Fig. 20.13 A scanning electron micrograph of natural killer cells from a pig (small round cells) attached to a target cell (a human tumor cell). Original magnification ×5400. From Yang, W.C., Schultz, R.D., Spano, J.S., 1987. Isolation and characterization of porcine natural killer [NK] cells. Vet. Immunol. Immunopathol. 14, 345–356.

increased production of reactive oxygen species. This trained immunity is dependent on epigenetic remodeling and rewiring of cellular metabolic pathways, resulting in a persistent inflammatory phenotype (Bekkering et al., 2018).

Species Differences

NK cell expression of KIR and Ly49 receptors is species-specific and mutually exclusive. A species may use either a diverse *Ly49* or a diverse *KIR* gene family, but not both. For example, humans have multiple polymorphic *KIR* genes but only a single, nonfunctional *Ly49* gene. Likewise, cattle, dogs, cats, and pigs also possess multiple *KIR* genes and a single functional *Ly49* gene. The use of multiple *Ly49* genes by rodents and horses is not typical of mammals in general (Fig. 20.12).

Cattle

NK cells constitute about 3.5% of blood lymphocytes in young calves and about 2% in older cattle (Kulberg et al., 2004; Graham et al., 2009). They are found in the highest concentrations in the spleen, lymph nodes, and peripheral blood. Bovine NK cells can kill cells infected with parainfluenza-3, bovine leukemia virus, or bovine herpesvirus type 1. They generate resistance to mycobacteria by preventing its replication within macrophages. They play a role in resistance to the protozoan parasite *Neospora caninum* by producing IFN-γ that kills infected cells. Three NK subpopulations have been described. For example, most bovine NK cells express both CD2 and NCR1, but subpopulations may be CD2 or NCR1 negative. Other NK cell surface molecules include CD16, perforins, CD5, CD94, WC1, and MHC class II (Boysen and Storset, 2009).

Cattle, sheep, and goat NK cells use KIR proteins as their MHC class I receptors (Storset et al., 2003). Of 18 bovine *KIR* genes, 8 are

functional while 10 have been inactivated by point mutations. Cattle NK cells also express NKG2D. They possess one *Ly49* gene (McQueen et al., 2002). Thus cattle NK cells are heterogeneous and express many different receptors for MHC class I (Sanderson et al., 2014). The single bovine *Ly49* (*KLRA*) gene encodes three alleles, so cattle are the only species known to express both polymorphic Ly49 and KIR receptors (Dobromylskyj et al., 2009).

Cattle NK cells are activated by IL-2, IL-12, IL-15, IFN-α, and IFN-γ. Activation by IL-2 enables them to express CD25 and CD8 and lyse tumor cell lines (Endsley et al., 2006). Cattle also produce NK-lysin and uniquely, have four functional *NK-lysin* genes (As opposed to one in other mammals) (Chen et al., 2016).

Sheep

Sheep have CD16+ and CD14− NK cells in their bloodstream. More than 80% of these cells also express perforin and NCR1 and are cytotoxic for mouse and sheep cell targets. They produce IFN-γ in response to IL-12 stimulation (Ehlmouzi-Younes et al., 2010).

Pigs

In contrast to other mammals in which NK cells are characteristically large, granular lymphocytes, in pigs they appear to be small to medium-sized cells that largely lack granules. NK cell numbers vary greatly among individual pigs ranging from 1% to 24% of circulating lymphocytes. They are found in spleen and peripheral blood, but very few are found in lymph nodes or thymus (Fig. 20.13). Pig NK cells are NCR1, CD25, CD8a, and CD16 positive but subsets exist.

Only a single gene encoding KIR and one for Ly49 have been reported in pigs. The Ly49 (*KLRA1*) gene has a mutation in the codon for a highly conserved cysteine residue and may therefore be a pseudogene. Despite this apparent lack of NK cell receptor diversity, it does not appear to affect their numbers. Thus, it remains uncertain how pig NK cells recognize their targets.

Porcine NK cells are effectively cytolytic against pseudorabies, swine fever, and coronavirus-infected cells. Their activities are enhanced by IFN-γ and IL-2. IL-2, IL-12, and IL-18 act synergistically to promote pig NK cell expression of perforin and IFN-γ.

Horses

In marked contrast to the other nonrodent mammals, the domestic horse and other members of the family Equidae employ multiple killer cell lectin-like Ly49-related receptors as a result of the significant expansion of their *LY49* gene locus (Futas and Horin, 2013). They do not appear to possess any functional *KIR* genes. Genomic analysis has shown the presence of six highly conserved polymorphic *LY49* genes in horses, donkeys, and zebras (Takahashi et al., 2004). Equine peripheral blood NK cells constitute about 10% of total blood lymphocytes. They are active against equine herpesvirus-1-infected equine embryonic kidney and embryonic lung cells (Viveiros and Antcak, 1999).

Dogs

Dog NK cells are medium to large-sized lymphocytes with electron-dense cytoplasmic granules that contain granzyme B and perforin (Huang et al., 2008). They account for up to 15% of blood lymphocytes. They are CD4$^-$ and CD20$^-$ thus distinguishing them from T and B cells. These NK cells are CD3$^-$, granzyme B$^+$, CD45$^+$, and MHC class I$^+$ (Grondahl-Rosado et al., 2016). It is unclear which MHC receptors they use, since they express both KIR and NKG2D receptors on their surface. IL-15 and IL-21 stimulate their proliferation, receptor expression, and cytotoxic functions. They can lyse distemper-infected target cells as well as cancer cells from thyroid adenocarcinomas, melanomas, osteosarcomas, and mammary carcinomas (Michael et al., 2013).

Cats

Feline NK cells are large granular lymphocytes found in the blood and spleen. In general, cat NK cell numbers and properties are similar to those in other domestic mammals. However, unlike other species, 10%–30% of feline NK cells are CD11b$^+$ and selectin CD62L$^+$. They are active against feline target cells infected with feline leukemia virus, herpesvirus, or vaccinia virus.

Both dogs and cats have a single *Ly49* gene. The cat *Ly49* is functional, but the dog *Ly49* product lacks a conserved cysteine in its C-type lectin domain and may therefore be defective (Vermeulen et al., 2012).

Rabbits

Such evidence as is available suggests that rabbits either do not possess NK cells or possess an NK cell system that differs significantly from that in other species. Thus, the use of classical approaches in rabbit peripheral blood and lymph node cells has failed to detect either NK or natural cytotoxic cell activity or even ADCC under conditions where NK cells from other species were highly effective. Nor have any large granular lymphocytes, the typical NK cells, been seen in rabbit blood. That said, there is a single published report regarding the antitumor cell activity of rabbit NK cells. In this study, positive staining with antirabbit CD56 was the criterion used to identify and separate the NK cell population by cell sorting.

NATURAL KILLER T CELLS

Natural killer T cells (NKT cells) combine the properties of NK cells and T cells. They are innate-like T cells that express both NK cell markers and a TCR of limited diversity. There are two functionally distinct NKT cell subsets. Type I NKT cells are T cells that express a TCR consisting of an invariant α-chain associated with diverse β-chains. These T cells respond to lipid, lipopeptide, and glycolipid antigens presented by the MHC class I-like molecule CD1. CD1 proteins are nonpolymorphic MHC molecules found on antigen-presenting cells (Fig. 20.14). The CD1-lipid presentation system allows the immune system to respond to lipid antigens. Some CD1 proteins present lipid antigens to conventional T cells while others present lipids to NKT cells (Zajonc, 2016). Type I NKT cells can

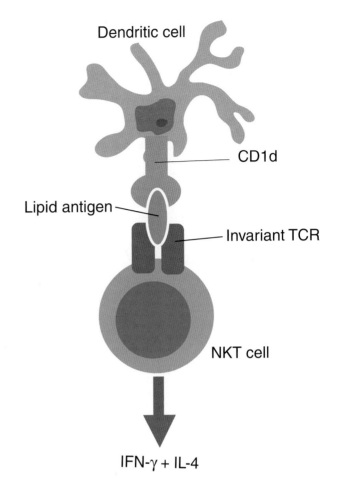

Fig. 20.14 Type I natural killer T cells (NKT) cells recognize and respond to lipid antigens by using CD1d as an antigen-presenting molecule. *IFN-γ,* Interferon-γ; *IL-4,* interleukin-4; *TCR,* T-cell antigen receptor.

promote immunity in response to lipid antigens from infectious agents and tumor cells. They are found in the liver, spleen, blood, and especially in adipose tissue where they may contribute to obesity (Bentley et al., 2019). Most are found in the sinusoids of the liver.

In the absence of prior antigenic stimulation, NKT cells respond more rapidly than conventional T cells. They produce proinflammatory cytokines such as IFN-γ and TNF-α as well as antiinflammatory cytokines such as IL-4 and IL-10. As a result, they can modulate immunity in a broad spectrum of diseases. NKT cells trigger chemokine and cytokine release, enhance NK function, and promote dendritic cell maturation and B cell responses. NKT cells inhibit the development of Th17 cells and regulate IL-17 production. NKT cells secrete IL-12 that acts on neutrophils to decrease their production of IL-10. They play a role in allergies, antitumor immunity, autoimmunity, and antimicrobial immunity, especially to Mycobacteria. Thus they link the T-cell system with the innate NK cell system.

Type II NKT cells, in contrast, use diverse TCRs where both α- and β-chains contribute equally to lipid recognition. Their functions are predominantly antiinflammatory, and they recognize diverse hydrophobic antigens. The type II cells also suppress the type I cells, suggesting that they have an immunoregulatory role (Dhodapkar and Kumar, 2017).

Species Differences

Equine type 1 NKT cells can recognize lipid antigens presented by CD1 molecules. The presence of a functional CD1 system appears to be critical for horse health (Porcelli and Modlin, 1999). Equine T cells recognize the cell wall lipids of *Prescotella* (*Rhodococcus*) *equi* when they are bound to CD1. The equine genome contains 13 complete CD1 genes located on chromosome 5 (Dossa et al., 2014). Twelve of these CD1 molecules have been shown to be expressed on antigen-presenting cells, including monocytes, macrophages, and dendritic cells. Horse NKT cells can, therefore, recognize many different lipid antigens. It is possible that this unusually large number of CD1 molecules reflects their key role in protection against *P. equi*. Other cells that express CD1 include dendritic cells, Kupffer cells, endothelial cells, and hepatocytes.

Although horses clearly possess functional NKT cells as well as the largest and most diverse CD1 gene family, they also differ in some respects from other mammals. For example, while the synthetic lipid, α-galactosylceramide (α-GalCer), is a potent NKT cell stimulator in most species examined, it is not an immunostimulatory NKT cell agonist in the horse (Dossa et al., 2015).

Cattle possess 12 CD1 genes. Most of these are nonfunctional pseudogenes (Van Rhijn et al., 2006). However, α-GalCer immunization of cattle does not trigger an immune response against this glycolipid which raises the question as to whether bovine NKT cells are functional. Cattle do, however, possess a novel T cell subset that has features of both T and NK cells. Thus these cells express both NCR1 and CD3. They can be activated by either the NKR or TCR pathways and can kill *Theileria parva*–infected cells. Presumably, these are the functional equivalents of NKT cells in other species.

Pigs also possess functional *CD1* genes. In pigs, type I NKT cells use a T-cell receptor with an invariant α chain to recognize α-GalCer. Their production is enhanced by IL-2, -15, and -33 (Yang et al., 2019). Dogs also have 13 CD1 genes.

REFERENCES

Artis, D., Spits, H., 2015. The biology of innate lymphoid cells. Nature 517, 293–301.

Bekkering, S., Arts, R.J.W., Novakovic, B., et al., 2018. Metabolic induction of trained immunity through the mevalonate pathway. Cell 172, 135–146.

Belz, G.T., 2016. ILC2s masquerade as ILC1s to drive chronic disease. Nat. Immunol. 17, 611–612.

Bentley, E.G., Pugh, G., Gledhill, L.R., Flynn, R.J., 2019. An analysis of the immune compartment within bovine adipose tissue. Dev. Comp. Immunol. 100, 103411.

Boysen, P., Storset, A.K., 2009. Bovine natural killer cells. Vet. Immunol. Immunopathol. 130, 163–177.

Chen, J., Huddleston, J., Buckley, R.M., Malig, M., Lawhon, S.D., Skow, L.C., Lee, M.O., Eichler, E.E., Andersson, L., Womack, J.E., 2015. Bovine NK-lysin: copy number variation and functional diversification. Proc. Natl. Acad. Sci. U.S.A. 112, E7223–7229.

Chen, J., Yang, C., Tizioto, P.C., Huang, H., Lee, M.O., Payne, H.R., Lawhon, S.D., Schroeder, F., Taylor, J.F., Womack, J.E., 2016. Expression of the Bovine NK-Lysin gene family and activity against respiratory pathogens. PLoS One 11, e0158882.

Colonna, M., 2018. Innate lymphoid cells: diversity, plasticiity, and unique functions in immunity. Immunity 48, 1104–1117.

Dhodapkar, M.V., Kumar, V., 2017. Type II NKT cells and their emerging role in health and disease. J. Immunol. 198, 1015–1021.

Dobromylskyj, M.J., Connelley, T., Hammond, J.A., Ellis, S.A., 2009. Cattle Ly49 is polymorphic. Immunogenetics 61, 789–795.

Dossa, R.G., Alperin, D.C., Hines, M.T., Hines, S.A., 2014. The equine CD1 gene family is the largest and most diverse yet identified. Immunogenetics 66, 33–42.

Dossa, R.G., Alperin, D.C., Garzon, D., Mealey, R.H., et al., 2015. In contrast to other species, α-galactosylceramide (α-GalCer) is not an immunostimulatory NKT cell agonist in horses. Dev. Comp. Immunol. 49, 49–58.

Dotiwala, F., Santara, S.S., Binker-Cosen, A.A., Li, B., et al., 2017. Granzyme B disrupts central metabolism and protein synthesis in bacteria to promote an immune cell death program. Cell 171, 1125–1137.

Ehlmouzi-Younes, J., Boysen, P., Pende, D., et al., 2010. Ovine CD16+/CD14- blood lymphocytes present all the major characteristics of natural killer cells. Vet. Res. 31, 04.

Endsley, J.J., Endsley, M.A., Estes, D.M., 2006. Bovine natural killer cells acquire cytotoxic/effector activity following activation with IL-12/15 and reduce *Mycobacterium bovis* BCG in infected macrophages. J. Leukocyte Biol. 79, 71–79.

Freud, A.G., Mundy-Bosse, B.L., Yu, J., Caligiuri, M.A., 2017. The broad spectrum of human natural killer cell diversity. Immunity 47 (5), 820–833.

Futas, J., Horin, P., 2013. Natural killer cell receptor genes in the family *Equidae*: not only Ly49. PLOS One. https://doi.org/10.1371/journal.pone.0064736

Govaerts, M.M., Goddeeris, B.M., 2001. Homologues of natural killer cell receptors NKG2-D and NKR-P1 expressed in cattle. Vet. Immunol. Immunopathol. 80, 339–344.

Graham, E.M., Thom, M.L., Howard, C.J., et al., 2009. Natural killer cell number and phenotype in bovine peripheral blood is influenced by age. Vet. Immunol. Immunopathol. 132, 101–108.

Grondahl-Rosado, C., Boysen, P., Johansen, G.M., Brun-Hansen, H., Storset, A.K., 2016. NCR1 is an activating receptor expressed on a subset of canine NK cells. Vet. Immunol. Immunopathol. 177, 7–15.

Hu, S., Xiang, D., Zhang, L., Wang, s., et al., 2022. The mechanisms and cross-protection of trained innate immunity. Virology J. https://doi.org/10.1186/s12985-022-01937-5.

Huang, Y.-C., Hung, S.-W., Jan, T.-R., et al., 2008. CD5-low expression lymphocytes in canine peripheral blood show characteristics of natural killer cells. J. Leukoc. Biol. 84, 1501–1510.

Jarick, K.J., Topczewska, P.M., Jakob, M.O., Yano, H., et al., 2022. Non-redundant functions of group 2 innate lymphoid cells. Nature 611, 794–799.

Katzmarski, N., Dominguez-Andres, J., Cirovic, B., Renieris, G., et al., 2021. Transmission of trained immunity and heterologous resistance to infections across generations. Nature Immunol. 22 (11), 1382–1390.

Kulberg, S., Boysen, P., Storset, A.K., 2004. Reference values for relative numbers of natural killer cells in cattle blood. Dev. Comp. Immunol. 28, 941–948.

Lane, P.J.L., McConnell, F.M., Withers, D., Gaspal, F., et al., 2009. Lymphoid tissue inducer cells: bridges between the ancient innate and the modern adaptive immune systems. Nature Immunol. 2 (6), 472–477.

Mace, E.M., 2023. Human natural killer cells: form, function, and development. J. Allergy Clin. Immunol. 151, 371–385.

McQueen, K.L., Wilhelm, B.T., Harden, K.D., Mager, D.L., 2002. Evolution of NK receptors: a single Ly49 and multiple KIR genes in the cow. Eur. J. Immunol. 32, 810–817.

Michael, H.T., Ito, D., Mccullar, V., Zhang, B., Miller, J.S., Modiano, J.F., 2013. Isolation and characterization of canine natural killer cells. Vet. Immunol. Immunopathol. 155, 211–217.

Mody, C.H., Ogbomo, H., Xiang, R.F., Kyei, S.K., et al., 2019. Microbial killing by NK cells. J. Leukoc. Biol. 105, 1285–1296.

Moorlag, S., Roring, R.J., Joosten, L.A.B., Netea, M.G., 2018. The role of the interleukin-1 family in trained immunity. Immunol. Revs. 281, 28–39.

Netea, M.G., Joosten, L.A., Latz, E., Mills, K.H., et al., 2016. Trained immunity: a program of innate immune memory in health and disease. Science 352, aaf1098.

Orange, J.S., 2008. Formation and function of the lytic NK-cell immunological synapse. Nat. Rev. Immunol. 28, 713–725.

Porcelli, S.A., Modlin, R.L., 1999. The CD1 system: antigen-presenting molecules for T cell recognition of lipids and glycolipids. Annu. Rev. Immunol. 17, 297–329.

Sanderson, N.D., Norman, P.J., Guethlein, L.A., Ellis, S.A., et al., 2014. Definition of the cattle killer cell Ig-like receptor gene family: comparison with aurochs and human counterparts. J. Immunol. 193, 6016–6030.

Splits, H., Mjosberg, J., 2022. Heterogeneity of type 2 innate lymphoid cells. Nature Rev. Immunol. 22, 701–712.

Storset, A.K., Slettedal, I.O., Williams, J.L., et al., 2003. Natural killer cell receptors in cattle: a bovine killer cell immunoglobulin-like receptor multigene family contains members with divergent signaling motifs. Eur. J. Immunol. 33, 980–990.

Takahashi, T., Yawata, M., Raudsepp, T., et al., 2004. Natural killer cell receptors in the horse: evidence for the existence of multiple transcribed LY49. Eur. J. Immunol. 34, 773–784.

Valle-Noguera, A., Ochoa-Ramos, A., Gomez-Sanchez, M.J., Cruz-Adalia, A., 2021. Type 3 innate lymphoid cells as regulators of the host-pathogen interaction. Front. Immunol. https://doi.org/10.3389/fimmu.2021.748851.

Van Rhijn, I., Koets, A.P., Im, J.S., et al., 2006. The bovine CD1 family contains group 1 CD1 proteins but no functional CD1d. J. Immunol. 176, 4888–4893.

Vermeulen, B.L., Devriendt, B., Olyslaegers, A., et al., 2012. Natural killer cells: frequency, phenotype and function in healthy cats. Vet. Immunol. Immunopathol. 150, 69–78.

Viveiros, M.M., Antczak, D.F., 1999. Characterization of equine natural killer and IL-2 stimulated lymphokine activated killer cell populations. Dev. Comp. Immunol. 23, 521–532.

Vivier, E., Tomasello, E., Baratin, M., et al., 2008. Functions of natural killer cells. Nat. Immunol. 9, 503–510.

Wang, S., Xia, P., Chen, Y., Qu, Y., et al., 2017. Regulatory innate lymphoid cells control innate intestinal inflammation. Cell 171, 201–216.

Withers, D.R., 2011. Lymphoid tissue Inducer cells. Curr. Biol. 21 (10), RR381–R382.

Yang, G., Artiaga, B.L., Lomelino, C.L., Jayaprakash, A.D., et al., 2019. Next generation sequencing of the pig ab TCR repertoire identifies the porcine invariant NKT cell receptor. J. Immunol. 202, 1981–1991.

Zajonc, D.M., 2016. The CD1 family: serving lipid antigens to T cells since the Mesozoic era. Immunogenetics 68 (8), 561–576.

21

Regulation of Adaptive Immunity

The adaptive immune system can recognize and respond to foreign invaders and can learn from the experience so that the body responds faster and more effectively when exposed to the invader a second time. There is, however, a risk associated with this—the risk of collateral damage. One of the reasons why the adaptive immune system is so complex is that much effort must be put into ensuring that lymphocytes will only attack invaders or abnormal cells and will ignore normal healthy cells and tissues. As might be anticipated, many different regulatory circuits act to minimize the chances of inappropriate or damaging responses. In addition, immune responses are regulated to ensure that they are appropriate with respect to both quality and quantity.

Since both T and B cells randomly generate antigen-binding receptors, it is clear that the initial production of self-reactive cells cannot be prevented. An animal cannot control the amino acid sequences and, hence, the binding specificity of these receptors. As a result, when first generated, as many as 50% of T cells and B cells may bind self-antigens. If autoimmunity is to be avoided, these lymphocytes must be destroyed.

TOLERANCE

Tolerance is the name given to the situation in which the immune system will not respond to a specific antigen. Tolerance is primarily directed against self-antigens from normal tissues. In 1948 two Australian immunologists, MacFarlane Burnet and Frank Fenner, recognized this need for self-tolerance and suggested that immature lymphocytes would become tolerant to an antigen if they first met it early in fetal life.

Support for this suggestion came from observations on chimeric calves. In 1945 Ray Owen noted that when cows are carrying twin calves, blood vessels in the two placentas commonly fuse. As a result, the blood of the twins intermingles freely, and bone marrow stem cells from one animal colonize the other. Each calf is born with a mixture of blood cells, some of its own and some originating from its twin. In dizygotic (nonidentical) twins, this is called a chimera. These "foreign" blood cells persist indefinitely because each chimeric calf is fully tolerant to the presence of its twin's cells (Fig. 21.1). Burnet and Fenner suggested that this could only happen because each calf

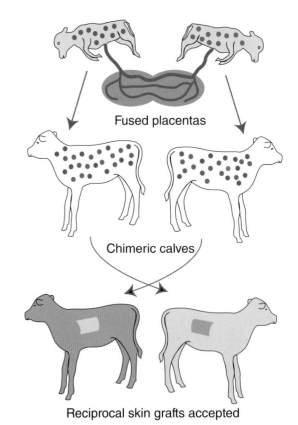

Fig. 21.1 Fusion of the placentas of dizygotic twin calves results in the development of calf chimeras. Hematopoietic stem cells from each animal colonize the bone marrow of the other. Each chimera is tolerant to its twin's cells and will accept a skin graft from its twin despite their genetic differences.

was exposed to the foreign cells early in fetal life at a time when lymphocytes become tolerant upon encountering antigens. Cells from an unrelated calf would be rejected normally if administered after birth. Thus, immune tolerance is not innate. It is established during fetal and postnatal development and relies on mechanisms that control lymphocyte development.

Subsequent studies have shown that self-tolerance is of two types, central and peripheral. In central tolerance, any self-reactive lymphocytes that develop within the thymus, bursa, or bone marrow are killed. In peripheral tolerance, mature lymphocytes that recognize self-antigens either die, are turned off, or are suppressed by Treg cells. By reconstituting lethally irradiated mice with T or B cells derived from normal or tolerant donors, tolerance can be shown to occur in both cell populations. However, their susceptibility to peripheral tolerance differs. T cells can be made tolerant rapidly and easily within 24 hours and remain in that state for more than 100 days (Fig. 21.2). In contrast, B cells develop tolerance in about 10 days and return to normal within 50 days.

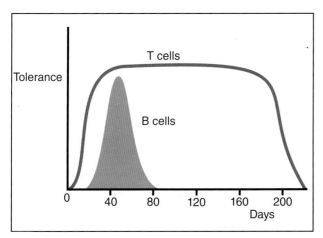

Fig. 21.2 The duration of tolerance in T cells and B cells. T cells are much more easily rendered tolerant than B cells. Once tolerant, they remain that way for much longer.

T-CELL TOLERANCE

Central T-Cell Tolerance

Developing T cells must undergo education in the thymus where they learn to discriminate between self and nonself antigens. Tolerance results when there are no functional T cells that can bind self-antigens (Fig. 21.3). (It should be pointed out here that an exception must be made for MHC molecules. T cells must be able to recognize them if they are to respond to foreign peptides.) Although lymphocytes can generate an enormous diversity of TCRs, far fewer receptors are actually used by mature T cells than might be anticipated. Several processes limit receptor diversity. First, the mechanisms used to generate TCRs inevitably result in the production of nonfunctional receptors. For example, two-thirds of possible gene arrangements will be out-of-frame. Cells with these nonfunctional TCRs die. As T cells mature within the thymus, positive selection ensures that the cells that can bind antigens survive. At this point, however, the cells whose receptors bind too strongly to self-antigens are killed (Fig. 21.4). The timing and extent of their apoptosis depend on the affinity of the TCR for a self-antigen. T cells that bind self-antigens strongly die earlier and more completely than weakly binding cells. Thus the T cells that eventually leave the thymus have been purged of dangerous, self-reactive cells. The survivors are both functional and safe.

This negative selection process is assisted by the expression of many different self-antigens in the thymus. Normally, each tissue possesses its own tissue-specific antigens. Thus "skin antigens" are usually restricted to the skin, whereas "liver antigens" are restricted to the liver, and so forth. However, the epithelial cells in the thymic medulla show uniquely "promiscuous" gene expression. Thymic epithelial cells use a transcription factor called the autoimmune regulator (AIRE), that promotes the expression of hundreds of nonthymic protein antigens (Anderson et al., 2002). Examples include insulin, thyroglobulin, and myelin basic protein. In this way, the thymic epithelial cells ensure that developing T cells are exposed to many normal tissue antigens and are eliminated if they respond too strongly. In addition, some normal tissue antigens may be taken up by macrophages and carried to the thymus. Immature T cells that respond to these antigens are also eliminated. However, this raises another question: What about self-antigens that are not expressed in, or do not enter, the thymus? Antigens from the

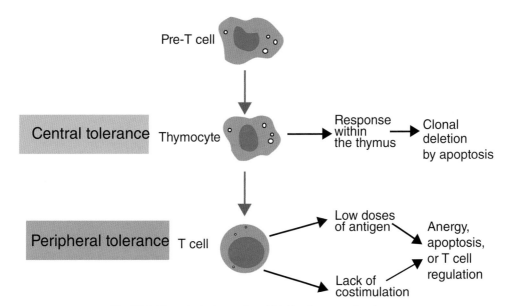

Fig. 21.3 The principal ways by which T cells are made tolerant.

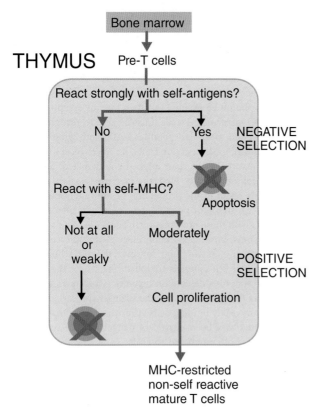

Fig. 21.4 How the thymus induces central T-cell tolerance by negative selection. Surviving T cells are unreactive to autoantigens yet can still respond to foreign antigenic peptides in association with Major histocompatibility complex (MHC), molecules as a result of positive selection.

eye, testis, or brain are not processed in this way, and as a result, central tolerance to these antigens does not develop. Mice genetically lacking the *aire* gene develop multiple autoimmune diseases (see Chapter 37; Passos et al., 2017).

An additional factor that determines thymocyte survival is the dose of antigen presented to the cells. If the amount of a specific antigen is high (as one might anticipate for a self-antigen), multiple TCRs will be occupied on each thymocyte and trigger apoptosis. In contrast, if the amount is low, this will occupy only a few TCRs, and the weak signal may result in positive selection and thymocyte proliferation (Ramsdell and Fowlkes, 1992).

These selection processes together ensure that T cells that respond strongly to self-antigens are eliminated. As a result, only the moderate-affinity clones survive and are available to recognize foreign antigens.

When the antigen receptors of a developing T cell bind to self-antigens, another strategy that prevents autoimmunity is receptor editing (see Chapter 37). Although cell maturation stops when a T cell leaves the thymus, its recombinase-activating genes (*RAG*) remain active, and as a result, V(D)J recombination continues. Consequently, their *TCR* genes continue to diversify, and these new receptors are expressed on the cell surface. This process is called receptor editing. If a cell successfully edits its receptors, its maturation can proceed. Failure to do so will result in its death. This is a potentially hazardous process since it may permit the development of self-reactive T cells that have not undergone selection within the thymus.

Peripheral T-Cell Tolerance

Low-affinity, self-reactive T cells survive the selection process and leave the thymus. Their responses must then be controlled by peripheral tolerance mechanisms. One form of peripheral tolerance is clonal anergy, the prolonged, antigen-specific suppression of T-cell function. Clonal anergy is triggered when T cells are exposed to an antigen in the absence of effective costimulation. As described previously, T cells normally require multiple costimulatory signals from several sources in order to respond to antigen. The binding of an antigen to a TCR is by itself insufficient to trigger a T-cell response. Indeed, occupation of the TCR in the absence of costimulation causes tolerance. For example, protein solutions normally contain some aggregated molecules. These aggregated molecules are readily taken up and processed by dendritic cells and thus are highly immunogenic. If a solution of such a protein, such as bovine γ-globulin, is ultracentrifuged so that all the aggregates are removed, then the aggregate-free solution will induce tolerance due to the absence of costimulation from APCs (Fig. 21.5; El Tanbouly and Noelle, 2021).

Binding to the TCR by an antigen in the absence of costimulation activates the tyrosine kinases and phospholipases of the T cell and raises its intracellular Ca^{2+}. This results in enhanced production of IκB that inhibits NF-κB. This, in turn, prevents the cell from making cytokines, especially IL-2. Tolerant Th1 cells produce less than 3% of normal IL-2 levels and much less IFN-γ and TNF-α. Once induced, this T-cell "anergy" can last for several weeks.

Triggering of T-cell responses normally requires prolonged interactions with antigen-presenting cells (APCs). Tolerance induction, on the other hand, is characterized by relatively short interactive episodes. Thus, a key difference between T-cell activation and anergy may simply be the duration of their encounter with APCs (Katzman et al., 2010).

Very high doses of an antigen can induce a form of clonal anergy called immune paralysis (Fig. 21.6). The high doses of the antigen probably bypass APCs, reach the Th cell receptors directly, and, in the absence of costimulation, trigger paralysis.

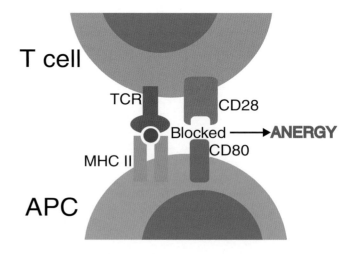

Fig. 21.5 Peripheral tolerance through clonal anergy will develop if a T-cell antigen receptor (TCR) is stimulated by antigen in the absence of simultaneous costimulation through the CD28/CD80 or CD28/CD86 pathway. *APC*, Antigen-presenting cell; *MHC*, major histocompatibility complex.

B-CELL TOLERANCE

Unlike the TCR repertoire, B-cell antibody diversity is generated in two phases. The first phase involves V(D)J rearrangement or gene conversion within the primary lymphoid organs; the second phase involves random somatic mutation in secondary lymphoid organs. B cells, therefore, have several opportunities to generate receptors that can bind self-antigens. It has been estimated that 55%–75% of early immature B cells may have self-reactive receptors, so suppression of these B cells must begin at an early stage in an animal's development.

Immature B cells in the bone marrow can be made tolerant once they have rearranged their V-region genes and are committed to express complete immunoglobulin M (IgM) molecules. When these immature cells encounter and bind antigen, the BCR transmits a signal that arrests cell development, blocks synapse formation, and triggers apoptosis. An immature B-cell population can be rendered tolerant by one-millionth of the dose of an antigen required to make mature B cells

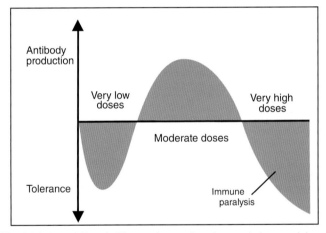

Fig. 21.6 The ability of different doses of antigen to induce peripheral tolerance. Both very low and very high doses can induce tolerance. Moderate doses, in contrast, induce an immune response.

tolerant. Immature B cells may also undergo receptor editing. If receptor editing fails to prevent self-reactivity, the B cell will die.

Peripheral B-cell tolerance is induced by multiple mechanisms including apoptosis, clonal anergy, clonal exhaustion, and blockage of BCRs. Because BCRs undergo random somatic mutation within germinal centers, self-reactive B cells will develop in secondary lymphoid organs. These cells will not, however, make autoantibodies if APCs and helper T cells are absent or if Treg cells are active (Fig. 21.7). This is not, however, a foolproof method of preventing self-reactivity. In the absence of T-cell help, B cells may be activated by PAMPs such as LPS, flagellins, or unmethylated CpG DNA acting through TLRs. B cells may also be activated by either cross-reacting epitopes or by foreign carrier molecules stimulating nontolerant helper T cells (see Fig. 37.4).

As with T cells, B-cell anergy occurs when the B cells encounter antigens in the absence of costimulation. B cells are difficult to maintain in a tolerant state, however, and will reactivate rapidly unless steps are taken to maintain tolerance. Self-reactive B cells must also bind to a critical threshold of self-antigen to be made tolerant. This results in selective silencing of high-affinity B cells. Presumably, the failure of low-affinity antiself B cells to become tolerant poses little threat of autoimmune disease because the low-affinity antibodies they produce will not cause tissue damage.

B cells subjected to repeated exhaustive antigenic stimulation may differentiate into short-lived plasma cells. If all B cells develop into such plasma cells, no memory B cells will remain to respond to antigen, and tolerance will result. Some polymeric antigens such as pneumococcal polysaccharide can also bind irreversibly to BCRs, freezing the B-cell membrane and blocking any further responses by these cells. The B cells recover once the antigen is removed.

DURATION OF TOLERANCE

The duration of tolerance depends on antigen persistence and on the ability of the bone marrow to generate fresh T or B cells. Once an antigen is completely eliminated, tolerance fades. If, however, the antigen is persistent, such as occurs with an animal's own self-antigens, tolerance also persists. In the continued presence of an antigen, newly

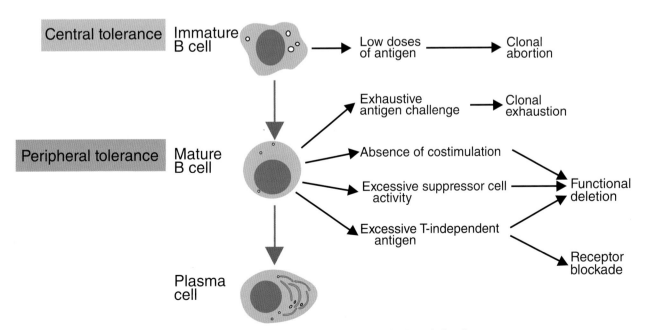

Fig. 21.7 Central and peripheral tolerance mechanisms in B cells.

formed antigen-sensitive cells will undergo apoptosis as soon as their receptors bind the self-antigen. Treatment that promotes bone marrow activity, such as low-dose X-irradiation, hastens the fading of tolerance, whereas immunosuppressive drug treatment has the opposite effect.

CONTROL OF IMMUNE RESPONSES

Tolerance is not the only mechanism of immune regulation employed by the body. The magnitude of immune responses must also be regulated. An inadequate immune response may lead to increased susceptibility to infection. An excessive immune response may result in the development of allergies or autoimmunity (Chapters 31 and 37). Failure to control the lymphocyte proliferation that occurs during immune responses may permit the development of lymphoid cell tumors. Failure to control the immune response to the fetus may lead to abortion (Chapter 35). The immune responses must therefore be carefully regulated to ensure that they are appropriate in both quality and quantity. As might be anticipated, many different control mechanisms exist (Box 21.1).

Antigen Regulation

Adaptive immune responses are antigen driven. They commence only on exposure to an antigen, and once its concentration drops below a critical threshold, they stop. If an antigen persists, the stimulus persists, and the immune response is prolonged. Prolonged responses occur after immunization with slowly degraded antigens such as the bacterial polysaccharides, or with antigens incorporated in oil or insoluble adjuvants. Antigens that do not reach organized lymphoid tissues, irrespective of their origin, may fail to induce either immunity or tolerance. Thus self-antigens restricted to sites such as the brain, or viruses such as papillomaviruses that never enter lymphoid organs, are often ignored by the immune system.

Antibody responses are also regulated by antigen structure. Rigid polymeric antigens such as those on a bacterial surface or antigens linked to BCR activators such as LPS can induce B-cell responses in the absence of T-cell help. On the other hand, nonpolymeric, flexible antigens such as soluble proteins induce B-cell responses only in the presence of CD4+ T cells. Antigen concentration also affects this because the lower the antigen concentration, the greater the need for T-cell help.

Antigen Processing and Immune Regulation

The nature of the immune response may vary in different parts of the body depending on dendritic cell populations. Langerhans cells in the skin seem especially suited for promoting T-cell responses, whereas follicular dendritic cells prime B cells. cDC1 cells are optimized to present antigens to Th1 cells, whereas cDC2 cells present antigens to Th2 cells. Adjuvants also influence the type of immune response induced through their effects on APCs (see Chapter 25).

Antibody Regulation

As a result of negative feedback, antibodies generally suppress B-cell responses. IgG antibodies tend to suppress the production of both IgM and IgG, whereas IgM antibodies suppress only the synthesis of IgM. Specific antibodies tend to suppress a specific immune response better than nonspecific immunoglobulins. An excellent example of this is seen in the method employed to prevent hemolytic disease of the newborn in humans (see Chapter 32). In this disease, a mother who lacks the Rhesus (Rh) antigen makes antibodies against the Rh antigens expressed on the red blood cells of her fetus. If the mother is administered antibodies against the Rh antigen at the time of her exposure to fetal red blood cells at birth, she will be completely prevented from responding to this antigen.

This negative feedback by antibodies on B-cell functions is mediated through the inhibitory B-cell receptor CD32b (FcγRIIb). In diseases where immunoglobulin levels are abnormally high, as in patients with myelomas (see Chapter 16), this feedback depresses normal antibody synthesis, and patients are immunosuppressed. A similar phenomenon occurs in newborn animals that acquire antibodies from their mother. The presence of maternal antibodies, while conferring protection, inhibits immunoglobulin synthesis and so prevents the successful vaccination of newborn animals (Fig. 21.8).

Serum IgG levels are also regulated through the neonatal immunoglobulin receptor (FcRn) (Fig. 24.6). Despite its name, it is present throughout life and is widely distributed on endothelial cells, in muscle, vasculature, and hepatic sinusoids. Because it binds IgG and albumin with high affinity, it regulates the serum half-lives of these proteins. When IgG binds to FcRn, it is protected from degradation and so has a longer half-life. If FcRn expression remains constant, IgG levels remain stable. If IgG levels rise, the surplus will fail to bind FcRn and be degraded. Conversely, if IgG levels drop, a greater proportion

BOX 21.1   Long Noncoding RNAs

Long noncoding RNAs (lncRNA) are transcripts that contain at least 200 nucleotides mainly derived from intergenic RNA located between the protein-coding regions. LncRNAs can interact with other nucleic acids or proteins to promote or restrain the expression of specific protein-coding genes. As described throughout this chapter, both innate and adaptive immune responses rely on the activation or inhibition of expression of hundreds of different genes. LncRNAs play a key role in regulating this gene expression. In effect, they form regulatory complexes with either proteins or with other RNA molecules that regulate immune cell activation and in so doing influence disease resistance, inflammation, and tissue repair. Thus they regulate myeloid and dendritic cell development and gene expression. They regulate the genes encoding IL-1α and β. They regulate STAT3 expression in DCs. They affect both Th1 and Th2 development and functions by influencing the NF-AT and NF-κB signaling pathways. Even some herpesviruses produce lncRNA that promotes their survival by acting as an immunosuppressant. LncRNAs can act within the cell cytoplasm by either binding to specific proteins or interacting with RNA. They can also act within the nucleus to interfere with gene translation.

From Agliano, F., Rathinam, V.A., Medvedev, A.E., et al., 2019. Long noncoding RNAs in host-pathogen interactions. Trends Immunol. 40 (6), 492–510; Atianand, M.K., Caffrey, D.R., Fitzgerald, K.A., 2017. Immunobiology of long noncoding RNAs. Annu. Rev. Immunol. 35, 177–198.

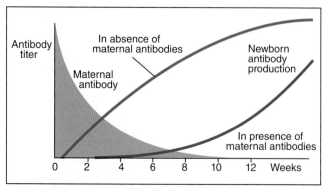

Fig. 21.8 The presence of maternal antibody in a newborn animal effectively delays the onset of immunoglobulin synthesis through a negative feedback process.

will bind to FcRn and be protected. This receptor also plays a key role in the transfer of maternal immunoglobulins to newborn mammals (see Chapter 24).

The class, as well as the quantity, of immunoglobulins produced during an immune response is also regulated. Most unstimulated B cells express both IgM and IgD BCRs. During an immune response, these cells switch to the production of IgM, IgG, IgA, or IgE. This class switch is controlled by helper T cells. In animals given T-independent antigens, there is no class switch, and a persistent low-level IgM response ensues.

INHIBITORY RECEPTORS

A key feature of the adaptive immune system is that, while poised to launch a potent array of destructive attacks against invaders, the body maintains control of the process. It is critically important to limit and eventually terminate a response by inactivating pathways that are no longer required. This regulation involves the extensive use of inhibitory receptors. These suppress the activity of lymphocytes once they have completed their task and so provide a crucial safeguard against inappropriate immune responses. Thus activation and inhibition must be paired to initiate and terminate immune responses. In some cases, activating and inhibitory receptors recognize similar ligands, so the net outcome is a product of the relative strength of these signals. Loss of inhibitory signals is often associated with autoimmunity or hypersensitivity.

An excellent example of an inhibitory receptor is CD32b (FcγRIIb) expressed on B cells. Any antibodies present will occupy these receptors. If these receptor-bound antibodies are cross-linked to a BCR through an antigen, the BCR and CD32 come together (Fig. 21.9). As a result, their signal transduction pathways interact, and BCR signaling is blocked. This prevents B-cell activation and triggers its apoptosis. The CD32 pathway is a feedback mechanism whereby B-cell activation is suppressed by antibody and uncontrolled B-cell responses are prevented. Since another receptor, FcγRIII, stimulates B cells, B-cell responses can be regulated by altering the ratio of FcγRIIb to FcγRIII.

Macrophage activation is regulated in a similar manner, and activated macrophages have a high FcγRIII-to-II ratio.

CD28 and CTLA4 on T cells both bind the same ligand (CD80) but deliver antagonistic signals. CD28 is an activator, whereas CTLA4 is an inhibitor. A deficiency of CTLA4 can lead to uncontrolled T-cell proliferation and autoimmunity (Buchbinder and Desai, 2016).

REGULATORY CELLS

Although much immune regulation is "passive" in that self-reactive lymphocytes are eliminated by central tolerance, cells in peripheral tissues also "actively" regulate the immune system. Cells with regulatory functions include T cells, B cells, macrophages, dendritic cells, and natural suppressor (NS) cells.

Regulatory T Cells

Regulatory T cells (Tregs) play a master role in regulating the immune system and maintaining the balance between peripheral tolerance and immunity (Fig. 21.10). In addition to suppressing autoimmunity, they are implicated in tissue repair, maintenance, and regeneration. In their absence, multiorgan autoimmune disease or uncontrolled inflammation results. Some of these Treg cells develop naturally, whereas others are induced by cytokine exposure (Belkaid and Tarbell, 2009).

Treg cells are typical lymphocytes that express CD4 and CD25 (the α-chain of the IL-2 receptor). All activated T cells express CD25, but Treg cells are the only ones that express it when naïve. Their most characteristic feature, however, is their use of a specialized transcription factor called FoxP3. This is yet another example of a situation in which cattle are different from mice and humans. FoxP3+, CD4+, and CD25+ cells are found in cattle, but these are not Tregs. The Treg cells in cattle are WC1.1+, WC1.2+, and γ/δ +T cells (Veiga-Parga, 2016).

There are many Treg subpopulations, and they employ multiple suppressive mechanisms (Dikiy and Rudensky, 2023). Natural Treg cells originate in the thymus (tTregs), whereas peripheral Treg cells (pTregs) are produced in secondary lymphoid organs, especially the

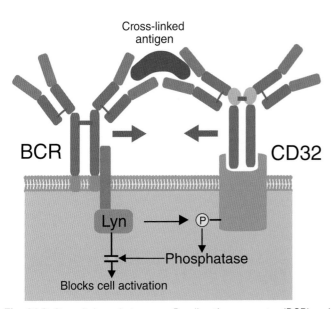

Fig. 21.9 Cross-linkage between a B-cell antigen receptor (BCR) and CD32, an Fc receptor, by antibody and antigen can turn off a B cell by activating a phosphatase that in turn blocks signaling by tyrosine kinase.

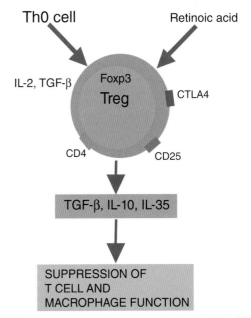

Fig. 21.10 The production and functions of regulatory T cells. They are generated by the combined actions of interleukin (IL-2) and transforming growth factor-β (TGF-β) as well as the presence of retinoic acid. They characteristically produce the suppressive cytokines, TGF-β, IL-10, and IL-35. *Treg*, Regulatory T cells.

intestine. The intestine is a major site of pTreg development, and specialized intestinal dendritic cells promote this through pathways that use a combination of transforming growth factor-β (TGF-β) and retinoic acid, a metabolite of vitamin A. Retinoic acid is generated by the bacterial microbiota in the gut and is required for normal T-cell function. Changes in the microbiota may therefore reduce the pTreg population while increasing the Th17 cell population. Intestinal pTreg cells develop from naïve T cells in response to antigen and costimulation by IL-2 and TGF-β. These signals induce the transcription of FoxP3. FoxP3 in turn induces transcription of the genes for CTLA4, TGF-β, and IL-10. pTregs are scattered throughout the body. They account for roughly 5% of circulating T cells and 10% of lymph node T cells in the dog.

Tregs suppress immune responses through multiple pathways (Fig. 21.11; Dikiy and Rudensky, 2023). Thus tTreg cells inhibit immune responses through direct cell-to-cell contact. This may be mediated by delivery of suppressive molecules through gap junctions, by binding of membrane-bound suppressive cytokines such as TGF-β, by producing cytotoxic granzymes and perforins, or by CTLA4-mediated reverse signaling through CD80. CD25 on Treg cells may bind and hence reduce the availability of IL-2. Galectin 1 on Tregs can bind receptors on effector T cells, resulting in cell cycle arrest. CTLA4 cells can induce apoptosis of effector T cells by releasing granzymes or tumor necrosis factor-related apoptosis-inducing ligand. A second mechanism—inhibition by suppressive cytokines—is used predominantly by pTreg cells. These cytokines include IL-10, TGF-β, and IL-35 as well as competitors for cytokine receptors. IL-10 is the most important of these suppressive cytokines (Fig. 21.12).

As a result of all these mechanisms, Treg cells suppress the response of helper T cells to antigens and prevent inappropriate T-cell activation in the absence of an antigen. Treg cells can also suppress CD4 and CD8 T-cell responses through pathways independent of IL-10 and TGF-β. For example, they appear to shorten the interaction time between T cells and APCs and thus prevent activation. Treg cells may also suppress immune responses indirectly by promoting dendritic cell IDO expression. Oral administration of an antigen may induce pTreg cells. Treg cells from the mesenteric lymph nodes of orally tolerant animals secrete TGF-β, IL-4, and IL-10. These cells account in large part for tolerance to food antigens.

Treg cells are not the only way in which cellular control of immune responses is exercised. Many of the regulatory activities of T cells reflect the antagonistic functions of Th1 and Th2 cells. For example, IFN-γ from Th1 cells can suppress IgE production, whereas IL-10 from Th2 cells is suppressive for dendritic cell IL-12 production and thus for the production of Th1 cytokines.

In cattle, γ/δ T cells are a major regulatory T-cell subset in peripheral blood. They spontaneously secrete IL-10 and proliferate in response to IL-10 and TGF-β. They can inhibit both antigen-specific and nonspecific proliferation of CD4+ and CD8+ T cells in vitro (Veiga-Parga, 2016).

In horses, Tregs are FoxP3+, CD4+, and CD25+. They act in a manner similar to other species by cell-cell contact and through IL-10 and TGF-β production. As in humans, their circulating CD4+ and CD25hi populations contain tTreg cells, while their pTreg cells can be induced in vitro by appropriate stimulation.

Pigs possess CD4+, CD25hi, and FoxP3+ Tregs that produce immunosuppressive IL-10. They require IL-2 stimulation for activation but excessive IL-2 stimulation may reduce their suppressive activity (Kaser et al., 2015).

In dogs, Treg cells play an important role in blocking resistance to some cancers (Biller et al., 2007).

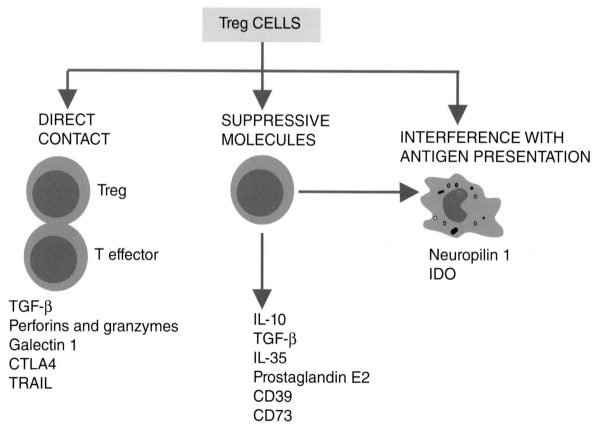

Fig. 21.11 The mechanisms by which regulatory T (Treg) cells can suppress other immune responses. *IDO*, Indoleamine 2,3-dioxygenase; *IL-10*, interleukin-10; *TGF-β*, transforming growth factor-β.

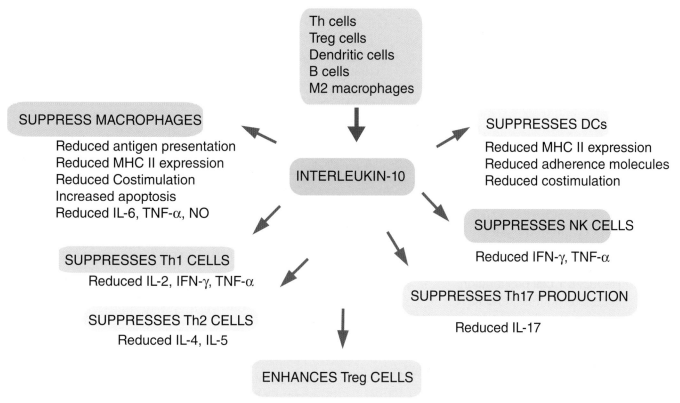

Fig. 21.12 The origins and properties of interleukin (IL)-10. *IFN-γ*, interferon-γ; *MHC*, major histocompatibility complex; *NK*, natural killer; *NO*, nitric oxide; *TNF-α*, tumor necrosis factor–α; *Treg*, regulatory T cells.

Interleukin-10

IL-10 is a regulatory cytokine that inhibits both innate and adaptive immune responses (Fig. 21.12). It is a protein of about 178 amino acids produced by macrophages (especially M2 macrophages) and classical dendritic cells in response to microbial products (Fickenscher et al., 2002). It is also produced by multiple T-cell subsets, including some populations of helper T cells in response to high antigen doses and IL-12. It is produced in especially large amounts by Treg cells in response to TGF-β. Small amounts of IL-10 may also be produced by B cells, mast cells, neutrophils, and natural killer (NK) cells (Ouyang and O'Garra, 2019).

IL-10 down-regulates MHC class II and costimulatory molecule expression on dendritic cells and macrophages and hence impairs antigen presentation. IL-10 or IL-10-treated dendritic cells can induce a long-lasting, antigen-specific, anergic state when T cells are activated in their presence. IL-10 inhibits the synthesis of the Th1 cytokines (IL-1, IFN-γ, and TNF-α) and the Th2 cytokines (IL-4 and IL-5). Thus it can regulate both Th1 and Th2 responses. IL-10 also inhibits the production of IL-5, CXCL8, IL-12, granulocyte-macrophage colony-stimulating factor (GM-CSF), and granulocyte colony-stimulating factor (G-CSF). It down-regulates the production of IFN-γ and TNF-α by NK cells (Castillo and Kolls, 2016).

Transforming Growth Factor-β

Among the immunosuppressive cytokines, the TGF-β family is one of the most important. It is a family of three glycoproteins (TGF-β1, TGF-β2, and TGF-β3) in mammals. They are secreted as inactive precursors that are activated on the cell surface by proteases after binding to integrins. TGFs are produced by platelets, activated macrophages, neutrophils, B cells, and T cells and act on T and B cells, dendritic cells, macrophages, neutrophils, and fibroblasts (Fig. 21.13).

TGF-β regulates macrophage activities. It may be either inhibitory or stimulatory, depending on the presence of other cytokines. Thus, it can enhance integrin expression as well as phagocytosis by blood monocytes. On the other hand, it suppresses the respiratory burst and NO production and blocks monocyte differentiation and the cytotoxic effects of activated macrophages. TGF-β is required for optimal dendritic cell development and regulates the interaction between follicular dendritic cells and B cells. TGF-β inhibits T- and B-cell proliferation and stimulates their apoptosis. Apoptotic T cells release TGF-β, contributing to the suppressive environment. TGF-β influences the differentiation of Th subsets. It tends to promote Th1 responses and the production of IL-2 in naïve T cells, but it also antagonizes the effects of IFN-γ and IL-12 on memory cells. It also controls the development and differentiation of B cells, inhibiting their proliferation, inducing apoptosis, and regulating IgA production. TGF-β also plays an important role in immunosuppression in animals bearing tumors (Batile and Massagué, 2019).

Regulatory Macrophages

Cytokines cause macrophage polarization. Thus exposure to IFN-γ from NK or Th1 cells generates classically activated M1 cells. Exposure of macrophages to IL-4 or IL-13 from Th2 cells, in contrast, results in the development of M2 cells (see Chapter 7; Gordon, 2003). Some M2 cells participate in tolerance induction, suppress inflammation, and participate in tissue repair. M2 cells increase expression of the macrophage mannose receptor, the β-glucan receptor, and CD163; they enhance endocytosis and antigen processing; and increase MHC class II expression. M2 macrophages produce large amounts of the Th2 and regulatory cytokines such as IL-4, IL-13, IL-10, TGF-β, and IL-1RA (see Fig. 7.8). In healthy animals, M2 cells may be found in the placenta and lung, where they inhibit dendritic cell antigen presentation and

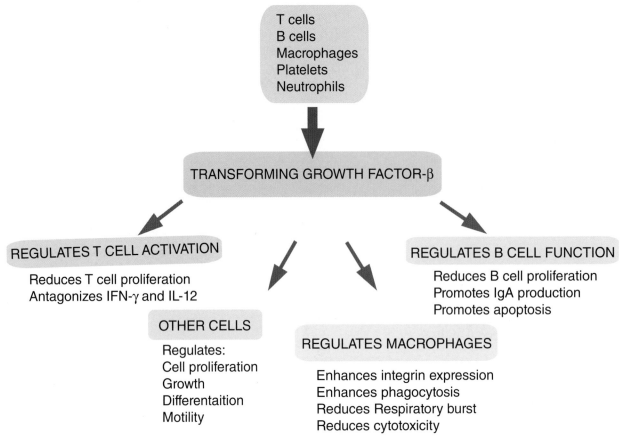

Fig. 21.13 The origins and properties of transforming growth factor-β. *IgA*, ImmunoglobulinA; *IFN-γ*, interferon-γ; *IL-12*, interleukin-12.

mitogen responses in lymphocytes. M2 macrophages are responsible for control of granuloma formation as well as for skin immune tolerance induced by ultraviolet B radiation. They can also be found in healing tissues, where they are associated with angiogenesis.

Indoleamine 2,3-Dioxygenase and Tolerance

Many regulatory cells, including Tregs, dendritic cells, some M2 macrophages, fibroblasts, trophoblast giant cells, endothelial cells, and some tumor cell lines produce indoleamine 2,3-dioxygenase (IDO) (Grohmann et al., 2003). This enzyme catalyzes the oxidative degradation of the amino acid tryptophan, resulting in its local depletion. Tryptophan is required for the mTOR pathway in T cells so that they undergo cell cycle arrest and apoptosis when deprived of tryptophan. IDO therefore inhibits T-cell activation, proliferation, and survival and promotes peripheral tolerance. Th1 cells appear to be more sensitive to tryptophan depletion than are Th2 cells. Treg cells may also induce IDO expression in some dendritic cells. IDO activity has been documented in T-cell tolerance to tumors, as a negative regulator in autoimmune diseases, and in some allergies (Mellor and Munn, 2004). IDO plays a key role in preventing immunological rejection of the fetus and of liver and corneal allografts (Chapter 35). IDO may also act as a defensive enzyme since by removing tryptophan it inhibits the growth of *Toxoplasma gondii*, *Chlamydia pneumoniae*, streptococci, and mycobacteria (Munn and Mellor, 2013).

Regulatory Dendritic Cells

The function of dendritic cells is to capture and process foreign antigens for presentation to T cells. However, the precise signals generated by dendritic cells depend on their state of maturity, on their costimulating molecules, and on the presence or absence of inflammatory cytokines. Thus, proteins from dead and dying cells that are captured by immature dendritic cells in the absence of inflammation may cause the dendritic cells to kill responding T cells or cause the T cells to differentiate into Treg cells. Treatment of dendritic cells with IL-10 can block their ability to activate Th1 cells while preserving their ability to promote Th2 responses.

Regulatory B cells

A subpopulation of B cells may secrete IL-10, IL-35, and TGF-β. As a result, they suppress the functions of Th17, Th1, and effector T cells and induce the differentiation of Treg cells (Rosser and Mauri, 2015).

Natural Suppressor Cells

NS cells are innate lymphocytes that produce cytokines with Treg-inducing activity. They suppress B- and T-cell proliferation as well as immunoglobulin production. NS cells occur normally in the adult bone marrow and neonatal spleen and possibly regulate innate immune responses.

When Do Regulatory Cells Work?

Regulatory cells control almost all aspects of immunity. Treg cells, for example, work constantly throughout an animal's life to prevent self-reactivity. They are responsible for the lack of immune responses in the newborn; immunosuppression following trauma, burns, or surgery; as well as prevention of autoimmunity and food tolerance. Regulatory cells are found in some tumor-bearing animals, where they may block tumor rejection, and in the placenta of pregnant animals, where they prevent rejection of the fetus.

NEURAL REGULATION OF IMMUNITY

The nervous and immune systems communicate through parasympathetic and sympathetic nerves and through soluble neurotransmitters. Neuroendocrine hormones, such as corticotrophin-releasing factor and α-melanocyte-stimulating hormone, as well as some neurotransmitters, act on the immune system to regulate cytokine production (Borgetti et al., 2009). Conversely, cytokines and chemokines modulate nervous system activities such as appetite, body temperature, and sleep behaviors. In addition, inflammation can lead to activation of sensory nerves (and cause pain) that then relay messages to the brain (Fig. 21.14). Many cytokines are produced by brain and meningeal macrophages—microglia. For example, IL-1 is produced in the brain in response to endotoxin.

Memory T cells may secrete acetylcholine in response to vagal nerve stimulation. Electrical stimulation of the vagus inhibits cytokine release from the spleen and reduces inflammation-mediated injury in endotoxemia and sepsis. This is called the "inflammatory reflex" and requires acetylcholine production. The acetylcholine inhibits inflammasome activity and thus reduces cytokine production. Both TNF-α and IL-1 also affect vagus nerve activity (Zanos et al., 2018). Immune cells employ a complete set of cholinergic receptors. Efferent activity in the vagus nerve activates a cholinergic antiinflammatory pathway. Vagal stimulation suppresses the systemic response to endotoxin by downregulating hepatic TNF-α synthesis. Activation of acetylcholine receptors on macrophages inhibits the production of IL-1 and TNF-α.

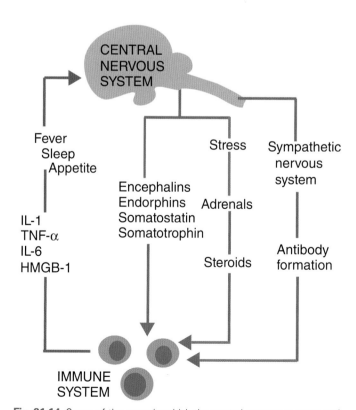

Fig. 21.14 Some of the ways in which the central nervous system and the immune system interact. *HMGB1*, High-mobility group band protein–1; *IL-1*, interleukin–1; *TNF-α*, tumor necrosis factor–α.

Autonomic Nervous System

Almost all primary and secondary lymphoid organs are supplied by nerves through the autonomic nervous system, and many cells of the immune system express receptors for the neurotransmitters released by both arms of the autonomic nervous system. This may occur either through adrenergic signals from the sympathetic nervous system or cholinergic signals from the parasympathetic nervous system (Kenney and Ganta, 2014).

The sympathetic nerves act through the neurotransmitter norepinephrine. They innervate the thymus, the splenic white pulp, and the lymph nodes. They influence blood flow, vascular permeability, and lymphocyte migration and differentiation. Surgical or chemical sympathectomy of the spleen enhances antibody production and can induce changes in the distribution of lymphocyte subpopulations. NK cell activity appears to be modulated directly by the hypothalamus through the splenic nerve. Autonomic nerves innervate Langerhans cells in the skin. By releasing neuropeptides, these nerves can depress their antigen-presenting ability. This might explain why "hot spots" in dogs worsen with anxiety. Denervated skin shows reduced inflammation after tissue damage and heals more slowly. Most importantly, sympathetic nerves innervate the adrenal medulla (Downing and Miyan, 2000).

Immune cells have a complete set of cholinergic receptors. Efferent activity in the vagus nerve activates a cholinergic antiinflammatory pathway. Vagal stimulation suppresses the systemic response to endotoxin by downregulating hepatic TNF-α synthesis. Activation of acetylcholine receptors on macrophages inhibits the production of IL-1 and TNF-α.

The production of antimicrobial proteins such as the defensins is also regulated by the autonomic nervous system, and stress reduces cutaneous epithelial antimicrobial activity. This appears to be a result of increased glucocorticoid and acetylcholine production (Bagath et al., 2019).

Both adrenergic and cholinergic stimulation increase noradrenaline signaling, leading to NF-κB activation in mononuclear cells. The sympathetic nervous system can alter the Th1/Th2 balance through the β-adrenergic receptor. Stimulation of sympathetic nerves enhances production of Th2 cytokines while inhibiting production of Th1 cytokines. Norepinephrine suppresses production of IL-6 and TNF-α.

Hypothalamic-Pituitary-Adrenal Cortical Axis

The adrenal cortex is stimulated by adrenocorticotropic hormone (ACTH) from the pituitary under the influence of corticotrophin-releasing hormone from the hypothalamus. As a result, in stressed animals, glucocorticoids are secreted and suppress T-cell function by blocking the NF-κB pathway. IL-1 and IL-6 act on both the hypothalamus and the pituitary to increase ACTH production and subsequent cortisol release. Stress can be profoundly immunosuppressive (see Chapter 41; Padgett and Glaser, 2003).

Neuropeptides and Lymphocytes

Lymphocytes have receptors for neuropeptides such as enkephalins and endorphins that thus can influence lymphocyte activity. The generation of cytotoxic T cells is enhanced by metenkephalin and β-endorphin, whereas α-endorphin suppresses antibody formation and β-endorphin reverses this suppressive effect. Other neuropeptides that influence the immune system include ACTH, oxytocin, vasoactive intestinal peptide, somatostatin, prolactin, and substance P (Brogden et al., 2005).

Many neuropeptides such as vasoactive intestinal peptide and neurokinin-1 (NK-1) have antimicrobial properties and may be involved in host defense. For example, NK-1 (also known as substance P) not only mediates pain and inflammation but also kills bacteria. Other neuropeptides have similar effects. As a result, appropriate nervous stimulation can promote neuropeptide release and enhance local antibacterial activity. The pain associated with acute inflammation may well reflect this local resistance to infection. Some neuropeptides can promote Th17 activity by triggering monocyte production of IL-23.

Immune responses are also modulated by environmental factors. Changes in day length (photoperiod) influence immunity. These effects can be complex, but in general reduced day length appears to promote immunity. The effect appears to be mediated through the hormone melatonin. Circadian rhythms also regulate some immune functions such as the activities of hematopoietic stem cells and lymphocyte recruitment from the blood. These appear to be a result of oscillations in chemokine levels and the expression of adhesion molecules on vascular endothelial cells (Scheiermann et al., 2013).

Finally, the innate immune system can influence nervous function. For example, cytokines such as IL-1, IL-6, and TNF-α as well as other inflammatory mediators induce "sickness behavior," including fever, fatigue, depressed activity, and excessive sleep. All these are closely associated with the systemic response to infectious agents and chronic inflammation (see Chapter 41). In cats, cytokines, including IL-1 and IL-2, have been implicated in causing aggressive behavior and defensive rage (Zalcman et al., 2006).

REFERENCES

Anderson, M.S., Venanzi, E.S., Klein, L., et al., 2002. Projection of an immunological self-shadow within the thymus by the AIRE protein. Science 298, 1395–1401.

Atianand, M.K., Caffrey, D.R., Fitzgerald, K.A., 2017. Immunobiology of long noncoding RNAs. Annu. Rev. Immunol. 35, 177–198.

Bagath, M., Krishman, G., Devaraj, C., Rashamol, V.P., et al., 2019. The impact of heat stress on the immune system of dairy cattle: a review. Res. Vet. Sci. 126, 94–102.

Batile, E., Massagué, J., 2019. Transforming growth factor-β signaling in immunity and cancer. Immunity 50, 924–940.

Belkaid, Y., Tarbell, K., 2009. Regulatory T cells in the control of host-microorganism interactions. Annu. Rev. Immunol. 27, 551–589.

Biller, B.J., Elmslie, R.E., Burnett, R.C., et al., 2007. Use of FoxP3 expression to identify regulatory T cells in healthy dogs and dogs with cancer. Vet. Immunol. Immunopathol. 116, 69–78.

Borghetti, P., Saleri, R., Mocchegiani, E., et al., 2009. Infection, immunity and the neuroendocrine response. Vet. Immunol. Immunopathol. 130, 141–162.

Brogden, K.A., Guthmiller, J.M., Salzet, M., Zasloff, M., 2005. The nervous system and innate immunity: the neuropeptide connection. Nat. Immunol. 6, 558–564.

Buchbinder, E.J., Desai, A., 2016. CTLA-4 and PD-1 pathways: similarities, differences and implications for their inhibition. Am. J. Clin. Oncol. 39, 98–106.

Castillo, P., Kolls, J.K., 2016. IL-10: a paradigm for counterregulatory cytokines. J. Immunol. 197, 1529–1530.

Dikiy, S., Rudensky, A.Y., 2023. Principles of regulatory T cell function. Immunity 56, 240–255.

Downing, J.E.G., Miyan, J.A., 2000. Neural immunoregulation: emerging roles for nerves in immune homeostasis and disease. Immunol. Today 21, 281–289.

El Tanbouly, M.A., Noelle, R.J., 2021. Rethinking peripheral T cell tolerance: checkpoints across a T cell's journey. Nat. Rev. Immunol 21, 257–267.

Fickenscher, H., Hor, S., Kupers, H., et al., 2002. The interleukin-10 family of cytokines. Trends Immunol. 23, 89–96.

Gordon, S., 2003. Alternative activation of macrophages. Nat. Rev. Immunol. 3, 23–34.

Grohmann, U., Fallarino, F., Puccetti, I., 2003. Tolerance, dendritic cells, and tryptophan: much ado about IDO. Trends Immunol. 24, 242–249.

Kaser, T., Mair, K.H., Hammer, S.E., Gerner, W., Saalmuller, A., 2015. Natural and inducible Tregs in swine: helios expression and functional properties. Dev. Comp. Immunol. 49, 323–331.

Katzman, S.D., O'Gorman, W.E., Villarino, A.V., et al., 2010. Duration of antigen receptor signaling determines T-cell tolerance or activation. Proc. Natl. Acad. Sci. U.S.A. 107, 18085–18090.

Kenney, M.J., Ganta, C.K., 2014. Autonomic nervous system and immune system interactions. Compr. Physiol. 4, 1177–1200.

Mellor, A.L., Munn, D.H., 2004. IDO expression by dendritic cells: tolerance and tryptophan catabolism. Nat. Rev. Immunol. 4, 762–774.

Munn, D.H., Mellor, A.L., 2013. Indoleamine 2,3 dioxygenase and metabolic control of immune responses. Trends Immunol. 34, 137–143. 2013

Ouyang, W., O'Garra, A., 2019. IL-10 family cytokines, IL-10 and IL-22. From basic science to clinical translation. Immunity 50, 871–891.

Padgett, D.A., Glaser, R., 2003. How stress influences the immune response. Trends Immunol. 24, 444–448.

Passos, G.A., Speck-Hernandez, C.A., Assis, F., Mendes-da-Cruz, D.A., 2017. Update on Aire and thymic negative selection. Immunology 153, 10–20.

Ramsdell, F., Fowlkes, B.J., 1992. Maintenance of in vivo tolerance by persistence of antigen. Science 257, 1130–1138.

Rosser, E.C., Mauri, C., 2015. Regulatory B cells: origin, phenotype, and function. Immunity 42, 607–612.

Scheiermann, C., Kunisaki, Y., Frenette, P.S., 2013. Circadian control of the immune system. Nat. Rev. Immunol. 13, 190–198.

Veiga-Parga, T., 2016. Regulatory T cells and their role in animal disease. Vet. Pathol. 53, 737–745.

Zalcman, S.S., Siegel, A., 2006. The neurobiology of aggression and rage: role of cytokines. Brain Behav. Immun. 20 (6), 507–514.

Zanos, T.P., Silverman, H.A., Levy, T., Tsaava, T., et al., 2018. Identification of cytokine-specific sensory neural signals by decoding murine vagus nerve activity. Proc. Natl. Acad. Sci. https://doi.org/10.1073/pnas.1719083115.

The Microbiota and the Immune System

The surfaces of the animal body consist of many stable, nutrient-rich ecosystems where microbes thrive. Each external surface is populated by enormous numbers of bacteria, archea, fungi, and viruses, collectively termed the microbiota. The bacteria are the best studied of these. Thus bacteria live on the skin, in the respiratory tract, in parts of the genitourinary tract, and sometimes within the body but mainly within the gastrointestinal tract. It has been estimated that in an animal body, at least half of all the cells are microbial. As a result of their life-long, intimate association with body surfaces, the microbiota can be considered to be an integral part of the body—"a virtual organ." As such, they influence both innate and adaptive immunity, and conversely, they are influenced by signals generated by their host. This has given rise to the concept that animals and their microbiota together form "superorganisms" that share nutrition and exchange energy and metabolites and whose complex interactions are regulated in large part by immune mechanisms (Rodrigues-Hoffmann et al., 2016).

It has been proposed that, as a result of "Western lifestyles" and "excessive hygiene," the intestinal microbiota has lost much of its diversity. This "dysbiosis," it is suggested, has altered the regulatory signals reaching T helper cells. As a result, excessive inflammatory and immune responses develop. The "Hygiene Hypothesis" therefore suggests that as a result of this decline in Treg cells, humans in Western societies have become more prone to develop allergic and autoimmune diseases (Xu et al., 2019; Lambrecht and Hammad, 2017; Bach, 2017).

By harnessing the immensely diverse genomes present in the complex microbiota, animals enhance their metabolic potential and obtain new ways to utilize food. (Mammals possess about 20,000 protein-encoding genes, while our microbiota may collectively possess about 10 million). As a result, the microbiota increase an animal's ability to extract energy from plant structural carbohydrates and obtain essential vitamins. Because of the microbiota, animals can utilize food sources that would otherwise be unavailable. Microbial metabolism permits animals to adapt to otherwise noncompetitive lifestyles. For example, mice with a conventional microbiota need to eat 30% fewer calories than germ-free mice to maintain their body weight. This is due to the ability of the microbiota to extract more energy from food.

Domestic mammals do, however, have some additional complexities associated with their diet and lifestyle. The large domestic herbivores contain massive amounts of microbial material in their rumen and large intestine. The evolution of these organs reflects the importance of the microbiota in providing nutrition by extracting energy from complex, plant-derived polysaccharides such as cellulose (Fig. 22.1). Carbohydrate digestion is the primary function of the gastrointestinal microbiota. Many members of the microbiota are optimized to ferment oligosaccharides and thus generate short-chain fatty acids (SCFAs). These fatty acids, in turn, can be used as energy sources by other, more specialized bacteria. It is estimated that in an omnivore such as a human, as much as 10% of daily energy needs are provided by colonic fermentation. This figure is much higher for herbivores such as ruminants and horses (Costa et al., 2015).

It is now well accepted that the intestinal microbiota both contribute to local host defenses and also have effects on the immune system and metabolism that extend throughout the body. Nutrients and microbial metabolites are continually released into the body where they influence both innate and adaptive immune functions.

The immunological defenses on body surfaces are therefore faced with the task of coexisting with the microbiota while at the same time preventing microbial invasion through breaks in the epithelial barriers (Belkaid and Hand, 2014).

THE LOCATIONS OF THE MICROBIOTA

The Skin

Normal skin harbors trillions of microorganisms. These are found on the keratinocyte surface and extend into sebaceous glands and hair follicles. The skin is not, however, a hospitable surface. The outer cell layers are constantly shed and replaced by new cells from below. It is cool in some areas and hot in others. Haired skin may be very different from mucocutaneous junctions. Some areas of skin may be very dry, with a high salt content, hydrophobic and acidic as well as being nutrient-poor. Other areas may be moist but bathed in a complex mixture of proteases, lysozyme, and antimicrobial peptides such as β-defensins and cathelicidins. Nevertheless, it has been estimated that up to a billion bacteria may live on a square centimeter of human skin. Given the sheltering effects of hairs or feathers, it is likely that the skin microbiota

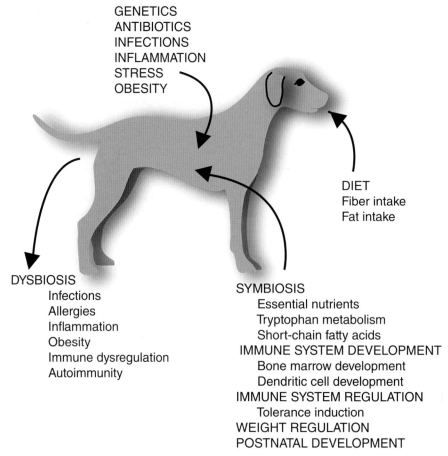

GENETICS
ANTIBIOTICS
INFECTIONS
INFLAMMATION
STRESS
OBESITY

DIET
Fiber intake
Fat intake

DYSBIOSIS
    Infections
    Allergies
    Inflammation
    Obesity
    Immune dysregulation
    Autoimmunity

SYMBIOSIS
    Essential nutrients
    Tryptophan metabolism
    Short-chain fatty acids
IMMUNE SYSTEM DEVELOPMENT
    Bone marrow development
    Dendritic cell development
IMMUNE SYSTEM REGULATION
    Tolerance induction
WEIGHT REGULATION
POSTNATAL DEVELOPMENT

Fig. 22.1 The importance of the microbiota to the proper functioning of the animal body, some of the factors that modify its composition, and the consequences of dysregulation.

in domestic animals may be even more dense and complex. The skin microbiota of dogs varies greatly between different dogs and different skin sites. For example, there is higher microbial diversity in hairy skin, compared to mucocutaneous junctions. The highest diversity has been found in the axilla and the dorsum of the nose. On average about 300 different bacterial species have been identified on the dorsal canine nose (Rodrigues-Hoffmann et al., 2014).

The skin microbiota can be divided into a resident population that is relatively stable and consistent—a true commensal population, and a changing population of transient bacteria that may only persist on the skin for hours or days. Both populations contain a mixture of commensals and potential pathogens, yet invasion and disease are relatively uncommon. Large populations of Proteobacteria and Oxalobacteriaceae predominate (Fig. 22.2). The precise composition of the skin microbiota thus depends on the location (hairy, wooly, or bald skin; back versus skin in the axilla or groin or ear) and the presence of disease such as seborrhea or atopic dermatitis. There is also great variation between individuals. Grooming activities will have some impact on these microbial populations, but their significance is unclear (Ross and Rodrigues-Hoffmann, 2019).

In mice, it has been shown that the skin microbiota influences local inflammatory and T-cell responses (Fig. 22.3). Epidermal Th17 and CD8+ T cells are especially affected. The microbiota controls the balance between effector and regulatory T cells within skin tissue. They influence keratinocyte production of IL-1 and its effects on epidermal dendritic cells and thus control local T-cell responses. Skin bacteria can activate antigen-specific T cells across intact epithelium. However, the presence of Treg cells in neonatal skin mediates tolerance to skin commensal bacteria at a time when the skin is establishing its microbiota. Wound healing in germ-free mice is significantly accelerated and scarring is much reduced. Skin bacteria certainly contribute to the failure of some wounds to heal promptly. It is also apparent that the microbiota may change significantly in pathological conditions such as atopic dermatitis, but it is unclear whether this reflects the cause or the effect of the disease (Rodrigues-Hoffmann, 2017; Older et al., 2017).

The Respiratory Tract

Like all body surfaces exposed to the external environment, the upper respiratory tract houses a dense, dynamic, and complex microbiota. It has been calculated that a human inhales 10^5 organisms/day just breathing normally. Many nasal bacteria are also found on the skin while others are common environmental bacteria. Deeper in the airways, in the lower respiratory tract, there is also a diverse bacterial population (O'Dwyer et al., 2016).

Contrary to previous belief, the lung is not sterile. Healthy lungs harbor a complex microbiota, closely related to, but much less dense than that found in the upper respiratory tract. The bronchi contain about 2000 bacterial genomes per cm². Lung tissues contain between 10 and 100 bacterial cells per 1000 lung cells. These include both aerobes and anaerobes, and like other surfaces, the populations differ greatly between individuals. The predominant phyla are Firmicutes with lesser numbers of Proteobacteria and Actinobacteria. The organisms generally live within the mucus layer and include bacteria, fungi (yeasts), and viruses such as bacteriophages. Pathobionts are also present and may induce

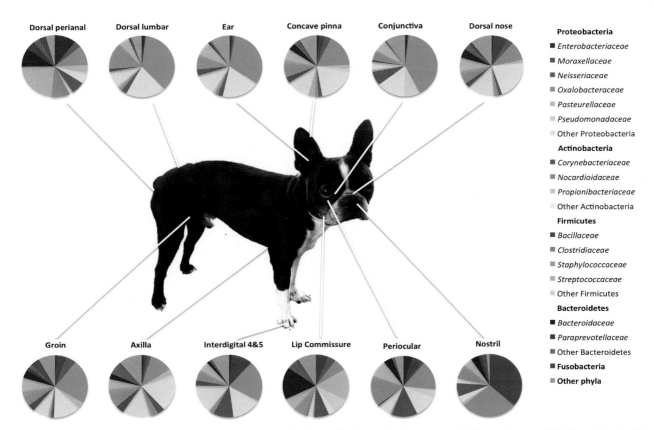

Fig. 22.2 The composition of the microbiota on canine skin. From Rodrigues-Hoffmann, A., Patterson, A.P., Diesel, A., et al., 2014. The skin microbiome in healthy and allergic dogs. PLoS One 9 (1), e83197.

ENVIRONMENTAL BACTERIA AND VIRUSES

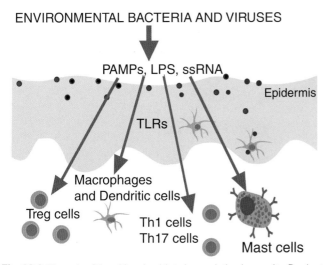

Fig. 22.3 The role of the skin microbiota in regulating immunity. Products from the commensal organisms influence many aspects of the immune system. *LPS,* Lipopolysaccharide; *PAMPs,* Pathogen-associated molecular patterns; *TLRs,* toll-like receptors; *Tregs,* regulatory T cells.

disease in immunodeficient individuals. Perhaps the best example of these are the fungi of the genus *Pneumocystis* (see Chapter 40). As might be expected, the microbiota of individuals with chronic respiratory disease differs from healthy individuals. The airway microbiota plays a role in resistance to respiratory infections as well as the development of asthma and hay fever (Zeineldin et al., 2019). Thus, in the absence of the microbiota, the airways are prone to mount exaggerated Th2 responses. The presence of a microbiota induces Treg activity that suppresses this. This

probably explains the protective effects of inhaled microbial antigens (as in a farming environment) on the development of allergies. Dietary fiber also has a protective effect on allergic airway inflammation in mice and this results from increased levels of circulating SCFAs. The intestinal microbiota also regulate pulmonary adaptive responses (Dang and Marsland, 2019). For example, segmented filamentous bacteria (SFBs) in the intestine regulate pulmonary immunity to bacteria and fungi. The gut microbiota directs ILC2 cells to migrate from the gut to the lung where they promote IL-33 production (Pu et al., 2021). Conversely, influenza infection in the lungs generates type I interferons. These, in turn, induce changes in the gut microbiota such as depletion of obligate anaerobic bacteria and an increase in Proteobacteria resulting in intestinal dysbiosis—a possible cause of "stomach flu."

The Genitourinary System

In adult women, the healthy cervicovaginal microbiota is usually dominated by lactobacilli and other lactic acid-producing bacteria. The vagina is also lined by a squamous epithelium composed of cells rich in glycogen. When these cells desquamate, the glycogen provides a substrate for the lactobacilli that, in turn, generate large quantities of lactic acid. This reduces the pH to a level that protects the vagina against invasion by many pathogenic bacteria and yeasts. Glycogen storage in the vaginal epithelial cells is stimulated by estrogens and thus occurs only in sexually mature individuals. The vaginal microbiota of other mammals, such as cows, is very different and almost totally lacking in *Lactobacilli.*

The Gastrointestinal Tract

The gut microbiota is a complex community containing bacteria, archea, fungi, and viruses. The most obvious of these are trillions of bacteria belonging to hundreds of different species. They are dominated by members of two phyla, the Firmicutes and the Bacteroidetes, with lesser numbers of Actinobacteria and Proteobacteria and many minor phyla, such as the Fusobacteria and the Verrucomicrobia. It has been estimated that the canine small intestine harbors more than 200 different bacterial species, while the canine colon may house up to a thousand (Fig. 22.4; Hooda et al., 2013). Bacterial counts in the canine and feline duodenum range from 10^2 to 10^9 per gram of content. In the colon, the count ranges from 10^9 to 10^{11} colony-forming units/g.

Each individual animal's microbiota is unique, and its composition is determined by management, diet, genetics, antibiotic exposure, and environmental factors. The composition of the microbiota also changes along the gastrointestinal tract under the influence of nutrient availability and the local microenvironment. The Firmicutes mainly consist of gram-positive bacteria. Many are spore-forming. Important members include the Clostridia that may be beneficial or pathogenic. They also include potentially pathogenic Streptococci and Staphylococci. The Actinobacteria are also gram-positive bacteria with a different G+C content than the Firmicutes. The Bacteroidetes are gram-negative bacteria that ferment indigestible plant carbohydrates to produce SCFAs. The Proteobacteria contain gram-negative enterobacteria such as *Escherichia coli* and Klebsiella. The canine stomach has a microbiome dominated by *Helicobacter* spp.

Foregut Fermenters
Herbivorous mammals are divided into those that digest cellulose in their foregut, the rumen, and those that do so in their hindgut, the cecum. The surface of the rumen is covered by stratified squamous epithelium. Thus its defenses have more in common with skin rather than with the rest of the gastrointestinal tract. Although this epithelium is largely leak-proof, the presence of such a large source of microbial antigens suggests that some provision must be made for defense against leakage and that it may have a profound influence on the innate and adaptive immune systems of ruminants.

Disturbances in rumen metabolism, often caused by feeding very high-energy diets, result in changes in the ruminal microbiota leading to an increase in fatty acid and ethanol production, a drop in rumen pH, and the development of subacute rumen acidosis. This, in turn, results in local inflammation, the opening of intercellular junctions, and a disruption in the barrier function of the ruminal squamous epithelium. This can permit bacterial PAMPs such as endotoxins, flagellae, and other microbial products to cross the ruminal wall and enter the bloodstream. This may lead to endotoxemia, a systemic innate immune response, an acute-phase response, and prolonged systemic inflammation.

While much is known about the relationships between the intestinal immune system and lymphoid tissues in simple-stomached animals, much less is known about the interactions between the rumen and the immune system. The ruminal lymphatics drain to many lymph nodes (Fig. 22.5). Toll-like receptors such as TLR-4 and cytokines such as IL-1β, IL-10, and caspase-1 can be found in the ruminal walls suggesting that inflammation can readily occur here. Interferon-γ is found in ruminal contents. It appears, that the ruminal microbiota may communicate with its associated lymphoid tissues and so promote regulatory responses. There is little evidence that the ruminal microbiota

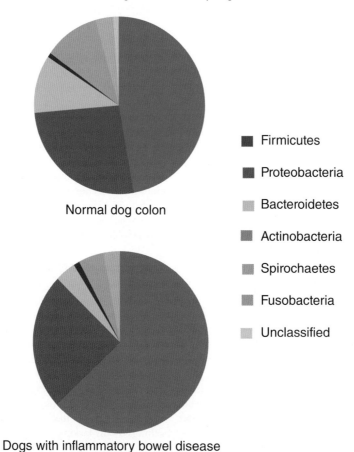

Normal dog colon

■ Firmicutes

■ Proteobacteria

▨ Bacteroidetes

■ Actinobacteria

▨ Spirochaetes

▨ Fusobacteria

▨ Unclassified

Dogs with inflammatory bowel disease

Fig. 22.4 The enormous diversity of the gut microbiota in the dog is well seen in this comparison of the composition of the colon microbiota in normal dogs and dogs with inflammatory bowel disease. Courtesy Dr. Panagiotis Xenoulis.

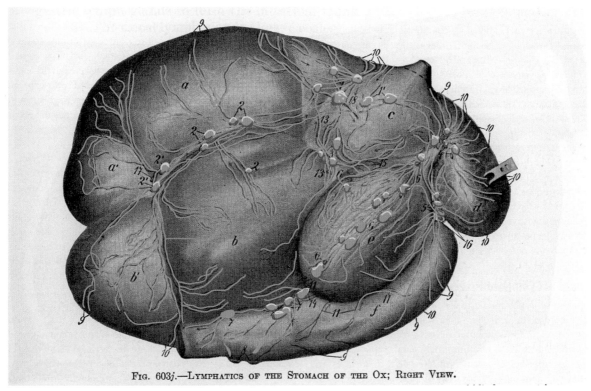

FIG. 603j.—LYMPHATICS OF THE STOMACH OF THE OX; RIGHT VIEW.

Fig. 22.5 The rumen is an organ specialized for the fermentation and digestion of complex plant polysaccharides. It is lined by stratified squamous epithelium and is thus generally impermeable to most invading microorganisms. However, leakage is inevitable and as a result, ruminants have large numbers of lymph nodes located where they can trap any ruminal escapees. The lymphatic drainage of the rumen. From Sisson, S., 1953. Anatomy of the Domestic Animals, fourth ed. Saunders, Philadelphia, PA. [Revised by Grossman JD.]

directly shapes the development of the immune system, but it has been suggested that the complex innate immune systems of ruminants, especially their highly diverse antimicrobial peptides, may have evolved in response to this source of microbial invasion.

Hindgut Fermenters

Hindgut fermenters such as the horse are monogastric herbivores that digest fibrous plant material by anaerobic fermentation in the cecum and colon (Costa et al., 2015). The SCFAs produced are absorbed through the mucosa. Firmicutes are the main bacterial phylum (especially Clostridia), but the predominant organism is a member of the Verrucomicrobia. Other phyla found in the equine large intestine include Spirochaetes, Fibrobacteres, Ruminococcus, and Bacteroidetes. Under certain conditions such as carbohydrate overload, the microbiota of the large gut change drastically as a result of which their pH drops and bacterial PAMPs escape into the bloodstream. This can result in the development of acute laminitis (see Chapter 8).

THE FUNCTIONS OF THE MICROBIOTA

Nutritional Efficiency

The composition and metabolism of the microbiota are critically dependent on diet. Thus the microbiota in animals fed a low-fat, high-plant polysaccharide diet is very different from that in animals on a high-fat, high-sugar, and low-plant polysaccharide diet. There are great differences in the microbiota of African children compared to European children or in Indian cattle compared to American cattle. Fluctuations in the intestinal microbiota may require an animal to adjust its metabolic and immunologic performance in response to nutritional and environmental changes.

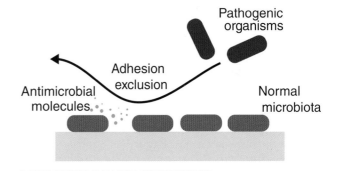

ACTIVATED INNATE DEFENSES
Upregulated mucus layer
Upregulated defensins
Upregulated IgA
Activated macrophages
Activation of Th17 and ILCs

Nutrient competition
Carbon source limitation
Nutrient availability
Micronutrient limitation
Oxygen consumption

Fig. 22.6 The mechanisms by which the microbiota protect body surfaces against colonization and invasion by pathobionts. *IgA*, Immunoglobulin A, *ILCs*, innate lymphoid cells.

The intestinal microbiota also changes during pregnancy. In mothers during the third trimester, there is a reduction in species richness. When transferred to germ-free mice, late-pregnancy microbiota induced greater adiposity and reduced insulin sensitivity. This effect is beneficial in a normal pregnancy since it supports fetal growth and the onset of lactation. The maternal microbiota also drives early postnatal immune development including the potential for young animals to develop type 2 immune responses and hence allergies (Liu et al., 2019).

Intestinal Protection

The microbiota protects the body against colonization by pathogens and prevents the overgrowth of pathobionts. They do this by competing for essential metabolites and nutrients, and by inducing intestinal immune responses (Fig. 22.6; Kamada et al., 2013a, 2013b). By fully occupying and exploiting the intestinal environment, commensal bacteria block subsequent colonization by pathogenic bacteria. (It is, for example, possible to prevent or reduce *Salmonella* colonization of the chicken intestine by feeding an appropriate mixture of commensal bacteria to birds.) The microbiota also modifies local environmental conditions by keeping the pH and oxygen tension low. This is also influenced by the diet; for example, the intestine of milk-fed animals contains many lactobacilli that produce bacteriostatic lactic and butyric acids. These acids inhibit colonization by *E. coli*, so young animals suckled naturally tend to have fewer digestive disturbances than animals weaned early in life. There is a strong negative correlation between the level of lactobacilli and the number of pathogens in the intestine (Blander et al., 2017).

Development of Lymphoid Organs

The development of the lymphoid tissues in the gastrointestinal tract begins well before birth. However, their complete maturation and the development of immunoglobulin A (IgA)-secreting B cells and T cells only occur after birth and intestinal colonization (Gensollen et al., 2016). The microbiota recruits immune cells to surfaces and drives the development and organization of all the major lymphoid tissues (Ennamorati et al., 2020).

It has long been possible to derive animals by cesarean surgery and raise them within sealed chambers in such a way that they are free of microbes. Compared to conventionally-raised animals, these "germ-free" animals have fewer and smaller Peyer's patches, smaller mesenteric lymph nodes, and fewer CD4+ T cells in the lamina propria of the gut wall. They have fewer intraepithelial T lymphocytes (IELs) within their intestinal epithelium. These IELs have reduced expression of TLR and MHC class II, as well as reduced cytotoxicity. Systemic immune defects are also apparent. Germ-free mice have fewer CD4+ T cells in their spleen, and fewer and smaller germinal centers as a result of reduced B-cell numbers. Their production of macrophages and neutrophils by bone marrow stem cells is impaired. Their immunoglobulin levels are only about 2% of normal so that if exposed abruptly to the external environment, they are vulnerable to bacterial invasion. The presence of the microbiota is also necessary for the production of tertiary lymphoid structures such as cryptopatches and isolated lymphoid follicles.

Mammals have evolved two strategies to generate B-cell populations with a diverse antibody repertoire (see Chapter 16). Thus mice and humans rely mainly on random rearrangements of the V, D, and J genes during B-cell development within the bone marrow. Other mammals such as cattle, sheep, pigs, and rabbits use an alternative strategy. These species undertake an initial burst of B-cell proliferation with limited diversification in utero. These newly produced cells then migrate to the gut-associated lymphoid tissues where after birth, they expand both their numbers and their diversity. As described in Chapter 13, in sheep the ileal Peyer's patch is the site of B-cell repertoire expansion, while the jejunal Peyer's patch is the source of antigen-specific IgA responses.

The process of microbial-driven B-cell diversification and IgA production appears to depend upon the presence of a select subgroup of bacteria within the microbiota. For example, a combination of *Bacteroides fragilis* and *Bacillus subtilis* can induce B-cell development and VDJ diversification in germ-free rabbits. Neither species alone has this effect, suggesting that two signals are needed. Once B-cell proliferation and diversification are triggered, the microbiota continue to regulate any additional diversification. It is believed that microbial molecules trigger these B-cell responses by binding to their TLRs and activating NF-κB pathways. Alternatively, soluble bacterial superantigens might trigger a polyclonal B-cell response and drive the process by preferentially stimulating the production of B cells expressing certain V_H regions. It may be relevant to note here that the distribution of TLRs on cells differs significantly between conventional and germ-free pigs.

Microbiota Signals to the Body

Bacteria, be they on the skin, respiratory tract, genital tract, or intestine, communicate directly and effectively with their host's immune system. Indeed, this interaction is essential to the proper functioning of the innate and adaptive immune responses. Alterations or imbalances in the microbiota therefore can have profound effects on the functions of the immune system. The proper interaction between the immune system and the microbiota is required for optimal health (Arpaia and Rudensky, 2014).

Dietary plant fibers contain complex carbohydrates. When digested by Clostridia in the cecum and colon, these complex carbohydrates generate large amounts of SCFAs) such as butyrate, propionate, and acetate that promote the production of intestinal Foxp3+ Treg cells (Fig. 22.7). Butyric acid has antiinflammatory effects since it acts on macrophages to enhance their antibacterial peptide production and prevents epigenetic changes by inhibiting histone deacetylases (Schulthess et al., 2019). Butyrate also increases barrier functions by stimulating enterocytes and increasing goblet cell differentiation, and mucus production. It can also stimulate some bovine neutrophil functions. As a result, SCFAs from

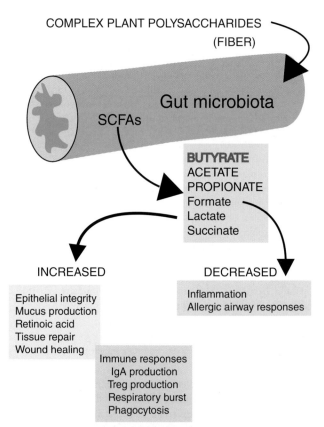

Fig. 22.7 The importance of short-chain fatty acids (SCFAs), especially butyrate, in promoting immunity. These fatty acids are generated by the digestion of complex carbohydrates and are also a major source of energy in herbivores. They are produced in large quantities by the microbial digestion of high-fiber diets. *IgA*, Immunoglobulin A; *Tregs*, regulatory T cells.

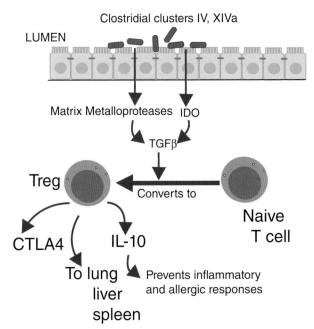

Fig. 22.8 The role of clostridial clusters in promoting both local and systemic Treg activity. *IDO*, Indoleamine 2,3-dioxygenase; *IL-10*, interleukin-10; *TGF-β*, transforming growth factor-β; *Treg*, Regulatory T cells.

high-fiber diets play a key role in regulating intestinal inflammation and physiology (van der Hee and Wells, 2021). If the intestinal microbiota generates increased production of acetate, then this will activate the parasympathetic nervous system and promote glucose-stimulated insulin production (Takeuchi et al., 2021). This stimulates the production of a hunger hormone called ghrelin that enhances appetite leading to increased food intake and obesity.

Among the intestinal microbiota, some species play a key role in regulating immune responses. One such group is classified as Clostridial clusters. Several of these bacteria (Clostridia clusters IV, XIVa, and XVIII) specifically induce Treg cells and IL-10 production in the gut. These Clostridia form a thick layer over the epithelium and enhance the release of TGF-β and IDO from enterocytes (Fig. 22.8). They also promote mucus production by goblet cells.

In addition to the Clostridia, the capsular polysaccharide-A of *B. fragilis* triggers IL-10 production through the TLR-2-MyD88 pathway. Numerous Clostridial species can also trigger IL-10 production by a non-MyD88 pathway involving TGF-β production by intestinal epithelial cells. Other mechanisms such as desensitization of TLRs to bacterial PAMPs and bacterial stimulation of IL-10 and IL-2 production by Treg cells also help minimize inflammation. Additionally, some commensal bacteria actively suppress intestinal inflammation. For example, *Lactobacilli* and *Bacteroides* inhibit the innate signaling pathways triggered by TLRs and NLRs. A common commensal, *Bacteroides thetaiotamicron* inhibits NF-κB signaling while intestinal lactobacilli prevent degradation of the NF-κB inhibitor IκB.

The presence of Clostridial clusters in the colon also results in an increase in the numbers of IL-10-producing Treg cells in distant tissues such as the spleen and lung, and they play a role in inhibiting allergic responses. Thus T cells educated by commensal bacteria may emigrate from the gut to remote tissues and determine the body's T-cell balance.

IMMUNE RESPONSES TO THE MICROBIOTA

For many years, it was believed that the role of the immune system was simply to ensure the complete exclusion of all invading microbes by distinguishing between self and not-self and eliminating foreign antigens. We now know, however, that that decision alone is insufficient to ensure health. The immune system must also determine the degree of threat posed by the microbes it encounters and adjust its response accordingly. It must maintain tolerance to microbiota or food antigens while, at the same time, being highly responsive to invading pathogens. This discrimination is determined in part by the way in which enteric antigens are processed and the behavior of enterocytes. It is also determined by intestinal T and B cells as well as by the gut microenvironment.

The presence of the intestinal microbiota must either be tolerated or ignored if an animal is to remain healthy. An animal cannot afford to act aggressively toward its own microbiota. The presence of all these bacterial products has the potential to trigger massive acute inflammation. But this inflammation must not happen unless necessary for the defense of the body.

Enterocytes

The intestinal epithelium is not simply a barrier. It is a highly responsive tissue that employs innate and adaptive immune cells to restrain the microbiota without triggering unnecessary inflammation but is always ready to activate more potent defensive responses should the need arise. Enterocytes interact with the intestinal microbiota. They produce many peptides that kill or inactivate bacteria and, as a result, shape their composition. Enterocytes block access of intact antigens to the lamina propria. They ensure that a balance exists between inflammation and tolerance. They secrete and respond to regulatory cytokines. They present antigens to dendritic cells. Within the epithelium and the underlying lamina propria are IELs that, upon appropriate stimulation by microbiota-induced IL-1 or IL-23, can regulate their differentiation into effector or regulatory cells.

Enterocytes express receptors for many microbial-associated molecular patterns (MAMPs) including TLRs-1, -2, -3, -5, and -9 as well as NOD-2. When exposed to MAMPs, recruitment of MyD88 and TRIF results in NF-κB and MAP kinase activation and cytokine synthesis. In practice, bacterial signals trigger the production of some antimicrobial peptides and cytokines but not inflammation. This is because the PRRs are not expressed on the luminal side of enterocytes, where they would normally come into contact with commensals. They are located at the base of the cells and at intracellular locations. Thus they are activated only after bacteria penetrate the epithelial barrier. By preventing microbial invasion, enterocytes also prevent the development of inflammation within the intestinal wall. Some of the cytokines produced by enterocytes also influence the regulatory activities of antigen-processing cells such as macrophages and dendritic cells. IL-10 inhibits the TLR-MyD88 pathway, whereas IL-2 inhibits TLR-independent pathways.

The antimicrobial peptides within the inner mucus layer keep most of the microbiota from contacting the enterocytes and thus ensure that the microbiota remains within the intestinal lumen. They not only protect the host from microbial invasion but also from the potentially harmful inflammatory response that would occur if MAMPs are absorbed into the body (see Chapter 4).

ILC3 Cells

Group 3 innate lymphoid cells also regulate the interactions between the microbiota and its host (see Fig. 20.4). They respond to IL-23, IL-1β, and TSLP from dendritic cells by producing IL-17 and IL-22. These attract neutrophils and promote the production of antimicrobial peptides, especially REGIIIγ in the small intestine. REGIIIγ interacts with the mucus layer to maintain a relatively bacteria-free zone adjacent to the mucosal surface. ILC3 cells also activate B cells and induce IgA

BOX 22.1   The Aryl Hydrocarbon Receptor

The aryl hydrocarbon receptor (AhR) was originally identified as a transcription factor in the liver where it controls cellular responses to aromatic hydrocarbons such as dioxanes and bisphenols. It also regulates the enzymes that metabolize xenobiotics such as cytochrome p450. Its endogenous ligands include derivatives of tryptophan, indoles, and lipoxins. Dietary tryptophan is metabolized by *Lactobacilli* to generate indole-3-aldehyde, tryptamine, and indole, all of which are AhR ligands.

AhR also plays an important role in regulating immune responses. Thus it is expressed at high levels in antigen-presenting cells, intraepithelial lymphocytes, Th17, and Treg cells. Ligand binding to the AhR stimulates IL-23 production and Th17 differentiation. IL-22 from these cells enhances the production of antimicrobial peptides. The development of ILC3 cells also depends on AhR expression and activation.

AhRs are essential for the formation of intraepithelial lymphocytes, cryptopatches, and isolated lymphoid follicles. Defective AhR signaling results in severe intestinal inflammation and the development of allergies. Thus AhR-knockout mice mount enhanced Th2 responses and higher levels of IgE and IgG1. Their dendritic cells express high levels of CD86 and MHCII molecules. AhR signaling negatively affects the type 1 interferon response.

AhR ligands such as indoles and flavonoids are naturally found in cruciferous vegetables (cabbage, cauliflower, lettuce). These act through AhRs to maintain IELs and promote normal intestinal lymphoid function. AhRs also play an important role in resistance to *Pseudomonas aeruginosa, Mycobacterium tuberculosis, Listeria, Toxoplasma, Leishmania* and *Trypanosoma cruzi.*

From Hahn, M.E., 2002. Aryl hydrocarbon receptors: diversity and evolution. Chem. Biol. Interact. 141, 131–160.

production. They can promote tolerance to food antigens by producing GM-CSF that, in turn, promotes Treg production. Their production is regulated by the aryl hydrocarbon receptor as well as by butyrate generated by the intestinal microbiota (Box 22.1; Kim et al., 2017).

B Cells

There is more immune activity in the intestine than in all other lymphoid tissues combined. It has been estimated that more than 80% of the body's activated B cells are found in the intestine. Their function is to defend against possible invasion by the microbiota (and any ingested pathogens).

Although the microbiota are separated by the inner mucus layer and glycocalyx from direct contact with enterocytes, intestinal dendritic cells can extend their processes into the intestinal lumen and sample the microbiota. These bacteria persist within the dendritic cells for several days while the cells carry them into the mucosa and mesenteric lymph nodes and process and present them to B cells. In addition, some bacteria are taken up by specialized antigen-capturing M cells, penetrate the Peyer's patches, and become resident within the tissues. Although most of these invading bacteria are killed by macrophages, some are also presented to B cells. The B cells produce IgA, which may modify the composition of the microbiota and block further mucosal penetration. Bacteria are thus prevented from breaching the mucosal barrier by the ongoing IgA response, and the mesenteric lymph nodes form an additional barrier that prevents the commensals from reaching the systemic immune system. (The role of IgA is discussed in detail in Chapter 23; Mu et al., 2021.)

T Cells

The key to successful accommodation with the intestinal microbiota depends on the body's ability to control inflammation in the gut wall. This is achieved by maintaining a balance between proinflammatory Th17 cells and antiinflammatory Treg cells (Fig. 22.9).

Intestinal helper T-cell phenotypes are "plastic," and precursor cells can differentiate into either Treg or Th17 cells, while Th17 cells may further differentiate into Th1 cells. This differentiation is regulated by signals from the microbiota. In effect, the microbiota program the T-cell system to optimize its function. Additionally, helper T-cell differentiation is determined by cytokines. For example, the development of both Tregs and Th17 cells is promoted by TGF-β. Treg cells require TGF-β plus retinoic acid and IL-2, whereas Th17 cells require TGF-β plus IL-6 and IL-23. The major transcription factors used by Tregs and Th17 are Foxp3 and RORγt, respectively, and these are coexpressed in naïve and effector CD4+ cells.

Treg cells. Intestinal Treg cells are required to maintain the body's commensal relationship with its microbiota. Treg cells produce IL-10 as well as expressing high levels of CTLA-4 (cytotoxic T lymphocyte antigen 4), the inhibitory ligand for CD80. Treg production occurs in response to signals from both the microbiota and enterocytes. These Treg cells, when acted on by proinflammatory cytokines, can convert to IL-17 or IFN-γ-expressing effectors and so "break" tolerance. Under some circumstances, Th17 cells can give rise to IFN-γ producers that functionally resemble Th1 cells, and it is likely that many intestinal Th1 cells develop through this pathway. Under other circumstances, the Treg cells may convert to helper cells and promote the switch to IgA production. Indeed about 75% of the IgA reactive to the microbiota is produced through a pathway controlled by Treg cells.

Mucosal inflammation is therefore actively suppressed by the production of large numbers of IL-10-producing Foxp3+ Tregs. Under stable conditions, the production of Treg cells is favored while that of Th17 cells is suppressed. In the absence of Treg cells, uncontrolled effector T cells will respond to microbial antigens and trigger inflammatory bowel disease. IL-10-deficient mice develop chronic unremitting colitis driven by IL-23 and the Th17 pathway. It is also clear, however, that this tolerance can only go so far. Should a potential pathogen seek to invade the body from the intestine, then the immune system must be prepared to act aggressively in response. This is mediated by proinflammatory Th17 cells.

Th17 cells. As described in Chapter 15, Th17 cells are a subset of CD4+ T cells that regulate inflammation and maintain the intestinal epithelial barrier. Under the influence of IL-23, they produce the proinflammatory cytokines IL-17A, IL-17F, and IL-22. They also produce the antibacterial cytokine IL-26 (Fig. 22.10). Like Treg cells, the development of Th17 cells is regulated by signals from the microbiota and from enterocytes. Th17 cell development is specifically stimulated by the attachment of SFBs to enterocytes. Enterocytes can sense this tight attachment (Fig. 22.11; Ivanov et al., 2009). The mechanism by which this affects enterocytes is unclear, but it causes enterocytes to produce serum amyloid A (SAA; see Chapter 8). The SAA acts as a cytokine and stimulates IL-23 production by macrophages, leading to ILC3 secretion of IL-22 and -17. This, in turn, triggers the development of Th17 cells. Lamina propria macrophages and dendritic cells can also detect SFB-derived molecules through their TLRs and produce IL-23 and TGF-β, promoting further Th17 cell differentiation. As a result, the T cells differentiate into RORγt—expressing Th17 cells. Th17 cells, in turn, regulate the abundance of SFBs by promoting the production of antibacterial peptides such as β-defensins, lipocalins, and calprotectin by enterocytes.

SFB are unique spore-forming, long filamentous gram-positive anaerobic commensals found in the small intestine of mammals and birds. Their scientific name is "*Candidatus savagella.*" They have a unique ability to stimulate the maturation of T and B cells and especially stimulate Th17 responses and IgA production. They can also stimulate the upregulation of host innate defense genes, inflammatory cytokines, and lymphokines (Wu et al., 2010). They attach very strongly

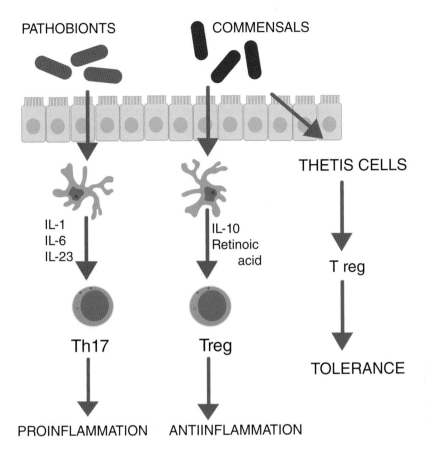

PATHOBIONTS

COMMENSALS

THETIS CELLS

IL-1
IL-6
IL-23

IL-10
Retinoic
acid

T reg

Th17

Treg

TOLERANCE

PROINFLAMMATION

ANTIINFLAMMATION

Fig. 22.9 The countervailing activities of regulatory T (Treg) and Th17 cells require a balanced microbiota to maintain health. Imbalances and dysbiosis can cause disturbances in both the digestive and immune systems. Note that Thetis cells are essential in promoting intestinal tolerance. *IL*, Interleukin.

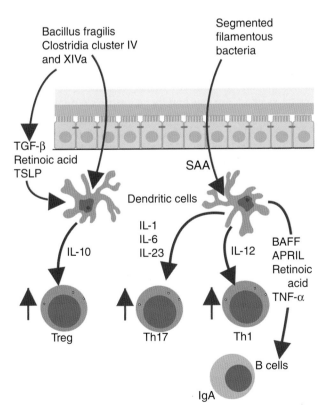

Bacillus fragilis
Clostridia cluster IV
and XIVa

Segmented
filamentous
bacteria

TGF-β
Retinoic acid
TSLP

SAA

Dendritic cells

IL-1
IL-6
IL-23

IL-12

BAFF
APRIL
Retinoic
acid
TNF-α

IL-10

Treg

Th17

Th1

B cells

IgA

Fig. 22.10 The role of segmented filamentous bacteria and Clostridial clusters in regulating T-cell subset formation and thus suppressing unwanted intestinal inflammation. *IgA*, Immunoglobulin A; *IL*, interleukin; *TGF-β*, transforming growth factor-β; *Tregs*, regulatory T cells; *TNF-α*, tumor necrosis factor-α.

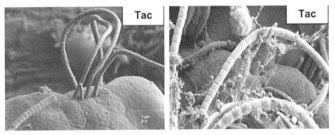

Fig. 22.11 A scanning electron micrograph of segmented filamentous bacteria in the terminal ileum of mice. From Ivanov, I.I., Atarashi, K., Manel, N., et al., 2009. Induction of intestinal Th17 cells by segmented filamentous bacteria. Cell 139, 485–498.

to the enterocytes of the terminal ileum and the cells overlying Peyer's patches where they are in a good position to be sampled by dendritic cells. (Most other bacteria remain within the mucus layer.) SFB induces the development of germinal centers in Peyer's patches and other intestinal lymphoid organs and increases the production of IgA and Th17 cells. In the absence of SFB, mice mount weaker IgA responses and poorer intestinal T-cell responses (Gaboriau-Routhiau et al., 2009).

Retinoic acid. Retinoic acid, the active metabolite of vitamin A, is a critical regulator of mucosal immunity. It is produced by intestinal epithelial cells. In association with transforming growth factor-β (TGF-β), it enhances T-cell proliferation and cytotoxicity and is especially important in promoting Th2 and Treg differentiation and in the homing of IgA+ B cells to mucosal surfaces (see Chapter 23). It is essential for maintaining the stability of Th1 cells and preventing their transition to Th17 cells. Retinoic acid normally suppresses Th17 responses and favors tolerance to food antigens. However, it also primes host defenses against intestinal infection (Woo et al., 2021).

Interleukin 22. IL-22 is produced by Th17 cells, activated T cells, and ILC3s in response to IL-23. IL-22-producing ILC3s are present in normal intestinal tissues, especially in cryptopatches (see Chapter 13). In herbivores, the IL-22 acts on nearby Paneth cells to release their granules rich in antimicrobial peptides (defensins, lipocalin, and calprotectin) and hence influences the composition of the microbiota. IL-22 acts on cells of the skin and the digestive and respiratory systems to increase the expression of several β-defensins and promotes innate immunity and repair in these tissues. It promotes enterocyte growth and survival.

DYSBIOSIS

It is clear from the above discussion that the gut microbiota exerts a significant influence on the systemic immune response. If this microbiota becomes unstable or imbalanced, dysbiosis occurs. Dysbiosis is a cause of equine laminitis, and ruminal acidosis, and has been implicated in the development of several immune-mediated diseases such as canine chronic enteropathy and inflammatory bowel diseases. Antibiotic treatment is an important cause of dysbiosis (Becattini et al., 2016). This can radically alter the composition of the intestinal microbiota and increase the risk of developing infections with organisms such as *Clostridium difficile* or overgrowth with other unwanted pathogens. Antibiotics alter the composition of the microbiota, resulting in an increased risk of obesity. (Obese individuals have more Firmicutes and fewer Bacteroides than lean ones). However, much remains to be learned about this very complex subject. Perhaps the most significant dysbiosis is that which leads to the development of allergies.

The role of the intestinal microbiota also extends to inflammatory diseases. For example, antibiotic-induced intestinal dysbiosis in mice affected circulating cytokine levels as well as the severity of ischemia/reperfusion injury on the heart. Oral vancomycin decreased circulating leptin levels, resulted in smaller myocardial infarcts, and improved functional recovery as compared to untreated controls. Modification of the gut microbiota by the probiotic *Lactobacillus plantarum* had a similar effect. Even oral antifungal drugs can disrupt the intestinal fungal microbiota in mice and increase the severity of airway allergic disease.

In critically ill animals, the breakdown of the intestinal epithelium and mucosal barriers may permit leakage of bacterial components into the body. Conversely, depletion of the gut microbiota, especially as a result of antibiotic treatment, can make the mucosal defenses vulnerable and perhaps reduce the priming of the systemic immune responses. It may therefore be advantageous to modulate the composition of the gut microbiota in some critically ill animals by the judicious use of probiotics (Box 22.2).

ODORS

Another way the microbiota affect their host is by increasing the diversity of the communication signals available to the host. Thus it is postulated that bacteria in mammalian scent glands as well as those in the mouth and the intestine, generate odorous metabolites such as SCFAs. Some of these odors are used for host communication. Variations in these host chemical signals may be a result of underlying variations in the microbiota of the scent glands. For example, surveys of the microbiota of hyaena scent glands suggest that variations in their microbiota correlate with the volume and fatty acid profiles of scent secretions. The bacterial populations also vary with species, gender, pregnancy, and reproductive state. In other mammals, odors are used for kin identification and mate choice. Given that genes for many odor receptors are linked to the MHC, it is not difficult to imagine how mammals recognize others of their species by the odors generated by their microbiota (Tizard and Skow, 2021).

BOX 22.2   Probiotics

Probiotics are cultures of live bacteria that when given orally may improve health by minimizing dysbiosis and its effects on the animal body. Provided the dose of these bacteria is large enough, the probiotics may change the composition of the microbiota at least for a time and thus influence the functions of the immune system. The results obtained depend not only on the dose of microbes administered but also on the specific strain or mixture of organism(s). *Lactobacilli* and *Bifidobacteria* are usually favored for probiotic use and appear to enhance resistance to diarrhea and respiratory tract infections. They possibly act by outcompeting pathogens. They may also reduce the severity of atopic disease. No single microbe is likely to solve all gastrointestinal problems, so it may be important to select the mixture of bacteria used with care. A widely employed technique involves oral administration of diluted feces or complex bacterial mixtures to outcompete Salmonellae in poultry and pigs. Fecal transplants have proven successful in treating *Clostridium difficile* infections in humans.

THE VIROME

The viral component of the microbiota is called the virome—the collection of all viruses found within an animal. They include not only eukaryotic viruses that cause infection and disease but also the endogenous viruses that are integrated into and form a significant component of mammalian genomes. This virome differs between individuals and may be even more diverse than the bacterial microflora. It has been estimated that the number of distinct viruses in human stool samples can range from 50 to almost 3000. In addition to mammalian viruses, the virome contains huge numbers of bacteriophages, perhaps as many as 100 phages for every bacterium. These phages prey on the bacteria and may play a role in transmitting genes between bacteria. When alterations in diet change the composition of the bacterial microflora, they also alter the composition of virome. This, in turn, can have effects on the host immune system (Neil and Cadwell, 2018).

Certain enteric viruses such as the noroviruses can influence the development of the enteric immune system. Thus they can restore intestinal morphology and lymphocyte function in germ-free mice. Conversely, the ability of noroviruses to persistently infect animals depends on the microbiota. Antibiotics prevent persistent norovirus infections by changing the composition of the microbiota. Removal of the virome with antiviral drugs can result in enteritis.

INFLAMMATORY BOWEL DISEASES

Chronic enteropathies with persistent clinical signs in domestic species such as dogs are a diverse group of diseases that result from a combination of genetic, microbial, nutritional, allergic, and environmental factors. Some resemble inflammatory bowel diseases in humans (Crohn's disease and ulcerative colitis), but most cases probably have a very different pathogenesis. Some result from dysbiosis and dysregulation of the immune responses to the intestinal microbiota (Xenoulis et al., 2008). As pointed out, commensal bacteria within the intestine are prevented from invading the intestinal wall by a glycocalyx, by high concentrations of defensins, and by an ongoing IgA response. They also suppress inflammation by blocking NF-κB activation and generating IL-10-secreting Treg cells. If these control mechanisms fail and the animal responds aggressively to its commensals, perhaps by increasing Th1 responses, then severe inflammation may result, making the intestine much more susceptible to bacteria-induced injury (Pilla and Suchodolski, 2021).

BOX 22.3 Thetis cells

As pointed out in the introduction, the immune system has to be selective in its responses. It must only respond to threats. It must not respond to normal body components otherwise autoimmunity will result. Likewise, strong immune responses to much of the intestinal microbiota and foods are best avoided. This gut immune tolerance to the microbiota and foods is mediated by a specialized population of antigen-presenting cells called Thetis cells. These Thetis cells are a unique class of RORγt⁺ antigen-presenting cells that are distinct from dendritic cells. When they present antigen, they induce the appearance of a population of peripheral Treg cells. (Fig. 22.9) They do this by removing self-reactive T cells in a manner similar to that in the thymus. As a result, the production of Th17 cells is suppressed hence maintaining oral tolerance and preventing the development of inflammatory bowel disease.

From Cannon, A.S., Sagadevan, A., Murugaiyan, G., 2022. Novel "Thetis" antigen-presenting cells promote early life immune tolerance. Immunol. Cell Biol. 1–4; Akagbosu, B., Tayyebi, Z., Shibu, G., et al., 2022. Novel-antigen presenting cell imparts Treg-dependent tolerance to gut microbiota. Nature 610, 752–760.

Canine chronic enteropathies are characterized by persistent or recurrent gastrointestinal inflammation of an undetermined cause. These diseases present with a history of chronic vomiting, diarrhea, and weight loss. There is a breed predisposition in Weimaranars, Rottweilers, German Shepherds, Border Collies, and Boxers. The most common form is a lymphocytic–plasmacytic enteritis.

Affected dogs may show an increase in Proteobacteria, especially *E. coli* or *Pseudomonas*, and a decrease in Firmicutes and Bacteroidetes. Other changes, such as increased bacterial adherence to the mucosa, reduced bacterial diversity, changes in the bacterial mixture, and overgrowth of other bacteria, may all contribute to the inflammation (Fig. 22.4).

Many cases are associated with an increase in T cells and IgA⁺ plasma cells in the small intestine. The T cells are primarily α/β CD4⁺ cells, although there may be an increase in intraepithelial γ/δ T cells as well. There may also be an increase in the number of intestinal mast cells. Some dogs with chronic enteropathy have reduced IgA levels in feces, duodenum, and blood. Hypoalbuminemia may reflect severe protein loss and carry a poor prognosis.

The affected small intestine shows increased messenger RNA for IL-12, IFN-γ, TNF-α, and TGF-β. In dogs, cases have been associated with altered expression or dysregulation of TLR-2, -4, and -5. Polymorphisms in TLR-4 and -5 have also been associated with disease susceptibility. Thus it has been suggested that excessive TLR activation might increase IL-1β levels. If this is accompanied by decreased production of its receptor antagonist, IL-1RA, then acute inflammation may result. The IL-1RA:IL-1 ratio in affected dogs is negatively correlated with disease severity. There is no evidence for changes in the IL-17 group of cytokines in these diseases in dogs. Likewise, there is no evidence of a Th1/Th2 imbalance in either dogs or cats. The expression of IL-12 does appear to be consistently increased.

It is convenient to divide these diseases into three subgroups based on their response to treatment.

Food-responsive enteropathies: In about 50% of cases, feeding a hypoallergenic or a novel-antigen diet may result in rapid clinical improvement within a few days and suggests that some forms of enteropathy result from food hypersensitivities.

Antibiotic-responsive enteropathies: Other forms may result from enteric infections, and some animals may respond well to antibiotic therapy. Drugs commonly used include oxytetracycline, metronidazole, and tylosin. These responsive dogs include young large-breed

animals and German Shepherds. The effects of antibiotic therapy may be short-lived.

Immunosuppression-responsive enteropathies: Some IBD cases are immunologically mediated, and dogs may respond well to glucocorticoids such as prednisolone and the immunosuppressive drugs such as cyclosporine or azathioprine. Unfortunately, the results of many clinical trials have been mixed and confusing, and long-term control remains difficult (Box 22.3).

REFERENCES

Arpaia, N., Rudensky, A.Y., 2014. Microbial metabolites control gut inflammatory responses. Proc. Natl. Acad. Sci. U.S.A. 111, 2058–2059.
Bach, J.-F., 2017. The hygiene hypothesis in autoimmunity: the role of pathogens and commensals. Nat. Rev. Immunol. https://doi.org/10.1038/nri.2017.111.
Becattini, S., Taur, Y., Pamer, E.G., 2016. Antibiotic-induced changes in the intestinal microbiota and disease. Trends Mol. Med. 22, 458–478.
Belkaid, Y., Hand, T.W., 2014. Role of the microbiota in immunity and inflammation. Cell 157, 121–141.
Blander, J.M., Longman, R.S., Iliev, I.D., Sonnenberg, G.F., Artis, D., 2017. Regulation of inflammation by microbiota interactions with the host. Nat. Immunol. 18, 851–860.
Costa, M.C., Silva, G., Ramos, R.V., Staempfli, H.R., et al., 2015. Characterization and comparison of the bacterial microbiota in different gastrointestinal tract compartments in horses. Vet. J. 205, 74–80.
Dang, A.T., Marsland, B.J., 2019. Microbes, metabolites, and the gut-lung axis. Mucosal Immunol. 12, 843–850.
Ennamorati, M., Vasudevan, C., Clerkin, K., et al., 2020. Intestinal microbes influence development of thymic lymphocytes in early life. Proc. Natl. Acad. Sci. U. S. A. 117, 2570–2578.
Gaboriau-Routhiau, V., Rakotobe, S., Lecuyer, E., Mulder, I., et al., 2009. The key role of segmented filamentous bacteria in the coordinated maturation of gut helper T cell responses. Immunity 31, 677–689.
Gensollen, T., Iyer, S.S., Kasper, D.L., Blumberg, R.S., 2016. How colonization by microbiota in early life shapes the immune system. Science 352, 539–544.
Hooda, S., Minamoto, Y., Suchodolski, J.S., Swanson, K.S., 2013. Current state of knowledge: the canine gastrointestinal microbiota. Anim. Health Res. Rev. 13, 78–88.
Ivanov, I.I., Atarashi, K., Manel, N., et al., 2009. Induction of intestinal Th17 cells by segmented filamentous bacteria. Cell 139, 485–498.
Kamada, N., Chen, G.Y., Inohara, N., Nunez, G., 2013a. Control of pathogens and pathobionts by the gut microbiota. Nat. Immunol. 14, 685–690.
Kamada, N., Seo, S.-U., Chen, G.Y., Nunez, G., 2013b. Role of the gut microbiota in immunity and inflammatory disease. Nat. Rev. Immunol. 13, 321–333.
Kim, S.-H., Cho, B.-H., Kiyono, H., Jang, Y.-S., 2017. Microbiota-derived butyrate suppresses group 3 innate lymphoid cells in terminal ileal Peyer's patches. Sci. Rep. https://doi.org/10.1038/s41598-017-02729-6.
Lambrecht, B.N., Hammad, H., 2017. The immunology of the allergy epidemic and the hygiene hypothesis. Nat. Immunol. 18, 1076–1083.
Liu, H., Hou, C., Li, N., Zhang, x, et al., 2019. Microbial and metabolic alterations in gut microbiota of sows during pregnancy and lactation. FASEB J. 33, 4490–4501.
Mu, Q., Swartwout, B.K., Edwards, M., Zhu, J., et al., 2021. Regulation of neonatal IgA production by the maternal microbiota. Proc. Natl. Acad. Sci. U.S.A. 118 (9) e2015691118
Neil, J.A., Cadwell, K., 2018. The intestinal virome and immunity. J. Immunol. 201, 1615–1624.
O'Dwyer, D.N., Dickson, R.P., Moore, B.B., 2016. The lung microbiome, immunity, and the pathogenesis of chronic lung disease. J. Immunol. 196, 4839–4847.
Older, C.E., Diesel, A., Patterson, A.P., et al., 2017. The feline skin microbiota: the bacteria inhabiting the skin of healthy and allergic cats. PLoS One 12 (6), E0178555. https://doi.org/10.1371/journal.pone.0178555.

Pilla, R., Suchodolski, J.S., 2021. The gut microbiome of dogs and cats and the influence of diet. Vet. Clin. Small Anim. https://doi.org/10.1016/j.cvsm.2021.01.002.

Pu, Q., Lin, P., Gao, P., Wang, Z., et al., 2021. Gut microbiota regulate gut-lung axis inflammatory responses by mediating ILC2 compartmental immigration. J. Immunol. 207, 1–11.

Rodrigues-Hoffmann, A., 2017. The cutaneous ecosystem: the roles of the skin microbiome in health and its association with inflammatory skin conditions in humans and animals. Vet. Dermatol. 28 60-e15.

Rodrigues-Hoffmann, A., Patterson, A.P., Diesel, A., et al., 2014. The skin microbiome in healthy and allergic dogs. PLoS One 9, e83197.

Rodrigues Hoffmann, A., Proctor, L.M., Surette, M.G., Suchodolski, J.S., 2016. The microbiome: the trillions of microorganisms that maintain health and cause disease in humans and companion animals. Vet. Pathol. 53, 10–21.

Ross, A.A., Rodrigues-Hoffmann, A., Neufeld, J.D., 2019. The skin microbiome of vertebrates. BMC Microbiome. https://doi.org/10.1186/s40168-019-0694-6.

Schulthess, J., Pandey, S., Capitani, M., Rue-Albrecht, K.C., et al., 2019. The short chain fatty acid butyrate imprints an antimicrobial program in macrophages. Immunity 50, 432–445.

Takeuchi, T., Miyauchi, E., Kanaya, T., Kato, T., et al., 2021. Acetate differentially regulates IgA reactivity to commensal bacteria. Nature 595, 560–564.

Tizard, I.R., Skow, L., 2021. The olfactory system: the remote sensing arm of the immune system. Anim. Health Res. Rev. https://doi.org/10.1017/s1466252320000262.

Van der Hee, B., Wells, J.M., 2021. Microbial regulation of host physiology by short-chain fatty acids. Trends Microbiol., 29. https://doi.org/10.1016/j.tim.2021.02.001.

Woo, V., Eshleman, E.M., Hashimoto-Hill, S., Whitt, J., et al., 2021. Commensal segmented filamentous bacteria-derived retinoic acid primes host defense to intestinal infection. Cell Host Microbe 29, 1744–1756.

Wu, H.-J., Ivanov, I.I., Darce, J., Hattori, K., et al., 2010. Gut-residing segmented filamentous bacteria drive autoimmune arthritis via helper Th17 cells. Immunity. https://doi.org/10.1016/j.immuni.2010.06.001.

Xenoulis, P.G., Palculict, B., Allenspach, K., Steiner, J., et al., 2008. Molecular phylogenetic characterization of microbial communities imbalances in the small intestine of dogs with inflammatory bowel disease. FEMS Microb. Ecol. 66, 579–589.

Xu, H., Liu, M., Cao, J., Li, X., et al., 2019. The dynamic interplay between the gut microbiota and autoimmune diseases. J. Immunol. Res. https://doi.org/10.1155/2019/7546047

Zeineldin, M., Lowe, J., Aldridge, B., 2019. Contribution of the mucosal microbiota to bovine respiratory health. Trends Microbiol. 27 (9), 753–770.

Immunity on Body Surfaces

Although mammals possess an extensive array of innate and adaptive defense mechanisms within tissues, it is at their surfaces that invading microorganisms are first encountered and largely repelled or destroyed (Fig. 23.1). Although the skin is the most obvious of these surfaces, it in fact represents only a small fraction of the area of the body exposed to the exterior. The surface areas of the mucous membranes of the intestine and respiratory tracts are at least 200 times larger. The majority of pathogens enter the body through mucosal surfaces when ingested or inhaled so respiratory and enteric infections are the major causes of death in young animals. While the immune system ensures that the interior of the body remains largely free of microbial invaders, it is not possible to keep the surfaces of the body sterile. Indeed, a huge microbiota live in a commensal relationship on body surfaces. As a result,

by far the greatest numbers of immune cells are found associated with the gastrointestinal tract or other body surfaces. The immune system functions on the basis that microorganisms that invade the body must be eliminated. Organisms that penetrate the epithelial barriers are promptly detected, attacked, and destroyed by innate and adaptive mechanisms.

IMMUNITY ON BODY SURFACES

The Defenses of the Skin

The skin is the first line of defense against many microbial invaders. Few bacteria can penetrate intact skin unaided. Skin forms a tough

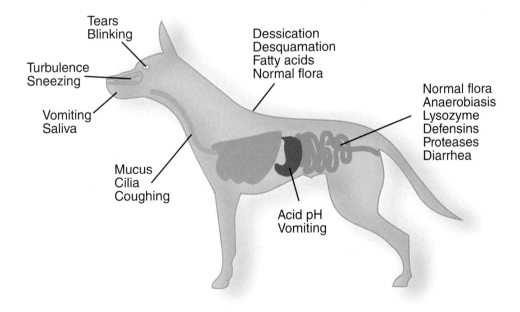

Fig. 23.1 The wide diversity of innate surface protection mechanisms.

physical barrier supplemented by continuous desquamation, desiccation, and a low pH because of the fatty acids in sebum. In addition, the skin carries a resident microbiota that excludes pathogenic bacteria and fungi. If the skin microbiota is disturbed, its protective properties are reduced, and microbial invasion may result. Thus skin infections tend to occur in areas such as the axilla or groin, where both pH and humidity are high. Similarly, animals forced to stand in water or mud show an increased frequency of foot infections as the skin becomes sodden, its structure breaks down, and its resident microbiota changes in response to alterations in the environment. Hair itself prevents desiccation and may protect against some fungal infections as well as being important in waterproofing and insulation.

Each layer of the skin has its own defensive mechanisms. For example, keratinocytes express multiple PRMs such as the toll-like receptors (TLRs), mannose receptors, and C-type lectins, so they are well able to recognize PAMPs associated with microbial invasion. Upon stimulation, keratinocytes produce a complex mixture of interleukins, interferons, chemokines, and other cytokines, growth factors, and antimicrobial peptides, all of which assist in excluding microbes seeking to penetrate the skin. Keratinocytes are the main source of cathelicidins and β-defensins (Wingate et al., 2009). Pigs, for example, have 11 different skin cathelicidins. Calprotectin is also produced in the skin. It is a metal chelator and restricts the availability of the essential trace elements Zn and Mn to bacteria. Mast cells and skin secretory cells such as sweat, apocrine, and sebaceous glands also contribute more antimicrobial peptides and lipids. Under normal conditions, keratinocyte precursor cells divide and continually renew the epidermis in a coordinated manner. If the skin is wounded or inflamed, alterations in adhesion molecules, surface receptors, and the cytokine environment change the behavior of these keratinocytes. Keratinocytes also express MHC class II molecules and can act as antigen-presenting cells (Afshar and Gallo, 2013).

Once they penetrate the skin, microbes are trapped by macrophages, neutrophils, and dendritic cells. Both the epidermis and dermis contain large numbers of antigen-trapping dendritic cells. The most important of these are Langerhans cells. Langerhans cells bind exogenous antigen and present it to nearby helper T cells. They account for 50%–70% of the dendritic cells in pig epithelium. The dermis also contains resident DCs, as does the subcutaneous adipose tissue layer (Coates et al., 2018).

Skin-resident T cells are mainly located in the basal layer associated with Langerhans cells. CD4+ and CD8+ cells are present in equal numbers. In humans and mice, these are predominantly α/β T cells. In some domestic mammals many are γ/δ T cells. The three major helper T-cell subsets are also present.

The microbiota regulates the development of immunity in the skin and intestine. For example, *Staphylococcus epidermidis* induces Th17 cells in the skin and these cells are regulated by the skin microbiota. A subset of circulating T cells that home to the skin and produce IL-22 (Th22 cells) have also been identified. IL-22 plays an important role in maintaining barrier function on exposed body surfaces (Sonnenberg et al., 2011). It promotes antimicrobial immunity, inflammation, and tissue repair. Treg cells are present in the skin where they facilitate cutaneous wound healing by enhancing local production of the epithelial growth factor receptor (Gallo and Hooper, 2012). They also promote tolerance to many skin commensal organisms, especially those living within hair follicles (Ali and Rosenblum, 2017).

Ruminant γ/δ T cells recirculate continuously between epithelial surfaces such as the skin or intestinal epithelium and the bloodstream. In sheep, they predominate in skin near the basal layer of the epidermis and in the dermis close to hair follicles and sebaceous glands. They are uncommon in wool-covered skin but are present in large numbers in bare and hairy skin. In cattle, for example, 44% of dermal T cells are γ/δ positive. They are also found in the epithelium of the tongue, esophagus, trachea, and bladder. γ/δ T cells are a major population in skin-draining afferent lymph. They can produce both interferon-γ (IFN-γ) and IL-17 and they express high levels of the skin-seeking molecule, E-selectin. They survey the skin and inflammatory sites when attracted by CCR6 and E-selectin ligands. B cells are also present in the skin so skin washings contain immunoglobulins. For example, in cattle, serum IgM, IgG1, and IgG2 cross the skin by transudation, but the IgA is locally synthesized.

Immunity in the Mammary Gland

The protective mechanisms of the udder are presumably not at their most effective in that biological anomaly, the modern dairy cow. Most infections result from invasion through the teat canal and subsequent bacterial growth in the teat cistern and mammary tissue. In a nonlactating animal, a keratin plug blocks the teat orifice and excludes bacteria. In a lactating animal, the flushing action of the milk helps to prevent invasion by some potential pathogens, while milk itself contains many innate antibacterial molecules (Wellnitz and Bruckmaier, 2012). These include complement, lysozyme, lactoferrin, and lactoperoxidase. Lactoferrin competes with bacteria for iron and makes it unavailable for bacterial growth. It also enhances the neutrophil respiratory burst. Milk contains lactoperoxidase and thiocyanate (SCN^-) ions. In the presence of exogenous hydrogen peroxide, lactoperoxidase can oxidize the SCN^- to bacteriostatic products such as $OSCN^-$.

$$H_2O_2 + SCN^- \rightarrow OSCN^- + H_2O$$

The hydrogen peroxide may be produced by bacteria such as streptococci or by the oxidation of ascorbic acid. Bacterial lipopolysaccharides can also trigger local production of lipopolysaccharide-binding protein and soluble CD14 in the mammary gland. As described in Chapter 2, both these proteins enhance LPS-induced cell activation by promoting its binding to TLR4.

The mammary gland epithelium consists not only of layers of epithelial cells but also intraepithelial leukocytes, dendritic cells, macrophages, and lymphocytes. The epithelial cells express pattern-recognition molecules such as TLRs and NODs and are able to respond to invading microbes. Defensive responses include the production of defensins as well as inflammatory cytokines and chemokines (Rainard et al., 2022).

Phagocytic cells that enter the gland in response to inflammation also contribute to antimicrobial resistance. They express PRMs, especially TLRs. Their activation by invading bacteria triggers the production of TNF-α, IL-1β, and IL-8 and results in clinical mastitis. Thus these cells are not only actively phagocytic (Fig. 6.11), but they also release lactoferrin, hydrogen peroxide, and lysosomal peroxidases. The binding of bovine lactoferrin to *Streptococcus agalactiae* can activate C1q. Experimental mastitis induced by inoculation of *E. coli* into the udder results in increased concentrations of IL-6, IL-22, TNF-α, and IL-10 in milk. There is also a significant increase in Th17 cells within infected glands. Infusion of IL-17A at the onset of infection is associated with decreased bacterial numbers, decreased IL-10 production, and increased neutrophil recruitment.

Milk also contains IgA, secretory component, and IgG1. The IgA and secretory component are closely associated with the milk fat globules. In simple-stomach animals, IgA predominates, whereas in ruminants, IgG1 does. IgA is synthesized in the mammary tissue, although many of the IgA-producing B cells in the gland are derived from precursors originating in the intestine. These cells are a source of antibodies against intestinal pathogens. Colostral IgG1, in contrast, is selectively transferred by active transport from serum using the FcRn receptor on mammary gland epithelial cells (see Fig. 24.6).

If an antigen is infused into a lactating mammary gland, it tends to be promptly flushed out again in the milk. If it is infused into a nonlactating gland, a local antibody response develops. Because of the continuous removal of milk, antibody concentrations remain low (<100 mg/dL) even though, over a period of time, the total amount of immunoglobulin produced in the udder may be considerable. In acute mastitis, the inflammatory response leads to the influx of actively phagocytic cells, especially neutrophils, and to the exudation of serum proteins. As a result, immunoglobulin levels in mastitic milk may rise to levels at which they can exert a protective effect (~8000 mg/dL).

Because the local immune response in the udder is relatively ineffective in preventing infection, attempts to vaccinate against mastitis-causing organisms have been generally unsuccessful. Nevertheless, recent advances have produced encouraging results. Thus a *Staphylococcus aureus* vaccine that stimulates the production of antibodies against the bacterial pseudocapsule appears to be effective. This pseudocapsule interferes with the ability of milk leukocytes to phagocytose *S. aureus*. Antibodies induced by the vaccine promote opsonization and destruction of the bacteria. A vaccine designed to stimulate antibody production against staphylococcal α toxin, as well as the pseudocapsule, is also effective. Encouraging results have also been obtained by the use of a J5 mutant vaccine against coliform bacteria (see Chapter 26). The vaccine is given to cattle at drying off, 30 days later, and at calving.

Colostrum is rich in macrophages and lymphocytes. These macrophages can process antigen, and when cultured, their supernatants can enhance IgA production from blood lymphocytes. Milk lymphocytes survive for a short time in the calf intestine and can transfer cell-mediated immunity to the newborn animal (see Chapter 24).

Immunity in the Respiratory Tract

The respiratory tract differs from other external surfaces in that it is in intimate connection with the interior of the body yet is required to allow unhindered access of air to the alveoli. The system obviously requires a filter. Particles suspended in inhaled air are largely removed by turbulence that directs them onto its mucus-covered walls, where they adhere. The turbulence is caused by the conformation of the turbinate bones, the trachea, and the bronchi. This turbulence filter serves to remove particles as small as 5 μm before they reach the alveoli (Fig. 23.2; Iwasaki et al., 2016).

A blanket of mucus gel produced by goblet cells lines the upper respiratory tract. The mucus contains soluble host defense molecules such as lysozyme, lactoferrin, surfactant proteins, and cationic peptides such as the defensins and cathelicidins (Christmann et al., 2009). Most microorganisms trapped in the mucus layer are killed rapidly. There are four major surfactant proteins in lung fluid (SP-A, -B, -C, -D) produced by alveolar type II cells. SP-B and -C are extremely hydrophobic. Their function is to reduce surface tension at the alveolar surface so that a thin film of fluid forms on the surface and prevents lung collapse. SP-A and -D, in contrast, are C-type lectins that bind to microbial surface carbohydrates and act as opsonins. SP-A and -D also activate macrophages, promote chemotaxis, enhance the respiratory burst, and the production of inflammatory cytokines. These surfactant proteins also enhance the clearance of apoptotic cells from the lung. This is especially important in the resolution of inflammation since apoptotic neutrophils must be removed by macrophages as promptly as possible. Surfactant proteins can also modulate the functions of dendritic cells and T cells. SP-A inhibits the maturation of dendritic cells, whereas SP-D enhances their uptake and presentation of antigen. Both SP-A and SP-D inhibit T-cell proliferation (Wright, 2005).

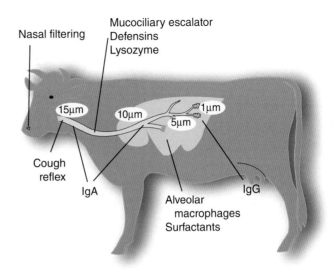

Fig. 23.2 Some of the innate mechanisms involved in the protection of the respiratory tract against infection and the influence of particle size on the site of deposition of particles within the respiratory tract. Note that only the smallest particles can penetrate deeply and gain access to the lung alveoli. *IgA*, Immunoglobin A.

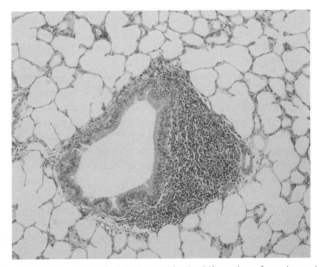

Fig. 23.3 A lymphoid follicle located in the bifurcation of an airway in a calf lung. This type of bronchus-associated lymphoid tissue is a key component of the defenses of the respiratory tract. From a specimen kindly provided by Drs. McArthur, N.H. and Abbott, L.C.

The respiratory mucus layer is in continuous flow, being carried from the bronchioles up the bronchi and trachea by ciliary action or backward through the nasal cavity to the pharynx. Here, the dirty mucus is swallowed and digested in the intestinal tract. Particles that bypass this mucociliary escalator and reach the alveoli are phagocytosed by alveolar macrophages. Once these cells have successfully ingested particles, they migrate to the mucus escalator and are also carried to the pharynx.

The respiratory tract contains bronchial lymphoid nodules as well as lymphocytes distributed diffusely throughout the lung and airways (Fig. 23.3). The mucosa of the larynx contains many immunologically active cells, including a large number of T cells. Antigen-sampling M cells may be associated with these lymphoid nodules as well as with

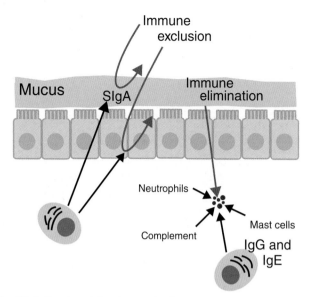

Fig. 23.4 Two key defensive mechanisms are employed on mucosal surfaces. The most important is immune exclusion, an effect primarily mediated by immunoglobin (Ig) A. If antigens gain access to the mucosa, they are destroyed through IgG- and IgE-mediated processes by immune elimination. *SIgA*, Secretory IgA.

TABLE 23.1   Composition of Cells in Canine Bronchoalveolar Lavage Fluid

Cell	Percentage (Range)
Macrophages	79.4 (71–87)
Lymphocytes	13.5 (7–20)
Eosinophils	3.6 (0–14)
Mast cells	2.1 (0–5)
Epithelial cells	0.8 (0–6)
Neutrophils	0.6 (0–2)
Lymphocyte Percentages	
T cells	52.0 (34–69)
CD4+	21.9 (10–32)
CD8+	17.8 (6–25)
CD4/CD8 ratio	1.3 (0.8–2.4)

From Vail, D.M., Mahler, P.A., Soergel, S.A., 1995. Differential cell analysis and phenotypic subtyping of lymphocytes in bronchoalveolar lavage fluid from clinically normal dogs. Am. J. Vet. Res. 56, 282–285.

nasal mucosal lymphoid tissues. Tonsils form a ring around the pharynx (Waldeyer's ring) (Barker et al., 2006). These tissues mainly produce secretory IgA, especially in the upper regions of the respiratory tract (Pabst and Gehrke, 1990). This IgA binds to mucus through secretory component and so enhances the clearance of adherent bacteria. The polymeric immunoglobulin receptor (pIgR) is expressed at low levels in bronchial epithelial cells. In the bronchioles and alveoli, however, the secretions contain a large proportion of IgG, the concentration of which is intermediate between the levels in the trachea and in serum. IgE is also synthesized in significant amounts in the lymphoid tissues of the upper respiratory tract. As on other body surfaces, IgA in the respiratory tract probably protects by immune exclusion, whereas IgG and IgE act by immune elimination (see Fig. 23.4).

Many cells may be washed out of the airways of the lung with saline. In normal dogs, about 80% of bronchoalveolar cells obtained in this way are macrophages, and 13% are lymphocytes, of which about half are T cells (Table 23.1). In healthy horses, about 50% of the cells in bronchoalveolar washes are macrophages, 40% are lymphocytes, and 2% are neutrophils. In sheep, B cells are less than 10% of the lung lymphocyte population. Lung T cells can produce cytokines, and alveolar macrophages are activated following infection with *Listeria monocytogenes*. Cell-mediated immune reactions are therefore readily provoked among the cells within the lower respiratory tract (Pickles et al., 2002).

Alveolar macrophages reside on alveolar surfaces where they are in direct contact with the air. When they respond to invaders, it is essential that they do not interfere with gas exchange. A full-scale inflammatory response is to be avoided whenever possible. Thus, in the absence of infection, alveolar macrophages are quiescent and tend to suppress local cytokine production. They are, however, highly phagocytic (Karagianni et al., 2013).

The lungs of most domestic species (pigs, horses, sheep, goats, cattle, and cats) differ from rodent, human, or dog lungs in that they contain large numbers of intravascular macrophages (see Chapter 7). It has been estimated that these macrophages cover 16% of the lung capillary surface in young pigs. As a result, the lungs of these species can remove more bacteria from the blood than can the liver and spleen. A dense network of dendritic cells is also found within the airway epithelium and alveoli (Iwasaki et al., 2016).

Although it has long been believed that the respiratory tract was sterile, it too has a normal bacterial microbiota. The composition of this microbiota has a direct influence on the development of allergic respiratory disease (see Chapter 22). The lung is exposed to an array of microorganisms with the very first breath an animal takes. Despite this, it does not develop extensive inflammation. The early defense of the lung is almost totally dependent on innate antimicrobial molecules. The inhaled organisms trigger signaling cascades that result in the generation of surfactants, defensins, interferons, lactoferrin, and oxidants. These are critical protective factors.

Immunity in the Urogenital Tract

In the urinary system, the flushing action and low pH of urine generally provide adequate protection; however, when urinary stasis occurs, urethritis and cystitis resulting from the unhindered ascent of pathogenic bacteria are not uncommon.

The female reproductive tract can be divided into a lower (vagina and cervix) and an upper part (uterus and fallopian tubes). The lower part is covered by stratified squamous epithelium, and the upper by columnar epithelium. All are covered by microbiocidal mucus (Johansson and Hansson, 2016). Within the lower part, the keratinocytes express PRMs and produce cytokines and antimicrobial peptides. The upper part contains large numbers of macrophages, dendritic cells, and innate lymphoid cells. The predominant immunoglobulin in cervicovaginal mucus is IgA, whereas within the uterus, it is IgG. If bacteria such as *Campylobacter fetus* infect the genital tract, vaginal IgA antibodies immobilize and agglutinate the organisms. If the mucous membrane becomes inflamed, IgG antibodies from serum will also assist in protection. Surfactant protein A is also important in protecting the vagina from infection. *C. fetus* infections are associated with the presence of many mononuclear cells as well as delayed skin reactions (type IV hypersensitivity) so that cell-mediated immunity is also involved in resistance to this local infection. Similar local immune responses may also be directed against other organisms that infect the cervix and vagina, and the presence of agglutinating antibodies in vaginal mucus may be used as a diagnostic test for brucellosis, campylobacteriosis, and trichomoniasis. (The local immune response to trichomoniasis is largely mediated by IgE; see Chapter 29.) IgG also reaches the uterine lumen and the vagina by active transport mediated by FcRn. This receptor is pH dependent. It binds IgG in the tissues where the pH is high and releases it in the vagina where the pH is very low.

A type I interferon, designated interferon-ε, is expressed in the epithelial cells of the female reproductive tract (Fung et al., 2013). IFN-ε induces typical IFN-regulated genes. It is not, however, induced by the conventional pattern-recognition pathways involving receptors such as the TLRs. Instead, it is constitutively expressed and hormonally regulated. IFN-ε-deficient mice show increased susceptibility to sexually transmitted infections such as herpes simplex 2 and *Chlamydia muridarum*, suggesting that this interferon plays a role in protecting the female reproductive tract. IFN-ε has been identified in humans, cattle, pigs, and dogs (Guo et al., 2015).

Antimicrobial peptides are found in the testes, seminal vesicles, and prostate. Epithelial cells lining the urethra express PRMs, while macrophages and dendritic cells are abundant. IgG is the predominant immunoglobulin in seminal plasma and IgA is also present. The B cells that produce these immunoglobulins are mainly found in the penile urethra and prostate. T cells are also abundant in the urethra, testes, and prepuce. Preputial washings of bulls infected with *C. fetus* may contain IgG1 antibodies with some IgM and IgA. IgA is present in small amounts in normal urine, produced presumably by B cells in the walls of the urinary tract.

Immunity in the Gastrointestinal Tract

The gastrointestinal mucosal defense system can be considered to consist of four components. The microbiota; the mucus layer, the mucosal epithelium, and the mucosal-associated lymphoid tissues. All four interact in such a way that the intestine serves as a barrier to infection while at the same time serving as a hospitable environment for the commensal microbiota.

The layer of enterocytes lining the gastrointestinal tract is the largest surface between the body and the external environment. Thus the gastrointestinal tract, from mouth to anus is a potential route of microbial invasion. This includes not only potential pathogens but also the commensals of the normal microbiota. It must be able to respond rapidly to enteric invaders while, at the same time being tolerant of some foreign proteins such as those in food and on beneficial commensals (Allensbach, 2011).

Saliva is rich in IgA and hence protects the mouth against infections. Small amounts of IgG are secreted into the crevicular groove between the gums and the base of the teeth. As a result, it has proved possible to make a vaccine against caries-causing bacteria (Box 23.1). Immunization of dogs with these organisms reduces microbial colonization of this area and prevents plaque formation and periodontitis. The flushing activity of saliva may be complemented by the generation of peroxidases from streptococci. The tonsils also produce much IgA, but because of the thin epithelium over the tonsillar clefts, they are very vulnerable to microbial invasion (Fig. 23.5).

In single-stomached animals, the gastric pH may be sufficiently low to have an antimicrobial effect, although this varies among species and among meals. The dog, for instance, has a low gastric pH relative to that of the pig. Similarly, the pH in the center of a mass of ingested food may not necessarily drop to low levels, and some foods such as milk are potent buffers. In addition to antimicrobial peptides, lysozyme is synthesized in the gastric mucosa and in macrophages within the intestinal mucosa. As a result, it is found in large quantities in intestinal fluid.

In the small intestine, the separation of the microbiota and enterocytes is maintained by a layer of mucus containing multiple antimicrobial peptides. In the large intestine, this separation is maintained by two distinct layers of mucus. The inner layer is almost bacteria-free. The outer loose layer contains large numbers of bacteria. In the developing

BOX 23.1 Periodontal Disease

Gingivitis and progressive chronic periodontitis are common diseases in animals. The tissue damage that occurs in periodontal disease is mediated by cells of the immune and inflammatory systems. The disease is triggered by many oral bacteria, the most important of which is *Porphyromonas gingivalis*. But the tooth microbiota are diverse, and the composition of the population varies over time. These bacteria form biofilms on the surface of dental plaque. The PAMPs from these bacteria act through TLRs and other PRRs to attract neutrophils. The neutrophils, however, cannot phagocytose biofilms, so they undergo abortive phagocytosis and release their contents into the tissues (see Chapter 33). These released enzymes, especially collagenases, initiate progressive tissue destruction. In addition, local mast cells secrete TNF-α that contributes to neutrophil immigration. The gingival fluid contains complement components, especially C3a and C5a. The biofilm ensures that inflammation persists, and chronic inflammation leads to chronic tissue destruction. Neutrophils are followed by macrophages and lymphocytes by about 4–7 days. By day 21, lymphocytes are 70% of the cellular infiltrate and are mainly T cells. CD4+ cells increase progressively through the course of the disease, and the lesion resembles a delayed hypersensitivity reaction (see Chapter 34). Th1 and Th17 populations predominate. The Th17 cells produce a cytokine mixture that promotes bone resorption. IL-17 especially promotes osteoclast activation, while IL-10 and TGFβ1 are downregulated. IL-1β and IFN-γ from the Th1 cells also promote osteoclast production and bone resorption. Since both Treg and Th17 cells are present in inflamed periodontal tissues, it is believed that an imbalance in these T-cell populations, especially a deficiency in Treg cells, contributes to the chronic inflammatory process. For example, both IL-17 and IL-35 are expressed in inflamed periodontal tissue, and it has been demonstrated that if Treg populations in dogs with experimental periodontal disease are enhanced, the progress of disease is slowed. The bone resorption and soft tissue destruction are mediated by host matrix metalloproteases and collagenases. The matrix metalloproteases degrade extracellular matrix especially type I collagen, and basement membrane components in the periodontal supporting tissues. Oxidative and proteolytic activation cascades develop that destroy both tissues and bone and give rise to the gross lesions associated with periodontal disease (Glowacki et al., 2013).

From Ohlrich, E. J., Cullinan, M. P., Seymour, G. J., 2009. The immunopathogenesis of periodontal disease. Aust. Dent. J. 54 (Suppl. 1), S2–10.

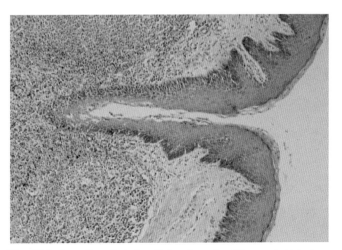

Fig. 23.5 A section of pig tonsil showing a tonsillar crypt. Note how thin the epithelium is at the base of the crypt. This is an easy invasion route for many organisms. Original magnification ×150. Courtesy Dr. S. Yamashiro.

animal, it takes time for these mucus layers to develop, and this provides a window of opportunity for organisms such as segmented filamentous bacteria (SFB) to reach and bind enterocytes.

The first cellular barrier to microbial invasion is the intestinal epithelium (Rescigno, 2011). This consists of enterocytes, goblet cells, and Paneth cells (in herbivores) (Fig. 23.6). Collectively, these cells form an effective physical barrier by having tight junctions between cells and a coating of mucin glycoproteins that form a glycocalyx. In addition to the goblet cells that produce the mucus, enterocytes can produce a diverse mixture of antimicrobial peptides that limit microbial exposure. In the small intestine, these are predominantly α-defensins and RegIIIα and β, while in the colon these are mainly β-defensins and cathelicidins (see Chapter 4).

Paneth cells are specialized intestinal epithelial cells in herbivores such as horses and cattle that express TLRs (Fig. 23.7). When triggered by MAMPs, they secrete large quantities of α-defensins. Most of these defensins are amphipathic molecules that act like detergents. They insert themselves into microbial cell walls, cause bacterial lysis, and interfere with bacterial lipid synthesis. One defensin, the α-6 defensin acts in a very different manner. It does not have direct antibacterial effects but when released from the Paneth cell granules, it assembles spontaneously into elongated molecular networks—nanonets—that surround, entangle, and entrap bacteria. Presumably, by so doing, they help protect the intestinal surface from bacterial invasion (Ouellette and Selsted., 2012).

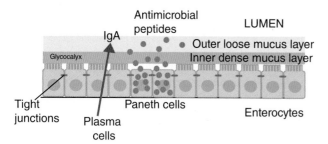

Fig. 23.6 Some of the mechanisms involved in the protection of mucosal surfaces. Paneth cells produce antimicrobial peptides, plasma cells produce Immunoglobin A (IgA) while enterocytes, mucus layers, and the glycocalyx form a protective barrier.

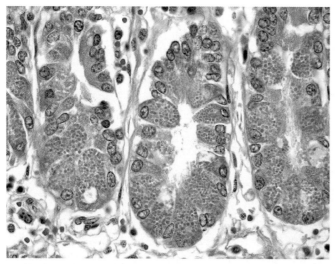

Fig. 23.7 Paneth cells from the intestine of a horse. The cells are filled with large eosinophilic granules and are the major source of intestinal defensins. Original magnification ×60. Courtesy Dr. Brian Porter.

Enteric defensins accumulate within intestinal crypts and achieve very high concentrations in the mucus layer closest to the epithelium. They serve a barrier function since they prevent commensals from entering the crypt space and so reduce microbial contact with enterocytes. The defensin mixture selectively kills some bacterial species and as a result also regulates the composition of the microbiota. In cattle, expression of defensin genes occurs throughout the small intestine and colon. Bovine defensins are secreted as active molecules, as opposed to the human and mouse molecules that are secreted as inactive precursors and subsequently activated by trypsin within the intestine. Parasitic or other intestinal infections may increase the production of α- and β-defensins (Vaishnava et al., 2008).

Enterocytes possess a complete set of PRRs and can sense signals coming from the microbiota. They can then pass on these signals to the immune cells in the lamina propria and are actively involved in shaping the intestinal immune environment. They help maintain balance between anti- and proinflammatory signals. They also block access of intact antigens to the lamina propria. Tight junctions between enterocytes help maintain this barrier. (Molecules larger than about 2 kDa are excluded.) Thus, they keep the intestinal microbes away from the intestinal immune system. Enterocytes secrete or respond to regulatory cytokines. They produce thymic stromal lymphopoietin (TSLP) that is required for the generation of Tregs. They also produce TGF-β and the B cell–stimulating molecules, BAFF and APRIL (see Box 16.2). The enterocytes form a major barrier against microbial invasion. If an enterocyte becomes infected, it can respond by releasing antimicrobial peptides and increasing mucin and cytokine production. It can also respond by undergoing pyroptosome-mediated cell death. This mechanism is used by enterocytes to block invasion of *Salmonella enterica* serovar Typhimurium. Pyroptosomes are protein activation complexes, that can trigger a form of cell death called pyroptosis (see Box 19.1). When *S. typhimurium* invades enterocytes, the number of intracellular bacterial colonies increases for the first twelve hours and then begins to decline at 18 hours. This decline is correlated with the shedding of infected enterocytes into the lumen. At the same time, pyroptosome activation also results in cytokine release that in turn activates Th17 cells and promotes local inflammation (Perez-Lopez et al., 2016).

The gastrointestinal mucus layer is also critical to the exclusion of both commensals and pathogens (Chase and Kaushik, 2019). The layer consists of a gel composed of mucins, glycoproteins, and lipids that prevent bacteria from contacting the epithelium. This mucus acts as a lubricant, blocks chemical insults, and can trap and then expel pathogens. The mucus forms an inner and outer layer. The inner layer next to the enterocytes consists of firm mucus rich in defensins and lysozyme and contains few bacteria. The looser mucus in the intestinal lumen is composed primarily of mucins produced by intestinal goblet cells. Many bacteria are embedded in this mucus, where it prevents their washout. Its thickness and composition vary, but it tends to be thickest where the microbiota is abundant. The enterocyte brush border is also covered by the glycocalyx, a layer of acidic polysaccharides and glycoproteins that binds to the apical surface of the cells and serve as a protective barrier while still permitting the absorption of nutrients.

Goblet cells are the source of intestinal mucus. Both the inflammasome and autophagy pathways control the production of this mucus. In the absence of inflammasomes, mucus production is reduced, and mice develop severe colonic inflammation. Upon consideration, this should not come as a surprise to most people, especially veterinarians. Mucus secretion increases greatly in response to mucosal inflammation—it's called a "runny nose".

Recent evidence suggests that some antigens can penetrate the intestinal epithelium by way of goblet cell–associated antigen passages (GAPs!).

MUCOSAL LYMPHOID TISSUES

Because of the importance of preventing invasion through the mucosa, these surfaces contain large amounts of lymphoid tissue. Mucosal lymphoid tissues fall into two groups; sites where antigens are processed and immune responses are initiated (inductive sites), and sites where antibodies and cell-mediated responses are generated (effector sites).

Inductive Sites

The mucosa-associated lymphoid tissues possess the three cell types required to initiate adaptive immune responses: T cells, B cells, and dendritic cells. These tissues include lymphoid tissues in the nasal mucosa, tonsils, pharynx, tongue, and palate; Peyer's patches; solitary lymphoid nodules; the appendix in some mammals; and numerous lymphoid nodules in the lung. These lymphoid tissues are known by their acronyms. Thus GALT (gut-associated lymphoid tissue) is the collective term for all the lymphoid nodules, Peyer's patches, and individual lymphocytes found in the intestinal walls. Similarly, BALT is the acronym used for the bronchus-associated lymphoid tissue in the lungs. These organized lymphoid tissues, unlike lymph nodes, do not react to foreign antigens delivered through afferent lymph but rather sample them directly from the mucosal surface (Liebler-Tenorio and Pabst, 2006).

The tonsils are especially important in inducing immunity on mucosal surfaces. Some organisms, however, can overcome the defenses of the tonsils and use them as a portal of entry into the body. For example, pathogens such as bovine herpesvirus-1, *Mannheimia hemolytica*, *Streptococcus suis*, and *Mycobacterium tuberculosis* can persist indefinitely within the tonsils.

Peyer's patches are the most significant of the mucosal lymphoid tissues. A newborn calf normally has about 100 Peyer's patches, and these may cover as much as half of the ileal surface. In ruminants and pigs, there are two types of Peyer's patch that differ in location, structure, and functions. The ileocecal Peyer's patches are primary lymphoid organs in some species, whereas the jejunal Peyer's patches are secondary lymphoid organs (see Fig. 13.7). In lambs, the ileocecal patches increase in size from birth to 6 months of age and then regress, leaving only a small scar. In contrast, the jejunal patches persist throughout adult life and continue to play a major role in intestinal defense. Both types of Peyer's patch consist of masses of lymphocytes arranged in follicles and covered with an epithelium that contains microfold (M) cells. M cells are specialized epithelial cells involved in antigen transportation. They have microfolds rather than microvilli on their surface (Fig. 23.8). The mucus layer tends to thin out over Peyer's patches so that the M cells protrude into the lumen. M cells endocytose the proteins and microbes they encounter, but rather than destroy them, they transport the antigens to their underlying lymphoid tissue. M cells may also transport soluble macromolecules such as IgA, small particles, and even whole organisms. (Some pathogens, such as salmonellae, *Yersinia* and *Listeria*, *M. avium* ssp. *paratuberculosis*, and the reoviruses may take advantage of the M cells and use them to gain access to the body.) The proportion of M cells in the follicle-associated epithelium varies from less than 10% in humans and mice to 50% in rabbits and 100% in the terminal ileum of pigs and calves.

Artiodactyls possess gut-associated lymphoid tissues that develop at the distal end of the ileum during fetal life. They contain ~90% B cells with very few T cells and involute within weeks after birth. A similar lymphoid organ called the sacculus rotundus is present in rabbits. It was long believed that these lymphoid organs in the lower hind gut are the primary lymphoid organs where B cells develop. However, recent studies on piglets have cast doubt on this. Removal of the piglet ileal Peyer's patch does not result in a B cell deficiency such as would occur

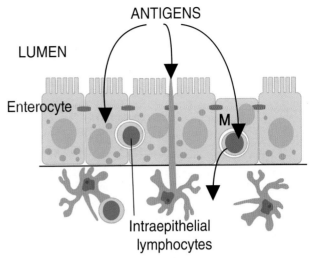

Fig. 23.8 The role of M cells and dendritic cells as antigen-processing cells in the intestinal wall. Antigen that enters enterocytes is usually rapidly degraded in lysosomes. Antigen that enters M cells is not degraded. It may be presented directly to intraepithelial lymphocytes within the M cell or, alternatively, permitted to pass along the intercellular space to the tissue fluid. From here, it will be carried to the draining lymph nodes.

in a bursectomized bird. There are no differences in B cell diversity, distribution or repertoire in piglets where this organ has been removed. In addition, there is no evidence that B cell diversification occurs within this organ. Evidence now suggests that in pigs at least, the ileal Peyer's patch is a secondary lymphoid organ that regulates the initial microbial colonization of the lower bowel. There may be no discrete organ equivalent to the bursa in this species.

Many dietary components have a profound effect on the organization and maintenance of intestinal immune tissues. For example, vitamin A metabolites play a role in the differentiation and functioning of B and T-cell subsets. Likewise, dietary vitamin D alters B and Th responses, inhibiting Th1 and enhancing Th2 activity. Dietary lipids influence prostaglandin and leukotriene synthesis and so modify inflammatory responses. Collectively, these and other dietary components play a key role in ensuring that the intestinal lymphoid tissues function optimally.

Effector Sites

Although Peyer's patches are full of lymphocytes, most IgA is produced in diffuse lymphoid nodules and in isolated plasma cells scattered throughout the walls of the intestine, in bronchi, in salivary glands, and in the gallbladder.

B Cells

B cells respond to antigen that penetrates the enterocyte barrier. Some of these responding B cells migrate to regional lymph nodes and into intestinal lymphatics, from which they reach the thoracic duct and enter the bloodstream. These circulating IgA-positive B cells have an affinity for all body surfaces. As a result, they colonize not only in the intestinal tract but also at the respiratory tract, urogenital tract, and mammary gland. Thus antigen priming at one location will permit antibodies to be synthesized and secondary responses to occur at locations remote from the priming site reflecting the existence of a common mucosal immune system (Fig. 23.9; Chase and Kaushik, 2019; Wilson and Obradovic, 2015). The movement of IgA-positive B cells from the Peyer's patches in the intestine to the mammary gland is especially important since it provides a route by which antibodies directed

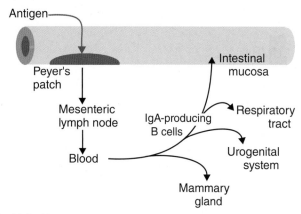

Fig. 23.9 When stimulated by antigen, immunohlobin A (IgA)-producing B cells are produced in inductive sites, such as the Peyer's patches. They then leave the intestine and circulate in the bloodstream. They all eventually settle on other surfaces, such as the lung, the mammary gland, and other regions of the gastrointestinal tract effector sites reflecting the existence of a common mucosal immune system. This transfer of antibody-producing cells in the mammary gland ensures that milk contains IgA antibodies directed against intestinal pathogens.

against intestinal pathogens can be transferred to the newborn through milk (Usami et al., 2021). Oral administration of antigen to a pregnant animal will thus result in the appearance of IgA antibodies in its milk. In this way, antibodies directed against intestinal pathogens will flood the intestine of the newborn animal when it suckles. T cells originating within the Peyer's patches also home specifically to the intestinal mucosa by using specialized vascular adhesive molecules. For example, mucosal addressin cell-adhesion molecule–1 is an adhesion molecule expressed on the high endothelial venules of Peyer's patches and on venules in intestinal lamina propria and the mammary gland. Its ligand is the lymphocyte integrin α4/β7. B and T cells that express this integrin migrate preferentially to the intestine and the mammary gland.

The IgA Receptor, CD89

The functions of IgA are in large part mediated through its receptor, (FcαR1 or CD89). FcαR1 is an activating receptor expressed on diverse myeloid cells such as neutrophils, monocytes, macrophages, dendritic cells, and eosinophils. As a result, signaling of IgA through this receptor can promote opsonization and phagocytosis, cytokine release, NETosis, the neutrophil respiratory burst, and macrophage antibody-dependent cell-mediated cytotoxicity. It also stimulates the release of leukotriene B$_4$ which serves as a neutrophil chemoattractant. These reactions generally occur at sites of IgA synthesis—the mucosal surfaces, and so mediate local inflammation. In addition to acting as an IgA receptor, CD89 also serves as a receptor for C-reactive protein and as a pattern-recognition receptor for bacteria such as *Streptococcus pneumoniae* and *Escherichia coli*. The CD89 gene, unlike the other major Fc receptors, is located along with the natural killer (NK) cell receptors of the leukocyte receptor complex. In dogs it may be a pseudogene and thus nonfunctional. CD89 appears to be more structurally related to the LRC-encoded receptors than to the other FcRs (Morton et al., 2005).

T Cells

Both α/β and γ/δ T cells are found in the intestinal wall but in two very different locations. Thus α/β T cells are mainly scattered throughout the lamina propria and in Peyer's patches. γ/δ T cells, in contrast, are embedded within the single layer of enterocytes on the mucosal surface, where they are known as intraepithelial lymphocytes (IELs)

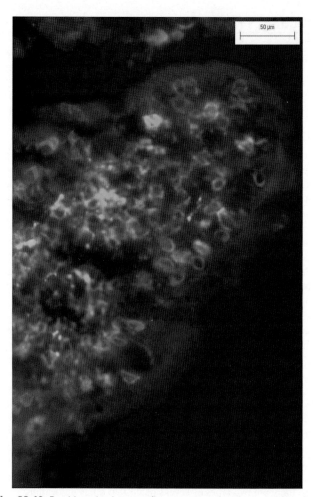

Fig. 23.10 Double-color immunofluorescence showing a canine duodenal villous tip stained with monoclonal antibodies to α/β T-cell antigen receptor (TCR) and γ/δ TCR. The α/β T cells are stained green and are located in the interior of the villus. The γ/δ T cells are stained red and are clearly located within the intestinal epithelium. From German, A.J., Hall, E.J., Moore, P.F., et al., 1999. The distribution of lymphocytes expressing alpha/beta and gamma/delta T-cell receptors, and the expression of mucosal addressin cell adhesion molecule-1 in the canine intestine. J. Comp. Pathol. 121, 249–263.

(Fig. 23.10). In the small intestine there is about one IEL for every 10 enterocytes. They do not recirculate. Their location suggests that they play a key role in maintaining the mucosal barrier. IELs regulate host-microbial interactions at the intestinal mucosal surface and are critical components in preventing invasion by the commensal microbiota. IEL function is in turn regulated by many different cytokines including IL-2, -7, -15, and TGF-β. While T cells predominate (90%), ILC1 cells are also found embedded in the epithelium (Van Kaer and Olivares-Villagomez, 2018).

γ/δ IELs originate in the bone marrow and mature within cryptopatches, clusters of cells located just under the enterocytes. Cryptopatches each contain several hundred immature T cells. Located between epithelial cells, IELs can recognize PAMPs directly, through the TLR-MyD88 pathway as well as through their antigen receptors (TCRs). In response, they secrete a variety of proinflammatory cytokines such as IL-1β, and IL-18 and defensive cytokines such as IFN-γ and IFN-λ. The interferons, in turn, stimulate macrophages and nearby enterocytes to secrete protective nitric oxide. They also secrete regulatory cytokines such as IL-25, TGF-β, TSLP, and retinoic acid (Wiarda and Loving, 2022).

There are major species differences in the properties of IELs. Five percent of IELs in humans, 50% in mice, and up to 90% in ruminants carry γ/δ TCR. A high proportion of the IELs are CD8+ (85% in humans, 77% in pigs, 24% in sheep). These CD8 molecules are α/α homodimers, in contrast to the CD8 α/β heterodimers found on conventional α/β T cells. IELs tend to use unusual TRGV and TRDV genes to form the TCR antigen binding site. These genes are not expressed in other lymphoid organs, suggesting that the intraepithelial T cells are specialized for epithelial surveillance. IELs are MHC class II positive and may act as antigen-presenting cells (Luckschander et al., 2009). They regulate B cell IgA responses. Some have NK cell activity, whereas others are cytotoxic T cells that may attack parasites within the intestinal lumen. They also play a role in the repair of damaged epithelia (Ismail et al., 2011).

ADAPTIVE PROTECTIVE MECHANISMS

Both antibody- and cell-mediated immune responses protect body surfaces. The antibodies produced on mucosal surfaces include IgA, IgD (In some species), IgM, IgE, and IgG. Some of these, most notably IgA and possibly IgM, act by immune exclusion (Fig. 23.4). The others, especially IgE and IgG, destroy antigen within the surface tissues by immune elimination.

Immune Exclusion
Immunoglobulin A

IgA predominates in surface secretions. At least 80% of all plasma cells are found in the lamina propria, and together they produce more immunoglobulin A than all other immunoglobulin isotypes combined. IgA is found in enormous amounts in saliva, intestinal fluid, nasal and tracheal secretions, tears, milk, colostrum, urine, and the secretions of the urogenital tract (Fig. 23.11; Table 23.2).

To undergo a class switch and thus produce IgA, mucosal B cells must receive signals from other cells as well as the microbiota and retinoic acid from dietary vitamin A (Chapter 22). Some IgA production is T cell independent and so requires cytokines from dendritic cells and epithelial cells. Other B cells require help from Th2 cells to make the switch to IgA production.

T cell–dependent IgA production mainly occurs in Peyer's patches. Dendritic cells take antigen from M cells, process it, and use it to generate Tfh cells. CD40-ligand and IL-21 from these Tfh cells induce the expression of activation-induced cytidine deaminase. This promotes IgA class switch recombination. This pathway is stimulated by bacteria such as the SFBs attached to the enterocytes. The B cells generated by this pathway are persistent. They can re-enter germinal centers and

undergo somatic mutation. As a result, this IgA may be of very high affinity for an antigen.

T-independent IgA production mainly occurs in the lamina propria and isolated lymphoid follicles under the influence of BAFF and APRIL. ILC3 cells also contribute to this process. The IgA produced is usually of low affinity and is directed primarily at the microbiota.

Follicular dendritic cells secrete soluble B cell–stimulating cytokines including BAFF and APRIL (see Chapter 16). The dendritic cells themselves are activated by intestinal neuropeptides, such as vasoactive intestinal peptide. Eosinophils are required for the maintenance of plasma cells in the lamina propria. They are also a major source of APRIL. As a result, they directly support the B cell class switch and are required for both T-independent and -dependent generation of IgA. These signals, together with CD40-CD154 interactions, trigger B cell IgA production in the absence of antigen. Enterocytes and IELs also produce APRIL and promote B cell differentiation. B cells that require both antigen and Th2 cells to make the switch to IgA are stimulated by TGF-β (Fig. 23.12). Other Th2 cytokines that promote this switch include IL-4, IL-5, IL-6, and even IL-10. The IgA response is relatively slow to develop and has a very high threshold for induction (10⁹ bacteria). When boosted, the IgA response does not increase exponentially but rather in an additive manner. The plasma cells that synthesize IgA have other unique properties in that they also produce TNF-α and iNOs and thus share some properties with monocytes.

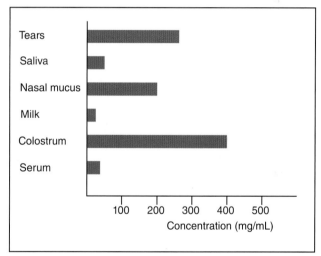

Fig. 23.11 Typical immunoglobulin A (IgA) levels in bovine body fluids. In other species, milk and colostral IgA concentrations may be considerably higher.

TABLE 23.2	Approximate Immunoglobulin A Levels in the Serum and Various Secretions of the Domestic Animals					
	SECRETION (mg/dL)					
Species	Serum	Colostrum	Milk	Nasal Mucus	Saliva	Tears
Horse	60–350	500–1500	50–1000	160	140	150
Cow	10–50	100–700	10–50	200	56	260
Sheep	10–50	100–700	5–12	50	90	160
Pig	50–200	1000	300–500	2–14	25–75	–
Dog	20–150	500–2200	110–620	–	–	–
Cat	30–150	150	240–620	–	54	–
Chicken	50	–	–	–	20	15

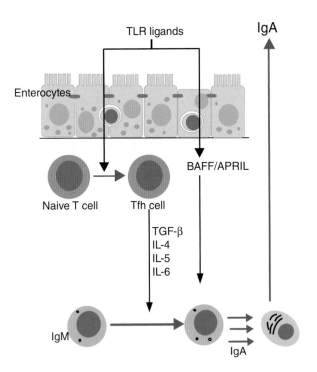

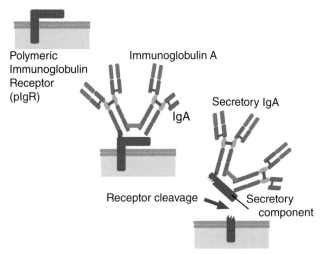

Fig. 23.13 Immunoglobin A (IgA) is secreted by mucosal plasma cells and binds to receptors on the interior surface of intestinal enterocytes. The bound IgA is taken into the enterocytes and passed in vesicles to the cell surface. Once in the intestinal lumen, the polymeric immunoglobulin receptor (pIgR) is cleaved from the cell and remains bound to the IgA. In this state, it is called secretory component and serves to protect the IgA from degradation.

Fig. 23.12 The control of immunoglobin A (IgA) production. Multiple T helper 2 cells cytokines, especially transforming growth factor–β (TGF-β), are primarily responsible for the IgM-to-IgA switch. Costimulation is provided by BAFF and APRIL from epithelial cells and dendritic cells as well as CD40-CD154 interactions. *IL-6*, Interleukin-6; *Tfh cell*, follicular helper T cells; *TLR*, toll-like receptors.

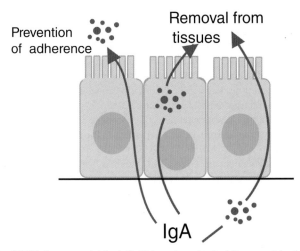

Fig. 23.14 Immunoglobin A (IgA) is unique in that it can act in three locations. It can bind antigen in tissue fluid or in enterocytes as well as in the intestinal lumen. The bound antigen in tissues or enterocytes is carried to the intestinal lumen.

IgA monomers are about 160 kDa in size and are typical four-chain, Y-shaped molecules (see Fig. 17.6). They are usually secreted as dimers or larger polymers linked by a J-chain. IgA has several extra cysteine residues in its heavy chains. As a result, the short interchain disulfide bonds compact the chains and shield vulnerable bonds from proteases.

IgA is synthesized and secreted by plasma cells in the intestinal submucosa, especially in the crypt region. This dimeric IgA binds to a glycoprotein receptor for pIgR on the basal surface of enterocytes (Fig. 23.13). The receptor binds covalently to the Cα2 domain of one of the IgA monomers. The membrane-bound IgA-pIgR complex is then endocytosed and actively transported across the enterocyte. When it reaches the exterior surface, the endocytic vesicle fuses with the plasma membrane and exposes the complex to the intestinal lumen. The extracellular domains of the pIgR are then cleaved by proteases so that the IgA, with the receptor peptide still attached (secretory IgA), is released into the lumen. The receptor peptide is called secretory component. The production, transport, and secretion of secretory component occur even in the absence of IgA, so that free secretory component is found in high concentrations in intestinal contents.

IgA is not bactericidal and does not activate complement. It can neutralize viruses and some viral and bacterial enzymes. IgA-antigen complexes bind to monocytes and macrophages, neutrophils, and eosinophils through CD89. When IgA-opsonized particles bind to this receptor, they trigger superoxide production, opsonization, antibody-dependent cell-mediated cytotoxicity, and the release of inflammatory mediators. Its most important function is to prevent the adherence of bacteria and viruses to epithelial surfaces—immune exclusion. If bacteria or viruses cannot adhere to enterocytes, they simply pass along with the intestinal contents and are expelled without doing any harm.

The presence of the gut microbiota also drives IgA production. Different commensals differ in their ability to induce SigA. The gut microbiota is constantly being sampled at the inductive sites and this triggers the generation of new IgA-secreting plasma cells. Thus the IgA system is constantly responding to the resident microbiota and in effect, is sculpted by the microbiota (Yang et al., 2022). Most, but not all, commensals are coated with IgA and this IgA affects their composition. It is likely that the IgA-coated organisms are potential mucosal pathogens. For example, it preferentially coats the Enterobacteriaceae while ignoring the Bacteroides and Lactobacilli. SFBs are especially potent at triggering IgA responses (Bunker and Bendelac, 2018).

Because IgA is transported through enterocytes, it can also act inside these cells (Fig. 23.14). Thus IgA can bind to newly synthesized viral proteins inside these cells and interrupt viral replication. In this way, the IgA can prevent viral growth before the integrity of the epithelium is damaged. This is a unique example of antibodies acting in an intracellular location. The second unique function of intracellular IgA is to excrete foreign antigens. Thus IgA can bind to antigens that have penetrated the submucosa. Once bound, the IgA-antigen complexes will bind to pIgR and be actively transported back across the enterocytes into the intestinal lumen. IgA can therefore acts at three different levels to exclude foreign antigens: within the submucosa, within enterocytes, and within the intestinal lumen.

Rabbit IgA. The European rabbit has at least fifteen *IGHA* genes and this is the most complex IgA system known in mammals. At least ten of the rabbit *IGHA* genes are expressed in the small intestine as well as in the appendix, mesenteric lymph nodes, and mammary gland. Each subclass appears to differ in its susceptibility to bacterial proteases. The ability of lagomorphs to produce so many diverse IgA subclasses likely has a significant effect on the diversity of their microbiota. In some ways, these may function as innate IgAs that control microbial colonization, especially in the large rabbit caecum. This IgA diversity may also encourage the diversification of the microbiota (Tizard, 2023).

Immunoglobulin M

The earliest immunoglobulins found in the intestine of the newborn are of the IgM class. IgM will also bind to pIgR and is carried through the enterocyte to the lumen. Because of its structure, however, secretory IgM is much more susceptible to proteases than secretory IgA.

Immune Elimination
Immunoglobulin E

In addition to immune exclusion, there is a second line of surface defense that destroys antigen that penetrates the mucosal barrier (immune elimination). This is mediated by IgE. Cells producing IgE are mainly found under epithelial surfaces rather than in the lymph nodes or spleen. IgE binds to mast cell Fc receptors in the mucosa of the intestine, respiratory tract, and skin. If invading organisms evade the IgA and gain access to the tissues, IgE-mediated inflammation will be triggered (Fig. 23.15). These responses involve rapid degranulation of mast cells and the release of their inflammatory mediators into the surrounding tissues. As described in Chapter 30, the mast cell contents

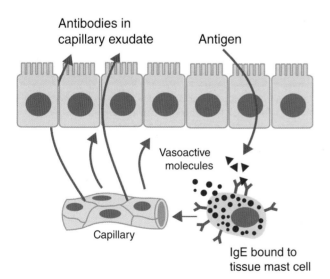

Fig. 23.15 The immunoglobulin E (IgE) response in the intestinal wall. Antigen reaches IgE-sensitized mast cells to cause their degranulation. As a result of this, vasoactive factors are released. These cause increased vascular permeability and exudation of serum Immunoglobulin G antibodies. This occurs in the "self-cure" phenomenon in parasitized sheep.

cause acute inflammation, increase the permeability of small blood vessels, and promote fluid leakage between enterocytes, leading to the outflow of mucus containing large quantities of IgG.

This process occurs, for example, when parasitic worms invade the intestinal mucosa. IgA has little effect on these invaders, so they have no difficulty in burrowing into the superficial layers of the mucosa. When sensitized mast cells encounter parasite antigens however, the release of vasoactive molecules, together with the intense local inflammation, changes in blood flow, and intestinal motility, may be sufficient to force the parasite to disengage—a phenomenon called "self-cure" (see Chapter 29).

IgA and IgE work in concert. IgA normally is the first line of defense, and IgE serves as a backup system. If IgA production is defective, the IgE response may be triggered to excess. As a result, dogs deficient in IgA have increased IgE production and commonly develop atopic dermatitis in response to food and inhaled antigens (see Chapter 40).

Immunoglobulin G

In ruminants (especially cattle), IgG1, not IgA, is the major secretory immunoglobulin in colostrum and milk. This is due to its selective transfer from the bloodstream into the mammary gland. On other body surfaces in ruminants, however, IgA remains the predominant immunoglobulin, although IgG1 is also present. IgG2 is also transferred into the intestine and saliva in ruminants. IgG may be of greater protective significance in the respiratory tract than in the intestine because there it is less likely to be degraded by proteases.

IMMUNITY TO FOOD

Normal animals are tolerant to the protein antigens in foods and as a result, are immunologically unresponsive to ingested proteins. Dietary proteins are not normally antigenic for two reasons. First, the ingested proteins are degraded by the gut proteases to small, nonimmunogenic peptides. Second, dietary proteins normally generate a strong intestinal Treg cell response (see Fig. 31.4). Tregs are abundant in the intestinal mucosa where they mediate tolerance to food antigens as well as to many of the microbiota. Treg cells suppress Th2 cells, decrease B cell IgE production, suppress effector T-cell emigration into tissues, induce IL-10 production by DCs, and inhibit the activation of mast cells, eosinophils, and basophils. A specialized subpopulation of intestinal dendritic cells (Thetis cells) stimulates this Treg production and hence triggers oral tolerance (Akagbosu et al., 2022). Secretory IgA responses are not usually generated against food antigens. Likewise, soluble food proteins are unlikely to trigger TLR responses. (Although TLR4-deficient mice readily develop food allergies.)

Another mechanism by which oral tolerance may be induced is through the production of "tolerosomes." These are exosomes produced by enterocytes. They carry MHC class II on their surface and this binds antigenic peptides from the gut lumen. Purified tolerosomes fed to animals induce tolerance. It is suggested that the presentation of food antigens by tolerosomes induces Treg formation (Ostman et al., 2005).

It has been estimated that about 2% of ingested food protein is absorbed as peptide fragments large enough to be recognized by the immune system, although a very much smaller fraction of these molecules (<0.002%) is absorbed intact. This protein reaches the portal circulation, but little passes the liver and enters the systemic circulation. Presumably, the Kupffer cells of the liver capture blood-borne food antigens. Antibodies produced locally may bind to this adsorbed antigen and generate immune complexes that are removed as the blood passes through the liver. If a calf is fed a defined dietary antigen such as soy protein, although it is initially well absorbed, the animal soon begins to make IgA antibodies to soy. Once antibodies are produced, immune exclusion occurs, and the amount of protein absorbed drops significantly. If another novel protein is introduced into the feed, it too will be initially absorbed until IgA is produced against it. Thus IgA may serve to exclude intact food antigens from the body. The extent to which normal animals make antibodies against proteins in their food has been unclear. Cats fed soy and casein produced high levels of IgG and IgA antibodies in their serum against both these proteins. For unknown reasons, proteins from canned food appear to be more immunogenic than unprocessed proteins (Cave and Marks, 2004).

VACCINATION ON BODY SURFACES

When animals are vaccinated against organisms that invade the intestinal or respiratory tracts, it makes sense to stimulate a mucosal IgA response. To do this, the vaccine antigen can simply be ingested or inhaled. Unfortunately, such vaccines are not always effective. Inactivated antigens fail to trigger an IgA response because they are immediately washed or sneezed off when applied to mucous membranes. Because of the abundant intestinal microbiota, intestinal IgA responses also have a high threshold, tend to lack memory, and tend to fade rapidly. The body tightly regulates antigen input across epithelial cells. Regulatory effects on IgA production constantly adapt the IgA response to the intestinal microbiota. The only way a significant IgA response can be triggered is to use live vaccines, in which the vaccine organism can invade mucous membranes. The vaccine must persist for a sufficient time to trigger an immune response yet not cause significant damage. Good examples of such vaccines are the respiratory tract vaccines against bovine or feline rhinotracheitis. Even some of these vaccines may cause a transient conjunctivitis or tracheitis. Other examples of effective live oral vaccines include polio vaccine and some influenza vaccines in humans and transmissible gastroenteritis vaccine in piglets. Oral tolerance also remains a challenge for mucosal vaccines. Thus the administration of some antigens to the respiratory or intestinal tracts may promote mucosal and T-cell unresponsiveness (Correa et al., 2022).

Systemic vaccination against surface infections may provide adequate immunity (as in human influenza and polio vaccines) since some IgG may be transferred from serum to the mucosal surface. Indeed, many available vaccines simply work by stimulating high levels of IgG antibodies in blood. These are effective because once an invading organism causes tissue damage and triggers inflammation; the site of invasion is flooded by IgG. Nevertheless, this is not the most efficient way of providing immunity.

Once a protective IgA response has been generated, other difficulties may arise. For example, secondary immune responses are sometimes difficult to induce on surfaces, and multiple doses of vaccine may not increase the intensity or duration of the local immune response. This is not caused by any intrinsic defect but occurs because high levels of IgA can block antigen absorption and so prevent it from reaching antigen-presenting cells (Chen and Cerutti, 2010).

REFERENCES

Afshar, M., Gallo, R.L., 2013. Innate immune defense system of the skin. Vet. Dermatol. 24 32-8.e8-9

Akagbosu, B., Tayyebi, Z., Shibu, G., et al., 2022. Novel antigen presenting cell imparts Treg-dependent tolerance to gut microbiota. Nature 610, 752–760.

Ali, N., Rosenblum, M.D., 2017. Regulatory T cells in skin. Immunology 152, 372–381.

Allensbach, K., 2011. Clinical immunology and immunopathology of the canine and feline intestine. Vet. Clin. Small Anim. 41, 345–360.

Barker, E., Haverson, K., Stokes, C.R., et al., 2006. The larynx as an immunological organ: immunological architecture in the pig as a large animal model. Clin. Exp. Immunol. 143, 6–14.

Bunker, J.J., Bendelac, A., 2018. IgA responses to microbiota. Immunity 49, 211–224.

Cave, N.J., Marks, S.L., 2004. Evaluation of the immunogenicity of dietary proteins in cats and the influence of the canning process. Am. J. Vet. Res. 65, 1427–1433.

Chase, C., Kaushik, R.S., 2019. Mucosal immune system of cattle: all immune responses begin here. Vet. Clin. Food Anim. 35, 431–451.

Chen, K., Cerutti, A., 2010. Vaccination strategies to promote mucosal antibody responses. Immunity 33, 479–491.

Coates, M., Blanchard, S., MacLeod, As, 2018. Innate antimicrobial immunity in the skin: a protective barrier against bacteria, viruses, and fungi. Plos Pathogens. https://doi.org/10.1371/journal.ppat.1007353.

Correa, V.A., Portilho, A.I., De Gaspari, E., 2022. Vaccines, adjuvants and key factors for mucosal immune response. Immunology 167, 124–138.

Christmann, U., Buechner-Maxwell, V.A., Witonsky, S.G., Hite, R.D., 2009. Role of lung surfactant in respiratory disease: current knowledge in large animal medicine. J. Vet. Intern. Med. 23, 227–242.

Fung, K.Y., Mangan, N.E., Cumming, H., et al., 2013. Interferon-ε protects the female reproductive tract from viral and bacterial infection. Science 339, 1088–1090.

Gallo, R.L., Hooper, L.V., 2012. Epithelial antimicrobial defense of the skin and intestine. Nat. Rev. Immunol. 12, 503–516.

Glowacki, A.J., Yoshizawa, S., Jhunjhunwala, S., Vieira, A.E., et al., 2013. Prevention of inflammation-mediated bone loss in murine and canine periodontal disease via recruitment of regulatory lymphocytes. Proc. Natl. Acad. Sci. U.S.A. 110, 18525–18530.

Guo, Y., Gao, M., Bao, J., Luo, X., Liu, Y., An, D., Zhang, H., Ma, B., Wang, J., 2015. Molecular cloning and characterization of a novel bovine IFN-epsilon. Gene 558, 25–30.

Ismail, A.S., Severson, K.M., Vaishnava, S., et al., 2011. γδ Intraepithelial lymphocytes are essential mediators of host-microbial homeostasis at the intestinal mucosal surface. Proc. Natl. Acad. Sci. U.S.A. 108 (21), 8743–8748.

Iwasaki, A., Foxman, E.F., Molony, R.D., 2016. Early local immune defenses in the respiratory tract. Nat. Rev. Immunol. https://doi.org/10.1038/nri.2016.117.

Johansson, M.E., Hansson, G.C., 2016. Immunological aspects of intestinal mucus and mucins. Nat. Rev. Immunol. 16, 639–649.

Karagianni, A.E., Kapetanovic, R., McGorum, B.C., et al., 2013. The equine alveolar macrophage: functional and phenotypic comparisons with peritoneal macrophages. Vet. Immunol. Immunopathol. 155, 219–228.

Liebler-Tenorio, E.M., Pabst, R., 2006. MALT structure and function in farm animals. Vet. Res. 37, 257–280.

Luckschander, N., Pfamatter, N.S., Sidler, D., et al., 2009. Phenotyping, functional characterization, and developmental changes in canine intestinal intraepithelial lymphocytes. Vet. Res. 40, 58.

Morton, H.C., Pleass, R.J., Storset, A.K., et al., 2005. Cloning and characterization of equine CD89 and identification of the CD89 gene in chimpanzees and rhesus macaques. Immunology 115, 74–84.

Ostman, S., Taube, M., Telemo, E., 2005. Tolerosome-induced oral tolerance is MKC dependent. Immunology 116, 464–476.

Ouellette, A.J., Selsted, M.E., 2012. HD6 defensin nanonets. Science 337 (6093), 420–421.

Pabst, R., Gehrke, I., 1990. Is the bronchus-associated lymphoid tissue(BALT) an integral structure of the lung in normal mammals, including humans? Am. J. Respir. Cell Mol. Biol. 3, 131–135.

Perez-Lopez, A., Behnsen, J., Nuccio, S.-P., Raffatellu, M., 2016. Mucosal immunity to pathogenic intestinal bacteria. Nat. Rev. Immunol. 16, 135–148.

Pickles, K., Pirie, R.S., Rhind, S., et al., 2002. Cytological analysis of equine bronchoalveolar fluid. Part 2: comparison of smear and cytocentrifuged preparations. Equine Vet. J. 34, 292–296.

Rainard, P., Gilbert, F.B., Germon, P., 2022. Immune defenses of the mammary gland epithelium in dairy ruminants. Front. Immunol. https://doi.org/10.3389/2022.1031785.

Rescigno, M., 2011. The intestinal epithelial barrier in the control of homeostasis and immunity. Trends Immunol. 32, 256–264.

Sonnenberg, G.F., Fouser, L.A., Artis, D., 2011. Border patrol: regulation of immunity, inflammation and tissue homeostasis at barrier surfaces by IL-22. Nat. Immunol. 12 (5), 383–390.

Tizard, I.R., 2023. Comparative Mammalian Immunology. Academic Press, San Diego, CA.

Usami, K., Niimi, K., Matsuo, A., Suyama, Y., et al., 2021. The gut microbiota induces Peyer's -patch-dependent dsecrcrtion of maternal IgA into milk. Cell Rep. https://doi.org/10.1016/j.celrep.2021.109655.

Van Kaer, L., Olivares-Villagomez, D., 2018. Development, homeostasis and functions of intestinal intraepithelial lymphocytes. J. Immunol. 200, 2235–2244.

Vaishnava, S., Behrendt, C.L., Ismail, A.S., et al., 2008. Paneth cells directly sense gut commensals and maintain homeostasis at the intestinal host-microbial interface. Proc. Natl. Acad. Sci. U.S.A. 105, 20858–20863.

Wellnitz, O., Bruckmaier, R.M., 2012. The innate immune response of the bovine mammary gland to bacterial infection. Vet. J. 192, 148–152.

Wiarda, J.E., Loving, C.L., 2022. Intraepithelial lymphocytes in the pig intestine: T cell and innate lymphoid cell contributions to intestinal barrier immunity. Front. Immunol. https://doi.org/10.3389/fimmu.2022.1048708.

Wilson, H.L., Obradovic, M.R., 2015. Evidence for a common mucosal immune system in the pig. Mol. Immunol. 66, 22–34.

Wingate, K.V., Torres, S.M., Silverstein, K.A.T., et al., 2009. Expression of endogenous antimicrobial peptides in normal canine skin. Vet. Dermatol. 20, 19–26.

Wright, J.R., 2005. Immunoregulatory functions of surfactant proteins. Nat. Rev. Immunol. 5, 58–68.

Yang, C., Chen-Liaw, A., Spindler, M.P., Tortorella, D., et al., 2022. Immunoglobulin A antibody composition is sculpted to bind the self-gut microbiome. Sci. Immunol. 7 (73) https://doi.org/10.1126/sciimmunol.abg3208.

24

Immunity in the Fetus and Newborn

CHAPTER OUTLINE

When a mammal is born, it emerges from the sterile uterus into an environment where it is immediately exposed to a host of microorganisms. Its surfaces, such as the gastrointestinal tract, acquire a complex microbial flora within hours (Box 24.1). If it is to survive, the newborn animal must be able to control this microbial colonization. In practice, the adaptive immune system takes some time to become fully functional, and innate mechanisms are responsible for initial resistance to infection. In species with a short gestation period, such as dogs, the adaptive immune system may not even be fully developed at birth. In animals with a long gestation period, such as the large domestic herbivores, the adaptive immune system is fully developed at birth but cannot function at adult levels for

several months. The complete functional development of the adaptive immune system depends on antigenic stimulation. The development of B cells and B-cell receptor (BCR) diversity requires clonal selection and antigen-driven cell multiplication (see Chapter 16). Thus newborn mammals are very vulnerable to infection for the first few weeks of life. They need assistance in defending themselves at this time. This temporary help is provided by the mother's colostrum in the form of antibodies and T cells. The passive transfer of immunity from mother to newborn is essential for survival.

DEVELOPMENT OF THE IMMUNE SYSTEM

The development of the immune system in the mammalian fetus follows a consistent pattern. The thymus is the first lymphoid organ to develop, followed by the secondary lymphoid organs. B cells appear soon after the development of the spleen and lymph nodes, but antibodies are not usually detectable until late in fetal life. The ability of the fetus to respond to antigens develops very rapidly once the lymphoid organs appear, but all antigens are not equally capable of stimulating fetal lymphoid tissue. The immune system develops in a series of steps, each step permitting the fetus to respond to more antigens. These steps are driven by a gradual increase in the use of gene conversion or somatic mutation to increase antibody diversity. The ability to mount cell-mediated immune responses develops at the same time as antibody production. T-cell antigen receptor diversity is also limited in the fetus and neonate, and their cytokine production may be low.

Species Differences

Foal

The gestation period of the mare is about 340 days. Lymphocytes are seen first in the thymus at about 60–80 days postconception. They are found

---

> ### BOX 24.1 The Microbiota of the Placenta
>
> It has been a widely held belief that the internal organs of the body are sterile. However, the rapid development of the microbiota in newborn infants in less than a week after birth has raised the possibility that they are somehow seeded by bacteria inside the body prior to birth. One possible source is the placenta. Gram-positive and -negative intracellular bacteria can be seen in the tissue layer at the maternal-fetal interface. Studies on placental tissues using DNA-based metagenomic studies have also detected a small but unique placental microbiome. It has generally been assumed that these bacteria originate in the lower genital tract and ascend into the uterus. However, this microbiota appears to be more closely related to the oral microbiota in nonpregnant subjects! *Escherichia coli* was the single most prevalent species in the placenta. It is no coincidence that *E. coli* can be found in meconium and is a major cause of early-onset sepsis in newborns.

From Aagaard, K., Ma, J., Antony, K.M., Ganu, R., Petrosino, J., Versalovic, J., 2014. The placenta harbors a unique microbiome. Sci. Transl. Med. 6, 237–246.

in the mesenteric lymph node and intestinal lamina propria at 90 days and in the spleen at 175 days. Blood lymphocytes appear at about 120 days. A few plasma cells may be seen at 240 days. Graft-versus-host disease, a cell-mediated response, has developed in immunodeficient foals transplanted with tissues from a 79-day-old fetus. The equine fetus can respond to coliphage T2 at 200 days postconception and to Venezuelan equine encephalitis virus at 230 days. V(D)J sequence diversity increases as the fetus develops and as the foal develops into an adult. Newborn foals have detectable quantities of IgM and IgG in their serum, but IgE production in the horse does not begin until foals are 9–11 months of age. Like other large herbivores, the foal has a well-developed ileal Peyer's patch that serves as a primary lymphoid organ and eventually involutes. Major B-cell markers are detectable by 90–120 days of gestation. *IGHM* and *IGLC* transcripts are expressed in the liver, bone marrow, and spleen at all ages (Talmadge et al., 2013). As a result, small amounts of IgM and IgG are detectable at birth. Despite this competence, B-cell functions may be actively suppressed by Treg cells during the first few months of a foal's life. Equine neonates tend to have a Th1-biased immune response, and their IFN-γ production is quantitatively similar to that of adult horses (Breathnach et al., 2006). However, other cytokine production is delayed (Liu et al., 2009).

Calf

Although the gestation period of the cow is 280 days, the fetal thymus is recognizable by 40 days postconception. The bone marrow and spleen appear at 55 days. Lymph nodes are found at 60 days, but Peyer's patches do not appear until 175 days (Fig. 24.1). Blood lymphocytes are seen in fetal calves by day 45, IgM+ B cells by day 59, and IgG+ B cells by day 135. The time of appearance of serum antibodies depends on the sensitivity of the techniques used. It is therefore no accident that the earliest detectable immune responses are those directed against viruses, using highly sensitive neutralization tests. Fetal calves have been reported to respond to rotavirus at 73 days, to parvovirus at 93 days, and to parainfluenza 3 virus at 120 days. Fetal blood lymphocytes can respond to mitogens between 75 and 80 days, but this ability is temporarily lost near the time of birth as a result of increased steroid production at that time. T-cell subpopulations are present in calves at levels comparable to adults, but B-cell numbers increase significantly during the first 6 months after birth.

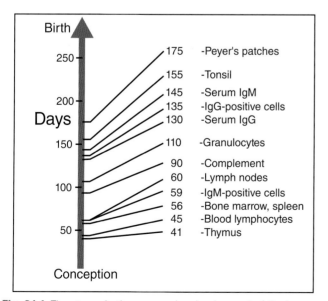

Fig. 24.1 The stages in the progressive development of the immune system in the fetal calf. *Ig,* Immunoglobin.

Calves acquire innate and IgM-mediated immune competence within the first week of life. IgA and IgG expression reach adult levels by 14–28 days.

Lamb

The gestation period of the ewe is about 145 days. MHC class I+ cells can be detected by day 19, and MHC class II+ cells can be found by day 25. The thymus and lymph nodes are recognizable by 35- and 50-day postconception, respectively. Gut-associated follicles appear in the colon at 60 days, jejunal Peyer's patches at about days 75–80, and ileal Peyer's patches at days 110–115. Blood lymphocytes are seen in fetal lambs by day 32, and CD4+ and CD8+ cells appear in the thymus by 35–38 days. B cells are detectable at 48 days in the spleen and by that time have already begun to rearrange their IGLV genes. C3 receptors appear by day 120, but Fc receptors do not appear until the animal is born. Fetal liver lymphocytes can respond to phytohemagglutinin by 38 days. Lambs can produce antibodies to phage φX174 at day 41 and reject skin allografts by day 77. Some fetal lambs can produce antibodies to Akabane virus as early as 50 days postconception. Antibodies to Cache Valley virus can be provoked by day 76, to SV40 virus by day 90, to T4 phage by day 105, to bluetongue virus by day 122, and to lymphocytic choriomeningitis virus by day 140. The proportions of α/β and γ/δ T cells change as lambs mature. Thus, 1 month before birth, 18% of blood T cells are γ/δ positive. By 1 month after birth, they constitute 60% of blood T cells.

Piglet

The gestation period of the sow is about 115 days. B cells appear in the yolk sac at day 20, in the fetal liver by day 30, and in the bone marrow by day 45. The first SWC3+ leukocytes can be found in the yolk sac and liver on day 17. The thymus develops by 40 days postconception and is colonized by two waves of T-cell progenitors beginning on day 38. γ/δ T cells appear first in the thymus and in peripheral blood about 10 days later. α/β T cells develop by day 55, but their numbers grow rapidly so that they predominate late in gestation. The intestinal lymphoid tissues are devoid of T cells at birth. CD4+ T cells appear in the intestine at 2 weeks of age, and CD8+ T cells appear at 4 weeks. Their proliferation appears to be driven by the intestinal microbiota. IgM+ B cells can be found in the fetal liver at 40 days, spleen by day 50, and bone marrow by day 60. Fetal piglets can produce antibodies to parvoviruses at 58 days gestation and can reject allografts at about the same time. Blood lymphocytes can respond to mitogens between 48 and 54 days. Natural killer (NK) cell activity does not develop until several weeks after birth, although cells with an NK phenotype can be identified at 45 days' gestation in spleen and umbilical blood.

B cells are the first lymphocytes to appear in peripheral blood. The number of circulating B cells rises significantly between 70 and 80 days' gestation. The response to antigens in the fetus is of the IgM type. It is interesting to note that B cells are present in the thymus of newborn pigs (Sinkora and Butler, 2009). Piglets are born with relatively limited B-cell diversity. B-cell numbers increase for the first 4 weeks after birth, but their antigen-binding repertoire does not begin to expand until 4–6 weeks of age (Butler et al., 2002).

The production of IgA is controlled by exposure to the intestinal microbiota (Box 24.2). A limited amount of B-cell class switching occurs in the developing fetus so that, as a result, newborn piglets already possess some intestinal IgA. Thus piglets at birth are exposed to new antigens from the growing microbiota as well as from colostrum and milk. It is these antigens that initiate IgA production. At weaning, the animal is exposed to new dietary antigens and must also develop oral tolerance. B-cell lymphogenesis and gene rearrangements continue for at least 5 weeks postpartum (Sun et al., 1998).

Puppy

The gestation period of the bitch is about 63 days. During that time her thymus shrinks significantly but recovers by the end of lactation (Pereira et al., 2019). The fetal thymus differentiates between days 23 and 33, and fetal puppies can respond to phage φX174 by day 40. Blood lymphocytes can respond to phytohemagglutinin by 45 days postconception, and these cells can be detected in lymph nodes by 45 days and in the spleen by 55 days. The ability to reject allografts also develops at about day 45, although rejection is slow at this stage, and fetal puppies may be made tolerant by intrauterine injection of an antigen before day 42. Thymic seeding of T cells to the secondary lymphoid organs and the development of humoral immune responses are therefore relatively late phenomena in dogs compared with the situation in other domestic mammals (Day, 2007). Their immune system continues to develop during the first 10–14 days after birth while the puppies are blind and only suckle and sleep.

Kitten

Lymphocytes are seen in fetal kitten blood at 25 days postconception. B cells are seen in the fetal liver at 42 days. Fetal kittens do make some IgG that can be detected in their serum before suckling, although this may be due to antibodies crossing the placenta. Nevertheless, newborn kittens are essentially agammaglobulinemic (Day et al., 2010).

BOX 24.2   The Inheritance of Fecal IgA Levels

In inbred mice, fecal IgA levels are highly variable. Some have high—while others have low-fecal IgA. If the microbiota of low-fecal IgA mice are transferred to high-fecal IgA mice, the recipient's fecal IgA levels promptly drop. So, the quantity of IgA in the feces is determined by the microbiota. The bacteria from IgA-low mice appear to be able to degrade both secretory component and IgA. It is generally recognized that a young animal receives its microbiome from its mother. As a result, fecal IgA levels are vertically transmitted from the mother and just appear to be inherited. If this process occurs in domestic mammals, it may explain many of the enteric disease problems associated with intensive production of pigs and other livestock.

The Immune System and Intrauterine Infection

Although a fetus is not totally defenseless, it is less capable than an adult of combating infection. Its adaptive immune system is not fully functional; as a result, some infections may be mild or unapparent in the mother but severe or lethal in the fetus. Examples include bluetongue, infectious bovine rhinotracheitis (bovine herpesvirus 1 [BHV-1]), bovine viral diarrhea, rubella in humans, and toxoplasmosis. Fetal infections commonly trigger an immune response as shown by lymphoid hyperplasia and elevated immunoglobulin levels. For this reason, the presence of any immunoglobulins in the serum of a newborn, unsuckled animal suggests infection in utero.

In general, the response to these viruses is determined by the state of immunological development of the fetus. For example, if the live bluetongue virus vaccine, which is nonpathogenic for normal adult sheep, is given to pregnant ewes at 50 days postconception, it causes severe lesions in the nervous system of fetal lambs, including hydranencephaly and retinal dysplasia, whereas if it is given at 100 days postconception or to newborn lambs, only a mild inflammatory response is seen. Bluetongue vaccine virus given to fetal lambs between 50 and 70 days postconception may be isolated from lamb tissues for several weeks, but if given after 100 days, re-isolation is not usually possible. Akabane virus acts in a similar fashion in lambs. If given before 30–36 days postconception, it causes congenital deformities. If given to older fetuses, it provokes antibody formation and is much less likely to cause malformations. Piglets that receive live parvovirus vaccine before 55 days postconception will usually be aborted or stillborn. After 72 days, however, piglets develop high levels of antibodies to the parvovirus and survive. Prenatal infection of calves with BHV-1 results in a fatal disease, in contrast to postnatal infections, which are relatively mild. The transition between these two types of infections occurs during the last month of pregnancy.

The effects of the timing of viral infection are well seen with bovine viral diarrhea virus (BVDV). If a cow is infected early in pregnancy (up to 50 days), she may abort. On the other hand, infections occurring between 50 and 120 days, before the fetus develops immune competence, lead to asymptomatic persistent infection because the calves develop tolerance to the virus (Fig. 24.2). These calves are viremic yet, because of their tolerance, fail to make antibodies or T cells against the

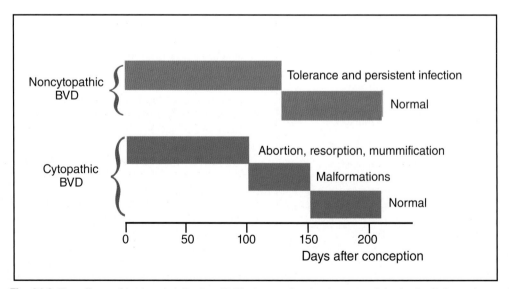

Fig. 24.2 The effects of bovine viral diarrhea (BVD) virus on the development of the fetal calf depend upon the timing of the infection. With adult cattle, there is considerable individual variation in resistance to infection. Persistently infected calves may develop minor neurologic problems or failure to thrive.

virus. Some of these calves may show minor neurologic problems and failure to thrive, but many are clinically normal. If the cow is infected with BVDV between 100 and 180 days postconception, calves may be born with severe malformations involving the central nervous system and eye, as well as jaw defects, atrophy, and growth retardation. Calves infected after 150–180 days' gestation are usually clinically normal.

Since they are tolerant to BVDV, persistently infected calves shed large quantities of the virus in secretions and excretions. These calves may also produce neutralizing antibodies if immunized with a live BVDV vaccine of a serotype different from that of the persistent virus. Despite this, the original virus will persist in these animals. These persistently infected calves grow slowly and often die of opportunistic infections such as pneumonia before reaching adulthood. (BVDV has a tropism for lymphocytes and is immunosuppressive.)

BVDV occurs in two distinct biotypes: cytopathic and noncytopathic. (The name derives from their behavior in cell culture, not their pathogenicity in animals.) Noncytopathic strains suppress type I interferon (IFN) production but permit type III (IFN-λ) production by plasmacytoid DCs. This type III interferon suppresses T-cell responses and enables the virus to survive in calves and causes persistent infections by depleting $WC1^+$ γ/δ T cells. Cytopathic strains induce type I IFN production and cannot cause persistent infection. These cytopathic strains, however, do cause mucosal disease (MD), a severe enteric disease leading to profuse diarrhea and death (Fig. 24.3). MD develops as a result of a mutation in a nonstructural viral gene that changes the BVDV biotype from noncytopathic to cytopathic, while the animal fails to produce neutralizing antibodies or T cells. The cytopathic strain can spread between tolerant animals and lead to a severe MD outbreak. Both cytopathic and noncytopathic viruses

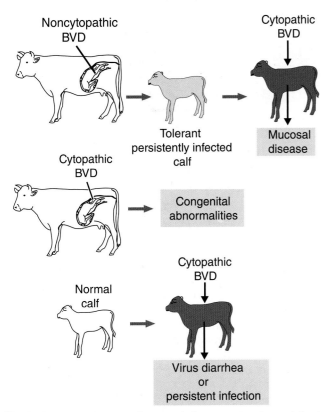

Fig. 24.3 The relationship of mucosal disease to persistent infection with bovine viral diarrhea virus (BVDV) in tolerant cattle. Calves persistently infected with noncytopathic BVDV and then superinfected with cytopathic BVDV develop mucosal disease.

can be isolated from these animals. Recombination may also occur between persistent noncytopathic strains and cytopathic strains in vaccines and lead to MD outbreaks. Although some of the lesions in MD are attributable to the direct pathogenic effects of BVDV, glomerulonephritis and other immune complex–mediated lesions also develop. This may reflect a superinfection or the production of nonneutralizing antibodies. Because persistently infected calves can reach adulthood and breed, it is possible for BVD infection to persist indefinitely within carrier animals and their progeny. Between 0.4% and 1.7% of cattle in the United States are persistently infected in this way.

IMMUNE RESPONSES OF NEWBORN MAMMALS

After developing in the sterile environment of the uterus, newborn mammals first encounter a diverse population of microbes during the birth process. They must be able to combat any attempted invasion immediately. Thus neonatal mammals are capable of mounting both innate and adaptive immune responses at birth. However, any adaptive immune response mounted by a newborn will be a primary response with a prolonged lag period and low antibody levels. Innate immune responses are therefore critical for survival in the first weeks of life.

Role of the Intestinal Microbiota

The development of the newborn immune system is driven by the first microorganisms that colonize body surfaces, especially the gastrointestinal tract and skin (see Chapter 22). These early-life microbial exposures have a profound effect on the development of the immune system. In their absence, "germ-free" mammals fail to fully develop their mucosal lymphoid tissues. The microbiota generates a complex mixture of pathogen-associated molecular patterns that act through enterocyte toll-like receptors. Likewise, microbial antigens are taken up by dendritic cells and presented to $CD4^+$ T cells. These signals collectively promote the functional development and regulatory control of the immune system. Thus the Bifidobacteria can produce immunoregulatory compounds that induce immune tolerance and minimize intestinal inflammation (Spreckels and Zhernakova, 2021). The intestinal and skin microbiota also play a key role in determining any Th1 or Th2 bias in immune function. This results in changes in the blood levels of IgE in adult life and their sensitivity to orally induced anaphylaxis. This is the basis of the "hygiene hypothesis," the concept that the development of allergies is influenced by microbial exposure early in life (see Chapter 31).

The Gut-Mammary Axis

Once established, the presence of the gut microbiota drives B-cell IgA production by plasma cells within the intestinal wall. The gut microbiota is constantly generating antigens that are sampled and processed by M cells and dendritic cells overlying inductive lymphoid sites such as the Peyer's patches. These processed antigens trigger B-cell responses and their differentiation into IgA-secreting plasma cells. Thus the IgA system is constantly responding to the microbiota. During pregnancy, many of these responding B cells leave the mother's Peyer's patches, enter her circulation, and eventually colonize the developing mammary glands under the influence of the chemokine CCL28. It is these IgA^+ B cells and plasma cells that subsequently produce the IgA that is found in milk. As a result, the suckling newborn will ingest large quantities of IgA. Some of this IgA is directed specifically against enteric pathogens, while some low-affinity antibodies may also promote the growth of beneficial commensals. Different commensals differ in their ability to induce secretory IgA (SIgA) production. In mice, organisms such as *Bacteroides acidfaciens* and *Prevotella buccalis* appear to be indispensable for programming this maternal IgA synthesis. Thus the intestinal microbiota is, in part, responsible for the production of much of the IgA in milk.

Innate Immunity

Newborns can produce a diverse array of antimicrobial molecules, including pentraxins and collectins, peptides such as the defensins, lactoferrin, and lysozyme. Surfactant proteins A and D as well as β-defensin 1 and TLR4 are produced in the preterm lamb lung. As a result, invaders can be killed relatively efficiently. TLRs are present and functional in the newborn. In the fetal pig, neutrophils at 90 days postconception are fully capable of phagocytizing bacteria such as *Staphylococcus aureus*. However, they are deficient in bactericidal activity, which only reaches adult levels 10 days later. Near birth, the phagocytic and bactericidal capacity of these neutrophils declines as a result of increased steroid production. The neutrophils of newborn foals move relatively slowly compared with their dams. The serum of newborn mammals, however, is deficient in some complement components, resulting in a poor opsonic activity. Serum C3 increases rapidly after birth in newborn piglets and reaches adult levels by 14 days of age.

Adaptive Immunity

Newborn mammals, generally mount adaptive responses skewed toward type 2 rather than type 1 responses. Thus they favor antibody responses over cell-mediated immunity. This imbalance results from the late development of IL-12-producing DC1 and the activities of IL-4 and IL-13 from DC2 cells. Mononuclear cells from newborn foals are unable to express IFN-γ. Their Th2 cells rapidly differentiate, whereas their Th1 cells are slow to develop. Excess IFN-γ may cause placental damage, so this skewing is not accidental. IFN-γ production gradually increases in foals through the first 6 months of life to reach adult levels within a year when the acquired responses revert to the balanced adult pattern.

During the first three months of life, puppies have a higher lymphocyte count than adult dogs. Much of the difference is due to CD21+ B cells. The proportion of puppy CD8+ T cells is low at birth but gradually climbs to reach adult levels. Thymic involution begins at around 6 months of age in dogs.

TRANSFER OF IMMUNITY FROM MOTHER TO OFFSPRING

Unless additional immunological assistance is provided, organisms that present little threat to an adult may kill newborn mammals. This immunological assistance is provided by antibodies transferred from the mother to her offspring through colostrum. Maternal lymphocytes may also be transferred to the fetus through the placenta or to newborn mammals through colostrum.

The placenta is also of major immunological significance since it is involved, not only in regulating fetal tolerance but also controls the transfer of antibodies from the mother to the developing fetus. The route by which maternal antibodies reach the fetus is determined by the structure of the placenta (Fig. 24.4).

TRANSFER OF IMMUNOGLOBULINS

Direct immunoglobulin transfer between the maternal and fetal circulations can only occur in species with endotheliochorial or hemochorial placentation. In effect, the placenta acts as a selective barrier preventing maternal leukocytes, proteins, and infectious agents from crossing from the mother to the fetus while in some species, permitting the selective passage of immunoglobulins (Langer, 2009).

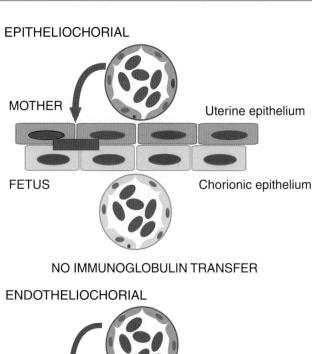

EPITHELIOCHORIAL

MOTHER   Uterine epithelium

FETUS   Chorionic epithelium

NO IMMUNOGLOBULIN TRANSFER

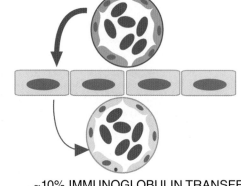

ENDOTHELIOCHORIAL

~10% IMMUNOGLOBULIN TRANSFER

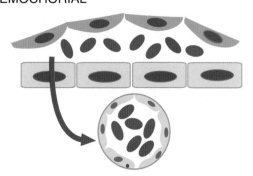

HEMOCHORIAL

~ 100% IMMUNOGLOBULIN TRANSFER

Fig. 24.4 The structure of the placentas of domestic mammals and their relationship to immunoglobulin transfer. The blue endothelial cells are on the maternal side of the placenta.

The human hemomonochorial placenta allows maternal IgG but not IgM, IgA, or IgE to transfer from the mother to the fetus. Thus maternal IgG can enter the fetal bloodstream, and as a result, the newborn human infant has circulating IgG levels comparable to those of its mother.

The polycotyledonary placentas of artiodactyls and perissodactyls are epitheliochorial and although differing in overall structure between species, still retain the six tissue layers separating the fetal and maternal blood systems. They do not permit the transfer of immunoglobulins. As a result, the newborn foal or piglet is completely dependent upon receiving immunoglobulins by way of maternal colostrum. The efficacy of such transfer depends upon adequate colostral intake and absorption from the gastrointestinal tract.

Dogs have an endotheliochorial placenta in which the chorionic epithelium is in contact with the endothelium of the maternal capillaries. In this species, about 5%–10% of normal serum IgG levels are directly transferred from the mother to the puppy, but the rest must be obtained through colostrum. Interestingly cats have a similar type of placenta, but very few immunoglobulins are transferred to kittens in utero.

The amount and composition of the first milk, the colostrum, very much depends on the nature of the maternal placentation and the ability of the mother to passively transfer immunity to her young. Species that have significant transplacental immunoglobulin transfer such as primates and lagomorphs do not require much additional transfer via the colostrum. Conversely in ungulates where placental transfer is minimal, then colostrum must be rich in immunoglobulins. Their young are agammaglobulinemic when born. In these species, the intake and absorption of sufficient colostrum is mandatory if the newborn are to be adequately protected against systemic infections. Their B cells have never had occasion to encounter or respond to foreign antigens. They are unexercised in this role and as a result require time to respond and

generate protective levels of immunoglobulin. They need immediate immunological assistance.

Secretion and Composition of Colostrum and Milk

Colostrum contains the accumulated secretions of the mammary gland over the last few weeks of pregnancy together with proteins actively transferred from the bloodstream under the influence of estrogens and progesterone. Neonatal immunoglobulin receptors (FcRn) are expressed in mammary gland ductal and acinar cells and mediate the active transfer of IgG from serum into colostrum. Colostrum is therefore rich in IgG and IgA and contains some IgM and IgE. In cows, colostral IgG concentration is 28.7-fold that in serum! In sows, it is 5.4-fold, while in dogs, it is 2.8-fold (Mila et al., 2015). The predominant immunoglobulin in the colostrum of most domestic mammals is IgG, which may account for 65%–90% of its total antibody content; IgA and the other immunoglobulins are usually minor but significant components. As lactation progresses and colostrum changes to milk, differences among species emerge. In primates, IgA predominates in both colostrum and milk. In pigs and horses, IgG predominates in colostrum, but its concentration drops rapidly as lactation proceeds so that IgA predominates in milk. In ruminants, IgG1 is the predominant immunoglobulin in both milk and colostrum (Fig. 24.5; Tizard, 2001).

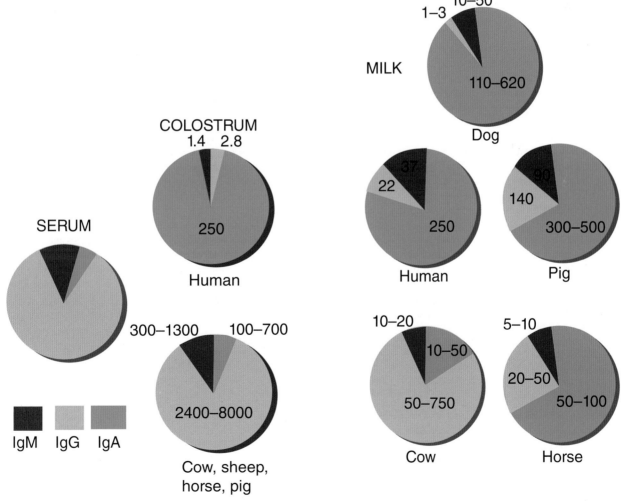

Fig. 24.5 The level of immunoglobulins (Ig) in colostrum and milk of selected domestic mammals and humans. While there is great variation in these levels between individuals, it is clear that the situation in bovine milk and colostrum is very different from that in humans and other single-stomached animals. The Ig levels in milk are expressed in mg/dL.

Horse

Mares use an epitheliochorial placenta. Six tissue layers separate the mother and her fetus. As a result, in order to provide sufficient oxygen and nutrition for the fetus, the entire surface of the placenta must be functional. In addition, only one fetus can usually be supported at a time. As another consequence, no immunoglobulins can cross the placenta and foals are therefore born agammaglobulinemic.

Normal equine colostrum contains, from 3000 to 12,000 mg/dL of IgG. It also contains about 150 mg/dL 1gM and 300 mg/dL IgA. An average of about 100 g of IgG is produced per lactation in the mare. There are significant amounts of IL-4 in mare's colostrum which may serve to compensate for the very low level of IL-4 production in the young foal (Perkins and Wagner, 2015). IL-13 has not been detected on the colostrum but IFN-γ is present in both colostrum and foal serum at birth. Equine colostrum has been shown to contain TNF-α and IL-8 (CXCL8). These cytokines may promote the development of the immune system in the young animals (Mariella et al., 2017). Equine colostrum is also rich in activated T cells (Perkins et al., 2014a, 2014b).

It is of interest to note that donkey foals are not totally agammaglobulinemic at birth. When born, they have a significant concentration of IgG (8.97 ± 0.5 mg/mL) in their serum. In contrast, IgG concentrations in the serum of neonatal horse foals average 0.3 mg/mL.

While neonatal foals have some functional innate immune responses at birth, their development of adaptive responses is uneven. For example, foals produce IgG1, IgG3, IgG5, and IgA at birth and these can reach adult levels by 3 months of age. Conversely, igG4, IgG7, and IgE production do not reach adult levels until one year of age (Perkins and Wagner, 2015). Similar issues affect the T-cell responses. Thus IFN-γ production begins at birth and progressively increases over the first year of life. Conversely, the Th2 cytokine IL-4 is largely undetectable during the first three months of life. This delayed onset of Th2 activity explains in part, why young foals respond very poorly to vaccination.

Bovine

Cows do not transfer immunoglobulins to their young in utero. Neonatal immunoglobulin receptors (FcRn) are expressed on mammary gland ductal and acinar cells and mediate the transfer of IgG from not totally agammaglobulineserum into colostrum (Baumrucker et al., 2022). The predominant immunoglobulin in the colostrum of ruminants is IgG1, which may account for 65%–90% of its total antibody content. IgG2 is present but in very much smaller quantities. IgA and the other immunoglobulins are usually minor but significant components, 7%–10% each. All of the IgG, most of the IgM, and about half of the IgA in bovine colostrum are transferred from the bloodstream. In milk, in contrast, only 30% of the IgG and 10% of the IgA are so derived; the rest is produced locally by lymphoid tissue within the udder. Colostrum also contains secretory component both in the free form and bound to IgA. Colostrum contains many cytokines. For example, bovine colostrum contains significant amounts of IL-1β, IL-6, TNF-α, and IFN-γ.

Piglet

As in the other artiodactyls, the sow placenta does not permit the transfer of immunoglobulins to developing piglets. As a result, newborn piglets are born agammaglobulinemic. They receive a concentrated solution of immunoglobulins when they suckle maternal colostrum. In other mammals, this maternal antibody is transported into the colostrum through the Fc receptor FcRn (Bandrick et al., 2014). FcRn does not, however, appear to be the responsible receptor in pigs since FcRn-knock-out pigs still accumulate IgG in their colostrum. Pig FcRn is however still responsible for the absorption of immunoglobulins from the piglet's intestinal tract (Ke et al., 2021).

Puppy

Dogs have an endotheliochorial placenta that limits the transfer of immunoglobulins to the developing fetus. In this case, it is a zonary placenta that forms a complete band around the developing puppy. In this form of placenta, the chorionic epithelium comes into contact with the endothelium of the maternal capillaries. As a result, about 5%–10% of required serum IgG is directly transferred from the mother to the puppy, but most must still be obtained through colostrum. Newborn puppies, while not totally agammaglobulinemic, have very low IgG levels in their blood (0.3 g/L) as compared to the adults 8–25 g/L (Walther et al., 2015).

Kittens

Cats have an endotheliochorial placenta. Thus their fetal chorionic epithelial cells are in direct contact with maternal endothelial cells. The placenta is of the zonary type that forms a complete band encircling the fetus. There may be hematomas located at the margins of the placenta. While endotheliochorial placentas are considered to permit limited immunoglobulin transfer to kittens in utero, in practice, the amount transferred is negligible. No IgG or IgA is detectable, and only trace amounts of IgM are present in newborn kittens. Periparturient cats do, however, produce colostrum containing a very high concentration of IgG. The neonatal kitten absorbs IgG from the maternal colostrum for up to 16 hours after birth. Once absorption ceases, their serum IgG drops steadily with a half-life of 4.4 ± 3.57 days for IgG and an IgA half-life of 1.93 ± 1.94 days. Serum IgM, presumably synthesized by the kitten itself, climbs steadily through the first weeks of life.

Absorption of Colostrum

Young mammals that suckle soon after birth ingest colostrum. Naturally suckled calves ingest an average of 2 L of colostrum, although individuals may ingest as much as 6 L. In these young mammals, protease activity in the digestive tract is low and is further reduced by trypsin inhibitors in colostrum. Therefore, colostral proteins are not degraded but can reach the small intestine intact. Colostral IgG is endocytosed by enterocytes and binds to FcRn within their endosomes (Fig. 24.6). Once bound to endosomal FcRn, immunoglobulin molecules are transported across the enterocytes and transferred to the lacteals and the intestinal capillaries. Eventually, the absorbed immunoglobulin reaches the bloodstream, and newborn mammals obtain a massive transfusion of maternal IgG (Fig. 24.7). Young pigs and probably other young mammals have large amounts of free secretory component in their intestine. Colostral IgA and, to a lesser extent, IgM can bind this secretory component, which may then prevent their absorption.

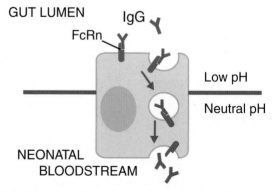

Fig. 24.6 The role of Fc receptor of the neonate (FcRn) in absorbing immunoglobulin (Ig) from the intestine. IgG binds FcRn at low pH and unbinds at neutral pH.

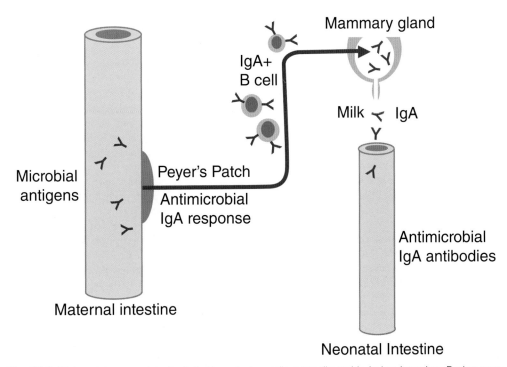

Fig. 24.7 Maternal immunoglobulin A (IgA) producing cells normally reside in her intestine. During pregnancy, these cells migrate to the developing mammary gland where they secrete IgA into the milk.

The duration of intestinal permeability also varies among species. In general, permeability is highest immediately after birth and declines after about 6 hours because of the replacement of FcRn-bearing enterocytes by cells that do not express this receptor. As a rule, absorption of all immunoglobulin classes drops to a very low level after about 24 hours. Feeding colostrum tends to hasten this closure, whereas a delay in feeding results in a slight delay in closure (up to 33 hours). In piglets, the ability to absorb immunoglobulins may be retained for up to 4 days if milk products are withheld. The presence of the mother may be associated with increased immunoglobulin absorption. For example, calves fed measured amounts of colostrum in the presence of the mother will absorb more immunoglobulins than calves fed the same amount in her absence. In laboratory studies in which measured amounts of colostrum are fed, there is a great variation (25%–35%) in the quantity of immunoglobulins absorbed. Management should ensure that foals or calves ingest at least 1 L of colostrum within 6 hours of birth.

Unsuckled mammals normally have very low levels of immunoglobulins in their serum. The successful absorption of colostral immunoglobulins immediately supplies them with serum IgG at a level approaching that found in adults (Fig. 24.8). Peak serum IgG levels are normally reached between 12 and 24 hours after birth. After absorption ceases, these passively acquired antibodies decline through normal metabolic processes. The rate of decline differs among immunoglobulin classes, and the time taken to decline to nonprotective levels depends on their initial concentration. In calves, the serum half-life of colostral-derived IgG is about 28 days.

As intestinal absorption is taking place, a simultaneous proteinuria may also occur. This is due to intestinal absorption of very small proteins, such as β-lactoglobulin that can be excreted in the urine. In addition, the glomeruli of newborn mammals are permeable so that the urine of neonatal ruminants contains intact immunoglobulin molecules. This proteinuria ceases with the termination of intestinal

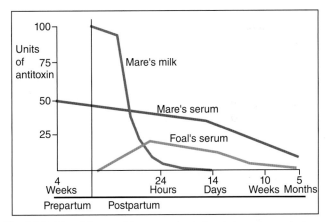

Fig. 24.8 *Clostridium perfringens* antitoxin levels in serum, colostrum, and milk of six pony mares and in the serum of their foals from birth to 6 months. (From Jeffcott, L.B., 1994. Studies on passive immunity in the foal. 1. G-globulin and antibody variations associated with the maternal transfer of immunity and the onset of active immunity. J. Comp. Pathol. 84, 93–101.)

absorption. Urine from puppies collected 24 hours after birth contains relatively large amounts of IgG, IgM, and IgA. The amount declines over time so that IgM is undetectable by 14 days, although there may still be significant amounts of IgG and IgA present. Over the first 2 weeks of life, the puppy's glomeruli mature and acquire the ability to retain macromolecules (Schaefer-Somi et al., 2005).

The secretions of the mammary gland gradually change from colostrum to milk. Ruminant milk is rich in IgG1 and IgA. Nonruminant milk is rich in IgA. For the first few weeks in life, while protease activity is low, these immunoglobulins can be found throughout the intestine and in the feces of young mammals. As the digestive ability of the intestine increases, eventually only SIgA molecules remain intact. The amount of IgA provided by milk can be large; for instance, a 3-week-old piglet may receive 1.6 g daily from sow's milk.

Although IgE is present in mare's milk and transmitted to the suckling foal, its level in foal serum drops to a very low level by 6 weeks of age. IgE synthesis by foals begins at about 9–11 months of age, and at that time a pattern of relatively high or low IgE levels is established. Total levels of IgE in young horses (and their susceptibility to allergies) are mainly determined by genetic factors and the microbiota. IgE is also transferred in sheep colostrum. Colostral IgE levels are significantly higher than in ewe's serum. IgE is absent from presuckling lamb serum but can rise to adult levels by 2 days after birth. It then declines steadily over several weeks (Marti et al., 2009).

The IgG transferred through a mother's colostrum represents the results of her history of antigen exposure, B-cell responses, and somatic mutation. This maternal IgG, in effect, reflects the immunological experiences of the mother. Maternal antibodies act on the immune system of the newborn during a critical imprinting period and exert a lifelong influence on the newborn's immune development. This influence may be stronger than some genetic predispositions! Thus maternal antibodies can enhance the newborn immune responses to some antigens and suppress their responses to others. They may also influence Th1/Th2 polarization and the subsequent development of allergies (Fink et al., 2008).

TRANSFER OF CELL-MEDIATED IMMUNITY

Bovine colostrum contains between 3×10^4 and 1×10^5 lymphocytes/mL; about half of which are T cells. These cells can penetrate the epithelium of Peyer's patches and reach the lacteal ducts or the mesenteric lymph nodes. As a result, cell-mediated immunity is transferred to newborn mammals.

Cell-containing and cell-free colostrum have been compared for their ability to protect calves against enteropathic *E. coli*. The calves receiving cells excreted significantly fewer bacteria than the mammals receiving cell-free colostrum. The concentration of IgA- and IgM-specific antibodies against *E. coli* in the serum of neonatal calves was higher in those that received colostral cells than in those that did not. The calves that received cells had better responses to the mitogen concanavalin A and foreign antigens such as sheep erythrocytes. The mechanisms of this protective effect are unclear. Transcriptome analysis of colostral T cells in sows, however, has indicated that they are more activated than peripheral blood T cells (Hagiwara et al., 2008).

The CD8⁺ T cells in bovine colostrum can produce large quantities of IFN-γ, which may influence the early development of Th1 responses in neonatal calves. Thus ingestion of maternal colostral cells appears to accelerate the development of activated calf lymphocytes. The monocytes of calves that received colostral cells are also more capable of processing and presenting antigens (Reber et al., 2006).

Transfer of cell-mediated immunity by bovine milk lymphocytes has been demonstrated (Donovan et al., 2007). Pregnant cows were vaccinated against BVDV. Blood lymphocytes from calves that received cell-free colostrum from these cows were unresponsive to BVDV antigen. In contrast, lymphocytes from calves that received colostrum-containing live cells showed enhanced responses to BVDV antigen at 1 and 2 days after colostral ingestion. The lymphocytes of calves that had received whole colostrum showed enhanced mitogenic responses to maternal and unrelated leukocytes after 24 hours. They also responded to the nonspecific stimulant staphylococcal enterotoxin B. In contrast,

the lymphocytes of calves that received acellular colostrum did not (Reber et al., 2008a, 2008b).

The mononuclear cells in mare's colostrum are mainly CD4⁺ and CD8⁺ T cells. CD8⁺ cells in colostrum are enriched when compared to blood. These cells are polarized towards IFN-γ and IL-17 production. This phenotype is generally considered to promote inflammation (Perkins et al., 2014a, 2014b).

Sow colostrum contains between 1×10^5 and 1×10^6 lymphocytes/mL. Of these, 70%–80% are T cells. Some of these cells may also be NK cells. Colostral lymphocytes can pass between the intestinal epithelial cells, enter the lymphatic vessels, and reach the mesenteric lymph nodes. Within two hours after receiving colostrum that contained radiolabeled cells, maternal lymphocytes appeared in the bloodstream of piglets. Piglets that received these colostral cells showed enhanced responses to mitogens compared with control animals. Transcriptome analysis of colostral T cells in sows, however, has indicated that they are more activated than peripheral blood T cells (Hlavova et al., 2014). Clearly, ingestion of maternal colostral leukocytes immediately after birth stimulates the development of the neonatal immune system (Ghosh et al., 2016).

MicroRNAs and Intestinal Development

MicroRNAs (miRNAs) are small single-stranded RNA molecules about 22 nucleotides in length that regulate gene expression. They bind to the 3′untranslated region or the coding regions of messenger RNAs and promote their degradation. miRNAs regulate many different biological processes including embryonic development, cell differentiation, and apoptosis. Their expression patterns and regulatory functions may be tissue-specific. Some miRNAs also regulate gut development and mucosal immunity in newborns. miRNAs are present in many body fluids including milk and colostrum. They are shed into the colostrum in microvesicles and exosomes. These colostral miRNAs are absorbed from the intestine and enter the circulation of newborn mammals. These miRNAs promote the development of the mucosal immune system in the neonatal calf, especially during the first week of life (Emam et al., 2019). The miRNAs likely regulate IL-6 and IL-17 signaling as well as T-cell differentiation in the jejunum and ileum at this early stage. The commensal microbiota also influences miRNA expression and coordinates intestinal colonization and immune system development. Thus the expression of miRNAs in the small intestine of neonatal dairy calves is correlated with the total bacterial load and the presence of specific bacterial phyla such as Lactobacilli and Bifidobacteria (Liang et al., 2015).

FAILURE OF PASSIVE TRANSFER

The absorption of IgG from colostrum is required for the protection of a newborn against septicemic disease. The continuous intake of IgA or IgG1 from milk is required for protection against enteric disease (Fig. 24.9). Failure of these processes predisposes a young animal to infection. There are three major reasons for the failure of passive transfer through colostrum. First, the mother may produce insufficient or poor-quality colostrum (production failure). Second, there may be sufficient colostrum produced but inadequate intake by the newborn animal (ingestion failure). Third, there may be a failure of absorption from the intestine despite an adequate intake of colostrum (absorption failure).

Production Failure

Since colostrum represents the accumulated secretions of the udder in late pregnancy, premature births may mean that insufficient colostrum has accumulated. Valuable colostrum may also be lost from mammals

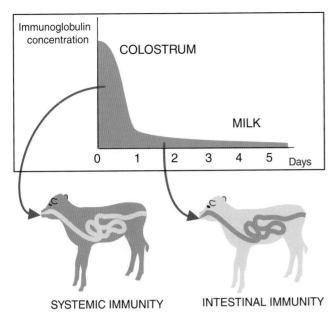

Fig. 24.9 Colostrum intake is required to provide the serum antibodies that protect young animals against septicemic disease. The prolonged intake of milk is necessary to provide persistent immunoglobulin A–mediated protection against enteric infection.

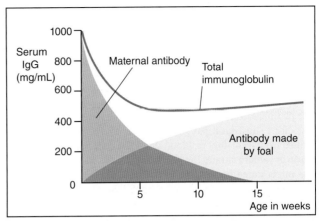

Fig. 24.10 Immunoglobulin (Ig) levels in newborn serum during the first 15 weeks of life indicating the relative contributions of maternal antibody and antibody synthesized by the newborn animal.

as a result of premature lactation or excessive dripping. Cows milked continuously (without a drying-off period) produce colostrum with reduced immunoglobulin concentrations. Colostral IgG levels also vary among individuals, with up to 28% of mares producing low-quality colostrum. It is not possible to assess colostral quality simply by looking at it. Its IgG content should be assessed using a colostrometer (a modified hydrometer) to measure its specific gravity. In mares, this is normally in the range of 1.060–1.085, equivalent to an IgG concentration of 3000–8500 mg/dL. Colostrum with an IgG level of less than 3000 mg/dL may be inadequate to protect a foal, and feeding supplemental, high-quality colostrum may become necessary.

Ingestion Failure

In sheep or pigs, an inadequate intake may result from multiple births simply because the amount of colostrum produced does not rise in proportion to the number of newborns. It may be due to poor mothering, an important problem among young, inexperienced mothers. It also may be due to weakness in the newborn, to a poor suckling drive, or to physical problems such as damaged teats or jaw defects.

Absorption Failure

Failure of intestinal absorption is a major cause for concern in any species. It is especially important in horses not only because of the value of many foals but also because even with good husbandry, about 25% of newborn foals fail to absorb sufficient quantities of immunoglobulins. Alpacas also appear to experience a disproportionate number of cases of failure of passive transfer. Foals require serum IgG concentrations of at least 800 mg/dL 18–24 hours after receiving colostrum to ensure protection (Fig. 24.10).

Diagnosis of Failure of Passive Transfer

The success of passive transfer cannot be evaluated in a foal until 18–24 hours after birth when antibody absorption is essentially complete. Several assays for serum immunoglobulins are available. The most rapid and economic procedure is the zinc sulfate turbidity test,

which involves mixing a zinc sulfate solution with foal serum. Zinc sulfate precipitates globulins and the amount of precipitate is proportional to the immunoglobulin concentration. In total failure of transfer, the reaction mixture remains clear. In sera with an IgG level of more than 400 mg/dL, the mixture becomes cloudy. As an alternative to visual inspection, the optical density of the mixtures can be read in a spectrophotometer and the IgG concentration read off a standard curve. The relative amount of precipitate can also be read in a hematocrit capillary (immunocrit). Similar techniques include precipitation by ammonium sulfate, glutaraldehyde, or sodium sulfite.

Single radial immunodiffusion is a more accurate method in that it is both quantitative and specific for IgG. As described in Chapter 43, known standards are compared with the test serum by measuring the diameter of precipitation produced in agar gel containing an antiserum to equine IgG. A diagnosis of failure of passive transfer is made in foals if IgG levels are less than 400 mg/dL and partial failure of passive transfer if IgG levels are between 400 and 800 mg/dL. Unfortunately, radial immunodiffusion is slow. It takes 18–24 hours to obtain a result and is thus impractical when a rapid diagnosis is required.

A third method of measuring IgG levels is by use of a latex agglutination test. The latex particles are coated with anti-equine IgG. In the presence of IgG, they agglutinate. This test can be performed in about 10 minutes using either whole foal blood or serum. It appears to be reliable and rapid but somewhat insensitive.

It is also possible to use a semiquantitative membrane-filter enzyme–linked immunosorbent assay (ELISA) test to measure IgG in a foal's serum. The color intensity of the reaction on the test filter is compared with color calibration spots. A variant technique uses a dipstick ELISA. Less satisfactory techniques include serum protein electrophoresis and refractometry. (Refractometry is an acceptable, rapid, and convenient test of colostral IgG in calves but is less reliable in foals, in which the wide range of values leads to inaccuracy. It may severely underestimate serum IgG levels in calves). Point-of-care portable analyzers also provide acceptable results in a timely manner (Denholm et al., 2022).

Management of Failure of Passive Transfer

Colostrum may be obtained from mares that have more than is needed for their own young. It can be stored frozen at −15°C to −20°C for up to 1 year (Nath et al., 2010). If stored colostrum is unavailable, fresh colostrum from primiparous mares can be used. If colostrum is not available, serum or plasma may be administered orally. A large volume (up to 9 L) may be required since serum IgG is rapidly catabolized, so that within 12 hours its concentration is much less than that found in colostrum-fed calves. The reasons for this are unknown (Vivrette, 2001).

In foals that are older than 15 hours, oral absorption ceases, and intravenous plasma infusion must be given. Ideally, the dose used can be calculated to attain an IgG level of at least 400 mg/dL. Frozen horse plasma is available commercially, although this may not contain antibodies against local pathogens. Alternatively, the plasma may be obtained from local donors. Blood should be collected aseptically with heparin or sodium citrate. The plasma is collected after the erythrocytes settle and is stored frozen until used. The plasma must be prechecked for antierythrocyte antibodies and must be free of bacterial contamination. The transfusion should be given slowly while the foal is monitored for untoward reactions. All foals receiving supplemental colostrum or plasma should have their IgG levels rechecked 12–24 hours later.

DEVELOPMENT OF ADAPTIVE IMMUNITY

Local Immunity

The intestinal lymphoid tissues of neonatal mammals respond rapidly to ingested antigens. For example, calves vaccinated orally with coronavirus vaccines at birth are resistant to virulent virus within 3–9 days. Likewise, piglets vaccinated orally 3 days after birth with transmissible gastroenteritis virus vaccines develop neutralizing antibodies in the intestine 5–14 days later (Levast et al., 2014). Much of this early resistance is attributable to the innate production of IFN-α/β, but they also mount an early intestinal IgM response that switches to IgA by 2 weeks. In the young calf, the IgA response appears earlier and reaches adult levels well before the other immunoglobulins.

Systemic Immunity

The antibodies acquired by a young animal from its mother's colostrum inhibit the ability of the newborn B cells to mount their own immune responses (Fig. 24.11). As a result, very young animals are unable to respond to systemic immunization. This inhibition is B cell specific, and T-cell responses are largely unaffected. For example, neonatal calf NK cells appear to be fully functional (Elhmouz1-Younes et al., 2009).

Several different mechanisms of this suppression have been suggested. The simplest is the rapid neutralization of live viral vaccines by maternal antibodies. This would prevent viral replication and provide insufficient antigen to prime neonatal B cells. However, data from human infants and domestic mammals indicate that there is usually sufficient antigen present to prime T cells. Likewise, neutralization cannot account for inhibition of the immune response to nonliving vaccines.

A second proposed mechanism suggests that the inhibition results from antibodies binding to B-cell inhibitory Fc receptors (CD32) and so blocking BCR signaling (see Fig. 21.9). However, studies of mice whose Fc receptors have been deleted (FcR knockout mice) have shown that the ability of maternal antibodies to inhibit antibody responses is unaffected. This clearly cannot be the mechanism involved.

A third suggested mechanism is that maternal antibodies simply mask the epitopes on vaccine antigens, preventing their recognition by the animal's B cells. This suggestion is compatible with the selective inhibition of B-cell responses, the lack of inhibition of T-cell responses, and the evidence that, at least in humans and mice, high doses of antigen can overcome maternal immunity. Thus, for a given vaccine dose, an immune response can be elicited only when maternal antibody titers fall below a critical threshold.

In the absence of maternal antibodies, newborn mammals are able to make antibodies soon after birth. For example, if calves fail to suckle

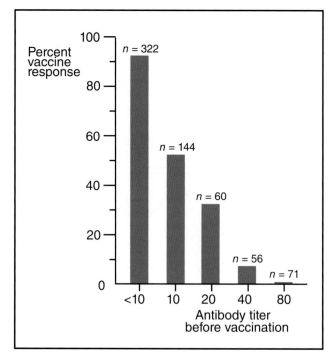

Fig. 24.11 Effect of the presence of maternal antibodies to canine parvovirus in 653 puppies on their response to a modified live parvovirus vaccine. The prevaccination antibody titer profoundly inhibits the response of the puppies to the vaccine. (From Carmichael, L.E., 1883. Compend Contin. Educ. Prac. Vet. 5, 1043–1054.)

and are therefore hypogammaglobulinemic, their endogenous IgM is detectable in blood by 4 days and reaches functional levels by 8 days. Serum IgG and IgA reach functional levels by 16–32 days. In calves that have suckled and thus possess maternal antibodies, antibody synthesis does not commence until about 4 weeks of age. Likewise, colostrum-deprived piglets respond to pseudorabies virus by 2 days after birth, but if they have suckled, antibody production does not begin until 5–6 weeks after birth. Colostrum-deprived lambs synthesize IgG1 at 1 week and IgG2 by 3–4 weeks. In colostrum-fed lambs, however, IgG2 synthesis does not occur until 5–6 weeks.

Passively acquired maternal antibodies not only protect newborns before their immune system becomes fully functional but they have a significant influence on the way in which a newborn's immune system develops. Mouse pups nursed by mothers producing antibodies to the vesicular stomatitis virus developed higher titers of protective antibody when infected as adults.

VACCINATION OF YOUNG ANIMALS

Because maternal antibodies inhibit neonatal antibody synthesis, they prevent the successful vaccination of young animals. This inhibition may persist for many months, its length depending upon the quantity of antibodies transferred and the half-life of the immunoglobulins involved. This problem can be illustrated using the example of vaccination of puppies against canine distemper.

Maternal antibodies, absorbed from the puppy's intestine, reach maximal levels in serum by 12–24 hours after birth. Their levels then decline slowly through normal protein catabolism. The catabolic rate of proteins is exponential and is expressed as a half-life. The half-life of antibodies to canine distemper and adenovirus 1 is 8.4 days, and the half-life of antibodies to feline panleukopenia is 9.5 days. Experience has shown that, *on average*, the level of maternal antibodies to distemper in puppies declines to insignificant levels by about 10–12 weeks, although this may range from 6 to 16 weeks. In a population of puppies, the proportion of susceptible animals, therefore, increases gradually from a very few or none at birth to almost all at 10–12 weeks. Rarely, a puppy may reach 15 or 16 weeks before it can be successfully vaccinated. If virus diseases were not so common, it would be sufficient to delay vaccination until all puppies were about 12 weeks old, when success could be almost guaranteed. In practice, a delay of this type means that an increasing proportion of puppies, fully susceptible to disease, would be without immune protection—an unacceptable situation. Nor is it feasible to vaccinate all puppies repeatedly at short intervals from birth to 12 weeks, a procedure that would ensure almost complete protection; therefore a compromise must be reached.

The earliest recommended age to vaccinate a puppy or kitten with a reasonable expectation of success is at 8 weeks (Day et al., 2010). Colostrum-deprived orphan pups may be vaccinated at 2 weeks of age. Essential vaccines for normal puppies should include distemper, two adenovirus, and parvovirus vaccines. In puppies, a second dose should be given 3–4 weeks after the first and a third at 14–16 weeks of age. Rabies is an essential vaccine that should be given at 14–16 weeks. In kittens an appropriate protocol would be to use three doses of the essential vaccines (viral rhinotracheitis [herpesvirus 1], calicivirus, and panleukopenia) at 8–9 weeks, 3–4 weeks later, and at 14–16 weeks; feline leukemia vaccine can be given at 8 weeks and 3–4 weeks later; and rabies vaccine can be given at 8–12 weeks depending on the type of vaccine used (Fig. 24.12).

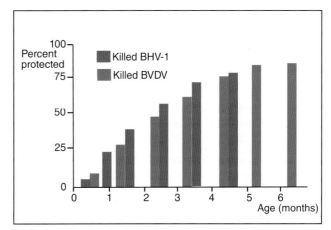

Fig. 24.13 Effectiveness of two inactivated bovine herpesvirus (BHV) vaccines in calves between birth and 6 months of age. It is clear that early vaccine is largely ineffective. *BVDV*, Bovine viral diarrhea virus. (Courtesy Dr. RJ. Schultz.)

Similar considerations apply when vaccinating large farm animals. The prime factor influencing the duration of maternal immunity is the level of antibodies in the mother's colostrum. Thus, in foals, maternal antibodies to tetanus toxin can persist for 6 months and antibodies to equine arteritis virus for as long as 8 months. Antibodies to BVDV may persist for up to 9 months in calves. The half-lives of maternal antibodies against equine influenza and equine arteritis virus antigens in the foal are 32–39 days. As in puppies, a young foal may have nonprotective levels of maternal antibodies long before it can be vaccinated. Maternal antibodies, even at low levels, effectively block immune responses in young foals and calves, so premature vaccination may be ineffective. The effectiveness of vaccines increases progressively after the first 6 months of life (Fig. 24.13). A safe rule is that calves and foals should be vaccinated no earlier than 3–4 months of age followed by one or two revaccinations at 4-week intervals. The precise schedule will depend on the vaccine used and the species to be vaccinated. Animals vaccinated before 6 months of age should always be revaccinated at 6 months or after weaning to ensure protection.

Some live recombinant vaccines such as canarypox-vectored distemper in dogs or influenza in horses appear to effectively prime young animals in the face of significant maternal immunity. DNA vaccines against pseudorabies also appear to be effective in priming cell-mediated responses in the face of maternal immunity, whereas a DNA vaccine against bovine respiratory syncytial virus vaccine is not. Thus the ability of DNA vaccines to overcome maternal immunity varies among species and infections.

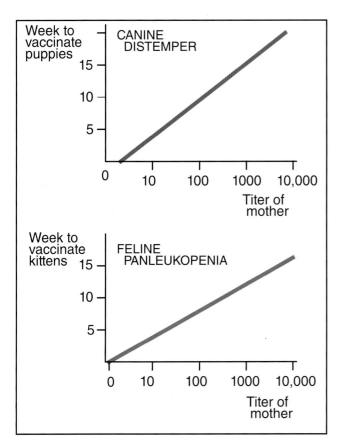

Fig. 24.12 Nomographs showing the relationship between the antibody titer of the mother and the age at which to vaccinate her offspring with modified live virus vaccine. (From Gillespie, J.H., et al., 1959. A nomograph that depicts the age to vaccinate puppies for distemper. Cornell. Vet. 49, 158–167 [CD].)

REFERENCES

Bandrick, M., Ariza-Nieto, C., Baidoo, S.K., Molitor, T.W., 2014. Colostral antibody-mediated and cell-mediated immunity contributes to innate and antigen-specific immunity in piglets. Dev. Comp. Immunol. 43, 114–120.

Baumrucker, C.R., Macrina, A.L., Bruckmaier, R.M., 2022. Clostrogenesis: role and mechanism of the bovine Fc receptor of the neonate (FcRn). J. Mammary Gland Biol. Neoplasia. https://doi.org/10.1007/s0911-021-09506-2.

Breathnach, C.C., Sturgill-Wright, T., Stiltner, J.L., et al., 2006. Foals are interferon gamma-deficient at birth. Vet. Immunol. Immunopathol. 112, 199–209.

Butler, J.E., Weber, P., Sinkora, M., et al., 2002. Antibody repertoire development in fetal and neonatal piglets. VIII. Colonization is required for newborn piglets to make serum antibodies to T-dependent and type 2, T-independent antigens. J. Immunol. 169, 6822–6830.

Day, M.J., 2007. Immune system development in the dog and cat. J. Comp. Pathol. 137, 810–815.

Day, M.J., Horzinek, M.C., Schultz, R.D., 2010. WSAVA guidelines for the vaccination of dogs and cats. J. Small Anim. Pract. 51, 338–356.

Denholm, K., Haggerty, A., Mason, C., Ellis, K., 2022. Comparison of testing for failure of passive transfer in calf serum using four different testing methods. Vet. J., 281. https://doi.org/10.1016/j.tvjl.2022.105812.

Donovan, D.C., Reber, A.J., Gabbard, J.D., et al., 2007. Effect of maternal cells transferred with colostrum on cellular responses to pathogen antigens in neonatal calves. Am. J. Vet. Res. 68, 778–782.

Elhmouz1-Younes, J., Storset, A.K., et al., 2009. Bovine neonatal natural killer cells are fully functional and highly responsive to interleukin-15 and to NK p46 receptor stimulation. Vet. Res. 40, 54–60.

Emam, M., Livernois, A., Paibomesai, M., Atalla, H., Mallard, B., 2019. Genetic and epigenetic regulation of immune response and resistance to infectious diseases in domestic ruminants. Vet. Clin. Food Anim. 35, 405–429.

Fink, K., Zellweger, R., Weber, J., et al., 2008. Long-term maternal imprinting of the specific B cell repertoire by maternal antibodies. Eur. J. Immunol. 38, 90–101.

Ghosh, M.K., Nguyen, V., Muller, H.K., Walker, A.M., 2016. Maternal milk T cells drive development of transgenerational Th1 immunity in offspring thymus. J. Immunol. 197, 2290–2296.

Hagiwara, K., Domi, M., Ando, J., 2008. Bovine colostral CD8-positive cells are potent IFN-γ-producing cells. Vet. Immunol. Immunopathol. 124, 93–98.

Hlavova, K., Stepanova, H., Faldyna, M., 2014. The phenotype and activation status of T and NK cells in porcine colostrum suggest these are central/effector memory cells. Vet. J. 202, 477–482.

Ke, C., Ma, Y., Pan, D., Wan, Z., et al., 2021. FcRn is not the receptor mediating the transfer of serum IgG to colostrum in pigs. Immunology 163, 448–459.

Langer, P., 2009. Differences in the composition of colostrum and milk in eutherians reflect differences in immunoglobulin transfer. J. Mammalol. 90 (2), 332–339.

Levast, B., Berri, M., Wilson, H.L., Meurens, F., Salmon, H., 2014. Development of gut immunoglobulin A production in piglet in response to innate and environmental factors. Dev. Comp. Immunol. 44, 235–244.

Liang, G., Malmuthuge, N., Guan Le, L., Griebel, P., 2015. Model systems to analyze the role of miRNAs and commensal microflora in bovine mucosal immune system development. Mol. Immunol. 66, 57–67.

Liu, T., Nerren, J., Liu, M., et al., 2009. Basal and stimulus-induced cytokine expression is selectively impaired in peripheral blood mononuclear cells of newborn foals. Vaccine 27, 674–683.

Mariella, J., Castagnetti, Prosperi, A., Scagliarini, A., Peli, A., 2017. Cytokine levels in colostrum and in foals' serum pre-and post-suckling. Vet. Immunol. Immunopathol. 185, 34–37.

Marti, E., Ehrensperger, F., Burger, D., et al., 2009. Maternal transfer of IgE and subsequent development of IgE responses in the horse (Equus caballus). Vet. Immunol. Immunopathol. 127, 203–211.

Mila, H., Feugier, A., Grellet, A., Anne, J., et al., 2015. Immunoglobulin G concentration in canine colostrum: evaluation and variability. J. Reprod. Immunol. 12, 24–28.

Nath, L.C., Anderson, G.A., Savage, C.J., McKinnon, A.O., 2010. Use of stored equine colostrum for the treatment of foals perceived to be at risk for failure of transfer of passive immunity. J. Am. Vet. Med. Assoc. 236, 1085–1090.

Pereira, M., Valério-Bolas, A., Saraiva-Marques, C., Alexandre-Pires, G., et al., 2019. Development of the dog immune system: from in uterus to elderly. Vet. Sci. https://doi.org/10.3390/vetsci040083.

Perkins, G.A., Goodman, L.B., Wimer, C., Freer, H., et al., 2014a. Maternal T-lymphocytes in equine colostrum express a primarily inflammatory phenotype. Vet. Immunol. Immunopathol. 161, 141–150.

Perkins, G.A., Goodman, L.B., Wimer, C., Freer, H., Babasyan, S., Wagner, B., 2014b. Maternal T-lymphocytes in equine colostrum express a primarily inflammatory phenotype. Vet. Immunol. Immunopathol. 161, 141–150.

Perkins, G.A., Wagner, B., 2015. The development of equine immunity: current knowledge on immunology of the young horse. Equine Vet. J. 47, 267–274.

Reber, A.J., Donovan, D.C., Gabbard, J., et al., 2008a. Transfer of maternal colostral lymphocytes promotes development of the neonatal immune system I. Effects on monocyte lineage cells. Vet. Immunol. Immunopathol. 123, 186–196.

Reber, A.J., Donovan, D.C., Gabbard, J., et al., 2008b. Transfer of maternal colostral lymphocytes promotes development of the neonatal immune system II. Effects on neonatal lymphocytes. Vet. Immunol. Immunopathol. 123, 305–313.

Reber, A.J., Lockwood, A., Hippen, A.R., Hurley, D.J., 2006. Colostrum induced phenotypic and trafficking changes in maternal mononuclear cells in a peripheral blood leukocyte model for study of leukocyte transfer in the neonatal calf. Vet. Immunol. Immunopathol. 109, 139–150.

Schaefer-Somi, S., Baer-Schadler, S., Aurich, J.E., 2005. Proteinuria and immunoglobulinuria in neonatal dogs. Vet. Rec. 157, 378–382.

Sinkora, M., Butler, J.E., 2009. The ontogeny of the porcine immune system. Dev. Comp. Immunol. 33, 273–283.

Spreckels, J.E., Zhernakova, A., 2021. Milk and bugs educate infant immune systems. Immunity. https://doi.org/10.1016/j.immune.2021.07.013.

Sun, J., Hayward, C., Shinde, R., et al., 1998. Antibody repertoire development in fetal and neonatal piglets. I. Four VH genes account for 80 percent of VH usage during 84 days of fetal life. J. Immunol. 161, 5070–5078.

Talmadge, R.L., Tseng, C.T., King, R.A., Felippe, M.J.B., 2013. Developmental progression of equine immunoglobulin heavy chain variable region diversity. Dev. Comp. Immunol. 41, 33–43.

Tizard, I.R., 2001. The protective properties of milk and colostrum in non-human species. In: Woodward, B., Draper, H.H. (Eds.), Advances in Nutritional Research: Immunological Properties of Milk, 10. Kluwer/Plenum Publishers, New York, pp. 139–166.

Vivrette, S., 2001. Colostrum and oral immunoglobulin therapy in newborn foals. Contin. Educ. Prac. Vet. 23, 286–291.

Walther, S., Rusitzka, T.V., Diesterbeck, U.S., Czarny, C.-P., 2015. Equine immunoglobulins and organization of immunoglobulin genes. Dev. Comp. Immunol. 53, 303–319.

25

Vaccines and Their Production

CHAPTER OUTLINE

Vaccination is by far the most efficient and cost-effective method of controlling infectious diseases. The eradication of smallpox and rinderpest from the globe, the elimination of hog cholera and brucellosis from many countries, and the control of diseases such as foot-and-mouth disease, canine distemper, rabies, influenza, and pseudorabies would not have been possible without the use of effective vaccines. Vaccines are among the greatest triumphs of modern veterinary medicine.

A BRIEF HISTORY

In the 12th century, the Chinese observed that people who recovered from smallpox were resistant to further attacks of this disease. They therefore deliberately infected infants with smallpox by blowing dried smallpox scab powder up their noses. Those infants who survived the resulting disease were protected in later life. After gaining experience with the technique, it was found that inserting scab material into superficial skin wounds (variolation) worked even better and minimized the hazards. As a result, mortality due to smallpox variolation dropped to about 1%, compared to a mortality of about 20% in clinical smallpox. Knowledge of variolation spread westward to Europe by the early 18th century and was soon widely employed.

In 1798 Edward Jenner, an English physician, demonstrated that material from cowpox (vaccinia) lesions could be substituted for smallpox in variolation. Since cowpox does not cause severe disease in humans, its use has reduced the risks incurred by variolation to insignificant levels. The effectiveness of this procedure, called vaccination (*vacca* is Latin for "cow"), was such that it was eventually used in the 1970s to eradicate smallpox from the globe.

The broader implications of Jenner's observations on vaccinia and the importance of reducing the ability of an immunizing organism to cause disease were not realized until 1879. In that year, Louis Pasteur in France investigated fowl cholera, a disease caused by the bacterium now called *Pasteurella multocida*. Pasteur had a culture of this organism that was accidentally allowed to age on a laboratory bench while his assistant was on vacation. When the assistant returned and tried to infect chickens with this aged culture, the birds remained healthy. Pasteur retained these chickens and subsequently used them for a second experiment in which they were challenged again, this time with a fresh culture of *P. multocida* known to be capable of killing chickens. To Pasteur's surprise, the birds were resistant to the infection and did not die. In a remarkable intellectual leap, Pasteur immediately recognized that this phenomenon was similar in principle to Jenner's use of cowpox for vaccination. Having established the general principle of vaccination, Pasteur first applied it to anthrax. He made the anthrax bacteria (*Bacillus anthracis*) avirulent by growing them at an unusually high temperature. Local vets were skeptical. A prominent veterinarian, Monsieur Rossignol, challenged Pasteur to prove his theories in public. Pasteur accepted his challenge and used his anthrax vaccine to protect sheep and cows against challenge with virulent anthrax bacteria. The result was a triumph for immunology. The vaccinated animals lived; the unvaccinated animals all died. Pasteur subsequently developed a successful rabies vaccine by drying spinal cords taken from rabies-infected rabbits and using the dried cords as his vaccine material. The drying process effectively rendered the rabies virus avirulent.

Although Louis Pasteur used only living organisms in his vaccines, it was not long before Daniel Salmon and Theobald Smith, in the United States, demonstrated that killed organisms could also make effective vaccines. A little later, Von Behring and Kitasato in Germany showed that filtrates taken from cultures of the tetanus bacillus (*Clostridium tetani*) could protect animals against tetanus even though they contained no bacteria. Thus bacterial products, in this case, tetanus toxin, were also protective. By 1900 many new vaccines had been developed, and the development of immunity to infectious diseases in animals was a well-recognized phenomenon.

TYPES OF IMMUNIZATION PROCEDURES

There are two procedures by which any animal may be made immune to an infectious disease: passive and active immunization (Fig. 25.1). Passive immunization produces temporary immunity by transferring antibodies from a resistant to a susceptible animal. These transferred antibodies (or antisera) give immediate protection, but since they are gradually catabolized, this protection wanes, and the recipient eventually becomes susceptible again.

Active immunization, in contrast, involves administering antigen to an animal so that it responds by mounting an adaptive immune response. Reimmunization or exposure to infection in the same animal will result in a secondary response and greatly enhanced immunity. The disadvantage of active immunization is, as with all adaptive immune responses, that protection is not conferred immediately. However, once established, active immunity is long-lasting and capable of restimulation (Fig. 25.2; Plotkin, 2010).

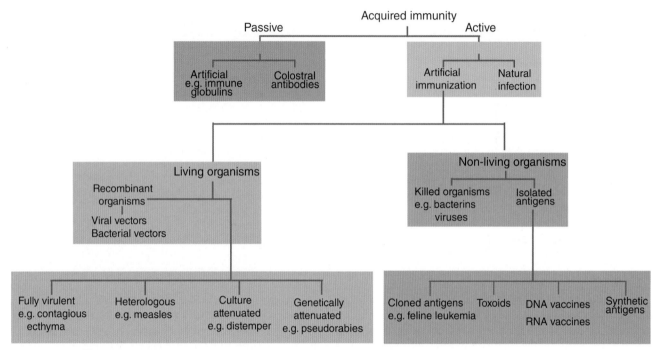

Fig. 25.1 A classification of the different types of adaptive immunity and of the methods employed to induce protection.

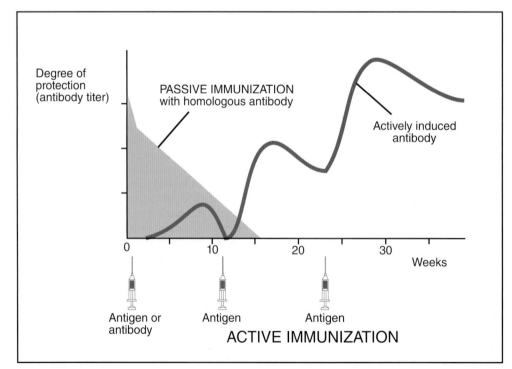

Fig. 25.2 The levels of serum antibody (and hence the degree of protection) conferred by active and passive methods of immunization.

PASSIVE IMMUNIZATION

Passive immunization requires that antibodies be produced in donor animals by active immunization and that these antibodies be administered to susceptible animals to confer immediate protection. Serum containing these antibodies may be produced against a wide variety of pathogens. For instance, they can be produced in cattle against anthrax, in dogs against distemper, or in cats against panleukopenia. They are most effective in protecting animals against toxigenic organisms such as *C. tetani* or *Clostridium perfringens*, using antisera raised in horses. Antisera made in this way are called immune globulins and are commonly produced in young horses by a series of immunizing injections. The clostridial toxins are proteins that can be denatured and made nontoxic by treatment with formaldehyde. Formaldehyde-treated toxins are called toxoids. Donor horses are initially injected with toxoids, but once antibodies are produced and the horses are immune, subsequent injections may contain purified toxin. The responses of the donors are monitored, and once their antibody levels are sufficiently high, they are bled. Bleeding is undertaken at intervals until the antibody level drops, when the animals are again boosted with antigen. Plasma is separated from the horse blood, and the globulin fraction that contains the antibodies is concentrated, titrated, and dispensed.

To standardize the potency of different immune globulins, a comparison must be made with an international biological standard. In the case of tetanus immune globulin, this is done by comparing the dose necessary to protect guinea pigs against a fixed amount of tetanus toxin with the dose of the standard preparation of immune globulin required to achieve the same. The international standard immune globulin for tetanus toxin is a quantity held at the State Serum Institute in Copenhagen. An international unit (IU) of tetanus immune globulin is the specific neutralizing activity contained in 0.03384 mg of the international standard. The US standard unit (AU) is double the IU.

Tetanus immune globulin is given to animals to confer immediate protection against tetanus. At least 1500 IU of immune globulin should be given to horses and cattle; at least 500 IU to calves, sheep, goats, and swine; and at least 250 IU to dogs. The exact amount should vary with the amount of tissue damage, the degree of wound contamination, and the time elapsed since injury. Tetanus immune globulin is of little use once the toxin has bound to its target receptor and clinical disease develops.

Although immune globulins provide immediate protection, some problems are associated with their use. For instance, when horse tetanus immune globulin is given to a cow or dog, the horse proteins are recognized as foreign, elicit an immune response, and are then rapidly eliminated (Fig. 25.3). To reduce their antigenicity, immune globulins

are usually treated with pepsin to destroy their Fc region and leave intact only the portion of the immunoglobulin molecule required for toxin neutralization, the F(ab)$'_2$ fragment.

If circulating horse globulins are still present by the time the recipient animal mounts an antihorse response, the immune-complexes formed may cause a type III hypersensitivity reaction called serum sickness (see Chapter 33). If repeated doses of horse immune globulin are given to an animal of another species, this may provoke immunoglobulin E production and so cause allergic reactions (see Chapter 30). Finally, the presence of high levels of circulating horse antibodies may interfere with active immunization against the same antigen. This is a phenomenon similar to that seen in newborn animals who are passively protected by maternal antibodies.

Monoclonal antibodies are another source of passive protection for animals. Initially, however, these were derived from mouse-mouse hybridomas and thus were mouse immunoglobulins. They were therefore antigenic. Nevertheless, mouse monoclonal antibodies against the K99 pilus antigens of *Escherichia coli* can be given orally to calves to protect them against diarrhea caused by this organism. A mouse monoclonal antibody to lymphoma cells has been used to treat affected dogs. Monoclonal antibodies, especially when engineered to match the immunoglobulins of the recipient species, are increasingly used to treat inflammatory diseases and cancer (see Chapters 38 and 36). Thus the US Department of Agriculture (USDA) has licensed a caninized monoclonal antibody directed against canine parvovirus. It has proven effective in reducing mortality and the severity of clinical signs such as vomiting.

Oral administration of specific chicken IgY to calves within the first two weeks of life can delay the onset of neonatal diarrhea and reduce its severity and duration. The IgY antibodies are produced by immunizing chickens against diverse bovine enteric pathogens (rotavirus, coronavirus, *E. coli*, and *Salmonella enterica* Dublin). The birds concentrate these antibodies in their egg yolks, so the eggs are harvested and the yolks spray-dried to produce a powdered product. The neonatal calves are fed milk supplemented with this egg IgY (Vega et al., 2020).

ACTIVE IMMUNIZATION

Active immunization has several major advantages over passive immunization. These include the prolonged period of protection and the recall and boosting of this protective response by repeated injections of antigen or by exposure to infection. An ideal vaccine for active immunization should therefore give prolonged strong immunity. This immunity should be conferred on both the animal immunized and any fetus carried by it. In order to obtain this strong immunity, the vaccine should be free of adverse side effects. (In effect, it should stimulate adaptive immunity without triggering the inflammation associated with innate immunity.) The ideal vaccine should be cheap, stable, and adaptable to mass vaccination; ideally, it should stimulate an immune response distinguishable from that due to natural infection so that immunization and eradication may proceed simultaneously.

In addition to these requirements, effective vaccines must have other critical properties. First, antigen must be delivered efficiently so that antigen-presenting cells can process the antigen and release appropriate cytokines. Second, both T and B cells must be stimulated so that they generate large numbers of memory cells. Third, helper and effector T cells must be generated to several epitopes in the vaccine so that individual variations in MHC class II polymorphism and epitope properties are minimized. Fourth, the immune response triggered by the vaccine must be appropriate to the infectious agent, in other words, antibodies or cell-mediated immunity as required. Finally, the antigen must be able to stimulate memory cells in such a way that protection will last for as long as possible.

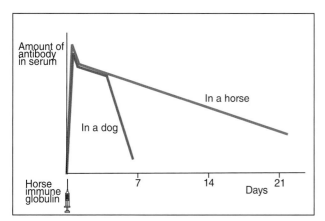

Fig. 25.3 The fate of passively administered equine immune globulin when given to a homologous species (horse) or to a heterologous species (dog).

Living and Killed Vaccines

Unfortunately, two of the prerequisites of an ideal vaccine, high antigenicity and absence of adverse side effects, are sometimes incompatible. Modified live viruses infect host cells and undergo replication. The infected cells then process the endogenous antigen. In this way, live viruses trigger a type 1 immune response dominated by CD8+ cytotoxic T cells. While protective, this approach may be hazardous because the vaccine viruses may themselves cause sickness or persistent infection as a result of residual virulence. In contrast, killed organisms act as exogenous antigens. As a result, they usually stimulate type 2 responses dominated by CD4+ T cells and antibodies. This may not be the most effective protective response to some organisms, but it may be safer (Table 25.1).

The practical advantages and disadvantages of vaccines containing living or killed organisms are well demonstrated in the search for effective and safe vaccines against *Brucella abortus* in cattle. *B. abortus* is a cause of abortion, and vaccination has been used successfully to control and eradicate the infection in many countries. Because it can grow within cells, Brucella infections are best controlled by type 1 immune responses involving macrophage activation, the production of IFN-γ by Th1 cells, and cytotoxic CD8+ T cells. A vaccine containing a living attenuated strain of *Brucella* is therefore required to induce a protective response. Many attempts have been made to produce the ideal attenuated vaccine strain but with limited success. Thus, the first, and most widely used vaccine is the modified strain 19 (S19) of *B. abortus*. This is a spontaneously generated smooth mutant strain. However, it is not highly protective, conferring only 65% protection against infection but 96% against abortion. As a smooth stain, it also contains the O-polysaccharide that stimulates continuous antibody production but, as a result, interferes with serologic tests used to identify infected cattle. S19 can also cause orchitis in bulls and may cause abortions if given to pregnant cows.

As a result of the shortcomings of S19, an attenuated streptomycin-resistant, smooth strain of *B. melitensis* called strain Rev.1 was developed. Rev.1 can be administered by the conjunctival route. Unfortunately, while effective, Rev.1 also has significant residual virulence and may cause abortions in pregnant cows. It also causes disease in humans and so poses a significant threat to the operator.

A rough attenuated strain of *B. abortus* called RB-51 has also been used in cattle in the United States. This is a mutant that lacks the lipopolysaccharide O antigen. It produces a strong Th1 response with production of IFN-γ and CD8+ cytotoxic T cells. Because of its rough phenotype, it can be distinguished serologically from wild-type infections and is thus appropriate for use in eradication programs. Unlike S19, it does not induce false-positive results in the standard diagnostic tests such as card agglutination, complement fixation, or tube agglutination tests. RB-51 is less pathogenic for cattle than S19, and it is not shed in nasal secretions, saliva, or urine. It will, however, cause disease in accidentally exposed humans, and because of its failure to stimulate antibody production, this may be difficult to diagnose (Ashford et al., 2004).

Another attenuated strain of *B. melitensis* is M5. M5 has been attenuated by serial passage in chicken cells. However, it can also revert to virulence. A smooth strain of *B. suis* has also been used with success in pigs and other species. It is widely used to prevent brucellosis in swine and has given satisfactory results (Hou et al., 2019). Multiple other smooth *B. abortus* vaccine strains have been developed, including strains H38 and S2. A smooth-rough strain of *B abortus* is SR82, widely used in Russia and the former Soviet republics.

Another rough strain of *B abortus* is 45/20. This was originally attenuated by serial passage through guinea pigs. As a result of its instability, it has been used as a killed vaccine with an oil adjuvant. Unfortunately, killed vaccines such as strain 45/20 protect cattle for less than a year.

Live vaccines always run the risk of contamination with unwanted organisms; for instance, outbreaks of reticuloendotheliosis in chickens in Japan and Australia have been traced to contaminated Marek's disease vaccines. An outbreak of bovine leukosis in Australia resulted from contamination of a batch of babesiosis vaccine containing whole calf blood. Abortion and death have occurred in pregnant bitches that received a canine parvovirus vaccine contaminated with bluetongue virus. Contaminating mycoplasma may also be present in some vaccines. Scrapie has been spread in mycoplasma vaccines. Finally, vaccines containing living attenuated organisms require much care in their preparation, storage, and handling to avoid killing the organisms. Maintaining the cold chain can account for up to 80% of the cost of a vaccine in the tropics.

Inactivation

Organisms killed for use in vaccines must remain as antigenically similar to the living organisms as possible. Therefore crude methods of killing that cause major changes in antigen structure as a result of protein denaturation are usually unsatisfactory. If chemicals are used, they must not alter the structure of the antigens responsible for stimulating protective immunity. One such chemical is formaldehyde, which cross-links proteins and nucleic acids and confers structural rigidity. Proteins can also be mildly denatured by acetone or alcohol treatment. Alkylating agents that cross-link nucleic acid chains are also suitable for killing organisms since, by leaving the surface proteins of organisms unchanged, they do not interfere with antigenicity. Examples of alkylating agents include ethylene oxide, ethyleneimine, acetyl ethyleneimine, and β-propiolactone, all of which have been used in veterinary vaccines. Many successful vaccines containing killed bacteria (bacterins) or inactivated toxins (toxoids) can be made relatively simply by the use of these agents. Some vaccines may contain mixtures of these components. For example, some vaccines against *Mannheimia hemolytica* contain both killed bacteria and inactivated bacterial leukotoxin.

The disadvantages of killed vaccines parallel the advantages of living vaccines. The use of adjuvants to increase effective antigenicity can cause severe inflammation or systemic toxicity, and multiple doses or high individual doses of antigen increase the risk of causing hypersensitivity reactions, as well as increasing costs (Table 25.1).

TABLE 25.1 The Relative Merits of Living and Inactivated Vaccines	
Living Vaccines	**Inactivated Vaccines**
Fewer doses required	Stable on storage
Adjuvants unnecessary	Unlikely to cause disease due to residual virulence
Less chance of hypersensitivity	Do not replicate in recipient
Induction of interferon	Unlikely to contain live contaminating organisms
Relatively cheap	Will not spread to other animals
Smaller dose needed	Safe in immunodeficient patients
Can be given by natural route	Easier to store
Stimulate both humoral and cell-mediated response	Lower development costs
Longer lasting protection	No risk of reversion

Attenuation

Virulent living organisms cannot normally be used in vaccines. Their virulence must be reduced so that, although still living, they can no longer cause disease. This process of reduction of virulence is called attenuation. Effective attenuation is critical to vaccine success. Underattenuation will result in residual virulence and disease; overattenuation may result in an ineffective vaccine. The traditional methods of attenuation were empirical, and there was little understanding of the changes induced by the attenuation process. They usually involved adapting organisms to growth in unusual conditions so that they lost their adaptation to their usual host. For example, the bacille Calmette-Guérin (BCG) strain of *Mycobacterium bovis* was rendered avirulent by being grown for 13 years on bile-saturated medium. Pasteur's vaccine strain of anthrax was rendered avirulent by growth in 50% serum agar under an atmosphere rich in CO_2, so that it lost its ability to form a capsule. *B. abortus* S19 vaccine was grown under conditions in which there was a shortage of nutrients. Unfortunately, genetic stability cannot always be guaranteed in these attenuated strains. Back-mutation or genome reassortment using genes from related organisms may occur, and the attenuated organisms may redevelop virulence.

A more reliable method of making bacteria avirulent is by genetic manipulation. For example, a modified live vaccine is available that contains streptomycin-dependent *M. hemolytica* and *P. multocida*. These mutants depend on the presence of streptomycin for growth. When they are administered to an animal, the absence of streptomycin will eventually result in the death of the bacteria, but not before they have stimulated a protective immune response.

Viruses have traditionally been attenuated by growth in cells or species to which they are not naturally adapted. For example, rinderpest virus, which was normally a pathogen of cattle, was first attenuated by growth in rabbits. Eventually, a successful tissue culture-adapted rinderpest vaccine devoid of residual virulence was developed. Similar examples include the adaptation of African horse sickness virus to mice and of canine distemper virus to ferrets. Alternatively, mammalian viruses may be attenuated by growth in eggs. For example, the

Flury strain of rabies was attenuated by prolonged passage in eggs and lost its virulence for normal dogs and cats.

The traditional method of virus attenuation has been prolonged tissue culture. In these cases, virus attenuation is accomplished by culturing the organism in cells to which they are not adapted. For example, virulent canine distemper virus preferentially attacks lymphoid cells. For vaccine purposes, therefore, this virus was cultured in canine kidney cells. In adapting to these culture conditions, it lost its ability to cause severe disease.

Under some circumstances, it is possible to use fully virulent organisms for immunization. Vaccination against contagious ecthyma of sheep is of this type. Contagious ecthyma (orf) is a viral disease of lambs that causes massive scab formation around the mouth, prevents feeding, and results in a failure to thrive. The disease has little systemic effect. Lambs recover completely within a few weeks and are immune from then on. It is usual to vaccinate lambs by rubbing dried, infected scab material into scratches made in the inner aspect of the thigh. The local infection at this site has no untoward effect on the lambs, and they become solidly immune. Because vaccinated animals may spread the disease, however, they must be separated from unvaccinated animals for a few weeks.

MODERN VACCINE TECHNOLOGY

Although both killed and modified live vaccines have been successful in controlling many infectious diseases, there is always a need to make them more effective, cheaper, and safer (Fig. 25.4). The use of modern molecular techniques has produced many new and improved vaccines. These vaccines can be classified into several categories (Table 25.2).

Antigens Generated by Gene Cloning (Category I)

Gene cloning can be used to produce large quantities of purified antigen in culture. In this process, DNA coding for the antigen of interest is first isolated from the pathogen. This DNA is then inserted into a bacterium or yeast in such a way that the gene is functional, and the recombinant

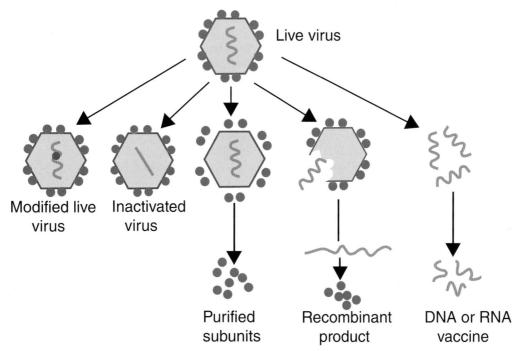

Fig. 25.4 A schematic diagram showing some of the different ways in which a virus and its antigens may be treated in order to produce a vaccine. *DNA*, Deoxyribonucleic acid; *RNA*, ribonucleic acid.

TABLE 25.2   USDA Classification of Genetically Engineered Veterinary Biologics

Category	Description
I	Vaccines that contain inactivated recombinant organisms or purified antigens derived from recombinant organisms
II	Vaccines containing live organisms that contain gene deletions or heterologous marker genes
III	Vaccines that contain live expression vectors expressing heterologous genes for immunizing antigens or other stimulants
IV	Other genetically engineered vaccines such as polynucleotide vaccines.

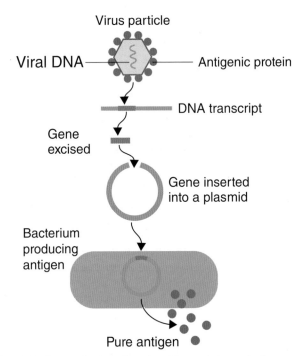

Fig. 25.5 The production of a recombinant viral protein for use in a vaccine. The gene coding for the viral antigen of interest is cloned into another organism, in this case, a bacterium, and expressed and produced in very large quantities. *DNA,* Deoxyribonucleic acid.

protein is expressed in large amounts (Shin and Yoo, 2013). The first successful use of a cloned protein in this way involved foot-and-mouth disease virus (Fig. 25.5). This virus is extremely simple. The protective antigen (VP1) is well recognized, and the genes that code for this protein have been mapped. The RNA genome of the foot-and-mouth disease virus was isolated and transcribed into DNA by the enzyme reverse transcriptase. The DNA was then carefully cut by restriction endonucleases so that it only contained the gene for VP1. This DNA was then inserted into a plasmid, the plasmid was inserted into *E. coli,* and the bacteria were grown. The bacteria synthesized large quantities of VP1, which was harvested, purified, and incorporated into a vaccine. The process is highly efficient since 4×10^7 doses of foot-and-mouth vaccine can be obtained from 10 L of *E. coli* grown to 10^{12} organisms per milliliter. Unfortunately, the immunity produced by the pure protein is inferior to that produced by killed whole virus and requires a 1000-fold higher antigen dose to induce comparable protection.

The first commercially available category I recombinant veterinary vaccine was made against feline leukemia virus. The major envelope protein of FeLV, gp70, is the antigen largely responsible for inducing a protective immune response in cats. Thus the gene for gp70 (a glycoprotein of 70 kDa) plus a small portion of a linked protein called p15e (a protein of 15 kDa from the envelope) was isolated and inserted into *E. coli,* which then synthesized large amounts of p70. This recombinant p70 is not glycosylated and has a molecular weight of just over 50 kDa. Once cloned, the recombinant protein is harvested, purified, mixed with a saponin adjuvant, and used as a vaccine.

Another example of a recombinant vaccine is that directed against the Lyme disease agent, *Borrelia burgdorferi.* Thus the gene for OspA, the immunodominant outer surface lipoprotein of *B. burgdorferi,* has been cloned into *E. coli.* The recombinant protein expressed by *E. coli* is purified and used as a vaccine when combined with adjuvant. This vaccine is unique since ticks feeding on immunized animals ingest host antibodies. The antibodies then kill the bacteria within the tick midgut and prevent their dissemination to the salivary glands. They thus prevent transmission by the vector.

Gene cloning techniques are useful in any situation where pure protein antigens need to be synthesized in large quantities. Unfortunately, very pure proteins are often poor antigens because they are not effectively delivered to antigen-sensitive cells and may not be correctly folded. An alternative approach to this problem is to chemically link multiple key protective epitopes of a virus into a single artificial protein. These so-called mosaic vaccines are theoretically much more potent than single epitopes or even the original organism. They are currently being developed for use against HIV and SARs coronaviruses. Mosaic-based vaccines formulated with polyanhydride nanoparticles have also been developed against H5 avian influenza in poultry. They appear to be safe and highly effective (Kingstad-Bakke et al., 2019).

Genetically Attenuated Organisms (Category II)

Molecular genetic techniques make it possible to deliberately alter the genes of an organism so that it becomes irreversibly attenuated. These are classified as category II vaccines. They are available against the herpesvirus that causes pseudorabies in swine. The enzyme, thymidine kinase (TK), is required by herpesviruses to replicate in nondividing cells such as neurons. Viruses from which the *TK* gene has been removed can infect nerve cells but cannot replicate and therefore cannot cause disease (Fig. 25.6). As a result, these vaccines not only confer effective protection but also block cell invasion by virulent pseudorabies viruses, preventing the development of a persistent carrier state. A similar deletion vaccine has been generated for equine herpesvirus–1. In this case, four virulence and immune evasive genes have been deleted resulting in a highly attenuated but immunogenic vaccine strain (Balena et al., 2022).

Genetic manipulation can also be used to make "marker vaccines." For example, pseudorabies virus synthesizes two glycoprotein antigens called gX and gI. These are potent antigens, yet neither is essential for viral growth or virulence. They are expressed by all field isolates of this virus, and so infected animals will make antibodies to both gX and gI. An attenuated pseudorabies vaccine has been produced that lacks these proteins. Vaccinated pigs do not make antibodies to gX or gI, but naturally infected pigs will. The vaccine will not cause positive serological reactions in assays for anti-gX or -gI, and the presence of antibodies to gX and gI in a pig is evidence that the animal has been exposed to field strains of pseudorabies virus. This type of vaccine, called a DIVA vaccine (Differentiate Infected from Vaccinated Animals), should assist in eradicating specific infectious diseases much more economically and rapidly than conventional methods. Another example of a DIVA vaccine is the insertion of an influenza B gene into an avian influenza A

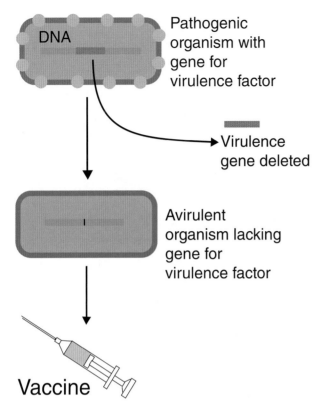

Fig. 25.6 The production of an attenuated virus by removal of a gene required for virulence. Genes coding for major antigens detected by serological techniques can also be removed, ensuring that vaccinated animals can be distinguished from naturally infected ones. *DNA*, Deoxyribonucleic acid.

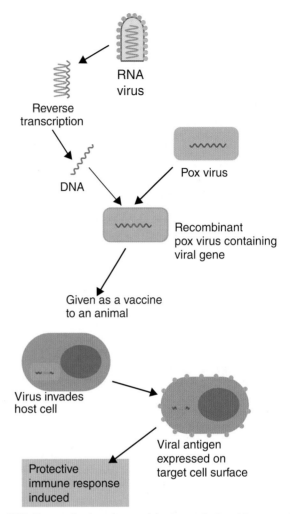

Fig. 25.7 The production of a vaccinia-vectored recombinant vaccine. Vaccinia is selected because it has room to spare in its genome, and it is easy to administer to an animal. Thus, rabies-vaccinia recombinants can be given orally. *DNA*, Deoxyribonucleic acid; *RNA*, ribonucleic acid.

vaccine. Since influenza B does not infect birds, the presence of anti-influenza B antibodies confirms vaccination.

Live Recombinant Organisms (Category III)

Genes coding for protein antigens can be cloned directly into a variety of organisms. Instead of being purified, the live recombinant organism itself may then be used as a vaccine. These are classified as category III vaccines (Fig. 25.7). Experimental recombinant vaccines have used adenoviruses, herpesviruses, and bacteria such as BCG or salmonella as vectors, but the organisms that have been most widely employed for this purpose are poxviruses such as vaccinia, fowlpox, and canarypox. These viruses are easy to administer by dermal scratching or by ingestion. They have a large, stable genome that makes it relatively easy to insert a new gene (up to 10% of its genome can be replaced by foreign DNA), and they can express high levels of the new antigen. Moreover, these recombinant proteins undergo appropriate processing, including glycosylation and membrane transport within the poxvirus. The Avian poxviruses, such as canarypox, are especially effective vectors in mammals. They do not replicate, and antigen expression only lasts about 6 hours. As a result, these vaccines are very safe, they cannot be transmitted by arthropods, and they are not excreted in body fluids. It is of interest to note that they do not stimulate immunity to the vector virus, a feature that occurs with the use of other vectors and hence can prevent subsequent immunizations. Canarypox-vectored vaccines appear to overcome blocking by maternal antibodies and can thus prime very young animals. They cannot revert to virulence and, as a result, are widely employed to prevent diseases caused by feline leukemia, the West Nile virus, canine parvovirus, canine distemper,

equine influenza, and rabies. Another example of a live recombinant vaccine is vaccinia-vectored rabies. The gene for the rabies envelope glycoprotein, or G-protein, can be inserted into vaccinia virus. This glycoprotein can induce virus-neutralizing antibody and thus confer protection against rabies. Infection with this rabies-vaccinia recombinant results in the production of antibodies to the G-protein and the development of immunity. This vaccine has been successfully used as an oral bait vaccine administered to wild carnivores. This form of the vaccine can be distributed by dropping baited vaccine packs from aircraft. It has been used in Ontario to prevent the spread of fox rabies, in New Jersey to prevent the spread of raccoon rabies, and in Texas to block the spread of coyote rabies. For example, since 1995, 17.5 million doses of vaccinia-vectored rabies vaccine have been air-dropped over 255,500 square miles (661,745 km²) of Texas with great success (Box 25.1; Weyer et al., 2009).

Highly effective category III vaccines were developed for rinderpest; these consisted of a vaccinia or capripox vector containing the hemagglutinin *(H)* or fusion *(F)* genes of rinderpest virus. These vaccines were so effective that their systematic use led to the global eradication of that disease. The recombinant capripox vaccine has also had the benefit of protecting cattle against lumpy skin disease. Another example of a category III vaccine involves the use of a yellow fever viral

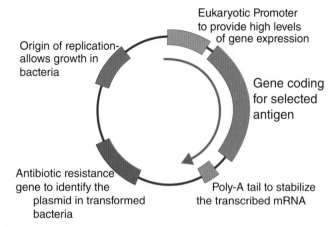

Fig. 25.8 The structure of a typical deoxyribonucleic plasmid used for vaccination purposes. In this case, the plasmid codes for protective antigens of the West Nile virus. In addition to coding for the specific protective antigen, the plasmid carries an antibiotic resistance marker so that its fate may be traced. *mRNA*, Messenger ribonucleic acid.

chimera to protect against the West Nile virus. This technology uses the capsid and nonstructural genes of the attenuated yellow fever vaccine strain 17D to deliver the envelope genes of other flaviviruses, such as the West Nile virus. The resulting virus is the yellow fever-West Nile virus chimera that is much less neuroinvasive and hence much safer than either of the parent viruses. The margin of safety can be increased even further by introducing targeted point mutations into the envelope genes. The first category III vaccine approved by the USDA was against the Newcastle disease virus. The vector is a fowlpox virus, into which Newcastle disease *HA* and *F* genes have been incorporated. It has the additional benefit of conferring immunity against fowlpox.

Oral vaccination has long been considered a desirable route of administration for animals but has been hindered by the ability of the gastrointestinal tract to digest and destroy oral antigens. Such vaccines have been delivered in the form of plant materials. Cloning of vaccine antigen genes into plants has been successfully achieved for viruses such as transmissible gastroenteritis, Norwalk virus, and Newcastle disease. The plants employed include tobacco, potato, soybean, rice, and corn. A Newcastle disease vaccine produced in suspension-cultured tobacco cells has been licensed in the United States. Rather than administering the antigen in plants, an alternative approach is to deliver it within yeast cells. Yeast-based vaccines show high expression levels, are considered very safe, may be "self-adjuvanting," and their antigens undergo appropriate posttranslational modification. Many potential yeast-based vaccines are currently under development, especially for poultry and swine vaccinations (Shin and Yoo, 2013).

Nucleic Acid Vaccines (Category IV)

An increasingly popular method of vaccination involves injection, not of a protein antigen, but of pure DNA or RNAs that encode the vaccine antigens (Dunham, 2002). These are, technically speaking, not vaccines; they simply turn an animal's cells into vaccine factories that produce large amounts of viral antigens. These nucleic acids have to be delivered directly into the animal's cells.

DNA Vaccines

To induce protective immunity an animal is administered DNA encoding the antigen of interest. This DNA is first inserted into a bacterial plasmid, a piece of circular DNA that acts as a vector (Moss, 2009). The

vaccine antigen gene is placed under the control of a strong mammalian promoter sequence. When the genetically engineered plasmid is injected intramuscularly into an animal, it is taken up by host cells. The DNA is then transcribed into messenger RNA (mRNA) and translated into endogenous vaccine protein (Fig. 25.8). Transfected host cells synthesize the vaccine protein and present it, as an endogenous antigen, in association with MHC class I molecules. This leads to the development of not only neutralizing antibodies but also cytotoxic T cells. Expressed antigens have an authentic tertiary structure and posttranslational modifications such as glycosylation. The immune response is also enhanced since the bacterial DNA contains unmethylated CpG motifs that are recognized by toll-like receptor 9 (TLR9) and activate dendritic cells. These, in turn, promote a strong Th1 response. The DNA sequence of a plasmid can be easily modified in order to manipulate the Th1-Th2 ratio in the induced response. Similarly, the DNA can be combined with genes for cytokines, as well as adjuvants, polymeric carriers or viral vectors. Thus it can be modified in many ways to improve antigen yield and immunogenicity (Gerdts et al., 2013). Some plasmids may be engineered to express more than one antigen or perhaps an antigen plus an immunostimulatory protein separated by a spacer. Alternatively, a mixture of two plasmids, one expressing the antigen gene and one expressing a cytokine gene, may be administered at the same time.

A DNA vaccine is used to protect horses against the West Nile virus infection. The commercial vaccine consists of a plasmid vector engineered to express high levels of the virus envelope (E) and premembrane proteins. In addition, the plasmid contains gene promoters and marker genes. Upon injection together with a biodegradable oil adjuvant, this plasmid enters cells and causes them to express the viral protein. Other DNA vaccines have been approved to prevent infectious hematopoietic necrosis in Atlantic salmon and melanomas in dogs (see Chapter 36). This approach has also been applied experimentally to produce vaccines against avian influenza, lymphocytic choriomeningitis, canine and feline rabies, canine parvovirus, bovine viral diarrhea, feline immunodeficiency virus, feline leukemia virus, pseudorabies, foot-and-mouth disease virus, bovine herpesvirus–1, and Newcastle disease (Fischer et al., 2003; Jiang et al., 1998). Although theoretically producing a response similar to that induced by attenuated live vaccines, these nucleic acid vaccines are ideally suited to protect against organisms that are difficult or dangerous to grow in the laboratory.

Some DNA vaccines can induce immunity even in the presence of very high titers of maternal antibodies. Although the maternal antibodies block serological responses, the development of strong memory responses is not impaired (Babiuk et al., 2003).

DNA vaccines must get inside the nuclei of target cells in order to be effective. This can be done by intramuscular injection or by "shooting" the DNA plasmids directly through the skin adsorbed onto microscopic gold beads fired by a "gene gun." Although intramuscular injection is very inefficient because the transfection rate is low (about 1%–5% of myofibrils in the vicinity of an intramuscular injection site), the expression can persist for at least 2 months. The use of a gene gun is more efficient than injection since some of this DNA is taken up by dendritic cells, and it minimizes degradation. By bypassing TLR9, the DNA preferentially stimulates a Th2 response. Viral DNA in eye drops can induce an IgA response in the tears and bile of recipients (Russell and Mackie, 2001).

Messenger RNA Vaccines

Messenger RNA vaccines have recently risen to prominence as a result of their effectiveness against the coronavirus that causes COVID-19. They have multiple advantages over DNA vaccines. Thus, if the amino acid sequence of the protective viral antigen is known, then the RNA encoding that sequence can be readily synthesized. Unlike DNA that must cross both the cell membrane and the nuclear membrane to gain access to the cell nucleus in order to be transcribed, RNA works in the cell cytoplasm. Antigens can be translated immediately after they enter the cytoplasm. Thus, the RNA is commonly delivered within stable lipid nanoparticles that are readily endocytosed by dendritic cells and macrophages. Once inside the cytoplasm, the RNA is released and efficiently translated into a protein that is processed and expressed on the cell surface (Fig. 25.9).

Messenger RNA is produced by transcription of DNA and is subsequently translated into proteins. Thus, when it enters cells, the mRNA triggers specific protein expression. This mRNA is only transiently expressed and, as a result, is potentially safer than persistent DNA. RNA can be synthesized so that it encodes complete proteins or even selected parts of proteins. The mRNA incorporates open reading frames that encode proteins combined with sequences at both termini that regulate translation and protein expression. While conventional vaccines require large and expensive production facilities, RNA synthesis is relatively simple. It can be readily manufactured using a standardized process, reducing both cost and time. Only information about the RNA sequence is required, and there is no need to handle dangerous pathogens.

RNA can be delivered to cells in two forms: either as conventional mRNA or as self-amplifying mRNAs, also called replicons. Both types of RNA are safe and well tolerated and induce antigen-specific immune responses. Conventional mRNA vaccines have largely been developed for use in human cancers. They encode tumor specific antigens that can trigger a protective immune response.

Much recent focus has however been on the use of self-amplifying vectors—replicons, derived from alphaviruses since these are highly effective and require a much lower dose of RNA to induce a protective immune response (Lundstrom, 2012). Replicons are defined as nucleic acids that contain the instructions for their own replication. This self-amplifying RNA has the potential to make more copies of the antigen for a longer time, making it more effective than conventional RNA vaccines. Given the success of RNA vaccines in combating COVID-19, it is unsurprising that mRNA vaccines are being investigated for use in many other diseases (Li et al., 2022). RNA replicon vaccines that have been investigated with encouraging results include those directed against swine influenza, avian influenza, foot-and-mouth disease, equine arteritis, porcine respiratory and reproductive syndrome, and Nipah virus. Three RNA replicon vaccines have been licensed by USDA. These are directed against porcine epidemic diarrhea, swine influenza H3N2, and highly pathogenic avian influenza H5N2.

Bacterial Ghosts

Bacterial "ghosts" are the empty cell envelopes of gram-negative bacteria. They have no cytoplasm and no chromosomal or plasmid DNA, but a conserved cellular morphology and all cell surface structures. They are constructed using the cloned bacteriophage lysis gene *E*. This protein fuses the inner and outer membranes of gram-negative bacteria to form a transmembrane pore through which the bacterial cytoplasm escapes. For safety reasons, any remaining DNA is destroyed by nucleases during the production process. Thus, these ghosts contain no genetic information. However, when used as vaccines, they are highly immunogenic. These ghosts appear to be excellent alternatives

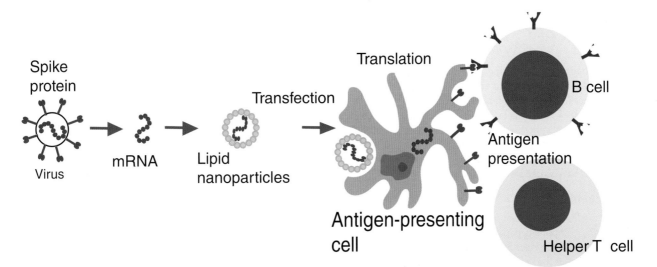

Fig. 25.9 Ribonucleic acid (RNA) vaccines may be delivered within stable lipid nanoparticles that are readily endocytosed by dendritic cells and macrophages. Once inside the cytoplasm, the RNA is translated into a protein sequence that is processed and the foreign expressed on the cell surface, where it is recognized by T and B cells. *mRNA*, Messenger RNA.

WHOLE VIRUS

VIRUS-LIKE PARTICLE

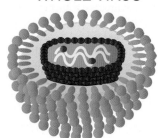
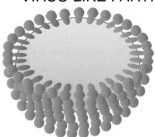

Fig. 25.10 The structure of virus-like particles. These are essentially virus particles that do not contain genetic material. These "empty shells" are fully immunogenic and trigger a protective response against the original virus.

to killed bacterial vaccines. Ghosts have also been generated against the bovine pathogens *P. multocida* and *Mannheimia haemolytica* and diverse gram-negative pathogens, such as Salmonellae and *E. coli*, with encouraging results.

Virus-Like Particles

In general, resistance to virus infections depends on immune responses directed against protein antigens on the surface of the virus or on virus-infected cells (Crisci et al., 2012). Subunit vaccines directed against isolated surface antigens tend to be poorly immunogenic. Virus-like particles (VLPs) are subunit vaccines that assemble into structures resembling the outer protein shell of viruses. They do not contain a viral genome and cannot spread the infection (Fig. 25.10). They have the same shape and size as native viruses, such as icosahedrons or rods (Liu et al., 2012). VLPs are diverse nanoparticles 20–100 nm in size. They may be constructed using viral protein subunits to form, in effect, a natural viral capsid. Subunit vaccines, as described above, are often poor immunogens because of incorrect folding or poor presentation to antigen-presenting cells. VLPs, in contrast, are the optimal size and present dense repeating protein arrays and conformational epitopes similar to those of intact viruses. Thus, VLPs can serve as modular vaccine platforms for a diverse range of viral diseases, such as influenza and bluetongue (Lee et al., 2013). VLPs and other nanoparticles are sufficiently small that they can penetrate tissue barriers, travel to draining lymph nodes and are readily taken up by antigen-presenting cells.

Virosomes

Virosomes are liposomes expressing viral antigens. Liposomes are lipid-based vesicles with an aqueous core surrounded by a phospholipid bilayer. Cationic liposomes bind antigenic proteins as a result of their surface charge. Viral antigens may be enclosed in the aqueous core, absorbed into the phospholipid bilayer or adsorbed onto the liposome surface. Thus purified viral antigens can be used to make antigenic virosomes. Experimental vaccines incorporating Newcastle disease virosomes have worked well in chickens.

Subunit Vaccines

The simplest method to produce a subunit vaccine is to break an organism into its component parts. For example, influenza vaccines are grown in eggs, and the virus membrane is disrupted by means of a surfactant. This releases the envelope as well as the internal nuclear and matrix proteins. The vaccines are further purified by centrifugation to remove the internal viral core. Split-virion vaccines do not undergo further purification, so they usually contain more protein and are thus more likely to cause local reactions. However, comparative efficacy

studies suggest that split-virion flu vaccines are more effective than subunit vaccines. It appears that the internal viral core proteins stimulate greater cell-mediated responses. It is also possible to isolate and use the two major influenza antigens, the hemagglutinin and neuraminidase, in a vaccine so as to minimize toxic effects.

Prime-Boost Strategies

It has long been normal practice to use exactly the same vaccine for boosting an immune response as was employed when priming an animal. This approach has many advantages, not the least of which is simplicity in manufacturing and regulating vaccine production. There is, however, no reason why different forms of a vaccine should not be used for priming and for boosting if this will induce a better response. This approach is known as a heterologous prime-boost strategy. Under some circumstances, this may result in improved vaccine effectiveness. Combinations may involve priming with one DNA plasmid but boosting with either another plasmid, perhaps in another vector, or with recombinant protein antigens. These strategies may increase the avidity and persistence of antibody responses as well as cytotoxic T-cell responses.

Reverse Vaccinology

Now that many complete microbial genomes are available, it is possible to identify all the proteins of a pathogen by computer analysis (Sette and Rappuoli, 2010). Artificial intelligence can then be used to select potential protective epitopes from this repertoire. This can lead to the identification of unique or unsuspected antigens that may then be experimentally tested, a process called reverse vaccinology (Fig. 25.11). The procedures involved include complete sequencing of the antigens of interest, followed by identification of their important epitopes, especially those that bind to common MHC molecules and are likely recognized by CD4[+] and CD8[+] T cells. These epitopes may be predicted by the use of computer models of the protein. Once identified, the protective epitopes may be chemically synthesized and tested in animals. Experimental reverse vaccines have been developed in this way against foot-and-mouth disease virus, canine parvovirus, and equine influenza (Ohta et al., 2022).

ADJUVANTS

To maximize the effectiveness of vaccines, especially those containing killed organisms or highly purified antigens, it has been common practice to add substances called adjuvants to the vaccine (*adjuvare* is the Latin verb for "to help") (Aucouturier et al., 2001). Adjuvants can increase the speed or the magnitude of the body's response to vaccines, permit a reduction in the amount of antigen injected or the

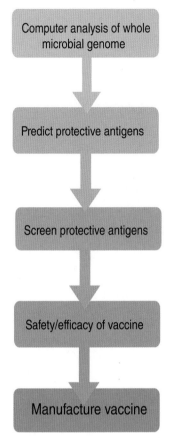

Fig. 25.11 Reverse vaccinology involves the use of our detailed knowledge of an organism's genome together with computer-based artificial intelligence to predict the structure of protective epitopes. These can then be synthesized and then tested in animals.

The flowchart in Fig. 25.11 shows the following steps:
- Computer analysis of whole microbial genome
- Predict protective antigens
- Screen protective antigens
- Safety/efficacy of vaccine
- Manufacture vaccine

TABLE 25.3	Types and Modes of Action of Some Common Adjuvants Employed in Veterinary Vaccines	
Type	**Adjuvant**	**Mode of Action**
Depot adjuvants	Aluminum phosphate	Slow-release antigen depot?
	Aluminum hydroxide	
	Alum	Slow-release antigen depot?
	Freund's incomplete adjuvant	Activate DAMPs
		Slow antigen release depot
Microbial adjuvants	Anaerobic corynebacteria	Macrophage stimulator
	BCG	Macrophage stimulator
	Muramyl dipeptide	Macrophage stimulator
	Bordetella pertussis	Lymphocyte stimulator
	Lipopolysaccharide	Macrophage stimulator
Immune stimulators	Saponin	Stimulates antigen processing
	Lysolecithin	
	Pluronic detergents	Stimulates antigen processing
	Glucans	
	Dextran sulfate	Stimulates antigen processing
		Macrophage stimulator
		Macrophage stimulator
Delivery systems	Liposomes	Stimulates antigen processing
	ISCOMS	
	Microparticles	Stimulates antigen processing
		Stimulates antigen processing
		Stimulates antigen processing
Mixed adjuvants	Freund's complete adjuvant	Depot plus immune stimulant

BCG, Bacille Calmette-Guérin; *DAMPs*, damage-associated molecular patterns.

number of doses administered, induce appropriate bias in the response (Th1 or Th2), trigger cell-mediated immunity, and are essential if long-term memory is to be established to soluble antigens. Many of the commonly employed adjuvants are TLR ligands. Their main mode of action is to promote antigen uptake, processing, and presentation by dendritic cells. In general, adjuvants trigger innate immune responses that in turn act on dendritic cells to enhance antigen presentation to T or B cells (Table 25.3; Coffman et al., 2010). Thus the growing use of particles coated with antigen, cytokines, and costimulatory molecules as adjuvants has led to encouraging improvements in vaccine efficacy (Brunner et al., 2010).

Aluminum Salts

These are by far the most widely employed adjuvants. They come in different forms including aluminum hydroxide gel (which is actually aluminum oxyhydroxide), aluminum phosphate gel, and aluminum potassium sulfate (alum), as well as calcium phosphate. Aluminum-adjuvanted vaccines induce inflammatory nodules at the injection site in the first 48 hours. These contain neutrophils with some eosinophils and lymphocytes. The neutrophils generate antigen-trapping extracellular traps (NETs). Similarly, activated macrophages are attracted to these sites, and these macrophages may develop into dendritic cells. Recruitment of mature myeloid dendritic cells to the sites of injection is also enhanced (HogenEsch, 2012).

Alum has multiple effects that serve to promote antigen processing and presentation. It appears to affect lipids in the plasma membrane and promotes DC homing to lymph nodes (Kool et al., 2008). Additionally, alum kills inflammatory cells such as neutrophils, resulting in DNA release and enhancing DC-T cell interactions (Fig. 25.12). Thus it enhances Th2 responses to protein antigens and generates large numbers of B cells. However, it is not good at generating Th1 CD8⁺ cells.

Saponin-Based Adjuvants

Saponins (triterpene glycosides), derived from the bark of the soapbark tree (*Quillaja saponaria*), are widely used as adjuvants. Crude saponins have both toxic and adjuvant activities, although it is possible to purify those with potent adjuvant activity and minimal toxicity. Saponin-based adjuvants selectively stimulate Th1 responses since they direct antigens into endogenous processing pathways and enhance IFN-γ release by dendritic cells. The saponins activate inflammasomes. Micelles may be constructed using protein antigens and a complex saponin mixture called Quil A. ISCOMs (Immune Stimulating Complexes) are stable constructs containing cholesterol, phospholipid, saponin, and antigen. ISCOMs are effective adjuvants with few adverse side effects. They are highly effective in targeting antigens to the professional antigen-processing cells, while the saponin activates these cells and promotes cytokine production and the expression of costimulatory molecules. Depending on the antigen employed, ISCOMs can stimulate either Th1 or Th2 responses.

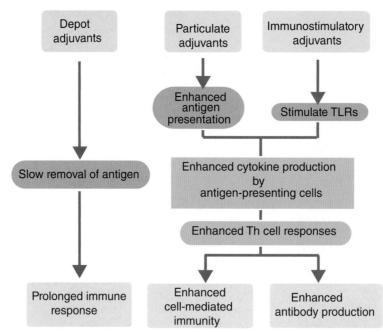

Fig. 25.12 The three major groups of adjuvants and the ways in which these may act to enhance immune responses triggered by vaccine antigens.

Water-in-Oil Emulsions

One method of forming a slow-release antigen depot is to incorporate the antigen in a water-in-oil emulsion (droplets of the aqueous phase plus a surfactant such as Tween, span or lecithin emulsified in an oil phase). The light mineral oil stimulates a local, chronic inflammatory response, and as a result, a small granuloma forms around the site of the inoculum. The antigen is slowly leached from the aqueous phase of the emulsion. These depot adjuvants may cause significant tissue irritation and destruction. Mineral oils are especially irritating. Nonmineral oils, although less irritating, are also less effective. Adjuvants with significant irritant activity are not, however, acceptable in modern vaccines, and it is essential to reduce this irritation while retaining adjuvant effectiveness. In humans, squalene-based oil-in-water emulsions have been licensed as vaccine adjuvants. (Squalene is a triterpene oil.) They are more potent than alum-based vaccines but may induce mild local reactions.

Particulate Adjuvants

The immune system can trap and process particles such as bacteria or other microorganisms much more efficiently than soluble antigens. As a result, successful adjuvants may incorporate antigens into readily phagocytosable particles (Fig. 25.13). These adjuvants include emulsions, microparticles, ISCOMs, and liposomes, and all are designed to deliver antigen efficiently to antigen-presenting cells. These particles are usually of similar size to bacteria and are readily endocytosed. Liposomes are lipid-based synthetic microparticles 200–1000 nm in size containing encapsulated antigens that are effectively trapped and processed yet are also protected from rapid degradation. All of these particulate adjuvants may be made more potent by incorporating microbial immunostimulants. They are not yet widely employed in veterinary vaccines. Especially when coupled to specific-cell targeting molecules, nanoparticles are much more effective than microparticles at being taken up by cells of the immune system. They promote DC activation and presentation of antigens to both MHC class I and class II. As a result, they can prime both CD4+ and CD8+ T cells.

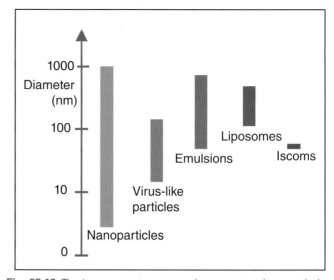

Fig. 25.13 The immune system responds more strongly to particulate than to soluble antigens. Particulate vaccines come in many different sizes, and this influences the nature of immune responses to these vaccines.

Nanoparticle adjuvants show considerable promise in new-generation vaccines. They can be made from many different compounds, such as poly amino acids, polysaccharides, polystyrene, and biodegradable polymers, as well as nondegradable elements such as gold, silver, iron, and silica. They can be engineered to display a mixture of antigens and costimulating molecules on their surface so that the immune response is optimized (Getts et al., 2015). By associating antigens with NLRs, TLRs, and other PRRs, nanoparticles can trigger cytotoxic lymphocyte responses to antigens that normally won't do this. Intradermal and intramuscular administration can induce strong immune responses, while intravenous administration may induce tolerance (Steinhagen et al., 2011).

Immunostimulatory Adjuvants

Immunostimulatory adjuvants exert their effects by promoting cytokine production. Many of them are complex microbial products that act by stimulating TLRs. Depending on the specific microbial product, they may enhance either Th1 or Th2 responses. Killed anaerobic Corynebacteria, especially *Propionibacterium acnes*, have an immunostimulatory effect. When used as adjuvants, these bacteria enhance antibacterial and antitumor activity. The TLR5 ligand bacterial flagellin is an adjuvant that promotes mixed Th1 and Th2 responses. Some synthetic ligands, such as the imidazoquinolines, and some guanosine and adenosine analogs may be effective adjuvants. Unmethylated CpG oligodinucleotides that bind TLR9 are potent immunostimulatory adjuvants for Th1 responses. There are multiple classes of CpG oligodinucleotides, each of which has slightly different immunostimulatory effects. In practice, it has been found that multiple innate stimuli may be more effective than a single stimulus and that combination adjuvants that have multiple mechanisms of action appear to be most effective.

Combined Adjuvants

Very powerful adjuvants can be constructed by combining a particulate or depot adjuvant with an immunostimulatory agent. For example, an oil-based depot adjuvant can be mixed with killed *Mycobacterium tuberculosis* incorporated into the water-in-oil emulsion. The mixture is called Freund's complete adjuvant (FCA). Not only does FCA form a depot, but the tubercle bacilli also contain muramyl dipeptide (*N*-acetylmuramyl-L-alanyl-D-isoglutamine), a molecule that activates macrophages and dendritic cells through NOD2. FCA works best when given subcutaneously or intradermally and when the antigen dose is relatively low. FCA promotes IgG production over IgM. It inhibits tolerance induction, favors delayed hypersensitivity reactions, accelerates graft rejection, and promotes resistance to tumors. FCA can be used to induce experimental autoimmune diseases, such as experimental allergic encephalitis and thyroiditis (see Chapter 37). It also stimulates activation to M1 cells, promoting their phagocytic and cytotoxic activities. Use of oil-based adjuvants in animals intended for human consumption is problematic since the oil may cause local lesions and spoil the meat. Use of FCA is unacceptable in cattle, not only because of the mineral oil but also because its mycobacteria may induce a positive tuberculin skin test. FCA is highly toxic in dogs and cats.

FURTHER INFORMATION

Tizard IR. Vaccines for Veterinarians. Elsevier, St. Louis, 2021. ISBN: 978-0-323-68299-2

REFERENCES

Ashford, D.A., di Pietra, J., Lingappa, J., et al., 2004. Adverse events in humans associated with accidental exposure to the livestock brucellosis vaccine RB51. Vaccine 22, 3435–3439.

Aucouturier, J., Dupuis, L., Ganne, V., 2001. Adjuvants designed for veterinary and human vaccines. Vaccine 19, 2666–2672.

Babiuk, L.A., Pontarollo, R., Babiuk, S., et al., 2003. Induction of immune responses by DNA vaccines in large animals. Vaccine 21, 649–658.

Balena, V., Pradhan, S.S., Bera, B.C., Anand, T., et al., 2022. Double and quadruple deletion mutant of EHV-1 is highly attenuated and induces optimal immune response. Vaccine. https://doi.org/10.1016/j.vaccine.2022.12.044

Brunner, R., Jensen-Jarolim, E., Pali-Scholl, I., 2010. The ABC of clinical and experimental adjuvants: a brief overview. Immunol. Lett. 128, 29–35.

Coffman, R.L., Sher, A., Seder, R.A., 2010. Vaccine adjuvants: putting innate immunity to work. Immunity 33, 492–503.

Crisci, E., Barcena, J., Montoya, M., 2012. Virus-like particles: the new frontier of vaccines for animal viral infections. Vet. Immunol. Immunopathol. 14, 211–225.

Dunham, S.P., 2002. The application of nucleic acid vaccines in veterinary medicine. Res. Vet. Sci. 73, 9–16.

Fischer, L., Barzu, S., Andreoni, C., et al., 2003. DNA vaccination of neonatal piglets in the face of maternal immunity induces humoral memory and protection against a virulent pseudorabies virus challenge. Vaccine 21, 1732–1741.

Gerdts, V., Mutwiri, G., Richards, J., Van Drunen Littel-Van Den Hurk, S., Potter, A.A., 2013. Carrier molecules for use in veterinary vaccines. Vaccine 31, 596–602.

Getts, D.R., Shea, L.D., Miller, S.D., King, N.J., 2015. Harnessing nanoparticles for immune modulation. Trends Immunol. 36, 419–427.

HogenEsch, H., 2012. Mechanism of immunopotentiation and safety of aluminum adjuvants. Front. Immunol. 3, 406–415.

Hou, H., Liu, X., Peng, Q., 2019. The advances in Brucellosis vaccines. Vaccine, 37. https://doi.org/10.1015/j.vaccine.2019.05.084

Jiang, W., Baker, H.J., Swango, L.J., et al., 1998. Nucleic acid immunization protects dogs against challenge with virulent parvovirus. Vaccine 10, 601–607.

Kingstad-Bakke, B.A., Chandrasekar, S.S., Phanse, Y., Ross, K.A., et al., 2019. Effective-mosaic-based nanovaccines against avian influenza in poultry. Vaccine 37, 5051–5058.

Kool, M., Soullie, T., van Nimwegen, M., et al., 2008. Alum adjuvant boosts adaptive immunity by inducing uric acid and activating inflammatory dendritic cells. J. Exp. Med. 205, 869–882.

Lee, D.H., Bae, S.W., Park, J.K., Kwon, J.H., et al., 2013. Virus-like particle vaccine protects against H3N2 canine influenza virus in dog. Vaccine 31, 3268–3273.

Li, J., Liu, Q., Liu, J., Wo, X., et al., 2022. An mRNA rabies vaccine induces strong protective immune responses in mice and dogs. Virology J., 19. https://doi.org/10.1186/s12985-022-01919-7

Liu, F., Ge, S., Li, L., Wu, X., Wang, Z., 2012. Virus-like particles: potential veterinary vaccine immunogens. Res. Vet. Sci. 93, 553–559.

Lundstrom, K., 2012. Alphavirus vectors in vaccine development. J. Vaccines Vaccin. 3 (3) https://doi.org/10.4172/2157-7560.1000139

Moss, R.B., 2009. Prospects for control of emerging infectious diseases with plasmid DNA vaccines. J. Immune Based Ther. Vacc. 7, 3–10.

Ohta, M., Kambayashi, Y., Mita, H., Kuroda, T., et al., 2022. Protective efficacy of a reverse genetics-derived inactivated vaccine against equine influenza virus in horses. Vaccine 40, 6362–6366.

Plotkin, S.A., 2010. Correlates of protection induced by vaccination. Clin. Vaccine Immunol. 17, 1055–1065.

Russell, P.H., Mackie, A., 2001. Eye-drop DNA can induce IgA in the tears and bile of chickens. Vet. Immunol. Immunopathol. 10, 327–332.

Sette, A., Rappuoli, R., 2010. Reverse vaccinology: developing vaccines in the era of genomics. Immunity 33, 530–541.

Shin, M.-K., Yoo, H.S., 2013. Animal vaccines based on orally presented yeast recombinants. Vaccine 31, 4287–4292.

Steinhagen, F., Kinjo, T., Bode, C., Klinman, D.M., 2011. TLR-based adjuvants. Vaccine 29, 3341–3355.

Vega, C.G., Bok, M., Ebinger, M., Rocha, L.A., et al., 2020. A new passive immune strategy based on IgY antibodies as a key element to control neonatal calf diarrhea in dairy farms. BMC Vet. Res. https://doi.org/10.1186/s12917-020-02476-3

Weyer, J., Rupprecht, C.E., Nel, L.H., 2009. Poxvirus-vectored vaccines for rabies: a review. Vaccine 27, 7198–7201.

The Use of Vaccines

CHAPTER OUTLINE

Although the principles of vaccination have been known for many years, vaccines and vaccination procedures are continuing to improve in both efficacy and safety. The earliest veterinary vaccines were often of limited efficacy, and some had significant adverse effects, although these were considered acceptable when measured against the risks of animals dying from disease. The vaccination protocols developed at that time reflected the inadequacies of these vaccines. Ongoing developments in vaccine design and production have resulted in great improvements in both safety and effectiveness. These improvements permit a reassessment of the relative risks and benefits of vaccination. Vaccination is not always an innocuous procedure. For this reason, the use of any vaccine should be accompanied by a risk-to-benefit analysis conducted by the veterinarian in consultation with the animal's owner. Vaccination protocols should be determined for each individual animal, giving due consideration to the seriousness of the disease, the zoonotic potential of the agent, the animal's susceptibility and exposure risk, and any legal requirements relating to vaccination (Squires et al., 2024).

The two major factors that determine vaccine use are safety and efficacy. We must always be sure that the risks of vaccination do not exceed those associated with the chance of contracting the disease. Thus it may be inappropriate to vaccinate against a disease that is rare, readily treated by other means, or has little clinical significance. Because the detection of antibodies is a common diagnostic procedure, unnecessary use of vaccines may complicate diagnosis based on serology and perhaps make eradication of a disease impossible. On the other hand, new serologic tests may make it possible to determine animal susceptibility and rationalize vaccine use decisions. The decision to use vaccines for the control of any disease must be based not only on the degree of risk associated with the disease but also on the availability of superior alternatives.

The second major consideration is vaccine efficacy. Vaccines may not always be highly effective. In some diseases, such as equine infectious anemia, Aleutian disease in mink, and African swine fever, poor or no protective immunity can be induced even with the best currently available vaccines. In other diseases, such as foot-and-mouth disease in pigs, the immune response is transient and relatively ineffective, and successful vaccination is sometimes difficult to achieve (Plotkin, 2010).

As a result of these considerations, animal vaccines should be ranked based on their importance. The first category consists of essential (or core) vaccines—those that are required because they protect against common, dangerous diseases and because a failure to use them would place an animal at significant risk of disease or death. Determination of which vaccines are essential will vary based on local conditions and disease threats. A second category consists of optional vaccines. These are directed against diseases for which the risks associated with not vaccinating may be low but are determined by an individualized risk/benefit assessment. In many cases, risks from these diseases are determined by the age and life stage, health status, degree of exposure, and the history of an animal. The use of these optional vaccines should be determined by a veterinarian on the basis of exposure risk. A third category consists of vaccines that may have no application in routine vaccination but may be used under special circumstances. These are vaccines directed against diseases of little clinical significance or vaccines whose risks do not significantly outweigh their benefits. Of course, all vaccine use should be conducted on the basis of informed consent. An animal's owner should be made aware of the risks and benefits involved before seeking approval to vaccinate (Ellis et al., 2022; Stone et al., 2020).

When vaccines are used to control disease in a population of animals rather than in individuals, a veterinarian should also consider the concept of herd immunity. This herd immunity is the resistance of an entire group of animals to a disease as a result of the presence, in that group, of many immune animals. Herd immunity reduces the probability of a susceptible animal meeting an infected one, so that the spread of disease is slowed or prevented. If it is acceptable to lose individual animals from disease while preventing epizootics, it may be possible to do this by vaccinating only a proportion of the population. Certainly, veterinarians should seek to ensure that as many animals as possible are vaccinated in order to maximize herd immunity.

ADMINISTRATION OF VACCINES

Most vaccines are administered by injection. Care must be taken not to injure or introduce infection into an animal. All needles used must be clean and sharp. Dirty or dull needles can cause tissue damage and infection at the injection site. The skin at the injection site must be clean and dry, although excessive alcohol swabbing should be avoided. Vaccines are provided in a standard dose, and this dose should not be divided to account for an animal's size. Doses are not yet formulated to account for body weight or age (Taguchi et al., 2012). There must be a sufficient antigen to trigger the cells of the immune system and provoke an immune response. This amount is not related to body size. (Unfortunately, the risk of an adverse event occurring is increased in smaller animals, so it may be necessary to make some adjustments in vaccine dose for safety reasons.) Vaccination by subcutaneous or intramuscular injection is the simplest and most common method of administration. This approach is obviously excellent for small numbers of animals and for diseases in which systemic immunity is important. In other diseases, however, systemic immunity is not as important as mucosal immunity, and it is perhaps more appropriate to administer a vaccine at the site of potential invasions. Therefore, intranasal vaccines are available for infectious bovine rhinotracheitis, parainfluenza 3, and respiratory syncytial virus of cattle; for *Streptococcus equi* infections in horses; for feline rhinotracheitis, *Bordetella bronchiseptica*, coronavirus, and calicivirus infections; for canine parainfluenza and *Bordetella* infection; and for infectious bronchitis and Newcastle disease in poultry (Bradley et al., 2012). These methods of administration require that each animal be dealt with on an individual basis. Whenever possible, a vaccination visit should include a physical examination and a client dialog discussing both risks and benefits, especially if the client evidences vaccine hesitancy.

When animal numbers are large, other methods of vaccination must be employed. For example, aerosolization of vaccines enables them to be inhaled by all the animals in a group. This technique is employed in vaccinating against canine distemper and mink enteritis on mink ranches and against Newcastle disease in poultry. Alternatively, the vaccine may be administered in the feed or drinking water, as is done with *Erysipelothrix rhusiopathiae* vaccines in pigs and against Newcastle disease, infectious laryngotracheitis, and avian encephalomyelitis in poultry. Alternative routes of vaccine administration that are in development or employed in humans include cutaneous vaccination using liquid-jet injectors, or topical skin application through microneedle patches or nanoparticles. Oral rabies vaccine in fish-meal bait has been air-dropped in many states in order to vaccinate wild animal carriers such as coyotes. Plague vaccine-coated M&M candies have been delivered to prairie dogs and black-footed ferrets in the western United States by means of drones that can shoot the candies in three directions simultaneously in order to ensure even coverage.

Multiple-Antigen Vaccines

For convenience, it is common to employ mixtures of organisms within single vaccines. In cattle, for example, vaccines are available that contain infectious bovine rhinotracheitis (BHV-1), bovine virus diarrhea (BVDV), parainfluenza 3 (P13), and even *Mannheimia haemolytica*. Dogs may be given vaccines containing all of the following organisms: canine distemper virus, canine adenovirus–1, canine adenovirus–2, canine parvovirus–2, canine parainfluenza virus, leptospira bacterin, and rabies vaccine. These mixtures may be used to protect animals against several diseases with economy of effort. However, it can also be wasteful to use vaccines against organisms that are unlikely to cause problems. When different antigens in a mixture are inoculated simultaneously, competition occurs between antigens. Manufacturers of multiple-antigen vaccines take this into account and adjust their components accordingly. Vaccines should never be mixed indiscriminately since one component may dominate the mixture or interfere with the response to the other components (Strasser et al., 2003).

Some veterinarians have questioned whether the use of complex vaccine mixtures leads to less than satisfactory protection or increases the risk for adverse side effects. They are concerned that the use of 5- or 7-component vaccines in pets will somehow overwhelm the immune system, forgetting that our animals encounter hundreds of different antigens in daily life. The suggestion that these multiple-antigen vaccines can overload the immune system is unfounded, nor is there any evidence to support the contention that the risk of adverse effects increases disproportionately when more components are added to vaccines. The success of a 21-component bluetongue vaccine in sheep or a 23-component pneumococcal vaccine in human AIDS patients should serve as a reassurance that multiple component vaccines are not overwhelming. Certainly, such vaccines should be tested to ensure that all components induce a satisfactory response. Licensed vaccines provided by a reputable manufacturer will generally provide satisfactory protection against all components.

Vaccination Schedules

Although it is not possible to give exact schedules for all veterinary vaccines, certain principles are common to all methods of active immunization. Most vaccines require an initial series in which protective immunity is initiated, followed by revaccination (booster shots) at intervals to ensure that this protective immunity remains at an adequate level.

Initial Series

Because maternal antibodies passively protect newborn animals, it is not usually possible to successfully vaccinate very young animals. If strong immunity is deemed necessary at this stage, the mother may be vaccinated during the later stages of pregnancy, with the vaccinations being timed so that peak antibody levels are achieved at the time of colostrum formation. Once an animal is born, successful active immunization is effective only after passive immunity has waned. Since it is impossible to predict the exact time of loss of maternal immunity, the initial vaccination series will generally require administration of multiple doses. Current guidelines for essential canine and feline vaccines, for example, indicate that the first dose of vaccine should be administered at 8–9 weeks of age, followed by a second dose 3–4 weeks later, and concluding at about 16 weeks of age. (These are not, strictly speaking, booster doses. They are simply designed to trigger a primary response as soon as possible after maternal immunity has waned.) All animals should then receive a booster dose 12 months later or at one year of age. Administration of vaccines to young animals is discussed in Chapter 24. It is unclear whether maternal antibodies can block responses to all intranasal vaccines. Despite high levels of circulating maternal antibodies, maternal interference does not always occur, and nasal antibody production is often unimpaired (Jas et al., 2009).

The timing of initial vaccinations may also be determined by epidemiology. Some diseases are seasonal, and vaccines may be given before outbreaks are expected. Examples of these include the vaccine against the lungworm *Dictyocaulus viviparus* given in early summer, just before the anticipated lungworm season; the vaccine against anthrax given in spring; and the vaccine against *Clostridium chauvoei* given to sheep before turning them out to pasture. Bluetongue of lambs is spread by midges (*Culicoides variipennis*) and is thus a disease of midsummer and early fall. Vaccination in spring will therefore protect lambs during the susceptible period.

Revaccination and Duration of Immunity

As pointed out in Chapter 16, it is the persistence of memory cells after vaccination that provides an animal with long-term protection. The presence of long-lived plasma cells is associated with persistent antibody production, so a vaccinated animal may have antibodies in its bloodstream for many years after exposure to a vaccine. It is these antibodies that are mainly responsible for long-term protection (Schultz, 2006).

Revaccination schedules depend on the duration of effective protection (Table 26.1). This in turn depends on specific antigen content, whether the vaccine consists of living or dead organisms, and its route of administration. In the past, relatively poor vaccines required frequent administration, perhaps as often as every 6 months, to maintain an acceptable level of immunity. Newer, modern vaccines can produce long-lasting protection, especially in companion animals. Many require revaccination only every 3 or 4 years, whereas for other diseases, immunity may persist for an animal's lifetime. Even killed viral vaccines may protect individual animals against disease for many years. Unfortunately, the minimal duration of immunity has, until recently, rarely been measured, and reliable figures are not available for many vaccines. Likewise, although serum antibodies can be monitored in vaccinated animals, few tests have been standardized, although there is a growing consensus regarding the interpretation

of these antibody titers (Egerer et al., 2022). Even animals that lack detectable antibodies may have significant resistance to disease. Nor is there much information available regarding long-term immunity on mucosal surfaces. In general, immunity against feline panleukopenia, canine distemper, canine parvovirus, and canine adenovirus is considered to be relatively long-lasting (>5 years). On the other hand, immunity to feline rhinotracheitis, feline calicivirus, and *Chlamydophila* is believed to be relatively short. One problem in making these statements is variability among individual animals and among different types of vaccines. Thus recombinant canine distemper vaccines may induce immunity of shorter duration than conventional, modified live vaccines. There may be a great difference between the shortest and longest durations of immunological memory within a group of animals. Duration of immunity studies is confounded by the fact that many older animals have increased innate resistance. Different vaccines within a category may differ significantly in their composition, and although all vaccines may induce immunity in the short term, it cannot be assumed that all confer long-term immunity. Manufacturers use different master seeds and different methods of antigen preparation. The level of immunity required for most of these diseases is unknown. A significant difference exists between the minimal level of immunity required to protect most animals and the level of immunity required to ensure protection of all animals.

Annual revaccination was once the rule for most animal vaccines, since this approach is administratively simple and has the advantage of ensuring that an animal is regularly seen by a veterinarian. It is clear, however, that modern vaccines such as those against canine distemper or feline herpesvirus induce protective immunity that can last for many years and that annual revaccination using these vaccines is inappropriate. A growing body of evidence now indicates that most modified live viral (MLV) vaccines induce lifelong sterile immunity in dogs and cats. In contrast, immunity to bacteria is of much shorter duration and often may prevent disease but not infection. Old dogs and cats rarely die from vaccine-preventable disease, especially if they have been vaccinated as adults (Schultz et al., 2010). Young animals, in contrast, may die from such diseases, especially if not vaccinated or if vaccinated prematurely. A veterinarian should always assess the relative risks and benefits to an animal in determining the timing of any vaccination. It is therefore good practice to use serum antibody assays such as rapid ELISA tests, if available, to provide guidance on revaccination intervals. Persistent antibody titers determine whether an animal requires additional protection. These tests not only identify those animals that have responded to vaccination, but they can also determine if an animal is a nonresponder (Twark and Dodds, 2000). They can determine if an animal that previously suffered from an adverse event really requires revaccination. They can determine whether an animal with an undocumented vaccine history needs to be vaccinated and with which vaccines. They can determine which animals in a shelter undergoing a disease outbreak are susceptible and so require vaccination. They can also determine whether revaccination is really necessary at three years. It should be pointed out however that animals with low or undetectable serum antibody levels may still be protected as a result of persistence of memory B and T cells capable of responding rapidly to reinfection. "Blind" revaccination should be avoided if appropriate serum antibody assays are available (Coyne et al., 2001a, 2001b).

Notwithstanding the previous discussion, animal owners should be made aware that protection against an infectious disease can only be maintained reliably when vaccines are used in accordance with the protocol approved by the vaccine-licensing authorities. The duration of immunity claimed by a vaccine manufacturer is the minimum duration of immunity that is supported by the data available at the time

TABLE 26.1 Estimated Minimum Duration of Immunity (DOI) of Select Commercially Available Canine Vaccine Antigens		
Vaccine	Estimated Minimum DOI (years)	Estimated Relative Efficacy (%)
Essential		
Canine distemper (modified live virus [MLV])	>7	>90
Canine distemper (recombinant [R])	>1	>90
Canine parvovirus–2 (MLV)	>7	>90
Canine adenovirus–2 (MLV)	>7	>90
Rabies virus (killed [K])	>3	>85
Optional		
Canine coronavirus (K or MLV)	N/A	N/A
Canine parainfluenza (MLV)	>3	>80
Bordetella bronchiseptica (ML)	<1	<70
Leptospira canicola (K)	<1	<50
Leptospira grippotyphosa (K)	<1	N/A
Leptospira icterohaemorrhagiae (K)	<1	<75
Leptospira pomona (K)	<1	N/A
Borrelia burgdorferi (K)	1	<75
Borrelia burgdorferi OspA (R)	1	<75
Giardia lamblia (K)	<1	N/A

From Paul, M.A., Appel, M., Barrett, R., et al., 2003. Report of the American Animal Hospital Association (AAHA) Canine Vaccine Task Force: executive summary and 2003 canine vaccine guidelines and recommendations, J. Am. Anim. Hosp. Assoc. 39, 119–131.

the vaccine license is approved. This must always be considered when discussing revaccination protocols with an owner (Squires et al., 2024).

VACCINATION STRATEGIES

Although vaccination is a powerful tool for the control of infectious disease, its potential to prevent the spread of, or eliminate, a disease depends on selecting correct control strategies. If an infectious disease outbreak, such as one caused by foot-and-mouth virus, is to be rapidly controlled, it is vitally important to select the correct population to be vaccinated. The success of any mass vaccination program depends both on the proportion of animals vaccinated and on the efficacy of the vaccine. Neither of these factors will reach 100%, so it is essential to target the vaccine effectively. It is also the case that vaccines do not confer immediate protection, so the strategy employed will depend on the rate of spread of an infection. Vaccines may thus be given prophylactically, in advance of an outbreak, or reactively, in response to an existing outbreak. Both strategies have advantages and disadvantages. In general, prophylactic vaccination greatly reduces the potential for a major epidemic of a disease such as foot-and-mouth disease by reducing the size of the susceptible population. The effectiveness of this approach can be greatly enhanced by identifying high-risk individuals and ensuring that they are protected in advance of an outbreak (Keeling et al., 2003).

It is generally not feasible to vaccinate an entire population of animals once a disease outbreak has occurred. However, two effective reactive vaccination strategies are *ring vaccination*, which seeks to contain an outbreak by establishing a barrier of immune animals around an infected area, and *predictive vaccination*, which seeks to vaccinate the animals on farms likely to contribute most to the future spread of disease. Reactive vaccination in this way can ensure that an epidemic is not unduly prolonged. A prolonged "tail" to an epidemic commonly results from the disease "jumping" to a new area. Well-considered, predictive vaccination may well prevent these jumps. Thus a combination of prophylactic and reactive vaccinations will likely yield the most effective results.

VACCINE ASSESSMENT

To assess the efficacy of a vaccine, animals must first be vaccinated and then challenged. The percentage of vaccinated animals that survive this challenge can then be measured. It is important, however, to determine the percentage of nonvaccinated control animals that also survive the challenge. The true efficacy of a vaccine, called the preventable fraction (PF), is calculated as follows:

$$PF = \frac{(\% \text{ of controls dying} - \% \text{ of vaccinates dying})}{(\% \text{ of controls dying})}$$

For example, a challenge that kills 80% of controls and 40% of vaccinates shows that the PF of the vaccine is as follows:

$$PF = \frac{80-40}{80} = 50\%$$

Good, effective vaccines should have a PF of at least 80%. Obviously, less effective vaccines are acceptable if safe and if nothing better is available. In determining vaccine efficacy, however, large challenge doses may overwhelm any reasonable level of vaccine-induced immunity. It is also important to determine what degree of protection is desired. It may be much easier to prevent deaths rather than illness.

FAILURES IN VACCINATION

There are many reasons why a vaccine may fail to confer protective immunity on an animal (Fig. 26.1).

Failure to Vaccinate

Most cases of vaccine failure result from unsatisfactory or incomplete administration of the vaccine or noncompliance with manufacturer's recommendations. For example, a live vaccine may have died as a result of poor storage, the use of antibiotics in conjunction with live bacterial vaccines, the use of chemicals to sterilize the syringe, or the excessive use of alcohol swabs on the skin. Sometimes animals given vaccines by unconventional routes may not be protected. When large flocks of poultry or mink are to be vaccinated, it is common to administer the vaccine either as an aerosol or in drinking water. If the aerosol is not evenly distributed throughout a building, or if some animals do not drink, they may receive insufficient vaccine. Premature vaccination of young animals prior to loss of maternal immunity remains a problem. Animals that subsequently develop disease may be interpreted as cases of vaccine failure (Heininger et al., 2012).

Failure to Respond

Occasionally, a vaccine may actually be ineffective. The method of production may have destroyed the protective epitopes, or there may simply be insufficient antigen in the vaccine. Problems of this type are uncommon and can generally be avoided by using only vaccines from reputable manufacturers.

More commonly, an animal may simply fail to mount an immune response. The immune response, being a biological process, never confers absolute protection and is never equal in all members of a vaccinated population. Since immunity is influenced by many genetic and environmental factors, the range of immune responses in a large random population of animals follows a normal distribution. This means that most animals respond to antigens by mounting an average immune response, whereas a few will mount an excellent response, and a few will mount a poor immune response (Figs. 26.2 and 26.3). These poor responders may not be protected against infection despite having received an effective vaccine. It is impossible to protect 100% of a large, outbred population of animals by vaccination. The size of this unreactive portion of the population will vary between vaccines, and its significance will depend on the nature of the disease. Thus, for highly infectious diseases against which herd immunity is poor and in which infection is rapidly and efficiently transmitted, such as foot-and-mouth disease, the presence of even a few unprotected animals can permit the spread of disease and disrupt control programs. Likewise, problems can arise if the unprotected animals are individually important, such as companion animals. In contrast, for diseases that are inefficiently spread, such as rabies, 70% protection may be sufficient to effectively block disease transmission within a population and may therefore be satisfactory from a community health viewpoint (Johnson et al., 2010).

Another type of vaccine failure occurs when the normal immune response is suppressed. For example, heavily parasitized or malnourished animals may be immunosuppressed and should not be vaccinated. Some virus infections induce profound immunosuppression. Animals with a major illness or high fever should not normally be vaccinated unless for a compelling reason. Stress may reduce a normal immune response, probably because of increased steroid production; examples of such stress include fatigue, malnutrition, and extremes of cold and heat (Richeson et al., 2019). Studies have shown that surgical neutering at or near the time of first vaccination does not impair the antibody responses of kittens (Reese et al., 2008). This type of immunosuppression is discussed in detail in Chapter 41. The most important cause of

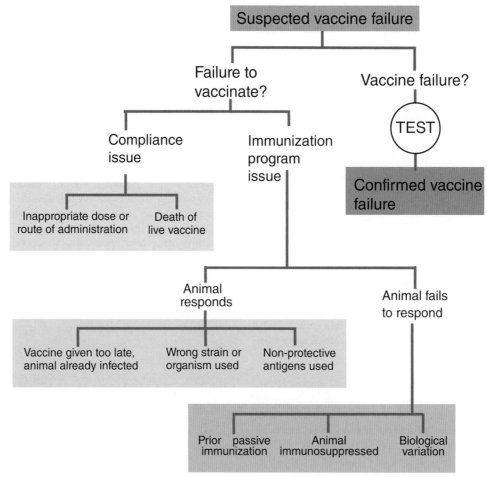

Fig. 26.1 A simple classification of the ways in which a vaccine may fail to protect an animal.

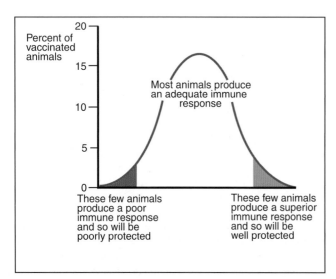

Fig. 26.2 The normal distribution of protective immune responses in a population of vaccinated animals. No vaccine can be expected to protect 100% of a population.

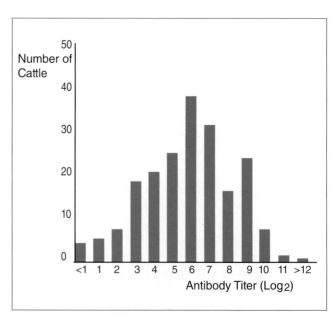

Fig. 26.3 The actual antibody responses in a herd of cattle vaccinated against Bovine Viral Diarrhea Type 1. Titers of less than 8 are not considered significant. Titers greater than 512 may reflect prior infection or previous vaccination. Note that these results represent a normal distribution and reflect the responses to most vaccines. Vaccination success is not guaranteed.

vaccine failure of this type is passively derived maternal immunity in young animals, as described in Chapter 24.

Analysis of an outbreak of influenza in racehorses has shown some interesting and important factors that appeared to determine vaccine effectiveness. Thus, when the effect of age was analyzed, it appears that 2-year-old horses were less susceptible to flu than other animals. Further analysis suggested that this increased resistance resulted from recent vaccination of this age cohort despite other age groups possessing similar antibody levels. There was evidence of gender differences in resistance (62% of females and 71% of males were infected). There was also some evidence that vaccination at a young age (<6 months) in the presence of maternal antibody had detrimental long-term effects on protection when compared to foals first vaccinated between 6 and 18 months of age (Barquero et al., 2007).

Recent studies have also analyzed data from 10,483 dogs of all ages and breeds vaccinated against rabies to determine the factors that influence seroconversion (Kennedy et al., 2007). It was found that a relationship exists between a dog's size and its antibody level. Smaller dogs produced higher antibody titers than large dogs. Vaccine effectiveness also varied among breeds. Thus significant failure rates were seen in German Shepherds and Labrador Retrievers. Young animals vaccinated before 1 year of age produced lower antibody levels than adults. The highest antibody titers were generated in dogs aged 3–4 years at time of the first vaccination. Primary vaccination of aged animals showed lower antibody levels and increased failure rates. Gender had no effect on failure rate or titer. Failure rates varied greatly between vaccines. They ranged from 0.2% in the worst case to 0.01% in the best, and some vaccines showed significant batch-to-batch variation in efficacy. Of the variation in antibody titers observed, 19% was due to vaccine differences, 8% was due to breed differences, 5% was attributed to size differences, and 3% to other differences. It is likely that similar variables influence the responses of animals to other vaccines. Perhaps vaccines should be reformulated to take these age, size, and breed differences into account (HogenEsch and Thompson, 2010)

Correct Administration and Response

Even animals given an adequate dose of an effective vaccine may fail to be protected. If the vaccinated animal was incubating the disease before inoculation, the vaccine may be given too late to affect the course of the disease. Alternatively, the vaccine may contain the wrong strain of organisms or the wrong (nonprotective) antigens. As in humans, some vaccine failures may be attributed to persistent parasitic infections, malnutrition, and the composition of the intestinal microbiota (Pabst and Hornef, 2014; de Jong et al., 2020).

ADVERSE CONSEQUENCES OF VACCINATION

Vaccination continues to be the only safe, reliable, and effective way of protecting animals against the major infectious diseases. Vaccine-related toxicity is usually rare, mild, and transient, and hypothetical side effects must not dominate our perceptions. Nevertheless, the use of vaccines is not free of risk. Residual virulence and toxicity, allergic responses, disease in immunodeficient hosts, neurological complications, and harmful effects on the fetus are the most significant risks associated with the use of vaccines (Fig. 26.4). Veterinarians should use only licensed vaccines, and the manufacturer's recommendations should be carefully followed. Before using a vaccine, the veterinarian should consider the likelihood that an adverse event will happen, as well as the possible consequences or severity of this event. These factors must be weighed against the benefits to the animal. A common but mild complication may require a different consideration than a rare, severe complication (Meyer, 2001).

The issue of the risk associated with vaccination remains in large part a philosophical one since the advantages of vaccination are well documented and extensive, whereas the risk for adverse effects is poorly documented and, in many cases, largely hypothetical.

Nevertheless, established facts should be recognized, misinformation rebutted with sound data, and uncertainties acknowledged. For example, there is absolutely no evidence that vaccination itself leads to ill health. Although it is difficult to prove a negative, competent statistical analysis has consistently failed to demonstrate any general adverse effect of vaccination (Edwards et al., 2004).

Identification of an adverse event is based on the clinical judgment of the attending veterinarian and is subject to bias. Standard case definitions of a vaccine-associated adverse event are not yet available. Traditionally, adverse events resulting from vaccine administration have been reported by veterinarians to manufacturers or government agencies. The resulting figures have been difficult to analyze satisfactorily for two major reasons. First, reporting is voluntary, so significant underreporting occurs. Many adverse events are regarded as insignificant, or it may be inconvenient to report them. Second, very little data has been available on the number of animals vaccinated. Although manufacturers know the number of doses of vaccine sold, they are unable to determine the number of animals vaccinated. Nevertheless, it has proved possible by examining the electronic records of a very large general practice to determine the prevalence of vaccine-associated adverse events in more than 1 million dogs. The use of a standardized reporting system within a very large population has permitted objective analysis of the prevalence of adverse events occurring within 3 days of vaccine administration. Out of 1,226,159 dogs vaccinated, there were 4678 adverse events recorded (38.2/10,000 dogs); 72.8% of these events occurred on the same day the vaccine was administered, 31.7% were considered to be allergic reactions, and 65.8% were considered "vaccine reactions" and were likely due to toxicity. Additional analysis indicated that the risk of adverse events was significantly greater for small than for large dogs (Fig. 26.5); for neutered than for sexually intact dogs; and for dogs that received multiple vaccines. Each additional vaccine dose administered increased the risk of an adverse event occurring by 27% in small dogs (<10 kg) and by 12% in dogs heavier than 12 kg. High-risk breeds included Dachshunds, Pugs, Boston Terriers, Miniature Pinschers, and Chihuahuas. Overall, the increased incidence of adverse events in small dogs and their relationship to multiple dosing suggests that veterinarians should look carefully at the practice of giving the same dose of vaccine to all dogs irrespective of their size (Moore et al., 2005).

A similar study examined the prevalence of vaccine-associated adverse events following the administration of 1,258,712 doses of vaccine to 496,189 cats. The investigators reported 2560 adverse events (51.6/10,000 cats vaccinated). The risk was greatest for cats 1 year old. For unknown reasons, risk was greater in neutered than in sexually intact cats. Lethargy was the most commonly reported event (Fig. 26.6). The number of adverse events increased significantly when multiple vaccines were given during a single visit (Moore et al., 2007).

In a report from Japan, 359 dogs showed an adverse event out of 57,300 vaccinated (62.7/10,000 doses) (Ohmori et al., 2005). Of these 351 dogs, 41 developed anaphylaxis, 244 had dermatological signs, and 160 had gastrointestinal signs. About half the anaphylaxis events occurred within 5 minutes of vaccination. Additional analysis of these anaphylaxis cases reported 87% collapse, 77% cyanosis, and both in 71% of affected dogs. These are higher rates than reported elsewhere. This adverse event rate (62.7/10,000 vaccinated dogs) was higher than in the United States (38.2/10,000) (Miyaji, et al., 2012).

"Normal" Toxicity

Vaccines commonly elicit transient innate immune responses, and some degree of inflammation is required for the efficient induction of protective immune responses (Moore and HogenEsch, 2010). This may cause pain. Thus the sting produced by some vaccines may present

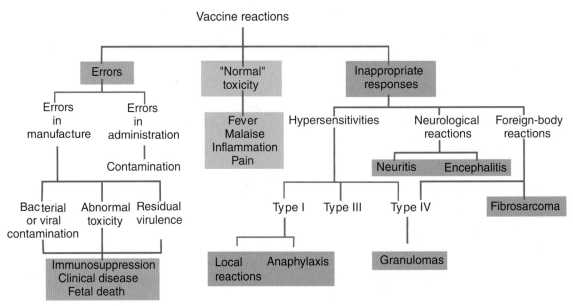

Fig. 26.4 A simple classification of the major adverse effects of vaccination.

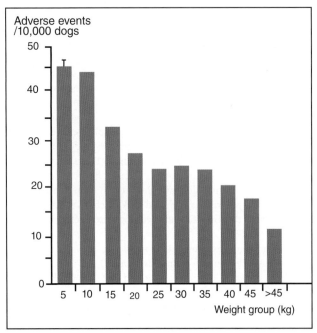

Fig. 26.5 Vaccine-associated adverse events are much more likely to occur in small rather than in large dogs. Mean ± SEM vaccine-associated adverse event rates by 5-kg weight groups in 1,226,159 dogs vaccinated at 360 veterinary hospitals from January 1, 2002 to December 31, 2003. These adverse events were diagnosed within 3 days of vaccine administration. From Moore, G.E., Guptill, L.P., Ward, M.P., et al., 2005. Adverse events diagnosed within three days of vaccine administration in dogs, J. Am. Vet. Med. Assoc. 227, 1102–1108.

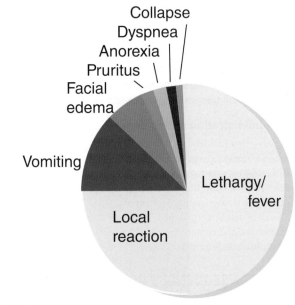

Fig. 26.6 The nature of vaccine-associated adverse events in cats occurring within 3 days postvaccination. Data from Moore, G.E., et al., 2007. J. Am. Vet. Med. Assoc. 231, 94–100.

problems not only to the animal being vaccinated but also, if the animal reacts violently, to the vaccinator. More commonly, swellings may develop at the reaction site. These may be firm or edematous, and they may be warm to the touch. They appear about a day after vaccination and can last for about a week. Unless an injection-site abscess develops, these swellings leave little trace. Vaccines containing killed gram-negative organisms may be intrinsically toxic owing to the presence of

endotoxins that can cause cytokine release, leading to shock, fever, and leukopenia (Richeson et al., 2019). Although such a reaction is usually only a temporary inconvenience to male animals, it may be sufficient to provoke abortion in pregnant females. It may be prudent to avoid vaccinating pregnant animals unless the risks of not giving the vaccine are considered to be too great (Broaddus et al., 2011). Vaccination with either ISCOM vaccines or live recombinant vectored vaccines against influenza and tetanus may induce an acute-phase response in horses.

Inappropriate Responses

Vaccines may cause rare but serious allergic reactions. For example, allergic responses may occur when an animal produces immunoglobulin E (IgE) in response not only to the immunizing antigen but also to other antigens found in vaccines, such as egg antigens or antigens from tissue culture cells. All forms of hypersensitivity are more commonly associated with multiple injections of antigens and therefore tend to be associated with the use of killed vaccines. It is important to emphasize that a type I hypersensitivity reaction is an immediate response to an antigen and occurs within a few minutes or hours after exposure to an antigen. Reactions occurring more than 2 or 3 hours after administration of a vaccine are likely not type I hypersensitivity reactions.

Type III hypersensitivity reactions are also potential hazards. These may cause intense local inflammation, or they may present as a generalized vascular disturbance such as purpura. A type III reaction can occur in the eyes of dogs vaccinated against infectious canine hepatitis (Chapter 33). Some rabies vaccines may induce a local complement-mediated vasculitis, leading to ischemic dermatitis and local alopecia. This type of reaction is most often seen in small dogs such as Dachshunds, Miniature Poodles, Bichon Frises, and Terriers.

Type IV hypersensitivity reactions may occur in response to vaccination, but a more common reaction is granuloma formation at the site of inoculation. This may be a response to depot adjuvants containing alum or oil. Vaccines containing a water-in-oil adjuvant produce larger and more persistent lesions at injection sites than vaccines containing alum and aluminum hydroxide. These lesions can be granulomas or sterile abscesses. If the skin is dirty at the injection site, these abscesses may become infected. For this reason, it is inappropriate to administer vaccines intramuscularly to animals used for human consumption (Asin et al. 2019).

Postvaccinal canine distemper virus encephalitis is a rare complication that may develop after administration of a modified live canine distemper vaccine. The affected animal may show aggression, incoordination, and seizures or other neurological signs. The pathogenesis of this condition is unknown, but it may be due to residual virulence, increased susceptibility, or triggering of a latent paramyxovirus by the vaccine.

Errors in Manufacture or Administration

Some problems associated with vaccine use may be due to poor production or administration. Thus some modified live vaccines may retain the ability to cause disease. For example, some modified live herpes vaccines or calicivirus vaccines given intranasally may spread to the oropharynx and result in persistent infection. Indeed, such a virus vaccine may infect (and protect) other animals in contact. Even if these vaccines do not cause overt disease, they may reduce the rate of growth of farm animals with significant economic consequences.

Some vaccines may trigger mild immunosuppression. For example, some modified live parvovirus vaccines may cause a transient decrease in lymphocyte responses to mitogens or even lymphopenia in some puppies, although not all strains of canine parvovirus–2 are immunosuppressive. Some polyvalent canine viral vaccines can cause a transient drop in absolute lymphocyte numbers and their responses to mitogens (see Fig. 41.1). This occurs even though the individual components of these vaccines may not have this effect. Several vaccine combinations may result in transient immunosuppression between 5 and 11 days after vaccination. For example, a combination of canine adenovirus type 1 or type 2 with canine distemper virus suppresses lymphocyte responses to mitogens. This T-cell suppression may be accompanied by simultaneous enhancement of B-cell responses and raised immunoglobulin levels. Rather than being a pure immunosuppressive effect, it may simply reflect a transient change in the Th1/Th2 balance.

A Live bluetongue vaccine has been reported to cause malformations in the offspring of ewes vaccinated while pregnant (Wilbur et al., 1994). The stress from this type of vaccination may also be sufficient to reactivate latent infections; for example, reactivation of equine herpesvirus has been demonstrated following vaccination against African horse sickness. Mucosal disease may develop in calves vaccinated against bovine virus diarrhea.

Vaccine-Associated Autoimmune Disease

It is widely believed that the prevalence of autoimmune disease in domestic pets, especially dogs, has risen in recent years. Some investigators have attributed this rise to excessive use of potent vaccines. This link is by no means proven; nevertheless, there is limited evidence that supports an association between vaccination and autoimmunity. A retrospective analysis of the history of dogs presenting with immune-mediated hemolytic anemia (IMHA) (see Chapter 38) showed that 15 of 70 dogs with IMHA had been vaccinated within the previous month, compared with a randomly selected control group in which none had been vaccinated. Dogs with IMHA that developed within a month of vaccination differed in some clinical features from dogs with IMHA unassociated with prior vaccination. Epidemiologic studies using very large databases tend to confirm this effect, in that they show an approximately threefold increase in diagnoses of autoimmune thrombocytopenia and a twofold increase in diagnoses of IMHA, in dogs in the 30 days following vaccination, compared with other time periods. The overall incidence of these diseases, however, is low, and they can be diagnosed at times not temporally associated with vaccination. Vaccination may therefore serve as a trigger for these diseases in some dogs, but other, undefined, stimuli must also exist.

Vaccine-associated neonatal pancytopenia of calves is a lethal hemorrhagic disease that has resulted from ingestion of maternal colostrum containing anti-BoLA antibodies. The antibodies were generated in response to a specific bovine vaccine. Its pathogenesis is discussed in detail in Chapter 32.

Contaminating thyroglobulin found in some vaccines (usually from the presence of fetal bovine serum) may lead to the production of antithyroid antibodies in vaccinated dogs. Lymphocytic thyroiditis has been found in 40% of Beagles on necropsy, but there was no association detected between vaccination and the development of this thyroiditis (Scott-Moncrieff et al., 2006).

It is well recognized that Guillain-Barré syndrome, an autoimmune neurological disease of humans, can be triggered by administration of some vaccines, such as influenza vaccine. At least one case has been reported in a dog following vaccination with a polyvalent distemper-hepatitis-parvovirus vaccine (see Chapter 38). In some animals, the administration of potent, adjuvanted vaccines may stimulate the transient production of autoantibodies to connective tissue components such as fibronectin and laminin.

Vaccine-Induced Osteodystrophy

Vaccination of some Weimaraner puppies may be associated with the development of a severe hypertrophic osteodystrophy. The disease appears within 10 days of administration of MLV canine distemper vaccine. Systemic signs include anorexia, depression, fever, and gastrointestinal, nervous, and respiratory symptoms, in addition to symmetrical metaphyseal lesions with painful swollen metaphyses. Radiological examination shows radiolucent zones in the metaphyses, flared diaphyses, and formation of new periosteal bone. Hind and forelimbs are equally affected. It is possible that the condition is triggered in genetically susceptible animals by the vaccine. The disease responds well to corticosteroid therapy. In many cases, these dogs show a preexisting immune dysfunction with low concentrations of one or more immunoglobulin classes, recurrent infections, and inflammatory disease (see Chapter 39). It has been suggested that Weimaraners are especially susceptible to this condition and that they therefore receive only killed virus vaccines.

A mild transient polyarthritis has been reported in some dogs following vaccination. The dogs show a sudden onset of lameness with swollen and painful joints within 2 weeks of vaccination. The dogs recover within 2 days. No specific breed or vaccine has been associated with this problem. Vaccination against calicivirus has been associated with polyarthritis and a postvaccination limping syndrome in cats.

Injection Site–Associated Sarcomas

The development of tumors (sarcomas) in cats at sites of vaccine injection is discussed in detail in Chapter 36.

ADVERSE EFFECT PRINCIPLES

In determining whether a vaccine causes an adverse effect, the following three principles should apply: First, is the effect consistent? The clinical responses should be the same if the vaccine is given to a different group of animals, by different investigators, and irrespective of the method of investigation. Second, is the effect specific? The association should be distinctive, and the adverse event should be linked specifically to the vaccine concerned. It is important to remember that an adverse event may be caused by vaccine adjuvants and components other than the major antigens. Finally, there must be a temporal relationship. Administration of the vaccine should precede the earliest manifestations of the event or a clear exacerbation of a continuing condition.

PRODUCTION, PRESENTATION, AND CONTROL OF VACCINES

The production of veterinary vaccines is controlled by the Animal and Plant Health Inspection Service of the USDA in the United States; by the Canadian Centre for Veterinary Biologics of the Canadian Food Inspection Agency; and by the Veterinary Medicines Directorate in the United Kingdom; as well as by appropriate government agencies in other countries. In general, regulatory authorities have the right to license establishments where vaccines are produced and to inspect these premises to ensure that the facilities are appropriate and that the methods employed are satisfactory (Erdman et al., 2020). All vaccines must be checked for safety and potency. Safety tests include confirmation of the identity of the organism used and of the freedom of the vaccine from extraneous organisms (i.e., purity), as well as tests for toxicity and sterility. Because the living organisms or antigens found in vaccines normally die or degrade over a period of time, it is necessary to ensure that they will be effective even after storage. It is therefore usual to use an antigen in generous excess of the dose required to protect animals under laboratory conditions, and potency is tested both before and after accelerated aging. Vaccines that contain killed organisms, although much more stable than living ones, contain an excess of antigens for the same reason. Vaccines approved for licensing on the basis of challenge exposure studies must usually show evidence of protection in 80% of vaccinated animals, whereas at least 80% of the unvaccinated controls must develop evidence of disease after challenge exposure (the 80:80 efficacy guideline). The route and dose of administration indicated on the vaccine label should be scrupulously heeded since these were probably the only route and dose tested for safety and efficacy during the licensing process. Vaccines must be correctly labeled and packaged appropriately. Vaccines usually have a designated shelf life, and although properly stored vaccines may still be potent after the expiration of this shelf life, this should never be assumed. Correct storage and handling are essential. All expired vaccines should be discarded. Adverse reactions should always be reported to the appropriate

licensing authorities as well as to the vaccine manufacturer. Because MLV vaccines carry with them the risks for residual virulence and for contamination with other agents, certain countries will not approve their use (Box 26.1).

Inactivated vaccines are commonly available in liquid form and usually contain suspended adjuvant. These should not be frozen, and they should be shaken well before use. The presence of preservatives such as phenol or thiomerosal will not control massive bacterial contamination, and multidose containers should be discarded after partial use. Many vaccines containing live virus are susceptible to heat inactivation but are much more resistant if lyophilized. Remember, however, that intense sunlight and heat can destroy even lyophilized vaccines. They store well but should be kept cool and away from light and should only be reconstituted with the fluid provided by the manufacturer.

BOX 26.1 Equine Serum Hepatitis

On rare occasions, horses may develop acute hepatic necrosis 30–70 days after vaccination. This disease, called Theiler's disease, has followed administration of horse plasma, equine immune globulin against tetanus, anthrax, strangles, influenza, and equine encephalitis. It has also occurred after active immunization against equine encephalitis and rhinopneumonitis when the vaccines were prepared using fetal equine cells. Certain serum mixtures or a single vaccine batch may be associated with a high incidence of the disease. Occasional cases have been described in untreated horses living with affected animals, suggesting that a virus transmits the disease. Theiler's disease is severe, with 53%–88% mortality. Clinical signs include anorexia, icterus, excessive sweating, and neurological abnormalities. Clinical chemistry confirms severe liver damage with high liver enzyme levels, ammonia, and bilirubin (Guglick et al., 1995).

This now appears to be a parvovirus-induced hepatitis. A specific parvovirus (Ungulate Copiparvovirus 6) is now considered to be the cause of equine serum hepatitis. It is readily transmissible through contaminated equine biologicals such as tetanus antitoxin. This virus appears to be endemic in some areas of the United States. An Equine Pegivirus had been identified as a potential cause. But this has now been disproven.

From Tomlinson, J.E., Wolfisberg, R., Fahnøe, U., Sharma, H., et al., Equine pegiviruses cause persistent infection of bone marrow and are not associated with hepatitis. PLOS Pathog. 16(7) doi:10.1371/journal.ppat.1008677; Divers, T.J., Tennant, B.C., Kumar, A., McDonough, S., et al., 2018. New parvovirus associated with serum hepatitis in horses after inoculation with a common biological product. Emerg. Inf. Dis. 24(2), 303–307.

REFERENCES

Asin, J., Molin, J., Perez, M., Pinczowski, P., et al., 2019. Granulomas following subcutaneous injection with aluminum adjuvant-containing products in sheep. Vet. Pathol. 56 (3), 418–428.

Barquero, N., Daly, J.M., Newton, J.R., 2007. Risk factors for influenza infection in vaccinated racehorses: lessons from an outbreak in Newmarket, UK in 2003. Vaccine 25, 7520–7529.

Bradley, A., Kinyon, J., Frana, T., Bolte, D., et al., 2012. Efficacy of intranasal administration of a modified live feline herpesvirus 1 and feline calicivirus vaccine against disease caused by *Bordetella bronchiseptica* after experimental challenge. J. Vet. Int. Med. 26, 1121–1125.

Broaddus, C.C., Balasuriya, U.B.R., White, J.L.R., et al., 2011. Evaluation of the safety of vaccinating mares against equine viral arteritis during mid or late gestation or during the immediate postpartum period. J. Am. Vet. Med. Assoc. 238, 741–750.

Coyne, M.J., Burr, J.H.H., Yule, T.D., et al., 2001a. Duration of immunity in dogs after vaccination or naturally acquired infection. Vet. Rec. 149, 509–515.

Coyne, M.J., Burr, J.H.H., Yule, T.D., et al., 2001b. Duration of immunity in cats after vaccination or naturally acquired infection. Vet. Rec. 149, 545–548.

De Jong, S.E., Olin, A., Polendran, B., 2020. The impact of the microbiome on immunity to vaccination in humans. Cell. Host. Microbe. https://doi.org/10.1016/j.chom.2020.06.014

Edwards, D.S., Henley, W.E., Ely, E.R., Wood, J.L.N., 2004. Vaccination and ill-health in dogs: a lack of temporal association and evidence of equivalence. Vaccine 22, 3270–3273.

Egerer, A., Schaefer, Z., Larson, L., 2022. A point-of-care dot blot ELISA assay for detection of protective antibody against canine adenovirus, canine parvovirus and canine distemper virus is diagnostically accurate. J. Am. Vet. Med. Assoc. https://doi.org/10.2460/javma.22.05.0224

Ellis, J., Marziani, E., Aziz, C., Brown, C.M., et al., 2022. 2022 AAHA Canine vaccination guidelines. J. Am. Anim. Hosp. Assoc. 58, 213–230. http://doi.org/10.5326/JAAHA-MS-Canine-Vaccination-Guidelines

Erdman, M.M., Clough, N.E., Hauer, P.J., 2020. Review of updated regulations and product license categories for veterinary vaccines in the United States. J. Am. Vet. Med. Assoc. 257 (11), 1142–1147.

Guglick, M.A., MacAllister, C.G., Ely, R.W., Edwards, W.C., 1995. Hepatic disease associated with administration of tetanus antitoxin in eight horses. J. Am. Vet. Med. Assoc. 206, 1737–1740.

Heininger, U., Bachtiar, N.S., Bahri, P., Dana, A., Dodoo, A., Gidudu, J., Santos, E.M., 2012. The concept of vaccination failure. Vaccine 30, 1265–1268.

HogenEsch, H., Thompson, S., 2010. Effect of ageing on the immune response of dogs to vaccines. J. Comp. Pathol. 142, S74–77.

Jas, D., Aeberle, C., Lacombe, V., et al., 2009. Onset of immunity in kittens after vaccination with a non-adjuvanted vaccine against feline panleukopenia, feline calicivirus and feline herpesvirus,. Vet. J. 182, 86–93.

Johnson, N., Cunningham, A.F., Fooks, A.R., 2010. The immune response to rabies virus infection and vaccination. Vaccine 28, 3896–3901.

Keeling, M.J., Woolhouse, M.E.J., May, R.M., et al., 2003. Modeling vaccination strategies against foot-and-mouth disease. Nature 421, 136–142.

Kennedy, L.J., Lunt, M., Barnes, A., et al., 2007. Factors influencing the antibody response of dogs vaccinated against rabies. Vaccine 25, 8500–8507.

Meyer, E.K., 2001. Vaccine-associated adverse events. Vet. Clin. North Am. 31, 493–515.

Miyaji, K., Suzuki, A., Shimakura, H., Takase, Y., et al., 2012. Large-scale survey of adverse reactions to canine non-rabies combined vaccines in Japan. Vet. Immunol. Immunopathol. 145, 447–452.

Moore, G.E., HogenEsch, H., 2010. Adverse vaccinal events in dogs and cats. Vet. Clin. Small Anim. 40, 393–407.

Moore, G.E., DeSantis-Kerr, A.C., Guptill, L.F., et al., 2007. Adverse events after vaccine administration in cats: 2,560 cases (2002–2005). J. Am. Vet. Med. Assoc. 231, 94–100.

Moore, G.E., Guptill, L.F., Ward, M.P., et al., 2005. Adverse events diagnosed within three days of vaccine administration in dogs. J. Am. Vet. Med. Assoc. 227, 1102–1108.

Ohmori, K., Masuda, K., Maeda, S., et al., 2005. IgE reactivity to vaccine components in dogs that developed immediate-type allergic reactions after vaccination. Vet. Immunol. Immunopathol. 104, 249–256.

Pabst, O., Hornef, M., 2014. Gut microbiota: a natural adjuvant for vaccination. Immunity 41, 349–351.

Plotkin, S.A., 2010. Correlates of protection induced by vaccination. Clin. Vaccine Immunol. 17, 1055–1065.

Reese, M.J., Patterson, E.V., Tucker, S.J., et al., 2008. Effects of anesthesia and surgery on serologic responses to vaccination in kittens. Am. J. Vet. Med. Assoc. 233, 116–121.

Richeson, J.T., Hughes, H.D., Broadway, P.R., Carroll, J.A., 2019. Vaccination management of beef cattle. Delayed vaccination and endotoxin stacking. Vet. Clin. Food Anim. 35, 575–592.

Schultz, R.D., 2006. Duration of immunity for canine and feline vaccines: a review. Vet. Microbiol. 117, 75–79.

Schultz, R.D., Thiel, B., Mukhtar, E., et al., 2010. Age and long-term protective immunity in dogs and cats. J. Comp. Pathol. 142, S102–S108.

Scott-Moncrieff, J.C., Glickman, N.W., Glickman, L.T., HogenEsch, H., 2006. Lack of association between repeated vaccination and thyroiditis in laboratory beagles. J. Vet. Int. Med. 200, 818–821.

Squires, R.A. Crawford, C. Marcondes, M. Whitley, N. 2024 guidelines for the vaccination of dogs and cats - compiled by the Vaccination Guidelines Group (VGG) of the World Small Animal Veterinary Association (WSAVA). J. Small. Anim. Pract., 65, (5), 2024, 275–357.

Stone, A.E.S., Brummet, G.O., Carozza, E.M., Kass, P.H., et al., 2020. 2020 AAFA/AAFP feline vaccination guidelines. J. Am. Anim. Hosp. Assoc. 56, 249–265.

Strasser, A., May, B., Teltscher, A., et al., 2003. Immune modulation following immunization with polyvalent vaccines in dogs. Vet. Immunol. Immunopathol. 94, 113–121.

Taguchi, M., Namikawa, K., Maruo, T., et al., 2012. Effects of body weight on antibody titers against canine parvovirus type 2, canine distemper virus, and canine adenovirus type 1 in vaccinated domestic adult dogs. Can. J. Vet. Res. 76, 221–225.

Twark, L., Dodds, W.J., 2000. Clinical use of serum parvovirus and distemper virus antibody titers for determining revaccination strategies in healthy dogs. J. Am. Vet. Med. Assoc. 217, 1021–1024.

Wilbur, L.A., Evermann, J.F., Levings, R.L., et al., 1994. Abortion and death in pregnant bitches associated with a canine vaccine contaminated with bluetongue virus. J. Am. Vet. Med. Assoc. 204, 1762–1765.

FURTHER INFORMATION

Tizard, I.R., 2021. Vaccines for Veterinarians. Elsevier, St. Louis, ISBN:978-0-323-68299-2.

27

Immunity to Bacteria and Fungi

CHAPTER OUTLINE

Although we animals live in a world densely populated with bacteria, most of these neither invade animal tissues nor cause disease. This is unsurprising for several reasons. First, the combined efforts of the innate and adaptive immune systems are sufficient to prevent invasion. Second, even organisms that successfully invade the animal body gain very little by harming their host. On the contrary, illness or death of the host animal reduces the survival of most bacteria and is therefore normally avoided. Indeed, as discussed in Chapter 22, the bacterial microbiota are essential for the animal's well-being since they protect against other invaders, assist in the digestion of foods such as cellulose, and promote the development of the immune system. Nevertheless, many commensal bacteria are also pathobionts. For example, *Clostridium tetani* and *Clostridium perfringens* are commonly found among the intestinal microbiota of horses, and *Bordetella bronchiseptica* is found in the nasopharynx of healthy swine. Bacterial disease is not, therefore, an inevitable consequence of the presence of pathogenic organisms on a body surface. The development of disease is related to many other factors, including the immunity of the host, the presence of damaged tissues, the location of the bacteria, and their disease-producing power (or virulence).

The ability of many bacteria to survive within an animal also depends on their virulence factors. Many of these virulence factors are encoded in mobile genetic elements that can be transmitted between bacteria (e.g., plasmids). These virulence factors permit the bacteria to adapt to a specific environment and promote their transmission between hosts. Depending on their niche within the body, bacteria can use virulence factors to penetrate surface epithelia, to bind to cell surfaces, to acquire iron, to evade immune responses, to hide within cells, and to promote transmission to another host. Some of these strategies result in damage to host tissues and must be prevented by the immune system. It should also be pointed out that many bacteria are unable to invade and cause disease in healthy normal hosts but will take advantage of the opportunity offered by immunosuppression or other weaknesses in host defenses to invade their body. Dead bodies have no defenses and decompose.

INNATE IMMUNITY

Antimicrobial immunity is effected by an early innate response followed by a sustained adaptive response. Recognition of invading bacteria through toll-like receptors (TLRs) and other PRRs induces cytokine release, complement activation, inflammation, and phagocytosis. If this is insufficient to eliminate the invaders, adaptive immune mechanisms take over. Thus dendritic cells and macrophages capture invading bacteria and initiate adaptive immunity by secreting cytokines and triggering both T and B cell responses. The importance of these innate defenses is emphasized by the observation that the resistance of chickens to *Salmonella enterica* Typhimurium appears to be linked to allelic variations in TLR4, and the resistance of foals to *Prescottella* (*Rhodococcus*) *equi* is linked to TLR2. TLRs are responsible, in large part, for the initial recognition of invading bacteria. Binding of microbial pathogen-associated molecular patterns (PAMPs) to TLRs triggers a signal cascade that activates genes encoding proteins that are critical in host defense.

The production of cytokines by horse neutrophils following invasion by *P. equi* provides an example of these responses. Thus, after detecting *P. equi*, neutrophils express increased amounts of interleukin-23 (IL-23). This IL-23 promotes Th17 cell differentiation. Driven by transforming growth factor–β (TGF-β) and IL-6, the Th17 cells then promote inflammation. Not only do these Th17 cells produce IL-17 but also IL-6, GM-CSF, G-CSF, chemokines, and metalloproteases. They thus trigger local inflammation and coordinate early neutrophil recruitment to infection sites, especially on epithelial surfaces (Curis and Way, 2009).

However, neutrophils alone cannot manage *Prescottella* since *P. equi* primarily replicates within alveolar macrophages that produce a robust type 1 interferon response in a manner similar to that induced by *Mycobacerium tuberculosis*. It does this by triggering the DNA sensing process mediated by the cGAS-STING pathway (Vail et al., 2021). *Borrelia burgdorferi*, the cause of Lyme disease, uses the same pathway to sense bacterial DNA and produce type 1 IFNs (Farris et al., 2023).

Type I interferons are also produced in response to bacterial PAMPs. IFN-α/β boosts macrophage cytotoxicity by enhancing their production of IFN-γ, nitric oxide, and TNF-α.

Natural killer (NK) cells also play a protective role in bacterial, protozoan, and fungal infections. For example, some bacteria may activate NK cells by upregulating expression of NKG2D ligands on infected cells. Activated NK cells produce a large amount of IFN-γ that in turn activates both macrophages and dendritic cells (Manusco et al., 2007).

BOX 27.1 Vitamin D and Immunity

When an intracellular bacterium such as *Mycobacterium tuberculosis* interacts with TLR1 or TLR2 on the surface of macrophages, it upregulates many different genes and enhances their antimicrobial activity. In mice, this is mainly mediated by nitric oxide. In humans, however, nitric oxide is not elevated, and other mechanisms must be involved (Fig. 27.1). One gene activated by TLR1/2 signaling in humans is that encoding the vitamin D receptor. This receptor is therefore upregulated in activated macrophages. Binding of vitamin D to its receptor upregulates expression of the gene for the antibacterial peptide cathelicidin. The cathelicidin, in turn, can kill intracellular *M. tuberculosis*. It is no coincidence, therefore, that resistance to tuberculosis is directly related to serum vitamin D levels and that humans with a deficiency of vitamin D show significantly decreased resistance to this infection. It is of interest to recall that sanatorium treatment of tuberculosis classically involved exposure to fresh air and sunlight, a procedure that would be expected to increase vitamin D levels in human patients. Conversely, mice are nocturnal mammals that would not be expected to have high vitamin D levels and must rely on other pathways. Vitamin D supplementation has been shown to reduce the incidence and severity of tuberculosis in wild boar and red deer,

Although many bacteria are destroyed by phagocytosis, others are killed when free in the circulation. Bacteria are destroyed by complement acting through the alternate or lectin pathways. Bacterial cell walls, lacking sialic acid, inactivate factor H and stabilize the alternate C3 convertase (C3bBbP). As a result, these bacteria are either opsonized or lysed. Activation leads to production of terminal complement complexes (TCCs). These TCCs alone may be unable to insert themselves into the carbohydrates of the microbial cell wall. However, lysozyme in the blood may partially digest the cell wall and so enable the TCCs to insert themselves into the lipid bilayer of the inner bacterial membrane and kill it.

Antimicrobial peptides are critical for the defense against bacteria such as the mycobacteria (Box 27.1). Pulmonary collectins and surfactant proteins play an important role against *Mycobacterium avium* infections in the lung. They probably act by binding to, agglutinating, and opsonizing the bacteria. Suppression of bacterial growth by withholding iron is discussed in Chapter 8 (Collins, 2008).

Once activated, platelets also release antibacterial peptides and reactive oxygen species (ROS). They also bind to bacteria to form heterotypic aggregates that are readily phagocytosed by neutrophils or captured in NETs. Horse platelets exposed to bacterial lipopolysaccharide from *Escherichia coli* and lipotechoic acid from *Staphylococcus aureus* can inhibit bacterial growth as a result of the release of ROS (Aktan et al., 2013).

ADAPTIVE IMMUNITY

There are five mechanisms by which the adaptive immune responses combat bacterial infections (Fig. 27.2): (1) neutralization of toxins or enzymes by antibodies; (2) killing of bacteria by the classical complement pathway; (3) opsonization of bacteria by antibodies and complement, resulting in their phagocytosis and destruction; (4) destruction of intracellular bacteria by activated macrophages; and (5) direct killing of bacteria by cytotoxic T cells and NK cells. The relative importance of each of these processes depends on the species of bacteria involved and on the mechanisms by which they cause disease.

Immunity to Toxigenic Bacteria

In diseases caused by toxigenic bacteria such as the clostridia or *Bacillus anthracis*, the immune response must not only eliminate the

Fig. 27.1 Immunity to tuberculosis is governed in many species by the availability of vitamin D. The vitamin D receptor is upregulated on activated macrophages. Binding of vitamin D to this receptor upregulates vitamin D hydroxylase, which in turn increases production of the antibacterial cathelicidins and enhances disease resistance. *NK*, Natural killer.

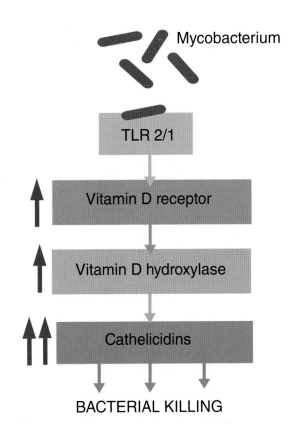

Fig. 27.2 Many and diverse mechanisms by which immune responses can protect the body against bacterial invasion. *TLR*, Toll-like receptors.

invading bacteria but also neutralize their toxins. Destruction of the bacteria, however, may be difficult if they are embedded in a mass of necrotic tissue, and toxin neutralization is a priority. Neutralization occurs when antibody prevents the toxin from binding to its receptors on a target cell. The neutralization process therefore involves competition between receptors and antibodies for the toxin molecule. Once a toxin has bound to its cell receptors, antibodies are relatively ineffective in reversing this combination.

Immunity to Invasive Bacteria

Protection against invasive bacteria is usually mediated by antibodies directed against their surface antigens. Efficient phagocytosis requires that the bacteria be coated with opsonins that can be recognized by phagocytic cells. These opsonins include antibodies and C3b in addition to the innate opsonins such as MBL. Antibodies not only are effective opsonins in their own right but also increase the binding of C3b by activating the classical complement pathway. Antibodies directed against capsular (K) antigens may neutralize the antiphagocytic properties of bacterial capsules, thus permitting their destruction. In bacteria lacking capsules, antibodies directed against O antigens act as opsonins. Protection also results when antibodies are produced against the *E. coli* pilus antigens F4 (K88) and F5 (K99). The antibodies may interfere with the expression of pili. Once expression of the adherence pili is suppressed, these strains of *E. coli* cannot bind to the intestinal wall and thus are no longer a threat.

The importance of bacterial capsules in immunity is seen in anthrax. *B. anthracis* possesses both a capsule and an exotoxin. Antitoxic immunity is protective but slow to develop. In addition, toxin production tends to be prolonged since the organism is encapsulated, and phagocytic cells have difficulty eliminating it. As a result, death is usually inevitable in unvaccinated animals. The vaccine commonly employed against animal anthrax contains an unencapsulated but toxigenic strain of *B. anthracis*. Given in the form of spores that can germinate, the unencapsulated bacteria are eliminated by phagocytic cells before dangerous amounts of toxin are synthesized but not before antitoxic immunity is established.

Molecule for molecule, immunoglobulin M (IgM) is about 500–1000 times more efficient than IgG in opsonization and about 100 times more potent than IgG in sensitizing bacteria for complement-mediated lysis. During a primary immune response, therefore, the quantitative deficiency of IgM is compensated for by its quality, ensuring early and efficient protection.

Many antibodies have direct antimicrobial activities. Antibodies against *E. coli* may be bacteriostatic since they interfere with production of the iron-binding protein enterochelin and thus prevent bacterial iron scavenging. IgM and IgG antibodies against *B. burgdorferi* damage surface proteins on the bacteria and are bactericidal in the absence of complement. Some antibodies are able to generate oxidants and may kill bacteria directly.

Heat Shock Protein Response

When bacteria are stressed, they produce many new proteins. These stressors include heat, starvation, and exposure to oxidants; toxins such as heavy metals; protein synthesis inhibitors; and viral infections. The heat shock proteins (HSPs) are the best understood of these new proteins. Low levels of HSPs are present in bacteria at normal temperatures. Mild stress, such as a low-grade fever induces HSP production. For example, HSP levels climb from 1.5% to 15% of the total protein in stressed *E. coli*. There are three major bacterial HSPs: HSP90, HSP70, and HSP60. (The number refers to their molecular weight in kDa.) When a bacterium is phagocytosed and exposed to the neutrophil respiratory burst, the resulting stress triggers the production of

bacterial HSPs. As a result, HSP60 is the dominant antigen in infections caused by Mycobacteria, *Coxiella burnetii*, Legionella, Treponema, and Borrelia species. These HSPs are highly antigenic for several reasons. First, they are produced in abundance within the infected host; second, they are readily processed by antigen-presenting cells; and third, the immune system may possess unusually large numbers of B and T cells capable of responding to HSPs. In addition, some γ/δ T cells may preferentially recognize bacterial HSPs. Thus anti-HSP responses may induce significant protection against many bacterial pathogens (Kaufmann and Dorhoi, 2016).

Immunity to Intracellular Bacteria

Some bacteria, such as *Brucella abortus*, *M. tuberculosis*, *Campylobacter jejuni*, *P. equi*, *Listeria monocytogenes*, *Corynebacterium pseudotuberculosis*, *C. burnetii*, and some serotypes of *S. enterica*, can grow readily inside resting macrophages. In addition, *L. monocytogenes* can travel from cell to cell without exposure to the extracellular fluid through cytoskeletal membrane protrusions (see Chapter 19).

Autophagy, as described in Chapter 6, is a key process in the destruction of intracellular bacteria. The same cellular machinery used to destroy unwanted organelles can be employed to eliminate intracellular organisms. Thus bacteria that escape into the cytosol may be surrounded by an autophagosome-like structure and subsequently destroyed by lysosomal enzymes. Autophagy (or more correctly, xenophagy) may also play a key role in delivering processed microbial antigens to major histocompatibility complex (MHC) molecules. That said, *B. abortus* can employ autophagy pathways to spread from cell to cell. The bacterium selectively suppresses some of the components of autophagosome formation so that it is not killed (Starr et al., 2012).

Protection against intracellular bacteria is mediated by cell-mediated mechanisms (Harris et al., 2009). Early in the immune response, activated M1 macrophages and cDC1 dendritic cells secreting IL-12 and TNF-α are most important (see Chapter 19; Benoit et al., 2008). Although macrophages from unimmunized animals cannot usually destroy these bacteria, this ability is acquired about 10 days after infection. Later in the response, IFN-γ from Th1 cells and the activities of cytotoxic CD8+ T cells become critical. IFN-γ, especially in association with TNF-α, greatly enhances the production of cytokines such as TNF-α, IL-6, IL-1β, IL-12, and IL-32, enzymes such as indoleamine 2,3-dioxygenase (IDO) and nitric oxide synthase 2 (NOS2), and the release of reactive oxygen and nitrogen species. Th17 cells may interact with Th1 cells to promote protection against Brucella. M1 macrophage activation has been shown to be important in resistance to *L. monocytogenes*, *S. enterica* Typhi and Typhimurium, *P. equi*, mycobacteria, and chlamydia. For example, IFN-γ and TNF-α produced by primed T cells generate M1 macrophages, acidify their phagosomes, and kill mycobacteria. Uncontrolled M1 activation by bacteria such as streptococci and *E. coli*, however, can contribute to disease pathology by inducing sepsis, tissue damage, and organ failure. The response of these activated macrophages tends to be nonspecific, particularly in listerial infections, and M1 activated macrophages are able to destroy many normally resistant bacteria. Thus an animal recovering from an infection with *L. monocytogenes* develops increased resistance to *M. tuberculosis*. The development of M1 macrophages often coincides with the appearance of delayed (type IV) hypersensitivity responses to intradermally administered antigen (see Chapter 34). *M. tuberculosis* can persist, in activated as well as resting macrophages. However, this persistence requires a bacterial dormant stage when its replication and many metabolic processes are suspended.

NK and CD8+ T cells also participate in immunity to intracellular bacteria such as *L. monocytogenes*. These cytotoxic cells bind to target cells and use perforins to generate pores that allow the delivery of lytic granule contents into the infected cells. Granulysin then penetrates the bacterial cell wall, and so permits granzymes to enter the bacteria. These granzymes generate ROS that disrupt key enzyme pathways. For good measure, the granzymes may also trigger apoptosis in the target cell, which further limits bacterial spreading. *P. equi*–infected macrophages can also be recognized and killed by cytotoxic T cells in an MHC class I unrestricted manner.

It has been observed that protective immunity against intracellular bacteria cannot be induced by vaccines containing killed bacteria. Only vaccines containing living bacteria are protective. This is because of the differential activation of helper T-cell populations by live and dead bacteria. Infection of mice with live *B. abortus* stimulates Th1 cells to secrete IFN-γ; a type 1 immune response. Conversely, immunization of these mice with purified *Brucella* proteins induces Th2 cells to secrete IL-4; a type 2 response. Likewise, live but not dead *L. monocytogenes* or *B. abortus* organisms induce macrophage production of TNF-α. Killed *Brucella* organisms stimulate IL-1 production to a greater extent than live bacteria. Resistance to these intracellular bacteria is generally short lived, persisting for only as long as viable bacteria remain in the body. (Tuberculosis is an exception, where memory is prolonged.)

If, in a bacterial disease, it is observed that dead vaccines do not give good protection, that serum cannot confer protection, that antibody levels do not relate to resistance, and that delayed hypersensitivity reactions can be elicited to the bacterial antigens, then type 1 immune responses probably play the major role in resistance, and the use of vaccines containing living bacteria should be contemplated.

Modification of Bacterial Disease by Immune Responses

The immune response influences the course and severity of an infection. At best, it will result in microbial destruction and a cure. In the absence of a cure, however, the infection may be profoundly modified. Much depends on whether a cell-mediated or antibody response is generated. Thus the type of helper T cells induced during infection affects the course of disease. As described in Chapter 19, type 1, cell-mediated responses are required to control intracellular bacteria since only activated macrophages can prevent their growth. Macrophage activation requires that Th1 cells produce IFN-γ. Once activated, the M1 cells may localize or cure these infections. If an animal mounts an inappropriate Th2 response so that M2 but not M1 macrophages are generated, chronic progressive disease may result. This is seen in Johne's disease of sheep. Some animals develop multibacillary (MB) disease, in which their intestinal lesions contain enormous numbers of bacteria (Fig. 27.3), and there is little histological evidence of a cell-mediated response. Their granulomas lack organization, containing large numbers of bacteria-laden macrophages intermixed with lymphocytes. In contrast, other sheep may develop paucibacillary (PB) disease, in which the lesions contain very few bacteria but large numbers of lymphocytes. These are organized nodular lesions with epithelioid cells and multinucleated giant cells at the center, surrounded by fibrous connective tissue (Smeed et al., 2010). The two forms of the disease are associated with differential expression of cytokine and chemokine receptors. Thus animals with the PB disease have increased numbers of CD25+ T cells that produce more IL-2 and much more IFN-γ than sheep with the MB form of the disease (Fig. 27.4). In contrast, sheep with the MB disease have higher antibody levels and a lack of cellular immune responses. Sheep with PB lesions mount a type 1 response, whereas those with MB disease mount a type 2 response (Gossner et al., 2017).

In bovine *M. bovis* infections, WC1+ γ/δ T cells accumulate within tuberculous lesions and play a role in granuloma development. They also affect the levels of IgG2 antibodies, the increase in IFN-γ, and the decrease in IL-4 levels, so they shape the character of the

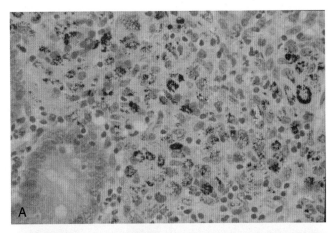

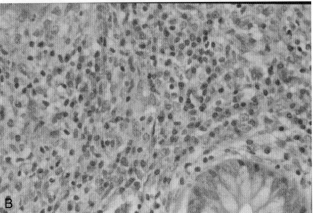

Fig. 27.3 The two forms of Johne disease in sheep. (A) Section of terminal ileum from a case of multibacillary Johne disease, showing abundant acid-fast organisms within large infiltrating macrophages. (B) Section of terminal ileum from a case of paucibacillary Johne disease, showing very few acid-fast bacteria and a significant lymphocyte infiltration. Ziehl-Nielsen stain. Courtesy Dr. C.J. Clarke.

antimycobacterial response. Expression of IFN-γ, IL-17A, and arginase are higher in lung granulomas (Shu et al., 2014). This arginase might facilitate the infection by reducing nitric oxide production.

IL-4 is a key cytokine that promotes Th2 responses while suppressing Th1 responses. In addition to normal IL-4, cattle produce two variants, called IL-4δ2 and IL-4δ3, by alternative splicing of pre–messenger RNA. These splice variants may bind and block IL-4 receptors and regulate their activity. As a result, they affect the resistance of cattle to tuberculosis. Animals showing significant resistance to tuberculosis produced high levels of IL-4δ3 compared to susceptible cattle (Rhodes et al., 2007).

The specific helper T-cell subset involved in immunity to tuberculosis can change once the response is established. Time-based studies have shown that immune responses to bacterial infections may swing between Th1 and Th2 responses, perhaps several times, before a final response is established. This final response may well be a Th1 or Th2 response, or even some intermediate point in the Th1/Th2 spectrum. This variability appears to be a common feature of chronic infections such as tuberculosis (Thacker et al., 2007).

EVASION OF THE IMMUNE RESPONSE

The outcome of any infection depends on the continuously evolving battle between the host and the microbe. To survive within an animal, bacteria must evade or inhibit the immune system's defenses.

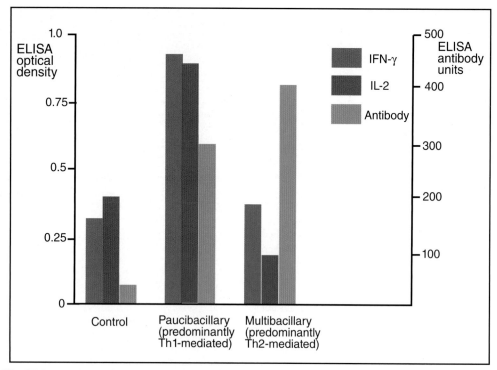

Fig. 27.4 The differences in peripheral blood lymphocyte interleukin-2 (IL-2), interferon-γ (IFN-γ), and antibody production between sheep with the paucibacillary (PB) form and sheep with the multibacillary (MB) form of Johne disease. Note that there is a marked tendency for the T cells from animals with the PB form of the disease to produce more Th1 cytokines than those with the MB form. Despite this, animals with the latter form appear to produce more antibodies. From data kindly provided by Chris Clarke and Charles Burrells.

The complex interrelationships between bacteria and their animal hosts, described in Chapter 22, include the role of commensal bacteria on mucosal surfaces in regulating the growth and development of the immune system. These commensal bacteria generally do not aggressively seek to invade the body, so equilibrium can be achieved. Nevertheless, an invading microorganism becomes a pathogen because it can invade the body, evade the immune defenses, and survive at least for a time within its host. Pathogenic bacteria, like all organisms, try to avoid destruction. They have evolved many different mechanisms to overcome host innate and adaptive immune responses.

Evasion of Innate Immunity

The key to successful microbial invasion, at least initially, is evading innate immunity. Bacteria employ diverse mechanisms to prevent or at least delay an unpleasant fate. Only a few selected examples can be mentioned here (Baxt et al., 2013).

For example, some bacteria interfere with TLR signaling pathways and inflammasome activation (Fig. 27.5). The methods used include the production of modified PAMPs that will not trigger TLRs, masking of PAMPs, blockage of TLR signaling pathways, destruction of signaling molecules, destruction of NF-κB, and misdirection of signaling pathways toward antiinflammatory pathways. Thus *M. tuberculosis* uses a masking lipid to cover its PRRs. *Leptospira* have lipopolysaccharides that are recognized by TLR2, but not by TLR4. *C. jejuni* makes a form of flagellin that is not recognized by TLR5 (Andersen-Nissen et al., 2005). *Yersinia pestis* reduces acetylation of lipid A so that it cannot be recognized by TLR4. Bacteria also differ in the amount of CpG dinucleotides in their DNA and, therefore, in their ability to trigger TLR9. Potent stimulators of TLR9 include *M. tuberculosis* and *Pseudomonas aeruginosa*. Weak TLR9 stimulators include *C. jejuni* and *Staphylococcus epidermidis*.

Many bacteria interfere with intracellular signaling pathways. *Brucella* synthesizes a protein called TcpB that closely resembles the mammalian Toll/IL-1 receptor. As a result, it accelerates degradation of an adaptor protein and blocks the TLR signaling pathway. *P. aeruginosa* secretes a protein that impairs the regulation of NF-κB. The *Mycobacterium avium paratuberculosis* (MAP) kinase pathway can be inhibited by proteolysis of MKK (anthrax), elimination of MAPK (Shigella), or acetylation of MAPK (Yersinia). Misdirection of signaling pathways occurs when products from Candida, Yersinia, or Mycobacteria trigger signaling through TLR2, leading to production of IL-10 (Reddick and Alto, 2014).

Another useful skill for a bacterium to possess is the ability to resist antibacterial peptides. For example, staphylokinase from *S. aureus* can bind and neutralize defensins. Another staphylococcal enzyme, aureolysin, destroys cathelicidins. Salmonella and *S. aureus* can produce proteins that change the negative charge and fluidity of the bacterial outer membrane, resulting in decreased defensin binding. *Klebsiella pneumoniae* capsular polysaccharide blocks β-defensin expression by airway epithelial cells. Proteases from *B. anthracis* can destroy defensins and cathelicidins.

Many bacteria can block phagocytosis (Fig. 27.6). For example, *S. aureus* expresses protein A. Protein A attaches to IgG Fc regions and so prevents antibodies from binding to Fc receptors on phagocytic cells or activating the classical complement pathway. Encapsulated bacteria, such as pneumococci, possess a hydrophilic capsule that cells cannot stick to. Many bacteria can evade opsonization by complement. For example, the M protein of streptococci binds fibrinogen and masks C3b-binding sites. It also binds factor H, which inactivates bound C3b. *S. aureus* produces a protein that blocks C3 convertases. Other bacteria produce proteases that can destroy complement components. *S. enterica* Typhimurium has a gene called *Rck* that confers resistance

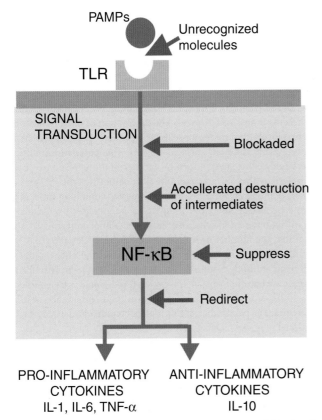

Fig. 27.5 Bacteria can interfere with toll-like receptor (TLR) signaling pathways in many different ways and at many different positions, as described in the text. This can include redirecting the nuclear factor kappa-B (NF-κB) signaling pathways from its normal proinflammatory state to antiinflammatory pathways. *IL*, Interleukin; *PAMPs*, pathogen-associated molecular patterns; *TNF-α*, tumor necrosis factor–α.

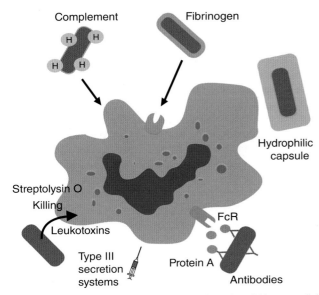

Fig. 27.6 Some of the many different mechanisms by which extracellular bacteria can avoid being phagocytosed and destroyed by phagocytic cells such as neutrophils. See text for details.

to complement-mediated lysis by preventing insertion of the terminal complement complex into the bacterial outer membrane (Garcia et al., 2016).

Strains of *Streptococcus pneumoniae* growing in suspension readily activate C3, leading to deposition of C3b on their surface and promoting their opsonization. This does not occur on pneumococci growing within biofilms where binding of C-reactive protein and C1q is reduced. Conversely, recruitment of factor H, the regulator of the alternative complement pathway, is enhanced in biofilms (Cerca et al., 2006). Thus biofilm formation is an efficient method of evading both the classical and alternative complement pathways. *S. aureus* and *P. aeruginosa* can also evade phagocytosis by switching from planktonic growth to biofilm production (Dominech et al., 2013).

Bacteria can, of course, avoid being eaten simply by killing phagocytic cells. For example, *Streptococcus canis* produces streptolysin O that lyses neutrophil cell membranes. Several gram-negative bacteria of veterinary importance, such as *Mannheimia haemolytica* and *Fusobacterium necrophorum*, secrete leukotoxins that kill leukocytes, especially granulocytes (Narayan et al., 2002). The most important leukotoxins are the RTX ("repeats in toxin") proteins. *M. haemolytica* secretes an RTX toxin that kills ruminant neutrophils, alveolar macrophages, and lymphocytes. This leukotoxin binds to CD18 as well as lipid rafts on leukocytes and induces their apoptosis. *Moraxella bovis* also secretes a leukotoxin for bovine neutrophils. *Actinobacillus pleuropneumoniae* secretes a toxin that kills porcine macrophages. *Mycoplasma mycoides* can kill bovine T cells. Other bacteria trigger lymphocyte death by apoptosis. These include *B. anthracis*, Streptococci, Shigella, *L. monocytogenes*, *S. aureus*, and Yersinia. Leukotoxins are a relatively crude method of assassination. Some bacteria use much more sophisticated methods, such as injecting toxins into their targets. Gram-negative bacteria such as *Salmonella*, *Pseudomonas*, and *E. coli* have developed an elaborate needle complex; a type III secretion system, to convey effector molecules directly into the cytosol of effector cells. These injection systems are turned on when a bacterium is ingested by a cell and exposed to a low pH within the phagosome. Once the needle complex enters the cytosol and detects its neutral pH, injection of effector molecules occurs. These molecules activate guanosine triphosphatases and disrupt intracellular signaling pathways. At high concentrations, they produce transmembrane pores and kill the cells.

Although killing leukocytes is an effective way to avoid being eaten, other bacteria are content to simply prevent intracellular destruction. Some bacteria generate a resistant cell wall to protect themselves against lysosomal enzymes. For example, the cell wall waxes of *C. pseudotuberculosis* make it resistant to lysosomal enzymes. *S. aureus* uses a cell wall peptidoglycan that is completely resistant to lysozyme. Some bacteria produce antioxidants that neutralize the products of the respiratory burst. For example, the carotenoid pigments responsible for the yellow color of *S. aureus* can quench singlet oxygen. *S. enterica* Typhimurium can prevent assembly of the NOX complex and downregulate host NOS2 activity. *Pasteurella multocida* and *Histophilus somni* are also able to inhibit the respiratory burst. Anthrax toxins LF and EF inhibit NAPDH oxidase activity. *S. aureus* produces catalase that inactivates hydrogen peroxide and the free radicals produced during the respiratory burst. It also produces lactate dehydrogenase that also helps it resist NO-mediated oxidation. Some bacteria can defend themselves against hypochloride through the actions of a molecular chaperone called Hsp33. This protein unfolds on exposure to HOCl and then binds and protects essential proteins against bleach-induced aggregation.

Bacteria such as enteropathogenic *E. coli*, *Y. pestis*, *M. tuberculosis*, and *P. aeruginosa* secrete molecules that can protect them against neutrophils. For example, *E. coli* produces lysozyme inhibitors. Other bacteria ensure that they are never exposed to these enzymes by interfering with phagosomal maturation (Fig. 27.7). Mycobacteria, *B.*

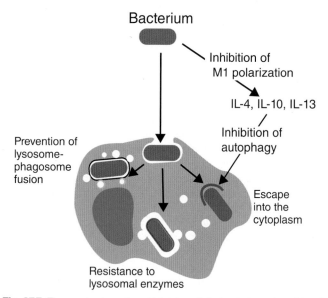

Fig. 27.7 The mechanisms by which intracellular bacteria such as *Listeria monocytogenes* or *Mycobacterium tuberculosis* can evade intracellular destruction by macrophages. *IL,* Interleukin.

abortus, and *Chlamydophila psittaci* can establish themselves within vacuoles that exclude proteases and oxidants by blocking lysosome-phagosome fusion. In the case of *M. tuberculosis,* the bacterium enters the macrophage through cholesterol-enriched membrane microdomains that are coated on the cytosolic side with a protein (tryptophan-aspartate-containing coat protein, or TACO) that prevents phagosome maturation. Thus lysosomes cannot fuse with the phagosome. They remain distributed within the cytosol, and the bacteria survive and grow (Pieters and Gatfield, 2002). Mycobacteria can also prevent acidification of phagosomes by preventing recruitment of the proton pump adenosine triphosphatase from the vacuolar membrane so that lysosomal cathepsins remain inactive. Another mechanism used by bacteria to avoid destruction is simply to escape from the phagosome by migrating into the cytosol, surrounded by a coat of polymerized actin. This method is employed by mycobacteria and by *L. monocytogenes.* Listeria secretes listeriolysin O that destroys cell membranes and so permits the organism to enter the cytosol.

Even extracellular killing can be inhibited by some bacteria. Neutrophils and macrophages can release intranuclear DNA and associated chromatin proteins, resulting in the formation of NETs and METs (see Fig. 6.15). This extracellular chromatin is studded with antimicrobial proteins, including granule components that can kill extracellular bacteria. However, bacteria such as *Mycoplasma bovis* and *S. aureus* can secrete endonucleases that degrade this chromatin scaffold (Thammavongsa et al., 2013). Additionally, the released phosphonucleotides can be dephosphorylated by another Staphylococcal enzyme and generate deoxyadenosine that then triggers apoptosis and eliminates any nearby macrophages!

Metabolic privation is the process by which animal hosts seek to sequester essential nutrients, thus preventing microbial growth. Thus tryptophan is one such nutrient. It is stored within macrophages and converted into IDO. This tryptophan depletion requires bacteria to activate tryptophan synthesis if they are to survive. Macrophages also sequester iron, as described in Chapter 8. As a result, pathogens must produce their own siderophores to capture any available iron. For example, pathogenic strains of *S. equi* produce equibactin, an iron-binding siderophore. Less pathogenic persistent strains do not.

Evasion of Adaptive Immunity

Bacteria also seek to avoid or modify adaptive immune responses—a more difficult task (Sansonetti and Di Santo, 2007).

The body will not respond effectively to organisms it cannot detect or to organisms that it encounters for the first time. *C. fetus* subspecies *venerealis,* an organism that normally colonizes the genital tract of cattle, prevents effective immune elimination by repeatedly changing the proteins in its surface layers. The destruction of most of these bacteria by a local immune response leaves a remnant population that possesses new and different surface antigens. This population multiplies but is largely eliminated in turn by another immune response, leaving the bacteria with a surface layer of a third antigenic type. This process of cyclical antigenic variation may be repeated for a long time, resulting in a persistent infection. *Anaplasma marginale,* a bacterium that lives within bovine red cells, also shows sequential antigenic variation. As a result, the number of Anaplasma in blood, cycles at 6- to 8-week intervals. Their numbers gradually increase and then fall rapidly as a result of an antibody response. This is followed by the growth of a new antigenic variant that repeats the cycle. *A. marginale* is transmitted by ticks, so its successful spread depends on the maintenance of a high bacteremia. The persistence of this high bacteremia is assisted by a dysfunctional memory CD4[+] T-cell response.

Some bacteria secrete proteases that can destroy immunoglobulins or cytokines. For example, proteases specific for IgA are produced by *Haemophilus influenzae,* and *S. pneumoniae.* These organisms can thus prevent opsonization and Fc receptor-mediated phagocytosis. *M. haemolytica* and *Mycoplasma bovis* secrete proteases specific for bovine IgG1. *P. aeruginosa* secretes a protease that destroys IL-2. B cells infected with *B. abortus* secrete IL-10. These cause transient immunosuppression and permit the bacterium to successfully establish a chronic infection (Goenka et al., 2011).

Pathogenic mycobacteria have evolved to survive within host macrophages, and MAP, the cause of Johne disease, is highly adept at such survival. MAP interacts with receptors on macrophages to initiate cell signaling and phagocytosis (Weiss and Sousa, 2008). Thus MAP crosses the intestinal epithelial barrier by triggering IL-1β production. This recruits macrophages to the apical side of the epithelium and facilitates entry into its macrophage habitat. MAP also traffics easily through M cells, where it can be picked up by DCs or macrophages and carried to the mesenteric lymph node. Mannosylated lipoarabinomannan (Man-lam) is a major component of the MAP cell wall. Man-lam binds to TLR2, triggering transcription of IL-10. The IL-10 suppresses production of proinflammatory cytokines and attenuates phagosome acidification and phagolysosome fusion. Thus Man-lam appears to be largely responsible for suppressing the inflammatory and antimicrobial responses against MAP. IDO is also generated in MAP infections and may downregulate the host's immune responses. Antigenic stimulation of mesenteric lymph node cells from cattle severely infected with MAP reveals upregulation of not only IL-10 but also IFN-γ, IL-13, IL-17A, and TNF-α. This suggests that cytokine synthesis is severely dysregulated. MAP also blocks macrophage activation by IFN-γ. Macrophage activation is required in order to kill the intracellular invader, and if this activation does not occur, then the bacterium can persist. The interferon blockage results from inhibition of the JAK-STAT pathway. MAP-infected cells cannot phosphorylate key peptides in the pathway (Arsenault et al., 2012).

Avirulent mycobacteria can be taken up by macrophages and induce their apoptosis. This produces a "cellular corpse" with an impermeable envelope that prevents the bacteria from escaping. As a result, the mycobacteria are killed only when the apoptotic cell is removed. Virulent mycobacteria, in contrast, when taken up by macrophages, cause necrosis. This produces a dead cell with a permeable cell membrane that enables the bacteria to escape and spread.

TABLE 27.1 Facultative Intracellular Bacteria and Their Mechanisms of Survival

Organism	Method of Intracellular Survival
Brucella abortus	Reduced PAMP expression Prevents phagosome maturation Suppression of autophagy
Corynebacterium pseudotuberculosis	Resistant cell wall
Listeria monocytogenes	Neutralizes respiratory burst Escapes into the cytosol
Mycobacterium tuberculosis	Lipid cell wall Prevents phagosome maturation Suppresses antigen presentation Detoxifies oxidants
Salmonella enterica	Prevents phagosome maturation Modifies endosomal trafficking Detoxifies oxidants Downregulates NOS2 and NOX
Prescottella equi	Survives in phagosomes

NOX, NADPH oxidase; *NOS2*, nitric oxide synthase; *PAMP*, pathogen-associated molecular pattern.

It has long been recognized that *M. tuberculosis* survives within macrophages by blocking fusion of the phagosome with lysosomes (Cambier et al., 2014a). IFN-γ can overcome this maturation block by triggering autophagy. As a result, a new autophagosome forms around the blocked phagosome, and this then fuses with lysosomes, permitting the killing of the mycobacteria. Conversely, Th2 cytokines such as IL-4 and IL-13 inhibit autophagy and permit mycobacterial survival. Several other intracellular bacteria are eliminated by autophagy. These include *Streptococcus pyogenes* and *S. enterica* Typhimurium. Other organisms such as *Brucella*, *Listeria*, and *Shigella* have evolved mechanisms to avoid autophagy and survive within autophagosomes (Table 27.1).

Bacteria may also interfere with macrophage polarization to promote their own survival. Some salmonella and mycobacteria can neutralize M1-related effectors or inhibit M1 cytokine secretion or expression. *S. enterica* Dublin suppresses IL-18, and *B. suis* inhibits TNF-α production. Proteins from *M. tuberculosis* can inhibit activation of NF-κB. Responding mycobacteria may induce the synthesis of IL-6, IL-10, and TGF-β and hence prolong their own survival. IL-10 is especially effective in inhibiting macrophage activation, suppressing oxidant production, and reducing MHC class II expression.

The evolution of bacterial diseases into persistent chronic infections is associated with a tendency to M2 polarization mediated by IL-10 (Weiss et al., 2005). This occurs in chronic brucellosis, Q fever, and tuberculosis. *B. abortus*–infected bovine monocyte-derived dendritic cells produce less IL-10, IL-12p40, and IFN-γ when compared to lipopolysaccharide-stimulated cells. Some pathogens, such as *Yersinia enterocolitica* and *C. burnetii*, actually stimulate M2 polarization.

SOME ANTIBACTERIAL VACCINES

Toxoids

The immunoprophylaxis of tetanus is restricted to toxin neutralization. Tetanus toxoid in an aluminum hydroxide suspension is given for routine prophylaxis, and a single injection will induce protective immunity in 10–14 days. Conventional immunological wisdom would suggest that the previous use of tetanus immune globulin should interfere with the immune response to toxoid and must therefore be avoided. This is not a problem in practice, however, and both may be successfully administered simultaneously (at different sites) without problems. This may be because of the relatively small amount of immune globulin usually needed to protect animals.

Some veterinary vaccines combine both toxoid and killed bacteria in a single dose by the simple expedient of adding formaldehyde to a whole culture. These products, sometimes called anacultures, are used to vaccinate against *Clostridium haemolyticum* and *C. perfringens*. Trypsinization of the anaculture may make it more immunogenic. Toxoids, usually incorporated with an alum adjuvant, are available for most clostridial diseases and for infections caused by toxigenic staphylococci.

Bacterins

Vaccines containing killed bacteria are called bacterins. It is usual to kill the bacteria with formaldehyde and to incorporate them with alum or aluminum hydroxide adjuvants. As with other dead vaccines, the immunity produced by bacterins is relatively short lived, usually lasting no longer than 1 year and sometimes considerably less. For example, formolized swine erysipelas (*Erysipelothrix rhusiopathiae*) vaccine protects for only 4–5 months, and *Streptococcus equi* bacterins give immunity for less than 1 year, even though recovery from a natural case of strangles may confer a lifelong immunity in horses.

Bacterins may be improved by adding purified antigens to the killed bacteria. *E. coli* bacterins against enteric colibacillosis may be enriched and made much more effective by the addition of K88 or K99 pilus antigens. Similarly, *Mannheimia* bacterins enriched with its leukotoxoid show improved efficacy over conventional bacterins. Purified bacterial components, such as the surface antigens of *M. haemolytica*, may also be effective vaccine components.

One problem encountered, especially when using coliform and *Campylobacter* vaccines, is strain specificity. Multiple different strains of each organism exist, and successful vaccination requires immunization with the appropriate strain. This is sometimes not possible if a commercial vaccine must be employed. One method of overcoming this difficulty is to use autogenous vaccines. These are vaccines that contain organisms obtained either from infected animals on the farm where the disease problem is occurring or from the infected animal itself. These can be very successful if carefully prepared, since the vaccine will contain all the antigens required for protection in that specific location. As an alternative to the use of autogenous vaccines, some manufacturers produce polyvalent vaccines containing a mixture of antigenic types. For example, leptospirosis vaccines commonly contain up to five different serovars. This practice, although effective, is inefficient since only a few of the antigenic types employed may be required to generate protection in any given location.

An alternative approach to the development of vaccines against gram-negative bacteria is the use of common core antigens. As pointed out in Chapter 2, the outer layer of the gram-negative bacterial cell wall consists of lipopolysaccharide. This lipopolysaccharide consists of a variable oligosaccharide (O antigen) bound to a highly conserved core polysaccharide and lipid A. The O antigens vary greatly among gram-negative bacteria, meaning that an immune response against one O antigen confers no immunity against bacteria expressing other O antigens. In contrast, the underlying core polysaccharide is similar between gram-negative bacteria of different species and genera. Thus an immune response directed against this common core structure has the potential to protect against a wide variety of different gram-negative bacteria.

Mutant strains of *E. coli* (J5) and *S. enterica* Minnesota and Typhimurium (Re) have been used as sources of core antigen. J5 is a rough mutant that is deficient in uridine diphosphate galactose 4-epimerase. As a result, the organism makes an incomplete oligosaccharide side chain, having lost most of the outer lipopolysaccharide structure (Fig. 2.2). Immunization with J5 thus provides protection against *E. coli*, *K. pneumoniae*, *A. pleuropneumoniae*, and *H. influenzae* (type B). J5 has been reported to protect calves against organisms such as *S. enterica* Typhimurium and *E. coli* and pigs against *A. pleuropneumoniae*. The most encouraging results have been obtained in protection against coliform mastitis.

Living Bacterial Vaccines

Successful living bacterial vaccines include strains 19 and RB51 of *B. abortus*. Another successful living vaccine is that employed for the prevention of anthrax. Older anthrax vaccines used Pasteur's technique of culturing the bacteria at a relatively high temperature (42°C–43°C) to reduce their virulence. The anthrax vaccines currently available for animals contain unencapsulated mutants that remain capable of forming spores. The vaccine is prepared as a spore suspension and is administered with saponin.

A rough strain of *S. enterica* Dublin (strain 51) is used in Europe to give good protection to calves when administered at 2–4 weeks of age. As discussed earlier, immunity to salmonellosis involves macrophage activation and is thus relatively nonspecific. For this reason, strain 51 may also provide good protection against *S. enterica* Typhimurium.

ADVERSE CONSEQUENCES

Although immune responses are beneficial in that they eliminate invading bacteria, this is not always the case. The immune responses can influence the course of a bacterial disease without producing a cure, and in some situations, they may increase its severity. The adverse consequences of the immune responses correspond in their mechanisms to the hypersensitivity types described in Chapters 30–34. For example, a local type I hypersensitivity reaction is sometimes seen in sheep vaccinated against foot rot by means of *Dichelobacter nodosus* vaccine, but in this case, it is believed that the hypersensitivity may assist in preventing reinfection.

Type II (cytotoxic) reactions may account for the anemia that occurs in animals with salmonellosis. In these infections, bacterial lipopolysaccharides from the bacteria are adsorbed onto erythrocytes. The subsequent immune response against the bacterium and its products therefore results in red cell destruction.

Type III (immune-complex) reactions may contribute to the development of arthritis in *E. rhusiopathiae* infections in pigs or to the development of intestinal lesions in Johne disease. In the former case, bacterial antigen tends to localize in joints, where local immune-complex formation then results in inflammation and arthritis. Passively administered antiserum may therefore exacerbate the arthritis in these infected animals. In Johne disease, type I or type III reactions occurring in the intestinal mucosa may increase the outflow of fluid and cause diarrhea. It is clear, however, that the intestinal lesions in this disease are etiologically complex since diarrhea can be transferred to normal calves by either plasma or leukocytes, and antihistamine drugs may reduce the diarrhea. Type III hypersensitivity reactions are involved in purpura hemorrhagica of horses, in which vascular immune-complex lesions result from *S. equi* infection (see Chapter 33).

Although cell-mediated (type IV) immune responses are manifestly beneficial, they do contribute to the development of granulomatous lesions in some chronic infections. Large granulomas such as tubercles, although serving to wall off invading bacteria and thus prevent their

spread, may also grow to involve uninfected tissues. If these granulomas invade essential structures such as airways in the lungs or large blood vessels, damage may be severe.

SEROLOGY OF BACTERIAL INFECTIONS

Bacterial infections may be diagnosed by detecting specific antibodies in serum. Thus the agglutination test is widely employed in the diagnosis of bacterial infections, particularly those involving gram-negative bacteria such as *Brucella* and *Salmonella*. The usual procedure in bacterial agglutination tests is to titrate serum (antibody) against a standard suspension of antigen. Bacteria are not, of course, antigenically homogeneous but rather are covered by a mosaic of many different antigens. Thus motile bacteria will have flagellar (H) antigens, and agglutination by antiflagellar antibodies will produce fluffy cotton-like floccules as the flagella stick together, leaving the bacterial bodies only loosely agglutinated. Agglutination of the somatic (O) antigens results in tight clumping of the bacterial bodies, so that the agglutination is finely granular in character. Many bacteria possess several O and H antigens, as well as capsular (K) and pilus (F) antigens. By using a set of specific antisera, it is possible to characterize the antigenic structure of an organism and consequently classify it. It is on this basis, for instance, that the 2400 or so different serovars of *S. enterica* are classified.

Flagellar (H) antigens are destroyed by heating, whereas O antigens are heat resistant and therefore remain intact on heat-killed bacteria. K antigens vary in their heat stability: the L antigen of *E. coli*, which is a capsular antigen, is heat labile, whereas another K antigen, antigen A, is heat stable. *S. enterica* Typhi possesses an antigen called Vi that, although heat stable, is removed from the bacterial cells by heating. The presence of K or Vi antigens in an organism may render them O-inagglutinable and thus complicate agglutination tests. It should also be pointed out that rough forms of bacteria do not form stable suspensions and therefore cannot be typed by means of agglutination tests.

Bacterial agglutination tests may be performed by mixing drops of reagents on glass slides or by titrating the reagents in tubes or wells in plastic plates. Tube agglutination tests are commonly used for such diseases as salmonellosis, brucellosis, tularemia, and campylobacteriosis. Slide agglutination tests are commonly used as screening tests. These include the *Brucella*-buffered antigen tests, in which killed, stained *Brucella* organisms are suspended in an acid buffer (pH 3.6). The dye used, either the red xanthene dye, rose-bengal, or a mixture of crystal violet and brilliant green, enables the test to be easily read. At this low pH, nonspecific agglutination by IgM antibodies is eliminated. The *Brucella*-buffered plate agglutination test has a specificity of as high as 99% and a sensitivity of 95%. The efficient and widespread use of these tests has eliminated bovine brucellosis from many countries.

S. enterica Pullorum infection in poultry can be diagnosed by a slide agglutination test, in which killed bacteria stained with gentian violet are mixed with whole chicken blood. Agglutination is readily seen if antibodies are present. Leptospirosis is diagnosed by a microscopic agglutination test, in which mixtures of living organisms and test serum are examined under the microscope for agglutination. This technique preferentially detects IgM antibodies and is thus an excellent test for detecting recent outbreaks as well as for distinguishing between infected and vaccinated animals.

It is not mandatory that serum be used as the source of antibody for diagnostic tests. The presence of antibodies in body fluids other than serum, such as milk whey, vaginal mucus, or nasal washings, may be of great significance, especially if the infection is of a local or superficial nature. One such example is the milk ring test used to detect the presence of antibodies to *B. abortus* in milk (Fig. 27.8). Fresh milk is shaken with bacteria stained with hematoxylin or triphenyl tetrazolium and

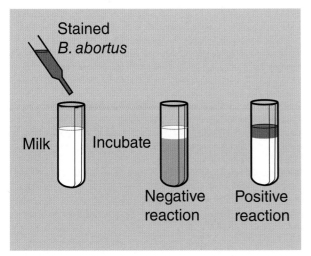

Fig. 27.8 The milk ring test. Stained *Brucella* organisms remain suspended in the milk in a negative test but rise with the cream in a positive reaction.

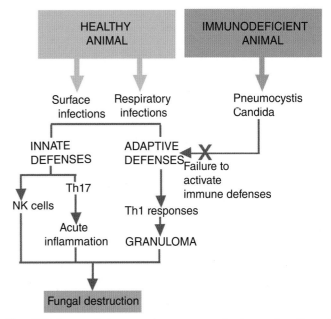

Fig. 27.9 Some of the most important mechanisms of antifungal immunity. *NK*, Natural killer.

allowed to stand. If antibodies, especially IgM or IgA, are present, the bacteria will clump and adhere to the fat globules of the milk and rise to the surface with the cream. If antibodies are absent, the stained bacteria will remain dispersed in the milk, and the cream, on rising, will remain white.

IMMUNITY TO FUNGAL INFECTIONS

Fungal infections are of three major types (Fig. 27.9). The first are primary infections by fungi that invade the skin or other surfaces, such as *Microsporum* or *Candida* species, and cause diseases such as ringworm or thrush. The second type includes primary infections by dimorphic fungi that mainly cause respiratory infections, for example, *Histoplasma capsulatum*, *Blastomyces dermatitidis*, and *Coccidioides immitis*. The third type consists of secondary infections by opportunistic fungi in immunodeficient animals, such as the Mucorales (*Rhizopus*, *Mucor*, and *Absidia*) and *Pneumocystis*. The body uses both innate and adaptive immune mechanisms to defend itself against primary infections. Thus innate immune mechanisms against invasive fungi such as *Candida* or *Aspergillus* species include activation of the alternate complement pathway, resulting in attraction of neutrophils and attempts by these neutrophils to destroy the invading hyphae or pseudohyphae. Neutrophils are also activated by the IL-23/IL-17 axis during fungal infections (Rivera, 2014).

Fungal PAMPs acting either through TLRs or NLRs or through cell-surface C-type lectins such as the dectins, mannose-binding lectins, and scavenger receptors such as DC-SIGN (CD209) (see Chapter 2) play a key role in early innate defenses (Plato et al., 2015). Thus dectin-1 (CD369) binds to fungal β-glucans and triggers IL-22 and IL-23 production. Both contribute to anti-aspergillus resistance. IL-23 activates Th17 cells. The IL-17 produced by these cells then activates both neutrophils and endothelial cells and promotes acute inflammation. Dectin-3 associates with dectin-1 while dectins 2 and 3 form a heterodimeric PRR on macrophages that can recognize the α-mannans in *Candida* hyphae. DC-SIGN binds mannose. It is of interest to note that culturing T cells and monocytes in the presence of *Candida* hyphae promotes the generation of Th17 cells. In contrast, culture in the presence of *Candida* yeast forms promotes production of IL-12 and a Th1 response. Because of their size, neutrophils cannot totally ingest invading fungi. Nevertheless, by releasing enzymes and oxidants into the tissue fluid, neutrophils may severely damage fungal hyphae. Small fungal

fragments or spores may be ingested and destroyed by macrophages or by NK cells.

Once established, fungal infections are mainly destroyed by Th1-mediated mechanisms. For example, some species of *Aspergillus* are facultative intracellular parasites, and chronic or progressive fungal diseases are commonly associated with defects in the T-cell system. Th1 cells function in fungal infections by activating macrophages and by promoting epidermal growth and keratinization. Some T and NK cells can exert a direct cytotoxic effect on yeasts such as *Cryptococcus neoformans* and *Candida albicans*. It is not uncommon for recovered animals to develop a type IV hypersensitivity to fungal antigens. The critical importance of adaptive immunity to fungi is seen in the way that fungal infections, such as the pneumonia caused by *Pneumocystis*, develop in immunosuppressed animals such as dogs with canine distemper. Although defense against *Pneumocystis canis* is critically dependent upon CD4+ T-cell function, it is also dependent on Th17 cells. Depletion of IL-17 or IL-23 increases the severity of *Pneumocystis pneumonia* (Danesi et al., 2022).

REFERENCES

Aktan, I., Dunkel, B., Cunningham, F.M., 2013. Equine platelets inhibit *E. coli* growth and can be activated by bacterial lipopolysaccharide and lipoteichoic acid although superoxide anion production does not occur, and platelet activation is not associated with enhanced production by neutrophils. Vet. Immunol. Immunopathol. 152, 209–217.

Andersen-Nissen, E., Smith, K.D., Strobe, K.L., et al., 2005. Evasion of toll-like receptor 5 by flagellated bacteria. Proc. Natl. Acad. Sci. U.S.A. 102, 9247–9252.

Arsenault, R.J., Li, Y., Bell, K., Doig, K., et al., 2012. *Mycobacterium avium* subsp. *paratuberculosis* Inhibits gamma interferon-induced signaling in bovine monocytes: insights into the cellular mechanisms of Johne's disease. Infect. Immun. 80, 3039–3048.

Baxt, L.A., Garza-Mayers, A.C., Goldberg, M.B., 2013. Bacterial subversion of host innate immune pathways. Science 340, 697–701.

Benoit, M., Desnues, B., Mege, J.L., 2008. Macrophage polarization in bacterial infections. J. Immunol. 181, 3733–3739.

Cambier, C.J., Falkow, S., Ramakrishnan, L., 2014a. Host evasion and exploitation schemes of *Mycobacterium tuberculosis*. Cell 159, 1497–1509.

Cerca, N., Jefferson, K.K., Oliviera, R., et al., 2006. Comparative antibody-mediated phagocytosis of *Staphylococcus epidermidis* cells grown in a biofilm or in the planktonic state. Infect. Immun. 74, 4849–4855.

Collins, H.L., 2008. Withholding iron as a cellular defense mechanism: friend or foe? Eur. J. Immunol. 38, 1803–1806.

Curis, M.M., Way, S.S., 2009. Interleukin-17 in host defense against bacterial, mycobacterial and fungal pathogens,. Immunology 126, 177–185.

Danesi, P., Petini, M., Falcaro, C., Bertola, M., et al., 2022. *Pneumocystis* colonization in dogs is as in humans. Int. J. Environ. Res. Public Health. https://doi.org/10.3390/ijerph19063192

Domenech, M., Ramos-Sevillano, E., Garcia, E., Moscoso, M., Yuste, J., 2013. Biofilm formation avoids complement immunity and phagocytosis of *Streptococcus pneumonia*. Infect. Immun. 81, 2606–2615.

Farris, L.C., Torres-Odio, S., Adams, L.G., West, A.P., et al., 2023. *Borrelia burgdorferi* engages mammalian type I IFN responses via the cGAS-STING pathway. J. Immunol. 210 (11), 1761–1770.

Garcia, B.L., Zwarthoff, S.A., Rooijakkers, S.H., Geisbrecht, B.V., 2016. Novel evasion mechanisms of the classical complement pathway. J. Immunol. 2016 (197), 2051–2060.

Goenka, R., Parent, M.A., Elzer, P.H., Baldwin, C.L., 2011. B-cell deficient mice display markedly enhanced resistance to the intracellular bacterium *Brucella abortus*. J. Infect. Dis. 203 (8), 1136–1146.

Gossner, A., Watkins, C., Chianini, F., Hopkins, J., 2017. Pathways and genes associated with immune dysfunction in sheep paratuberculosis. Sci. Rep. https://doi.org/10.1038/srep46695

Harris, J., Master, S.S., DeHaro, S.A., et al., 2009. Th1-Th2 polarization and autophagy in the control of intracellular Mycobacteria by macrophages. Vet. Immunol. Immunopathol. 128, 37–43.

Kaufmann, S.H., Dorhoi, A., 2016. Molecular determinants in phagocyte-bacteria interactions. Immunity 44, 476–491.

Mancuso, G., Midiri, A., Biondo, C., et al., 2007. Type I IFN signaling is crucial for host resistance against different species of pathogenic bacteria. J. Immunol. 178, 3126–3133.

Narayanan, S.K., Nagaraja, T.G., Chengappa, M.M., Stewart, G.C., 2002. Leukotoxins of gram-negative bacteria. Vet. Microbiol. 84, 337–356.

Pieters, J., Gatfield, J., 2002. Hijacking the host: survival of pathogenic mycobacteria inside macrophages. Trends Microbiol. 3, 142–146.

Plato, A., Hardison, S.E., Brown, G.D., 2015. Pattern recognition receptors in antifungal immunity. Semin. Immunopathol. 37, 97–106.

Reddick, L.E., Alto, N.M., 2014. Bacteria fighting back: how pathogens target and subvert the host innate immune system. Mol. Cell 54, 321–328.

Rhodes, S.G., Sawyer, J., Whelan, A.O., Dean, G.S., et al., 2007. Is interleukin-4δ3 splice variant expression in bovine tuberculosis a marker of protective immunity? Infect. Immun. 76 (5), 3006–3013.

Rivera, A., 2014. Protective immune responses to fungal infections. Parasite Immunol. 36, 453–462.

Sansonetti, P.J., Di Santo, J.P., 2007. Debugging how bacteria manipulate the immune response. Immunity 26, 149–161.

Shu, D., Heiser, A., Wedlock, D.N., Luo, D., de Lisle, G.W., Buddle, B.M., 2014. Comparison of gene expression of immune mediators in lung and pulmonary lymph node granulomas from cattle experimentally infected with *Mycobacterium bovis*.. Vet. Immunol. Immunopathol. 160, 81–89.

Smeed, J.A., Watkins, C.A., Gossner, A.G., Hopkins, J., 2010. Expression profiling reveals differences in immuno-inflammatory gene expression between the two disease forms of sheep paratuberculosis,. Vet. Immunol. Immunopathol. 135, 218–225.

Starr, T., Child, R., Wehrly, T.D., Hansen, B., et al., 2012. Selective subversion of autophagy complexes facilitates completion of the Brucella intracellular cycle. Cell Host Microbe 11, 33–45.

Thacker, T.C., Palmer, M.V., Waters, W.R., 2007. Associations between cytokine gene expression and pathology in *Mycobacterium bovis* infected cattle. Vet. Immunol. Immunopathol, 119, 204–213.

Thammavongsa, V., Missiakas, D.M., Schneewind, O., 2013. *Staphylococcus aureus* degrades neutrophil extracellular traps to promote immune cell death. Science 342, 863–865.

Vail, K.J., da Silveira, B.P., Bell, S.L., Cohen, N.D., et al., 2021. The opportunistic intracellular pathogen *Rhodococcus equi* elicits type 1 interferon by engaging cytosolic DNA sensing in macrophages. Plos Pathogens. https://doi.org/10.13471/journal.ppat.1009888

Weiss, D.J., Evanson, O.A., Souza, C.D., 2005. Expression of interleukin-10 and suppressor of cytokine signaling-3 associated with susceptibility of cattle to infection with *Mycobacterium avium* subsp paratuberculosis. J. Am. Vet. Med. Assoc. 66, 1114–1120.

Weiss, D.J., Souza, C.D., 2008. Review paper: modulation of mononuclear phagocyte function by *Mycobacterium avium* subsp. *paratuberculosis*,. Vet. Pathol. 45, 829–841.

28

Immunity to Viruses

Since viruses are obligate intracellular organisms, their very existence is threatened if they are destroyed by the immune system or by the death of their host. Because of this, both viruses and their hosts have been subjected to rigorous selection and adaptation. Viruses are selected for their ability to evade the host's immune responses, while at the same time, animals are selected for resistance to virus-induced disease. Viruses that are eliminated before they replicate cannot spread. Hosts eliminated by viruses can no longer serve as hosts. An "oversuccessful" virus will reduce the availability of susceptible hosts, whereas a very successful host will be the largest target for the next generation of viruses. As a result, there can never be a "solution" to the problem of viruses.

For example, in infections where virus-host adaptation is poor, diseases tend to be lethal. Rabies is an excellent example of this. The virus is inevitably lethal in dogs, cats, horses, and cattle because they are unnatural hosts. On the other hand, in its natural hosts, especially bats and skunks, rabies virus persists and may be shed in saliva for a long period without causing disease. From the virus's "point of view," infection of dogs, cattle, or horses is unprofitable since those animals almost never transmit rabies to skunks. Other diseases of this type include feline panleukopenia, canine parvovirus–2, and the virulent forms of Newcastle disease. Vaccination is relatively successful in this type of infection since the virus has not adapted to the host's defenses.

When the virus and its host are more adapted, although disease may be severe, mortality may not be high, and the virus may be persistent. In this type of disease, further attacks may occur as a result of infection by variants of the same virus. Examples of this type of virus infection include foot-and-mouth disease, coronaviruses, and influenza. Vaccination against diseases of this type is complicated by the diversity of these viruses.

Even more adapted viruses can result in persistent infection because the immune system is unable to eliminate these viruses completely.

Diseases of this type include the lentivirus infections, equine infectious anemia, and maedi-visna in sheep. Vaccination against these diseases is essentially unsuccessful. As their adaptation increases, viruses may cause latent infections and relatively mild, nonlethal disease. Some herpesvirus infections also fall into this category. The most extreme examples of virus adaptation are those in which the viral nucleic acid becomes stably integrated into the host genome. These endogenous viruses are common in the genomes of both domestic and wild mammals.

In studying the nature of the host responses to viruses, it is important to recognize that this continuing selective pressure on both host and virus exists and profoundly influences the outcome of all viral infections.

VIRUS STRUCTURE AND ANTIGENS

Virus particles, called virions, consist of a nucleic acid core surrounded by a layer of proteins (see Figs. 10.2 and 41.2). This protein layer, called the capsid, is made up of subcomponents called capsomeres. The virions may also be covered by a lipid envelope. The complexity of viruses varies. Some, such as poxviruses, are very complex, whereas others, such as foot-and-mouth disease virus (FMDV), are relatively simple. Antibodies can be produced against epitopes on all the proteins situated inside and on the surface of the virion. Antibodies against the nucleoprotein components are not usually protective, but they may be useful for serologic diagnosis.

PATHOGENESIS OF VIRUS INFECTIONS

Adsorption, the first step in the invasion of a cell by a virus, occurs when a virus binds to cell-surface receptors. These receptors are not there for the convenience of viruses but have some other physiological function.

Thus, rabies virus binds to the receptor for acetylcholine, a neurotransmitter. The Epstein-Barr virus (the cause of infectious mononucleosis) binds to a receptor for C3. Rhinoviruses that cause the common cold bind to cell-surface integrins. The chemokine receptor CCR5 is also the receptor used by the West Nile virus. The nature, number, and distribution of cell receptors determine the host range and tissue tropism of a virus. Once bound, the virion is taken into the cell through endocytosis or by fusion with the plasma membrane. Once inside a cell, the capsid is dismantled so that its nucleic acid is released into the cell cytoplasm, a process called uncoating. Once the virus genome is uncoated, replication begins (Fig. 28.1). Host cell DNA transcription is usually inhibited so that only viral genetic information is processed. If the virus, for example, a herpesvirus, contains DNA, this viral DNA is replicated. The new viral DNA is then transcribed into viral messenger RNA (mRNA), and this mRNA is translated into new capsid proteins. These new proteins are then assembled into virions. The host cell also replicates the viral nucleic acid so that large quantities of viral DNA are produced. The viral DNA is packaged inside the new capsids so that complete virions are formed. If the virus is unenveloped, the infected cells rupture, and the virions are released into the environment. If the virions are enveloped, they leave the cell by budding through the cell surface. The cell membrane that encloses them serves as the new envelope. The released virions may then spread to nearby cells and invade them in turn.

If a virus contains RNA rather than DNA, its replication takes a slightly different course. For most RNA viruses, such as Newcastle disease or FMDV, viral DNA is not used. Thus, in FMDV infection, the viral single-stranded RNA (the "plus strand") is used as a template to synthesize a complementary "minus strand" of RNA. These minus strands are then used to generate new plus strands that can be translated into viral proteins. Some viruses contain double-stranded RNA (dsRNA) and use only one of the strands generated during replication. In other RNA viruses, the infecting virus RNA may be complementary to the newly synthesized viral RNA that will translate into viral proteins.

A different replication mechanism is employed in the case of some RNA tumor viruses and immunodeficiency viruses (Fig. 28.2). These are called retroviruses since their RNA is first reversely transcribed into DNA by a reverse transcriptase. The new viral DNA is then integrated into the host cell genome as a provirus. This proviral DNA can then be transcribed into RNA, as well as being able to copy itself. The proteins and RNA can then be packaged into new virions.

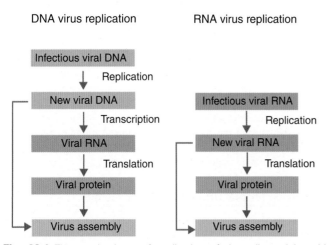

Fig. 28.1 The mechanisms of replication of deoxyribonucleic acid (DNA) and ribonucleic acid (RNA) viruses.

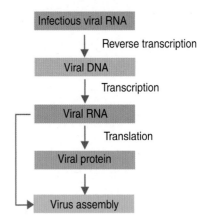

Fig. 28.2 The mechanism of replication of the retroviruses. *DNA,* Deoxyribonucleic acid; *RNA,* ribonucleic acid.

Changes in virus-infected cells may be minimal, perhaps only detectable by the expression of new proteins on the cell surface. Sometimes, however, the changes may be extensive and result in either cell death or malignant transformation.

INNATE IMMUNITY

Rapid, powerful innate immune responses limit many viral infections. Interferons are especially important in this process. Lysozyme can destroy several viruses, as can many intestinal enzymes and bile. C-type lectins bind to viral glycoproteins and block virus interaction with host cells. For example, conglutinin, MBL, SP-A, and SP-D can all inactivate influenza viruses. Defensins from leukocytes and mucosal epithelial cells play a dual role in antiviral defenses since they can act both on the virus and on the host cell. Thus, defensins can inactivate enveloped virions by disrupting their envelopes or by interacting with their glycoproteins. Some defensins can block intracellular signaling pathways in infected cells and interfere with transcription of viral RNA. Finally, cells invaded by viruses may undergo premature apoptosis, preventing successful viral invasion and replication (Klotman and Chang, 2006).

Pattern-Recognition Receptors: Nucleic Acid Sensors

Viruses, unlike bacteria and fungi, do not contain easily recognizable microbe-specific structures since they are constructed from host-derived components. For this reason, animal cells have evolved the ability to recognize the only virus-specific components, their nucleic acids (Ranjan et al., 2009). Three pattern-recognition receptor systems recognize viral nucleic acids. One system consists of nucleic acid receptors found within the cytosol of all nucleated cells. These PRRs are called RIG-1 and melanoma differentiation-associated protein 5. Both proteins detect viral dsRNA and then signal through several adaptor proteins to activate the interferon-β (IFN-β) gene. The second system is mediated by toll-like receptors. TLR3 recognizes dsRNA. TLR7 and TLR8 recognize single-stranded RNA viruses such as vesicular stomatitis and influenza viruses (Lund et al., 2005). TLR9 detects unmethylated CpG motifs in DNA. These motifs are common in both DNA viruses and bacteria. Mice deficient in either TLR7 or TLR9 or their adaptor protein, MyD88, have a reduced ability to defend themselves against viruses. Plasmacytoid dendritic cells (pDCs) use a specialized signaling pathway that links TLR7 and TLR9 to the production of very large amounts of type I interferons. The third PRR system uses receptors with nucleotide-binding oligomerization–like (NOD) domains.

Interferons

Interferons protect cells against viral, bacterial, and protozoan invasion. They are glycoproteins of 20–34 kDa classified into three types: I, II, and III.

Type I interferons include multiple forms of IFN-α and IFN-β as well as multiple single gene products such as IFN-ω, -δ, -ε, -ν, τ-, -κ, and -ζ. There are 18 isoforms of IFN-α in humans, 12 in pigs, 13 in cattle, 4 in horses, and 2 in dogs. IFN-α is produced in large quantities by pDCs and in much smaller amounts by lymphocytes, monocytes, and macrophages. IFN-β can be produced by almost any virus-infected cell. (There are 5 isoforms in cattle and pigs and 1 in dogs and humans.) IFN-ω is produced by lymphocytes, monocytes, and human, horse, pig, rabbit, and dog trophoblast cells (8 functional genes in pigs, 1 in humans, 2 in horses, 24 in cattle, 13 in cats, and none in dogs or mice). IFN-δ is found in the placental tissues of pigs, sheep, and horses (2 in horses). IFN-δ is only distantly related to the other type I interferons. IFN-κ is produced by keratinocytes. Bovine IFN-κ has been characterized and acts through JAK/STAT pathways in a manner similar to the other type I interferons. IFN-ζ is found in mice, where it is also called limitin. IFN-ε is a member of the type I family whose expression is limited to reproductive and brain tissues. It plays a role in protecting the female reproductive tract, where it is expressed constitutively. It has been detected in humans, dogs, cattle, sheep, and pigs. In most cases, these molecules act on virus-infected cells to inhibit viral growth. The trophoblast interferons also regulate the maternal immune response to the fetus (see Fig. 35.8; Guo et al., 2017).

Interferon τ is a type 1 interferon encoded by the *IFNT* gene loci and has only been detected in ruminants. It is secreted by trophoblast and endometrial cells during days 10–24 of pregnancy in the sheep. It plays a key role as a signal for the maternal recognition of pregnancy by maintaining progesterone production in the corpus luteum at that time and thus preventing a return to ovarian cyclicity. IFN-τ has many effects on the endometrium ensuring that the uterus is receptive to the fetus and has antiinflammatory effects that aid in preventing maternal rejection of her semiallogeneic fetus. It acts on cultured trophoblast cells to regulate their production of IL-6 and IL-8. Multiple IFN-τ polymorphisms and variants exist. Although not detected in humans and mice, they do respond to its effects. IFN-τ binds to the same receptor as IFN-α (IFNAR) and induces intracellular signaling through the JAK/STAT pathway. As a result, it promotes the production of the typical interferon-stimulated genes (ISGFs) that encode antiviral proteins as well as the regulatory cytokines IL-4, IL-6, and IL-10. Despite this, it is not, however, virally inducible.

Interferon-chi is encoded by a newly identified multigene family (*IFNX*) of four IFN-χ members, one of which appears to be a pseudogene. It is restricted to cattle (Guo et al., 2020). Two of the subtypes are functional genes whose products have antiviral and antiproliferative activities. They bind to type I IFN receptors, induce production of IRF7, and signal through the JAK-STAT pathway. They also appear to be involved in positive feedback of interferon production.

There is only a single type II interferon, IFN-γ, produced by antigen-stimulated Th1 cells. It is also produced in the pig trophoblast.

Four type III interferons have been identified: IFN-λ1,–2, and -3 (also known as interleukin-29 [IL-29], IL-28A, and IL-28B) and IFN-λ4. These are mainly produced by epithelial cells located on mucosal surfaces (pigs lack IFN-λ2) (Sang et al., 2010). They signal through a unique receptor complex consisting of IL-10Rβ and IL-28Rα. While structurally unrelated to type I interferons, they share signaling pathways and induce a similar gene response profile (Ichihashi et al., 2013). Their effects are most apparent at intestinal and respiratory epithelia and at the blood-brain barrier. They thus serve as a first line of defense against viral invasion (Lazear et al., 2019).

Antiviral Activities

The two major type I interferons (IFN-α and IFN-β) are produced within a few hours of viral invasion, and high concentrations are achieved long before adaptive immunity develops. For example, in cattle infected with bovine herpesvirus-1 (BHV-1), peak interferon levels in serum are reached 2 days later and then decline, but they are still detectable by 7 days (Fig. 28.3). In contrast, antibodies are not usually detectable in serum until 5–6 days after the onset of a virus infection (Stetson and Medzhitov, 2006).

IFN-α and IFN-β are produced when viral nucleic acids bind TLRs-7 and -9 or RIG-1. Both bind to heterodimeric receptors (IFNAR) on nearby cells and activate JAK/STAT signaling pathways (see Figs. 9.8 and 28.4). These pathways turn on at least 300 genes, many of which

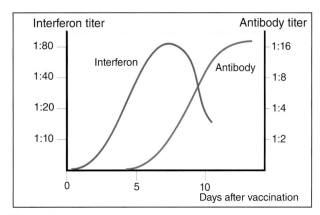

Fig. 28.3 The sequential production of interferon and antibody following intranasal vaccination of calves with infectious bovine herpesvirus vaccine (BHV-1). From data kindly provided by Dr. M. Savan.

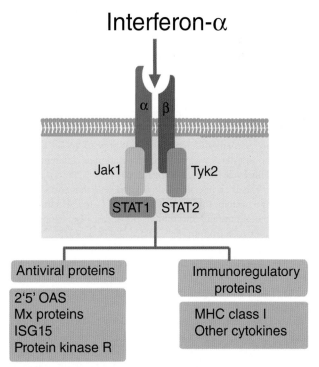

Fig. 28.4 The receptor for the type I interferons. Ligand binding triggers the JAK-STAT (Janus kinase-signal transducers and activators of transcription) transduction pathway and eventually activates both antiviral and immunoregulatory pathways. *ISG,* Interferon-stimulated gene; *MHC,* major histocompatibility complex.

encode antiviral proteins. The result is the development of an "antiviral state" within a few minutes that peaks by 5–8 hours.

IFN-stimulated genes act through many different pathways and have diverse effects on viruses. Some broadly inhibit viral growth, while others target specific viruses. They may target different stages of viral replication, such as viral entry, envelope uncoating, genome replication, protein assembly or viral release. The existence of diverse IFN-α isoforms, even though they signal through a common receptor, suggests that they have different functional roles. Interferons also target cells to promote viral clearance or induce apoptosis. These include increased neutrophil survival, activation of macrophages, and regulation of NK cells, DCs, B cells, CD8+T cells, and Th1 cells. They are, in effect, broad-spectrum antivirals.

Here are six of the most important pathways.

- *The 2′5′ A pathway:* Type I interferons upregulate transcription of the genes coding for 2′5′-oligoadenylate synthetases (2′5′-OAS). These enzymes are then activated by exposure to long dsRNA from viruses in the cytoplasm. They act on adenosine triphosphate to form 2′5′ adenylate oligomers. These oligomers bind and activate a ribonuclease called RNAase L (Fig. 28.5). RNAase L degrades viral RNA and so inhibits viral growth.
- *The Mx guanosine triphosphatase (GTPase) pathway:* Mx proteins are large interferon-induced GTPases that accumulate as oligomers on intracellular membranes. Following viral infection, Mx monomers are released. These bind and trap viral nucleocapsids and other essential viral components, thereby blocking the assembly of new viruses. Mx proteins are expressed in many different cell types, such as hepatocytes, endothelial cells, and immune cells. They inhibit a wide range of RNA viruses, including the influenza viruses (Verhelst et al., 2013).
- *The protein kinase R (PKR) pathway:* PKR is induced by type I interferons. The inactive kinase accumulates in the cell nucleus and cytoplasm, where it is activated by viral RNA. Activated PKR regulates several cell signaling pathways and phosphorylates an initiation factor called eIF2α, which then prevents translation initiation by viral mRNA.
- *The ISG15 pathway:* ISG15 codes for a ubiquitin-like protein that binds to many different proteins and enhances their destruction. It is not known how this results in increased antiviral resistance and reduced viral replication.
- *The viperin pathway:* Viperin is a protein that has direct antiviral activity. It is induced by all three classes of interferon, dsRNA and RNA and by many different viruses. It appears to act on cellular lipids and interferes with lipid raft formation at different stages in the viral life cycle (Helbig and Beard, 2014).
- *Tetherin.* This is an interferon-stimulated gene that encodes a small membrane protein. It physically crosslinks (tethers!) virions to the plasma membrane and thus inhibits the release of enveloped viruses such as influenza from the cell surface (Xu et al., 2023).

The ability of cells to produce interferons varies. Virus-infected leukocytes, especially pDCs directly interact with virus-infected cells to produce large amounts of IFN-α; almost any virus-infected cell can produce IFN-β; and antigen-stimulated T cells are the major source of IFN-γ (see Chapter 19; Assil et al., 2019).

Natural killer (NK) cells can kill virus-infected cells (see Chapter 20). NK cell cytotoxicity is stimulated by type I interferons and, as a result, is important early in a virus infection. Indeed, NK cells provide the first line of defense against many viruses. NK cells also produce large amounts of IFN-γ and perforins, and these too have direct antiviral effects. NK cells may therefore reduce the severity of viral infections long before the development of adaptive immunity and the appearance of specific cytotoxic T cells (Scalzo, 2002).

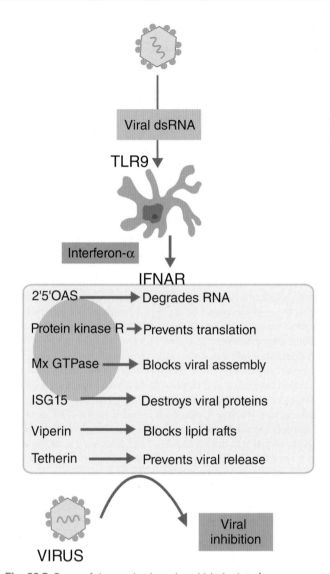

Fig. 28.5 Some of the mechanisms by which the interferons can exert their antiviral activities. *ISG,* Interferon-stimulated gen; *IFNAR,* IFN-τ binds to the same receptor; *Mx GTPase,* Mx guanosine triphosphatase pathway; *RNA,* ribonucleic acid; *TLR,* toll-like receptors.

IFN-α not only activates NK cells but most other immune cell populations as well. Thus, it stimulates the differentiation of monocytes into dendritic cells, as well as the maturation and activity of dendritic cells. IFN-α stimulates memory T-cell proliferation, activates naïve T cells in chronic viral diseases, and enhances antigen-specific T-cell priming. It promotes B-cell functions such as IgG production and MHC expression.

RNA Interference

RNA interference (RNAi) is an innate antiviral pathway that is important in plants and many invertebrates. It has recently been recognized in mammals (Sagan and Sarnow, 2013). Viral dsRNA is broken up by an intracellular nuclease called DICER into small interfering RNAs (siRNAs). These siRNAs are loaded into an RNA-induced silencing complex that then binds to the viral RNA and destroys it, thus preventing viral growth. These siRNAs have been detected in a mouse germ cell line. Conversely, they are absent from somatic cells from adult mice. Embryonic cell lines cannot produce type 1 interferons, but adult somatic cells can. It has been suggested, therefore, that germ cell lines rely on RNAi, but as they develop, they lose this pathway and replace it with the interferon response (Maillard et al., 2013). Small interfering RNAs appear to play an important role in the pathogenesis of feline coronavirus infections (Anis et al., 2014).

ADAPTIVE IMMUNITY

Antibody-Mediated Immunity

Virus proteins are antigenic, and it is against these proteins that antiviral antibody responses are largely mounted (Fig. 28.6). Antibodies can prevent cell invasion by blocking the adsorption of virions to target cells, by stimulating virus phagocytosis, by triggering complement-mediated virolysis, or by causing viral clumping and thus reducing the number of infectious units available for cell invasion. Binding of antibodies alone does not destroy viruses since splitting of virus-antibody complexes releases infectious virions.

Antibodies are not only directed against virion proteins but are also against viral proteins expressed by infected cells. As a result, these infected cells may also be destroyed. Antibody-mediated destruction of virus-infected cells occurs in Newcastle disease, rabies, bovine virus diarrhea, infectious bronchitis of birds, and feline leukemia. Antibodies may kill infected cells using complement or antibody-dependent cell–mediated cytotoxicity (ADCC). The cytotoxic cells include lymphocytes, macrophages, and neutrophils using their Fc receptors to bind to antibody-coated target cells.

Virus-neutralizing antibodies include IgG and IgM in serum and IgA in secretions. As in antibacterial immunity, IgG is quantitatively the most significant immunoglobulin, whereas IgM is qualitatively superior.

Although most viruses infect cells by binding directly to target cell receptors, some use an intermediate molecule. For instance, some antibody-coated viruses bind to cells through Fc receptors. This triggers viral endocytosis and enhances virus infection. Complement may enhance virus infections in a similar fashion. Examples of virus infections that are enhanced by antibodies include feline infectious peritonitis, Aleutian disease of mink, African swine fever, and human immunodeficiency virus.

Cell-Mediated Immunity

Although antibodies and complement can neutralize free virions and destroy virus-infected cells, cell-mediated immune responses are much more important in controlling virus diseases. This is readily seen in immunodeficient humans (see Chapter 41). Those who cannot mount an antibody-mediated response suffer from overwhelming bacterial infections but tend to recover from the common viral diseases. In contrast, humans with T-cell deficiencies are commonly resistant to bacterial infection but highly susceptible to virus diseases.

Viral antigens may be expressed on infected cells long before progeny viruses are produced. When this endogenous antigen is presented by MHC class I molecules to CD8+ T cells, the infected cells are recognized as foreign and killed. Viruses require host cells in which to replicate. Elimination of infected cells prevents viral spread. Although antibodies and complement or ADCC can assist, T cell–mediated cytotoxicity is the major protective mechanism. Cytotoxic T cells recognize peptide-MHC complexes and kill the presenting cells. Type I interferons can sensitize virus-infected cells to this cytotoxic effect. Under some circumstances, cytotoxic T cells may kill intracellular viruses without killing the infected cells. This effect is mediated by T cell–derived IFN-γ and TNF-α. These cytokines activate two virucidal pathways. One pathway eliminates viral nucleocapsid particles, including their contained genomes. The second pathway destabilizes viral RNA.

Some viral antigens may act as superantigens by binding directly to TCR Vβ chains. For example, rabies virus nucleocapsid binds to mouse Vβ8 T cells. By stimulating helper T-cell activity, rabies viruses can switch on Th2 cells. This in turn can result in an enhanced immune response to rabies viruses, as well as a polyclonal B-cell response.

Macrophages develop antiviral activity following activation. Viruses are readily endocytosed by macrophages and are then usually destroyed. If the viruses are noncytopathic and can grow inside macrophages, a persistent infection may result. Under these circumstances, the macrophages must be activated to eliminate the virus. Thus, macrophage activation mediated by IFN-γ is a feature of some virus diseases (see Chapter 19). For example, macrophages from birds immunized against fowlpox show an enhanced antiviral effect against Newcastle disease virus and will prevent the intracellular growth of *Salmonella gallinarum*, a feature that is not a property of normal macrophages.

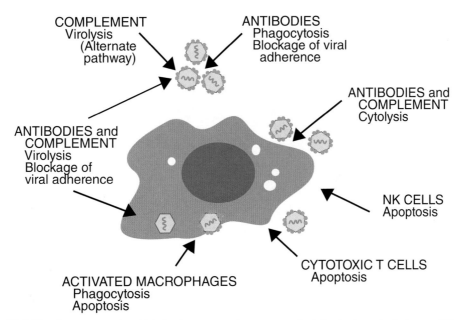

Fig. 28.6 The diverse ways in which the immune systems can protect the body against viruses. *NK cells,* Natural killer cells.

The duration of immunological memory to viruses is highly variable. Antiviral antibodies may persist for many years in the absence of the virus. On the other hand, cytotoxic T cells die soon after virus elimination, while memory T cells can persist for many years (Chapter 15).

EVASION OF THE IMMUNE RESPONSE

As discussed above, during the millions of years they have coexisted with animals, viruses have evolved numerous methods of evading host immune responses (Fig. 28.7;Alcami and Koszinowski, 2000). RNA viruses have a very small genome with little room to spare for genes dedicated to suppressing immunity. As a result, RNA viruses tend to rely on antigenic variation as their principal mechanism of immune evasion. On the other hand, DNA viruses have a larger genome and can afford to devote many different genes to immune evasion. In large DNA viruses such as the poxviruses and herpesviruses, as much as half the total genome may be devoted to immunoregulatory genes (Haig, 2001).

Negative Cytokine Regulation

Viruses can block interferon activity. Methods range from blocking interferon receptor signal transduction to synthesizing soluble interferon receptors. Some viruses inhibit IFN-γ production by blocking the activities of IL-18 and IL-12, both of which are required for its production. Myxoma and poxviruses produce a protein related to the IFN-γR. By binding free IFN-γ, this prevents its binding to cell receptors. Equine herpesvirus-1 suppresses IFN-β production, and as a result, expression of viperin was also suppressed. Interestingly, however, it does not suppress IFN-α production.

Some viruses make their own versions of cytokines and chemokines and their receptors. These have been called virokines or immunoevasins. For example, equine herpesvirus makes CCR3, the receptor for CCL11. Marek's disease virus makes a protein related to CXCL8. Poxviruses make a version of the immunosuppressive cytokine IL-10. Cowpox virus also makes an IL-1β-binding protein that reduces its availability (Iannello et al., 2006). African swine fever virus can interact with the intracellular innate adaptor molecule STING to block interferon production (Zhu et al., 2023).

Interference with Antigen Processing

Many viruses interfere with the expression of MHC class I molecules and so inhibit antigen presentation (Rigden et al., 2002). They use many different suppressive techniques, including reducing transcription of MHC genes; blocking TAP function and the transport of peptides into the endoplasmic reticulum; inhibiting proteasomal degradation of viral proteins; inhibiting the intracellular transport of MHC class I α chains; preventing delivery of the loaded MHC to the cell surface; and ubiquinating and hence destroying MHC molecules. Thus bovine herpesvirus suppresses the expression of MHC class I molecules by interfering with transporter protein functions and downregulating the expression of mRNA for MHC class I molecules. Other viruses may cause MHC class I molecules to be retained within a cell; they may prevent peptide binding to transporter proteins, prevent proteasomal degradation, redirect MHC molecules to lysosomes for degradation, or even encode inhibitors that block caspase activity. Influenza A viruses can stimulate the production of glucocorticosteroids resulting in profound immunosuppression and secondary infections (Jamieson et al., 2010). They can also block macrophage differentiation into dendritic cells. Other viruses may downregulate the expression of costimulating molecules such as ICAM-1, B7-2, CD4, and CD28.

Evasion of Natural Killer Cells

NK cells kill virus-infected cells at an early stage of infection before T and B cells are fully activated. Cytotoxic T cells kill targets that express foreign antigens on MHC class I molecules. NK cells kill targets that fail to express these MHC class I molecules. For a virus to survive, it must induce the selective down-regulation of some MHC class I molecules, enabling the virus-infected cells to evade destruction by T cells while at the same time preventing NK cell activation (Lanier, 2008). Some viruses may decrease the expression of the stress-related protein MIC-B and so inhibit NK cell–mediated cytotoxicity (Shekhar and Yang, 2015).

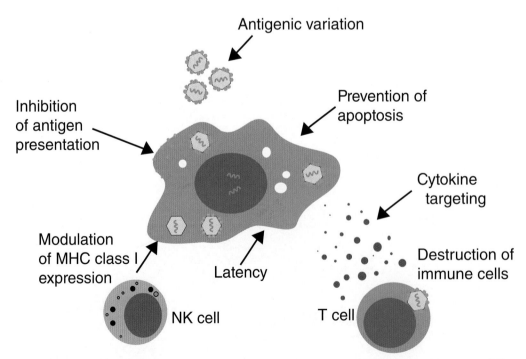

Fig. 28.7 Some of the ways by which viruses evade immune destruction. *MHC,* Major histocompatibility complex; *NK cell,* Natural killer cell.

Alterations in the B Cell System

One of the simplest mechanisms of viral immune evasion involves antigenic variation of RNA viruses. Multiple point mutations accompanied by poor editing functions of RNA polymerases permit the generation of many closely related but distinct viruses. The most significant examples of this occur among the influenza A viruses, the coronaviruses, and the lentiviruses.

Influenza A viruses express envelope proteins called hemagglutinins and neuraminidases. There are at least 18 different hemagglutinins and 9 neuraminidases found among the type A influenza viruses; they are identified according to a standard nomenclature system. The hemagglutinin of the swine influenza virus is called H1, and its neuraminidase is called N1. The two subtypes of the equine influenza viruses are typified by A/equine/Prague/56, which has H7 and N7, and A/equine/Hong Kong/92, which has H3 and N8. H3N8 and H3N2 strains are circulating in dogs in the United States (Table 28.1).

Since 2021, a highly pathogenic bird flu strain, H5N1, originating from A/goose/Guangdong/1/1996, has been circulating in wild birds, especially waterfowl, and has spilt over to poultry in Europe and North America. It has sporadically infected carnivorous mammals, such as foxes, that feed on infected birds. More importantly, it has infected dairy cattle in Texas and spread to other states. It colonizes the udder and can be detected in milk. Fortunately, it is readily destroyed by pasteurization. While it has infected some dairy workers, this clade cannot yet bind to the types of sialic acid receptors that are found in the upper respiratory tract of most humans. As a result, these human cases have been relatively mild.

As influenza viruses spread through a population, they undergo mutation and gradually change the structure of their hemagglutinins and neuraminidases. These changes alter the antigenicity of the virus. This gradual change is called antigenic drift, and it permits the virus to persist in a population for many years. In addition, influenza viruses sporadically undergo a sudden, major genetic change in which a new strain develops whose hemagglutinins show no apparent relationship to the hemagglutinins of prior strains. Such a major change, called an antigenic shift, is not due to mutation but results from recombination between two virus strains. This occurs readily since the influenza virus has a segmented genome. It is the development of these naturally recombinant influenza viruses with a completely new antigenic structure that accounts for the periodic pandemics of influenza in humans and poultry. In horses and pigs, in contrast, the rapid turnover of the population and the constant production of large numbers of susceptible young animals ensure the persistence of influenza viruses without the necessity for extensive antigenic drift. As a result, the antigenic structure of equine and swine influenza viruses has changed only slowly since they were first described. For example, the H3N8 equine influenza virus strains changed very little between 1963 and 1988. In 1989, they split into two clades. These two clades, one European and one American, differ in the structure of the HAI domain of their hemagglutinin. Viruses of both clades can circulate in horse populations at the same time. Examples of the European clade include A/Italy/99 and A/Richmond/07. The American clade includes A/Ohio/03 and A/South Africa/03. The two clades are sufficiently antigenically different as to require the presence of both in vaccines. Both are distinctly different from the original strain A/Miami/1/63 (Lewis et al., 2011).

A second form of immune evasion by viruses is seen in Caprine arthritis-encephalitis (CAE), Aleutian disease of mink, and African swine fever. Although infected animals respond to these viruses, their antibodies are incapable of virus neutralization. Thus, parvovirus-antibody complexes from Aleutian disease-infected mink are fully infectious. Goats with CAE make large amounts of antienvelope antibodies, but they develop negligible levels of neutralizing antibodies. In this case, goats fail to recognize and respond to the virus-neutralizing epitopes. If rabbits are immunized with CAE virus, they can readily produce virus-neutralizing antibodies; even goats will produce these antibodies if immunized with large amounts of an adjuvanted viral antigen. The antibodies produced in these hyperimmunized goats are very specific and will react only with the immunizing strain of the virus. Notwithstanding the absence of neutralizing antibodies, other antibodies can bind to CAE virions, and the opsonized virions are endocytosed by macrophages. Unfortunately, this virus grows within macrophages, so that opsonizing antibodies merely speed up virus replication, an example of antibody-mediated enhancement. Attempts to vaccinate goats against CAE lead only to more severe disease.

A third mechanism by which viruses can evade destruction by antibodies is seen in yet another lentiviral infection, maedi-visna, in sheep (maedi is a chronic pneumonia; visna is a chronic neurological disease caused by the same virus). In maedi-visna infections, neutralizing antibodies are produced slowly. These neutralizing antibodies are unable to reduce the viral burden in infected sheep, and cyclical relapses do not occur. The antibodies have a low affinity for viral epitopes and take at least 20 minutes to bind to the virus and 30 minutes to neutralize it. In contrast, it takes only 2 minutes for this virus to infect a cell. Thus, the virus can spread between cells much faster than it can be neutralized. The Maedi-visna virus also invades monocytes and macrophages. In most of these cells, the replication of the virus stops after its RNA has been reversely transcribed into proviral DNA. As a result, the cells are persistently infected by the virus without expressing viral antigens. The virus may therefore be disseminated without provoking immunological attack. Maedi-visna is associated with extensive infiltration of the lungs, mammary gland, and central nervous system with T cells and macrophages. This virus does not infect lymphocytes so there is no immunosuppression due to a loss of CD4+ T cells. Immunosuppression reduces the severity of the lesions, whereas immunization against the virus increases their severity. It is suggested that virus-infected macrophages stimulate the T cells to release cytokines. These cytokines delay the maturation of monocytes

TABLE 28.1 Examples of Influenza A Virus Strains and Their Antigenic Structure

Species	Virus Strain	Antigenic Structure
Human	A/New Caledonia/20/99[a]	H1N1
	A/California/7/09 (swine flu)	H1N1
	A/Perth/16/09	H3N2
Canine	A/Canine/Florida/04	H3N8
	A/Canine/Beijing/359/09	H3N2
Equine	A/Equine/Prague/1/56	H7N7
	A/Equine/Miami/1/63	H3N8
	A/Equine/South Africa/4/03	H3N8
	A/Equine/Richmond/1/07	H3N8
Swine	A/Swine/Iowa/15/30	H1N1
Avian	A/Fowl Plague/Dutch/27	H7N7
	A/Duck/England/56	H11N7
	A/Turkey/Ontario/6118/68	H8N4
	A/Chicken/Hong Kong/258/97	H5N1
Bovine	A/Goose/Guangdong/1996	H5N1

[a]The first number is the isolate number; the second is the year of isolation.

and restrict virus replication. They also enhance macrophage MHC class II expression and trigger T-cell proliferation and chronic lymphoid hyperplasia (Zhang et al., 2002).

Alterations in the T-Cell System

Viruses may, of course, use the cells of the immune system as their hosts. Viruses like HIV, feline immunodeficiency virus (FIV), canine distemper (CDV), and feline leukemia virus infect lymphocytes and either kill them or otherwise impair their ability to function normally. Glucocorticoids are profoundly suppressive for T cells and T-cell responses. Influenza virus triggers a generalized stress response leading to a sustained increase in serum glucocorticoid levels and resulting immunosuppression.

Viral Evasion Through Latency

If viruses cause a state of reversible nonproductive infection, this is called latency. It is a consistent feature of the herpesviruses. During latency, viruses express only the absolute minimum number of genes. Because they do not express viral antigens, they are not detected by the immune system and may remain in that state for many years.

In contrast to the short-lived immune response against bacteria, antiviral immunity is, in many cases, very long-lasting. The reasons for this are unclear, but they are often related to virus persistence within cells, perhaps in a slowly replicating or a nonreplicating form as typified by latent herpesviruses. It is usually difficult to isolate viruses from an animal that has recovered from a herpesvirus infection. Sometime later, however, especially when the individual is stressed, the herpesvirus may reappear and may even cause disease. During the latent period, when it is present in the host but cannot be reisolated, the virus nucleic acid persists in host cells, but its transcription is blocked, and no viral proteins are made. The persistent virus may periodically boost the immune response of the infected animal and, in this way, generate long-lasting immunity to superinfection. The immune responses in these cases, although unable to eliminate viruses, may prevent the development of clinical disease and therefore serve a protective role. Immunosuppression or stress may permit disease to occur in persistently infected animals. The association between stress and the development of some viral diseases is well recognized. It is likely that the increased steroid production in stressful situations may be sufficiently immunosuppressive to permit activation of latent viruses or infection by exogenous ones.

Sometimes viruses may interact with bacteria to overcome the immune system. For example, *Mannheimia hemolytica* and BHV-1, acting together, cause severe respiratory disease in cattle. BHV-1 infection increases expression of the β_2-integrin LFA-1 on lung neutrophils. The leukotoxin of *M. hemolytica* binds to this integrin and then kills the neutrophils, permitting growth of the invading bacteria.

Inhibition of Apoptosis

Apoptosis may be considered a protective response since viruses also die when a cell dies. This is especially significant if a cell dies before virions are released. It is therefore to a virus's advantage to delay apoptosis until progeny viruses can be released. Thus, cowpox and some herpesviruses (including equine herpesvirus-2) encode apoptosis inhibitors in their genomes. Viruses may also benefit by killing cells of the immune system. Rapidly dividing lymphocytes are susceptible to death signals. For example, lymphoid cell apoptosis is a feature of canine distemper, a disease characterized by severe immunosuppression.

ADVERSE CONSEQUENCES OF IMMUNITY TO VIRUSES

The immune response to viruses can, on occasion, be a disadvantage. Indeed, there are many virus diseases in which disease results from inappropriate or excessive immune responses. For example, bovine respiratory syncytial virus induces a type 2 response in infected cattle with production of IL-4 and specific IgE antibodies in the lungs. This may result in a type I hypersensitivity reaction since there is a direct correlation between lung IgE levels and the severity of clinical disease in these animals.

The destruction of virus-infected cells by antibody is classified as a type II hypersensitivity reaction (see Chapter 32) and, although normally beneficial, may exacerbate virus diseases. Thus, viruses are removed at the cost of cellular destruction. The severity and significance of this destruction depend on how widespread the infection becomes. In some diseases in which the virus causes little cell destruction, most of the tissue damage may result from immunological attack. A good example of this is seen in postdistemper encephalitis, in which neurons are demyelinated as a result of an antiviral immune response. Macrophages in these brain lesions ingest immune complexes and infected cells leading to the release of oxidants and other toxic products. These toxic products damage nearby cells, especially oligodendroglia, causing demyelination.

Type III (immune-complex) lesions (see Chapter 33) are associated with viral diseases, especially those in which viremia is prolonged. For example, a membranoproliferative glomerulonephritis resulting from the deposition of immune complexes is a common complication of equine infectious anemia, Aleutian disease of mink, feline leukemia, chronic hog cholera, bovine virus diarrhea-mucosal disease, canine adenovirus infections, and feline infectious peritonitis. A generalized vasculitis due to deposition of immune complexes throughout the vascular system is seen in equine infectious anemia, Aleutian disease of mink, malignant catarrhal fever, and possibly, equine viral arteritis.

In dogs infected with canine adenovirus 1 (infectious canine hepatitis), an immune-complex-mediated uveitis and a focal glomerulonephritis both develop. The uveitis, commonly called "blue-eye", is seen both in dogs with natural infections and in those vaccinated with live attenuated adenovirus vaccine (Fig. 28.8). The uveitis results from the formation of virus-antibody complexes in the anterior chamber of the eye and in the cornea with complement activation and consequent neutrophil accumulation. The neutrophils release enzymes and oxidants that damage corneal epithelial cells, leading to edema and opacity. The condition resolves spontaneously in about 90% of affected dogs.

In Borna disease, a lethal viral encephalitis, the noncytopathic virus does not kill neurons. Infected animals do, however, mount a strong Th1 response, which results in neuronal destruction by T cells. The development of clinical bornaviral disease in both birds and mammals can be prevented therefore by treatment with immunosuppressive drugs such as cyclosporine.

Antibody-Dependent Enhancement

There are many examples of virus infections in which the presence of antibodies results in increased susceptibility or severity of infection. Several mechanisms are involved in this, and many are poorly understood. One important mechanism observed in cats with feline coronavirus, or FIV, is antibody-dependent enhancement. This can involve, as described previously, antibody coating of virions so that their entry into cells through Fcγ receptors is facilitated. This FcR-mediated entry may be less effective than other routes in triggering

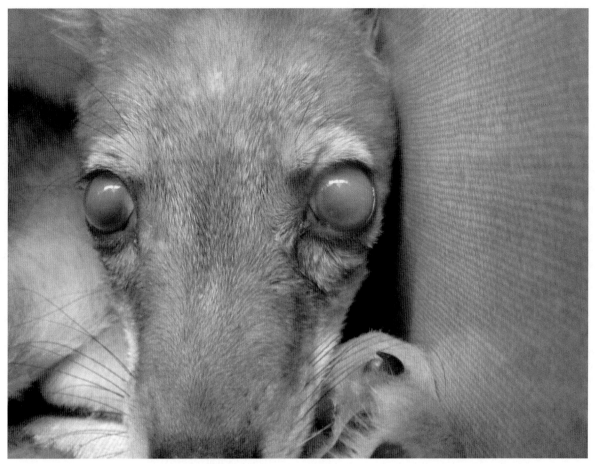

Fig. 28.8 A case of blue-eye in a coyote puppy. This is a type III hypersensitivity reaction to canine adenovirus 1 (ICH) occurring in the cornea. Courtesy Dr. Gregory J. Costanzo.

interferon production. Some experimental FIV, simian immunodeficiency virus, and equine infectious anemia virus (EIAV) vaccines may increase disease susceptibility by a similar mechanism. FIV envelope-specific antibodies appear especially effective in enhancing infection.

SOME SELECTED VIRAL DISEASES

Viruses, if they are to survive, must evade the immune responses. They use many different mechanisms, including, but not limited to, severe immunosuppression. These may result in significant immunopathology.

Feline Infectious Peritonitis

While feline coronaviruses commonly cause mild diarrhea, a mutant strain of feline enteric coronavirus (FECV) is the cause of feline infectious peritonitis (FIP). FIP is a fatal granulomatous disease of wild and domestic cats (Barker and Tasker, 2020). There are two distinct genotypes of FECV, avirulent and virulent. The avirulent genotype prefers to replicate within intestinal epithelial cells, whereas the virulent genotype prefers to replicate within macrophages. Macrophages also spread the virus throughout the body. FIP tends to infect relatively young cats between 6 months and 3 years of age (Pedersen et al., 2014). The disease presents in two major forms: (1) an effusive ("wet") form with peritonitis or pleuritis characterized by the presence of large amounts of proteinaceous fluid in the body cavities and associated with a vasculitis, and (2) a noneffusive ("dry") form characterized by multiple small granulomas on the surface of the major abdominal organs.

Pleural lesions are uncommon in the noneffusive form of FIP. Some cats may show central nervous system involvement and ocular lesions. Both forms of the disease are uniformly lethal, with affected cats dying between 1 week and 6 months (Pedersen, 2014).

The pathogenesis of FIP differs between the two forms of the disease (Brown et al., 2009). After invading a cat, the virus first replicates in intestinal epithelial cells. The virus shed by epithelial cells is then spread by monocytes and taken up by phagocytic cells in the target tissues. These target tissues include the serosa of the peritoneum and the pleura, as well as the meninges and the uveal tract. The course of the infection then depends on the nature of the immune response to the virus—a phenomenon also seen in several bacterial diseases (see Chapter 27). Immunity to FIP virus is entirely cell mediated, and a Th1 response is protective. A cat that mounts a good Th1 response will become immune, regardless of the quantity of antibodies it produces. Some cats, however, mount a Th2 response to the viral spike proteins. In these animals, antibodies enhance virus uptake by macrophages, in which they then replicate. Virus-laden macrophages accumulate around the blood vessels of the omentum and serosa (Fig. 28.9). These macrophages are activated in that they are strongly positive for CD18 and produce tumor necrosis factor-α (TNF-α) and IL-1β. Endothelial cells upregulate MHC class II expression. These antibodies also generate immune complexes that are deposited in the serosa, causing pleuritis or peritonitis, and in glomeruli, leading to glomerulonephritis. The serosal vasculitis is responsible for the effusion of fibrin-rich fluid into the serosal cavities. This massive production of immune complexes may also be responsible for the disseminated intravascular

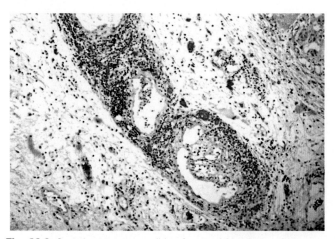

Fig. 28.9 Granulomatous vasculitis of serosal blood vessels in a cat with feline infectious peritonitis. Note the marked cellular infiltration of the vessel adventitia and media. This lesion may be due to the deposition of virus-antibody complexes in the vessel walls. Courtesy Dr. R.C. Weiss.

coagulation seen in these cats. IL-1 and IL-6 are found in unusually high concentrations in the peritoneal fluid from cats with effusive FIP. Cats with preexisting high levels of antibodies against FECV develop effusive FIP rapidly on challenge. Administering antiserum to FECV before FIP challenge may also enhance the peritonitis. Compared to cats with FIP, FECV-infected cats without FIP express higher levels of IL-10 and macrophage colony-stimulating factor (M-CSF) in their spleen, higher levels of IL-12 p40 in their lymphoid tissues, lower levels of IL-1β, IL-6, granulocyte colony-stimulating factor, and M-CSF, and higher levels of TNF-α in their mesenteric lymph nodes. It has been suggested that these FECV-infected cats do not develop FIP since they avoid excessive macrophage activation by upregulating IL-10 (Pedersen, 2014).

A modified live intranasal vaccine is available against the FIP virus. The vaccine contains a temperature-sensitive (ts) mutant virus that can only replicate in the upper respiratory tract and thus induces a local IgA response in the mucosa. This local mucosal response should prevent viral invasion without inducing high levels of serum antibodies. This vaccine, however, will only be effective if administered before coronavirus exposure. In highly endemic situations in which kittens are infected at a young age, vaccination at 16 weeks of age may be too late to prevent infection (Tizard, 2020).

Aleutian Disease of Mink

Although immune-complex-mediated lesions are usually only of passing interest in many infectious diseases, they generate the major pathological lesions in Aleutian disease of mink. Aleutian disease, due to a parvovirus infection, was first recognized in mink with the Aleutian coat color. Although all strains of mink are susceptible to this virus, Aleutian mink are genetically predisposed to the development of severe lesions since they are affected by the Chédiak-Higashi syndrome (see Chapter 40). Persistently infected mink develop a slowly progressive lymphoproliferative disease with a plasmacytosis that has been compared to a myeloma since it results in a polyclonal or monoclonal gammopathy (Fig. 28.10). They also develop immune-complex lesions (see Chapter 33). They make autoantibodies to their own immunoglobulins (rheumatoid factors) and to DNA (antinuclear antibodies). Their serum IgG concentration increases, sometimes to very high levels. On occasion, these elevated immunoglobulins are monoclonal in origin.

They are directed against the Aleutian disease virus. The virus transforms B cells so that they proliferate and differentiate excessively.

The immune-complex-mediated lesions of Aleutian disease include an arteritis, in which IgG, C3, and viral antigen are found within vessel walls, and a glomerulonephritis, in which deposits of immune complexes occur in the kidney. In addition, infected mink are anemic because their red cells are coated with antiviral antibodies. The red cells of infected animals adsorb virus-antibody complexes from plasma. These coated red cells are then removed from the circulation by macrophages. As might be predicted, the use of immunosuppressive agents such as cyclophosphamide or azathioprine prevents the development of many of these lesions and prolongs survival, whereas experimental vaccination with inactivated Aleutian disease virus increases the severity of infections.

Equine Infectious Anemia

This disease is caused by a lentivirus, EIAV. The disease may be acute, chronic, or inapparent (McGuire et al., 2002). Waves of viremia are associated with clinical disease. Following recovery from the first attack of disease characterized by anemia, fever, thrombocytopenia, weight loss, and depression, horses may remain healthy for weeks or months. However, three or four relapses at 2–8-week intervals may occur before the horse either develops a chronic wasting disease or becomes clinically normal. Each episode of disease tends to be milder than the previous one. The fevers are lower and the anemia less severe. EIAV, like other lentiviruses, undergoes random mutation, and new, antigenically different variants are produced at intervals. The elimination of each variant is determined by both CD4+ and CD8+ MHC–restricted cytotoxic T cells. Later, as new variants are produced, infected horses make neutralizing antibodies to that variant, and as a result, the viremia ends. Variants of EIAV, however, appear rapidly and randomly. The appearance of a new nonneutralizable variant leads to a viremic wave and clinical relapse. After the virus has undergone several of antigenic variations and the horse has responded to them all, the neutralizing antibody spectrum of the horse's serum becomes very broad, and viremia drops to a low level.

In addition to evading the immune response through antigenic variation, EIAV triggers immune-mediated tissue damage. The red cells of viremic horses adsorb circulating the virus onto their surface. Antibodies and complement then bind to the virus, as a result of which the red cells are cleared from the circulation more rapidly than normal. Infected horses may also develop a membranoproliferative glomerulonephritis as a result of immune-complex deposition on glomerular basement membranes. Horses infected with EIAV have unusually low levels of IgG3, although their circulating lymphocytes appear to be unaffected and respond normally to mitogens such as phytohemagglutinin.

Porcine Respiratory and Reproductive Syndrome

Porcine respiratory and reproductive syndrome virus (PRRSV) is a single-stranded, positive-sense RNA virus belonging to the family Arteriviridae. It causes a syndrome characterized by reproductive failure, infertility, abortions, anorexia, and secondary pneumonia (Gomez-Laguna et al., 2013). New strains are continually emerging worldwide (Du et al., 2017). When PRRSV invades the respiratory tract, it damages the mucociliary transport system, kills alveolar macrophages, and induces apoptosis of immune cells. Some PRRSV isolates downregulate TNF-α and IFN-γ while others induce Foxp3+ Tregs, and IL-10, both of which can suppress the immune response within the lungs. Enhanced IL-10 secretion and suppressed TNF-α and IFN-γ production result in a Th1/Th2 imbalance. As a result

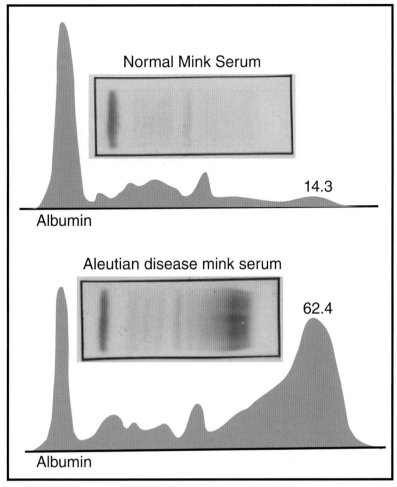

Fig. 28.10 The serum protein electrophoretic patterns seen in normal and Aleutian disease-infected mink. The serum of the infected animal shows a polyclonal gammopathy (the broad red band), so the γ-globulins account for 62.4% of the serum proteins in contrast to the normal level of 14.3%. Courtesy Dr. S.H. An.

of all this, PRRSV causes an increase in secondary pneumonias (Thanawongnuwech et al., 2000).

When PRRSV infects neonatal piglets, it stimulates their B cells. The piglets therefore present with polyclonal B-cell activation, autoimmunity (antibodies specific for Golgi antigens and dsDNA), grossly enlarged lymph nodes, and hypergammaglobulinemia (a 100- to 1000-fold increase in IgG; a 10- to 100-fold increase in IgM and IgA). The immunoglobulins produced are not directed against PRRSV, but the B-cell proliferative response is not purely polyclonal. The antibodies produced are derived from a limited number of dominant B-cell clones and are not neutralizing. It is speculated that the virus produces a B-cell superantigen. Affected pigs also have decreased CD4+ T cells and increased CD8+ cells. Cell-mediated responses and virus-neutralizing antibodies to PRRSV do not develop for about 4 weeks as a result of this loss of CD4+ cells. Because of this immunosuppression, PRRSV may cause persistent infections lasting for up to 6 months. The levels of IL-1, IL-6, TNF-α, and IFN-α are upregulated earlier and to a greater extent in pigs infected with a highly pathogenic strain of PRRSV than in pigs infected with less virulent strains. These cytokines are produced by alveolar macrophages, and they may reduce immunity to this virus. When PRRSV infects mature dendritic cells, it reduces their expression of CD80/86 and MHC class II molecules and increases their production of IL-10 (Flores-Mendoza et al., 2008).

Canine Distemper

Canine distemper is caused by a negative-sense, single-stranded RNA morbillivirus that evolved from the measles virus. Although distemper affects many organs, one of its prime targets is the lymphoid system. The virus invades lymphocytes through its receptor CD150 and then induces apoptosis of CD4+ T cells. Thus, there is a viremia-associated loss of CD4+ T cells. Lymphocytes are depleted in spleen, lymph nodes, and tonsils. Thymic atrophy occurs. There is a complete loss of secondary follicles. The bone marrow, in contrast, is minimally affected. The most affected lymphocyte populations are CD4+ T, CD8+ T, and CD21+ B cells. Subsequent regeneration of the lymphoid organs leads to a recovery of double-negative T-cell subsets. The numbers of CD5- and immunoglobulin-positive cells remain low. The CDV N-protein interacts with FcγR (CD32) to suppress IL-12 production and B-cell maturation. This leads to reduced plasma cell formation and immunoglobulin production. Even after CDV has cleared, affected dogs remain profoundly immunosuppressed.

CDV also causes a demyelinating leukoencephalomyelitis. This is a two-stage process. The initial lesion is probably due to direct viral activity, but this is followed by progression triggered by a strong Th1 response and the production of pro-inflammatory cytokines (IL-6, IL-8, IL-12, and TNF-α). Thus the damage may be secondary to excessive macrophage function and bystander mechanisms. Cytotoxic CD8+ cells may also contribute to the loss of myelin.

SOME ANTIVIRAL VACCINES

Because of the lack of antiviral drugs, vaccination is the only effective method for the control of most viral diseases in domestic animals. As a result, the development of viral vaccines is, in many ways, more advanced than the development of their bacterial counterparts. It has, for example, proved relatively easy to attenuate many viruses so that effective vaccines containing modified live virus (MLV) are readily available.

As discussed in Chapter 26, MLV vaccines are usually good immunogens, but their use may involve certain risks. The most important problem encountered is residual virulence. One serious example of this was the development of clinical rabies in some dogs and cats following administration of older strains of MLV rabies vaccine. Some strains of infectious bovine rhinotracheitis and equine herpesvirus-1 vaccines may cause abortion when given to pregnant cows or mares, respectively, and MLV bluetongue vaccines may cause disease in fetal lambs if given to pregnant ewes (see Chapter 24). More commonly, the residual virulence in these vaccines causes a mild disease. Thus intraocular or intranasal rhinotracheitis or calicivirus vaccines may cause a transient conjunctivitis or rhinitis in cats. MLV infectious bursal disease vaccines, some canine parvovirus–2 vaccines, and some bovine viral diarrhea vaccines can cause a mild immunosuppression.

Transient side effects such as these, which may otherwise be regarded as inconsequential, can be of major significance in the broiler chicken industry, where even a minor slowing in growth can have major economic results. Two strains of infectious bronchitis vaccine are available. The Massachusetts strain is mildly pathogenic but a good immunogen, whereas the Connecticut strain is nonpathogenic but a poor immunogen. It is common, therefore, in order to minimize complications, to use the Connecticut strain for primary vaccination and, if boosters are required, to use the Massachusetts strain subsequently. Similarly, of the two major vaccine strains of Newcastle disease, the LaSota strain is a good immunogen but may provoke mild adverse reactions. In contrast, the B1 strain is considerably milder but is less immunogenic, especially if given in drinking water. In other situations, birds may be primed with the very mild G2 Newcastle disease strain. Then, in the face of severe challenge, they may be boosted with a relatively virulent live vaccine.

Because of problems of this nature, persistent attempts have been made to minimize residual virulence in vaccines. One method involves the use of ts mutants. Ts strains of BHV-1, for example, will grow only at temperatures a few degrees lower than normal body temperature. When this organism is administered intranasally, it is able to colonize the relatively cool nasal mucosa but is unable to invade the rest of the body. Thus, the vaccine can stimulate local immunity without incurring the risk for a systemic invasion. (It also has the advantage that its activity is not blocked by maternal immunity). Some vaccine viruses may persist in vaccinated animals and cause a prolonged carrier state. Although this is a problem largely associated with herpesviruses, concerns have been expressed that the widespread use of MLV vaccines may serve to seed viruses into animal populations and that untoward consequences may develop in the future. This is a threat not to be taken lightly.

An alternative approach to overcoming the problems caused by MLV involves the increasing use of inactivated and subunit vaccines. Excellent inactivated vaccines are available against diseases such as foot-and-mouth disease, equine herpesvirus-4 (rhinopneumonitis), pseudorabies, feline panleukopenia, feline herpes (rhinotracheitis), and rabies. At their best, these vaccines confer immunity comparable in strength and duration to that induced by MLV vaccines, with the assurance that they are free of residual virulence. Virus-like particles are synthetic structures that resemble viruses in structure and

morphology and express viral antigens. In effect, they are viruses without a contained genome. They hold great potential for generating superior vaccines and are described in more detail in Chapter 26.

The rapid development and effectiveness of mRNA vaccines in combatting COVID-19 in humans has resulted in many new investigations into their use in preventing other viral diseases, including animal diseases.

SEROLOGY OF VIRAL DISEASES

Tests to Detect and Identify Viruses

Historically, serological tests were used to identify the presence of viruses within tissues. The tests commonly employed for this purpose included fluorescent antibody tests, enzyme-linked immunosorbent assay (ELISA), hemagglutination inhibition, virus neutralization, complement fixation, and gel precipitation. The precise tests employed depended on the nature of the unknown virus. The development of the polymerase chain reaction (PCR) has made many of these techniques obsolete. Exquisitely sensitive, the PCR can be used to detect viral DNA. A reverse-transcriptase PCR can be used to detect RNA viruses. The PCR is best suited for use in well-equipped laboratories. For animal-side testing or in situations in which the equipment is not available, more suitable techniques for the detection of viral antigen or antiviral antibodies are the membrane filter ELISA tests or lateral chromatography tests (see Chapter 43). (These are the tests widely employed in COVID-19 diagnosis.) These tests have the advantage that both positive and negative controls can be incorporated with the test serum in one well. In addition to serum, whole blood, plasma, nasal washings, or saliva may be employed as a source of antigen or antibody.

If the precise location of a virus needs to be determined in, for example, infected tissues, immunofluorescence or enzyme-linked immunohistochemical techniques may be employed. Specific antibodies can be used to enrich virus suspensions before electron microscopy. For example, a fecal sample may be centrifuged, leaving a clear supernatant that contains a small number of many different viruses. After sonication to break up clumps, antibody specific for the virus of interest is added to the supernatant, and after a brief incubation, the fluid is centrifuged again. Virus particles clumped by antibody are spun to the bottom, where they can be removed and examined by electron microscopy after negative staining. The antibody, by clumping only the virus of interest, renders it much easier to see by electron microscopy, and the presence of visible antibody within the virus clumps provides direct confirmation of the identity of the virus.

Tests to Detect and Identify Antiviral Antibodies

In general, the most widely employed techniques for detecting antibodies to viruses are hemagglutination inhibition, indirect ELISA, immunofluorescence, gel diffusion, Western blotting, complement fixation, and virus neutralization. The first four of these are technically simple and are thus preferred. Complement fixation and virus neutralization tests are complex, restricting the circumstances in which they may be used. Virus neutralization tests are also extremely specific, which, as discussed earlier, tends to reduce their value as screening tests.

REFERENCES

Alcami, A., Koszinowski, U.H., 2000. Viral mechanisms of immune evasion. Trends Microbiol. 8, 410–418.
Anis, E.A., Wilkes, R.P., Kania, S.A., Legendre, A.M., Kennedy, M.A., 2014. Effect of small interfering RNAs on in vitro replication and gene expression of feline coronavirus. Am. J. Vet. Res. 75, 828–834.

Assil, S., Coléon, S., Dong, C., Decembre, E., et al., 2019. Plasmacytoid dendritic cells and infected cells form an interferogenic synapse required for antiviral responses. Cell Host Microbe 25, 730–745.

Barker, E., Tasker, S., 2020. Update on feline infectious peritonitis. In Practice. https://doi.org/10.1136/inp.m3187

Brown, M.A., Troyer, J.L., Pecon-Slattery, J., et al., 2009. Genetics and pathogenesis of feline infectious peritonitis virus. Emerg Infect Dis 15, 1445–1452.

Du, T., Nan, Y., Xiao, S., Zhao, Q., Zhou, E.-M., 2017. Antiviral strategies against PRSSV infection. Trends Microbiol. 25, 968–979.

Flores-Mendoza, L., Silva-Campa, E., Resendiz, M., et al., 2008. Porcine reproductive and respiratory syndrome virus infects mature porcine dendritic cells and up-regulates interleukin-10 production. Clin. Vaccine Immunol. 15, 720–725.

Gomez-Laguna, J., Salguero, F.J., Pallares, F.J., Carrasco, L., 2013. Immunopathogenesis of porcine reproductive and respiratory syndrome in the respiratory tract of pigs. Vet. J. 195, 148–155.

Guo, Y., An, D., Liu, Y., Bao, J., Luo, X., Cheng, X., Wang, Y., Gao, M., Wang, J., 2017. Characterization and signaling pathway analysis of interferon-kappa in bovine. Dev. Comp. Immunol. 67, 213–220.

Guo, Y., Song, Z., Li, C., Yu, Y., et al., 2020. A novel type I interferon family, Bovine interferon-chi, is involved in positive-feedback regulation of interferon production. Front. Immunol. 11 https://doi.org/10.3389/fimmu.2020.528854

Haig, D.M., 2001. Subversion and piracy: DNA viruses and immune evasion. Res. Vet. Sci. 70, 205–219.

Helbig, K.J., Beard, M.R., 2014. The role of viperin in the innate antiviral response. J. Mol. Biol. 426, 1210–1219.

Iannello, A., Debbeche, O., Martin, E., et al., 2006. Viral strategies for evading antiviral cellular immune responses of the host. J. Leukoc. Biol. 79, 16–35.

Ichihashi, T., Asano, A., Usui, T., Takeuchi, T., Watanabe, Y., Yamano, Y., 2013. Antiviral and antiproliferative effects of canine interferon-λ1. Vet. Immunol. Immunopathol. 156, 141–146.

Jamieson, A.M., Yu, S., Annicelli, C.H., Medzhitov, R., 2010. Influenza virus-induced glucocorticoids compromise innate host defense against a secondary bacterial infection. Cell Host Microbe 18, 103–114.

Klotman, M.E., Chang, T.L., 2006. Defensins in innate antiviral immunity. Nat. Rev. Immunol. 6, 447–456.

Lanier, L.L., 2008. Evolutionary struggles between NK cells and viruses. Nat. Rev. Immunol. 8, 259–268.

Lazear, H.M., Schoggins, J.W., Diamond, M.S., 2019. Shared and distinct functions of Type I and Type III interferons. Immunity 50, 907–923.

Lewis, N.S., Daly, J.M., Russell, C.A., Horton, D.L., et al., 2011. Antigenic and genetic evolution of equine influenza A (H3N8) virus from 1968 to 2007. J. Virol. 85, 12742–12749.

Lund, J.M., Alexopoulou, L., Sato, A., et al., 2005. Recognition of single-stranded RNA viruses by toll-like receptor 7. Proc. Natl. Acad. Sci. U S A 101, 5598–5603.

Maillard, P.V., Ciaudo, C., Marchais, A., Li, Y., Jay, F., Ding, S.W., Voinnet, O., 2013. Antiviral RNA interference in mammalian cells. Science 342, 235–238.

McGuire, T.C., Fraser, D.G., Mealey, R.H., 2002. Cytotoxic T lymphocytes and neutralizing antibody in the control of equine infectious anemia virus. Viral Immunol. 15, 521–531.

Pedersen, N.C., 2014. An update on feline infectious peritonitis: virology and Immunopathogenesis. Vet. J. 201, 123–132.

Pedersen, N.C., Liu, H., Gandolfi, B., Lyons, L.A., 2014. The influence of age and genetics on natural resistance to experimentally induced feline infectious peritonitis. Vet. Immunol. Immunopathol. 162, 33–40.

Ranjan, P., Bowzard, J.B., Schwerzmann, J.W., Jeisy-Scott, V., Fujita, T., Sambhara, S., 2009. Cytoplasmic nucleic acid sensors in antiviral immunity. Trends Mol. Med. 15, 359–368.

Rigden, R.C., Carrasco, C.P., Summerfield, A., McCullough, K.C., 2002. Macrophage phagocytosis of foot-and-mouth disease virus may create infectious carriers. Immunology 106, 537–548.

Sagan, S.M., Sarnow, P., 2013. RNAi, Antiviral after all. Science 342, 207–208. 2013.

Sang, Y., Rowland, R.R.R., Blecha, F., 2010. Molecular characterization and antiviral analyses of porcine type III interferons. J. Interferon Cytokine Res. 30, 801–807.

Scalzo, A.A., 2002. Successful control of viruses by NK cells-a balance of opposing forces? Trends Microbiol. 10, 470–474.

Shekhar, S., Yang, X., 2015. Natural killer cells in host defense against veterinary pathogens. Vet. Immunol. Immunopathol. 168, 30–34.

Stetson, D.B., Medzhitov, R., 2006. Type I interferons in host defense. Immunity 25, 373–381.

Thanawongnuwech, R., Halbur, P.G., Thacker, E.L., 2000. The role of pulmonary intravascular macrophages in porcine reproductive and respiratory syndrome virus infection. Anim. Health Res. Rev. 1, 95–102.

Tizard, I.R., 2020. Vaccination against Coronaviruses in domestic animals. Vaccines. https://doi.org/10.1016/j.vaccine.2020.06.026.

Verhelst, J., Hulpiau, P., Saelens, X., 2013. Mx proteins: antiviral gatekeepers that restrain the uninvited. Microbiol. Mol. Biol. Rev. 77 (4), 551–566.

Xu, L., Ou, J., Hu, X., Zheng, Y., 2023. Identification of two isoforms of canine tetherin in domestic dogs and characterization of their antiviral activity against canine influenza virus. Viruses. https://doi.org/10.3390/v15020393.

Zhang, Z., Harkiss, G.D., Hopkins, J., Woodall, C.J., 2002. Granulocyte macrophage colony-stimulating factor is elevated in alveolar macrophages from sheep naturally infected with maedi-visna virus and stimulates maedi-visna virus replication in macrophages in vitro. Clin. Exp. Immunol. 129, 240–246.

Zhu, Z., Li, S., Ma, C., Yang, F., et al., 2023. African swine fever virus E184L protein interacts with innate immune adaptor STING to block IFN production for viral replication and pathogenesis. J. Immunol. 210, 442–458.

29

Immunity to Parasites

CHAPTER OUTLINE

Infectious diseases, as pointed out earlier, rarely result from the deliberate activities of a malicious microorganism. In most cases, disease occurs because of the host's reaction to the infection or because the invader inadvertently causes damage to its host. Well-adapted parasites do not make these mistakes. They exploit the host's resources without causing irreparable damage or triggering a destructive defensive response. A consistent feature of all parasite infestations, however, is that they block or delay host defenses so that they may survive for sufficient time to reproduce. Some parasites may simply delay their destruction until they complete a single life cycle. Other well-adapted parasites may contrive to survive for the life of their host protected from immunological attack by highly evolved evasive mechanisms (Fig. 29.1).

Ideally, a successful parasite will influence its host's immune responses by selectively suppressing those that reduce parasite survival, while at the same time allowing other responses to proceed and thus minimizing immunosuppression. In addition, many parasites use their host's metabolic or control pathways for their own purposes. For example, epithelial growth factor and IFN-γ enhance the growth of *Trypanosoma brucei*, whereas IL-2 and GM-CSF promote the growth of *Leishmania amazonensis*. This sharing of cytokines by host and parasites reflects the long history of their association and their success in adapting to a parasitic lifestyle.

Vaccination against parasitic diseases has therefore faced two hurdles. One is the complexity of the immune responses to these agents, compounded by the fact that they, by definition, have successfully evolved to evade the immune system. Thus, any antiparasite vaccine has to induce a protective immune response that is superior to the natural response. The second problem is economic. Many diverse drug treatments are available for parasite infestations, and newly developed vaccines are often much less effective. This is especially true of parasitic helminths.

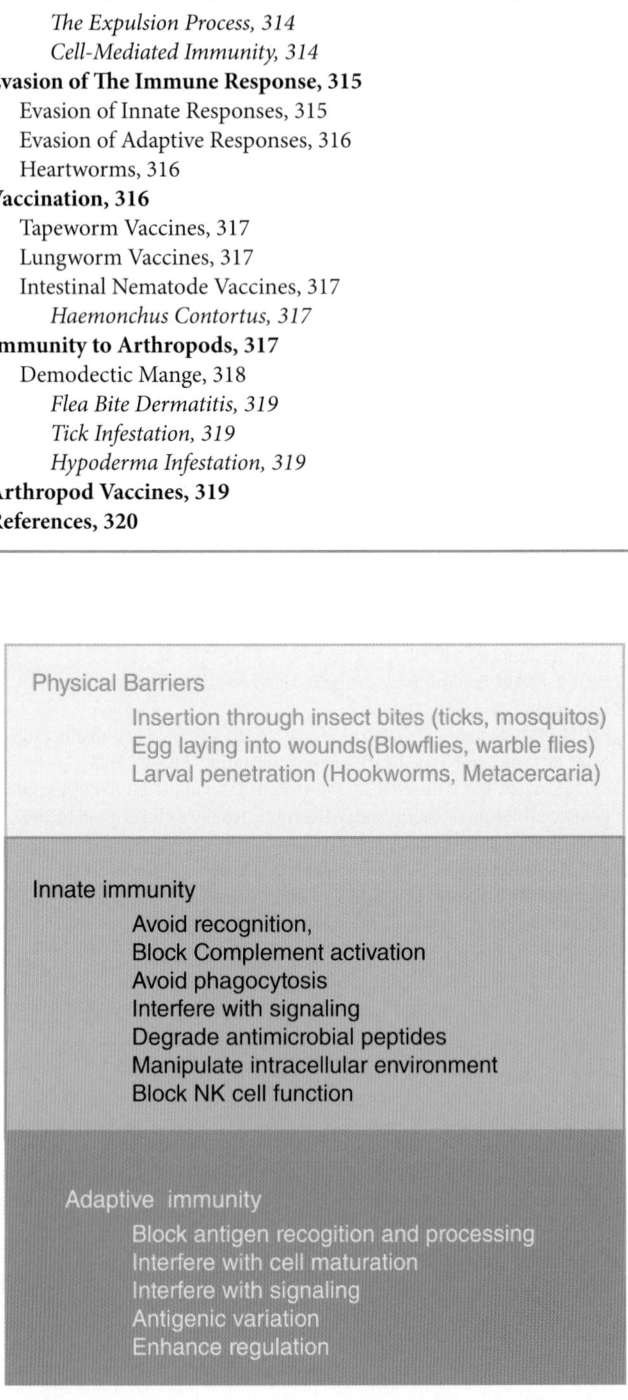

Fig. 29.1 Evasion of the immune response is critical to parasite survival. Some of the many ways by which parasites evade immune destruction or exclusion are shown. *NK,* Natural killer.

IMMUNITY TO PROTOZOA

Innate Immunity

The mechanisms of innate resistance to protozoa are similar to those that prevent bacterial and viral invasion, although species- and genetic influences may be of greater significance. For example, *T. brucei*, *Trypanosoma congolense*, and *Trypanosoma vivax* do not cause disease in the wild ungulates of East Africa but will kill domestic cattle, presumably as a result of lack of mutual adaptation. Similarly, the coccidia are extremely host specific; for example, *Toxoplasma gondii* tachyzoites can infect any species of mammal, but their coccidian stages affect only felids (e.g., cats).

Some breeds of African taurine cattle, most notably N'Dama, are resistant to trypanosomiasis. This "trypanotolerance" results from selection of the most resistant animals over many generations so that they develop a greater ability to resist the pathological effects of the parasite. The γ/δ T cells of N'Dama cattle are much more responsive to trypanosome antigens than are the γ/δ T cells of susceptible cattle. Trypanotolerant animals produce more IL-4 and less IL-6 than susceptible animals. At the same time, they show neither the severe anemia nor the production loss seen in susceptible cattle. Trypanotolerant animals produce high levels of IgG against *T. congolense* cysteine protease. Since this enzyme contributes to the pathology of infection, these antibodies may partially account for trypanotolerance.

Adaptive Immunity

Like other invaders, protozoa stimulate both antibody- and cell-mediated immune responses. In general, antibodies control extracellular parasites in blood and tissue fluids, whereas cell-mediated responses are directed against intracellular protozoa.

Serum antibodies directed against protozoan surface antigens may opsonize, agglutinate, or immobilize them. Antibodies together with complement and cytotoxic cells may kill them, and some antibodies (called ablastins) may inhibit their division. In genital infections of humans, *Trichomonas vaginalis* stimulates a local IgE response. This allergic reaction increases vascular permeability, permitting IgG antibodies to reach the site of infection and immobilize and eliminate the organisms.

In babesiosis the sporozoites invade red blood cells, and the infected red cells incorporate *Babesia* antigens into their membranes. These antigens induce antibodies that opsonize the red cells and cause their removal by phagocytosis. Macrophages and cytotoxic lymphocytes recognize the *Babesia* antigen-antibody complexes on the surface of infected red cells and destroy them by antibody-dependent cell–mediated cytotoxicity.

Intracellular parasites use many strategies to invade cells and avoid destruction. Most gain entry by employing host-mediated processes such as phagocytosis. Apicomplexans such as *Toxoplasma* and *Cryptosporidium*, however, actively penetrate cells. Once inside, they persist within specially modified vacuoles. Protective immunity against apicomplexan protozoa, such as *Cryptosporidium*, *Eimeria*, *Neospora*, *Plasmodia*, and *Toxoplasma*, is generally mediated by Th1 responses. For example, *T. gondii* is an obligate intracellular parasite whose tachyzoites live within cells, especially macrophages (Fig. 29.2). They penetrate these cells by "gliding" through molecular junctions in the cell membrane and so do not trigger phagosome formation. *Toxoplasma* tachyzoites are therefore not destroyed since their "parasitophorous vacuoles" do not mature and fuse with lysosomes. *Toxoplasma* can thus persist inside cells in an environment free of antibodies, oxidants, and lysosomal enzymes. The parasites eventually produce perforin-like molecules that permeabilize the cell membrane

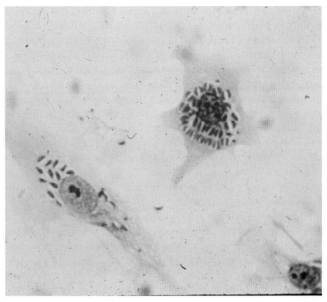

Fig. 29.2 Mouse macrophages containing healthy, growing tachyzoites of *Toxoplasma gondii*. After an immune response develops, these cells become activated and acquire the ability to destroy ingested tachyzoites. Courtesy Dr. C.H. Lai.

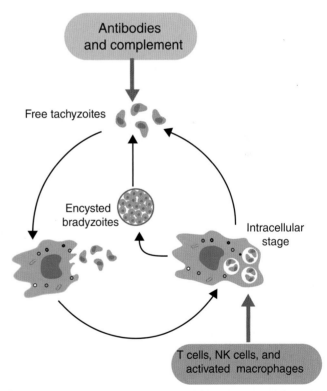

Fig. 29.3 The points in the life cycle of *Toxoplasma gondii* at which the immune system can exert a controlling influence. *NK*, Natural killer.

and permit the tachyzoites to escape and invade other cells. Antibodies and complement can destroy extracellular Toxoplasma and prevent its spread between cells (Fig. 29.3). Antibodies, however, have little or no influence on the intracellular forms of the parasite. These intracellular organisms can only be destroyed by a Th1 response.

An apicomplexan protein, called profilin found in Toxoplasma and Neospora, is a ligand for TLR11. Ligation of TLR11 on dendritic cells signals through the MyD88 pathway and stimulates IL-12 and IFN-γ production by NK and T cells. The IL-12 and IFN-γ in turn trigger a strong Th1 response. Activated Th1 cells secrete more IFN-γ in response to *Toxoplasma* ribonucleoproteins. This IFN-γ activates macrophages, permitting lysosome-vacuole fusion and killing the intracellular organisms. Cytotoxic T cells can also destroy *Toxoplasma* tachyzoites and *Toxoplasma*-infected cells on contact. *Toxoplasma*-infected dendritic cells are attacked and killed by natural killer (NK) cells. The *T. gondii* tachyzoites, however, may convert into cysts containing bradyzoites and so cause chronic infection. These cysts are weakly immunogenic and do not stimulate inflammation. As a result, they can persist indefinitely within tissues.

Th1-mediated macrophage activation is important in many protozoan diseases where the organisms are resistant to intracellular destruction. The most significant destructive molecules in these M1 cells are reactive nitrogen radicals. However, protozoa are also experts in surviving within macrophages; for example, *Leishmania*, *Toxoplasma*, and *Trypanosoma cruzi*, can migrate into safe intracellular vacuoles by blocking phagosome maturation. *Leishmania* and *T. cruzi* can suppress the production of oxidants or cytokine production, while *T. gondii* can promote macrophage apoptosis. *T. gondii* tachyzoites also inhibit inflammatory cytokine production by preventing the nuclear translocation of NF-κB.

In *Theileria parva* infection of cattle (East Coast fever), sporozoites invade α/β and γ/δ T cells, as well as B cells. These parasites activate NF-κB by continuously phosphorylating its inhibitor proteins, Iκ-Bα and Iκ-Bβ (see Chapter 9). This persistent NF-κB maintains the cell in an activated state and prevents its apoptosis. These activated cells produce both IL-2 and IL-2R. As a result, a loop is established, by which infected cells secrete IL-2, which in turn stimulates their growth. As *Theileria* schizonts grow within lymphocytes, the infected cells enlarge and proliferate. The parasite divides with its host cell, and its schizonts bind to the mitotic spindle. Thus, they infect both daughter cells leading to a rapid increase in parasitized cells, overwhelming infection, and death. Some animals, however, may recover from infection and become solidly immune. In these animals, CD8+ T cells kill infected lymphocytes by recognizing parasite antigens in association with MHC class I. In susceptible animals, the parasites interfere with MHC class I expression.

Infection of chickens or mammals with *Eimeria* oocysts generally leads to strong, species-specific immunity that can prevent reinfection. The immune response inhibits the growth of trophozoites, the earliest invasive stage, within intestinal epithelial cells. This growth inhibition is reversible since if the arrested stages are transferred to normal animals, they can complete their development. Resistance to primary infection is mediated by multiple mechanisms that involve CD4+ T cells, IL-12 and IFN-γ, macrophages, and NK cells. In contrast, resistance to secondary challenge by *Eimeria* is mediated by CD8+ T cells. In chickens, IFN-γ, tumor necrosis factor-α (TNF-α), and transforming growth factor-β (TGF-β), as well as intraepithelial CD8+ α/β T cells, are essential for anticoccidial immunity.

For many years, it was thought that a common feature of many protozoan infections was *premunition*, a term used to describe resistance that develops after the primary infection has become chronic and is only effective if the parasite persists in the host. It was believed, for example, that only cattle actually infected with *Babesia* were resistant to clinical disease. If all organisms were removed from an animal, resistance was believed to wane immediately. This is not entirely true. Cattle cured of *Babesia* infection by chemotherapy are resistant to challenge with the homologous strain of that organism for several years. Nevertheless, the presence of infection does appear to be mandatory for protection against heterologous strains. Babesiosis is also of interest since splenectomy of chronically infected animals, results in clinical

disease. The spleen not only serves as a source of antibodies in this disease but also removes infected erythrocytes.

Leishmaniasis

The importance of different adaptive responses in determining the course and nature of a protozoan disease is well seen in canine leishmaniasis. This disease is caused by *Leishmania infantum* or its New World synonym *Leishmania chagasi* and transmitted by biting sandflies (Baneth et al., 2008). When a sandfly injects the promastigotes of this parasite into the skin of dogs, they are phagocytosed by neutrophils. When the neutrophils undergo apoptosis, the parasites are released and are then engulfed by macrophages and dendritic cells. In these cells, the organisms differentiate into amastigotes. They divide within the macrophages until the cells rupture, and neighboring cells then phagocytose the released organisms. Depending on the degree and type of host immunity, the parasites may be restricted to the skin (cutaneous disease); alternatively, infected dendritic cells may carry the parasite to lymph nodes or enter the circulation and lodge in internal organs, leading to disseminated visceral disease. Although infection is widespread in endemic areas, most dogs are resistant to *Leishmania*, and only 10%–15% develop visceral disease (Toepp and Petersen, 2020).

Macrophages are the main host cells for *Leishmania* but are also responsible for parasite killing. Parasites divide within the phagolysosomes of infected macrophages. Their resistance to intracellular destruction results from multiple mechanisms. A study of 245 macrophage genes showed that 37% were suppressed by *Leishmania* infection. *Leishmania* lipophosphoglycan delays phagosome maturation, preventing the production of NO and inhibiting macrophage responses to cytokines. The parasite also reduces the antigen-presenting ability of macrophages by suppressing MHC class II expression. As a result of their persistence, the parasites trigger chronic inflammation. Initially characterized by granulocyte invasion, this is followed by macrophages, lymphocytes, and NK cells that collectively form granulomas (Baneth et al., 2008).

Clinical leishmaniasis is directly linked to the type of immune response mounted by the infected dog. In susceptible animals, the organisms may spread from the skin to the local lymph node, spleen, and bone marrow within a few hours. In resistant dogs, the parasites are restricted to the skin and draining lymph node so that the animals either remain healthy or develop a mild, self-limited disease. These resistant dogs mount a weak antibody response but a strong and effective Th1 response. They may have low antibody titers, but they produce IFN-γ in response to parasite antigens, generate type I granulomas, mount strong delayed hypersensitivity responses, and eventually destroy most of the parasites.

Resistance to *Leishmania* has a strong genetic component; for example, Ibizian hounds appear to be resistant to this parasite. There is also an association between resistance and certain MHC class II alleles, as well as some Slc11a1 (Nramp) alleles in dogs. Susceptible dogs, in contrast, mount a Th2 response characterized by high antibody levels but poor cell-mediated immunity. These differences have been attributed to the activities of IL-10 produced by Treg cells. In addition, the parasite may actively suppress transcription of the *IL-12* gene, ensuring that a Th2 response predominates (Altet et al., 2002).

Chronic, visceral disease develops in susceptible dogs. Parasite-laden macrophages accumulate, but the organism continues to multiply. These macrophages spread throughout the body, resulting in disseminated infection. Dogs develop severe generalized nodular dermatitis, granulomatous lymphadenitis, splenomegaly, and hepatomegaly. They show polyclonal (occasionally monoclonal) B cell activation involving all four IgG classes, as well as hypergammaglobulinemia, and they develop lesions associated with type II and type III hypersensitivity. Thus, polyclonal immunoglobulin production can lead to development of an immune-mediated hemolytic anemia, thrombocytopenia, and the production of antinuclear antibodies. Glomerulonephritis, uveitis, and synovitis may result from chronic immune complex deposition, leading to renal failure and death (Toepp and Petersen, 2020).

Evasion of the Immune Response

Despite their antigenicity, parasitic protozoa survive by using evasion mechanisms acquired over millions of years of evolution.

Immunosuppression

One approach is simply to suppress the immune system of affected animals. For example, *T. gondii* can avoid neutrophil attachment and phagocytosis. *T. parva* invades and destroys T cells. Other protozoa such as the African trypanosomes employ multiple suppressive mechanisms, such as promoting the development of regulatory macrophages and Treg cells, reducing complement activation, depleting dendritic cells or stimulating the B cell system to exhaustion. It is unsurprising that death in bovine trypanosomiasis is commonly due to bacterial pneumonia or sepsis as a result of this immunosuppression. Parasite-induced immunosuppression may assist parasite survival. For example, *Babesia bovis* is immunosuppressive for cattle. As a result, infected cattle have more ticks than noninfected animals, and the efficiency of transmission of *B. bovis* is enhanced. It must be pointed out, however, that parasite-induced immunosuppression may kill the host as a result of secondary infection, so it is not always beneficial to the parasite.

In addition to immunosuppression, protozoa have evolved two very effective evasive techniques. One involves becoming less antigenic, and the other involves the ability to alter surface antigens rapidly and repeatedly. An example of a nonantigenic organism is the encysted bradyzoite stage of *T. gondii*, which, as mentioned previously, does not appear to stimulate a host inflammatory response. Some protozoa may mask themselves with host antigens. Examples of these include *Trypanosoma theileri* in cattle and *Trypanosoma lewisi* in rats, both nonpathogenic trypanosomes that survive in the bloodstream because they are masked by host serum proteins and are not recognized as foreign. *T. brucei*, a pathogenic trypanosome of cattle, may also adsorb host serum proteins or soluble red cell antigens, thus reducing its antigenicity.

Protozoa often trigger a very robust T-cell response. Unfortunately, this may fail to eliminate the pathogen that then persists in the form of a chronic infection. Over time, this can lead to T-cell exhaustion. The T cells may be functionally impaired or even eliminated. These defects tend to follow a consistent pattern with an initial inability to produce IL-2 followed by loss of cytotoxicity and proliferative ability followed by impaired TNF-α and IFN-γ production. T-cell exhaustion and loss of function occur in chronic protozoan diseases such as Toxoplasmosis and Leishmaniasis (Gigley et al., 2012).

Antigenic Variation

Many protozoa successfully employ repeated antigenic variation (Barbour and Restrepo, 2000). If cattle are infected with the pathogenic trypanosomes *T. vivax, T. congolense*, or *T. brucei* and their parasitemia measured, it is found that periods of high parasitemia alternate regularly with periods of low or undetectable parasitemia (Fig. 29.4). Serum from infected animals contains antibodies against trypanosomes isolated prior to each bleeding but not against those that develop subsequently. Each period of high parasitemia corresponds to the expansion of a population of trypanosomes with new surface glycoprotein antigens. The elimination of this population by antibodies leads to a rapid fall in parasite numbers. Among the survivors, however, are parasites that express new surface glycoproteins and grow without hindrance. As a result, a fresh population arises to produce yet another period of high parasitemia (Fig. 29.5). This cyclical parasitemia, with each peak

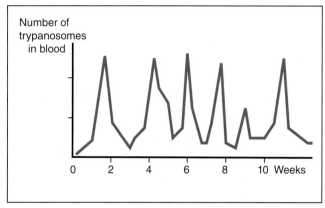

Fig. 29.4 The time course of *Trypanosoma congolense* parasitemia in an infected calf. Each parasitemic peak represents the development of a new, antigenically original population of organisms.

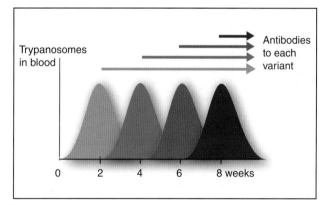

Fig. 29.5 A diagram showing how repeated antigenic variation accounts for the cyclical parasitemia observed in African trypanosomiasis. Each peak represents the growth and destruction of a new antigenic variant.

reflecting the appearance of a new population with new surface glycoproteins, can continue for many months.

The major antigens of these trypanosomes are known as variant surface glycoproteins (VSGs). The VSGs form a thick coat on the surface of the trypanosome that hides other cell surface antigens. VSGs are therefore targeted by host antibodies. As previous VSGs are recognized by the immune system and the organisms are destroyed, new VSGs emerge, giving rise to waves of parasitemia. The VSGs produced early in trypanosome infections tend to develop in a predictable sequence. However, as the infection progresses, the production of VSGs becomes more random. When antigenic change occurs, the VSGs in the old coat are shed and replaced by a different VSG. These trypanosomes possess about 2000 *VSG* genes, with an additional 1600 silent genes, of which two-thirds are pseudogenes. Antigenic variation occurs as a result of repeated DNA breaking and repair, replacing an active *VSG* gene with one from the silent gene pool. Each parasite expresses one VSG at a time. Since only a small part of the tightly packed VSG is exposed to host antibodies, it is not even necessary for the complete molecule to change. Replacement of exposed epitopes by gene conversion is sufficient for effective variation (see Chapter 18). Early in infections, complete *VSG* gene replacement occurs. Later on, partial replacement and point mutations can create new antigenic specificities. In some cases, the expressed *VSG* gene can be a mosaic derived from several archival pseudogenes. The potential for recombination-based variation is therefore absolutely enormous. Just to make sure, it appears that *T. brucei* also has an invariant surface glycoprotein that inhibits the alternative complement pathway by accelerating C3b degradation.

Trypanosomiasis is not the only protozoan infection in which variation of surface antigens occurs. It has also been recorded in infections by *B. bovis*, the plasmodia, and the intestinal parasite *Giardia lamblia*.

Since parasitic protozoa must evade the immune responses, it is not surprising that they preferentially invade immunosuppressed individuals. Organisms that are normally well controlled by the immune response, such as *T. gondii* or *Cryptosporidium bovis*, can grow and produce severe disease in immunosuppressed animals. For this reason, acute toxoplasmosis and cryptosporidiosis commonly occur in humans immunosuppressed for transplantation purposes or for cancer therapy and in those infected with human immunodeficiency virus.

Adverse Consequences

The immune responses to protozoa may result in hypersensitivity reactions. Type I hypersensitivity is a feature of trichomoniasis and results in local irritation and inflammation in the genital tract. Type II cytotoxic reactions are of significance in babesiosis and trypanosomiasis, in which they contribute to the anemia. In babesiosis, red cells express parasite antigens on their surfaces and are thus recognized as foreign and eliminated by hemolysis and phagocytosis. In trypanosomiasis, either fragments of disrupted organisms or possibly preformed immune complexes bind to red cells and cause their removal, causing anemia. Immune complex formation on circulating red cells is not the only problem of this type in trypanosomiasis. In some cases, excessive immune complex formation can result in a vasculitis or glomerulonephritis (type III hypersensitivity; see Chapter 33). Immune complex lesions are a marked feature of visceral leishmaniasis, as described previously.

Trypanosome infections may trigger an enormous increase in IgM-secreting cells, so that very high levels of polyclonal IgM develop in the blood of infected animals. Some of these antibodies are directed against autoantigens. These include rheumatoid factor-like molecules and antibodies against thymocytes, single-stranded DNA, red cells, and platelets. The mechanism of this polyclonal B cell activation is unknown.

It is probable that a type IV hypersensitivity reaction contributes to the inflammation that occurs when *Toxoplasma* cysts break down and release fresh tachyzoites. Extracts of *T. gondii* (toxoplasmin), if administered intradermally to infected animals, will cause a delayed hypersensitivity response (see Chapter 34).

Vaccination

Successful vaccination against protozoan infections is currently limited to coccidiosis, giardiasis, leishmaniasis, babesiosis, theileriosis, and toxoplasmosis (Brake, 2002).

Coccidiosis: Several live coccidial vaccines are given to poultry. These vaccines typically contain multiple species and strains of coccidia. Some consist of virulent, drug-sensitive organisms administered repeatedly in very low doses (trickle infection). Other vaccines have been attenuated by repeated passage through eggs, or they have been selected for precocity. Precocious strains mature very rapidly and, as a result, have less time to replicate, are less invasive, and are thus less virulent. All of these vaccines provide solid immunity to coccidia when applied carefully under good conditions. Nevertheless, the dose of vaccine must be carefully controlled, and the vaccines must be harvested from the feces of infected birds. Vaccinated birds shed oocysts that are transmitted to other birds.

Giardiasis: A vaccine has been available to protect dogs and cats against the intestinal parasite *Giardia duodenalis*. The vaccine contained disrupted cultured *Giardia* trophozoite extracts administered subcutaneously. It protected experimentally challenged dogs and cats against infection and clinical disease. It has now been withdrawn from the market.

Leishmaniasis: Several different vaccines are available against canine leishmaniasis. All are designed to stimulate T cell–mediated responses. One such vaccine consists of a *Leishmania* component called the fucose-mannose ligand adjuvanted with saponin. This vaccine may also serve as an immunotherapeutic agent, producing clinical improvement in dogs with disseminated disease. It has recently been withdrawn from the market.

An alternative vaccine containing a recombinant protein from several different Leishmania species (A2) with a saponin adjuvant also appears to be effective. Experimental vaccines, including killed vaccines and DNA vaccines, have shown encouraging results (Calzetta et al., 2020; Fernandez Cotrina et al., 2018). Another vaccine is available in Europe. It contains *L. infantum* excreted/secreted proteins with a saponin adjuvant (QA-21). Its efficacy is about 68%.

Another *L. infantum* vaccine contains a recombinant chimeric protein (protein Q). Four highly antigenic proteins from *L. infantum*, were identified as LiP2A, Lip2B, Lip0, and a histone H2A. The genes for five antigenic determinants from these four antigens were fused and expressed in *Escherichia coli* to form the recombinant protein Q. It is given subcutaneously to dogs over 6 months of age.

Babesiosis: Many factors contribute to the resistance of animals against babesiosis, including genetic factors (Zebu cattle are more resistant to disease than European cattle) and age (cattle show a significant resistance to babesiosis in the first 6 months of life). Animals that recover from acute babesiosis are resistant to further clinical disease. It is therefore possible to deliberately infect young calves when they are still relatively insusceptible to disease, so that they become resistant to reinfection. The organisms employed for this procedure are first attenuated by repeated passage through splenectomized calves and then administered to recipient animals in whole blood. The spleen is important in removing infected erythrocytes, so splenectomy permits very high parasitemias and thus high parasite yields. Rapid serial passage in splenectomized calves therefore selects parasite populations enriched for faster growing avirulent phenotypes. As might be anticipated, the side effects of this type of controlled infection may be severe, and drug therapy may be required to control them. The transfer of blood from one calf to another may also trigger the production of antibodies against the foreign red cells. These antibodies complicate any attempts at blood transfusion in later life and may provoke hemolytic disease of the newborn (see Chapter 32).

Two vaccines against canine babesiosis have been marketed in Europe. They contain soluble parasite antigens obtained from the supernatants of in vitro cultures of *B. canis* and *B. rossi*. The antigens are treated with formaldehyde and then freeze-dried. The lyophilized vaccine is adjuvanted with saponin (Schetters, 2005).

Theileriosis: Theileria infections, because they are intracellular parasites, must be controlled by cytotoxic T cells, and these can only be induced by live parasites. For *Theileria annulata*, a vaccine is prepared from schizonts attenuated by culture in vitro. Vaccination against *T. parva* is based on infection, followed by treatment. Thus cattle are infected by subcutaneous injection of a mixture of three different strains of tick-derived sporozoites, "The Muguga cocktail," and simultaneously treated with a long-acting tetracycline. As a result, the cattle get a mild infection followed by an immune response and recovery. Recovered animals develop a strong, persistent immunity to homologous challenge (Florin-Christensen et al., 2014).

Toxoplasmosis: *T. gondii* causes a placentitis leading to abortions, mummified fetuses, and weak lambs in sheep and goats. Since a primary infection with *T. gondii* will confer strong protective immunity on an animal, protective immunization is a real possibility. A live *Toxoplasma* vaccine containing the S48 incomplete strain has been used successfully for the control of toxoplasmosis in sheep. The strain was developed by passing it over 3000 times through laboratory mice and has lost the ability to develop bradyzoites or to initiate the sexual stages of the life cycle in cats. A single dose will provide lifetime immunity.

Trichomoniasis: Tritrichomonas is caused by *Tritrichomonas fetus*. Convalescent cows are usually resistant to reinfection for about 2 years. Whole cell–killed Tritrichomonas vaccines only confer a relatively short period of immunity and are not highly effective. As a result, they should be administered to heifers and cows immediately prior to the breeding season. They are not effective in bulls.

Neosporosis: *Neospora caninum*, an apicomplexan parasite related to Toxoplasma, is also an important cause of bovine abortion. An effective killed tachyzoite vaccine has been developed (Horcajo et al., 2016; Weber et al., 2013).

IMMUNITY TO HELMINTHS

Intestinal helminths have coevolved with the bacterial populations in the gut. Thus, the bacteria and helminths interact with each other in addition to interacting with their host's immune system. Parasite antimicrobial peptides may control bacterial numbers. The host's bacteria will also colonize worm guts. Their interactions with the host also influence intestinal inflammation and motility. The major defense against gastrointestinal helminths is a type 2 adaptive immune response, but the microbiota also plays an immunosuppressive role that may promote helminth colonization and survival (Box 29.1).

The effectiveness of the host's defenses depends on the animal's age, nutritional status, genetics, and the site of infection, as well as the species of worm involved and whether the infection is sudden and large or a much slower trickle infection. Thus, lambs infected with *Nematodirus battus* rapidly develop resistance, while immunity to *Teladorsagia circumcincta* is slow to develop. It takes up to a year for lambs to fully develop their resistance to nematodes. Adult sheep generally harbor only a few adult nematodes, but periodic re-exposure is required to maintain their immunity. Resistance to abomasal worms develops more slowly than resistance to intestinal worms. A reduction in resistance to nematodes is seen in ewes from 2 weeks prior, to 6 weeks after lambing as a result of periparturient immunosuppression. One consistent feature of intestinal nematode infestations is the very wide variation in parasite load within a population. Most animals harbor a few worms, but a few animals harbor a lot of worms.

Innate Immunity

Innate factors of host origin that influence helminth burdens include the age, sex, and most important, the genetic background of the host.

BOX 29.1 Parasites, Microbiota, and Host Immunity

Intestinal helminth parasites are members of the microbiota. Their presence alters the composition of the microbiota because the worms release metabolites and excretory/secretory products and stimulate their host's immune system. The composition of the bacterial microbiota also influences helminth colonization. Both helminths and the bacterial microbiota influence the Th17-Treg cell balance as well as an animal's Th2 responses. Alterations in the Th17-Treg cell balance, especially those that reduce intestinal inflammation, promote helminth survival. For example, premature initiation of Treg responses in *Trichuris muris* infections can inhibit protective immunity. Conversely, Treg depletion reduces the worm burden and intestinal Th1 inflammatory responses. Tregs appear to limit Th2 cell expansion, especially early in worm infestations.

From Hayes, K.S., Bancroft, A.J., Goldrick, M., et al., 2010. Exploitation of the intestinal microflora by the parasitic nematode *Trichuris muris*. Science 328, 1391–1394.

The influence of sex on helminth burdens appears to be largely hormonal. In animals whose sexual cycle is seasonal, parasites tend to synchronize their reproductive cycle with that of their hosts. For instance, ewes show a "spring rise" in fecal nematode ova, which coincides with lambing and the onset of lactation. Similarly, the development of helminth larvae in cattle in early winter tends to be inhibited until spring in a phenomenon called hypobiosis. The larvae of *Toxocara canis* may migrate from an infected bitch to the liver of the fetal puppy, resulting in a congenital infection. Once born, the infected pups can re-infect their mother by the more conventional fecal-oral route.

Inherited resistance to helminths is seen in the superior resistance of sheep with hemoglobin A (HbA) to *Haemonchus contortus* and *T. circumcincta* compared with sheep with hemoglobin B. The reasons for this are unclear, but sheep with HbA mount a more effective self-cure reaction and a better immune response to many other antigens as well. Polymorphisms in the IFN-γ gene affect the inflammatory response in sheep and may interfere with Th2 responses to helminths. Another example is the enhanced resistance to *Cooperia oncophora* seen in Zebu cattle compared to European cattle. In many cases, resistance to parasites is linked to MHC polymorphisms. Thus, cattle possessing BoLA-Aw7 and A36 tend to have low fecal egg counts, whereas animals with Aw3 tend to have high counts. Some BoLA haplotypes may also be associated with high antibody levels against *Ostertagia*. The effects of the SLA complex on parasite immunity in pigs have also been assessed. Thus, there was a 50% lower muscle larval burden in *Trichinella spiralis*-infected *cc* minipigs compared with pigs with the *dd* or *aa* haplotype. Resistance was characterized by a predominance of lymphocytes and macrophages in the cellular reaction around each larva.

Other innate factors that influence resistance to helminth infestations include the effects of other parasites within the same host. For example, calves infected with *Cysticercus bovis* show increased resistance to further infestation by this parasite. Similarly, lambs can acquire resistance to *Echinococcus granulosus* so that repeated dosing with large numbers of ova does not result in the development of massive worm burdens. The original dose of ova may stimulate rejection of subsequent doses. Interspecies competition among helminths for mutual habitats and nutrients in the intestinal tract will also influence the numbers, location, and composition of an animal's helminth population.

Adaptive Immunity

Helminths present the immune system with a challenge. Most parasitic worms migrate through the tissues as larvae and eventually reach the intestine or lungs, where they develop into adults. Clearly, the mechanisms that destroy these migrating larvae in the tissues must be very different from those used to expel large adult worms from the intestine or airways. The expulsion of adult worms from the intestine requires a coordinated response by multiple cell types under the control of T-cell-derived cytokines. These cells, especially tuft cells, collectively trigger a strong type 2 response that results in mast cell degranulation, eosinophil infiltration, acute inflammation, and ideally, expulsion of the parasites (Díaz and Allen, 2007).

In general, antigens derived from larvae and adult worms within tissues trigger type 2 immune responses and, as a result, are attacked by eosinophils and basophils. Adult worms attached to mucosal surfaces are less vulnerable to direct attack but also trigger similar responses and so can be expelled by IgE and cytokine-mediated mechanisms. Type 1, cell-mediated responses are relatively less important. Type 2 immunity to helminths involves the production of IL-4, -5, -9, and -13.

Because nematode antigens trigger type 2 responses, IgE levels and eosinophil numbers are usually elevated in parasitized animals. Additionally, many helminth infestations are associated with the characteristic signs of type I hypersensitivity, including eosinophilia, edema, asthma, and urticarial dermatitis. For example, pigs infested with *Ascaris suum* show cutaneous allergic reactions to injected parasite antigens, as well as degranulation of intestinal mucosal mast cells. Mammals eventually develop limited immunity to tissue helminths after several months. One parasite, *Ostertagia ostertagi*, is an exception. Cattle remain susceptible to reinfection by *Ostertagia* for many months, and immunity that can inhibit the production of viable larvae is not seen until an animal is more than 2 years old. It is not surprising that this is the most economically important bovine helminth parasite.

Eosinophils and Parasite Destruction

Invading parasites attract eosinophils, key cells mediating type 2 immunity. Eosinophils are attracted by mast cell and parasite-derived products, as well as by IL-5 and other cytokines from Th2 cells. IL-5 from Th2 cells and GM-CSF from Th17 cells mobilize bone marrow eosinophils, releasing large numbers into the circulation. Chemokines such as the eotaxins also attract eosinophils (Fig. 29.6). Eosinophils exposed to helminth antigens can increase their expression of MHC class II and become antigen-presenting cells. These antigen-presenting eosinophils are highly effective in promoting Th2 responses against worm antigens (Wildblood et al., 2005). Eosinophils express many

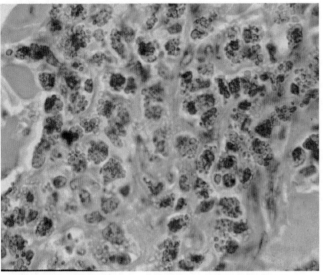

Fig. 29.6 Photomicrograph of a lesion in horse skin caused by allergy to migrating parasitic helminth larvae. The granular cells are eosinophils, and their presence indicates the occurrence of a type I hypersensitivity reaction.

different PRRs, including TLR1-5, TLR7, TLR9, NOD1, NOD2, and dectin 1. When these are stimulated, they trigger an oxidative burst, increase adhesiveness, and release IL-1, IL-6, TNF-α, and GM-CSF, as well as their cytotoxic granule contents (see Fig. 30.18).

Eosinophils employ Fc receptors to bind antibody-coated parasites; they then degranulate, and release their granule contents directly onto the worm cuticle (Fig. 29.7). These contents include oxidants, nitric oxide, lysophospholipase, and phospholipase D. Major basic protein, the crystalline core of the eosinophil-specific granules, can damage the cuticles of schistosomula, *Fasciola*, and *Trichinella*. Eosinophil cationic protein and eosinophil neurotoxin are ribonucleases that are lethal for helminths. It is important to point out, however, that some larval parasites may evade destruction by eosinophils. For example, larvae of *T. canis*, simply shed their outer coat together with the attached cells.

Eosinophil granules released from cells remain functional. These free granules express membrane receptors for IFN-γ and eotaxins, which when triggered, stimulate the granules to secrete their contents. Thus eosinophil granules function autonomously to contribute to the defenses against helminths. Eosinophils can also generate extracellular traps using released mitochondrial DNA (Meeusen and Balic, 2000).

Many nematodes are damaged or killed by eosinophil toxic products, supporting the idea that eosinophils serve a protective function. Nevertheless, this may not apply to all parasites. For example, both *T. circumcincta* and *H. contortus* produce chemoattractants for eosinophils, whereas the free-living nematode *Caenorhabditis elegans* does not. This suggests that some nematodes actively encourage eosinophil recruitment. Likewise, when *Trichinella spiralis* survival was studied in mice lacking eosinophils, it was found that the larvae in the muscles of these mice died in much larger numbers than in wild-type mice (Fabre et al., 2009).

Although the IgE-dependent eosinophil-mediated response is the most significant mechanism of resistance to larval helminths, other antibodies also play a protective role. The mechanisms involved include antibody-mediated neutralization of larval proteases, blocking of the anal and oral pores of larvae by immune complexes and prevention of molting and inhibition of larval development by antibodies directed against exsheathing antigens. Antibodies to the enzyme glutathione-S-transferase protect sheep against *Fasciola hepatica*. Antibodies against adult worms may stop egg production or interfere with worm development (Fig. 29.8). Thus, female *Ostertagia ostertagi* worms fail to develop vulvar flaps when grown in immune calves. Similarly, spicule morphology may be altered in *Cooperia* males from immune hosts.

Immunity to Migrating Larvae

Larvae and some adult worms migrate through tissues where they are attacked by inflammatory cells and molecules. Unlike bacteria

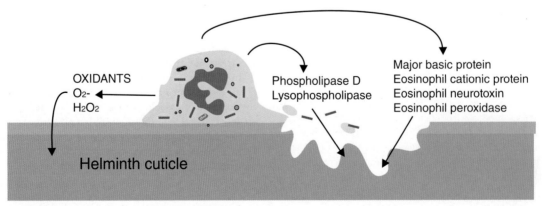

Fig. 29.7 Some of the molecules released from eosinophils that cause damage to the cuticle of parasitic helminths.

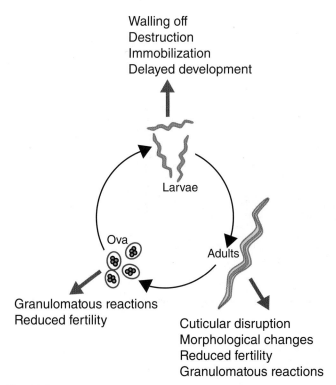

Fig. 29.8 Some effects of the immune responses on the stages of helminth development.

or protozoa, however, larval worms have a thick cuticle that protects their vulnerable hypodermal plasma membrane. As larvae develop and undergo periodic molts, damaged cuticles may be shed to be replaced with new ones. These cuticles cannot be penetrated by the terminal complement complex or by T-cell perforins. Thus eosinophils and macrophages are the key to destroying migrating larvae. Both possess FcεR (CD23) and can therefore bind and kill IgE-coated parasites. Chitinases can degrade helminth cuticles. Chitinases are produced by mast cells, macrophages, and neutrophils. Some mammalian chitinases may lack enzyme activity but can bind to helminth cuticles and serve as opsonins or chemoattractants.

If migrating worms cannot be killed, at least they can be walled off. M2 cells produce arginase. Arginase generates proline and polyamines. Proline and the polyamines are required for collagen synthesis and can induce fibroblast proliferation. The granulomas that develop around tissue helminths such as schistosomes or liver fluke are driven by arginase from M2 macrophages (Adams et al., 2014).

Immunity to Adult Helminths

Parasitic worms in the intestine are relatively invulnerable to immune attack. As a result, they must be forced to disengage from the gut wall and be expelled in the feces. While embedded in the intestinal and abomasal mucosa, worms secrete multiple antigens (Fig. 29.9), and these stimulate production of both IgA and IgE. IgE responses are probably more important than IgA since they play the key role in expelling adult worms from mucosal surfaces. This is most evident in the "self-cure" reaction in sheep infected with gastrointestinal nematodes, particularly *H. contortus* (McRae et al., 2015). Less is known about the role of IgA. It is associated with resistance to *T. circumcincta* affecting both worm size and fecundity.

The presence of adult worms and their excretory and secretory products in the intestinal wall will trigger some PRRs on enterocytes. Some helminth products can trigger TLRs, and the mannose receptor is known to bind the excretory/secretory proteins of *Trichuris muris*.

Parasite-mediated tissue damage triggers the release of all three Th2-stimulating cytokines, TSLP, IL-25, and IL-33, from enterocytes and tuft cells. These cytokines target both DC2s and ILC2s. For example, TSLP activates dendritic cells. IL-25 stimulates the production of type 2 cytokines by ILC2 cells and facilitates differentiation of Th2 cells. IL-33 acts on Th2 cells, ILC2 cells, basophils, and mast cells to drive their production of IL-4, IL-5, and IL-13 (Humphreys et al., 2008).

In response to this flood of cytokines, T cells release their own effector cytokines. For example, γ/δ T cells in the intestinal epithelium produce IL-4 and IL-25. Likewise, Th2 cells produce more IL-4 in a positive feedback loop generating the other Th2 cytokines and IL-25. The IL-4 activates STAT6, which upregulates GATA3 that causes differentiation into Th2 cells and suppresses Th1 responses. IL-6 acts with TGF-β to induce Th17 responses. IL-13 repairs epithelia, enhances mucus production, and together with IL-9 recruits and activates mucosal mast cells. Both IL-4 and IL-13 activate enterocytes, smooth muscle cells, and macrophages. Increased enterocyte proliferation and turnover may cause parasite disengagement (Cliffe et al., 2005). These cytokines also increase intestinal permeability and fluid secretion. The Th2 cytokines stimulate Paneth cells and the consequent increase in intestinal defensins may damage helminth cuticles. The cytokines also stimulate goblet cells to produce a resistin-like molecule that interferes with worm feeding (Gerbe and Jay, 2016). Mucins and other goblet cell products may also promote worm expulsion. IL-4 and -13, as well as IL-9, promote smooth muscle contractility (Zaph et al., 2014).

Mast Cells and Basophils

Mast cells and basophils are also required for helminth expulsion. They can be activated directly by PAMPs through PRRs, although it is unclear which parasite PAMPs do this. In response, the mast cells produce IL-4, -13, and -5 plus chemotactic factors. Mast cell proteases degrade tight junctions and allow fluid efflux into the intestine. Some mast cell products, such as chitinases, may be directly toxic to helminths. Basophils are also attracted to attached worms and are a major source of IL-4. Basophils can act as antigen-presenting cells in helminth (*T. muris*) infections. Eosinophils are attracted to these worms by IL-5 plus the eotaxins as described above (Voehringer, 2009).

Tuft Cells

Tuft cells are a specialized population of chemosensory cells found among the epithelial cell layer of the nasal mucosa, traches, salivary glands, stomach, and intestine (Grencis and Worthington, 2016). Tuft cells are so-called because they have a tuft of long microvilli at one pole that extends into the intestinal lumen. These cells play a key role in initiating type 2 immune responses to helminths. Tuft cells apparently use their microvilli to sense the fatty acid, succinate, produced by intestinal helminths. Tuft cells can also detect the protozoan parasite, *Tritrichomonas fetus*. In response, they produce large amounts of IL-25 (Fig. 29.10). In the presence of parasitic helminths, the IL-25 promotes the proliferation of tuft cells and mucus-producing goblet cells. Tuft cell IL-25 also recruits eosinophils and activates both Th2 cells and ILC2 cells (Schneider et al., 2019).

ILC2 Cells

ILC2 cells are a major source of acetylcholine and prostaglandin E2 during parasitic nematode infections. Their production is triggered by exposure to the activating cytokines, IL-33 and IL-25 from tuft cells. IL-13 and IL-4 from ILC2 cells stimulate further tuft cell proliferation and IL-25 production. The acetylcholine appears to have anthelmintic properties (Roberts et al., 2021). ILC2 cells are also an important source of IL-5, IL-9, and IL-13 (Coakley and Harris, 2020). IL-13 and IL-4 from the activated ILC2 cells also increase gut motility and mucus production (Gronke and Diefenbach, 2016; see Fig. 5.10).

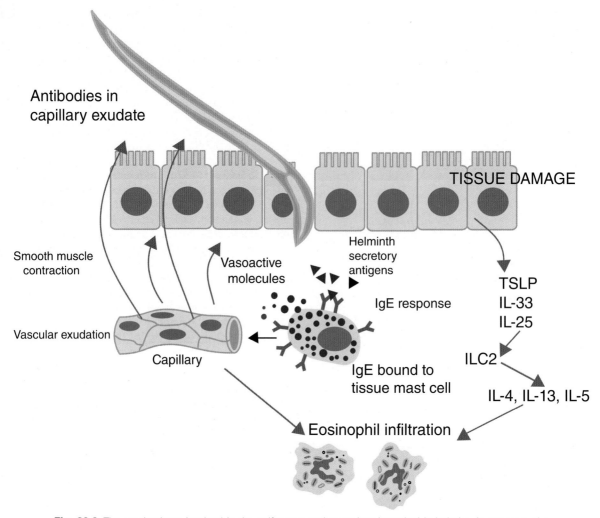

Fig. 29.9 The mechanisms involved in the self-cure reaction against intestinal helminths. In essence, the animal mounts an allergic response to the salivary antigens of attached nematodes. This acute inflammatory response causes the worms to detach from the intestinal wall and pass out in the feces. *IgE*, Immunoglobulin E; *ILC2*, innate lymphoid cells 2; *IL-4*, interleukin-4; *TSLP*, thymic stromal lymphopoietin.

The Expulsion Process

The combination of helminth antigens with mast cell and basophil-bound IgE triggers mast cell degranulation and the release of vasoactive amines such as histamine, cytokines such as IL-13 and IL-33, chitinases, and proteases. These molecules stimulate vigorous smooth muscle contraction and increase vascular permeability in the intestinal wall. The IL-13 also promotes parasite expulsion by stimulating epithelial cell proliferation. Presumably, the rapid epithelial cell turnover acts as an "epithelial elevator" to assist in disconnecting the parasites. IL-33 also induces the expulsion of adult worms. Tissue edema can inhibit parasite attachment. Increased permeability, epithelial cell proliferation, smooth muscle contraction and mucus production all contribute to worm expulsion. This expulsion is accompanied by mucosal mast cell infiltration, intestinal eosinophilia, elevated serum IgE, and high parasite-specific IgG1 levels.

The violent contractions of the intestinal muscles caused by histamine and acetylcholine, and the increase in the permeability of intestinal capillaries, cause an efflux of fluid into the intestinal lumen, resulting in dislodgment and expulsion of many worms. (This has been characterized as "weep and sweep"). In sheep that have just undergone self-cure, IgE antibody levels are high, and experimental administration of helminth antigens can cause acute anaphylaxis at that time (see

Chapter 30). A similar reaction is seen in fascioliasis in calves, where peak PCA antibody titers coincide with expulsion of the parasite.

Variations among worms. Tissue helminths may be thought of as xenografts. That is, grafts between individuals of two different species. The intensity of the graft rejection process can vary between individual hosts and between individual worms. Inbred mouse strains differ in their ability to expel intestinal nematodes such as *T. muris*. Since inbred mice are genetically homogeneous, these variations in resistance to *T. muris* must be due to differences among the worms. We know that strains of worms differ in their ability to trigger Th1 and Th2 responses. This may be due to manipulation of the immune response by each worm. For example, *T. muris* can produce a protein related to IFN-γ that suppresses Th2 responses and, therefore, enhances worm survival. Alternatively, these differences may be due to parasite numbers. Thus, low-level trickle infestations of *T. muris* provoke a Th1 response, and the parasites persist. If higher doses of parasites are administered, mice mount Th2 responses and expel the parasites. A threshold of infection is likely critical for the development of resistance.

Cell-Mediated Immunity

Live cysts of the tapeworm *Taenia solium* trigger a Th2 response and thus IgE production. However, after the cysts die, they stimulate a Th1

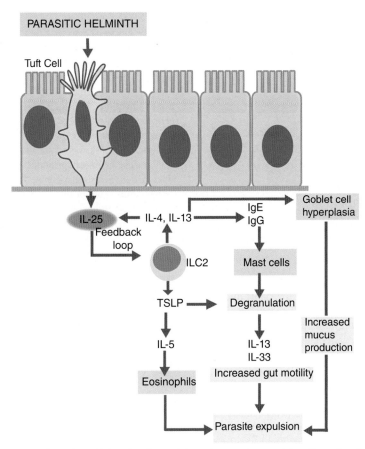

Fig. 29.10 The mechanisms by which tuft cells participate in parasite expulsion. The tuft cells produce inter-leukin (IL-25) that activates innate lymphoid cells2 (ILC2s). These cells produce IL-4 and IL-13 that promotes a strong type 2 immune response that results in tuft and goblet cell. *IgE,* Immunoglobulin E; *TSLP,* thymic stromal lymphopoietin.

response and granuloma formation. Biopsies show that IL-12, IL-2, and IFN-γ are associated with the granulomas surrounding dying tapeworm cysts. It may be that the Th1 response occurs only when the parasite can no longer influence the host's immune response.

Sensitized T cells attack tissue helminths by two pathways. First, mononuclear cells are attracted to the site of larval invasion and render the local environment unsuitable for growth or migration. Second, cytotoxic lymphocytes may kill the larvae. Thus, treatment of experimental animals with the T-cell stimulant, bacille Calmette-Guérin (BCG) vaccine (see Chapter 25), inhibits the metastases of hydatid cysts (*E. granulosus*). In tapeworm infestations in which the parasite cyst (metacestode) grows within the host, the parasite must obtain protein for nourishment. However, the cysticerci of *T. ovis* grow larger in the presence of immune serum than nonimmune serum. The parasites possess Fc receptors, and it is possible that host immunoglobulins may feed the parasite. Since cyst fluid contains lymphocyte mitogens, it has also been suggested that these might stimulate the production of immunoglobulins that may then be used by the parasite.

The complexity of resistance to helminths is well demonstrated in sheep bred for resistance to *H. contortus*. Compared with susceptible sheep, they show differences in B cell function; resistant sheep have significantly more IgA- and IgG1-containing cells. There is also evidence for differences in T-cell function because resistant sheep respond better to a T-dependent antigens. Treatment of resistant lambs with a monoclonal antibody to CD4 completely blocks their resistance to *H. contortus*. Mucosal mast cell numbers and tissue eosinophilia are also reduced in these treated sheep. In contrast, depletion of CD8+ cells has no effect on resistance.

EVASION OF THE IMMUNE RESPONSE

Although there are multiple mechanisms whereby animals resist helminth infection, it is obvious, even to a casual observer, that these defenses are not very effective. Successful helminth parasites survive and function in the presence of a fully functional host immune system. In general, helminths are most vulnerable to immunological attack while migrating through tissues. Thus, most evasion strategies work at the larval stage.

Evasion of Innate Responses

Brugia malayi secretes serpins that inhibit neutrophil serine proteases. *E. granulosus* secretes an elastase inhibitor that blocks neutrophil attraction by C5a or platelet-activating factor (PAF). Many helminths express surface antioxidants such as superoxide dismutase, glutathione peroxidase, and glutathione-S-transferase that neutralize the host's respiratory burst and protect their surfaces from oxidation (Fig. 29.11). A secreted antioxidant from *F. hepatica* called peroxiredoxin causes alternative activation of bovine macrophages, resulting in high arginase activity, low nitric oxide, low IFN-γ, and high IL-10 production. This, plus elevated IL-4, IL-5, and IL-13 production, promotes Th2 responses.

Many parasites interfere with the complement system. For example, schistosomes can neutralize the alternative complement pathway by

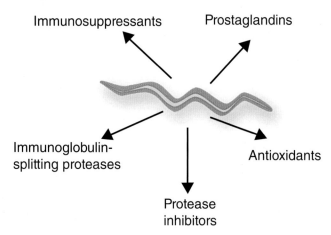

Fig. 29.11 Some methods by which migrating helminth larvae evade host defenses.

inserting decay-accelerating factor (CD55) from their host into their outer lipid bilayer. Tapeworms can secrete sulfated proteoglycans, which activate complement in the tissue fluid. Parasites such as *Necator americanus* and *H. contortus* secrete calreticulin homologs that bind C1q and block its activities.

Evasion of Adaptive Responses

Helminths become progressively less antigenic as they evolve in the presence of a functioning immune system. Presumably, natural selection favors the survival of individuals with reduced antigenicity. *H. contortus* is much less antigenic in sheep, its natural host, than in rabbits, which it does not normally infect. Sheep therefore respond to fewer *H. contortus* antigens than do rabbits. Larval helminths living within tissues may reduce their antigenicity by adsorbing host antigens onto their surface and masking parasite antigens. This occurs in *T. solium* infestations in swine, where the parasites are coated with IgG. Cysticerci can also adsorb MHC molecules to their surface.

Another mechanism of immune evasion is the use of sequential antigenic variation. Although helminths have not evolved a system as complex as that in trypanosomiasis, gradual antigenic variation is recognized. The cuticular antigens of *T. spiralis* larvae change after each molt. Even during their growth phase, these larvae change the expression of surface antigens. Some parasites such as *F. hepatica* shed their glycocalyx and hence their surface antigens when exposed to antibodies.

Some worms can interfere with antigen processing. Macrophages from schistosome-infested animals are incompetent antigen-presenting cells. Filarial worms secrete inhibitors that block macrophage proteases. *Taenia taeniaeformis* secretes taeniastatin, a protease inhibitor that inhibits neutrophil chemotaxis, complement activation, T-cell proliferation, and IL-2 production.

Immunosuppression is a consistent feature of parasitized animals. This may be due to the production of immunosuppressive molecules. For example, *F. hepatica* secretes proteases that destroy immunoglobulins. These proteases generate Fab fragments that bind and mask parasite antigens. In addition, *F. hepatica* tegumental protein suppresses production of IFN-γ and IL-12 by acting directly on dendritic cells and possibly suppressing signaling by NF-κB.

Many helminths suppress host immunity by promoting the production of Treg cells and IL-10. Because *F. hepatica* infestation is such a strong inducer of Th2 responses, it can adversely affect an animal's ability to mount Th1 responses and interfere with diagnostic tests such as the whole blood IFN-γ assay used to diagnose bovine tuberculosis

(see Chapter 34). Sheep infected with *H. contortus* may become specifically suppressed so that they are unreactive to *H. contortus*, even though they remain responsive to unrelated parasites. *O. ostertagi* and *Trichostrongylus axei* infestations depress calf lymphocyte responses to mitogens. *Oesophagostomum radiatum* secretes molecules that inhibit the responses of lymphocytes to antigens and mitogens. In other helminth infections, such as trichinosis, infected animals are nonspecifically immunosuppressed. This immunosuppression is reflected in a lowered resistance to other infections, a poor response to vaccines, and prolongation of skin graft survival.

Parasitic helminths produce a family of immunomodulatory peptides called helminth defense molecules that resemble mammalian cathelicidins. One of these molecules produced by *F. hepatica* can be endocytosed by host macrophages in a way that it prevents endosomal maturation, impedes antigen presentation and inhibits antigen carriage to the cell surface in conjunction with MHC class II molecules (Flynn and Mulcahy, 2008).

Heartworms

Canine heartworm disease is primarily caused by *Dirofilaria immitis*. Adult *D. immitis* live within the cardiopulmonary arteries and are thus continuously exposed to the cells and antibodies of the immune system. Nevertheless, they may live for years. In order to do this, the worms employ multiple evasive strategies so that adult worms effectively neutralize the immune system. However, it is also clear that the dog can control its heartworm burden to a limited extent by mounting an immune response against migrating larvae.

Dogs make IgM, IgG, and IgE directed against the larval stages. These antibodies mediate neutrophil adhesion to the surface of the microfilariae. This can kill larvae, but not adult worms. However, many larvae avoid this fate by shedding their major surface antigens (Simon et al., 2012).

Cysteine protease inhibitors (cystatins) are present in the heartworm cuticle and the gut. These cystatins can act on canine monocytes to induce the production of large quantities of IL-10 while downregulating production of TNF-α, IL-4, IL-5, IL-12, and IL-13 (Dong et al., 2019). They can also inhibit the proliferation of blood T cells in response to mitogens. Adult worms are coated with nonimmunogenic glycolipids and have surface proteases that destroy immunoglobulins. *D. immitis* adults are covered by a cuticle that is rich in glycans that can bind C-reactive protein but inhibit IgM binding (Martini et al., 2019).

Both adult and larval heartworms house the commensal bacterium *Wolbachia* within their intestinal tracts. These bacteria are also antigenic and can trigger an immune response in their canine host. Thus, when *Wolbachia* escape from dead worms into the bloodstream, they trigger antibody production. It has long been recognized that some dogs with heartworms develop an immune complex-mediated glomerulonephritis. Originally blamed on worm antigens, it now appears to be due in part to *Wolbachia* antigens (Morchon et al., 2012).

VACCINATION

It is not surprising, considering the nature of the host response to parasitic worms and the availability of cheap and effective anthelmintics, that vaccines against helminth parasites are not widely available. Nevertheless, the emergence of anthelmintic resistance and environmental concerns raised by excessive chemical use have resulted in an increased interest in antiparasite vaccines. Vaccine use is predicated on the assumption that a host's immune response can control or prevent an infestation. This is not always obvious in helminth infestations, and traditional vaccines may be of little use.

Tapeworm Vaccines

A recombinant *T. ovis* vaccine has been produced that can induce protective immunity in sheep. This vaccine contains a cloned oncosphere antigen (To45W) with a saponin-based adjuvant. It stimulates a response that prevents parasite penetration of the intestinal wall. A vaccine directed against *T. solium* has also been licensed in India (Lightowlers, 2013).

E. granulosus is the causative agent of hydatidosis, an important disease in sheep and humans in endemic areas. Sheep may be protected against *Echinococcus granulosus* using either oncospheres or secretory products from cultured oncospheres. An outer membrane protein called EG95 from activated oncospheres appears to be highly effective as an immunogen (Petavy et al., 2008).

Lungworm Vaccines

Protection against some helminths has been induced by vaccination using live irradiated organisms. The most important of these is the vaccine used to protect calves against pneumonia caused by the lungworm *Dictyocaulus viviparus*. In this vaccine, third-stage larvae hatched from ova in culture are exposed to 40,000 R X-irradiation, and two doses of these larvae are then fed to calves. The irradiated L3 larvae can penetrate the calf's intestine, but since they are unable to develop to the fourth stage, they cannot reach the lung and are thus nonpathogenic. During their exsheathing process, the larvae stimulate the production of antibodies that can block reinfection.

Intestinal Nematode Vaccines

Haemonchus Contortus

H. contortus, the "barber's pole" worm, is a major cause of sheep mortality. A vaccine against *H. contortus* that makes use of antigens derived from the worm's digestive tract is now available for use in sheep in Australia and South Africa. As the worm feeds, it ingests the sheep's blood. Antibodies in the blood of vaccinated sheep are directed against antigens expressed on the worm's intestinal enterocytes. These antibodies interfere with the worm's digestion and growth resulting in decreased egg output and a reduction in worm numbers by about 70% (Fig. 29.12; Ekoja and Smith, 2010). Field trials indicate that the vaccine induces a 75%–95% drop in egg output (Bassetto et al., 2014).

In general, helminth vaccines are not yet widely employed. There has been reluctance on the part of farmers to change established control procedures, especially when the major financial burden of these infestations is often borne by others. However, if highly effective, multivalent vaccines ever become available, they will revolutionize helminth parasite control (Ehsan et al., 2020).

IMMUNITY TO ARTHROPODS

When arthropods, such as ticks, fleas, or mosquitos, bite an animal, they inject saliva. This saliva contains digestive enzymes that assist the parasite in obtaining its blood meal. The saliva also contains components designed to minimize host responses; however, many are also antigenic (Fig. 29.13).

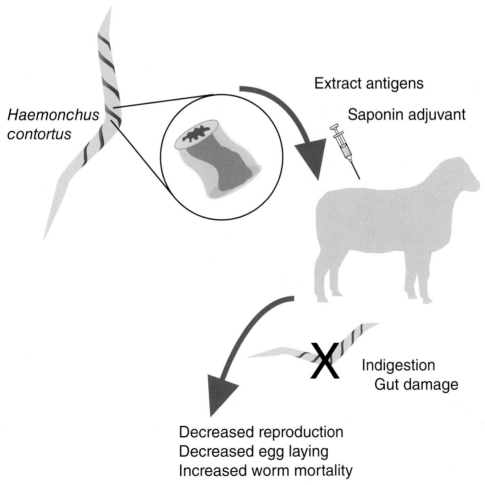

Fig. 29.12 The mechanism of action of the vaccine against *Haemonchus contortus*.

Host immune responses to injected arthropod salivary antigens are of three types. Some salivary components are of low molecular weight, bind to skin proteins such as collagen, and then act as haptens, stimulating Th1 responses. On subsequent exposure, these haptens may induce a delayed hypersensitivity response. Other salivary antigens may bind to epidermal Langerhans cells and induce cutaneous basophil hypersensitivity, a Th1 response associated with the production of IgG antibodies and a basophil infiltration. If these basophils are destroyed by antibasophil serum, resistance to biting arthropods is reduced. The third type of response to arthropod saliva is a Th2 response, leading to eosinophil infiltration, IgE production, mast cell degranulation, and type I hypersensitivity. This response may induce local inflammation, leading to urticaria, pain, and pruritus (Fig. 29.14). Each of these three types of response may modify the skin in such a way that the feeding of the offending arthropod is impaired, and the animal becomes a less attractive source of food. Unfortunately, natural selection and evolution ensure that the biting arthropod is well able to withstand such responses.

Demodectic Mange

The mange mites *Demodex folliculorum*, *Demodex canis*, and *Demodex injai* are common commensals that live within mammalian hair follicles and sebaceous glands. Normally present in low numbers, generalized demodicosis results from mite overgrowth. Under normal circumstances, an innate immune response to mite chitin and an adaptive response to mite antigens maintain mite populations at a low level. The development of generalized demodicosis results from defects in host immunity. The inflammatory reaction around mites and mite fragments contains mononuclear cells with a few plasma cells. The infiltrating lymphocytes are predominantly CD8+ T cells. There are also many ILC2 cells in these tissues, and recent studies suggest that it is these cells together with the IL-13 that they produce, that maintains stability within the parasitized hair follicles (Box 20.1). Dogs do, however, make

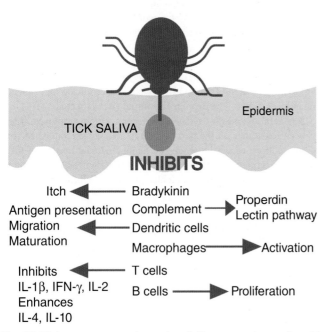

Fig. 29.13 Immunosuppressive and antiinflammatory factors found in tick saliva. Collectively, they act to permit prolonged tick attachment and feeding. *IL*, Interleukin; *IFN-γ*, interferon-γ.

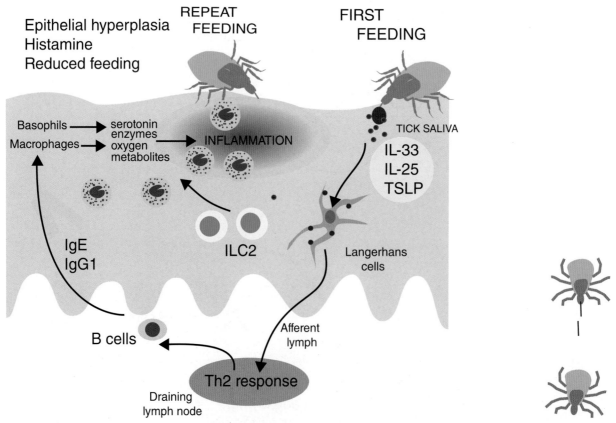

Fig. 29.14 The immune responses to tick bites. *IgE*, Immunoglobulin E; *IL*, interleukin; *ILC*, innate lymphoid cells; *TSLP*, thymic stromal lymphopoietin.

antibodies to mite proteins. The absence of eosinophils and edema in the lesion suggests that type I hypersensitivity is relatively unimportant. It is of interest to note that immunosuppressive agents such as antilymphocyte serum, azathioprine, or prolonged steroid therapy predispose animals to the development of demodectic mange. Animals with generalized demodicosis have normal neutrophil function and respond normally to vaccines or other foreign proteins. Nevertheless, their T-cell response to mitogens such as phytohemagglutinin and concanavalin A is depressed.

Flea Bite Dermatitis

Biting fleas secrete saliva into the skin wound. Some of the components of flea saliva are of low molecular weight and act as haptens after binding to dermal collagen. As a result, a local type IV hypersensitivity reaction characterized by a mononuclear cell infiltration occurs at the bite site. In some sensitized animals, this type IV reaction is gradually replaced over a period of months by a type I reaction, and the mononuclear cell infiltration gradually changes to an eosinophil infiltration. The immune response mounted by flea-allergic animals is protective. Thus, fleas produce fewer eggs on flea-allergic cats than on flea-naïve cats. Experimental vaccines containing the major antigens from the cat flea midgut have been able to reduce flea populations on dogs, and the female fleas recovered from these immunized animals produced significantly fewer eggs. This suggests that vaccination may eventually be effective in controlling flea populations (Jin et al., 2010).

Immune defenses also play a role in preventing invasion by other skin-penetrating arthropods. Body strike occurs when the larvae of the fly *Lucilia cuprina* attack the skin of a sheep. Sheep can be bred for low and high resistance to body strike. The resistant sheep have greater numbers of IgE-positive B cells in their skin than do susceptible sheep. Resistant sheep also mount a greater inflammatory response and produce more fluid exudate when injected with larval excretory and secretory products. On the other hand, larval proteases inhibit complement activation and degrade immunoglobulins.

Some success has been achieved with a recombinant salivary gland protein vaccine to disrupt blood feeding by horn flies (*Haematobia irritans*). It reduced blood meal size and delayed egg development in flies feeding on vaccinated animals.

Tick Infestation

Ticks are unique among arthropods in the way they attach and feed from their hosts for several days. This provides time for immune responses to occur and for ticks to employ countermeasures. For example, their saliva contains kininases that destroy bradykinin and histamine-binding proteins, thus reducing pain and itch. The salivary protein sialostatin-L2 inhibits inflammasome activation. The saliva of the tick *Ixodes scapularis* contains a protein that regulates the alternative complement pathway. It displaces properdin and enhances the degradation of C3bBb convertase. Tick saliva also contains an inhibitor of the complement-lectin pathway. As a result, host scratching and grooming responses are minimized.

Because tick salivary proteins are antigenic, they would be expected to induce adaptive immune responses that impair a tick's ability to feed. Ticks, however, have evolved immunosuppressive and antiinflammatory countermeasures that permit them to feed more effectively.

The saliva of *Ixodes ricinus* impairs the antigen-presenting abilities of dendritic cells. Tick saliva also inhibits the migration of dendritic cells from inflamed skin to draining lymph nodes and decreases their ability to present antigens to T cells. Furthermore, the treated dendritic cells preferentially stimulate Th2 responses. All these effects serve to facilitate the prolonged attachment and feeding of ticks.

Tick saliva impairs macrophage function and suppresses T-cell responses to mitogens, as well as the production of IL-1β and the Th1 cytokines IFN-γ and IL-2. It suppresses NK cell activity and macrophage nitric oxide production. Saliva from the ticks *Dermacentor andersoni* and *I. ricinus* increases the production of the Th2 cytokines IL-4 and IL-10. A tick salivary protein binds specifically to T-cell CD4 and blocks antigen-induced signaling and T cell responses. Saliva from *I. ricinus* also inhibits host B cell proliferation. Additionally, a serpin from *I. ricinus* interferes with the IL-6 pathway and consequently inhibits Th17 cell differentiation. A salivary protein from *I. scapularis* inhibits the proliferation of B cells exposed to the Osp proteins from the Lyme disease bacterium *Borrelia burgdorferi* but has no effect on T cells. It is abundantly clear that ticks have evolved many mechanisms to prevent immunological attack while they are feeding. Evasins are tick salivary proteins that inhibit mammalian chemokines and effectively inhibit leukocyte recruitment (Bhusal et al., 2020).

Basophils appear to play a critical role in immunity to tick infestation (Eberle and Voehringer, 2016). Initial sensitization by tick saliva stimulates an IgE response, and this IgE is bound by circulating basophils. Once sensitized, these basophils are recruited to tick attachment sites. Memory CD4+ T cells in the skin release IL-3 that attracts yet more basophils (Figure 34.3). The tick salivary antigens trigger basophil degranulation and histamine release. This histamine together with other mediators acts on keratinocytes to promote epidermal hyperplasia that enhances resistance by interfering with tick attachment (Karasuyama et al., 2018).

Thus, tick saliva contains components that suppress pain and itch, hemostasis, inflammation, adaptive immunity, and wound healing. Nevertheless, it has been observed that ticks on nonimmune animals are larger than those on immune animals. Although the nature of this resistance is unclear, it has been suggested that local hypersensitivity reactions to tick saliva may restrict the blood flow to the tick bite site, reduce its food supply, and stunt its growth. It is possible to immunize guinea pigs with tick homogenates and show that ticks feeding on these animals have reduced fecundity (Box 29.2).

Hypoderma Infestation

Unlike the arthropods described above, the larvae of the warble flies (*Hypoderma bovis* and *Hypoderma lineatum*) actually migrate through body tissues. These larvae must therefore evade the host's xenograft response. In fact, the first instar larvae of these flies do not trigger significant inflammation and are also immunosuppressive. Hypodermin A, the protease secreted by these larvae, can inhibit responses to mitogens and reduce IL-2 production, probably by destroying cell surface receptors. Vaccination with a cloned *Hypoderma* protein has effectively protected cattle against subsequent infestations.

ARTHROPOD VACCINES

If an animal is immunized with intestinal antigens from ticks, the ingested antibodies may cause intestinal damage. These internal antigens have been called "hidden" or "concealed" antigens since, under normal circumstances, the host would not usually encounter them. Vaccines can therefore be made containing a gut membrane-bound glycoprotein from the intestine of the tick *Rhiphicephalus microplus*. Vaccines made against antigens from the intestine of the tick *R. microplus* can inhibit tick reproduction. Indeed, a tick vaccine using a recombinant antigen, Bm86, is available in Australia and Central America. The antibodies produced bind to the brush border of tick intestinal cells, inhibit endocytosis, and prevent the tick from engorging fully. Thus, its digestive processes are impaired, and the tick experiences starvation, loss of fecundity, and weakness and may disengage

BOX 29.2 Alpha-Gal Allergy

About 28 million years ago, an ancestral primate underwent a mutation in the gene that encodes the galactosyl transferase that makes galactose alpha-1,3-galactose (alpha-gal)-linked carbohydrates. As a result, this enzyme was functionally inactivated. Ever since then, their descendants (including humans, apes, and old-world monkeys) lack the ability to make glycoproteins and glycolipids with alpha-gal side chains. All other mammals have retained the enzyme. As a result, alpha-gal is expressed on cell surfaces in nonprimates. It is found in skeletal muscle, organs, milk, and gelatin. Most humans make "natural" IgM and IgG antibodies against this foreign oligosaccharide because of continuous exposure to it from the gut microbiota.

Alpha-gal is present in the saliva of some ticks. As a result, some humans make IgE against alpha-gal in response to a tick bite. (This is somewhat unusual since it is the only carbohydrate known to act as a major allergen. All the other allergens are proteins.) Alpha-gal allergens have been detected in the salivary glands of two North American tick species, *Amblyomma americanum* and *Ixodes scapularis*. There are three theories as to its origin. It may be produced directly by the tick salivary glands. It may represent residual antigen left over in ticks that have recently fed on the blood of another mammal. Or it may be produced by commensal microbes within the tick. Tick bites preferentially attract large numbers of basophils (Eberle and Voehringer, 2016). These basophils establish a local environment that favors type 2 responses. Thus the combination of alpha-gal and an environment that promotes type 2 responses may trigger the IgE response. Dogs are an alpha-gal-positive species so alpha-gal allergies would not be expected to occur in dogs. However, it has been reported that healthy dogs may develop IgM antibodies to alpha-gal in response to bites of the tick, *Ixodes ricinus*. In this case, it has been speculated that something in the tick saliva results in a breakdown in tolerance.

When tick-sensitized individuals encounter the alpha-gal oligosaccharide by eating beef, pork, venison, lamb, goat, or rabbit, for example, they may develop a delayed onset anaphylaxis. This occurs not only in response to meats but also to vaccines that contain gelatin or to drugs ingested in gelatin capsules. As a result, allergic responses to alpha-gal are unusually common. Although mediated by IgE, the onset of symptoms may be delayed for 4–8 hours or longer after ingesting the meat. About 70% of victims develop respiratory distress, urticaria, and possible anaphylaxis. The unusual delay in the allergic response to alpha-gal is a result of slow passage of allergenic glycolipids across the intestinal epithelium. These sensitizing molecules will only cross the epithelial barrier when bound to lipids. While glycoproteins can cross into the bloodstream in 1–2 hours, it takes 4–5 hours for dietary lipids to reach the circulation carried by chylomicrons. Thus, the slower digestion and absorption of the glycolipids causes a delay in the onset of clinical signs.

Tick bites also induce anti-α-Gal antibodies in dogs, and these may be protective against *Anaplasma phagocytophilum*. (From Hodžic, A., et al., 2019. Tick bites induce anti-α-Gal antibodies in dogs. Vaccines 7, 114–128.)

from its host. As a result, the number of ticks on vaccinated animals is reduced. Experimental multicomponent tick vaccines show even more encouraging results (De La Fuente et al., 2016; Rodriguez-Mallon, 2016).

There is a commercially available vaccine against aquatic sea lice, a major problem in marine aquaculture. This is an oil-adjuvanted recombinant subunit vaccine against a protein (vitellogenin-1) of the louse *Caligus rogercresseyi*. Encouraging results have also been obtained with experimental vaccines directed against the red poultry mite (*Dermanyssus gallinae*). Initial studies with crude mite extracts have been followed by identification of candidate vaccine antigens (Jin et al., 2010).

REFERENCES

Adams, P.N., Aldridge, A., Vukman, K.V., Donnelly, S., O'neill, S.M., 2014. *Fasciola hepatica* tegumental antigens indirectly induce an M2 macrophage-like phenotype in vivo. Parasite Immunol. 36, 531–539.

Altet, L., Francino, O., Solano-Gallego, L., et al., 2002. Mapping and sequencing of the canine *NRAMPI* gene and identification of mutations in leishmaniasis-susceptible dogs. Infect. Immun. 70, 2763–2771.

Baneth, G., Koutinas, A.F., Solano-Gallego, L., et al., 2008. Canine leishmaniosis: new concepts and insights on an expanding zoonosis: part one. Trends Parasitol. 24, 324–330.

Barbour, A.G., Restrepo, B.I., 2000. Antigenic variation in vector-borne pathogens. Emerg. Infect. Dis. 6, 449–456.

Bassetto, C.C., Picharillo, M.É., Newlands, G.F., Smith, W.D., Fernandes, S., Siqueira, E.R., Amarante, A.F., 2014. Attempts to vaccinate ewes and their lambs against natural infection with *Haemonchus contortus* in a tropical environment. Int. J. Parasitol. 44, 1049–1054.

Bhusal, R.P., Eaton, J.R.O., Chowdhury, S.T., Power, C.A., et al., 2020. Evasins: tick salivary proteins that inhibit mammalian chemokines. Trends Biochem. Sci. https://doi.org/10.1016/j.tibs.2019.10.003.

Brake, D.A., 2002. Vaccinology for control of apicomplexan parasites: a simplified language of immune programming and its use in vaccine design. Int. J. Parasitol. 32, 509–515.

Calzetta, L., Pistocchini, E., Ritondo, B.L., Roncada, P., et al., 2020. Immunoprophylaxis pharmacotherapy against canine leishmaniosis: a systematic review and meta-analysis on the efficacy of vaccines approved in European Union. Vaccine. https://doi.org/10.1016/j.vaccine.2020.08.051.

Cliffe, L.J., Humphreys, N.E., Lane, T.E., et al., 2005. Accelerated intestinal epithelial cell turnover: a new mechanism of parasite expulsion. Science 308, 1463–1465.

Coakley, G., Harris, N.L., 2020. The intestinal epithelium at the forefront of host-helminth interactions. Trends Parasitol. 36 (9), 761–772.

De La Fuente, J., Kopacek, P., Lew-Tabor, A., Maritz-Olivier, C., 2016. Strategies for new and improved vaccines against ticks and tick-borne diseases. Parasite Immunol. https://doi.org/10.1111/pim.12339 2016.

Díaz, A., Allen, J.E., 2007. Mapping immune response profiles: the emerging scenario from helminth immunology. Eur. J. Immunol. 37, 3319–3326.

Eberle, J.U., Voehringer, D., 2016. Role of basophils in protective immunity to parasitic infections. Semin. Immunopathol. 38 (5), 605–613.

Ehsan, M., Hu, R.-S., Liang, Q.-L., Hou, J.-L., et al., 2020. Advances in the development of anti-*Haemonchus contortus* vaccines: challenges, opportunities, and perspectives. Vaccines 8, 555. https://doi.org/10.3390/vaccines8030555.

Ekoja, S.E., Smith, W.D., 2010. Antibodies from sheep immunized against *Haemonchus contortus* with H-gal-GP inhibit the haemoglobinase activity of this protease complex. Parasite Immunol. 32, 11–12.

Fabre, V., Beitin, D.P., Bliss, S.K., et al., 2009. Eosinophil deficiency compromises parasite survival in chronic nematode infection. J. Immunol. 182, 1577–1583.

Fernandez Cotrina, J., et al., 2018. A large-scale field randomized trial demonstrates safety and efficacy of the vaccine LetiFend(R) against *Canine leishmaniosis*. Vaccine 36 (15), 1972–1982.

Florin-Christensen, M., Suarez, C.E., Rodriguez, A.E., Flores, D.A., Schnittger, L., 2014. Vaccines against *Bovine babesiosis*: where we are now and possible roads ahead. Parasitology 141, 1563–1592.

Flynn, R.J., Mulcahy, G., 2008. Possible role for toll-like receptors in interaction of *Fasciola hepatica* excretory/secretory products with bovine macrophages. Infect. Immun. 76, 678–684.

Gerbe, F., Jay, P., 2016. Intestinal tuft cells: epithelial sentinels linking luminal cues to the immune system. Mucosal Immunol. 9, 1353–1359.

Gigley, J.P., Bhardra, R., Moretto, M.M., Khan, I.A., 2012. T cell exhaustion in protozoan disease. Trends Parasitol. 28, 377–384.

Grencis, R.K., Worthington, J.J., 2016. Tuft cells: a new flavor in innate epithelial immunity. Trends Parasitol. 32, 583–585.

Gronke, K., Diefenbach, A., 2016. Tuft cell-derived IL-25 activates and maintains ILC2. Immunol. Cell. Biol. 94, 221–223.

Horcajo, P., Regidor-Cerrillo, J., Aguado-Martinez, A., Hemphill, A., Ortega-Mora, L.M., 2016. Vaccines for *Bovine neosporosis*: current status and key aspects for development. Parasit Immunol. 38, 709–723.

Humphreys, N.E., Xu, D., Hepworth, M.R., et al., 2008. IL-33, a potent inducer of adaptive immunity to intestinal nematodes. J. Immunol. 80, 2443–2449.

Jin, J., Ding, Z., Meng, F., et al., 2010. An immunotherapeutic treatment against flea allergy dermatitis in cats by co-immunization of DNA and protein vaccines. Vaccine 28, 1997–2004.

Karasuyama, H., Tabakawa, Y., Ohta, T., Wada, T., Yoshikawa, S., et al., 2018. Crucial role for basophils in acquired protective immunity to tick infestation. Front. Physiol. 9 https://doi.org/10.3389/fphys.2018.01769

Lightowlers, M.W., 2013. Control of *Taenia solium* taeniasis/cysticercosis: past practices and new possibilities. Parasitology 140, 1566–1577.

Martini, F., Eckmair, B., Stefanic, S., Jin, C., et al., 2019. Highly modified and immunoactive N-glycans of the canine heartworm. Nat. Commun. https://doi.org/10.1038/s41467-018-07948-7

McRae, K.M., Stear, M.J., Good, B., Keane, O.M., 2015. The host immune response to gastrointestinal nematode infection in sheep. Parasite Immunol. 37, 605–613.

Meeusen, E.N.T., Balic, A., 2000. Do eosinophils have a role in the killing of helminth parasites? Parasitol Today 16, 95–101.

Morchón, R., Carretón, E., Grandi, G., González-Miguel, J., et al., 2012. Anti-Wolbachia surface protein antibodies are present in the urine of dogs naturally infected with *Dirofilaria immitis* with circulating microfilariae but not in dogs with occult infections. Vector Born Zoonotic Dis. 12 (1), 17–20.

Petavy, A.F., Hormaeche, C., Lahmar, S., Ouhelli, H., et al., 2008. An oral recombinant vaccine in dogs against *Echinococcus granulosus*, the causal agent of human hytadid disease: a pilot study. PLoS Negl. Trop. Dis. 2, e125. https://doi.org/10.1371/journal.pntd.0000125

Roberts, L.B., Schnoeller, C., Berkachy, R., Darby, M., et al., 2021. Acetylcholine production by group 2 innate lymphoid cells promotes mucosal immunity to helminths. Sci. Immunol. 6 eabd0359.

Rodriguez-Mallon, A., 2016. Developing anti-tick vaccines. Methods Mol. Biol. 1404, 243–259.

Schetters, T., 2005. Vaccination against canine babesiosis. Trends Parasitol. 21, 179–184.

Schneider, C., O'Leary, C.E., Locksley, R.M., 2019. Regulation of immune responses by tuft cells. Nat. Rev. Immunol. 19 (9), 584–593. https://doi.org/10.1038/s41577-019-0176-x.

Simón, F., Siles-Lucas, M., Morchón, R., González-Miguel, J., et al., 2012. Human and animal Dirofilariasis: the emergence of a zoonotic mosaic. Clin. Microbiol Rev. 25 (3), 507–544.

Toepp, A.J., Petersen, C.A., 2020. The balancing act: immunology in Leishmaniosis. Res. Vet. Sci. 130, 19–25.

Voehringer, D., 2009. The role of basophils in helminth infection. Trends Parasitol. 25, 551–556.

Weber, F.H., Jackson, J.A., Sobecki, B., Choromanski, L., Olsen, M., et al., 2013. On the efficacy and safety of vaccination with live tachyzoites of *Neospora caninum* for prevention of Neospora-associated fetal loss in cattle. Clin. Vacc. Immunol. 20, 99–105.

Wildblood, L.A., Kerr, K., Clark, D.A.S., et al., 2005. Production of eosinophils chemoattractant activity by ovine gastrointestinal nematodes,. Vet. Immunol. Immunopathol. 107, 57–65.

Zaph, C., Cooper, P.J., Harris, N.L., 2014. Mucosal immune responses following intestinal nematode infection. Parasite Immunol. 36, 439–452.

Mast Cell– and Eosinophil-Mediated Hypersensitivity

Adverse reactions triggered by the immune responses are called hypersensitivity reactions. They are classified into four major types based on their pathogenesis. Type I hypersensitivity reactions are inflammatory diseases that result from the release of the contents of mast cell, basophil, and eosinophil cytoplasmic granules. This granule release is triggered when antigens bind to IgE on the surface of mast cells or basophils. The granule contents consist of a mixture of molecules that trigger inflammation and attract eosinophils (Fig. 30.1). This inflammation plays an important role in resistance to parasitic helminths and arthropods. It is also, however, a cause of unwanted inflammatory disease and thus of major significance in veterinary medicine. Immunoglobulin E production is characteristic of type 1 hypersensitivity responses.

INDUCTION OF TYPE I HYPERSENSITIVITY

Animals are continuously exposed to environmental antigens (the exposome) in food, through skin contact, and in inhaled air. Most individuals will respond to these antigens by producing IgG or IgA antibodies, and there are no obvious clinical consequences. Some animals, however, respond by mounting an exaggerated Th2 response and so produce excessive IgE. It is these animals that develop type I hypersensitivity reactions or allergies. The excessive production of IgE is called atopy, and affected individuals are said to be atopic. The development of atopy and type I hypersensitivity results from the interaction between genes and environmental factors, especially the intestinal microbiota. The genetics of atopy and allergy are complex. If both parents are atopic, most of their offspring will also be atopic and will suffer from allergies. If only one parent is atopic, the percentage of atopic offspring varies. There is also a breed predisposition to atopy in dogs. For example, atopic dermatitis is most commonly observed in Terriers (Bull, Welsh, Cairn, West Highland White, Scottish), Dalmatians, and Irish Setters, although nonpurebred dogs may also be affected. The heritability of atopic dermatitis in Labrador and Golden Retrievers is estimated to be a relatively high 0.47. In horses, high levels of IgE and allergic responses are associated with certain ELA-DRB haplotypes.

Normal animals infested by parasitic worms and insects also produce IgE and it is believed that the IgE response may have evolved specifically to counteract these organisms. Chitin, the biopolymer that confers structural rigidity on fungi, insects, and parasitic helminths, induces the accumulation of eosinophils and basophils in tissues and may be a key trigger of some allergic reactions (Burton and Zaccone 2007). Indeed, the "self-cure" reaction seen in parasitized sheep has long been the only recognized benefit of type I hypersensitivity. It is of interest to note that both atopic and parasitized dogs may have reduced IgA levels, an observation supporting the concept that a deficiency of IgA may predispose to a compensatory increase in IgE (see Chapter 40) (Tizard, 2022).

IMMUNOGLOBULIN E

IgE is an immunoglobulin of conventional four-chain structure and about 200 kDa (see Fig. 17.7). It is found in serum in exquisitely small quantities (24–410 μg/mL in dogs), and its serum half-life is only 2 days (Table 30.1). Most IgE is firmly bound to Fcε receptors on tissue mast cells, where it has a half-life of 11–12 days. Some mast cells situated close to blood vessels can extend their cytoplasmic processes between the endothelial cells and into the vascular lumen to "fish" for IgE that then binds to their receptors. Some IgG subclasses may also bind to mast cell FcR and mediate type I hypersensitivity reactions. For example, IgG4 has been associated with some cases of canine atopic dermatitis. However, the affinity of IgG4 for Fc receptors is much lower than that of IgE, and it is of much less clinical significance.

Immunoglobulin E Production

Atopic individuals are predisposed to mount type 2 immune responses. Their Th2 cells produce interleukin-4 (IL-4), IL-5, and IL-13. The production of IgE appears to be driven by a specific subset of follicular helper T cells that produce this IL-13 (Gowthaman et al., 2019).

These, together with costimulation by CD40, trigger B cell IgE synthesis (Fig. 30.2).

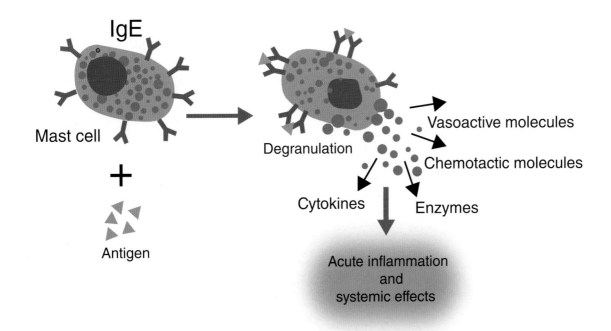

Fig. 30.1 The mechanism of type I hypersensitivity reactions. Numerous biologically active molecules and inflammatory mediators are released by mast cells when antigen cross-links two immunoglobulin E (IgE) molecules on the mast cell surface. Some are produced immediately. Others may be synthesized within minutes or hours.

TABLE 30.1 Serum Immunoglobulin E (IgE) Levels in Domestic Mammals and Humans

Species	"NORMAL" IgE (Range)	Range in Allergic or Parasitized Animals
Human[a]	5–513 ng/mL	<240 ng/mL
Dog[b]	182 ± 112 µg/mL (24–410)	195 ± 108 µg/mL (85–550)
Cat[c]	46 ± 19 µg/mL	328 ± 124 µg/mL
Horse[d]	84 ± 90.9 µg/mL	109 ± 69 µg/mL
Sheep[e]	1.8 ± 1.3 µg/mL	15–30 µg/mL
Pig[f]	2 µg/mL	~5 µg/mL

[a]From Martins, T.B., Bandhauer, M.E., Bunker, A.M., et al., 2013. New childhood and adult reference intervals for total IgE. J. Allergy Clin. Immunol. 33(2), 589–591.
[b]From Nimmo Wilkie, J.S., Yager, J.A., Eyre, P., Parker, W.M., 1990. Morphometric analysis of the skin of dogs with atopic dermatitis and correlations with cutaneous and plasma histamine and total serum IgE. Vet. Pathol. 27(3), 179–186.
[c]From Delgado, C., Lee-Fowler, T.M., DeClue, A.E., Reinero, C.R., 2010. Feline-specific serum total IgE quantitation in normal, asthmatic and parasitized cats. J. Feline Med. Surg. 12, 991–994.
[d]From Wagner B., 2009. IgE in horses: occurrence in health and disease. Vet. Immunol. Immunopathol. 132, 21–30.
[e]From Shaw, R.J., McNeill, M.M., Gatehouse, T.K., Douch, P.G., 1997. Quantitation of total sheep IgE concentration using anti-ovine IgE monoclonal antibodies in an enzyme immunoassay. Vet. Immunol. Immunopathol. 57, 253–265.
[f]From Wu, J.J., Cao, C.M., Meng, T.T., Zhang, Y., et al., 2016. Induction of immune responses and allergic reactions in piglets by injecting glycinin. Ital. J. Anim. Sci. (1), 166–173.

Immunoglobulin E Receptors

Mammals have two types of IgE receptors: high-affinity FcεRI and low-affinity FcεRII (CD23). FcεRI occurs in two forms. One form is expressed on mast cells, basophils, neutrophils, and eosinophils. It consists of four peptide chains, one α, one β, and two γ chains (αβγγ) (Fig. 30.3). The α chain binds IgE, the β chain stabilizes the complex, and the γ chains serve as signal transducers. (This same γ chain is also a signal transducer in FcγRI, FcγRIII, and γ/δ TCR.) The affinity of FcεRI for IgE is very high (10^{-10} M), so they bind almost irreversibly and thus ensure that mast cells are constantly coated with IgE. An important feature of these receptors is their range of expression. Once expressed on the cell surface, their half-life is about 24 hours. Some are recycled, while most are internalized and degraded. In the absence of IgE, there are about 8000 FcεRI per cell (on circulating basophils). Binding of IgE to these receptors stabilizes them, slows their degradation, and reduces their turnover. As a result, receptor numbers can climb to an average of 250,000/cell in allergic subjects. Receptor numbers cannot, however, keep pace with IgE production, and they can be readily swamped by high levels of nonantigen-specific IgE. A second form of FcεRI contains only three chains: one α- and two γ-chains (αγγ). It is expressed on antigen-presenting dendritic cells and monocytes. When an antigen-IgE complex binds to this receptor, it is ingested and treated as exogenous antigen. The expression of FcεRI on antigen-presenting cells is enhanced by IL-4 from Th2 cells. Thus, a positive feedback loop (the allergy loop) develops (Fig. 30.4). The antigen processing cells present antigen more effectively to Th2 cells. The Th2 cells then secrete IL-4 and enhance IgE production.

The second IgE receptor, FcεRII (CD23), is a selectin expressed on B cells, NK cells, macrophages, dendritic cells, eosinophils, and platelets. In addition to binding IgE, FcεRII also binds to the complement receptor CR2 (CD21) (Fig. 30.5). Thus B cells expressing FcεRII can

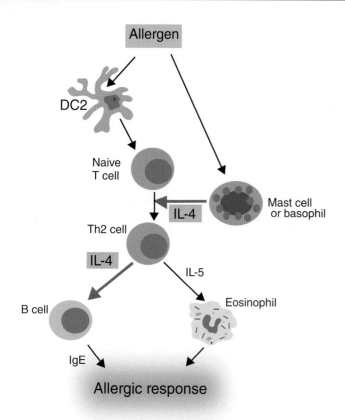

Fig. 30.2 The central role of interleukin-4 (IL-4) in induction of immuno-globin E (IgE) responses. IL-4 is produced by Th2 cells. Once released, it promotes the development of more Th2 cells, which are major sources of this cytokine and promote IgE responses. The degranulation of mast cells also releases IL-4, which further promotes this reaction. Nature killer cells may serve as an initial source of IL-4. The response to IL-4 is inhibited by interferon-γ and IL-12.

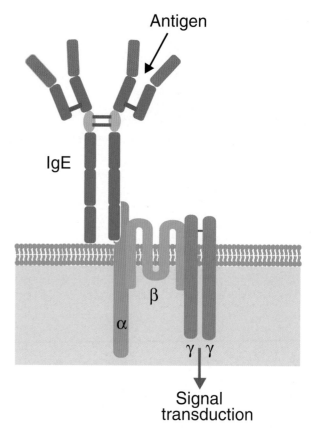

Fig. 30.3 The structure of FcεRI with a bound Immunoglobin E (IgE) molecule. This tetrameric form of the IgE receptor containing two γ chains is found on mast cells and basophils.

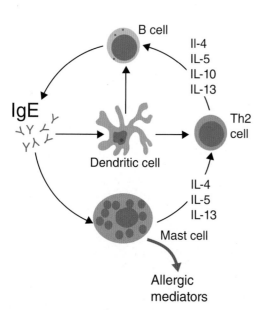

Fig. 30.4 The allergy loop. Dendritic cells express FcεRI and, as a result, can bind antigen-immunoglobin E (IgE) complexes. This antigen, once processed, stimulates Th2 responses. These Th2 cells in turn secrete cytokines, which further promote the IgE response. *IL*, Interleukin.

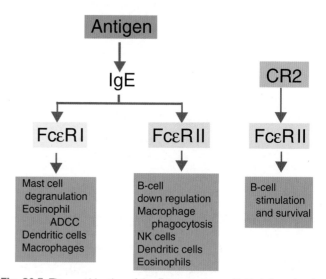

Fig. 30.5 The combination of the Fcε receptors with their ligands stimulates many different responses in mast cells depending on the nature of these stimuli. FcεRII also acts as a complement receptor. *ADCC*, Antibody-dependent cell-mediated cytotoxicity; *IgE*, immunoglobin E; *NK*, natural killer.

link to CR2 on other B cells, T cells, and dendritic cells. By linking B cells to dendritic cells, FcεRII enhances B cell survival and promotes IgE production.

MAST CELLS

Mast cells play an essential role in allergic diseases and innate immunity (Voehringer, 2013). They are located close to body surfaces and act as sentinel cells. They recognize pathogen-associated molecular patterns (PAMPs) and damage-associated molecular patterns (DAMPs) through their PRRs and, in response, release inflammatory cytokines within minutes (see Chapter 3). This release normally occurs in a controlled manner and ensures that the severity and type of inflammation are appropriate to the body's immediate needs—but not always!

Structure and Location

Mast cells are large, ovoid cells (15–20 μm in diameter) scattered throughout the body in connective tissue, under mucosal surfaces, and around nerves (Fig. 30.6). They are found in greatest numbers under the skin or in the intestine and airways. They are easily recognizable because their cytoplasm is densely packed with large granules that stain strongly with dyes such as toluidine blue. These granules often mask the large, bean-shaped nucleus (Fig. 30.7). (Mast cells are so called because, being full of granules, they were considered to be "well-fed cells" [German *Mastzellen*].)

Life History

There are two distinct mast cell populations in rodents. One occurs in the mucosa, the other is found in connective tissues (Table 30.2).

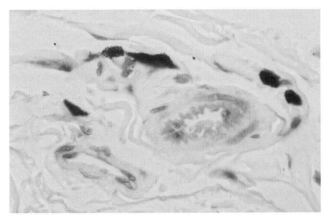

Fig. 30.6 A section of canine skin stained to show mast cells. The mast cells stain intensely because of the heparin in their cytoplasmic granules.

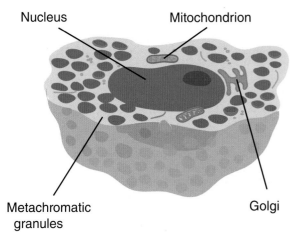

Fig. 30.7 The structural features of a connective tissue mast cell. The term *metachromatic* simply means that the granules stain intensely.

Mucosal mast cells arise from bone marrow–derived stem cells and are present in the intestinal mucosa and the lung. They are located beneath the epithelial cells lining the mucosal surfaces of the intestine and lung. They contain chondroitin sulfate but little histamine. Connective tissue mast cells, in contrast, arise from fetal liver stem cells. They are found in the skin, around blood vessels, and in the peritoneal cavity. They are rich in histamine and heparin. Connective tissue mast cell numbers remain relatively constant, but mucosal mast cells proliferate in the presence of intestinal worms. Induced mucosal mast cells disappear within a few weeks after the parasites have been eliminated (Gurish and Boyce, 2002).

Many different stimuli can trigger mast cell degranulation. The best recognized of these are IgE-plus-specific allergens. Allergies, however, are a special type of inflammation. Numerous other signals can cause mast cells to degranulate, including cytokines, chemokines, chemical agents, physical stimuli, insect and animal venoms, and viruses. Many alarmins, including the defensins, anaphylatoxins, IL-33, neuropeptides, adenosine, and endothelins (small peptides from endothelial cells), can also trigger mast cell degranulation.

Most mast cells express pattern-recognition receptors including TLRs, NLRs, RLRs, complement receptors, and the mannose receptor (CD48) (Agier et al., 2018). Triggering of these TLRs causes mast cells to release different mixtures of cytokines, chemokines, and lipid mediators. Thus, bacterial peptidoglycans acting through TLR2 may stimulate histamine release, whereas lipopolysaccharides acting through TLR4 do not. Bacterial binding to mast cell TLRs triggers TNF-α and IL-6 production. Mast cells can thus use these receptors to distinguish between different pathogens and release a select mixture of cytokines, chemokines, and other inflammatory mediators, depending on the nature of the stimulus. The inflammatory mediators released by mast cells activate nearby immune cells. They facilitate local neutrophil and eosinophil recruitment, activation, and bactericidal activity (Sandig and Bulfone-Paus, 2012).

MAST CELLS AND ANTIGENS

Although there are numerous ways by which mast cells can degranulate, the best studied of these is mediated by IgE bound to FcεRI on the cell surface (Fig. 30.8). Mast cells coated in this way are primed to bind antigen. The mast cell can reside in tissues, with its attached IgE acting like a mine in a minefield. If an antigen encounters the bound antibody, the receptor is activated, and the mast cell releases its granules into the surrounding tissues.

Perivascular dendritic cells continually probe nearby blood vessels by extending their processes (dendrites) through blood vessel walls

TABLE 30.2	Comparison of the Two Major Types of Mast Cell	
	Mucosal Mast Cells	**Connective Tissue Mast Cells**
Structure	Few, variable-sized granules	Many uniform granules
Size	9–10 μm diameter	19–20 μm diameter
Proteoglycan	Chondroitin sulfate	Heparin
Histamine	1.3 pg/cell	15 pg/cell
Lifespan	<40 days	>6 months
Location	Intestinal wall, lung	Peritoneal cavity, skin

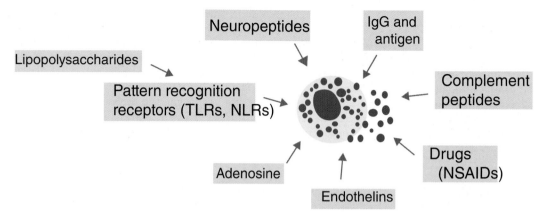

Fig. 30.8 Some of the stimuli that make mast cells degranulate. Antigen bound through IgE causes rapid complete degranulation. The other stimuli shown cause a more gradual, piecemeal degranulation. Thus, in normal inflammatory responses, the degree of mast cell degranulation is tailored to local defensive needs. *IgG*, Immunoglobulin G; *NLRs*, NOD-like receptors; *NSAIDs*, nonsteroidal antiinflammatory drugs; *TLRs*, toll-like receptors.

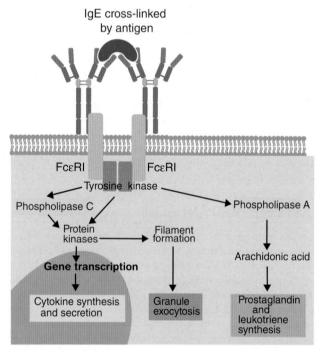

Fig. 30.9 A simplified view of mast cell signal transduction. The process is triggered by cross-linking two bound Immunoglobin E (IgE) molecules with antigen. The combined signal eventually leads to degranulation (granule exocytosis), leukotriene and prostaglandin synthesis, and cytokine production.

and directly sample any allergens they encounter. By using nonspecific mannose-binding receptors, these DCs can readily capture a broad range of circulating allergens. These allergens are not internalized or processed, but they are incorporated into microvesicles. The microvesicles, ranging from 50 to 1000 nm in size, then bud off from the membrane of the DC2 cells into the perivascular space. Direct cell-cell contact between the DCs, and mast cells may also occur, although it is not essential for the triggering of anaphylaxis. When mast cells coated with high-affinity IgE encounter, and their receptors are cross-linked by, allergen-loaded vesicles, they respond by rapid degranulation (Fig. 30.9; Valenta et al., 2018; Choi et al., 2018).

Thus allergens do not have to leave blood vessels or enter tissues to come into contact with mast cells (Cheng et al., 2013).

Mast Cell Degranulation

Mast cell degranulation is initiated when an antigen molecule cross-links IgE on two FcεRI receptors and activates their tyrosine kinases. These, in turn, activate phospholipase C, leading to the production of diacylglycerol and inositol triphosphate. These second messengers then increase intracellular calcium and activate more protein kinases. The protein kinases phosphorylate myosin in the cytoskeleton so that the granules move to the cell surface. Granule membranes then fuse with the plasma membrane, and their contents are released into the extracellular fluid (Fig. 30.10; MacGlashan, 2008).

Cross-linking of two FcεRI by an antigen also activates phospholipase A. This acts on membrane phospholipids to produce arachidonic acid. Other enzymes then convert the arachidonic acid to the inflammatory lipids, leukotrienes, and prostaglandins (Fig. 3.9). Finally, the protein kinases promote transcription of genes coding for many different cytokines as well as for cyclooxygenases and lipoxygenase. The degranulation of mast cells is the central event in the development of allergic reactions.

Mast cell granules contain a complex mixture of potent proinflammatory molecules. Some granules in mouse mast cells contain serotonin or cathepsin D, whereas others contain histamine and TNF-α. Different stimuli determine which granule subsets are exocytosed and, thus, which mediators are released. It is likely that different clinical forms of allergy may be determined by the mixtures of mediators released. The speed of these responses also differs among mast cells. For example, degranulation occurs within seconds after antigen binds to receptor-bound IgE (Fig. 30.10).

Mast Cell–Derived Mediators

Mast cell granules are loaded with amines such as histamine, serotonin, and dopamine; lipids such as prostaglandins, and leukotrienes; lysosomal enzymes including tryptases, chymases, and cathepsins; cytokines such as TNF-α, IL-4, -5, -6, -15; and some chemokines (Fig. 30.11). Mast cells can capture and store IL-17 by endocytosis. It is then released in allergic reactions. Mucosal mast cells secrete IL-9 in response to IL-33 and mast cell proteases, which can help drive food allergies (Chen et al., 2015; Mukai et al. 2018).

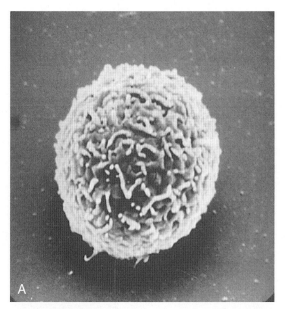

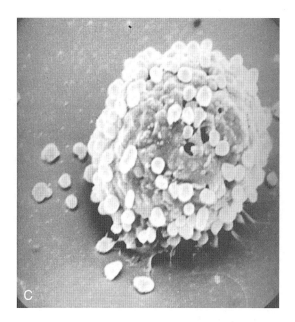

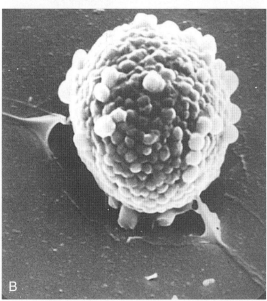

Fig. 30.10 Scanning electron micrographs. (A) A normal rat mast cell. (B) A sensitized mast cell fixed 5 s after exposure to antigen. (C) A sensitized mast cell fixed 60 s after exposure to antigen. Original magnification × 3000. From Tizard, I.R., Holmes, W.L., 1974. Degranulation of sensitised rat peritoneal mast cells in response to antigen, compound 48–80 and polymyxin B. A scanning electron microscope study. Int. Arch. Allergy. Appl. Immunol. 46, 867–879.

Mast cells also release small heparin-containing granules that are especially rich in TNF-α. These granules are carried in afferent lymph to draining lymph nodes, where they trigger changes in cell behavior. The presence of heparin stabilizes the TNF-α so that it persists after delivery (Mukai et al., 2018).

Mast cells also produce chitinases. Chitin is characteristically found in insects, fungi, and helminths, and the production of chitinases supports the suggestion that allergic reactions may have evolved to combat these invaders. Chitin itself is a key allergen in some helminth infections.

The Master Cytokines

Three cytokines play a critical role in triggering and regulating allergic inflammation. These are IL-33, IL-25 and TSLP. All three promote Th2 and ILC2 activation as well as cytokine production (Stanbery et al., 2022).

Interleukin-33

IL-33 is a 30 kDa protein belonging to the IL-1 family and found in many different cell types, especially the cells that act as epithelial barriers. These include keratinocytes, bronchial epithelial cells, and enterocytes. It is present in endothelial cells lining blood vessels (Haraldsen et al., 2009). IL-33 is not secreted like a conventional cytokine but is stored in the cell nucleus where it regulates DNA transcription. It is only released by cell death, injury, or stress. It can also be released by living cells following activation of their protease-activated receptors (Enoksson et al., 2011). It promotes allergic diseases while playing a protective role in helminth infections (Liew et al., 2016).

IL-33 functions as an alarmin when it escapes from damaged or dying cells (Fig. 30.12) (Lunderius-Andersson et al., 2012). It is especially potent at activating ILC2 cells, but it also activates DC2 cells, Th2,

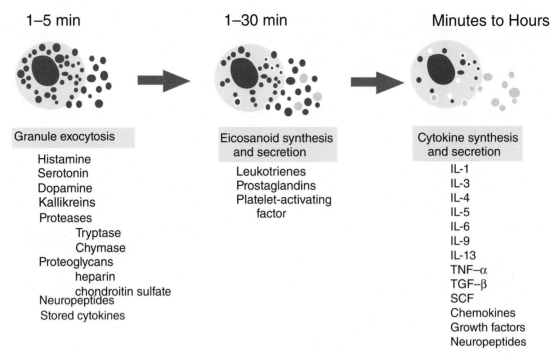

Fig. 30.11 The soluble mediators released from degranulating mast cells. These fall into three categories: molecules released from exocytosed granules, lipids (eicosanoids) synthesized within minutes, and proteins synthesized over several hours. *IL,* Interleukin; *SCF,* stem cell factor; *TGF-β*, transforming growth factor–β; *TNF-α,* tumor necrosis factor–α.

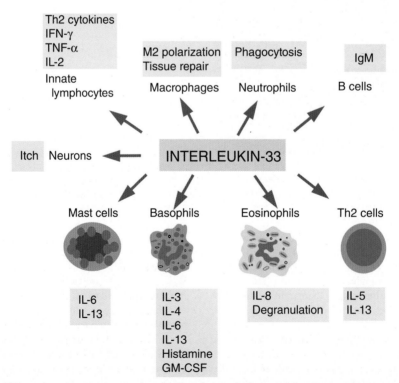

Fig. 30.12 The biological properties of interleukin-33 (IL-33). Interleukin-33 is released by dying cells as well as epithelial cells in response to pathogen-associated molecular patterns. It stimulates the production of inflammatory cytokines and chemokines from many different cell types. It stimulates the production of eosinophils. It acts on sensory neurons to induce itch. *GM-CSF,* Granulocyte-macrophage colony-stimulating factor; *IFN-γ,* interferon-γ; *TNF-α,* tumor necrosis factor–α.

and Tfh cells as well as Tregs and mast cells. The release of IL-33 therefore results in the development of type 2 allergic inflammation. IL-33 is a key inducer of the type 2 cytokines, IL-4, -5 and -13. When IL-33 is exposed to neutrophil and mast cell proteases, it is broken into short peptides. These peptides promote type 2 activity by stimulating mast cell and ILC2 cell production of IL-5, IL-6, and IL-13, and thus triggering an eosinophilia (Aoki et al., 2016).

IL-33 promotes IgE-mediated degranulation of mast cells as well as IgE production, eosinophilia and goblet cell proliferation. Additionally, it induces mast cell production of leukotrienes and cytokines and, as a result, can trigger acute allergic attacks in the absence of allergen. IL-33 also binds to sensory neurons triggering intense pruritus and scratching behavior. IL-33 is thus a key mediator of atopic disease.

TSLP

Thymic stromal lymphopoietin (TSLP) is a 15 kDa member of the IL-2 family that regulates type 2 inflammation at mucosal barriers. It is expressed by bronchial and colonic epithelial cells, mast cells, keratinocytes, tuft cells, and lung fibroblasts. Its highest expression is in bronchial smooth muscle cells and in keratinocytes. TSLP production is upregulated in inflamed skin. Its release is stimulated by contact with allergens (especially those with protease activity), infections, and some chemicals.

TSLP may be considered a master regulator that triggers and maintains allergic inflammation at barrier surfaces. (Ebina-Shibuya and Leonard, 2023) Its activities overlap significantly with IL-33 and IL-25. Like IL-33, TSLP activates DC2 cells. It stimulates their cytokine production and so promotes IgE production. The activated DC2s also secrete chemokines that attract neutrophils and eosinophils. TSLP also causes DC2 cells to release CCL17 and CCL22 that specifically attract Th2 cells. TSLP stimulates basophil production in the bone marrow and over 70% of activated basophils express TSLP receptors. TSLP receptors are expressed on the dorsal root ganglia neurons and sensory nerve endings. Thus, when keratinocytes release TSLP, it can causes severe itching (Ziegler et al., 2013).

Interleukin-25

The third important cytokine, IL-25, is an 18 kDa member of the IL-17 family (Its alternative name is IL-17E). Its major sources are Th2 cells, mast cells, basophils, epithelial cells, tuft cells, and innate lymphoid cells. Its release is triggered by exposure to proteases such as tryptase. Mast cells and basophils produce IL-25 after cross-linking of their FcɛRI (Borowczyk and Shutova, 2021).

IL-25 induces dendritic cell responses that initiate and sustain type 2 responses. Unlike other members of the IL-17 family that attract neutrophils, IL-25 attracts eosinophils as well as inducing an eosinophilia and promoting IgE production. It is a major activator of ILC2 cells. Eosinophils produce IL-25 after treatment with IL-5 and GM-CSF. Repeated intranasal application of IL-25 results in the production of IL-5 and -13 and the induction of airway hypersensitivity. IL-25 also activates Th2 cells and ILC2 cells and induces their IL-9 production.

Regulation of Mast Cell Degranulation

Mast cells express two catecholamine receptors called the α- and β-adrenoceptors. These receptors have opposing effects. Molecules that stimulate the α-adrenoceptors (such as norepinephrine and phenylephrine) or block the β-adrenoceptors (such as propranolol) enhance mast cell degranulation. Conversely, molecules that stimulate the β receptors or block the α receptors inhibit mast cell degranulation. β-stimulators include isoproterenol, epinephrine, and salbutamol and are widely used in the treatment of allergies. β-receptor blockers enhance mast cell degranulation and promote allergies. Some respiratory pathogens such as *Bordetella pertussis* and *Haemophilus influenzae* can cause β-blockade. As a result, the airways of infected animals are more likely to become inflamed because of mast cell degranulation. These infections may also predispose animals to the development of respiratory allergies.

Alpha- and β-adrenoceptors are found not only on mast cells but also on secretory and smooth muscle cells throughout the body. α-stimulators cause vasoconstriction and may be of use treating severe allergic reactions, in reducing edema, and raising blood pressure. β-stimulators mediate smooth muscle relaxation and may therefore reduce the severity of smooth muscle contraction. Pure α- and β-stimulators are of only limited use in the treatment of allergic diseases because each alone is insufficient to counteract all the effects of mast cell–derived factors. Epinephrine (or adrenalin), on the other hand, has both α- and β-adrenergic activity. In addition to causing vasoconstriction in skin and viscera, its β effects cause smooth muscle to relax. This combination of effects is well suited to combat the vasodilation and smooth muscle contraction produced in type I hypersensitivity reactions. Ideally, epinephrine should be available whenever potential allergens are administered to animals.

Other Causes of Degranulation

G-protein-mediated activation. In addition to the high-affinity IgE receptor FcɛRI, mast cells express numerous G-protein-coupled receptors. These receptors regulate vital cellular functions. They are called Mas-related G-protein-coupled receptors, and their acronym is MRGPR (Wedi et al., 2020). MRGPRX2 is the most important of these receptors. It is found on the plasma membrane as well as intracellularly in connective tissue mast cells. Cationic peptides, including the neuropeptides, substance P, vasointestinal peptide, and neurotensin, as well as antimicrobial peptides, such as beta-defensins, cathelicidins, and eosinophil-derived molecules such as MBP, and EPO, can act through MRGPRX2 to trigger mast cell degranulation. MRGPRX2 is expressed at high levels on skin mast cells but not on lung or intestinal mast cells (Redegeld et al., 2018).

Complement-mediated activation. Activation of the serum complement system generates two peptides called C3a and C5a. They induce mast cell degranulation on binding to their receptors on mast cell surfaces. They are called anaphylatoxins because of their ability to cause an anaphylaxis-like response.

Mast Cells in Infections

Mast cells play important roles in both antimicrobial and antiparasite immunity (Abraham and St. John, 2010). They can respond within seconds or minutes to microbial invasion. They possess a large array of PRRs as well as being able to recognize antigen indirectly through IgE and their Fc receptors. Lipopolysaccharide stimulation of mast cell TLR4 can induce cytokine production in the absence of degranulation. Increased vascular permeability due to mast cell–derived mediators promotes inflammation. They also release preformed antimicrobial peptides such as the cathelicidins. Mast cell tryptase and chymases have antibacterial and antiparasite activity. As a result, mast cells appear to play an important role in controlling the bacterial burden and the healing of infected wounds. Mast cell-deficient mice show significant delays in the closure of Pseudomonas-infected wounds (Zimmermann et al., 2019).

Late-Phase Reaction

When antigen is injected into the skin of an allergic animal, two waves of inflammation occur. There is an immediate acute inflammatory response that occurs within 10–20 minutes as a result of the release of preformed mast cell mediators. This is followed several hours later by a second wave of inflammation, called the late-phase reaction, which peaks at 6–12 hours and then gradually diminishes. The late-phase reaction is characterized by redness, edema, and pruritus. It is believed that the late reaction results from the release of inflammatory mediators by basophils, T cells, endothelial cells, neutrophils, and macrophages attracted by mast cell chemotactic factors. Th17 cells also play a role in this late process (see Chapter 15).

BASOPHILS

Basophils are functionally similar to mast cells, although their origins and gene expression profiles are different (St John et al., 2023). Basophils are polymorphonuclear granulocytes, 10–14 μm in diameter, whose cytoplasmic granules stain intensely with hematoxylin (Fig. 30.13). Their granules are fewer and smaller than those in mast cells. Basophils constitute about 0.5% of blood leukocytes. Unlike mast cells, they have a short lifespan of about 60 hours in mice and are actively replenished by stem cells. They are not normally found outside the bloodstream and only enter tissues under the influence of some T cell–derived chemokines (Karasuyama and Yamanishi, 2014).

Basophils bind IgE through FcεRI. Antigens binding to this IgE will cause basophil degranulation and the release of their granule contents (Nakashima et al., 2018). Basophil granules contain a mixture of molecules similar to those in mast cells, including proteases, amines, and cytokines such as IL-4 and lipid mediators. When activated, they produce IL-4, IL-6, IL-13, and TSLP. Basophils release platelet-activating factor (PAF), a lipid, in response to IgG1-mediated stimulation. PAF is about 10,000 times more effective than histamine in increasing vascular permeability (Cara et al., 2004).

Although mast cells induce acute inflammation, basophils probably mediate more long-term allergic states such as chronic allergic dermatitis as well as the late-phase reaction. Basophils can function as antigen-presenting cells. Basophils can capture antigen through FcR-bound antibodies. They can endocytose, process, and present soluble antigens but not particulate antigens (Maddur et al., 2010). Basophils play a protective role in helminth, tick, and bacterial infections; they degrade toxins in venoms; and they contribute to tumor cell rejection (Schwartz et al., 2016).

EOSINOPHILS

Tissues undergoing type I hypersensitivity reactions are characteristically infiltrated by large numbers of eosinophils. These eosinophils are attracted to sites of mast cell degranulation, where they release their granule contents. Eosinophils are polymorphonuclear leukocytes, slightly larger than neutrophils or basophils (12–17 μm in diameter), with cytoplasmic granules that stain intensely with the red dye eosin (Figs. 30.14–30.16). They normally originate in the bone marrow and

spend about 30 minutes circulating in the bloodstream before migrating into the tissues, where they have a half-life of about 12 days. The proportion of eosinophils among the blood leukocytes varies greatly since it is affected by the presence of parasites. Normal values range from about 2% in dogs to about 10% in cattle (Ramirez et al., 2018; Box 30.1).

Activation

Eosinophils arise from bone marrow stem cells under the influence of IL-3, IL-5, and GM-CSF (Fig. 30.17). They share a common progenitor with basophils and mast cells. The great majority of the body's eosinophils are located in the intestine. Both Th2 cells and mast cells produce IL-5 and the chemokines known as eotaxins that stimulate the release of eosinophils from the bone marrow. IL-25, IL-33, and TSLP all induce IL-5 production (Johnston et al., 2016). Thus Th2 cells mobilize eosinophils while promoting IgE responses. These eosinophils are attracted to sites of mast cell degranulation by eotaxins, histamine, and its breakdown product imidiazoleacetic acid, leukotriene B$_4$, 5-hydroxytryptamine (5-HT), and by PAF. Eosinophils are especially attracted by CXCL8 (IL-8) complexed to IgA. Some allergens directly activate eosinophils, stimulating their chemotaxis and upregulating CR3 expression. The mobilization and activation of eosinophils enhances their ability to kill parasites and supports the belief that the major function of the IgE-mediated responses is the generation of type 2 responses, resulting in the control of helminth parasites (see Chapter 29). Activated eosinophils express MHC class II molecules and can serve as antigen-presenting cells (Rosenberg et al., 2013).

Degranulation and Mediators

Eosinophils express many PRRs that recognize PAMPs and DAMPs. When triggered, the eosinophils release multiple cytokines, chemokines, and their granule contents. Although eosinophils can phagocytose small particles, they are much more suited to extracellular destruction of large parasites since they can degranulate into the surrounding fluid. Eosinophils may release intact granules by exocytosis, or, more commonly, undergo piecemeal degranulation. In this process small vesicles bud off the secondary granules and are released into the extracellular tissues. This occurs in response to IgE-coated parasites, many chemokines, PAF, and C5a. Once free in extracellular fluid, eosinophil granules can function as independent structures capable of releasing their proteins in response to IFN-γ or CCL11. Activated eosinophils can also eject extracellular traps containing mitochondrial DNA and granule cationic proteins. They do this in response to bacterial products such as endotoxins. The release of these traps is not accompanied by cell death.

Eosinophils contain two types of granules (Figs. 30.15 and 30.16). Their small, primary granules contain arylsulfatase, peroxidase, and acid phosphatase. Their large crystalloid granules have a

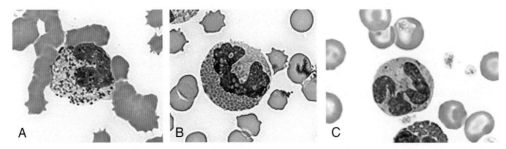

Fig. 30.13 Photomicrographs of peripheral blood basophils from a horse (A), a cat (B), and a dog (C). These cells are about 10 μm in diameter; all were photographed at the same magnification. Giemsa stain. Courtesy Dr. M.C. Johnson.

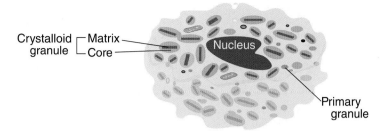

Fig. 30.14 The major structural features of an eosinophil.

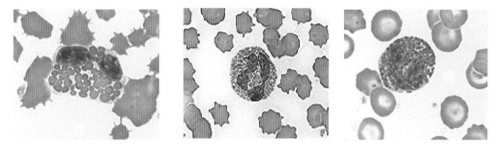

Fig. 30.15 Photomicrographs of peripheral blood eosinophils from left to right: horse, cat, and dog. Each cell is about 12 μm in diameter. Giemsa stain. Courtesy Dr. M.C. Johnson.

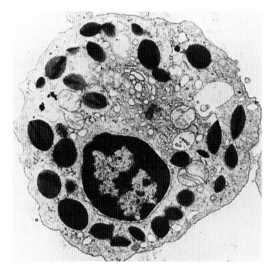

Fig. 30.16 A transmission electron micrograph of a rabbit eosinophil. Courtesy Dr. S. Linthicum.

core of major basic protein (MBP) surrounded by a matrix containing eosinophil cationic protein, eosinophil peroxidase (EPO), and eosinophil-derived neurotoxin (Fig. 30.18; Fondati et al., 2004). Eosinophils also produce lipid mediators such as leukotrienes and PAF. Particles bound to eosinophil receptors trigger a powerful respiratory burst. The EPO uses bromide in preference to chloride, thus producing OBr⁻ It also generates nitric oxide and nitrotyrosine, both potent oxidizing agents. Eosinophil granule proteins can kill helminths and bacteria and are important mediators of tissue pathology. They all, for example, damage respiratory epithelium. The production by eosinophils of multiple Th2 cytokines as well as indoleamine dioxygenase inhibits local Th1 responses and ensures

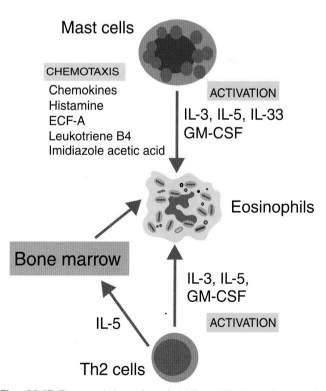

Fig. 30.17 The regulation of eosinophil mobilization, chemotaxis, and activation. *ECF-A*, Eosinophil chemotactic factors of anaphylaxis; *GM-CSF*, granulocyte-macrophage colony-stimulating factor; *IL*, interleukin.

that a "Th2 environment" is maintained where eosinophils accumulate (Melo and Weller, 2018).

Mast cells and eosinophils interact. Thus, eosinophil MBP causes mast cells to release histamine. Mast cells, in turn, release eosinophil chemotactic agents, activate eosinophils, and enhance the expression of eosinophil receptors. Mast cells can synthesize and secrete IL-3, IL-5, and GM-CSF, all of which promote eosinophil accumulation, degranulation, and survival.

Eosinophils also play a key role in the regulation of humoral immunity. Thus they are the major source of the B cell survival cytokine, APRIL (activation and proliferation-induced ligand). They are required for the homing of plasma cells to the bone marrow and for their long-term survival. An absence of eosinophils prevents efficient B cell class switching to IgA within Peyer's patches. In effect, eosinophils generate and maintain mucosal IgA plasma cells (Berek, 2015).

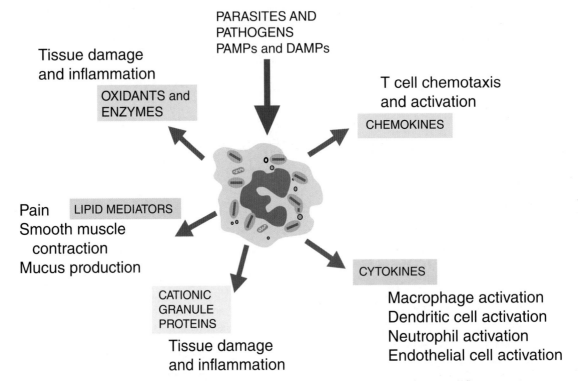

Fig. 30.18 Eosinophils release a complex array of molecules that contribute to the acute inflammatory process. It is clear that, on balance, eosinophils exacerbate the inflammation triggered by mast cells. *DAMPs*, Damage-associated molecular patterns; *PAMPs*, pathogen-associated molecular patterns.

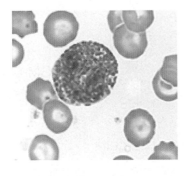

Normal eosinophil

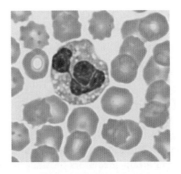

A "gray" eosinophil

Fig. 30.19 A normal canine eosinophil and a "gray" eosinophil in a blood smear from a golden retriever. It is possible that these "gray" cells are simply prematurely degranulated cells. Courtesy Dr. MC. Johnson.

In conclusion, type 1 hypersensitivity reactions are mediated by IgE and recruit three key cells, mast cells, eosinophils, and basophils, to participate in the reaction. Their biological role is likely to mediate antiparasite responses, but under modern conditions they also mediate allergic diseases.

REFERENCES

Abraham, S.N., St. John, A.L., 2010. Mast cell-orchestrated immunity to pathogens. Nat. Rev. Immunol. 10, 440–452.

Aoki, R., Kawamura, T., Goshima, F., Ogawa, Y., et al., 2016. The alarmin IL-33 derived from HSV-2-infected keratinocytes triggers mast cell-mediated antiviral innate immunity. J. Invest. Dermatol. 136, 1290–1292.

Agier, J., Pastwinska, J., Brzezinska-Blaszczyk, E., 2018. An overview of mast cell pattern recognition receptors. Inflamm. Res. 67, 737–746.

Berek, C., 2015. Eosinophils: important players in humoral immunity. Clin. Exp. Immunol. 183, 57–64.

Borowczyk, J., Shutova, M., 2021. IL-25 (IL-17E) in epithelial immunology and pathophysiology. J. Allergy. Clin. Immunol. 148, 40–52.

Burton, O.T., Zaccone, P., 2007. The potential role of chitin in allergic reactions. Trends Immunol. 28, 419–422.

Cara, D.C., Ebbert, K.V.J., McCafferty, D.-M., 2004. Mast cell-independent mechanisms of immediate hypersensitivity: a role for platelets. J. Immunol. 172, 4964–4971.

Chen, C.-Y., Lee, J.-B., Liu, B., Ohta, S., et al., 2015. Induction of interleukin-9-producing mucosal mast cells promotes susceptibility to IgE-mediated experimental food allergy. Immunity 43 (4), 788–802.

Cheng, L.E., Hartmann, K., Roers, A., Krummel, M.F., Locksley, R.M., 2013. Perivascular mast cells dynamically probe cutaneous blood vessels to capture immunoglobulin E. Immunity 38, 166–175.

Choi, H.W., Suwanpradid, J., Kim, I.H., Staats, H.F., et al., 2018. Perivascular dendritic cells elicit anaphylaxis by relaying allergens to mast cells via microvesicles. Science 362, 656–667.

Ebina-Shibuya, R., Leonard, W.J., 2023. Role of thymic stromal lymphopoietin in allergy and beyond. Nat. Rev. Immunol. https://doi.org/10.1038/s41577-022-00735-y.

Enoksson, M., Lyberg, K., Moller-Westerberg, C., Fallon, P.C., Nilsson, G., Lunderius- Andersson, C., 2011. Mast cells as sensors of cell injury through IL-33 recognition. J. Immunol. 186, 2523–2528.

Fondati, A., Carreras, E., Fondevila, D., Ferrer, L., Cuchillo, C.M., Nogues, V., 2004. Characterization of biological activities of feline eosinophil granule proteins. Am. J. Vet. Res. 65, 957–963.

Giori, L., Gironi, S., Scarpa, P., Anselmi, A., et al., 2011. Grey eosinophils in sighthounds: frequency in 3 breeds and comparison of neutrophil counts determined manually and with 2 hematology analyzers. Vet. Clin. Pathol. 40 (4), 475–483.

Gowthaman, U., Chen, J.S., Zhang, B., Flynn, W.F., et al., 2019. Identification of a T follicular helper cell subset that drives anaphylactic IgE. Science. https://doi.org/10.1126/science.aaw6433

Gurish, M.F., Boyce, J.A., 2002. Mast cell growth, differentiation and death. Clin. Rev. Allergy Immunol. 22, 107–118.

Haraldsen, G., Balogh, J., Pollheimer, J., et al., 2009. Interleukin-33: cytokine of dual function or novel alarmin? Trends Immunol. 30, 227–233.

Iazbik, M.C., Couto, C.G., 2005. Morphologic characterization of specific granules in Greyhound eosinophils. Vet. Clin. Pathol. 34, 140–143.

Johnston, L.K., Hsu, C.L., Krier-Burris, R.A., Chhiba, K.D., et al., 2016. IL-33 Precedes IL-5 in regulating eosinophil commitment and is required for eosinophil homeostasis. J. Immunol. 197, 3445–3453.

Karasuyama, H., Yamanishi, Y., 2014. Basophils have emerged as a key player in immunity. Curr. Opin. Immunol 31, 1–7.

Liew, F.Y., Girard, J.P., Turnquist, H.R., 2016. Interleukin-33 in health and disease. Nat. Rev. Immunol. 16, 676–689.

Lunderius-Andersson, C., Enoksson, M., Nilsson, G., 2012. Mast cells respond to cell injury through the recognition of IL-33. Front. Immunol. 3, 82–90. 2012

MacGlashan, D., 2008. IgE receptor and signal transduction in mast cells and basophils. Curr. Opin. Immunol. 20, 717–723.

Maddur, M.S., Kaveri, S.V., Bayry, J., 2010. Basophils as antigen presenting cells. Trends Immunol. 31, 45–48.

Melo, R.C.N., Weller, P.F., 2018. Contemporary understanding of the secretory granules in human eosinophils. J. Leukoc. Biol. 104, 85–93.

Mukai, K., Tsai, M., Saito, H., Galli, S.J., 2018. Mast cells as sources of cytokines, chemokines and growth factors. Immunol. Rev. 282, 121–150.

Nakashima, C., Otsuka, A., Kabashima, K., 2018. Recent advancement in the mechanism of basophil activation. J. Derm. Sci. 91, 3–8.

Ramirez, G.A., Yacoub, M.-R., Ripa, M., Mannina, D., Cariddi, A., Saporiti, N., et al., 2018. Eosinophils from physiology to disease: a comprehensive review. Biomed. Res. Int. https://doi.org/10.1155/2018/9095275.

Redegeld, F.A., Yu, Y., Kumari, S., Charles, N., Blank, U., 2018. Non-IgE-mediated mast cell activation. Immunol. Rev. 282, 87–113.

Rosenberg, H.F., Dyer, K.D., Foster, P.S., 2013. Eosinophils: changing perspectives in health and disease. Nat. Rev. Immunol. 13, 9–22.

Sandig, H., Bulfone-Paus, S., 2012. TLR signaling in mast cells: common and unique features. Front. Immunol. 3 https://doi.org/10.3389/fimmu.2012.00185.

Schwartz, C., Eberle, J.U., Voehringer, D., 2016. Basophils in inflammation. Eur. J. Pharmacol. 778, 90–95.

St John, A.L., Rathore, A.P.S., Ginhoux, F., 2023. New perspectives on the origins and heterogeneity of mast cells. Nat. Rev. Immunol. 23, 55–68.

Stanbery, A.G., Smita, S., von Moltke, J., Wojno, T., Ziegler, S.F., 2022. TSLP, IL-33, and IL-25: not just for allergy and helminth infection. J. Allergy Clin. Immunol. 150, 1302–1313.

Tizard, I.R., 2022. Allergies and Hypersensitivity disease in Animals. Elsevier, St Louis, MO, ISBN: 978-0-323-76393-6

Valenta, R., Karaulov, A., Niederberger, V., Gattinger, P., et al., 2018. Molecular aspects of allergens and allergy. Adv. Immunol. 138, 195–255.

Voehringer, D., 2013. Protective and pathological roles of mast cells and basophils. Nat. Rev. Immunol. 13, 362–375.

Wedi, B., Gehring, M., Kapp, A., 2020. The pseudoallergen receptor MRGPRX2 on peripheral blood basophils and eosinophils: expression and function. Allergy 75, 2229–2242.

Ziegler, S.F., Roan, F., Bell, B.D., Stoklasek, T.A., et al., 2013. The biology of thymic stromal lymphopoietin (TSLP). Adv. Pharmacol. 66, 129–150.

Zimmermann, C., Troeltzsch, D., Gimenez-Rivera, V.A., Galli, S.J., et al., 2019. Mast cells are crtitical for controlling the bacterial burden and the healing of infected wounds. Proc. Natl. Acad. Sci. https://doi.org/10.1073/pnas.1908816116.

Selected Allergic Diseases

The development of allergic diseases has long been considered to result from the release of inflammatory mediators by mast cells, basophils, and eosinophils. Disease severity depends on the number and location of these cells, the degree of sensitization of an animal, the amount of antigen involved, and its route of administration. Not all animals develop these hypersensitivity diseases. Nevertheless, their prevalence is increasing, and it has been suggested that this increase is due to a reduction in the diversity of the body's microbiota—the hygiene hypothesis (Gershwin, 2009; Tizard, 2022).

THE HYGIENE HYPOTHESIS

The prevalence of allergic disease has increased significantly in Western societies over the past 50 years. While most obvious in humans, this has also affected domestic species, especially dogs and cats. It is believed that this increase is a result of changes in the body's microbiota (Fig. 31.1). The hygiene hypothesis suggests that alterations in Western diets, environmental cleanliness, an urban lifestyle, and the overuse of antibiotics collectively have resulted in long-term changes in the intestinal microbiota that have driven these increases in allergic and inflammatory disease (Hakanen et al., 2018). Since the intestinal microbiota influences the Th1/Th2 balance, it is suggested that as diversity is lost, Th2 responses come to predominate. Thus the composition of the intestinal microbiota exerts a significant influence on allergy development. The skin and lung microbiota also have a significant effect on the development of allergies in those organs as well (Lambrecht and Hammad, 2017).

The hygiene hypothesis has received support from studies on piglets. Major differences can be found in their gut microbiota depending upon the environment in which piglets are raised. These differences also influence the expression of immune system genes. For example, piglets raised in a very clean environment have reduced microbial diversity and express more genes involved in inflammation, such as those encoding type 1 interferons, MHC class I, antibacterial peptides, and many chemokines. Conversely, outdoor pigs with a more diverse microbiota express more genes linked to T cell function, including the TCR, CD8, and pIgR.

Similar effects have been observed in rodents. Germ-free mice have high serum IgE levels in early life. These can be greatly reduced by bacterial colonization. If low doses of the antibiotic vancomycin are fed to neonatal mice, the diversity of their gut microbiota is reduced, Treg numbers are also reduced, and they suffer from an increased severity of allergic lung disease. Adult mice treated with oral antibiotics have

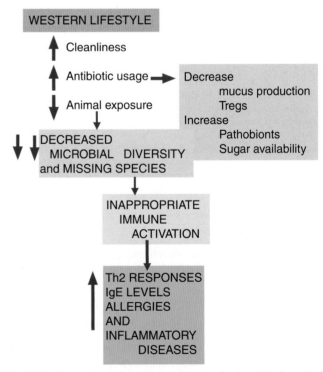

Fig. 31.1 The hygiene hypothesis. A lack of microbial diversity in the intestinal microbiota results in a dominant T helper 2 cells (Th2) response resulting in immunoglobin E (IgE) production and a predisposition to developing allergic and inflammatory diseases.

increased IgE levels and blood basophil numbers. They suffer from increased airway inflammation following allergen challenge.

Conversely, an appropriately balanced microbiota generates antiinflammatory molecules such as short-chain fatty acids (SCFAs), polysaccharide A, and peptidoglycans. SCFAs (formate, acetate, butyrate, and succinate) are produced in abundance in animals fed high-fiber diets. Humans that consume large amounts of fiber have a lower prevalence of colitis and inflammatory disease. Among the SCFAs, butyrate has potent antiinflammatory properties (see Fig. 22.7; Petersen et al., 2019). In general, therefore, a balanced and healthy microbiota suppresses inflammation by stimulating Treg activity. They inhibit the NF-κB pathway and block type 2 immune responses.

SPECIFIC ALLERGIC DISEASES

The severity of allergic diseases can range from lethal anaphylaxis to minor skin irritation based on the dose and route of exposure to an allergen.

Anaphylaxis

In its most extreme form, antigen administered rapidly to an allergic animal can cause generalized mast cell degranulation and massive mediator release. If the rate of release of vasoactive molecules from these mast cells exceeds their ability to adjust to the changes in their vascular and respiratory systems, an animal may collapse and die.

Anaphylaxis is a severe, life-threatening systemic hypersensitivity reaction triggered by rapid exposure to an antigen in a highly sensitized animal. Its clinical signs are determined by organ system involvement, which differs among the domestic mammals (Table 31.1). Overall, the signs of anaphylaxis result from smooth muscle contraction in the bronchi, some blood vessels, the gastrointestinal tract, uterus, and bladder mediated by large amounts of histamine and other amines released from degranulating mast cells and basophils.

The major shock organs of horses are the lungs and the intestine. Bronchial and bronchiolar smooth muscle constriction leads to coughing, dyspnea, and, if severe, apnea. On necropsy, severe pulmonary emphysema and peribronchiolar edema are commonly seen. In addition to the lung lesions, edematous hemorrhagic enterocolitis may result in severe diarrhea. The major mediators of anaphylaxis in horses are histamine and serotonin.

In cattle the major shock organs are the lungs (Fig. 31.2). Bovine anaphylaxis is characterized by profound systemic hypotension and pulmonary hypertension. The pulmonary hypertension results from constriction of the pulmonary vein, leading to pulmonary edema and severe dyspnea. The smooth muscles of the bladder and intestine contract, causing urination, defecation, and bloating. The main mediators of anaphylaxis in cattle are serotonin, kinins, and the leukotrienes. Histamine is of lesser importance in this species. Dopamine enhances histamine and leukotriene release from the lung, thus exerting a form of positive feedback. Because of the anticoagulant properties of heparin released by mast cells, blood from affected animals does not coagulate. In cattle, in contrast to the other species, β-stimulants such as isoproterenol potentiate histamine release from leukocytes, whereas α-stimulants such as norepinephrine inhibit histamine release. In addition, epinephrine potentiates histamine release in the bovine. The significance of these anomalous effects is unclear.

In sheep, pulmonary signs also predominate in anaphylaxis as a result of constriction of the smooth muscle in the bronchi and pulmonary vessels. Smooth muscle contraction also occurs in the bladder and intestine with predictable results. The major mediators of anaphylaxis in sheep are histamine, serotonin, leukotrienes, and kinins.

In pigs, anaphylaxis is largely the result of systemic and pulmonary hypertension, leading to dyspnea and death. In some pigs, the intestinal smooth muscle is involved, whereas in others, no gross intestinal lesions are observed. The most significant mediator identified in this species is histamine.

TABLE 31.1 Anaphylaxis in the Domestic Species and Humans

Species	Shock Organs	Symptoms	Pathology	Major Mediators
Horse	Respiratory tract Intestine	Cough Dyspnea Diarrhea	Emphysema Intestinal hemorrhage	Histamine Serotonin
Ruminants	Respiratory tract	Cough Dyspnea Collapse	Lung edema Emphysema Hemorrhage	Serotonin Leukotrienes Kinins Dopamine
Swine	Respiratory tract Intestine	Cyanosis Pruritus	Systemic hypotension	Histamine
Dog	Hepatic veins	Collapse Dyspnea Diarrhea Vomiting	Hepatic engorgement Visceral hemorrhage	Histamine Leukotrienes Prostaglandins
Cat	Respiratory tract Intestine	Dyspnea Vomiting Diarrhea Pruritus	Lung edema Intestinal edema	Histamine Leukotrienes
Human	Respiratory tract	Dyspnea Urticaria	Lung edema Emphysema	Histamine Leukotrienes
Chicken	Respiratory tract	Dyspnea Convulsions	Lung edema	Histamine Serotonin Leukotrienes

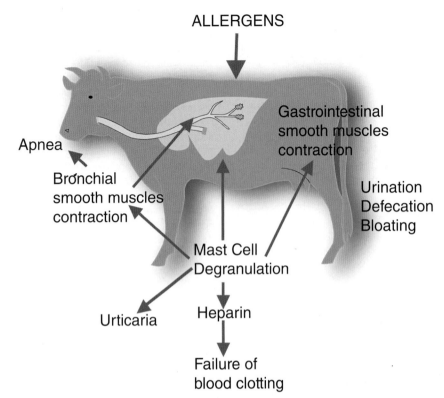

Fig. 31.2 The basic mechanisms of anaphylaxis in the bovine. The proximal cause of death in most but not all species results from extreme constriction of the bronchial smooth muscle and subsequent asphyxiation.

Dogs differ from other domestic mammals in that the major shock organ is not the lung but the liver. Dogs undergoing anaphylaxis show initial excitement, followed by vomiting, defecation, and urination. As the reaction progresses, dogs collapse with weakness and depressed respiration, become comatose, convulse, and die. On necropsy, the liver and intestine are massively engorged, perhaps holding up to 60% of the animal's total blood volume. All these signs result from occlusion of the hepatic veins. Dogs possess multiple sphincters on these veins. Blockage is due to a combination of smooth muscle contraction and hepatic swelling. This results in portal hypertension and visceral blood pooling, as well as a decrease in venous return, cardiac output, and arterial pressure. Identified mediators in the dog include histamine, prostaglandins, and leukotrienes.

In cats, the major shock organs are the lungs. Cats undergoing anaphylaxis show vigorous scratching around the face and head as histamine is released into the skin. This is followed by dyspnea, salivation, vomiting, incoordination, collapse, and death. Necropsy reveals severe bronchoconstriction, emphysema, pulmonary hemorrhage, and edema of the glottis. The major mediators in the cat are histamine and the leukotrienes.

Although anaphylaxis is the most dramatic and severe allergic reaction, it is more usual to observe local allergic reactions, the sites of which are referable to the route of administration of antigens. For example, inhaled antigens (allergens) provoke acute inflammation in the upper respiratory tract, trachea, and bronchi, resulting in fluid exudation from the nasal mucosa (hay fever/rhinitis) as well as tracheobronchial constriction (asthma). Aerosolized antigen will also contact the eyes and provoke conjunctivitis and intense lacrimation. Ingested antigens may provoke diarrhea and colic as intestinal smooth muscle contracts violently. If sufficiently severe, the resulting diarrhea may be hemorrhagic. Antigen penetrating the skin results in a local dermatitis. The skin reaction is erythematous and edematous and is described as

an urticarial type (*Urtica dioica* is the name of the "stinging nettle," a plant that has hollow stinging hairs that inject histamine into the skin when touched) (Fig. 31.3). Urticarial lesions are extremely pruritic; consequently, scratching may mask the true nature of the lesion. The inflammatory cell infiltrate in urticarial lesions reflects this type 2 response.

Milk Allergy

Jersey cattle may develop an allergy to the α-casein of their own milk. Normally, this protein is synthesized in the udder, and provided that the animals are milked regularly, it is removed by milking or suckling and nothing untoward occurs. If milking is delayed, however, the increased intramammary pressure forces milk proteins into the bloodstream. In sensitized cows, this may result in reactions ranging from mild discomfort with urticarial skin lesions to acute anaphylaxis and death (Campbell, 1970). Prompt milking can treat the condition, although some seriously affected animals may have to go for several lactations without drying-off because of the severe reactions that occur on cessation of milking.

Food Allergies

The healthy immune system is normally tolerant to foods and unresponsive to food allergens (see Chapter 23). Oral tolerance is a natural process by which ingested antigens are sampled by dendritic cells (Thetis cells), macrophages, and M cells, and presented to intestinal T cells in such a way that they drive the development of IL-10-producing Treg cells. Other tolerance-promoting molecules include retinoic acid, IDO, and TGF-β. The microbiota appears to play a minor role in oral tolerance since it develops in germ-free animals. If this tolerance breaks down, type 2 response triggered by IL-33 and ILCs may occur. IL-33 increases mucosal permeability and promotes Th2 skewing of the immune response. This results in the production of IgE and

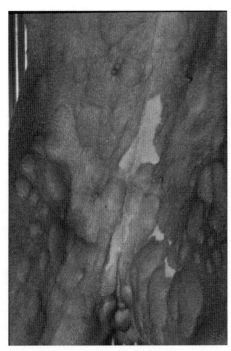

Fig. 31.3 Severe urticaria in a boxer stung by three wasps. Courtesy Dr. G. Elissalde.

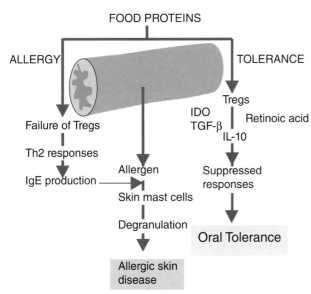

Fig. 31.4 The major mechanisms of food tolerance and food allergies. *IDO*, Indoleamine 2,3-dioxygenase; *IgE*, immunoglobin E; *IL-10*, interleukin-10; *TGF-β*, transforming growth factor–β; *Th2*, T helper 2 cells.

the development of food allergies. Type 2 responses to foods may also occur if Tregs are destroyed or dysfunctional, as induced by segmented filamentous bacteria (Johnston et al., 2014). The clinical consequences of food allergies are seen both in the digestive tract and on the skin (Fig. 31.4; Chesney, 2002). Antigens may enter the bloodstream and reach skin mast cells within a few minutes. It has been estimated that allergic food responses may account for 1% of cutaneous disease in dogs and cats.

The intestinal reaction to ingested allergens may be mild, perhaps showing only as an irregularity in the consistency of the feces, or it may be severe, with vomiting, cramps, and violent, sometimes hemorrhagic diarrhea occurring soon after feeding. Most food allergic dogs show

cutaneous symptoms, and these tend to be indistinguishable from atopic dermatitis. The skin reactions are usually papular and erythematous and may involve the feet, eyes, ears, and axillae or perianal area. Analysis of the skin infiltrate in these dogs shows that CD8+ T cells predominate and that expression of IL-4, IL-13, and FoxP3 is increased. The lesions themselves are highly pruritic and are commonly masked by self-inflicted trauma and secondary bacterial or yeast infections. In chronic cases the skin may be hyperpigmented, lichenified, and infected, leading to pyoderma. Chronic pruritic otitis externa may also develop. The foods involved vary but are usually protein rich, such as dairy products, wheat meal, fish, chicken, beef, or eggs. Food allergies have been reported in the horse but are uncommon. Wild oats, white clover, and alfalfa have been recognized as allergens in this species. In pigs, fishmeal and alfalfa have been incriminated. Analysis of serum from dogs that are allergic to beef and cow's milk shows that the major allergens are bovine IgG heavy chains. A second major antigen in lamb and beef extracts is phosphoglucomutase. The most common food allergens in cats are beef, fish, and chicken (Sampson et al., 2018).

The most reliable test for suspected food allergies is to remove all potential allergens and then feed a hypoallergenic diet. Several commercial hypoallergenic diets are available to facilitate this diagnosis. These diets usually contain meat and carbohydrates from sources to which the animal is unlikely to have been exposed. Examples include mutton, duck, venison, or rabbit with brown rice or potatoes. An alternative solution is to feed a hydrolyzed protein diet that contains smaller and less allergenic protein fragments. Elimination diet trials generally show evidence of remission by 5–6 weeks but should be fed for at least 8 weeks. These diets may subsequently be supplemented by adding other ingredients until the allergen is identified by a recurrence of clinical signs. Treatment involves eliminating the responsible allergen from the diet (Jackson, 2023).

Intestinal dysbiosis may play a role in inflammatory skin diseases such as atopic dermatitis in addition to food allergies. Metabolites from the intestinal microbiota can reach the skin and affect local inflammatory responses (Iweala and Nagler, 2019). Parasitized cats develop significantly higher levels of antibodies to food antigens than unparasitized cats. Most importantly, they develop higher levels of IgE antibodies, suggesting that the presence of parasitic worms in the intestine may provoke food allergies (Gilbert and Halliwell, 2005).

Allergic Respiratory Disease

While common in humans, nasolacrimal urticaria (hay fever) is an uncommon manifestation of respiratory allergy in dogs and cats. Pollens usually provoke a rhinitis and conjunctivitis, characterized by a profuse, watery nasal discharge and excessive lacrimation. If the allergenic particles are sufficiently small, they may reach the bronchi or bronchioles, where the resulting reaction can cause bronchoconstriction, wheezing, and recurrent paroxysmal dyspnea—asthma (Fig. 31.5; Lambrecht and Hammad 2015). It should be noted that some Basenji dogs may have unusually sensitive airways and experience a disease similar to some types of human asthma (Hirshman et al., 1980). Cats are also recognized as suffering from asthma with paroxysmal wheezing, dyspnea, and coughing. It is of interest to note that there is a concordance between asthma in cats and in their owners, suggesting the involvement of similar allergens (Padrid, 2000).

Asthma in humans is now recognized as a syndrome mediated by several different pathogenic processes. Thus the majority of cases are eosinophilic (>3% eosinophils in sputum) and regulated by ILC2s and basophils. These cases are commonly allergic in origin and steroid responsive. About 30% of human asthma cases are neutrophilic (>60% in sputum), associated with high Th17 cell levels and are often steroid unresponsive. Other asthma subtypes may have both neutrophils and

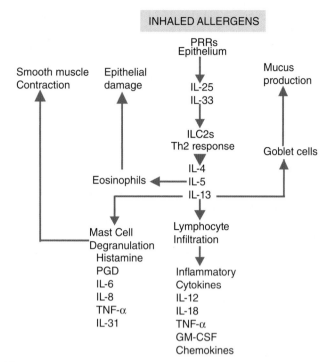

INHALED ALLERGENS

PRRs
Epithelium

Smooth muscle
Contraction

Epithelial
damage

IL-25
IL-33

Mucus
production

ILC2s
Th2 response

Goblet cells

IL-4
Eosinophils ← IL-5
IL-13

Mast Cell
Degranulation
Histamine
PGD
IL-6
IL-8
TNF-α
IL-31

Lymphocyte
Infiltration

Inflammatory
Cytokines
IL-12
IL-18
TNF-α
GM-CSF
Chemokines

Fig. 31.5 The pathogenesis of allergic asthma. *GM-CSF*, Granulocyte-macrophage colony-stimulating factor; *IL-6*, interleukin-6; *ILC2s*, Group 2 innate lymphoid cells; *PGD*, Prostaglandin D; *PRRs*, pattern recognition receptor; *Th2*, T helper 2 cells; *TNF-α*, tumor necrosis factor–α.

TABLE 31.2 The Diagnostic Criteria for Canine Atopic Dermatitis

The International Task Force on Canine Atopic Dermatitis has listed eight diagnostic criteria for this disease:

1. The disease mainly occurs in indoor dogs.
2. Disease onset occurs in animals under 3 years of age.
3. Animals develop a corticosteroid-responsive pruritus.
4. This pruritus is initially without obvious lesions.
5. The pruritus eventually affects the front feet.
6. The ear pinnae are affected next.
7. The ear margins are affected next.
8. The dorsolumbar area remains unaffected.

Any combination of five criteria from this set will diagnose atopic dermatitis with a sensitivity of 85% and a specificity of 79% (see Chapter 43).

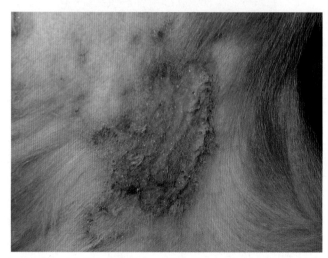

Fig. 31.6 A moist "Hot Spot" on a Golden Retriever. Courtesy Dr. Robert Kennis.

eosinophils or even neither, in sputum. Interleukin-33 is also generated in the lungs of many asthmatics. It activates ILC2 cells, basophils, and mast cells to promote type 2 inflammation (Lambrecht et al., 2019).

Asthma is common in horses. The term encompasses two distinct syndromes, inflammatory airway disease and recurrent airway obstruction. These are primarily type III hypersensitivity diseases (see Chapter 33). A familial allergic rhinitis characterized by extreme nasal pruritus, violent sneezing, dyspnea, mucoid nasal discharge, and excessive lacrimation has been observed in cattle. Depending on the allergen, it may be seasonal. The antigens involved are inhaled and come from a variety of plant and fungal sources. Diagnosis may be confirmed by skin testing. Nasal granulomas may form in chronically affected cattle. These consist of numerous polypoid nodules, 1–4 mm in diameter, situated in the anterior nasal mucosa. The nodules contain large numbers of mast cells, eosinophils, and plasma cells (Gail and Tsai, 2013).

Atopic Dermatitis

Atopic dermatitis (AD) is a complex, multifactorial syndrome characterized by chronically inflamed and itchy skin. It is very common in humans and dogs (as many as 15% are affected) and has been recognized in cats, horses, and goats. It is not simply an allergic disease driven by allergen exposure because it also involves immune dysregulation, skin barrier defects, and microbial colonization. It is better considered to be a manifestation of multiple diseases, mainly driven by local Th2/Th22 responses with some contributions from Th17 and Th1 cells (Pucheu-Haston et al., 2015a).

Transcriptome profiles of the blood lymphocytes from dogs with AD showed increases in CD8+, γ/δ+, and Treg cells. Likewise, there is increased expression of IL-13 and TNF-α, as well as decreased expression of IL-10 and TGF-β. The increase in Tregs together with a decline in IL-10 and TGF-β suggests that Treg function is somehow impaired (Sparling et al., 2022).

Th22 cells also promote skin inflammation especially epithelial cell proliferation and the production of antimicrobial peptides. IL-22 can be detected in chronic skin lesions, and its genes are upregulated in acute AD lesions (Pucheu-Haston et al., 2015b).

Some forms of AD are due to IgE-mediated allergic responses to environmental allergens and so can be classified as extrinsic AD. Conversely, other cases are not due to IgE responses and are classified as intrinsic AD or "atopic-like" dermatitis. Extrinsic AD cases develop high serum IgE levels, and this IgE is directed against environmental and food allergens. Intrinsic IgE cases usually have normal IgE levels.

Clinical Disease

Atopic dogs commonly present with pruritus. Initially, there may be no obvious skin lesions, but this progresses to diffuse erythema. Animals may present with the allergic triad: face rubbing, axillary pruritus, and foot licking (Table 31.2). Lesions occur most commonly on the front feet, the ventral abdomen, and in the inguinal and axillary regions, although they may be found anywhere on the body. These lesions are secondary to the intense pruritus and vary from acute erythema and edema to chronic secondary changes including crusting, scaling, hyperpigmentation, lichenification, and pyoderma. Some animals also develop rhinitis, otitis externa, or conjunctivitis. Dogs may also develop focal "hot spots" or urticaria (Fig. 31.6). Secondary bacterial or yeast infections (especially Malassezia yeasts) complicate the disease.

Depending on the inducing allergen, the extrinsic disease may or may not be seasonal and relapsing. Once it starts, it tends to get progressively more severe unless treated (Marsella et al., 2012).

Genetic Background

The development of canine AD is determined in part by genetic factors. Both susceptibility and protective gene loci have been identified in dogs (Wood et al., 2009). While not highly heritable, disease occurrence differs between breeds. AD is most common in West Highland White Terriers, Labrador and Golden Retrievers, German Shepherds, Cocker Spaniels, Boxers, French Bulldogs, and Shar-Peis (Shaw et al., 2004). Careful clinical evaluation has recognized several disease phenotypes that differ in such features as age of onset, the presence of hot spots, gastrointestinal disorders, flexural dermatitis, and the distribution of the skin lesions. Some breeds may develop lesions in specific areas. Thus French Bulldogs develop lesions in the axillae, eyelids, and flexural surfaces. German Shepherds, in contrast, tend to develop lesions in the elbows, hind limbs, and thorax.

Environmental Influences

Extrinsic AD is commonly associated with responses to environmental allergens such as molds, tree, weed, and grass pollens (especially pollens that are small and light and are produced in very large quantities) and, as a result, may be seasonal. Nonseasonal AD is mainly associated with allergies to house dust mites (*Dermatophagoides farinae* and *Dermatophagoides pteronyssinus*) and fleas; as well as to animal danders; and the yeast *Malassezia pachydermatis*. There are no significant clinical differences between food-induced AD and that associated with environmental allergens (Miller, 2018).

Skin Lesions, Cells, Cytokines, and Chemokines

It was long believed that canine AD was an allergic reaction to inhaled antigens despite the fact that respiratory signs are not commonly associated with the disease. It is now considered more likely, however, that allergen sensitization occurs through the skin. Antigens are trapped by Langerhans cells and then presented to γ/δ T cells. T cells play a critical role in the pathogenesis of AD, with type 2 responses predominating in the first 24 hours and mixed type 1 and 2 responses in the later, chronic disease (48–96 hours; Fig. 31.7). Lesions from patients with both forms of AD are infiltrated with T cells and dendritic cells. However, Th17- and Th22-derived cytokines are elevated only in those with intrinsic AD. Conversely, lesions from patients with extrinsic AD have more Th2 cytokines (IL-4, IL-13, and IL-5). The suppressive cytokine TGF-β is underexpressed in both types of AD. Thymic stromal lymphopoietin (TSLP) is upregulated in inflamed skin, especially when associated with epidermal barrier dysfunction. This TSLP is produced by Th2 cells, keratinocytes, and mast cells, in response to antimicrobial peptides such as β-defensins and cathelicidins. TSLP is a potent stimulator of Th2 cytokine production, and these in turn promote IgE production (Ziegler et al., 2013).

Pruritus

Chronic severe itching is one of the most important and distressing features of canine AD. It is caused by mediators released from skin cells (Fig. 31.8). These mediators bind to itch-specific neuronal receptors (pruriceptors). Itch mediators include histamine, some prostaglandins and leukotrienes, some neuropeptides, and IL-31. In addition, keratinocytes can communicate directly with cutaneous sensory neurons using TSLP. It is unclear what the relationship is between itch induced

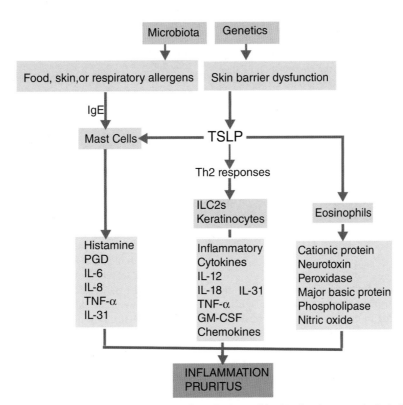

Fig. 31.7 A simplified view of the pathogenesis of atopic dermatitis showing the central role believed to be played by the cytokine, thymic stromal lymphopoietin. *GM-CSF*, Granulocyte-macrophage colony-stimulating factor; *IgE*, Immunoglobin E; *IL-6*, interleukin-6; *ILC2s*, Group 2 innate lymphoid cells; *Th2*, T helper 2 cells; *TNF-α*, tumor necrosis factor–α; *TSLP*, thymic stromal lymphopoietin.

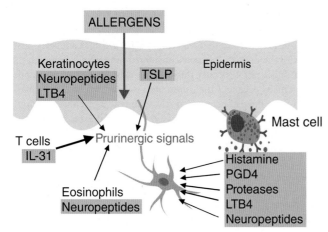

Fig. 31.8 The major mediators associated with pruritus. The most significant of these include histamine, thymic stromal lymphopoietin (TSLP), and interleukin 31 (IL-31). These act on specialized nerve receptors within the skin to induce itch. *LTB4*, Leukotriene B4; *PGD4*, prostaglandin D.

by TSLP and itch induced through immune-cell neuronal communication and histamine (Elmariah and Lerner, 2013).

Since canine mast cells contain histamine, it has long been assumed that histamine is the primary mediator of AD. It is known to cause vasodilatation, pain, and itching. However, histamine levels do not correlate well with disease severity and plasma histamine levels do not differ significantly between normal and itchy dogs.

The cytokine, IL-31, causes severe pruritus in dogs (McCandless et al., 2014). TGF-β induces IL-31 expression in dermal dendritic cells, and this in turn, activates sensory neurons (Xu et al., 2020). Peripheral blood mononuclear cells from dogs exposed to allergen (house dust mites) plus Staphylococcal enterotoxin B also produce high levels of IL-31. The IL-31 receptor is expressed on canine mononuclear cells, keratinocytes, and dorsal root ganglia. Thus, the combination of allergens and the presence of bacteria may stimulate T cells, keratinocytes, and neurons, to trigger the pruritus of atopic dermatitis using IL-31 (Gonzales et al., 2013). The synthetic Janus kinase (JAK) inhibitor, oclacitinib maleate, can reduce pruritus in many dogs and cats with AD (Gonzales et al., 2014). It blocks signal transduction by JAK 1 and JAK3 receptors and, as a result, inhibits the activities of IL-31 and several other cytokines. It can therefore reduce both the pruritus and the severity of the dermatitis and improve the quality of life for many animals (Fukuyama et al., 2015). Excessive blocking of IL-31 function may be undesirable since IL-31 regulated genes are also involved in forming an intact skin barrier and IL-31 stimulates the production of antimicrobial peptides (Nakashima et al., 2018; Box 31.1).

The Role of IgE

The division of AD into intrinsic and extrinsic disease stems from the observation that there is no consistent correlation between IgE levels and the severity of clinical AD in dogs and not all AD cases are associated with IgE antibodies to environmental antigens. Serological assays that measure serum IgE antibodies rarely correlate with disease severity or the levels of IgE in the skin. Blood IgE levels may drop to undetectable levels, whereas levels in skin and skin reactivity remain high. Intradermal testing of pruritic dogs shows that many are sensitive to house dust mites, various pollens (trees, weeds, grasses), as well as some seasonal allergens such as molds (Fig. 31.9). However, skin testing of clinically normal dogs also elicits positive reactions to these same antigens. For example, 50%–90% of clinically normal dogs react

BOX 31.1 Monoclonal Antibody Therapy for Atopic Dermatitis

As noted in the text, interleukin 31 is the major cause of the severe itching observed in atopic dermatitis in dogs. The production of IL-31 in affected skin can be inhibited by the JAK inhibitor oclacitinib. It can also be neutralized by administration of a caninized monoclonal antibody—Lokivetmab, directed specifically at canine IL-31. The antibody is injected subcutaneously. It binds to circulating IL-31 and inhibits its binding to the IL-31 receptor. In double-blind, placebo-controlled trials, a single dose has provided relief from itch and a reduction in disease severity in dogs with chronic AD.

From Michels, G.M., Ramsey, D.S., Walsh, K.F., et al., 2016. A blinded, randomized, placebo-controlled, dose determination trial of lokivetmab (ZTS-00103289), a caninized, anticanine IL-31 monoclonal antibody in client owned dogs with atopic dermatitis. Vet. Dermatol. 27, 478–e129.

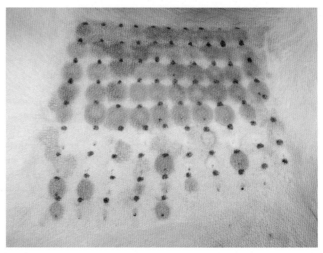

Fig. 31.9 A panel of intradermal skin tests performed on a dog. Each spot denotes a position where a small volume of dilute allergen was injected intradermally. If the dog is allergic to that allergen a local reaction characterized by redness and swelling occur around the injection site. Courtesy Dr. Robert Kennis.

to house dust mite allergens. Allergen-specific IgE may also be detected in dogs that have no clinical signs of AD, while IgE levels cannot discriminate between normal dogs, dogs with intestinal parasites, or dogs with AD. Additionally, about a quarter of canine cases are unreactive to intradermal antigens and lack any allergen-specific IgE.

Epidermal Barrier Dysfunction

In some cases of canine AD, the initial lesion is a defect in epithelial cells leading to skin barrier dysfunction. This permits loss of water as well as the penetration of allergens and microbes and increases contacts between the skin immune system and environmental allergens (Fig. 31.10). Defects in either the skin barrier protein filaggrin, or in skin lipids such as ceramides or sphingosine-1-phosphate, may increase skin water loss and its susceptibility to irritation. Atopic dogs may also be defective in the expression of tight junction proteins such as occludin and zonula occludens 1.

Filaggrin is a filament-associated protein involved in cross-linking keratin fibers in epidermal cells. It is a major barrier protein that helps the skin retain fluid. Single nucleotide polymorphisms within the canine filaggrin gene have been associated with some forms of atopic dermatitis. The importance of filaggrin in canine atopic dermatitis is

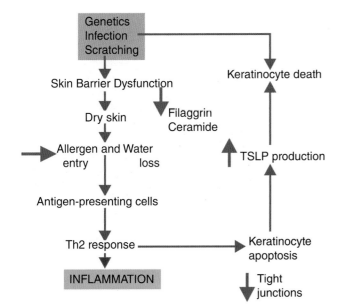

Fig. 31.10 A key contributor to the development of atopic dermatitis is skin barrier dysfunction. This is influenced by genetic, climatic, and allergic factors, and exacerbated by scratching. *Th2*, T helper 2 cells; *TSLP*, thymic stromal lymphopoietin.

unclear. It is possible that filaggrin defects only account for a subset of canine AD cases, or alternatively, filaggrin defects may be secondary to some other cause of AD. Likewise, there is no clear evidence as yet that improving skin barrier function is of clinical benefit in the treatment of atopic dogs (Palmer et al., 2006; Marsella, 2013).

Infections

The severity of canine AD is influenced by (and influences) the skin microbiota. The skin microbiota is altered in allergen-induced canine atopic dermatitis. This is associated with a relative increase in *Staphylococcus pseudintermedius*. Recurrent Staphylococcal skin infections are associated with canine AD. These Staphylococci may release toxins or superantigens (see Chapter 27) that promote skin inflammation.

Malassezia skin and ear infections are also common in canine AD cases. The yeast, *M. pachydermatis*, produces a phospholipase that may disrupt skin cell membranes and initiate a secondary dermatitis either by directly triggering inflammation or by acting as an allergen. Dogs with atopic dermatitis have higher expression of β-defensins in infected, atopic skin, but this may simply reflect the presence of secondary infections. Environmental pollutants also influence the development of AD (Box 31.2).

Allergies to Vaccines and Drugs

An IgE response may result from the administration of any antigen, including those in vaccines. These are most likely to be triggered by vaccines that contain trace amounts of fetal calf serum (specifically bovine serum albumin), gelatin, or casein (Gershwin et al., 2012). Severe allergic responses have been associated with the use of killed foot-and-mouth disease, rabies, and contagious bovine pleuropneumonia vaccines in cattle.

IgE responses may also occur following administration of drugs. Most drug molecules are too small to be antigenic, but many can bind to host proteins and then act as haptens. Penicillin allergy, for example, may be triggered either by therapeutic exposure or by ingestion of penicillin-contaminated milk. The penicillin molecule is degraded in vivo to several compounds; the most important of these contains a penicilloyl group. This penicilloyl group can bind to proteins and provoke an immune response. In sensitized animals, injection of penicillin may cause acute systemic anaphylaxis or milder forms of allergy. Feeding of penicillin-contaminated milk to these animals can lead to severe diarrhea.

Allergies to many drugs, especially antibiotics and hormones, have been reported in the domestic animals (Voie et al., 2012). Even substances contained in leather preservatives used in harnesses, in catgut sutures, or compounds such as methylcellulose or carboxymethylcellulose used as stabilizers in vaccines may provoke allergies (Ohmori et al., 2005).

Allergies to Parasites

The beneficial role of the IgE-mast cell-feosinophil system in immunity to parasitic worms was first observed in the self-cure phenomenon in sheep (see Chapter 29). Helminths preferentially stimulate IgE responses, and helminth infestations are commonly associated with many of the signs of allergy and anaphylaxis; for example, animals with tapeworms may show respiratory distress or urticaria. Anaphylaxis may be provoked by rupture of a hydatid cyst during surgery or through transfusion of blood from a dog infected with *Dirofilaria immitis* to a sensitized animal.

Allergies are also commonly associated with exposure to arthropod antigens. Chitin, the major component of arthropod exoskeletons and fungal cell walls is an effective trigger of immediate hypersensitivity. Insect stings account for many human deaths each year as a result of acute anaphylaxis following sensitization to venom. Anaphylaxis can also occur in cattle infested with the warble fly (*Hypoderma bovis*) if their subcutaneous pupae rupture and the animal reacts to the released coelomic fluid (Burton and Zaccone, 2007).

In horses and cattle, hypersensitivity to insect bites causes an allergic dermatitis variously called Gulf Coast itch or sweet itch. The insects involved include midges (*Culicoides* species), black flies (*Simulium* species), stable flies (*Stomoxys calcitrans*), and mosquitoes. If animals are allergic to antigens in the saliva of these insects, biting results in the development of urticaria accompanied by intense pruritus. The itching may provoke severe self-mutilation with subsequent secondary infection that may mask the original allergic nature of the lesion. Some horses may also develop airway hyperreactivity (Lanz et al., 2017). There is a major genetic component to this type of hypersensitivity.

Animals do not inevitably respond to arthropod allergens with a type I hypersensitivity. Thus responses to *Demodex* mites may be mediated by ILC2 cells, while responses to flea saliva may be T cell mediated (see Chapter 34).

Flea-bite allergic dermatitis is the single most important allergic skin disease in companion animals. There is no breed or gender predisposition, but atopic animals as well as those exposed to fleas on an intermittent basis tend to get more severe disease. Continual exposure to fleas at an early age appears to result in hyposensitization. Pruritus is a consistent feature, as is a history of flea infestation. Affected animals, in addition to the characteristic clinical signs, show a reaction to intradermally injected flea salivary antigen. Most sensitive animals will respond within a few minutes, but up to 30% may show a delayed skin response at 24–48 hours. Hyposensitization therapy has not been shown to be successful in treating flea allergy. Flea allergy can be successfully treated only by total flea control.

Eosinophilic Granuloma Complex

The presence of large numbers of eosinophils in skin is often associated with the development of pathological lesions. Thus, when purified eosinophil cationic protein (ECP) or eosinophil-derived neurotoxin (EDN) are injected into guinea pig or rabbit skin, they disrupt skin integrity and cause inflammation. ECP produces ulcers, whereas EDN produces cellular exudates. Purified eosinophil peroxidase and the chemokine MBP-1 produce induration and erythema. The activities of these proteins may explain the development of lesions in eosinophil-associated skin diseases (Bloom, 2006).

A seasonal eosinophilic lesion in cats has been associated with mosquito bites. This may present as scattered individual crusted papules. The eosinophilic plaques in the skin are intensely pruritic. As a result, the lesions may be masked by self-inflicted trauma and secondary bacterial infection. Histologically, they are associated with a local mast cell and eosinophil infiltration, as well as an eosinophilia. They contain elevated levels of IL-4, IL-5, IL-13, and IL-17A, as well as Th2-attracting chemokines (Vargo et al., 2023).

The eosinophilic granuloma complex is a group of diseases associated with various types of skin lesions (ulcer, plaque, and granuloma) in cats. Although their cause is unknown, they have been associated with flea or food allergies, or atopic dermatitis. (Fig. 31.11). Eosinophilic granulomas are not pruritic and present as a line of raised pink plaques on the skin. Some may present as scattered individual crusted papules. Linear eosinophilic ulcers (sometimes called indolent or rodent ulcers) are commonly located in the oral cavity or on the lips. Removal of the offending allergen may result in clinical improvement, and corticosteroid treatment is usually of benefit. The linear form and indolent ulcers may be difficult to treat and may require more aggressive therapy.

An idiopathic hypereosinophilic syndrome has been described in humans, cats, and dogs. It is characterized by a prolonged, unexplained eosinophilia, the infiltration of many organs with eosinophils, organ dysfunction (affecting especially the heart, but also the lungs, spleen, liver, skin, bone marrow, gastrointestinal tract, and central nervous system), and death. An eosinophilic enteritis may result from canine hookworm infestation. Eosinophilic lung diseases such as bronchitis and bronchopneumopathy also occur in dogs. Their initiating trigger(s) are unknown (Johnson et al., 2019).

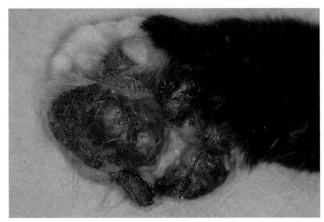

Fig. 31.11 An eosinophilic granuloma on the footpad of a dog. Courtesy of Dr. Robert Kennis.

DIAGNOSIS OF TYPE I HYPERSENSITIVITY

Diagnosis of allergic disease is based on clinical history and, if possible, the identification of the offending allergens by direct skin testing, or serology, and the exclusion of other similar conditions (Hensel et al., 2015).

The term *hypersensitivity* is used to denote inflammation that occurs in response to normally harmless material. For example, animals normally do not react to antigens injected intradermally. If, however, an allergic animal is given an intradermal injection of allergen, it will provoke local skin inflammation. Vasoactive molecules are released to produce redness (erythema) as a result of capillary dilation, as well as circumscribed edema (a wheal) due to increased vascular permeability. The reaction may also generate an erythematous flare due to arteriolar dilation caused by a local axon reflex. This wheal-and-flare response to an allergen reaches maximal intensity within 30 minutes and then disappears within a few hours. A late-phase reaction sometimes occurs 6–12 hours later.

Intradermal skin testing using very dilute aqueous solutions of allergens has been widely used for the diagnosis of allergies, especially canine atopic dermatitis. Following injection, the site is examined for an inflammatory response. The results obtained must be interpreted carefully since both false-positive and false-negative responses may occur. For example, the concentration of antigen in commercial skin testing solutions may be too low. Dogs may be up to 10 times less sensitive than humans to intradermal allergens such as pollens, fungi, or animal danders. False-positive reactions may be due to the presence of preservatives in allergen solutions. False-negative responses may be due to steroid treatment. The mixture of allergens used for intradermal skin testing commonly includes allergens from trees, grasses, fungi, weeds, danders, feathers, house dust mites, and insects. Intradermal skin testing is less commonly performed in cats because they fail to develop a significant wheal, and the reaction is therefore difficult to evaluate.

A research technique used to detect IgE antibodies is called the passive cutaneous anaphylaxis test. In this test, dilutions of test serum are injected at different sites into the skin of a normal animal. After waiting 24–48 hours, the antigen solution is administered intravenously. In a positive reaction, each injection site will show an immediate inflammatory response. The injected antibodies may remain fixed in the skin for a very long period of time. In the case of the calf, this may be up to 8 weeks. Because it is sometimes difficult to detect very mild inflammatory responses, they can be made more visible by injecting the test

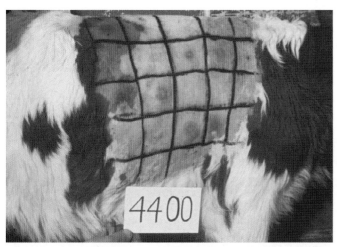

Fig. 31.12 PCA reactions in a calf. Several different sera were tested for PCA activity on the flank of a normal calf. *PCA*, Passive cutaneous anaphylaxis. Courtesy Dr. P. Eyre.

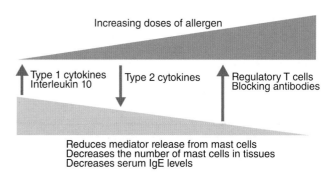

Fig. 31.13 The principles of allergen-specific immunotherapy. Increasing doses of allergen promote a T helper 1 cells response, while at the same time reducing the T helper 2 cells response and regulating antibody production. *IgE*, Immunoglobin E.

animal intravenously with Evans blue dye. The dye binds to serum albumin and does not normally leave the bloodstream. At injection sites where vascular permeability is increased, the dye-labeled albumin enters the tissue fluid and forms a striking blue patch (Fig. 31.12).

Serological methods of measuring the level of specific IgE in body fluids include the RAST (radioallergosorbent test), chemiluminescence assays, Western blotting, and ELISAs (see Chapter 43). These are not subject to clinical bias, but there may be a poor correlation between the results obtained by serology or skin testing and clinical severity. There is also a poor correlation between ELISA results and intradermal testing. Serological assays are especially prone to a high level of false-positive results (low specificity). A negative ELISA will generally rule out extrinsic disease. Heavily parasitized dogs may have elevated IgE levels, and this may result in false-positive serological results. For these reasons, many veterinary dermatologists prefer intradermal skin testing to serology.

TREATMENT OF TYPE I HYPERSENSITIVITY

By far the most satisfactory treatment of extrinsic allergic disease is avoidance of exposure to the allergen. Specific immunotherapy gives good responses in up to 80% of cases, but secondary infections such as bacterial or yeast (*Malassezia*) infections or flea infestations must also be controlled. Allergen-specific immunotherapy may also be used. This has the potential to induce stable, long-term remissions but is not a substitute for avoidance. Topical therapy, such as bathing with mild shampoos helps considerably. Diets enriched in the omega-3 fatty acids eicosapentaenoic acid and docosahexaenoic acid may be beneficial when fed to dogs with chronic allergic dermatitis. Omega-3 (fish) oil or omega-6 (evening primrose) oil probably promotes the synthesis of antiinflammatory eicosanoids (LeBlanc et al., 2008).

The principal indications for drug therapy include short-term, temporary relief either while waiting to begin immunotherapy or while waiting for it to take effect. Drugs may also be useful for relief of transient recurrences or in animals in which immunotherapy is not possible.

Topical or oral corticosteroids are most commonly used to reduce the irritation and inflammation associated with the acute allergic response. These drugs can suppress all aspects of inflammation by inhibiting NF-κB and blocking the production of inflammatory mediators (see Chapter 42). Other immunosuppressants, such as the calcineurin inhibitors, cyclosporine and tacrolimus may have similar benefits.

Epinephrine is the most important drug used to treat anaphylaxis. It is rapidly absorbed following intramuscular injection and thus can rapidly reverse the clinical signs of shock. Another group of drugs widely employed in the treatment of type I hypersensitivity reactions are the specific pharmacological inhibitors. These drugs, by mimicking the structure of the active mediators, stimulate inhibitory receptors. Thus H1 antihistamines such as diphenhydramine can effectively inhibit the activities of histamine. However, since histamine is only one of a large number of mast cell-derived mediators, and its levels do not correlate well with skin disease severity, antihistamines are of limited effectiveness in controlling allergic diseases in animals.

Treatment of chronic pruritus and skin lesions includes oral and topical corticosteroids, oral cyclosporine, and topical tacrolimus, in addition to oclacitinib and possibly oral interferons. Allergen-specific immunotherapy should be offered when feasible. Cytokine-inhibiting monoclonal antibodies are being widely tested for the treatment of atopic dermatitis in humans with encouraging results (see Chapter 42; Saridomichelakis and Olivry, 2016).

Allergen-Specific Immunotherapy

Allergies may be controlled in dogs and cats by allergen-specific immunotherapy. This involves administering gradually increasing quantities of an allergen to the animal in order to reduce the severity of subsequent allergic disease. In veterinary medicine multiple open studies have suggested that this therapy is effective in the treatment of atopic dermatitis, although few randomized controlled trials have been published (Shida et al., 2004).

Immunotherapy injections promote IgG rather than IgE production and reduce the recruitment of inflammatory cells. This reduces mast cell and eosinophil numbers in the lung, as well as the infiltration of CD4+ T cells and eosinophils in the skin. It induces a shift in the dominant helper cell response from Th2 to Th1 (Fig. 31.13). For example, the IFN-γ/IL-4 ratio is low in atopic dogs, indicating a Th2 cytokine profile. After immunotherapy, the ratio rises, IFN-γ levels increase, and the balance shifts toward a Th1 response. It also stimulates Tregs to produce IL-10, inhibiting IgE production, mast cell activation, and histamine and leukotriene release (Mueller, 2023).

In immunotherapy, small amounts of dilute aqueous solutions of antigen are administered. The first injections contain very little allergen. Over a number of weeks, the dose is progressively increased. If an animal's allergy is of the seasonal type, the course of injections should be timed to reach completion just before the anticipated antigen exposure. It has been estimated that up to 80% of dogs have a good to excellent response to this procedure. This includes clinical improvement and a reduction in the amount of medication required. It may take several months before the benefits of immunotherapy become apparent. Cats may respond even better than dogs. On the other hand, horses with hypersensitivity to biting flies have a poor response to allergen-specific immunotherapy. Sublingual immunotherapy may also be an effective treatment modality. It appears to work well against dust mite and food allergy in dogs (Maina and Cox, 2016).

REFERENCES

Bloom, P.B., 2006. Canine and feline eosinophilic skin diseases. Vet. Clin. Small Anim. 36, 141–160.

Burton, O.T., Zaccone, P., 2007. The potential role of chitin in allergic reactions. Trends Immunol. 28, 419–422.

Campbell, S.G., 1970. Milk allergy, an autoallergic disease of cattle. Cornell Vet. 60, 684–721.

Chesney, C.J., 2002. Food sensitivity in the dog: a quantitative study. J. Small Anim. Pract. 43, 203–207.

Elmariah, S.B., Lerner, E.A., 2013. The missing link between itch and inflammation in atopic dermatitis. Cell 155, 267–269.

Fukuyama, T., Ehling, S., Cook, E., Baumer, W., 2015. Topically administered Janus-kinase inhibitors to facitinib and oclacitinib display impressive anti-pruritic and anti-inflammatory responses in a model of allergic dermatitis. J. Pharmacol. Exp. Ther. 354, 394–405.

Gail, S.J., Tsai, M., 2013. IgE and mast cells in allergic disease. Nat. Med. 18 (5), 693–704.

Gershwin, L.J., 2009. ed A special issue dedicated to reviews of IgE and allergy in domestic animals. Vet. Immunol. Immunopathol. 132, 1–84.

Gershwin, L.J., Netherwood, K.A., Norris, M.S., Behrens, N.E., Shao, M.X., 2012. Equine IgE responses to non-viral vaccine components. Vaccine 30, 7615–7620.

Gilbert, S., Halliwell, R.E.W., 2005. The effects of endoparasitism on the immune response to orally administered antigen in cats. Vet. Immunol. Immunopathol. 106, 113–120.

Gonzales, A.J., Bowman, J.W., Fici, G.J., Zhang, M., et al., 2014. Oclacitinib (APOQUEL®) is a novel Janus kinase inhibitor with activity against cytokines involved in allergy. J. Vet. Pharmacol. Ther. 37, 317–324.

Gonzales, A.J., Humphrey, W.R., Messamore, J.E., Fleck, T.J., et al., 2013. Interleukin-31: its role in canine pruritus and naturally occurring canine atopic dermatitis. Vet. Dermatol. 24, 48–e12.

Hakanen, E., Lehtimäki, J., Salmeda, E., Tiira, K., et al., 2018. Urban environment predisposes dogs and their owners to allergic symptoms. Sci. Rep. https://doi.org/10.1038/s41598-018-19953-3

Hensel, P., Santoro, D., Favrot, C., Hill, P., Griffin, C., 2015. Canine atopic dermatitis: detailed guidelines for diagnosis and allergen identification. BMC Vet. Res. 11, 196–220.

Hirshman, C.A., Malley, A., Downes, H., 1980. Basenji-Greyhound model of asthma reactivity to *Ascaris suum*, citric acid and methacholine. J. Appl. Physiol. 49, 953–957.

Iweala, O.I., Nagler, C.R., 2019. The microbiome and food allergy. Ann. Rev. Immunol. 37, 377–403.

Jackson, H.A., 2023. Food allergy in dogs and cats: current perspectives on etiology, diagnosis and management. J. Am. Vet. Med. Assoc. https://doi.org/10.2460/javma.22.0548

Johnson, L.R., Johnson, E.G., Hulsebosch, S.E., Dear, J.D., Vernau, W., 2019. Eosinophilic bronchitis, eosinophilic granuloma, and eosinophilic bronchopneumopathy in 75 dogs (2006–2016). J. Vet. Intern. Med. 33, 2217–2226.

Johnston, L.K., Chien, K.B., Bryce, P.J., 2014. The immunology of food allergy. J. Immunol. 192, 2529–2534.

Lambrecht, B.N., Hammad, H., 2015. The immunology of asthma. Nat. Immunol. 16, 45–56.

Lambrecht, B.N., Hammad, H., 2017. The immunology of the allergy epidemic and the hygiene hypothesis. Nat. Immunol. 18 (10), 1076–1083.

Lambrecht, B.N., Hammad, H., Fahy, J., 2019. The cytokines of asthma. Immunity 50, 975–991.

Lanz, S., Brunner, A., Graubner, C., Marti, E., Gerber, V., 2017. Insect bite hypersensitivity in horses is associated with airway hyperreactivity. J. Vet. Intern. Med. https://doi.org/10.1111/jvim.14817

LeBlanc, C.J., Horohov, D.W., Bauer, J.E., et al., 2008. Effects of dietary supplementation with fish oil on in vivo production of inflammatory mediators in clinically normal dogs. Am. J. Vet. Res. 69, 486–493.

Maina, E., Cox, E., 2016. A double blind, randomized, placebo controlled trial of the efficacy, quality of life and safety of food allergen-specific sublingual immunotherapy in client owned dogs with adverse food reactions: a small pilot study. Vet. Dermatol. 27, 361–e91.

Marsella, R., Sousa, C.A., Gonzales, A.J., Fadok, V.A., 2012. Current understanding of the pathophysiologic mechanisms of canine atopic dermatitis. JAVMA 241, 194–207.

Marsella, R., 2013. Does filaggrin expression correlate with severity of clinical signs in dogs with atopic dermatitis? Vet. Dermatol. 24, 266–e59.

McCandless, E.E., Rugg, C.A., Fici, G.J., Messamore, J.E., Aleo, M.M., Gonzales, A.J., 2014. Allergen-induced production of IL-31 by canine Th2 Cells and identification of immune, skin, and neuronal target cells. Vet. Immunol. Immunopathol. 157, 42–48.

Miller, J.D., 2018. The role of dust mites in allergy. Clin. Revs. Allergy Immunol. https://doi.org/10.1007/s12016-018-8693-0.

Mueller, R.S., 2023. A systematic review of allergen immunotherapy, a successful therapy for canine atopic dermatitis and feline atopic skin syndrome. J. Amer. Vet. Med. Assn. https://doi.org/10.2460/javma.22.0576.

Nakashima, C., Otsuka, A., Kabashima, K., 2018. Interleukin-31 and interleukin-31 receptor: new therapeutic targets for atopic dermatitis. Exp. Dermatol. 27, 327–331.

Ohmori, K., Masuda, K., Maeda, S., Kaburagi, Y., et al., 2005. IgE reactivity to vaccine components in dogs that developed immediate-type allergic reactions after vaccination. Vet. Immunol. Immunopathol. 104, 249–256.

Padrid, P., 2000. Feline asthma. Vet. Clin. NA: Small Anim. Pract. 30, 1279–1292.

Palmer, C.N., Irvine, A.D., Terron-Kwiatkowski, A., et al., 2006. Common loss-of-function variants of the epidermal barrier protein filaggrin are a major predisposing factor for atopic dermatitis. Nat. Genet. 38, 441–446.

Petersen, E.B.M., Skov, L., Yhyssen, J.P., Jensen, P., 2019. Role of the gut microbiota in atopic dermatitis: a systemic review. Acta Derm. Venereol. 99, 5–11.

Pucheu-Haston, C.M., Bizikova, P., Eisenschenk, M.N., Santoro, D., et al., 2015a. Review: the role of antibodies, autoantigens and food allergens in canine atopic dermatitis. Vet. rDermatol. 26, 115–e130.

Pucheu-Haston, C.M., Bizikova, P., Marsella, R., Santoro, D., et al., 2015b. Review: lymphocytes, cytokines, chemokines and the T-helper 1-T-helper 2 balance in canine atopic dermatitis. Vet. Dermatol. 26, 124–e132.

Sampson, H.A., O'Mahony, L., Burks, A.W., Plaut, M., et al., 2018. Mechanisms of food allergy. J. Allergy Clin. Immunol. 141, 11–19.

Saridomichelakis, M.N., Olivry, T., 2016. An update on the treatment of canine atopic dermatitis. Vet. J. 207, 29–37.

Shaw, S.C., Wood, J.L., Freeman, J., et al., 2004. Estimation of heritability of atopic dermatitis in labradors and golden retrievers,. Am. J. Vet. Res. 65, 1014–1020.

Shida, M., Kadoya, M., Park, S.J., et al., 2004. Allergen-specific immunotherapy induces Th1 shift in dogs with atopic dermatitis. Vet. Immunol. Immunopathol. 102, 19–31.

Sparling, B.A., Moss, N., Kaur, G., Clark, D., et al., 2022. Unique cell populations and disease progression markers in canines with atopic dermatitis. J. Immunol. 209, 1379–1388.

Tizard, I.R., 2022. Allergies and Hypersensitivity Disease in Animals. Elsevier, St Louis, MO, ISBN: 978-0-323-76393-6

Vargo, C., Howerth, E.W., Banovic, F., 2023. Transcriptome analysis of selected cytokine and chemokines in the eosinophilic plaques of cats with atopic skin syndrome. Vet. Dermatol. 34, 40–45.

Voie, K.L., Campbell, K.L., Lavergne, S.N., 2012. Drug hypersensitivity reactions targeting the skin in dogs and cats. J. Vet. Intern. Med. 26, 863–874.

Wood, S.H., Ke, X., Nuttall, T., McEwan, N., et al., 2009. Genome-wide association analysis of canine atopic dermatitis and identification of disease related SNPs. Immunogenetics 61, 765–772. 2009

Xu, J., Zanvit, P., Tseng, P.-Y., Liu, N., et al., 2020. The cytokine TGF-β induces interleukin-31 expression in dermal dendritic cells to activate sensory neurons and stimulate wound itching. Immunity 53, 1–134.

Ziegler, S.F., Roan, F., Bell, B.D., Stoklasek, T.A., Kitajima, M., Han, H., 2013. The biology of thymic stromal lymphopoietin (TSLP). Adv. Pharmacol. 66, 129–155.

32

Red Cell Antigens and Antibody-Mediated Hypersensitivity

CHAPTER OUTLINE

Red blood cells, like nucleated cells, express many different glycoproteins and glycolipids on their surface. Unlike the major histocompatibility complex (MHC) molecules, these molecules are not involved in antigen processing, although they do influence graft rejection (allografts between blood group-incompatible animals are rapidly rejected). Most are functional components of the cell membrane. For example, the ABO glycoproteins in humans are anion and glucose transporter proteins, while the molecules of the M and C systems of sheep red cells are associated with the membrane potassium pump and amino acid transport, respectively.

If blood is transfused from one animal to another, unrelated individual, these red cell molecules may act as powerful antigens and stimulate antibody responses in the recipient. These antibodies will then cause the rapid elimination of the transfused red cells by complement-mediated intravascular hemolysis and by extravascular destruction by the mononuclear phagocyte system. Cell destruction by antibodies in this way is classified as a type II hypersensitivity reaction.

BLOOD GROUPS

The antigenic molecules expressed on the surface of red blood cells are called blood group antigens or erythrocyte antigens (EAs). There are many different blood group antigens, and they vary in their antigenicity, some being more potent and therefore of greater importance than others. The expression of blood group antigens is controlled by genes and inherited in conventional fashion. For each blood group system, there are a variable number of alleles. The complexity of erythrocyte blood group systems varies greatly. They range from simple systems like the L system of cattle, which consists of one gene with two alleles coding for a single protein antigen, to the highly complex B system of cattle. The B system contains several hundred alleles that, together with the other cattle blood groups, may yield millions of unique blood group combinations. Although most blood group antigens are integral cell membrane components, some are also found free in serum, saliva, and other body fluids and passively adsorbed onto red cell surfaces. Examples of such soluble antigens include the J antigens of cattle, the R antigens of sheep, the A antigens of pigs, and the DEA7 antigens of dogs (Tizard, 2022).

BOX 32.1 The Intestinal Microbiota and Blood Groups

Intestinal mucus is "decorated with" blood group antigens. These are synthesized by enterocytes, but only in certain individuals (secretors). These blood group antigens influence the composition of the intestinal microbiota. Thus, Bifidobacteria depend on these blood group antigens to colonize the gut, which is much less common in nonsecretors. Nonsecretor humans are more susceptible to necrotizing enterocolitis and gram-negative sepsis in premature infants. Presumably because they lack the protective benefits of the Bifidobacteria. On the other hand, noroviruses can also attach through these glycans when they colonize the gut so nonsecretors are resistant to these agents!

Animals may make antibodies against foreign blood group antigens even though they may never have been exposed previously to foreign red cells. For example, J-negative cattle have anti-J antibodies in their serum, and A-negative pigs have anti-A antibodies. These "natural" antibodies (or isoantibodies) are derived not from previous contact with foreign red cells but from exposure to cross-reacting epitopes that are commonly encountered in nature (Fig. 10.8; Maynard et al., 2012). Many blood group antigens, for example, are also common structural components of plants, the intestinal microbiota, or parasitic helminths. The presence of these natural antibodies is not, however, a uniform phenomenon, and not all blood group antigens are accompanied by the production of natural antibodies to their alternative alleles (Box 32.1).

BLOOD TRANSFUSIONS

Blood is easily transfused from one animal to another. If the donor's red cells are identical to those of the recipient, no immune response results. If, however, the recipient possesses preexisting antibodies to donor's red cell antigens, the transfused cells will be attacked immediately. The preexisting antibodies are usually of the IgM class. When these antibodies bind red cell antigens, they can cause agglutination or hemolysis, or stimulate opsonization and phagocytosis of the transfused cells. In these cases, acute reactions occur within 24 hours. In the absence of preexisting antibodies, the transfused red cells will stimulate an immune response in the recipient. The transfused cells will circulate until antibodies are produced and will then be eliminated in a delayed response. A second transfusion with identical foreign cells results in their immediate destruction.

The rapid destruction of large numbers of foreign red cells can lead to serious illness. The severity of hemolytic transfusion reactions ranges from a mild febrile response to rapid death, depending on the amount of incompatible blood transfused. Early recognition of the problem may avert the most severe consequences. The most severe reactions occur when large amounts of incompatible blood are transfused to a sensitized recipient. This results in complement activation and lysis of the transfused cells. Large amounts of free hemoglobin escape, resulting in hemoglobinemia and hemoglobinuria. The lysed red cell membranes may trigger blood clotting and disseminated intravascular coagulation. Complement activation also results in anaphylatoxin production, mast cell degranulation, and the release of vasoactive molecules and cytokines. These molecules may provoke shock with hypotension, bradycardia, and apnea. The animal may show sympathetic responses such as sweating, salivation, lacrimation, diarrhea, and vomiting. This may be followed by a second stage in which the animal is hypertensive, with cardiac arrhythmias as well as increased heart and respiratory rates.

If such a reaction is suspected, the transfusion must be stopped immediately. It is important to maintain urine flow with fluids and a diuretic because the free hemoglobin may cause renal tubular destruction. Recovery follows elimination of the foreign red cells. Transfusion reactions can be almost totally prevented by blood typing the donor and recipient and prior testing of the recipient's serum for antibodies against the donor's red cells. The procedure is called cross-matching.

Blood typing in dogs and cats has been greatly simplified by the availability of commercial blood testing kits. These include testing cards, immunochromatography tests, and the use of typing gels. Testing cards have shallow wells containing lyophilized monoclonal antibodies such as anti-DEA1.1. A drop of anticoagulated whole blood is dropped into a well, and after about 2 minutes, a positive response is revealed by agglutination. Cats can also be effectively blood typed in this way. In immunochromatography, whole blood is allowed to perfuse across a membrane in which a line of monoclonal antibody has been printed. Positive cells will thus form a colored line when captured by the monoclonal antibody (see Chapter 43). As described later, typing gels in small tubes contain a blood group-specific monoclonal antibody. If the test is positive, the antibody prevents the tested blood cells from passing through the gel.

Blood typing kits are generally unavailable for large animal species. In this case, typing is best done in a laboratory. Blood from the donor is centrifuged, and the plasma is discarded. The red cells are then resuspended in saline and recentrifuged. This washing procedure is repeated (usually three times), and eventually a 2%–4% suspension of red cells in saline is made. These donor's red cells are mixed with recipient serum and incubated at 37°C for 15–30 minutes. If the donor's red cells are lysed or agglutinated by the recipient's serum, no transfusion should be attempted with those cells. It is occasionally found that the donor's serum may react with the recipient's red cells. This is not of major clinical significance because transfused donor antibodies are rapidly diluted within the recipient. Nevertheless, blood giving such a reaction is best avoided.

HEMOLYTIC DISEASE OF THE NEWBORN

Female animals may become sensitized to foreign red cells not only by incompatible blood transfusions given for clinical purposes but also by leakage of fetal red cells into their bloodstream through the placenta during pregnancy. Once sensitized, these anti-red cell antibodies may then be concentrated in maternal colostrum. When a newborn animal suckles, these colostral antibodies will be absorbed through the intestinal wall and enter its bloodstream. These antibodies, directed against the blood group antigens of the newborn, then cause rapid destruction of their red cells. The resulting disease is called hemolytic disease of the newborn (HDN) or neonatal isoerythrolysis (Whiting and David, 2000).

Four conditions must be met for HDN to occur: the young animal must inherit a red cell antigen from its sire that is not present in its mother. The mother must be sensitized to this red cell antigen. The mother's response to this antigen may be boosted repeatedly by transplacental hemorrhage or repeated pregnancies. Finally, a newborn animal must ingest colostrum containing high-titered antibodies to its red cells.

DOMESTIC ANIMALS

All mammals possess red cell antigens that can affect blood transfusions and, on occasion, cause HDN in newborn animals (Table 32.1). Although historically they were named alphabetically in order of their discovery, there is a growing tendency to add the prefix EA to reduce confusion with MHC antigens.

Horses

Horses possess seven internationally recognized blood group systems (EAA, EAC, EAD, EAK, EAP, EAQ, and EAU). The alleles within each system are denoted by lowercase letters. Some, such as EAC, EAK, and EAU, are simple, one-gene, two-allele, two-phenotype systems. EAA contains 7 alleles, EAO has 4, and EAQ has 3. On the other hand, the EAD system is very complex, with at least 25 alleles identified to date. About 10% of normal horses have natural antibodies against foreign blood groups, especially EAAa and EACa. These antibodies can cause severe reactions following incompatible transfusions. Their major

TABLE 32.1 Domestic Animal Blood Groups

Species	Blood Group Systems	Serology
Horse	EAA, EAC, EAD, EAK, EAP, EAQ, EAU	Agglutination Hemolytic
Bovine	EAA, EAB, EAC, EAF, EAJ*, EAL, EAM, EAR', EAS, EAT', EAZ	Hemolytic
Sheep	EAA, EAB, EAC, EAD, EAM, EAR*, EAF30, EAF41	Hemolytic Agglutination (D only)
Goat	EAA, EAB, EAC, EAE, EAF, EAR*	Hemolytic
Pig	EAA*, EAB, EAC, EAD, EAE, EAF, EAG, EAH, EAI, EAJ, EAK, EAL, EAM, EAN, EAO, EAP	Agglutination Hemolytic Antiglobulin
Dog	DEA1, 3, 4, 5, 6, 7*, 8, Dal, Kai	Agglutination Hemolytic Antiglobulin
Cat	AB, Mik	Agglutination Hemolytic

*Soluble blood group substances.

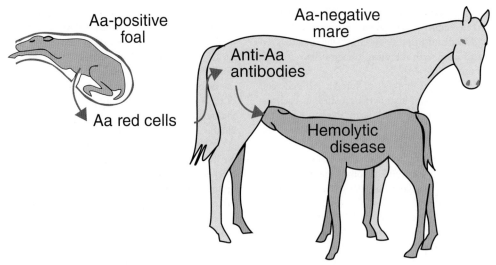

Fig. 32.1 The pathogenesis of hemolytic disease of the newborn in foals. In the first stage, fetal red cells leak into the mother's circulation and sensitize her. In the second stage, these antibodies are concentrated in colostrum and are then ingested by the suckling foal. These ingested antibodies enter the foal's circulation and cause red cell destruction.

significance lies in the fact that HDN in foals is relatively common (Fig. 32.1). In mules, in which the antigenic differences between dam and sire are great, about 8%–10% of foals may be affected (McClure et al., 1994). In thoroughbreds and standardbreds, the prevalence of HDN is considerably less, ranging from 0.05% to 2% of foals. This is despite the fact that in up to 14% of pregnancies, the mare and the stallion have incompatible red cells (Bailey, 1982).

HDN may occur in foals born from mares that have been sensitized by previous blood transfusions or by administration of vaccines containing equine tissues. Most commonly, however, mares are sensitized by exposure to fetal red cells as a result of repeated pregnancies. The mechanism of this sensitization is unclear, but fetal red cells are assumed to gain access to the maternal circulation as a result of transplacental hemorrhage. Mares have been shown to respond to fetal red cells as early as day 56 after conception. The greatest leakage probably occurs during the last month of pregnancy and during foaling as a result of the breakdown of placental blood vessels (Becht, 1983).

Maternal sensitization is usually minimal following a first pregnancy. However, if repeated pregnancies result in exposure to the same red cell antigens, the maternal response will be boosted. Hemolytic disease is, therefore, usually only a problem in mares that have had several foals. The most severe form of the disease results from the production of antibodies directed against the Aa antigen of the EAA system. Anti-Qa (EAQ system) produces a less severe disease of slower onset. In practice, 90% of clinical cases are attributable to anti-Aa and anti-Qa. Other minor antigens, such as Pa, Ab, Qc, Ua, Dc, and Db, have been implicated in some cases. Mares that lack Aa and Qa are therefore most likely to produce affected foals. Pregnant mares may also produce antibodies to Ca (EAC system), but these are rarely associated with clinical disease. Indeed, preexisting antibodies to Ca may reduce sensitization by Aa. The presence of this anti-Ca in a mare may eliminate any fetal red cells that enter her bloodstream and so prevent further sensitization.

Antibodies produced by mares do not cross the placenta but reach the foal through the colostrum. Affected foals are therefore born healthy but sicken several hours after suckling. The severity of the disease is determined by the amount of antibody absorbed and by the sensitizing antigen. The earliest signs are weakness and depression.

The mucous membranes of affected foals may be pale and may eventually show a distinct jaundice. Some foals sicken by 6–8 hours and die from shock so rapidly that they may not have time to develop jaundice. More commonly, the disease presents as lethargy and weakness between 12 and 48 hours of age, although it may be delayed for as long as 5 days. Icterus of the mucous membranes and sclera is consistent in foals that survive for at least 48 hours. Hemoglobinuria, although uncommon, is diagnostic in a newborn foal. As a result of anoxia, some foals in the terminal stages of the disease may convulse or become comatose. The most common causes of death in these foals are liver failure, brain damage, and bacterial sepsis.

Hemolytic disease is readily diagnosed by clinical signs alone. Hematological examination is of little diagnostic use but may be of assistance in indicating appropriate treatment. Definitive diagnosis requires that immunoglobulin be demonstrated on the surface of the red cells of the foal. In the case of anti-Aa or anti-Qa, addition of a source of complement (fresh normal rabbit serum) causes rapid hemolysis. If hemolytic disease is anticipated, the serum of a pregnant mare may be tested for antibodies by an indirect antiglobulin test (see Chapter 43). By using red cells from horses with a major sensitizing blood group, it is possible to show that the mare's antibody titer increases significantly in the month before parturition.

A test that may be useful for detecting the presence of antierythrocyte antibodies in colostrum is the jaundiced foal agglutination test. This involves making serial dilutions of colostrum in saline. A drop of anticoagulated foal blood is then added to each tube, and the tubes are centrifuged so that the red cells form a pellet at the bottom. In the presence of antibodies, the cells clump tightly, and the pellet remains intact when the tubes are emptied. Nonagglutinated red cells, in contrast, flow down the side of the tube. Concentrated colostrum is viscous and tends to induce rouleaux formation that mimics agglutination. However, if the mare's blood is used as a negative control, this can be accounted for. The foal's blood should also be diluted in saline to ensure that the foal has not already absorbed antibodies and that false-positive results are not obtained.

Mildly affected foals, with a packed cell volume (PCV) of 15%–25% and a red cell count greater than 4×10^6, will continue to nurse. Those with a PCV of less than 10% will stop nursing and become recumbent.

The prognosis of uncomplicated hemolytic disease is good, provided the condition is diagnosed sufficiently early and the appropriate treatment is instituted rapidly. Management of HDN includes prevention of further antibody absorption, adequate nutrition, oxygen therapy, fluid and electrolyte therapy, and maintenance of the acid-base balance. Warmth, adequate hydration, and antimicrobial therapy are also critically important. In acute cases, blood transfusion is necessary. A red cell count of less than $3 \times 10^6/\mu L$ or a PCV of less than 15% warrants a blood transfusion. Transfused equine red cells have a half-life of only 2–4 days, so transfusion is only a temporary life-saving measure. Compatible blood may be difficult to find because of the high prevalence of Aa and Qa in the normal equine population. A donor should not only be Aa or Qa negative but should also lack antibodies to these antigens. Exchange transfusion, although efficient, requires a donor capable of providing at least 5 L of blood as well as a double intravenous catheter and an anesthetized foal. A much simpler procedure that avoids many difficulties is the transfusion of washed red cells from the mare. About 3–4 L of blood is collected in sodium citrate and centrifuged, after which the plasma is discarded. The red cells are washed once in saline and transfused slowly into the foal. The blood is usually given in divided doses about 6 hours apart. Milder cases of hemolytic disease may require only careful nursing.

If hemolytic disease is anticipated as a result of either a rising antibody titer or the previous birth of a hemolytic foal, stripping off the mare's colostrum and giving the foal colostrum from another mare will prevent its occurrence. The foal should not be allowed to suckle its own mare for 24–36 hours. Once suckling is permitted, the foal should only be allowed to take small quantities at first and should be observed carefully for adverse side effects.

Neonatal thrombocytopenia has been recorded in the foal. Immunoglobulins can be detected on the foal's platelets, and antibodies to these platelets can be found in the mare's serum (Buechner-Maxwell et al., 1997).

Horse blood groups may be identified by tube agglutination, hemolytic, and antiglobulin tests. Gel-based agglutination tests and immunochromatographic techniques have produced encouraging results (Luethy et al., 2016). Each blood group system has a preferred test system. The complement used in the hemolytic test comes from rabbits, but it must be absorbed before use to remove any antihorse antibodies.

Cattle

Eleven blood group systems—EAA, EAB, EAC, EAF, EAJ, EAL, EAM, EAR, EAS, EAT, and EAZ—have been identified in cattle. Two of these (EAB and EAJ) are of the greatest importance. The EAB blood group system is one of the most complex systems known since it is estimated to contain more than 60 different alleles. These alleles are not inherited independently but rather in specific combinations called phenogroups. Because of the complexity of the EAB system, it is practically impossible to obtain absolutely identical blood from any two unrelated cattle. Indeed, it has been suggested that the complexity of the EAB system is such that there exist sufficient different antigenic combinations to provide a unique identifying character for every bovine in the world. Naturally, such a system provides an ideal method for the accurate identification of individual animals, and breed societies may use blood grouping to check the identity of registered animals. The EAC system is also complex, with 10 alleles combining to form about 90 phenogroups (Thomsen et al., 2002).

The EAJ antigen is a lipid found free in body fluids and passively adsorbed onto red cells (Wagner et al., 1984). It is absent from the red cells of newborn calves but is acquired within the first 6 months of life. J-positive cattle are of two types. Some possess J antigen in high concentration, and this may be readily detected both on their red cells

and in serum. Other animals may have low levels of J in serum, and it is detected only with great difficulty on red cells. (It is probable that a secretor gene controls the expression of EAJ in cattle.) Anti-J is the only natural blood group antibody found in cattle. J-negative cattle, lacking the J antigen completely, may possess natural antiJ antibodies, although the level of these antibodies shows seasonal variation, being highest in the summer and fall. Because of the presence of these antibodies, transfusion of J-positive red cells into J-negative recipients may result in a transfusion reaction even in the absence of known previous sensitization.

HDN in calves is rare but has resulted from vaccination against anaplasmosis or babesiosis. These vaccines contain red cells from infected calves. In the case of *Anaplasma* vaccines, for example, the blood from a large number of infected donors is pooled, freeze-dried, and mixed with adjuvant before being administered to cattle. The vaccine against babesiosis consists of fresh, infected calf blood. Both vaccines cause infection and, consequently, the development of immunity in recipients. They may also stimulate the production of antibodies against blood group antigens of the EAA and EAF systems. Cows sensitized by these vaccines and then mated with bulls carrying the same blood groups can transmit colostral antibodies to their calves, which may then develop hemolytic disease.

The severity of HDN in calves is related to the amount of colostrum ingested. Calves are usually healthy at birth but begin to show symptoms 12 hours to 5 days later. In acute cases, death may occur within 24 hours after suckling, with the animals developing respiratory distress and hemoglobinuria. On necropsy, these calves have severe pulmonary edema, splenomegaly, and dark kidneys. Less severely affected animals develop anemia and jaundice and may die during the first week of life. The red cells of affected calves have antibodies on their surface (detected by an antiglobulin test) and may sometimes be lysed by the addition of complement in the form of fresh normal rabbit serum. Death is due to disseminated intravascular coagulation as a result of activation of the clotting system by red cell ghosts.

Bovine blood groups are detected by hemolytic tests. Washed red cells are incubated in specific antisera, and rabbit serum is used as a source of complement.

Bovine Neonatal Pancytopenia

Beginning in 2007 multiple outbreaks of an unexplained hemorrhagic disease of newborn beef calves were reported from many countries in Western Europe (Bastian et al., 2011). This is called bovine neonatal pancytopenia. Affected calves showed sudden onset bleeding, including nasal hemorrhage, petechiation on mucus membranes, internal bleeding, and excessive bleeding from minor wounds such as injection or ear-tag sites. The disease appeared 7–28 days after birth, and affected calves could die within 48 hours of disease onset. Investigation showed an early drop in granulocytes, followed by erythrocytes and lymphocytes. The net result was a profound pancytopenia, including thrombocytopenia, anemia, and leucopenia. The bone marrow was often completely aplastic. Mortality was as high as 90% in clinically affected calves, but there were clearly many subclinical cases as well. Since the disease only occurred in suckled calves and developed within hours of the first suckling, it appeared to result from the consumption of colostrum (Benedictus et al., 2014). Further investigations showed that the colostrum from cows known to produce affected calves contained antibodies directed against the MHC class I molecules expressed on neonatal leukocytes and bone marrow stem cells (Bell et al., 2015). (Precursors and committed cells of the thrombocyte, lymphocyte, and monocyte lineages and precursors of neutrophil, erythrocyte, and eosinophil lineages.) These antibodies also mediated phagocytosis of blood cells since they bound both the α-chain of MHC class I antigens

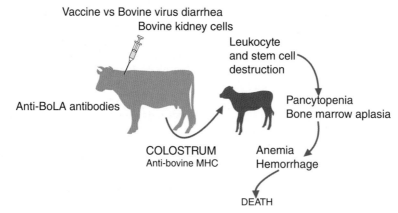

Fig. 32.2 The pathogenesis of bovine neonatal pancytopenia. It was triggered by a vaccine containing adjuvanted bovine kidney cells. *MHC*, Major histocompatibility complex.

and β2-microglobulin. These antibodies were not present in the serum or colostrum of cows that delivered healthy calves (Demasius et al., 2014).

The disease is now known to have been triggered by the administration of a specific vaccine against bovine virus diarrhea virus (BVDV) (Fig. 32.2; Kasonta et al., 2014). This vaccine—Pregsure; contained inactivated BVDV grown in a bovine kidney cell line. A potent, oil-in-water adjuvant containing Quil A was added (see Chapter 25). Immunization with this vaccine induced high levels of antibodies against the class I MHC antigens on the kidney cells. These antibodies, when transferred to calves via colostrum bound to their leukocytes and bone marrow stem cells and killed them. This resulted in the pancytopenia and bone marrow destruction. Not all of the calves born from cows that received this specific vaccine developed clinical disease. The reasons for this are unknown but most likely depend on their MHC haplotype. Antibody levels remain high in cows for many years and could be boosted by each pregnancy. As a result, BNP cases have occurred many years after the offending vaccine was removed from the market.

Sheep

The blood groups of sheep resemble those of cattle. Eight blood group systems (EAA, EAB, EAC, EAD, EAM, EAR, EAF30, and EAF41.) are currently recognized. The ovine equivalent of bovine EAB is also termed EAB and, like the bovine system, is complex, containing at least 52 different alleles. Sheep also possess an ovine equivalent of the bovine EAJ system, called the EAR system. Two soluble antigens are found in this system, R and O, coded for by alleles R and r. The production of R and O substances is controlled by a gene called I and its recessive allele I. If a sheep is homozygous for I, it expresses neither R nor O antigens. This interaction between the I/i genes and the R-O system is called an epistatic effect (Fig. 32.3). R and O antigens are soluble antigens found in the serum of II or Ii sheep and are passively adsorbed onto red cells. Natural antiR antibodies may be found in EAR-negative sheep. Sheep also fall into two groups according to whether their red cells have high or low potassium levels. This is regulated by the EAM blood group system. The Mb antigen is an inhibitor of potassium transport. Goats possess six recognized blood group systems, EAA, EAB, EAC, EAE, EAF, and EAR.

Sheep blood groups are detected by hemolytic tests. One exception to this rule is the EAD system, which is detected by agglutination.

Pigs

Sixteen blood group systems have been identified in the pig (EAA to EAP). Most are one-gene, two-allele systems. The most important exceptions are EAE with 17 alleles and EAM with 20. The most

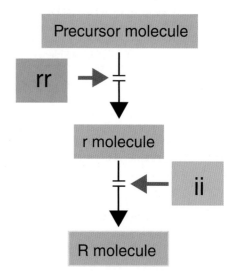

Fig. 32.3 The regulation of expression of EAR blood group antigens in sheep. The *I* gene controls expression of the EAR system.

important is the EAA system. EAA, like the human ABO system, controls the expression of two carbohydrate antigens, A and O, through the use of glycosyltransferases (Nguyen et al., 2011). Their expression is regulated by a gene called *S* (suppressor) with two alleles, S and s. In the homozygous recessive state (ss), this gene can prevent the production of the A and O substances (Fig. 32.4). As a result, the amount of these antigens bound to red cells in these animals is reduced to an undetectable level (Box 32.2). A and O substances, like J in cattle and R and O in sheep, are not true red cell antigens but rather soluble carbohydrates found in serum and saliva and passively adsorbed onto red cells after birth. Natural anti-A antibodies may be present in A-negative pigs, and transfusion of A-positive blood into such an animal may cause transient collapse and hemoglobinuria.

HDN in piglets formerly occurred as a result of the use of a hog cholera vaccine containing pig blood. This vaccine consisted of pooled blood from viremic pigs inactivated with the dye crystal violet. Sensitization of sows by this vaccine led to the occasional occurrence of hemolytic disease of their offspring. There appeared to be a breed predisposition to this disease, which was most commonly seen in the offspring of Essex and Wessex sows. Affected piglets did not necessarily show clinical disease, although their red cells were sensitized by antibody. Other piglets showed rapidly progressive weakness and pallor of mucous membranes preceding death, and those animals that survived

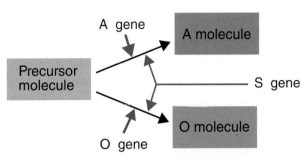

Fig. 32.4 The production of A or O blood group substances by a pig requires the presence of the *S* gene. Pigs that lack this gene (ss animals) produce neither of these blood group substances.

BOX 32.2 Inheritance of the EAA Blood Group System in Pigs

In pigs, the expression of the EAA blood group is regulated by two gene loci. One locus, the A locus, contains two alleles, A and O, of which A is dominant. The other, the S locus, also contains two alleles, S and its recessive allele s. The S locus controls the expression of the A system, so that A or O blood groups can only be expressed if the animal carries at least one S gene. Possible genotypes are, therefore, AA, AO, and OO, as well as SS, Ss, and ss.

These may be combined thus:

- Animals that are AASS, AASs, AOSS, or AOSs will have A red cells.
- Animals that are OOSS or OOSs will have O red cells.
- Animals that are AAss, Aoss, or Ooss will express neither A nor O and so will have "null" red cells.

---

the longest showed hemoglobinuria and jaundice. The severity of the reaction did not appear to be directly related to the anti-red cell antibody titer in the piglet serum. Since the withdrawal of all blood-based hog cholera virus vaccines, the problems associated with their use have disappeared.

True HDN has also been recorded in the pig. The antibodies responsible are usually directed against antigens of the EAE system. In addition to the development of hemolytic anemia in newborn piglets, the presence of antibodies to platelet antigens may cause thrombocytopenia. This is seen clinically as a bleeding problem on tail docking and a tendency to bruise easily (neonatal purpura). On blood smears, the platelets may be clumped, and antiglobulin testing of them will yield a positive result (Dimmock et al., 1982). Deprivation of colostrum in an attempt to prevent piglets from absorbing anti-red cell antibodies may result in the newborn animals being highly susceptible to infection.

Pig blood groups are detected by agglutination, hemolytic, and antiglobulin tests.

Dogs

In dogs, seven red cell antigens are internationally recognized (DEA1, 3, 4, 5, 6, 7, 8), but others have been described. (An older nomenclature called them by the traditional alphabetic system, A, Tr, B, C, D, F, J, K, L, M, and N) (Colling and Saison, 1980). Most of these appear to be inherited as simple Mendelian dominants. Only the DEA1 antigens are sufficiently antigenic to be of clinical significance. Based on polyclonal antibody testing, DEA1 dogs were initially divided into 1.1 and 1.2, but DEA type 1.2 is now recognized as just a very strong 1.1. About 60% of dogs express DEA1 antigens on their red cells. Naturally occurring antibodies to DEA1 do not occur. DEA3, 4, 5, and 6 are one-gene, two-allotype systems, with expression dominant over the

negative phenotype. DEA3 is relatively rare with only about 10% of North American dogs being DAE3-positive. Conversely, 97% of dogs are DEA4-positive. DEA5-positive dogs are usually less than 25% of the population while 60%–75% are DEA6-positive. DEA7 (Tr) is a two-allele, three-phenotype system. Its prevalence is highly variable ranging from 8% to 80%. DEA8 has not been extensively studied.

Natural antibodies to DEA7 are found in 20%–50% of DEA7-negative dogs. Antibodies to DEA3, and 5 are found in about 10% of negative dogs, but these are usually of low titer and not of clinical significance (Symons and Bell, 1992). Therefore, it is recommended that canine blood donors be negative for DEA1, 3, 5, and 7. A universal donor would be an animal negative for all the DEA groups except DEA4. Unless the blood type of the recipient is known, only universal donor blood should be used, and a cross-match should be performed on all recipients.

In practice, the most important canine blood type is DEA1. About 50% of the dog population is DEA1 positive, and in general, these dogs can be considered to be universal recipients. Dogs that are DEA1 negative can also be considered to be universal donors. DEA1-positive blood should never be transfused into a DEA1-negative dog. If so, the recipient will become sensitized to DEA1, and high-titered antibodies will be produced. Subsequent transfusion of positive blood into such an animal may lead to a severe hemolytic reaction (Harrell et al., 1997). Similarly, if a negative bitch is sensitized by incompatible transfusions and mated to a positive dog, hemolytic disease may occur in her puppies. The puppies develop a hemolytic anemia 3–10 days after they are born (Blais et al., 2009).

The DEA7 system (Tr system) is a soluble antigen system related to the human A, cattle J, sheep R, and pig A systems. Two alleles belong to the system—Tr and O. An epistatic secretor gene controls their expression. Anti-DEA7 occurs naturally in some DEA7-negative dogs. When healthy female dogs with a prior history of pregnancies were examined, the only antibodies detected were directed against DEA7. However, the prevalence of these antibodies was similar in dogs with a prior history of pregnancy and control dogs. This suggests that pregnancy does not sensitize dogs to these antigens and that females with a prior pregnancy can be employed as blood donors. Surveys have reported the prevalence of DEA7 can range from 6% to 82% in different canine populations (Spada et al., 2017).

A blood group antigen called Dal has been identified on the basis of antibodies produced in Dalmatians following blood transfusion (Goulet et al., 2017). Surveys have shown that about 85%–100% of Dalmatians and 43%–78% of Dobermans are Dal+ depending upon location. The Dal+ phenotype is inherited in an autosomal dominant fashion. No natural antibodies to Dal have been identified.

Two additional blood groups (Kai 1 and Kai 2) unrelated to DEA have been identified through the use of monoclonal antibodies. About 94% of North American dogs are Kai 1+/Kai 2−. 5% are Kai 1−/Kai 2- and 1% are Kai 1−/Kai 2+. Their significance in blood transfusion is unclear.

Agglutination at 4°C as well as hemolytic and antiglobulin tests have been used for the detection of canine blood groups. The source of complement can be either fresh dog or rabbit serum. There are also several commercial blood typing kits available for dogs. One is a card agglutination test that uses monoclonal DEA1 antibodies to detect positive dogs (Seth et al., 2012). The other is an immunochromatographic strip technique (see Chapter 43). This test uses a monoclonal antibody against DEA1 to detect the antigen in a blood sample. A third method involves placing a suspension of the red cells on top of a matrix gel column containing specific antiblood group antibodies. Matrix gel agglutination relies on performing the agglutination test on top of a viscous gel layer. Nonagglutinated red cells will sink through the gel,

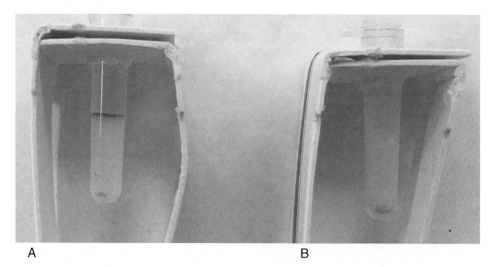

Fig. 32.5 A gel agglutination test. Blood is layered on top of a gel that contains anticanine antibodies and the tube is gently centrifuged. If the cells are coated in antierythrocyte antibodies, they cannot penetrate the gel (A) and remain on top. Nonantibody coated control cells (B), in contrast, can pass through the gel. (Courtesy Dr. Unity Jeffery.)

whereas agglutinated cells remain as a layer on top of the gel (Kessler et al., 2010; Fig. 32.5).

Cats

Cats have only single major blood group system, the AB system. Cats may be either type A, type B, or AB. A is completely dominant over B. The AB antigens are glycolipids found on multiple cell types (Symons and Bell, 1985). The differences between the blood groups are due to differences in the expression of neuraminic acid on the erythrocyte surfaces. Type A cells have predominantly glycolylneuraminic acid, while type B cells have acetylneuraminic acid. This difference results from mutations in the cytidine monophospho-*N*-acetylneuraminic acid hydroxylase gene that disrupts the enzyme function. This enzyme converts acetylneuraminic acid to glycolylneuraminic acid. The genetic basis of type AB is unknown.

About 75%–95% of cats are A positive, about 5%–25% are B positive, and fewer than 1% are AB positive. However, this distribution differs among countries and among different purebred cat breeds. In the United States, more than 99% of domestic short-hair and long-hair cats are type A, in western Canada, 94% are type A, whereas in the United Kingdom only about 40% of short-hair breeds are type A (Bücheler and Giger, 1993). Severe transfusion reactions have been described in group B cats that received very small quantities of group A blood since 95% of B cats possess IgM anti-A (Norsworthy, 1992). (Interestingly, only about 35% of A cats possess antiB, and it is of the IgG and IgM classes and of much lower titer.) If completely matched blood is transfused into cats, its half-life is about 4–5 weeks. If, however, group B blood is transfused into cats of blood group A, its half-life is only a few days. If group A blood is transfused into a cat of blood group B, its half-life is just over 1 hour. It is this very rapid destruction that results in severe clinical reactions. Thus a group B cat given as little as 1 mL of group A blood will go into shock, with hypotension, apnea, and atrioventricular block, within a few minutes. Cross-matching is essential in this species (Auer et al., 1982).

Occasionally, hemolytic transfusion reactions occur between AB blood group-matched cats. These appear to be due to natural antibodies against a blood group antigen called Mik (discovered in a cat called Mike!). Its mode of inheritance is undefined (Weinstein et al., 2007).

HDN has been recorded in Persian and related (Himalayan) breeds but is very rare. It occurs in kittens from queens of blood group B bred to sires of blood group A. The queens subsequently develop hightitered anti-A antibodies. Although healthy at birth, these kittens develop severe anemia as a result of intravascular hemolysis. Affected kittens show depression and possibly hemoglobinuria. Necropsy may reveal splenomegaly and jaundice. Antibodies to the sire's and the kitten's red cells are detectable in the queen's serum (Jonsson et al., 1990).

Agglutination and immunochromatographic tests are used for feline blood typing. Serum from type B cats has strong anti-A activity. Anti-B reagents can use the lectin from *Triticum vulgaris* (wheat germ) or increasingly, monoclonal antibodies. The agglutination tests can be performed in several different formats, such as in tubes, on cards, in matrix gel columns, or on glass slides. Results are comparable (Seth et al., 2011).

Humans

In humans, HDN is due almost entirely to immunization of the mother against the antigens of the Rhesus (Rh) system (now classified as CD240). The condition should be of historical interest only because a very simple but effective technique is available for its prevention. This depends on preventing a Rh-negative mother from reacting to the Rh-positive fetal red cells that escape from the placenta into her circulation at birth. Strong human antiRh globulin is obtained from male volunteers and given to mothers at risk soon after birth. It acts by specifically inhibiting the B-cell response to that antigen (see Chapter 21). Routine use of this material therefore prevents maternal sensitization, antibody production, and hemolytic disease. The use of a similar system in the domestic mammals is unnecessary because deprivation of colostrum is sufficient to prevent the disease.

PARENTAGE TESTING

Under some circumstances, it is necessary to confirm the parentage of an animal. One way of doing this is by examining the blood group antigens of an animal and its alleged parents (Table 32.2). The method is based on the principle that since blood group antigens are inherited, they must be present on the red cells of one or both parents. If a blood

TABLE 32.2 Use of Blood Groups to Assign Paternity

	DEA1	DEA6	DEA7	DEA8
Possible Sire 1	+	−	+	−
Possible Sire 2	+	−	−	+
Dam	−	+	+	−
Puppy 1	+	−	−	−
2	+	−	+	−
3	−	−	+	+*
4	−	+	+	−

*This puppy possesses Dog erythrocyte antigen (DEA8), which could not have come from sire 1 or its dam. Sire 1 could not have sired this litter. Courtesy Dr. D. Colling.

group antigen is present in a tested animal but absent from both its putative parents, parentage must be reassigned. Similarly, if one parent is homozygous for a specific blood group antigen, this antigen must inevitably appear in the offspring. However, it must be recognized that blood typing procedures can only exclude, never prove, parentage.

HEMOPHAGOCYTIC SYNDROME

Hemophagocytic syndrome is a disorder of activated macrophages associated with multiple cytopenias in the blood (Weiss, 2007). These cytopenias result from excessive phagocytic activity by macrophages. The syndrome has been described in humans, dogs, and cats. In humans, it may be either inherited or acquired. Diagnostic criteria include the presence of pancytopenia or bicytopenia and the presence of more than 2% macrophages containing ingested red cells in a bone marrow aspirate. About one-third of canine cases are associated with autoimmune diseases such as lupus or immune-mediated thrombocytopenia (see Chapter 38). These animals are commonly anemic, neutropenic, and thrombocytopenic, and it may be argued that autoantibodies opsonized the blood cells leading to their phagocytosis. Other affected dogs suffer from infectious diseases such as pyometra, pleuritis, ehrlichiosis, blastomycosis, or Lyme disease. In some cases, affected dogs recover once their underlying infection is treated. The disease is also associated with some neoplastic diseases, such as malignant lymphoma or myelodysplastic syndrome. Canine hemophagocytic syndrome may also occur in the absence of any obvious associated disease. Affected dogs are anemic, neutropenic, thrombocytopenic, febrile, anorexic, and lethargic.

TYPE II HYPERSENSITIVITY REACTIONS TO DRUGS

Red cells may be destroyed in drug hypersensitivities by three mechanisms. First, the drug and antibody may combine directly and activate complement, and nearby red cells will be destroyed in a bystander effect.

Second, some drugs may bind to cell surface glycoproteins. For example, penicillin, quinine, L-dopa, aminosalicylic acid, and phenacetin may bind to red cells. Since these cells are then modified, they may be recognized as foreign and eliminated by antibodies, resulting in hemolytic anemia. Penicillin-induced hemolytic anemia is not uncommon in horses (Blue et al., 1987). These conditions can be suspected based on recent treatment with penicillin and improvement when its use is discontinued. It may also be possible to detect antibodies against penicillin or penicillin-coated red cells in these animals (McConnico et al., 1992). Sulfonamides, phenylbutazone, aminopyrine, phenothiazine,

and possibly chloramphenicol may cause agranulocytosis by binding to granulocytes, and phenylbutazone, quinine, chloramphenicol, and sulfonamides can result in thrombocytopenia as they bind to platelet surface glycoproteins (Warkentin, 2007). If the cells of affected animals are examined using a direct antiglobulin test, antibody may be demonstrated on their surface. If these antibodies are eluted, they can be shown to be directed against the offending drug.

Third, drugs such as the cephalosporins may modify red cell membranes in such a way that the cells passively adsorb antibodies and then are removed by phagocytic cells. The red cells are thus antiglobulin-positive, although this rarely results in hemolytic anemia.

TYPE II HYPERSENSITIVITY IN INFECTIOUS DISEASES

Just as drugs can be adsorbed onto red cells and render them immunologically foreign, so too can bacterial antigens such as the lipopolysaccharides, viruses such as equine infectious anemia virus and Aleutian disease virus, bacteria such as *Anaplasma*, and protozoa such as the trypanosomes and *Babesia*. These altered red cells are regarded as foreign and are either lysed by antibody and complement or phagocytosed by mononuclear phagocytes. Clinically severe anemia is, therefore, characteristic of all these infections.

REFERENCES

Auer, L., Bell, K., Coates, S., 1982. Blood transfusion reactions in the cat. J. Am. Vet. Med. Assoc. 180, 729–730.

Bailey, E., 1982. Prevalence of anti-red blood cell antibodies in the serum and colostrum of mares and its relationship to neonatal isoerythrolysis. Am. J. Vet. Res. 43, 1917–1921.

Bastian, M., Holsteg, M., Hanke-Robinson, H., et al., 2011. Bovine neonatal pancytopenia: is this an alloimmune syndrome caused by vaccine-induced alloreactive antibodies? Vaccine 29, 5267–5275.

Becht, J.L., 1983. Neonatal isoerythrolysis in the foal. I. Background, blood group antigens and pathogenesis. Compend. Contin. Educ. Pract. Vet. 5, 591–599.

Bell, C.R., Machugh, N.D., Connelley, T.K., Degnan, K., Morrison, W.I., 2015. Haematopoietic depletion in vaccine-induced neonatal pancytopenia depends on both the titre and specificity of alloantibody and levels of MHC I expression. Vaccine 33, 3488–3496.

Benedictus, L., Otten, H.G., Van Schaik, G., Van Ginkel, W.G., et al., 2014. Bovine neonatal pancytopenia is a heritable trait of the dam rather than the calf and correlates with the magnitude of vaccine induced maternal alloantibodies not the MHC haplotype. Vet. Res. 45, 129–135.

Blais, M.-C., Rozanski, E.A., Hale, A.S., et al., 2009. Lack of evidence of pregnancy-induced alloantibodies in dogs. J. Vet. Intern. Med. 23, 462–465.

Blue, J.T., Dinsmore, R.P., Anderson, K.L., 1987. Immune-mediated hemolytic anemia induced by penicillin in horses. Cornell. Vet. 77, 263–276.

Bücheler, J., Giger, U., 1993. Alloantibodies against A and B blood types in cats. Vet. Immunol. Immunopathol. 38, 283–295.

Buechner-Maxwell, V., Scott, M.A., Godber, L., Kristensen, A., 1997. Neonatal alloimmune thrombocytopenia in a quarter horse foal. J. Vet. Intern. Med. 11, 304–308.

Colling, D.T., Saison, R., 1980. Canine blood groups. I. Description of new erythrocyte specificities. Anim. Blood Groups Biochem. Genet. 11, 1–12.

Demasius, W., Weikard, R., Kromik, A., Wolf, C., et al., 2014. Bovine neonatal pancytopenia (BNP): novel insights into the incidence, vaccination-associated epidemiological factors and a potential genetic predisposition for clinical and subclinical cases. Res. Vet. Sci. 96, 537–542.

Dimmock, C.K., Webster, W.R., Shiels, I.A., Edwards, C.L., 1982. Isoimmune thrombocytopenic purpura in piglets. Aust. Vet. J. 59, 157–159.

Goulet, S., Giger, U., Arsenault, J., Abrams-Ogg, A., et al., 2017. Prevalence and mode of inheritance of the Dal blood group in dogs in North America. J. Vet. Intern. Med. 31, 751–758.

Harrell, K., Parrow, J., Kristensen, A., 1997. Canine transfusion reactions. Compend. Contin. Educ. Pract. Vet. 19, 181–199.

Jonsson, N.N., Pullen, C., Watson, A.D.J., 1990. Neonatal isoerythrolysis in Himalayan kittens. Aust. Vet. J. 67, 416–417.

Kasonta, R., Holsteg, M., Duchow, K., Dekker, J.W., et al., 2014. Colostrum from cows immunized with a vaccine associated with bovine neonatal pancytopenia contains allo-antibodies that cross-react with human MHC-I molecules. PLoS One 9, e109239.

Kessler, R.J., Reese, J., Chang, D., Seth, M., et al., 2010. Dog erythrocyte antigens 1.1, 1.2, 3, 4, 7, and Dal blood typing and cross-matching by gel column technique. Vet. Clin. Pathol. 39 (3), 306–316.

Luethy, D., Owens, S.D., Stefanovski, D., Nolen-Walston, R., Giger, U., 2016. Comparison of tube, gel, and immunochromatographic strip methods for evaluation of blood transfusion compatibility in horses. J. Vet. Intern. Med. 30, 1864–1871.

Maynard, C.L., Elson, C.O., Hatton, R.D., Weaver, C.T., 2012. Reciprocal interactions of the intestinal microbiota and immune system. Nature 489, 231–241.

McClure, J.J., Kohn, C., Traub-Dargatz, J.L., 1994. Characterization of a red cell antigen in donkeys and mules associated with neonatal isoerythrolysis. Anim. Genet. 25, 119–120.

McConnico, R.S., Roberts, M.C., Tompkins, M., 1992. Penicillin-induced immune-mediated hemolytic anemia in a horse. J. Am. Vet. Med. Assoc. 201, 1402–1403.

Norsworthy, G.D., 1992. Clinical aspects of feline blood transfusions. Compend. Contin. Educ. Pract. Vet. 14, 469–475.

Nguyen, D.T., Choi, H., Jo, H., et al., 2011. Molecular characterization of the human ABO blood group orthologous system in pigs,. Anim. Genet. 42, 325–328.

Seth, M., Jackson, K.V., Winzelberg, S., Giger, U., 2012. Comparison of gel column, card, and cartridge techniques for dog erythrocyte antigen 1.1 blood typing. Am. J. Vet. Res. 73, 213–219.

Seth, M., Jackson, K.V., Giger, U., 2011. Comparison of five blood typing methods for the feline AB blood group system. Am. J. Vet. Res. 72, 203–209.

Spada, E., Proverbio, D., Priolo, V., Ippolito, D., et al., 2017. Dog erythrocyte antigens (DEA) 1, 4, 7 and suspected naturally occurring anti-DEA7 antibodies in Italian Corso dogs. Vet. J. 222, 17–21.

Symons, M., Bell, K., 1992. Canine blood groups: description of 20 specificities. Anim. Genet. 23, 509–515.

Symons, M., Bell, K., 1985. The occurrence of feline A blood group antigens on lymphocytes. Anim. Blood Groups Biochem. Genet. 16, 77–84.

Thomsen, H., Reinsch, N., Xu, N., et al., 2002. Mapping of the bovine blood group systems J, N′, R′, and Z show evidence for oligo-genetic inheritance. Anim. Genet. 33, 107–117.

Tizard, I.R., 2022. Allergies and Hypersensitivity Disease in Animals. Elsevier, St Louis, MO, ISBN: 978-0-323-76393-6

Wagner, R., Oulevey, J., Thiele, O.W., 1984. The transfer of bovine J blood group activity to erythrocytes: evidence of a transferable and of a non-transferable J in serum. Anim. Blood Groups Biochem. Genet. 15, 223–225.

Warkentin, T.E., 2007. Drug-induced immune-mediated thrombocytopenia: from purpura to thrombosis. N. Engl. J. Med. 356, 891–893.

Weinstein, N.M., Blais, M.-C., Harris, K., Oakley, D.A., et al., 2007. A newly recognized blood group in domestic shorthair cats: the mik red cell antigen. J. Vet. Intern. Med. 21 (2), 287–292.

Weiss, D.J., 2007. Hemophagocytic syndrome in dogs: 24 cases (1996–2005). J. Am. Vet. Med. Assoc. 230, 697–701.

Whiting, J.L., David, J.B., 2000. Neonatal isoerythrolysis. Compend. Contin. Educ. Pract. Vet. 22, 968–976.

33

Immune Complexes and Neutrophil-Mediated Hypersensitivity

CHAPTER OUTLINE

Immune complexes formed by the combination of antibodies with antigen activate the classical complement pathway. As a result, when these complexes are deposited in tissues, the activated complement generates chemotactic peptides that attract neutrophils. The accumulated neutrophils may then release oxidants and enzymes, causing acute inflammation and tissue damage. Lesions generated in this way are classified as type III or immune complex–mediated hypersensitivity reactions.

CLASSIFICATION

The severity and significance of type III hypersensitivity reactions depend, as might be expected, on the amount and site of deposition of immune complexes. For example, one form of reaction occurs locally when immune complexes are generated within tissues. Another form results when large quantities of immune complexes are produced within the bloodstream. This can occur, for example, when an antigen is administered intravenously to an immune recipient. Immune complexes generated within the bloodstream are deposited in glomeruli in the kidney, and so the development of glomerular lesions (glomerulonephritis) is characteristic of this type of hypersensitivity. If the complexes bind to blood cells, anemia, leukopenia, or thrombocytopenia may result. Immune complexes may also be deposited in blood vessel walls and so cause vasculitis, or in joints to cause arthritis (Tizard, 2022).

It might reasonably be pointed out that the combination of an antigen with antibody always produces immune complexes. However, the occurrence of clinically significant type III hypersensitivity reactions results from the formation of excessive amounts of these immune complexes in the wrong places over a long time period. For example, several grams of an antigen are needed to sensitize an animal, such as a rabbit, to produce experimental type III reactions. Minor and transient immune complex–mediated lesions probably develop relatively frequently following an antibody response but resolve without causing clinically significant disease or tissue damage.

LOCAL TYPE III HYPERSENSITIVITY

Arthus Reactions

If an antigen is injected subcutaneously into an animal that already has a high level of antibodies in its bloodstream, inflammation will develop at the injection site within several hours. This is called an Arthus reaction after the French scientist who first described it. It starts as a red, edematous swelling; eventually hemorrhage and thrombosis occur at the site; and if severe, it culminates in local tissue destruction (Kier et al., 1988).

Immediately following antigen injection and immune complex formation in tissues, neutrophils adhere to vascular endothelium and then emigrate into the site. By 6–8 hours, when the reaction has reached its greatest intensity, the injection site is densely infiltrated by these cells (Fig. 33.1). Eventually, damage to blood vessel walls results in hemorrhage and edema, platelet aggregation, and thrombosis. By 8 hours, mononuclear cells appear in the lesion, and by 24 hours or later, depending on the amount of antigen injected, they become the predominant cell type. Eosinophils are not a significant feature of this type of hypersensitivity.

The fate of the injected antigen can be followed if it is labeled with a fluorescent dye. The antigen first diffuses from the injection site through tissue fluid. When small blood vessels are encountered, the antigen diffuses into the vessel walls, where it encounters circulating antibodies. Immune complexes form and are deposited between and beneath the vascular endothelial cells. Complement components activated by the classical pathway will be deposited here as well.

Immune complexes formed in tissues must be removed. They first bind to Fc- and complement receptors on cells. The most widespread of these Fc receptors is FcγRIIa (CD32a) expressed on neutrophils. Immune complexes binding to these receptors activate the neutrophils and stimulate their production of oxidants, leukotrienes, prostaglandins, cytokines, and chemokines. Immune complexes also bind to mast

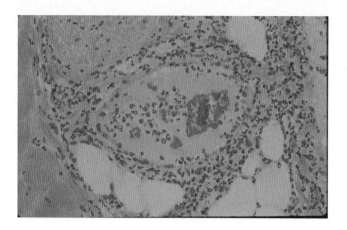

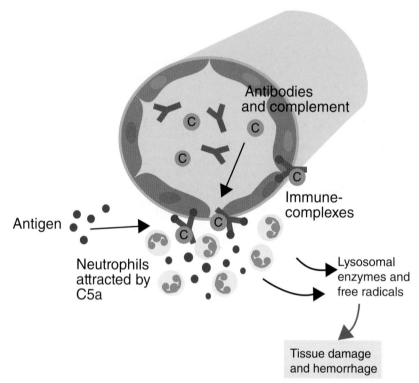

Fig. 33.1 The mechanisms of an Arthus reaction as well as a histological section of an Arthus reaction in the skin of a cat 6 h after intradermal inoculation of chicken red blood cells. *C5a,* Complement component 5a. Courtesy Dr. A. Kier.

cells through FcγRII and trigger them to release their granule contents. Among the molecules released by mast cells are chemoattractants and proteases, cytokines, kinins, and lipid mediators. All these mediators promote inflammation by acting on vascular endothelium and stimulating neutrophil adherence and emigration (Kohl and Gessner, 1999).

Immune complexes activate complement and generate the chemotactic peptide C5a (Fig. 33.2). Neutrophils, attracted by C5a and mast cell–derived chemokines, emigrate from the blood vessels, adhere to the complexes, and promptly phagocytose them. Eventually, the immune complexes are digested and destroyed. During this process, however, more proteases and oxidants are released into the tissues. When neutrophils attempt to ingest immune complexes attached to large structures, such as basement membranes, they release their granule contents directly into the surrounding tissues. Neutrophil proteases disrupt collagen fibers and destroy ground substances, basement membranes, and elastic tissue. Normally, tissues contain antiproteinases that inhibit neutrophil enzymes. However, neutrophils can subvert

these inhibitors by secreting OCl⁻. The OCl⁻ destroys the inhibitors and allows tissue destruction to proceed.

Though it has long been assumed that immunoglobulins do not themselves damage antigens, evidence has shown that they can kill microorganisms and cause tissue damage. When provided with singlet oxygen from phagocytic neutrophils, antibodies can catalyze the production of oxidants such as ozone. This ozone kills not only bacteria but also nearby cells.

Neutrophil proteases also act on C5 to generate C5a, which promotes further neutrophil accumulation and degranulation. Other enzymes released by neutrophils make mast cells degranulate or generate kinins. As a result of all this, inflammation and destruction of blood vessel walls results in the edema, vasculitis, and hemorrhage characteristic of an Arthus reaction.

Although the classical direct Arthus reaction is produced by local administration of an antigen to hyperimmunized animals, any technique that generates immune complexes in tissues will stimulate a

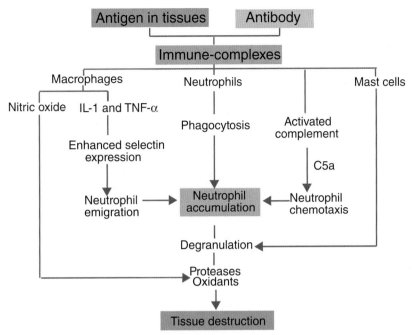

Fig. 33.2 Some of the mechanisms involved in the pathogenesis of the Arthus reaction. *IL-1*, Interleukin-1; *TNF-α*, tumor necrosis factor–α.

similar response. A reversed Arthus reaction can therefore be produced if antibodies are administered intradermally to an animal with a high level of circulating antigen. Injected, preformed immune complexes, especially those containing a moderate excess of an antigen, will provoke a similar reaction, although, as might be anticipated, there is less involvement of blood vessel walls, and the reaction is less severe. A passive Arthus reaction can be produced by giving antibody intravenously to a nonsensitized animal, followed by an intradermal injection of an antigen, and real enthusiasts can produce a reversed passive Arthus reaction by giving antibody intradermally followed by intravenous antigen.

Although it is unusual for pure hypersensitivity reactions of only a single type to occur under natural conditions, there are diseases in domestic animals in which type III reactions play a major role. Experimentally, Arthus reactions are usually produced in the skin since that is the most convenient site at which to inject the antigen. However, local type III reactions can occur in any tissues, with the precise site depending on the location of the inducing antigen (Powell et al., 2013).

Blue Eye

"Blue eye" is a condition seen in a small proportion of dogs that have been either infected or vaccinated with live canine adenovirus type 1 (see Fig. 28.8). These animals develop an anterior uveitis leading to corneal edema and opacity. The cornea is infiltrated by neutrophils, attracted by virus-antibody complexes that are deposited in tissue. Blue eye develops about 1–3 weeks after the onset of infection and usually resolves spontaneously once the virus is eliminated.

Hypersensitivity Pneumonitis

Type III hypersensitivity reactions may occur in the lungs when sensitized animals inhale antigens. For example, cattle housed during the winter are exposed to dust from hay. Normally, these dust particles are relatively large and are trapped in mucus in the upper respiratory tract and eliminated. If, however, hay is stored when damp, bacterial growth and metabolism will result in heating. As a result of this warmth, thermophilic actinomycetes will grow. One of the most important of

these thermophilic actinomycetes is *Saccharopolyspora rectivirgula*, an organism that produces large numbers of very small spores (~1 μm diameter). When inhaled, these spores can penetrate as far as the alveoli. If cattle are fed moldy hay for long periods, constant inhalation of *S. rectivirgula* spores will result in the development of high-titered antibodies to *S. rectivirgula* antigens in serum. Eventually inhaled spore antigens will encounter antibodies within the alveolar walls, and the resulting immune complexes and complement activation will cause a pneumonia (or pneumonitis), the basis of which is a type III hypersensitivity reaction (Spagnolo et al., 2015).

Hypersensitivity pneumonitis consists of an acute alveolitis together with vasculitis and exudation of fluid into the alveolar spaces. The alveolar septa may be thickened, and the entire lesion is infiltrated with inflammatory cells. Since many of these cells are eosinophils and lymphocytes, it is clear that the response is not a pure type III reaction. Examination of the lungs of affected cattle by immunofluorescence demonstrates deposits of immune complexes with complement. In animals inhaling small amounts of an antigen over a long period, a proliferative bronchiolitis and fibrosis may be observed.

Clinically, hypersensitivity pneumonitis presents as a pneumonia occurring between 5 and 10 hours after acute exposure to grossly moldy hay. The animal may have difficulty breathing and develop a severe cough. In chronically affected animals, the dyspnea may be continuous. The most effective method of managing this condition is by removing the source of the antigen. Administration of steroids may be beneficial.

A hypersensitivity pneumonitis also occurs in farmers chronically exposed to *S. rectivirgula* spores from moldy hay and is called farmer's lung. Many other syndromes in humans have an identical pathogenesis and are usually named after the source of the offending antigen. Thus, pigeon breeder's lung is due to exposure to the dust from pigeon feces, mushroom grower's disease is due to inhaling spores from actinomycetes in the soil used for growing mushrooms, and librarian's lung results from inhalation of dusts from old books! Hay sickness is a hypersensitivity pneumonitis seen in horses in Iceland that is probably an equine equivalent of farmer's lung (Asmundsson et al., 1983).

Equine Asthma

It has long been recognized that asthma in humans consists of several distinctly different diseases. Some are associated with high eosinophil counts in bronchoalveolar washes, others are characterized by high neutrophil counts. Some human cases have both neutrophils and eosinophils while others have neither. A similar spectrum and complexity are seen in equine asthma (Lavoie-Lamoureux et al., 2012). Thus, two forms of chronic obstructive respiratory disease are recognized in horses. They consist of recurrent airway obstruction (RAO) or "heaves," and inflammatory airway disease (IAD) (Couëtil et al., 2016; Bond et al., 2018).

Inflammatory Airway Disease

IAD is a mild respiratory disease of horses in which breathing appears normal at rest. It has minimal clinical signs such as a nasal discharge, cough, and decreased performance. It affects up to 30% of young horses (<5 years old) in training. Although commonly linked to bacterial or viral infections, in many cases, no infectious agent can be isolated. Horses with IAD show poor performance, exercise intolerance, and a chronic, intermittent cough. Excessive airway mucus production is apparent. Cytological evaluation of their bronchiolar lavage fluid shows evidence of inflammation. Cytokine transcripts show elevated IL-1β, -5, -6, -8, -10, -17, and -23 as well as TNF-α and IFN-γ, in affected horses compared to controls. However, these differences are influenced by the presence of mast cells, eosinophils, or neutrophils. Thus, in washes with high neutrophil numbers, IL-17 is also elevated, while IL-4 is depressed compared to those with high mast cell numbers. Its pathogenesis is uncertain, but IAD is associated with the inhalation of organic dusts, molds, and aeroallergens and may be seasonal.

Recurrent Airway Obstruction

RAO resembles severe asthma in humans (Sheats et al., 2019). It includes obstructive pulmonary disease seen in stabled horses and summer pasture-associated obstructive pulmonary disease. RAO occurs most obviously in horses that inhale large amounts of organic dusts, such as those generated in dusty stables. It is defined as a severe debilitating disease characterized by coughing and an increased breathing effort due to bronchoconstriction, airway hyperreactivity, neutrophil infiltration, and mucus accumulation in the airways. Characteristically, horses with RAO suffer from labored breathing even while at rest.

RAO is typically seen in horses over 9–12 years of age. Affected animals suffer from episodes of severe respiratory distress triggered by inhalation of airborne allergens. During these episodes, horses develop airflow obstruction as a result of bronchospasm, increased mucus production, airway hyperplasia, and airway hyperresponsiveness (Fig. 33.3). Neutrophil recruitment is apparent 4–6 hours after antigen challenge and precedes the development of airway obstruction. Th2 cytokines appear to contribute to the recruitment and activation of these neutrophils and the release of extracellular NETS (see Chapter 6; Henriquez et al., 2014). During remissions horses may be clinically normal and their airway function and bronchial cytology appear normal (Leguillette, 2003).

RAO is probably a hypersensitivity disease associated with an enhanced Th2 response. Thus, lung biopsies show significant increases in type 2 cytokines, IL-1β, IL-8, TNF-α, and transforming growth factor–β (TGF-β), as well as TLR4 and NF-κB transcripts. Similar but less marked trends occur in IL-17 and IFN-γ. High concentrations of the chemokine CXCL8 (interleukin-8 [IL-8]) are found in the bronchoalveolar washings of affected animals (Lavoie et al., 2011). Exposure of cultured equine bronchial epithelial cell cultures to hay dust or lipopolysaccharide increases their IL-8, CXCL2, and IL-1β expression. The percentage of CD4[+], Foxp3[+] Treg cells increases in the bronchoalveolar

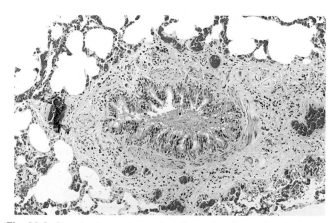

Fig. 33.3 Chronic airway obstructive disease in a horse showing mucus in the lumen, epithelial hyperplasia, smooth muscle hypertrophy and mildly increased numbers of submucosal inflammatory cells. Courtesy Dr. Brian Porter.

washings of horses with RAO suggesting that these also influence the course of this disease (Ainsworth et al., 2009).

Horses with RAO may show positive skin reactions to intradermal inoculation of actinomycete and fungal extracts (such as *Rhizopus nigricans*, *Candida albicans*, *S. rectivirgula*, *Aspergillus fumigatus*, or *Geotrichum deliquescens*). Affected horses may respond to aerosol challenge with extracts of these organisms by developing respiratory distress. Clinical signs may resolve on removal of the moldy hay and reappear on re-exposure. There is no evidence of IgE involvement in RAO, and there is little correlation between skin test results and severity of disease. There is, however, evidence for a genetic predisposition perhaps involving the gene for the IL-4 receptor. The prevalence of RAO is increased threefold when one parent is affected and fivefold when both are affected (Houtsma et al., 2015).

Affected animals usually have large numbers of neutrophils or eosinophils in their small bronchioles and high titers of antibodies to equine influenza in their bronchial secretions. The significance of the latter is unclear. It has been suggested that continuous prolonged activation of bronchoalveolar epithelial cells by dust particles and airborne endotoxins leads to excessive production of neutrophil-attracting chemokines. These neutrophils then cause damage by producing proteases, peroxidases, and oxidants. Removal of clinically affected horses to air-conditioned stalls results in improvement of the disease, but this is reversed if the horses are returned to dusty stables. In some cases, RAO may persist even when horses are moved to low-dust environments, probably as a result of chronic airway remodeling.

Staphylococcal Hypersensitivity

Staphylococcal hypersensitivity is a pruritic pustular dermatitis of dogs. Skin testing with staphylococcal antigens suggests that types I, III, and IV hypersensitivity may be involved. Histological findings of neutrophilic dermal vasculitis suggest that the type III reaction may predominate.

IMMUNOTHROMBOSIS

Circulating immune complexes can bind and activate Fc receptors on neutrophils. This will trigger the release of neutrophil extracellular traps (NETs). These traps consist of DNA strands "decorated" with antibacterial proteins such as elastases and myeloperoxidase. The activated neutrophils also release cytokines, proteases, peptides, and oxidants, as well as antimicrobial cathelicidins.

Immune complexes

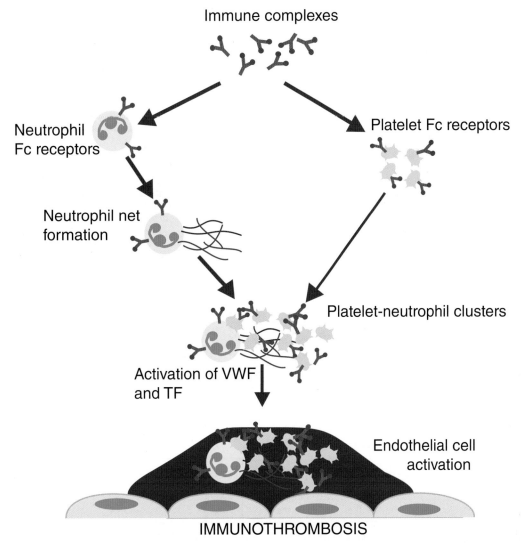

Neutrophil
Fc receptors

Platelet Fc receptors

Neutrophil net
formation

Platelet-neutrophil clusters

Activation of VWF
and TF

Endothelial cell
activation

IMMUNOTHROMBOSIS

Fig. 33.4 The mechanism of immunothrombosis. Immune complexes activate neutrophils resulting in neutrophil extracellular traps (NET)osis. Immune complexes also activate platelets so that they bind to NETs. The neutrophil-platelet clusters bind to vascular endothelial cells, activate von Willebrand factor (VWF) and tissue factor (TF), and a thrombus develops on the vessel wall.

Immune complexes can also interact with Fc receptors on blood platelets to cause their activation and aggregation. This platelet aggregation together with their release of clotting factors such as Von Willebrand factor (VWF), platelet-activating factor, platelet factor 1, and HMGB-1, can promote additional neutrophil NET release.

Aggregated platelets can then bind to neutrophil NETs to form NET-platelet complexes. Thus, the NETS provide a scaffold to which VWF, platelets, and fibronectin can attach. The NETs interact with VWF and may circulate or even bind to nearby blood vessel walls. NETs are also potent activators of the alternate complement pathway (Martinod and Deppermann, 2020).

NETosis is usually beneficial since the NETs trap and kill invading organisms. However, large NET-platelet complexes can also cause damage if they are generated in excess or in critical blood vessels (Goggs et al., 2020). Thus, the interaction of these NETS together with platelets can result in intravascular thrombus formation and the development of an associated vasculitis—a phenomenon called immunothrombosis (Nichols et al., 2001). NET-platelet complexes may also circulate within the bloodstream and trigger uncontrolled thrombin and fibrin generation leading to disseminated intravascular coagulation (see Chapter 8;

Innera, 2013). The commonest cause of immunothrombosis and vasculitis in small animals is a type III hypersensitivity reaction but the offending antigens may be difficult to identify, and at least half of canine vasculitis cases are idiopathic (Morris, 1987; Fig. 33.4).

GENERALIZED TYPE III HYPERSENSITIVITY

If an antigen is administered intravenously to animals already possessing antibodies, immune complexes form in the bloodstream. These immune complexes are removed by binding to either erythrocytes or platelets, or if very large, by macrophages (Fig. 33.5). If, however, complexes are produced in excessive amounts, they are also deposited in the walls of blood vessels, especially medium-sized arteries, and in vessels where there is a physiological outflow of fluid, such as glomeruli, synovia, and the choroid plexus (Fig. 33.6). An example of this type of hypersensitivity is serum sickness (Scherlinger et al., 2023).

Serum Sickness

During the First World War, when the use of antisera for passive immunization was in its infancy, it was observed that wounded soldiers who

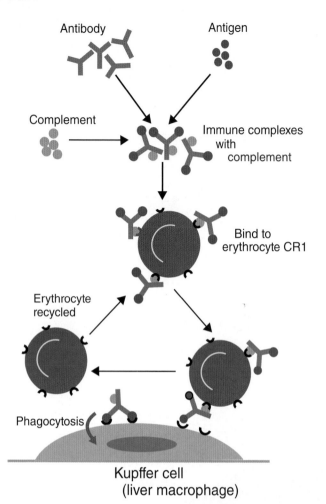

Fig. 33.5 In primates, immune complexes are removed by binding to complement receptors on red blood cells. They are then carried to the liver, where they are transferred to Kupffer cells for phagocytosis. In the absence of complement components, significant accumulation of immune complexes occurs in tissues. In other mammals immune complexes bind to receptors on platelets. *CR1*, Complement receptors 1.

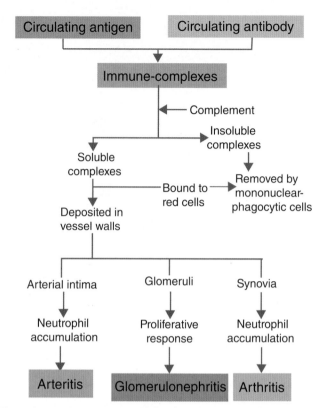

Fig. 33.6 The mechanisms involved in the pathogenesis of acute serum sickness.

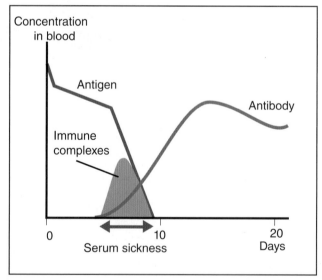

Fig. 33.7 The time course of acute serum sickness. The appearance of the disease coincides with the generation of immune complexes in the bloodstream.

had received a very large dose of equine antitetanus serum developed a characteristic illness about 10 days later. This was called serum sickness and consisted of a generalized vasculitis with erythema, edema, and urticaria of the skin; neutropenia; lymph node enlargement; joint swelling; and proteinuria. The reaction was usually of short duration and subsided within a few days. A similar reaction can be produced experimentally in rabbits by administration of a large intravenous dose of antigen. The development of sickness coincides with the formation of large amounts of immune complexes in the circulation (Fig. 33.7). The experimental disease may be acute if it is caused by a single, large injection of an antigen, or chronic if it is caused by multiple small injections. In either case, animals develop glomerulonephritis and arteritis (Fig. 33.8; Lee et al., 2019).

Glomerulonephritis

When immune complexes are deposited in the vessels of the renal glomeruli, they cause basement membrane thickening and stimulate glomerular cells to proliferate. Any or all of the three glomerular cell populations, epithelial cells, endothelial cells, and mesangial cells, can proliferate. The lesion is therefore called membranoproliferative glomerulonephritis (MPGN). MPGN lesions are classified

based on the site of immune complex deposition (Fig. 33.9; Sethi and Fervenza, 2012).

Membranoproliferative Glomerulonephritis

MPGN is caused by immune-complex deposition in glomerular blood vessels. The complexes can usually penetrate the vascular endothelium but not the basement membrane and are therefore trapped on the inside, where they stimulate endothelial cell swelling and

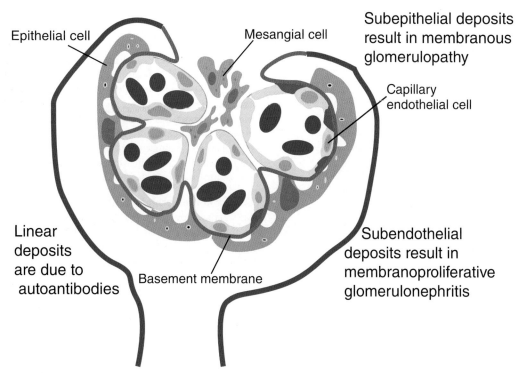

Fig. 33.8 The structure of a typical glomerulus. Immune complexes may be deposited on either side of, or within, the glomerular basement membrane.

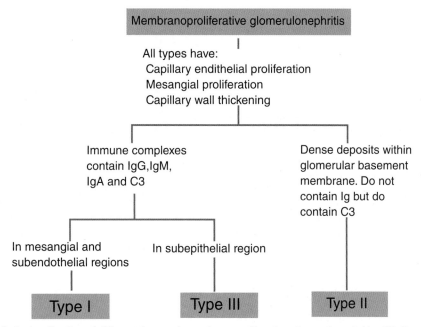

Fig. 33.9 A classification of different forms of membranoproliferative glomerulonephritis. *C3*, Complement component 3; *IgA*, immunoglobin A.

proliferation (Fig. 33.10; Slauson and Lewis, 1979). Experimentally, if an animal is given repeated injections of small doses of an antigen over a long period, continued damage to the glomerular cells by immune complexes leads to production of TGF-β. This cytokine stimulates nearby cells to produce fibronectin, collagen, and proteoglycans. This results in a thickening of the basement membrane to form a so-called "wire-loop" lesion (also called a membranous glomerulonephritis). Alternatively, the immune complexes and complement may be deposited in the mesangial region of glomeruli (Aresu

et al., 2008). Mesangial cells are modified smooth muscle cells. As such they can respond to immune complexes by proliferating and producing IL-6 and TGF-β. The IL-6 stimulates autocrine growth of the mesangial cells. The TGF-β stimulates production of extracellular matrix. The resulting cell growth eventually interferes with glomerular function. By using immunofluorescence, it can be shown that lumpy aggregates of immune complexes are deposited in capillary walls and on the epithelial side of the glomerular basement membrane (Fig. 33.11; Trang et al., 2014).

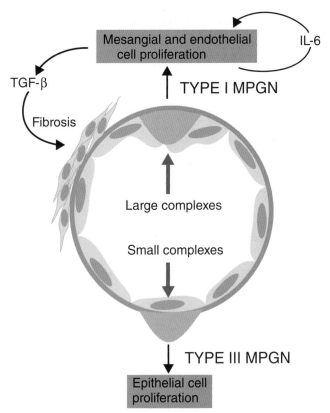

Fig. 33.10 The pathogenesis of membranoproliferative glomerulonephritis. Remember, however, that more than one type of lesion may be present in an animal at the same time. *MPGN*, Membranoproliferative glomerulonephritis; *TGF-β*, transforming growth factor–β.

A variant form of MPGN (dense deposit disease) is characterized by the presence of homogeneous, dense deposits within the glomerular basement membrane (in the lamina densa) rather than on its surface (see Fig. 4.18). These deposits may contain C3 but not immunoglobulin. This type of MPGN results from uncontrolled complement activation and is seen in factor H deficiency in pigs (see Chapter 5). In a third variant, immune complexes are deposited on both sides of the basement membrane. It is believed that very small immune complexes penetrate the basement membrane and are deposited where they stimulate epithelial cell swelling and proliferation. If excessive, these proliferating cells may fill the glomerular space to form epithelial crescents. A single case of unknown cause has been described in a cat (Inoue et al., 2001).

Causes of Glomerulonephritis

MPGN develops when prolonged antigenemia persists in the presence of antibodies (Grant and Forrester, 2001). As a result, it is a feature of many chronic infectious diseases. These include viral diseases such as equine infectious anemia, infectious canine hepatitis, bovine virus diarrhea, feline leukemia, Aleutian disease of mink, distemper encephalitis, and African swine fever. It occurs in parasitic diseases such as leishmaniasis, dirofilariasis, and generalized demodicosis. It also develops in chronic bacterial diseases such as pyometra, chronic pneumonia, acute pancreatic necrosis, bacterial endocarditis, Lyme disease, Ehrlichiosis, and recurrent staphylococcal pyoderma (Table 33.1).

In animals with tumors, large amounts of tumor antigen may be shed into the bloodstream and result in an MPGN. This has been associated with lymphosarcomas, osteosarcomas, and mastocytomas.

MPGN is also an important feature of many chronic autoimmune diseases. Circulating immune complexes resulting in renal lesions occur in dogs with systemic lupus erythematosus (see Chapter 39), discoid lupus, and rheumatoid arthritis. Some MPGN cases may be due

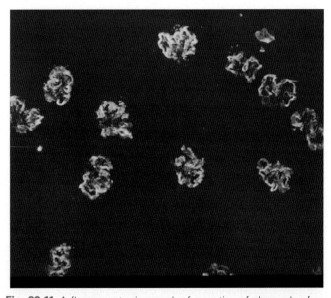

Fig. 33.11 A fluorescent micrograph of a section of glomerulus from a Finnish-Landrace lamb with immune complex–mediated glomerulonephritis. The labeled antisheep globulin reveals the presence of "lumpy-bumpy" deposits characteristic of type I membranoproliferative glomerulonephritis in many glomeruli. From Angus, K.W., Gardiner, A.C., Morgan, K.T., et al. 1974. Mesangiocapillary glomerulonephritis in lambs. II. Pathological findings and electron microscopy of the renal lesions. J. Comp. Pathol. 84, 319–330.

TABLE 33.1	Infectious Diseases With a Significant Type III Hypersensitivity Component
Organism or Disease	**Major Lesion**
Erysipelothrix rhusiopathiae	Arthritis
Mycobacterium johnei	Enteritis
Streptococcus equi	Purpura
Staphylococcus aureus	Dermatitis
Borrelia burgdorferi	Glomerulonephritis
Leishmania	Glomerulonephritis
Ehrlichiosis	Glomerulonephritis
Canine adenovirus–1	Uveitis, glomerulonephritis
Canine adenovirus–2	Glomerulonephritis
Feline leukemia	Glomerulonephritis
Feline infectious peritonitis	Peritonitis, glomerulonephritis
Aleutian disease	Glomerulonephritis, anemia, arteritis
Hog cholera	Glomerulonephritis
African swine fever	Glomerulonephritis
Bovine virus diarrhea	Glomerulonephritis
Equine viral arteritis	Arteritis
Equine infectious anemia	Anemia, glomerulonephritis
Visceral leishmaniasis	Glomerulonephritis
Dirofilaria immitis	Glomerulonephritis

to complement deficiencies. As a result of these deficiencies, removal of immune complexes is impaired, and they accumulate in glomeruli. Many cases of MPGN develop in the absence of any obvious predisposing cause (Murray and Sharpe, 2009).

Clinical Features of Glomerulonephritis

The presence of immune complexes within glomeruli stimulates neutrophils, mesangial cells, macrophages, and platelets to release thromboxanes, nitric oxide, and platelet-activating factor. These increase basement membrane permeability so that plasma proteins, especially albumin, are lost in the urine. This loss, if severe, may exceed the body's ability to replace the protein. As a result, albumin levels drop, the plasma colloid osmotic pressure falls, fluid passes from blood into tissue spaces, and the animal may become edematous and ascitic. The loss of fluid into tissues results in a reduction of blood volume, a compensatory increase in secretion of antidiuretic hormone, increased sodium retention, and accentuation of the edema. The decreased blood volume also results in a drop in renal blood flow, reduction in glomerular filtration, retention of urea and creatinine, azotemia, and hypercholesterolemia. Although all these may occur as a result of immune-complex deposition in glomeruli, the development of this nephrotic syndrome is not inevitable. Many animals may be clinically normal despite the presence of immune complexes in their glomeruli, and immune complexes are commonly observed in old, apparently healthy dogs, horses, and sheep. The most common initial signs are anorexia, weight loss, and vomiting. Polyuria and polydipsia occur when about two-thirds of glomeruli are destroyed. Azotemia occurs when 75% of the glomeruli are destroyed. Development of nephrotic syndrome (proteinuria, hypoproteinemia, edema, or ascites) only occurs in about 15% of affected dogs but in up to 75% of affected cats. Some dogs become hypertensive. Thromboembolic disease may also develop. It has been usual to treat affected animals with corticosteroids and immunosuppressive drugs, but the rationale and effectiveness of this treatment are unclear, except when the glomerulonephritis is associated with concurrent autoimmune disease such as systemic lupus erythematosus (Grauer, 2005). Recently, encouraging responses have been obtained with angiotensin-converting enzyme inhibitors and experimental thromboxane synthase inhibitors. Dietary protein restriction may help reduce the clinical signs of renal failure. The glomerular lesion is not inflammatory, and although the lesion contains immunoglobulins, there is no evidence to suggest that it is caused by hyperactivity of the immune system. For disease associated with a profound proteinuria, nephrotic syndrome, or progressive azotemia, mycophenolate alone or in combination with prednisolone has been recommended (see Chapter 42; Segev et al., 2013). For stable or slowly progressive disease, mycophenolate or chlorambucil alone or in combination with azathioprine on alternate days is appropriate (Goldstein et al., 2013). Therapeutic effectiveness should be assessed serially by changes in proteinuria, renal function, or serum albumin concentrations. In the absence of adverse side effects, therapy of at least 8–12 weeks should be provided before altering or abandoning a treatment (Cianciolo et al., 2013).

Immunoglobulin A Nephropathy

By far the most important cause of renal failure in humans is IgA nephropathy. In this form of type I MPGN, patients have elevated serum IgA, and IgA-containing immune complexes are deposited in the glomeruli. The resulting glomerulonephritis can lead to renal failure. Recent studies have identified the presence of IgA antimesangial autoantibodies in these patients (Nihei et al., 2023). IgA deposits can be found in the glomeruli of up to 35% of some human populations and up to 47% of dogs. In these dogs, the IgA is deposited in the mesangial and paramesangial areas and is associated with mesangial proliferation. Dogs with enteritis or liver diseases showed the highest

prevalence of glomerular IgA deposition. A slightly different condition has also been described in dogs aged 4–7 years. The animals developed a MPGN with mild hematuria, proteinuria, and hypertension. IgA-containing immune complexes were present in both the subepithelial and subendothelial locations (Harris et al., 1993).

Swine Glomerulopathy

Spontaneous MPGN is observed in pigs. It is especially common in Japan, where it appears to be due to deposition of immune complexes containing IgG (and IgA) antibodies against *Actinobacillus pleuropneumoniae* (Shirota et al., 2002). In other cases, it may be secondary to chronic virus infections such as hog cholera or African swine fever. Occasionally, however, proliferative glomerulonephritis develops spontaneously. (Bourgault and Drolet, 1995). In most cases, epithelial crescent formation suggests that the proliferating cells are epithelial in origin. There is usually strong staining for C3 and weaker staining for IgM using immunofluorescence assays. Pigs rarely have IgG or IgA deposits. Affected pigs are relatively young (<1 year). There is a high prevalence of gastric ulcers in affected animals, but whether this is related or not is unclear. An inherited complement factor H deficiency in Yorkshire pigs results in the development of a lethal MPGN called porcine dense deposit disease (see Chapter 5) (Jansen, 1993).

Finnish-Landrace Glomerulopathy

Some newborn lambs of the Finnish-Landrace breed die within a few weeks as a result of renal failure due to MPGN. The lesions develop in utero and are present at birth. The glomerular lesions are similar to those seen in chronic serum sickness, with mesangial cell proliferation and basement membrane thickening (Fig. 33.12). In extreme cases, epithelial cell proliferation may result in epithelial crescent formation. Neutrophils may be present in small numbers within glomeruli, and the rest of the kidney may exhibit diffuse interstitial lymphoid infiltration and necrotizing vasculitis. Deposits containing IgM, IgG, and C3 are found in the glomeruli and choroid plexus, but serum C3 levels are

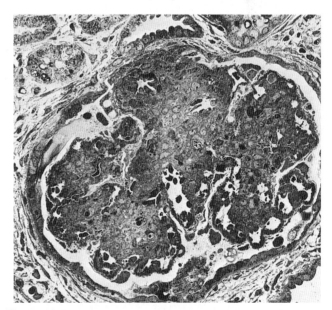

Fig. 33.12 A thin section of glomerulus from a Finnish-Landrace lamb with membranoproliferative glomerulonephritis. The primary lesion in this case is mesangial proliferation with some basement membrane thickening. From Angus, K.W., Gardiner, A.C., Morgan, K.T., et al. 1974. Mesangiocapillary glomerulonephritis in lambs. II. Pathological findings and electron microscopy of the renal lesions. J. Comp. Pathol. 84, 319–330.

low. It appears likely that this disease is a result of an inherited complement deficiency.

Canine Glomerulopathy

C3 deficiency inherited as an autosomal recessive condition has been described in Brittany Spaniels (see Chapter 5). Many of these dogs develop MPGN, which may lead to renal failure (Cork et al., 1991). The lesions are typical with mesangial proliferation, thickening of the glomerular capillary wall, and deposition of electron-dense deposits in the mesangium and subendothelial space. The deposits contain both IgG and IgM. A familial glomerulopathy has been observed in Bernese Mountain Dogs. It is associated with MPGN and interstitial nephritis.

Cutaneous and Renal Vascular Glomerulopathy

Cutaneous and renal vascular glomerulopathy is a disease of dogs of unknown etiology (Hope et al., 2019). It was first reported in racing Greyhounds in Alabama in the 1980s—hence its colloquial name—*Alabama rot*. It has subsequently been reported in other areas of North America and Europe. Its immediate cause is disseminated microvascular thrombosis resulting in widespread infarction and tissue necrosis. Affected dogs develop ulcerative necrotic lesions in the mouth, distal limbs, belly, and muzzle. Some dogs recover; however, many rapidly develop acute glomerulonephritis resulting in renal failure and death. Histologically, the dogs develop a thrombotic microangiopathy. This results in a thrombocytopenia, hemolytic anemia, and eventually multiorgan damage. Its etiology is unknown, and no infectious agents have yet been identified, nor have immune complexes been detected in the vascular lesions. The disease is certainly genetically influenced by being restricted to certain litters of Greyhounds. However, it is widely believed that the disease trigger is an infectious or environmental factor that has yet to be identified since disease outbreaks occur in clusters, have the highest incidence from November to May, and appear to be associated with walking in forested areas (Holm et al., 2020). A similar disease has been identified in Great Danes, English Springer Spaniels, Golden Retrievers, Vizslas, and Whippets.

Dirofilariasis

Dogs infested with the heartworm *Dirofilaria immitis* develop a proteinuria associated with a glomerulopathy. The lesions generally consist of a "wire-loop" thickening of the basement membrane with minimal cellular proliferation. Large amounts of IgG1 are deposited on the epithelial side of the basement membrane. Originally believed to be caused by immune complexes containing microfilarial antigens, these lesions are now believed to be a result of an immune response to their commensal bacterium *Wolbachia*. When heartworms die their intestinal bacteria are released, and these trigger an immune response. Antibodies to *Wolbachia* are detectable in the urine of heartworm-infected dogs, and the glomerular immune complexes contain *Wolbachia* surface protein (Morchón et al., 2012).

OTHER IMMUNE COMPLEX–MEDIATED LESIONS

Purpura Hemorrhagica

Two to four weeks after an acute *Streptococcus equi* infection (or vaccination against *S. equi*), horses may develop urticaria, followed by severe subcutaneous edema, especially involving the limbs, and the development of hemorrhages in the mucosa and subcutaneous tissues. Affected horses are anorexic, depressed, and have a high fever. Immune complexes containing *S. equi* antigens (M-protein or R-protein) are found in the bloodstream of affected animals (Galan and Timony, 1985). These immune complexes cause an acute vasculitis as well as

a type I MPGN with resulting proteinuria and azoturia (Divers et al., 1992; Delph et al., 2019). Other triggers of purpura hemorrhagica in the horse include infections with *Corynebacterium pseudotuberculosis*, *Prescottella equi*, equine influenza virus, and equine herpesvirus type 1. In some cases, it develops in the absence of any obvious infection. Horses usually recover when aggressively treated with systemic glucocorticosteroids (Pusterla et al., 2003).

Pigs also suffer from sporadic cases of an immune complex–mediated thrombocytopenic purpura syndrome. The animals have thrombocytopenia, anemia, excessive bleeding, and membranoproliferative lesions in their glomeruli. The cause is unknown (Carrasco et al., 2003).

Dietary Hypersensitivity

If an antigenic milk replacer, such as soy protein, is fed to very young calves before the development of ruminal function, the foreign antigen may be absorbed and stimulate antibody formation and type III hypersensitivity. As a result, the calves become unthrifty and lose weight. However, the precise pathogenesis of this condition is unclear. A small proportion of calves develop an IgE response and a type I hypersensitivity.

Polyarthritis

Immune complexes can be readily found in the blood and synovial fluid of animals with rheumatoid arthritis and in many with osteoarthritis. In rheumatoid arthritis, they are believed to have a major role in the etiologic progression of disease. Their role in osteoarthritis is unclear, but they may be secondary to local trauma. Important examples of this type of arthritis are the nonerosive polyarthritides seen in foals and puppies and described in Chapter 39.

REFERENCES

Ainsworth, D.M., Matychak, M., Reyner, C.L., et al., 2009. Effects of in vitro exposure to hay dust on the gene expression of chemokines and cell-surface receptors in primary bronchial epithelial cell cultures established from horses with chronic recurrent airway obstruction. Am. J. Vet. Res. 70, 365–372.

Aresu, L., Pregel, P., Bollo, E., et al., 2008. Immunofluorescence staining for the detection of immunoglobulins and complement (C3) in dogs with renal disease. Vet. Rec. 163, 679–683.

Asmundsson, T., Gunnarsson, E., Johannesson, T., 1983. "Haysickness" in Icelandic horses: precipitin tests and other studies. Equine Vet. J. 15, 229–232.

Bond, S., Leguillette, R., Richard, E.A., Couetil, L., et al., 2018. Equine asthma: integrative biologic relevance of a recently proposed nomenclature. J. Vet. Intern. Med. 32, 2088–2098.

Bourgault, A., Drolet, R., 1995. Spontaneous glomerulonephritis in swine. J. Vet. Diagn. Invest. 7, 122–126.

Carrasco, L., Madsen, L.W., Salguero, F.J., Nunez, A., Sanchez-Cordon, P.J., Bollen, P., 2003. Immune complex-associated thrombocytopenic purpura syndrome in sexually mature Gottingen minipigs. J. Comp. Pathol. 128, 25–32.

Cianciolo, R.E., Brown, C.A., Mohr, F.C., Spangler, W.L., et al., 2013. Pathologic evaluation of canine renal biopsies: methods for identifying features that differentiate immune-mediated glomerulonephritides from other categories of glomerular diseases. J. Vet. Intern. Med. 27, S10–S18.

Cork, L.C., Morris, J.M., Olson, J.L., et al., 1991. Membranoproliferative glomerulonephritis in dogs with a genetically determined deficiency of the third component of complement. Clin. Immunol. Immunopathol. 60, 455–470.

Couëtil, L.L., Cardwell, J.M., Gerber, V., Lavoie, J.P., Leguillette, R., Richard, E.A., 2016. Inflammatory airway disease of horses—revised consensus statement. J. Vet. Intern. Med. 30, 503–515.

Delph, K.M., Beard, L.A., Trimble, A.C., Sutter, M.E., et al., 2019. Strangles, convalescent *Streptococcus equi* subspecies equi M antibody titers and the presence of complications. J. Vet. Intern. Med. 33, 275–279.

Divers, T.J., Timoney, J.F., Lewis, R.M., Smith, C.A., 1992. Equine glomerulonephritis and renal failure associated with complexes of group-C streptococcal antigen and IgG antibody. Vet. Immunol. Immunopathol. 32, 93–102.

Galan, J.F., Timony, J.F., 1985. Immune complexes in purpura hemorrhagica of the horse contain IgA and M antigen of *Streptococcus equi*. J. Immunol. 135, 3134–3137.

Goggs, R., Jeffery, U., LeVine, D.N., Li, R.H.L., 2020. Neutrophil extracellular traps, cell-free DNA, and immunothrombosis of companion animals: a review. Vet. Pathol. 57 (1), 6–23.

Goldstein, R.E., Brovida, C., Fernandez-Del Palacio, M.J., Littman, M.P., et al., 2013. Consensus recommendations for treatment for dogs with serology positive glomerular disease. J. Vet. Intern. Med. 27 (Suppl. 1), S60–66.

Grant, D.C., Forrester, S.D., 2001. Glomerulonephritis in dogs and cats: glomerular function, pathophysiology, and clinical signs. Compend. Contin. Educ. Pract. Vet. 23, 739–743.

Grauer, G.F., 2005. Canine glomerulonephritis: new thoughts on proteinuria and treatment. J. Small Anim. Pract. 46, 469–478.

Harris, C.H., Krawiec, D.R., Gelberg, H.B., Shapiro, S.Z., 1993. Canine IgA glomerulopathy. Vet. Immunol. Immunopathol. 36, 1–16.

Henriquez, C., Perez, B., Morales, N., Sarmiento, J., et al., 2014. Participation of T regulatory cells in equine recurrent airway obstruction. Vet. Immunol. Immunopathol. 158, 128–134.

Holm, L.P., Stevens, K.B., Walker, D.J., 2020. Pathology and epidemiology of cutaneous and renal glomerular vasculopathy in dogs. J. Comp. Pathol. 176, 156–161.

Hope, A., Martinez, C., Cassidy, J.P., Gallagher, B., Mooney, C.T., 2019. Canine cutaneous adrenal glomerular vasculopathy in the Republic of Ireland: a description of three cases. Irish Vet. J. 72, 13. https://doi.org/10.1186/s13620-019-0151-7.

Houtsma, A., Bedenice, D., Pusterla, N., Pugliese, B., et al., 2015. Association between inflammatory airway disease of horses and exposure to respiratory viruses: a case control study. Multidiscip. Respir. Med. 10, 33–40.

Innera, M., 2013. Cutaneous vasculitis in small animals. Vet. Clin. North Am. Small Anim. Pract. 43, 113–134.

Inoue, K., Kamieie, J., Ohtake, S., et al., 2001. Atypical membranoproliferative glomerulonephritis in a cat. Vet. Pathol. 38, 468–470.

Jansen, J.H., 1993. Porcine membranoproliferative glomerulonephritis with intramembranous dense deposits (porcine dense deposit disease). APMIS 101, 281–289.

Kier, A.B., McDonnell, J.J., Stern, A., et al., 1988. The Arthus reaction in domestic cats. Vet. Immunol. Immunopathol. 18, 229–235.

Kohl, J., Gessner, J.E., 1999. On the role of complement and Fc gamma-receptors in the Arthus reaction. Mol. Immunol. 36, 893–903.

Lavoie, J.P., Cesarini, C., Lavoie-Lamoureux, A., et al., 2011. Bronchoalveolar lavage fluid cytology and cytokine messenger ribonucleic acid expression of racehorses with exercise intolerance and lower airway inflammation. J. Vet. Intern. Med. 25, 322–329.

Lavoie-Lamoureux, A., Leclere, M., Lemos, K., Wagner, B., Lavoie, J.P., 2012. Markers of systemic inflammation in horses with heaves. J. Vet. Intern. Med. 26, 1419–1426.

Lee, B.M., Zersen, K.M., Schissler, J.R., Sullivan, L.A., 2019. Antivenin-associated serum sickness in a dog. J. Vet. Emerg. Crit. Care (San Antonio) 29 (5), 558–563. https://doi.org/10.1111/vec.12874

Léguillette, R., 2003. Recurrent airway obstruction—heaves. Vet. Clin. Equine 19, 63–86.

Martinod, K., Deppermann, C., 2020. Immunothrombosis and thromboinflammation in host defense and disease. Platelets. https://doi.org/10.1080/09537104.2020.1817360.

Morchon, R., Carreton, E., Grandi, G., Gonzalez-Miguel, J., et al., 2012. Anti-Wolbachia surface protein antibodies are present in the urine of dogs naturally infected with *Dirofilaria immitis* with circulating microfilariae but not in dogs with occult infections. Vector Born Zoonotic Dis. 12 (1), 17–20.

Morris, D.D., 1987. Cutaneous vasculitis in horses: 19 cases (1978–1985). J. Am. Vet. Med. Assoc. 191, 460–464.

Murray, G.M., Sharpe, A.E., 2009. Nephrotic syndrome due to glomerulopathy in an Irish dairy cow. Vet. Rec. 164, 179–180.

Nichols, P.R., Morris, D.O., Beale, K.M., 2001. A retrospective study of canine and feline cutaneous vasculitis. Vet. Dermatol. 12, 255–264.

Nihei, Y., Haniuda, K., Higashiyama, M., Asami, S., et al., 2023. Identification of IgA autoantibodies targeting mesangial cells redefines the pathogenesis of IgA nephropathy. Sci. Adv. https://doi.org/10.1126/sciadv.add6734.

Powell, C., Thompson, L., Murtaugh, R.J., 2013. Type III hypersensitivity reaction with immune complex deposition in two critically ill dogs administered human serum albumin. J. Vet. Emerg. Crit. Care (San Antonio) 23, 598–604.

Pusterla, N., Watson, J.L., Affolter, V.K., et al., 2003. Purpura haemorrhagica in 53 horses. Vet. Rec. 153, 118–121.

Scherlinger, M., Richez, C., Tsokos, G.C., Boilard, E., Blanco, P., 2023. The role of platelets in immune-mediated inflammatory diseases. Nat. Rev. Immunol. https://doi.org/10.1038/s41577-023-00834-4.

Segev, G., Cowgill, L.D., Heiene, R., Labato, M.A., Polzin, D.J., 2013. Consensus recommendations for immunosuppressive treatment of dogs with glomerular disease based on established pathology. J. Vet. Intern. Med. 27, S44–S54.

Sethi, S., Fervenza, F.C., 2012. Membranoproliferative glomerulonephritis—a new look at an old entity. N. Engl. J. Med. 366, 1119–1131.

Sheats, M.K., Davis, K.U., Poole, J.A., 2019. Comparative review of asthma in farmers and horses. Curr. Allergy Asthma Reps. https://doi.org/10.1007/s11882-019-0882-2.

Shirota, K., Ohtake, S., Inoue, K., et al., 2002. Reactivity of immunoglobulins eluted from the isolated renal glomeruli of nephritic pigs with *Actinobacillus pleuropneumoniae* antigen. Vet. Rec. 151, 390–392.

Slauson, D.O., Lewis, R.M., 1979. Comparative pathology of glomerulonephritis in animals. Vet. Pathol. 16, 135–164.

Spagnolo, P., Rossi, G., Cavazza, A., et al., 2015. Hypersensitivity pneumonitis: a comprehensive review. J. Investig. Allergol. Clin. Immunol. 25 (4), 237–250.

Trang, N.T., Hirai, T., Nabeta, R., Fuke, N., Yamaguchi, R., 2014. Membranoproliferative glomerulonephritis in a calf with nephrotic syndrome. J. Comp. Path. 151, 162–165.

Tizard, I.R., 2022. Allergies and Hypersensitivity Disease in Animals. Elsevier, St Louis, MO, ISBN: 978-0-323-76393-6

T Cell–Mediated Hypersensitivities

Certain antigens, when injected into the skin of sensitized animals, only provoke inflammation at the injection site after a delay of 12–24 hours. These delayed hypersensitivity reactions are classified as type IV hypersensitivities and result from interactions between the injected antigen and T cells. An important example of a delayed hypersensitivity reaction is the tuberculin response. This is an inflammatory response that develops in the skin of an animal infected with tuberculosis following intradermal injection of tuberculin. Delayed hypersensitivity reactions can be considered T cell–mediated inflammatory responses directed against organisms that are resistant to elimination by conventional antibody responses (Tizard, 2022).

THE TUBERCULIN REACTION

Tuberculin is the name given to extracts of mycobacteria used to skin-test animals in order to identify those suffering from tuberculosis. Several types of tuberculin have been employed for this purpose. The most important is purified protein derivative (PPD) tuberculin, prepared by growing organisms in synthetic medium, killing them with steam, and filtering. The PPD tuberculin is precipitated from this filtrate with trichloroacetic acid, washed, and resuspended in buffer ready for use. Thus, PPD tuberculin is a crude mixture of proteins, carbohydrates, and lipids. Its major antigenic component is probably heat-shock protein (HSP) 65. Many of its proteins are shared among different mycobacterial species, so tests that use PPD tuberculin are relatively nonspecific. It is possible to increase the specificity of the tuberculin test with a defined mycobacterial protein such as early secretory antigenic target–6 (ESAT-6). ESAT-6 is a mycobacterial virulence factor that is recognized strongly by T cells (Pollock et al., 2000). However, the reactions induced by very pure proteins tend to be minimal and require greater amounts of antigen to induce a satisfactory skin response (Brodin et al., 2004; Srinavasan et al., 2019).

When tuberculin is injected into the skin of a normal animal, there is no obvious response. On the other hand, if it is injected into an animal sensitized to mycobacteria, a delayed hypersensitivity response occurs. In these animals, a red, indurated (firm) swelling develops at the injection site. The inflammation begins after 12–24 hours, reaches its greatest intensity by 24–72 hours, and may persist for several weeks before fading gradually.

In very severe reactions, tissue necrosis may occur at the injection site. The lesion is infiltrated with lymphocytes and macrophages, although neutrophils are present in the first hours of the reaction (Fig. 34.1).

The tuberculin reaction is mediated by T cells. When an animal is infected with *Mycobacterium tuberculosis*, the organisms are readily phagocytosed by macrophages. Some of this mycobacterial antigen triggers a Th1 response and generates memory cells. These memory T cells will respond to injected mycobacterial antigens, such as tuberculin. Since a positive tuberculin test can be elicited many years after exposure to an antigen, some of these memory T cells must be very long lived.

When tuberculin is injected intradermally, it is taken up by Langerhans cells, which then migrate to the draining lymph node (Fig. 34.2). Here they present processed antigen to memory T cells that respond by generating Th1 effector cells. The Th1 cells recognize the antigen and accumulate around the antigen deposit. By 12 hours the injection site is infiltrated with T cells. In humans and mice, α/β T cells

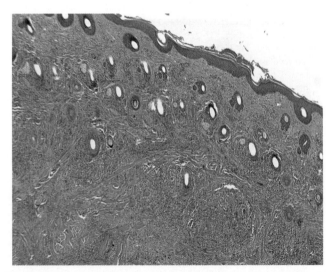

Fig. 34.1 A histological section of a positive tuberculin reaction in bovine skin. Note the perivascular mononuclear cell infiltration as well as the lack of neutrophils or edema. Courtesy Dr. Garry Adams.

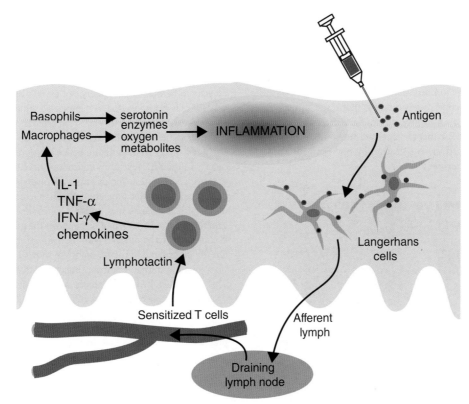

Fig. 34.2 A schematic diagram depicting the mechanism of a delayed hypersensitivity reaction. *IFN-γ*, Interferon-γ; *IL-1*, interleukin-1; *TNF-α*, tumor necrosis factor–α.

tend to predominate, whereas in sheep and cattle, γ/δ WC1 T cells predominate (Kennedy et al., 2002). There are no B cells in the lesion (Doherty et al., 1993).

The γ/δ T cells recruit other Th1 lymphocytes and macrophages to the site. The Th1 cells secrete interferon-γ (IFN-γ), interleukin-2 (IL-2), and IL-16. The first two act on endothelial cells to increase expression of adherence molecules. IL-2 stimulates production of chemokines that attract and activate more T cells. IL-16 attracts CD4+ T cells. These macrophages also release serotonin and chemokines that attract basophils. Basophil-derived vasoactive amines, cause yet more inflammation and enhance the migration of mononuclear cells into the lesion. The T cell–derived chemokines can also induce mast cell degranulation, whereas some CD4+ T cells activate mast cells directly through MHC class II-bound antigen (Askenase and Van Lovern, 1983).

T cell–derived chemokines cause inflammation and attract even more T cells. Most of these new T cells are not specifically sensitized to the inducing antigen. Only a very small proportion, perhaps 5%, of the lymphocytes seen in a delayed hypersensitivity reaction are specific for the antigen. Most are attracted nonspecifically by the chemokine XCL1 (lymphotactin) (Kelner et al., 1994). By 60–72 hours, the predominant lymphocytes are α/β+, CD4+, and CD8+. Macrophages accumulate in the lesion attracted by CXCL8 and may be activated by IFN-γ. The tissue damage in intense delayed hypersensitivity reactions may be due to the release of proteases and oxidants from these activated macrophages. The macrophages ingest and eventually destroy the injected antigen. This, plus the migration of regulatory cells into the lesion, permits the tissues to eventually return to normal.

Cutaneous Basophil Hypersensitivity

Feeding ticks can trigger a form of delayed inflammatory response in the skin where basophils and mast cells predominate (Fig. 34.3). This type of reaction is called cutaneous basophil hypersensitivity (CBH) (Karasuyama, et al., 2018). Tick salivary antigens are taken up by dendritic cells and presented to Th2 cells. These trigger local IgE and IgG responses that recruit and activate basophils. The basophils accumulate around the tick mouthparts and presumably interfere with tick feeding (Carvalho et al., 2010). Similar reactions occur in chickens in response to intradermal Rous sarcoma virus, in rabbits in response to schistosomes, and in humans with allergic contact dermatitis, and renal allograft rejection. CBH reactions may also contribute to the development of flea allergy dermatitis in dogs (Halliwell and Schemmer, 1987).

Tuberculin Reactions in Cattle

Because a positive tuberculin reaction occurs only in animals that have, or have had, tuberculosis, skin testing may be used to identify animals affected by this disease. Indeed, the tuberculin test has provided the basis for all tuberculosis eradication schemes that involve the detection and subsequent removal of infected animals (Bezos et al., 2014).

Skin testing of cattle may be performed in several ways (Table 34.1). The simplest is the single intradermal (SID) test. In this test, 0.1 mL of PPD tuberculin derived from *Mycobacterium tuberculosis* or *M. bovis* is injected into one caudal fold (the folds of skin underneath the tail), and the injection site is examined 72–96 hours later. A comparison is easily made between the injected and the uninjected folds, and a positive response consisting of a firm lump or marked discoloration at the injection site is readily detected.

In the United States, two separate tests are performed. Thus, two injections of tuberculin are made. One into the mucocutaneous junction of the vulva and the other into a caudal fold; in other countries, tuberculin is injected into the skin on the side of the neck. The neck site is more sensitive than the caudal folds, but restraint of the animal may be more difficult, and good injection technique is critical.

The advantage of the SID test is its simplicity and low cost, but it has significant limitations. Interpretation of results may be inconsistent, plus the need for a second visit and low accuracy. Its main disadvantage is that, because of poor specificity, it cannot distinguish between tuberculosis and infection by related mycobacteria such as *Mycobacterium avium*, *Mycobacterium avium* ssp. *paratuberculosis*, or the *Nocardia* group of organisms. A second disadvantage is that some animals react positively to the test but, on necropsy, do not have detectable tuberculosis lesions. The reasons for this are unclear, but some of these false positives probably result from sensitization by environmental mycobacteria such as *Mycobacterium phlei*.

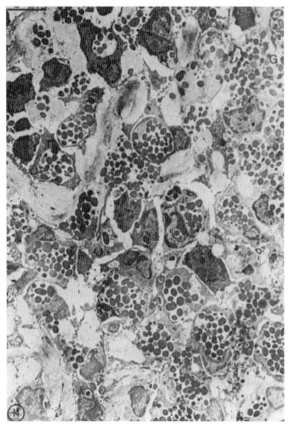

Fig. 34.3 A section of guinea pig skin 18h after attachment of a tick in an animal sensitized by prior infestation with tick larvae. The skin is infiltrated with large numbers of basophils. From McLaren, D., Worms, M.J., Askenase, P.W., 1983. Cutaneous basophil associated resistance to ectoparasites (ticks). Electron microscopy of *Rhipicephalus appendiculatus* larval feeding sites in actively sensitized guinea pigs and recipients of immune serum J. Pathol. 139, 289.

False-negative SID tests may occur in animals with advanced tuberculosis, in animals with a very early infection, in animals that have calved within the preceding 4–6 weeks, in very old cows, and in animals tested during the preceding 1–10 weeks. This lack of reaction (anergy) seen in advanced cases of tuberculosis also occurs in clinical Johne's disease and appears to be due to the presence of an IgG-blocking antibody that prevents T cells from reacting to the injected antigen. There is also evidence for suppression by regulatory cells. Repeated short-interval tuberculin testing leads to desensitization associated with elevated IL-10 and decreased IL-1β responses. (It does not influence IFN-γ responses.) Because of these defects in the SID, several modifications have been developed. The comparative cervical test, for example, involves intradermal inoculation of both avian and bovine tuberculins. Each tuberculin is injected into the side of the neck at separate sites, and these sites are examined 72 hours later. In general, if the avian tuberculin site shows the greatest reaction, the animal is considered to be infected with *M. avium* or *M. avium paratuberculosis*. On the other hand, if the *M. bovis* site shows a significantly greater reaction, then the animal is probably infected with *M. bovis* or *M. tuberculosis*. This test is useful when a high prevalence of avian tuberculosis or Johne's disease is anticipated in a herd. PPD from *M. bovis* is more specific in cattle than *M. tuberculosis*, giving less cross-reaction with *M. avium* as well as being more appropriate for use in cattle, and is therefore preferred. In practice, the comparative test has a sensitivity of 90% (10% false negatives) and a specificity of greater than 99% (<1% false positives); however, much depends on the criteria used to read the results (Whipple et al., 1995).

Another modified tuberculin test is the short thermal test, in which a large volume of tuberculin solution is given subcutaneously and the animal is examined for a rise in temperature between 4 and 8 hours later. (The tuberculin acts on T cells that then provoke the release of IL-1 and other pyrogenic cytokines from macrophages.) The Stormont test relies on the increased sensitivity of a test site, which occurs after a single injection; it is performed by giving two doses of tuberculin at the same injection site 7 days apart. Both tests are relatively sensitive. As a result, they may be used in postpartum cows as well as for the testing of heavily infected animals. Repeated tuberculin skin testing results in a period of decreased reactivity and the induction of antibodies against some *M. bovis* antigens such as HSP 70 and HSP 83 (Coad et al., 2010).

Tuberculin Reactions in Other Species

Tuberculin skin testing has never been a widely employed procedure in domestic animals other than cattle, so information on this is scant. Nevertheless, it appears that the ability of different species to mount a classic tuberculin reaction varies greatly. In pigs and cats, for example, the tuberculin test is positive for only a short period following infection. In pigs and dogs, the best test is an SID test given in the skin behind the ear, whereas in cats, the short thermal test is probably best. In sheep and goats, the antigen is usually given in the caudal fold, but the results can be unreliable in these species as well. Horses appear to be unusually

TABLE 34.1	**Tuberculin Tests Used in Cattle**		
Test	**Use**	**Advantages**	**Disadvantages**
Single intradermal	Routine testing	Simple	Prone to false positives Poor sensitivity
Comparative	When avian TB or Johne disease is prevalent	More specific than SID	More complex than SID
Short thermal	Use in postpartum animals and in infected animals	High efficiency	Time-consuming Risk for anaphylaxis
Stormont	Use in postpartum animals and in advanced cases	Very sensitive and accurate	Three visits required May sensitize an animal

SID, Single intradermal.

sensitive to tuberculin, and the dose used must be reduced accordingly. Nevertheless, the results obtained do not always correlate well with the disease status of the animal. In birds, good reactions may be obtained by inoculating tuberculin into the wattle or wing web.

Johnin Reactions

Animals infected with *M. avium* ssp. *paratuberculosis*, the cause of Johne's disease, develop a delayed hypersensitivity reaction following intradermal inoculation of an extract of this organism called Johnin. The injection site contains a mixed mononuclear cell infiltrate, possibly with multinucleated giant cells or plasma cells (Gulliver et al., 2015). Sheep with paucibacillary intestinal lesions tend to have greater induration, and greater cellular infiltration than animals with multibacillary lesions (see Chapter 27). Johnin can be used in a SID test but, like tuberculin, may give a negative result in animals with clinical disease. An intravenous Johnin test will be positive in these cases and is a preferable alternative to the SID test. In this test, the antigen is administered intravenously, and the animal's temperature is noted 6 hours later. A rise in temperature of 1°C or a neutrophilia is considered a positive result. These tests are of limited usefulness in individual animals but may help identify infected herds.

Other Skin Tests

Positive delayed hypersensitivity skin reactions may be obtained in any infectious disease in which T cell–mediated immunity has a significant role. Thus, extracts of *Brucella abortus* have been used in attempts to diagnose brucellosis. These include brucellin, a filtrate of a 20-day broth culture, and brucellergen, a nucleoprotein extract. Because these injected extracts may induce antibodies to brucella, they cannot be employed in areas where eradication is monitored by serological tests. In equine glanders, a culture filtrate of the organism *Burkholderia mallei*, termed mallein, is used for skin testing. Mallein can be used in either a short thermal test or an ophthalmic test. The ophthalmic test, also occasionally employed in tuberculosis, is performed by dropping the antigen solution into an eye. A transient conjunctivitis develops if the test is positive. Another method of testing for glanders is the intrapalpebral test. In this test, mallein is injected into the skin of the lower eyelid, where a positive reaction results in swelling and ophthalmia.

Intradermal skin testing with microbial extracts is also employed in the diagnosis of many fungal diseases; thus, histoplasmin is used for histoplasmosis, coccidioidin for coccidioidomycosis, and so on. In these cases, the tests are not very specific, and the injected antigen may sensitize the tested animal, causing it to become serologically positive. This problem also arises when toxoplasmin is used in attempts to diagnose toxoplasmosis (see Chapter 29).

Tuberculosis Serology

It must not be assumed that *M. bovis* stimulates only T cells. As the infection progresses, antibodies are produced. These are directed against the immunodominant antigens MPB83 and MBP70 released by *M. bovis* in advanced infections. The greatest and earliest immune response is directed against MPB83. These antibodies can be detected using ELISA tests or lateral flow assays (see Chapter 43). These assays are useful in the identification of infected animals missed by intradermal skin testing. Their sensitivity is often low, but they are simple, rapid, and inexpensive.

PATHOLOGICAL CONSEQUENCES OF TYPE IV HYPERSENSITIVITY

Tubercle Formation

Although the tuberculin reaction induced by intradermal inoculation is artificial in that antigen is administered by injection, a similar inflammatory response occurs when living tubercle bacilli lodge in tissues and sensitize an animal. However, *M. tuberculosis* is resistant to intracellular destruction until M1 macrophages are activated by Th1 cells (see Chapter 19), and dead organisms are very slowly removed because they contain large quantities of poorly metabolized waxes. As a result, the reaction to whole organisms is prolonged, and macrophages accumulate in very large numbers. Many of these macrophages ingest the bacteria but fail to prevent its growth, and so they die. Other macrophages fuse to form multinucleated giant cells. After 4–5 weeks of infection, granulomas enlarge and coalesce. The lesion that develops around invading tubercle bacilli therefore consists of a mass of caseous (cheesy!) debris containing both living and dead organisms surrounded by layers of fibroblasts, lymphocytes, and macrophages, which in this location are called epithelioid cells (see Chapter 27). The entire lesion forms a type 1 granuloma called a tubercle (Fig. 34.4). The mycobacteria are unable to multiply within the necrotic tissue because of its low pH and lack of oxygen. Nevertheless, some bacteria may survive in a dormant state. If the host mounts an adequate immune response of the correct (Th1) type, this may be sufficient to control the infection. However, if immunity is insufficient or inappropriate (e.g., a Th2 response), the organisms may escape from the tubercle and spread to local lymph nodes and nearby tissues. When the response is inadequate, the multiplying organisms continue to spread, and the resulting lung damage, together with liquefaction of the caseous center of the tubercle, leads to rapidly progressive lethal disease (Bold and Ernst, 2009).

During the early stages of granuloma formation, macrophages are highly mobile and provide the pathogen with fresh cells to infect. These infected macrophages continue to recruit uninfected macrophages to the site of infection. They phagocytose old macrophages and their bacterial contents. This process leads to the progressive growth of the bacterial population. Thus, virulent mycobacteria exploit the process by which macrophages promote tissue repair.

Allergic Contact Dermatitis

If certain reactive chemicals are painted onto the skin of an animal, they can trigger delayed inflammation. Allergic contact dermatitis (ACD) is, as a result, the most common occupational skin disease in humans. For example, TLR4 is a receptor for multiple contact sensitizers such as nickel ions or trinitrochlorobenzene. These chemicals

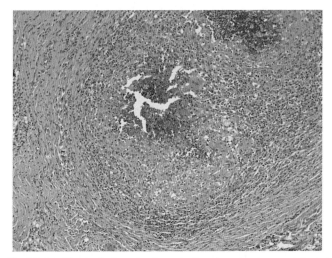

Fig. 34.4 A histological section from the lymph node of a cow infected with *Mycobacterium bovis* showing a small tubercle. The dark central mass is caseous material. It is surrounded by layers of macrophages and lymphocytes and walled off by fibroblasts. Courtesy Dr. John Edwards.

therefore trigger inflammation by stimulating IL-1β and TNF-α release (Ho et al., 2015). Additionally, they may bind to skin proteins such as keratin and act as strong haptens. The resulting hapten-protein complexes are captured by Langerhans cells in the dermis (Fig. 34.5; Wang et al., 2002). The Langerhans cells migrate to draining lymph nodes and present the antigen to T cells. Subsequent exposure to the sensitizing chemical may elicit a T cell–mediated inflammatory response. Thus, when encountering these hapten-protein complexes for a second time, activated Langerhans cells generate an NLRP3 inflammasome (see Chapter 3) and secrete large amounts of IL-12, IL-18, and IL-23 that activate both Th1 and Th17 cells. These hapten-specific helper cells produce large amounts of IFN-γ and IL-17 and promote the activities of cytotoxic T cells. Following exposure to a sensitizing chemical, activated M1 macrophages and CD8+ lymphocytes infiltrate the dermis, taking about 24 hours to generate a response. Eventually, the cytotoxic T cells kill the chemically altered cells, resulting in the development of intraepithelial vesicles. This destructive reaction, together with the production of IL-33 and accompanying inflammation, presents as an intensely pruritic skin reaction (Fig. 34.6; Liu et al., 2016). In addition to α/β T cells, other cell types, such as γ/δ T cells, B-1 cells, mast cells, and NKT cells, may contribute to the reaction. The inflammation is eventually moderated by IL-10 and TGF-β from Treg cells (He et al., 2009).

The inflammatory infiltrate in ACD also contains numbers of ILC2 cells, NK cells, and NKT cells (<10%). They are attracted to the site by multiple chemokines. They exacerbate the inflammation by producing more IFN-γ and TNF-α, and by killing modified keratinocytes by apoptosis. These NK cells can survive for at least 28 days in mice and form a trained cell population. It is also of interest to note that contact dermatitis will not occur in skin that lacks functional nerve fibers. Clearly, ACD has a complex and poorly understood etiology (Brys et al., 2020).

Contact Sensitizers

The chemicals that induce allergic contact dermatitis are usually highly reactive molecules that combine covalently with skin proteins to act as haptens; they include formaldehyde, picric acid, aniline dyes, plant resins and oils, organophosphates, some topical medications such as neomycin, and salts of metals such as nickel, cobalt, and beryllium

(Fig. 34.7). Thus allergic contact dermatitis can occur on pathologists' fingers as a result of exposure to formaldehyde; on the ears of dogs treated with neomycin for otitis externa; on the footpads, scrotum, and ventral abdomen of dogs on exposure to some carpet dyes and deodorizers; on parts of the body exposed to the oils (urushiols) of the poison ivy plant (*Rhus radicans*) and mango skin; and around the neck of animals as a result of exposure to dichlorvos (2,2-dichlorovinyldimethylphosphate) in flea collars (Box 34.1; Cronce and Alden, 1968). Severe lesions may develop on the teats of dairy cattle as a result of a contact dermatitis to a component of milking machine rubber

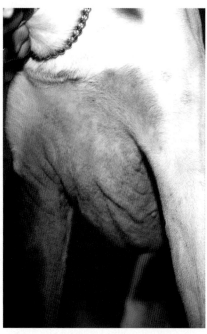

Fig. 34.6 A severe case of allergic contact dermatitis in a Great Dane. The contact sensitizer was not identified, but it appeared to originate in the concrete surrounding a newly constructed swimming pool. Chloride ions appear to release a contact sensitizer from concrete. Courtesy Dr. R. Kennis.

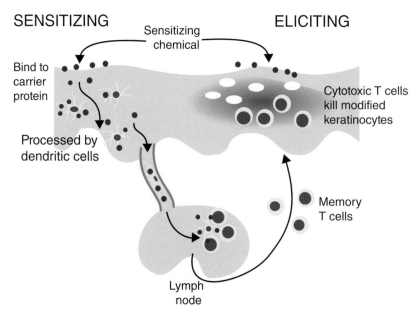

Fig. 34.5 The pathogenesis of allergic contact dermatitis.

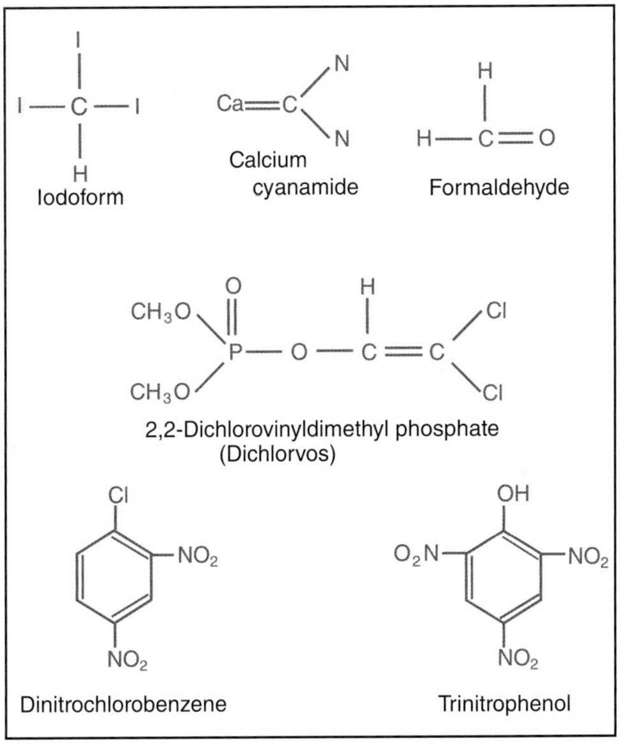

Fig. 34.7 Some of the simple chemicals that can cause allergic contact dermatitis.

BOX 34.1 Some Sources of Contact Allergens in Animals

Insecticides in flea collars
  In sprays
  In dips
Wood preservatives
Floor waxes
Carpet dyes
Some pollens
Dermatological drugs (creams, ointments)
Leather products
Paints
House plants

(N-isopropyl-N-phenyl diamine) (Holzhauer et al., 2004). Calcium cyanamide (CaCN$_2$) is used to reduce *Escherichia coli* levels in bedding. Dairy cattle have developed severe ACD on contact with calcium cyanamide spread on the floor of a cattle shed to prevent mastitis (Onda et al., 2008).

ACD involving the muzzle of dogs has been reported to result from sensitivity to plastics in food bowls. Some dogs, instead of developing the more usual type I hypersensitivity to pollen proteins, experience an allergic contact dermatitis as a result of a type IV hypersensitivity to pollen resins. It is unusual for ACD to affect the haired areas of the skin unless the allergen is in a liquid. Thus allergic contact dermatitis to shampoo components may result in total-body involvement. The period required for sensitization ranges from 6 months to several years. Hairless dogs are especially susceptible to developing contact dermatitis (Kimura, 2007, 2009).

The lesions of allergic contact dermatitis range from a mild erythema to severe erythematous vesiculation. However, because of the intense pruritus, self-trauma, excoriation, ulceration, and secondary

staphylococcal pyoderma often mask the true nature of the lesion. If the exposure to the allergen persists, hyperkeratosis, acanthosis, and dermal fibrosis may eventually occur. Histologically, the lesion is marked by a mononuclear cell infiltration and vacuolation of skin cells under attack by cytotoxic T cells (Table 34.2; Godfrey et al., 1983).

ACD is diagnosed by removal of the suspected antigen and by patch testing. In "closed" patch tests, allergen-impregnated gauze swabs are attached to shaved skin with tape. After 48–72 hours, the dressing is removed, and the areas in contact with the swabs are examined. A positive reaction is indicated by local erythema and vesiculation. Closed patch tests may be impractical for some dogs and cats. An "open" patch test may therefore be employed. In this procedure, a solution of the suspected allergen is applied to a small area of shaved, normal skin, and the area is examined daily for up to 5 days. Identification of the offending allergen and its avoidance by the animal is the optimal therapy for ACD. Hyposensitization therapy is not effective. Steroids are used to treat acute cases, with antibiotics to control secondary infections.

Mucocutaneous Diseases

Three related mucocutaneous disorders—erythema multiforme, Stevens-Johnson syndrome, and toxic epidermal necrolysis—occur in dogs and cats. The three diseases are characterized by skin loss of increasing severity. Erythema multiforme is characterized by patchy skin loss and low morbidity; Stevens-Johnson syndrome is more severe but involves less than 10% of the body surface; and toxic epidermal necrolysis is much more serious, with affected individuals losing more than 30% of their epidermis. Mortality is high.

Stevens-Johnson syndrome and toxic epidermal necrolysis are believed to involve a T cell–mediated hypersensitivity to drugs. Erythema multiforme is not associated with drug administration. Affected animals develop vesicles, shed large areas of epidermis, and develop skin ulcers as a result of widespread keratinocyte apoptosis. The apoptosis is believed to result from drugs binding to the epidermal cells and triggering their destruction by cytotoxic T cells. The skin lesions are infiltrated mainly by CD8$^+$ T cells. Many different drugs may trigger these responses, but common inducers in dogs include trimethoprim-potentiated sulfonamides, β-lactam antibiotics, penicillin, and cephalexin. Beginning about 14 days after drug exposure, the skin begins to blister and slough. Animals develop dyspnea, vomiting, fever, and weight loss. In dogs, sloughing of the epidermis occurs over

TABLE 34.2 Comparison of the Major Forms of Allergic Dermatitis

	Atopic Dermatitis	Allergic Contact Dermatitis
Pathogenesis	Type I hypersensitivity	Type IV hypersensitivity
Clinical signs	Hyperemia, urticaria, pruritus	Hyperemia, vesiculation, alopecia, erythema
Distribution	Face, nose, eyes, feet, perineum	Hairless areas, usually ventral abdomen and feet
Major allergens	Foods and pollens, fleas, inhaled allergens	Reactive chemicals, dyes in contact with skin
Diagnosis	Intradermal testing, immediate response	Delayed response on patch testing
Pathology	Eosinophilic infiltration, edema	Mononuclear cell infiltration, vesiculation
Treatment	Steroids, antihistamines, hyposensitization	Steroids

the nasal planum, the footpads, and the oral, pharyngeal, nasal, conjunctival, and preputial mucosa. Life-threatening secondary infections are common (Nuttall and Malham, 2004).

MEASUREMENT OF CELL-MEDIATED IMMUNITY

Although diagnostic immunology is based largely on the detection of serum antibodies, measurement of cell-mediated immunity may be desirable under some circumstances. For example, in determining the effectiveness of a vaccine, one must consider that serum antibody levels may not truly reflect the degree of immunity possessed by an animal. Animals without detectable antibodies may still possess significant cell-mediated immunity. The term "cell-mediated immunity" encompasses a diverse set of mechanisms that employ T cells and macrophages for protection. Currently, both in vivo and in vitro techniques are used for these assays (Sanbulte and Roth, 2004).

In Vivo Techniques

The simplest in vivo test of cell-mediated immunity is an intradermal skin test such as the tuberculin test. The inflammation and swelling that occur in response to intradermally injected antigens may be considered cell mediated, provided that they have the characteristic time course and histological features of a type IV reaction. Intradermal skin tests are not always convenient, they are difficult to quantitate, and injection of an antigen may sensitize an animal, thus preventing further testing.

It is sometimes useful to measure the ability of an animal to mount cell-mediated immune responses in general rather than the response to one specific antigen. One way to do this is to give the animal a small skin allograft and measure its survival time. A much simpler technique is to paint a small area of the animal's skin with a contact sensitizer such as dinitrochlorobenzene. The intensity of the resulting allergic contact dermatitis provides a rough estimate of the animal's ability to mount a cell-mediated immune response (Schultz and Maguire, 1982).

If the T cell–stimulating lectin, phytohemagglutinin is injected intradermally, it provokes a local tissue reaction with many features of a delayed hypersensitivity response. In pigs, for example, this reaction is characterized by infiltration with γ/δ⁺, CD4⁺, and CD8⁺ T cells. This is a very convenient and rapid method of assessing an animal's ability to mount a cell-mediated response without the need for first sensitizing the animal to an antigen. However, the response to phytohemagglutinin is nonspecific, and interpretation of the results may be difficult (Whyte et al., 1994).

In Vitro Techniques

In vitro tests are designed to measure the antigen-specific activation and proliferation of T cells. These also include their cytotoxic activities and their production of cytokines. All of these tests require that T cells be grown in cell culture and must be performed in a laboratory.

To measure T-cell proliferation in response to an antigen, a suspension of purified peripheral blood lymphocytes from the animal to be tested is mixed with the antigen and cultured for 48–96 hours (Fig. 34.8). Twelve hours before harvesting, thymidine labeled with the radioactive isotope tritium and antigen is added to the cultures. Normal, nondividing lymphocytes do not take up thymidine, but cells dividing in response to an antigen do. Thus, if the T cells are proliferating, they will take up the tritiated thymidine. The greater their proliferation, the greater will be their radioactivity. The ratio of the radioactivity in the stimulated cultures to the radioactivity in the controls is called the stimulation index. A related technique is to measure the proliferation of lymphocytes in response to mitogenic lectins such as concanavalin A (see Box 14.2). The intensity of the lymphocyte proliferative response, as measured by tritiated thymidine uptake, provides an estimate of the reactivity of an animal's lymphocytes.

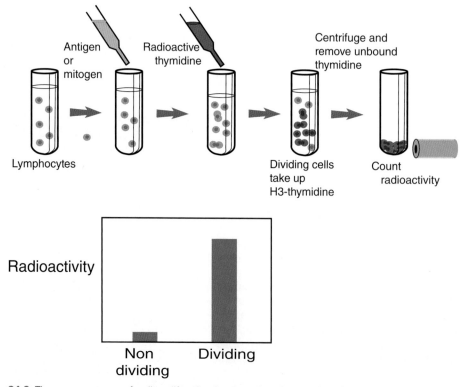

Fig. 34.8 The measurement of cell proliferation by detecting the uptake of tritiated thymidine. Cells are stimulated to divide by a specific antigen or a mitogen. The thymidine is incorporated into the DNA of the dividing cells. The uptake is simply measured by the radioactivity of the cells.

Radioactive tritium may be replaced in proliferation assays by a simple colorimetric enzyme assay. Methylthiazoldiphenyltetrazolium bromide (MTT) is a pale-yellow compound that serves as a substrate for active mitochondrial enzymes. The enzymes change the MTT color to dark blue. The intensity of this color change is a measure of the number of living cells in a culture. In proliferation assays, the number of living cells increases, and this can be measured colorimetrically. The test is sufficiently sensitive to quantify the increase in T-cell numbers triggered by antigen or mitogens.

To measure T cell–mediated cytotoxicity, it is necessary to have a simple method of measuring cell death. This is usually based on the fact that living cells take up and retain chromium ions. When a cell dies, the chromium is released into the extracellular fluid. Radioactive sodium chromate (^{51}Cr) is used to label target cells (Fig. 34.9). Lymphocytes from an immune animal are mixed in an appropriate ratio with ^{51}Cr-labeled target cells. The mixture is then incubated for 4–24 hours at 37°C. At the end of this time, the cell suspension is centrifuged, and the presence of free ^{51}Cr in the supernatant is measured. The amount of chromium released is directly related to the number of target cells killed. The amount of chromium released in the absence of cytotoxic cells must also be measured and subtracted from that released in the presence of cytotoxic cells to obtain a true reading.

A third in vitro assay is the measurement of cytokine release by T cells. One important example of this technique involves measuring the release of IFN-γ by peripheral blood lymphocytes following exposure to tuberculin or purified mycobacterial antigens (Fig. 34.10).

This method has been developed as an alternative or supplement to the tuberculin test for the diagnosis of tuberculosis in cattle and deer (Wood et al., 1990, 1991). It involves adding tuberculin PPD to heparinized blood and incubating the mixture for 24–48 hours at 37°C. The plasma is then removed and assayed for any interferon produced, either by means of a simple bioassay or preferably by use of a sandwich enzyme-linked immunosorbent assay (ELISA) employing monoclonal antibodies (see Chapter 43; Roupie et al., 2018). Three tubes are commonly tested: no antigen (negative control), *M. bovis* PPD, and *M. avium* PPD. The *M. avium* PPD is used to detect false-positive cross-reactions. The use of purified, recombinant mycobacterial proteins such as ESAT-6 can reduce the incidence of false-positive results even further. This technique has advantages over conventional tuberculin tests in that it does not sensitize the animal under testing by injection of antigen. In addition, the animal does not have to be held for several days for the test to be read. The assay is at least as sensitive as the SID test and, if purified recombinant mycobacterial proteins are employed, is highly specific and is also much simpler. (Its sensitivity is about 85%, and its specificity is as high as 90%–99%.) Positive results are obtained earlier than by skin testing. However, it does appear to detect tuberculosis cases in a slightly different population of animals than the skin test (Schiller et al., 2010). It has also been successfully used to diagnose Johne's disease in sheep as well as tuberculosis in cats and dogs.

It is possible to use a variation of a sandwich ELISA assay (see Chapter 43) to determine the frequency of cytokine-secreting cells in a

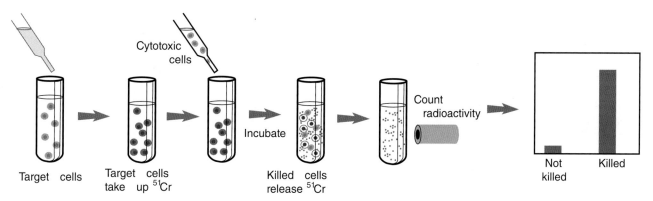

Fig. 34.9 The measurement of cell death by detecting the release of chromium-51 by dying cells. This release may be triggered by cytotoxic T cells or natural killer cells.

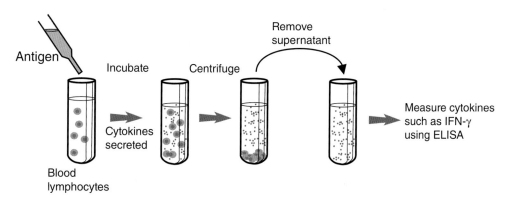

Fig. 34.10 The release of interferon-γ (IFN-γ) by peripheral blood lymphocytes following exposure to tuberculin or to purified mycobacterial antigens. This technique can be used for the diagnosis of tuberculosis in cattle and deer. Tuberculin purified protein derivative is added to blood, and the mixture is incubated for 24–48 h. The plasma is then removed and assayed for any interferon produced.

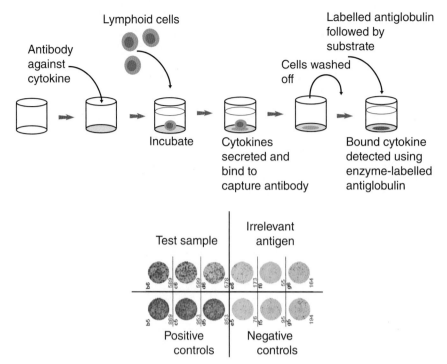

Fig. 34.11 The principles of the enzyme-linked immunospot assay. The photograph shows the interferon-γ response of bovine peripheral blood mononuclear cells exposed to a defined *Anaplasma marginale* antigen. Courtesy Dr. W. Mwangi.

tissue (Fig. 34.11). In the enzyme-linked immunospot (ELISpot) assay, a capture antibody directed against the cytokine of interest coats the bottom of plastic tissue culture wells. The cells to be tested are cultured on this surface and exposed to the antigen. If the cells secrete the cytokine of interest, it will bind to nearby capture-antibodies. Once the culture period is completed, the presence of this bound cytokine can be detected by a conventional sandwich ELISA using specific detection antibody and enzyme-labeled antiglobulin. This results in the development of a pattern of colored spots that each correspond to the location of a cytokine-secreting cell. These spots can be counted, and the frequency of specific cytokine-producing cells can be determined. This assay can also be used to quantitate cytotoxic cells by detecting granzyme or perforin production.

Although all of the assays described previously can be used to measure at least some aspects of cell-mediated immunity, none provide a complete picture. The investigator may, of course, simply be interested in the response to a single antigen or organism. In these cases, either a skin test or an in vitro assay may be appropriate. This is best exemplified by the tests available for the diagnosis of tuberculosis. In vitro tests are also useful if the time course of a cell-mediated immune response is to be examined. Repeated testing can be performed simply by obtaining more lymphocytes. If, on the other hand, an investigator wishes to obtain an overview of an animal's abilities in this area, one of the nonspecific in vivo assays may be more appropriate. These can be useful, for example, in assessing immune function in young animals thought to be immunodeficient. However, it is important to point out that in these animals, a complete hematological examination should be performed before more complex assays are considered. It is also prudent to measure the important lymphocyte subpopulations by flow cytometry. An animal that has no T cells is unlikely to mount any sort of cell-mediated response.

REFERENCES

Askenase, P.W., Van Loveren, M., 1983. Delayed-type hypersensitivity: activation of mast cells by antigen-specific T-cell factors initiates the cascade of cellular interactions. Immunol. Today 4, 259–264.

Bezos, J., Casal, C., Romero, B., Schroeder, B., et al., 2014. Current antemortem techniques for diagnosis of bovine tuberculosis. Res. Vet. Sci. 97 (Suppl), S44–52.

Bold, T.D., Ernst, J.D., 2009. Who benefits from granulomas, mycobacterias or host? Cell 136, 17–19.

Brodin, P., Rosenkrands, I., Andersen, P., et al., 2004. ESAT-6 proteins: protective antigens and virulence factors? Trends Microbiol. 12, 500–508.

Brys, A.K., Rodriguez-Homs, L.G., Suwanpradid, J., Atwater, A.R., et al., 2020. Shifting paradigms in allergic contact dermatitis: the role of innate immunity. J. Invest. Dermatol. 140 (1), 21–28.

Carvalho, W.A., Franzin, A.M., Abatepaulo, A.R., Freire de Oliviera, C.J., More, D.D., da Silva, J.S., et al., 2010. Modulation of cutaneous inflammation induced by ticks in contrasting phenotypes of infestation in bovines. Vet. Parasitol. 167, 260–273.

Coad, M., Clifford, D., Rhodes, S.G., et al., 2010. Repeat tuberculin skin testing leads to desensitisation in naturally infected tuberculous cattle which is associated with elevated interleukin-10 and decreased interleukin-1 beta responses. Vet. Res. 41, 14–20.

Cronce, P.C., Alden, H.S., 1968. Flea-collar dermatitis. J. Amer. Med. Assn. 206 (7), 1563–1564.

Doherty, M.L., Monaghan, M.L., Bassett, H.F., et al., 1993. The sequential cellular changes which characterize the tuberculin reaction in cattle. Vet. Immunol. Immunopathol. 35 (Suppl), 70–71.

Godfrey, M.P., Phillips, M.E., Askenase, P.W., 1983. Histopathology of delayed-onset hypersensitivities in contact-sensitive guinea pigs. Int. Arch. Allerg. Appl. Immunol. 70, 50–58.

Gulliver, E.L., Plain, K.M., Begg, D.J., Whittington, R.J., 2015. Histopathological characterization of cutaneous delayed-type hypersensitivity and correlations with intestinal pathology and systemic immune responses in sheep with paratuberculosis. J. Comp. Pathol. 153, 67–80.

Halliwell, R.E.W., Schemmer, K.R., 1987. The role of basophils in the immuno-pathogenesis of hypersensitivity to fleas (*Ctenocephalis felis*) in dogs. Vet. Immunol. Immunopathol. 15, 203–213.

He, D., Wu, L., Kim, H.K., et al., 2009. IL-17 and IFN-gamma mediate the elicitation of contact hypersensitivity responses by different mechanisms, and both are required for optimal responses. J. Immunol. 183, 1463–1470.

Ho, K.K., Campbell, K.L., Lavergne, S.N., 2015. Contact dermatitis: a comparative and translational review of the literature. Vet. Dermatol. 26, 314–327.

Holzhauer, M., Sampimon, O.C., Sol, J., et al., 2004. Allergic contact dermatitis of bovine teat skin caused by milking machine cluster rubber. Vet. Rec. 154, 208–209.

Karasuyama, H., Tabakawa, Y., Ohta, T., Wada, T., Yoshikawa, S., 2018. Crucial role for basophils in acquired protective immunity to tick infestation. Front. Physiol. 9, 1769–1776.

Kelner, G.S., Kennedy, J., Bacon, K.B., et al., 1994. Lymphotactin: a cytokine that represents a new class of chemokine. Science 266, 1395–1397.

Kennedy, H.E., Welsh, M.D., Bryson, D.G., et al., 2002. Modulation of immune responses to *Mycobacterium bovis* in cattle depleted of WC1+ γδ T cells. Infect. Immun. 70, 1488–1500.

Kimura, T., 2007. Contact dermatitis caused by sunless tanning treatment with dihydroxyacetone in hairless descendants of Mexican hairless dogs. Environ. Toxicol. 22, 176–184.

Kimura, T., 2009. Contact hypersensitivity to stainless steel cages (Chromium metal) in hairless descendants of Mexican hairless dogs. Environ. Toxicol. 24, 506–512.

Liu, B., Tai, Y., Achanta, S., Kaelberer, M.M., et al., 2016. IL-33/ST2 signaling excites sensory neurons and mediates itch response in a mouse model of poison ivy contact allergy. Proc. Natl. Acad. Sci. U.S.A. 113, E7572–e7579.

Nuttall, T.J., Malham, T., 2004. Successful intravenous human immunoglobulin treatment of drug-induced Stevens-Johnson syndrome in a dog. J. Small Animal Pract. 45, 357–361.

Onda, K., Yagisawa, T., Matsui, T., et al., 2008. Contact dermatitis in dairy cattle caused by calcium cyanamide. Vet. Rec. 163, 418–422.

Pollock, J.M., Girvin, R.M., Lightbody, K.A., et al., 2000. Assessment of defined antigens for the diagnosis of bovine tuberculosis in skin test reactor cattle. Vet. Rec. 146, 659–665.

Roupie, V., Alonso-Velasco, E., Van Der Heyden, Holbert, S., et al., 2018. Evaluation of mycobacteria-specific gamma interferon and antibody responses before and after a single intradermal test in cattle naturally exposed to *M. avium* subsp *paratuberculosis* and experimentally infected with *M. bovis*. Vet. Immunol. Immunopathol. 196, 35–47.

Sanbulte, M.R., Roth, J.A., 2004. Methods for analysis of cell-mediated immunity in domestic animal species. J. Am. Vet. Med. Assoc. 225, 522–530.

Schiller, I., Vordermeier, H.M., Waters, W.R., et al., 2010. Bovine tuberculosis: effect of the tuberculin skin test on in vitro interferon gamma responses. Vet. Immunol. Immunopathol. 136, 1–11.

Schultz, K.T., Maguire, H.C., 1982. Chemically-induced delayed hypersensitivity in the cat. Vet. Immunol. Immunopathol. 3, 585–590.

Srinavasan, S., Jones, G., Veerasami, M., Steinbach, S., et al., 2019. A defined antigen skin test for the diagnosis of bovine tuberculosis. Sci. Adv. 5, eaax4899.

Tizard, I.R., 2022. Allergies and Hypersensitivity Disease in Animals. Elsevier, St Louis, MO, ISBN: 978-0-323-76393-6

Wang, B., Feliciani, C., Howel, B.G., et al., 2002. Contribution of Langerhans cell-derived IL-18 to contact hypersensitivity. J. Immunol. 168, 3303–3308.

Whipple, D.L., Bolin, C.A., Davis, A.J., et al., 1995. Comparison of the sensitivity of the caudal fold skin test and a commercial γ-interferon assay for diagnosis of bovine tuberculosis. Am. J. Vet. Res. 56, 415–419.

Whyte, A., Haskard, D.O., Binns, R.M., 1994. Infiltrating γδ T-cells and selectin endothelial ligands in the cutaneous phytohemagglutinin-induced inflammatory reaction. Vet. Immunol. Immunopathol. 41, 31–40.

Wood, P.R., Corner, L.A., Plackett, P., 1990. Development of a simple, rapid in vitro cellular assay for bovine tuberculosis based on the production of γ-interferon. Res. Vet. Sci. 49, 46–49.

Wood, P.R., Corner, L.A., Rothel, J.S., et al., 1991. Field comparison of the interferon-gamma assay and the single intradermal tuberculin test for the diagnosis of bovine tuberculosis. Aust. Vet. J. 68, 286–290.

Organ Graft Rejection and Pregnancy

Although the immune responses first attracted the attention of scientists because of their ability to prevent infections, the observation that animals reject foreign organ grafts led to a much broader view of the immune system in that it indicated that the immune system had a surveillance function. The rejection of a foreign organ graft simply reflects the role of the immune system in identifying and destroying "abnormal" cells.

ORGAN GRAFTING

Advances in surgery have permitted the transfer of many tissues or organs between different parts of the body or between different individuals. When moved to a different part of an animal's own body, such transplants do not trigger an immune response. This type of graft within an individual is called an autograft (Fig. 35.1). Examples of autografting include the use of a skin graft to cover a burn in plastic surgery and the use of a segment of vein to bypass blocked cardiac arteries. Since autografts do not express foreign antigens, they do not trigger an immune response.

Isografts are grafts transplanted between two genetically identical individuals. Thus, a graft between identical (monozygotic) twins is an isograft. Similarly, grafts between two inbred mice of the same strain are isografts and present no immunological difficulties. Since the animals are identical, the immune system of the recipient cannot differentiate between the graft and normal body cells.

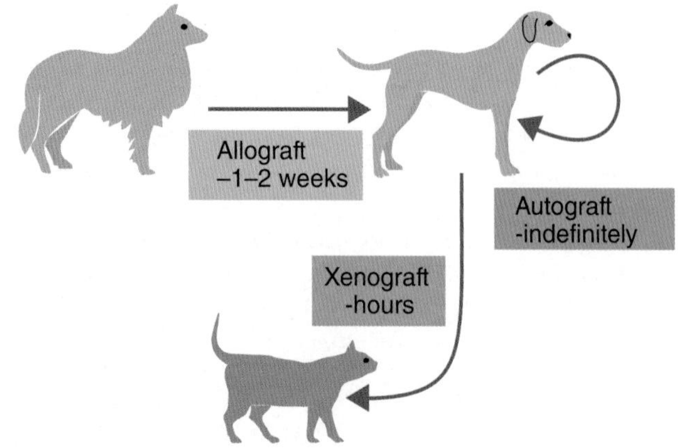

Allografts are transplanted between genetically different members of the same species. Most grafts performed on animals or humans for therapeutic reasons are of this type because tissues are obtained from a donor who is usually unrelated to the graft recipient. Because the major histocompatibility complex (MHC) and blood group molecules on the allograft are usually different from those of their host, allografts induce a strong immune response that results in graft rejection. This rejection process must be suppressed if the grafted organ is to survive.

Xenografts are organ grafts transplanted between animals of different species. Thus, the transplant of a pig liver into a human is a xenograft. Xenografted organs differ from their host both biochemically and immunologically. As a result, they provoke a rapid, intense rejection response that is very difficult to suppress.

Clinical grafting in domestic animals is now routine in dogs and cats, and bone marrow allografts promise to be very useful in some forms of tumor therapy. Most current organ grafts are obtained from healthy donor animals. This raises ethical issues as to whether it is appropriate to subject a donor animal to major surgery in order to provide an organ for another animal. Although the benefits of allografting to the recipient are obvious, it is unclear how the donor animal might benefit. Unlike human donors driven by altruism, an animal donor is given no choice in the matter. It is possible, however, to justify organ donation if, thereby, an animal would be saved from inevitable euthanasia and if the donor could be provided with a good home. For this reason, many animal transplantation centers require that the donor animal be adopted and cared for by the owner of the recipient animal.

ALLOGRAFT REJECTION

The identification and destruction of foreign molecules are central to the body's defense. Allografted organs represent a major source of foreign molecules. They contain not only antigens such as the foreign

Fig. 35.1 The differences among autografts, allografts, and xenografts and their approximate survival times.

blood group glycoproteins and MHC molecules expressed on the grafted cells but also endogenous antigens on the MHC class I molecules of these same cells. The mechanisms of allograft rejection are the same irrespective of the organ grafted, and both antibodies and T cells participate in the rejection process (Nankivell and Alexander, 2010).

Histocompatibility Antigens

When an organ is transplanted into a genetically dissimilar animal, the recipient will mount an immune response against many different antigens in and on the cells of the allograft. These are thus called histocompatibility antigens. Three types of histocompatibility antigens trigger graft rejection. These are the MHC class I molecules, the MHC class II molecules, and the major blood group molecules. All are expressed on the surface of the graft cells, but their distribution varies. MHC class I antigens are found on almost all nucleated cells. The major blood group antigens are found both on red cells and nucleated cells. MHC class II antigens, in contrast, have a restricted distribution that varies between species (see Chapter 12). For example, in rats and mice, MHC class II molecules are expressed only on their professional antigen-presenting cells (APCs): macrophages, dendritic cells, and B cells. In other mammals, such as humans and pigs, MHC class II molecules are also expressed on the endothelium of renal arteries and glomeruli, the sites where host cells first contact the graft. It is important to note that, as a result of these differences, it is much easier to prolong renal allograft survival in laboratory rodents than in humans or pigs.

As would be expected, grafts that differ minimally from the recipient will generally survive longer than grafts that are highly incompatible. When blood group A-O-compatible pigs are given renal allografts, median survival is about 12 days for MHC-unmatched grafts, 25 days for grafts compatible for MHC class I alone, 32 days for grafts compatible for MHC class II alone, and 80 days for grafts compatible for both class I and class II (Fig. 35.2). When dogs are given MHC-unmatched renal allografts, the grafts survive for about 10 days. Completely matched allografts in dogs survive for about 40 days. A more impressive result is obtained with canine liver grafts, which survive for about 8 days in unmatched animals and for 200–300 days in DLA-matched recipients (Kenmochi et al., 1994). The failure of MHC and blood group-compatible grafts to survive indefinitely is a result of the cumulative effects of many other minor antigenic differences. For example, skin grafts from male donors placed on histocompatible females are usually rejected, although the reverse is not the case. This is because male cells carry antigens encoded by genes on the Y chromosome, called H-Y antigens.

During the rejection process, the grafted tissue gradually becomes infiltrated with cytotoxic T cells, which first cause damage to the endothelial cells lining small blood vessels (Fig. 35.3). The T cells roll along the endothelial surface and bind using leukocyte function-associated antigen–1. T cell–mediated damage releases chemokines that attract more T cells into the graft. Cellular destruction, stoppage of blood flow, hemorrhage, and death of the grafted organ follow thrombosis of these vessels. The blood vessels of second organ grafts become blocked even more rapidly as a result of the action of antibodies and complement-triggering immunothrombosis on the vascular endothelium. This secondary reaction is specific for any graft from the original donor. It is not restricted to any particular site nor to any specific organ since MHC and blood group molecules are present on most nucleated cells (Krensky et al., 1990).

In practice, it is usually not difficult to ensure that the donor and recipient have identical major blood group antigens. MHC compatibility is much harder to achieve because extensive MHC polymorphism ensures that individuals differ widely in their MHC haplotypes. In general, the closer the donor and recipient are related, the less their MHC difference will be. For this reason, it is preferable that grafts be obtained from a recipient's parents or siblings. If this is not possible, a donor must be selected at random and the inevitable rejection responses suppressed by powerful drugs such as cyclosporine or tacrolimus (Chapter 42).

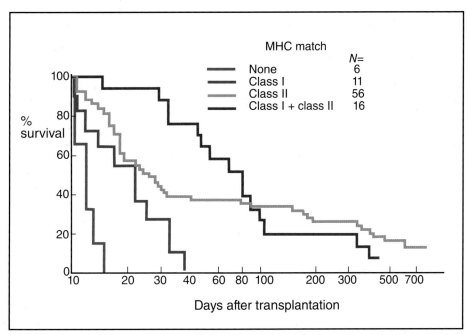

Fig. 35.2 Survival time of organ allografts between swine leukocyte antigen–incompatible minipigs clearly depends on the degree of major histocompatibility complex (MHC) compatibility between donor and host. From Pescovitz, M.D., Thistlethwaite, J.R., Jr, Auchincloss, H., Jr, Ildstad, S.T., Sharp, T.G., Terrill, R., Sachs, D.H., 1984. Effect of class II antigen matching on renal allograft survival in miniature swine. J. Exp. Med. 160, 1495–1508.

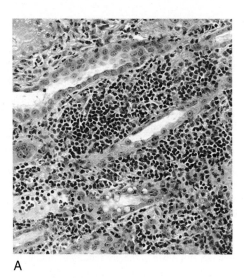
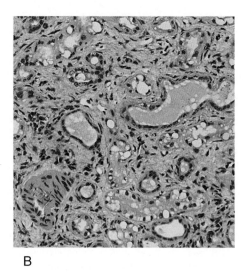

A   B

Fig. 35.3 (A) Section of a canine kidney that has been acutely rejected and as a consequence is densely infiltrated with lymphocytes. (B) Section of a kidney that has undergone chronic allograft rejection. In this case, the section shows interstitial fibrosis with tubular atrophy and a mild lymphocytic infiltration. Courtesy Dr. A.E. Kyles.

RENAL ALLOGRAFTS

Renal allograft rejection is of major clinical importance in humans and has been widely studied in animals. It therefore serves as a good example of the allograft response. In humans, for whom a great deal of experience with transplantation has been gained, four distinct clinical rejection syndromes are recognized. *Hyperacute rejection* occurs within 48 hours after grafting. Rejection occurring up to 7 days after grafting is called *accelerated rejection*. Rejection after 7 days is called *acute rejection*. *Chronic rejection* develops several months or years after grafting. It is unclear whether a similar classification is useful in animals.

When kidneys are allografted, the blood supply to the transplanted kidney is established at the time of transplantation. The graft and recipient leukocytes come into contact almost immediately. In an unsensitized host, a primary immune response is mounted, and renal allografts are only rejected after about 10 days and possibly much longer. In sensitized animals in which the immune system is already primed, hyperacute rejection occurs, and the graft can be destroyed within days or even hours without ever becoming functional. Acute rejection should be suspected when the recipient shows rapidly rising blood creatinine associated with an enlarged, painful kidney accompanied by signs of depression, anorexia, vomiting, proteinuria, hematuria, and ultrasonography showing an enlarged, hypoechoic kidney. In contrast, chronic rejection should be suspected if the creatinine and urea levels rise gradually, and this is associated with proteinuria, microscopic hematuria, and a small, hyperechoic kidney. This is also associated with a slow decline in renal function related to interstitial fibrosis and the proliferation of vascular endothelium. A renal biopsy is necessary to confirm rejection. Interestingly, a significant number of feline renal allograft recipients may also develop retroperitoneal fibrosis resulting in ureteral obstruction.

Pathogenesis of Allograft Rejection

The allograft rejection process is directed against the dominant antigens on the cells of the graft. The MHC molecules tend to trigger a T cell–mediated rejection response, whereas the blood group antigens tend to trigger antibody formation. The rejection process may be divided into two phases. First, the host's lymphocytes encounter the antigens of the graft and trigger a response. Second, cytotoxic T cells and antibodies from the host enter the graft and destroy graft cells (Fig. 35.4; Thomas et al., 2015).

Innate Mechanisms

Damage to the graft as a result of surgical trauma and ischemia followed by reperfusion upregulates MHC expression and generates cytokines and inflammatory mediators that attract neutrophils and macrophages into the graft. If large quantities of damage-associated molecular patterns, such as high mobility group box protein-1, are generated, they will activate toll-like receptors and other pattern-recognition receptors. An increase in expression of the stress protein MIC-A, on graft endothelial cells can activate natural killer cells (NK cells). Complement components such as C5a and C3a may also activate APCs within the graft.

Adaptive Mechanisms

Donor antigens are presented to the T cells of the recipient by APCs. The graft recipient may be sensitized by a direct pathway in which recipient T cells circulating through the graft encounter antigens presented by donor APCs. These donor APCs may also carry antigens to draining lymph nodes and the spleen. Alternatively, recipients may be sensitized when their own APCs enter the graft and encounter and process donor antigens (the indirect pathway). The direct pathway operates early in the rejection process but is replaced by the indirect pathway once the donor APCs have died. In humans, the direct pathway is responsible for the vigorous immune response that occurs in acute rejection, whereas the indirect pathway is more important in chronic rejection. Although macrophages and dendritic cells are important APCs, donor B cells and tubular epithelial and endothelial cells can also process antigen, and activate recipient T cells (Alegre et al., 2016).

In laboratory rodents, MHC class II molecules are expressed on professional APCs. In these species, the intensity of graft rejection is related to the number of donor B cells, macrophages, and dendritic cells transplanted within the graft. Removal of these cells by careful

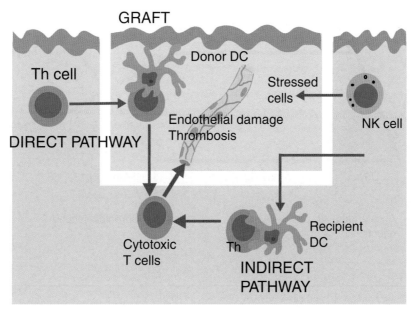

Fig. 35.4 Some of the mechanisms involved in the rejection of an allograft (see text for details). *NK cells*, Natural killer cells; *Th*, T helper.

flushing of the graft before surgery or by pretreatment of the donor with cytotoxic drugs greatly reduces the intensity of the rejection process. In other mammals in which MHC class II molecules are also expressed on vascular endothelial cells, these "passenger" cells are of less significance. Additionally, shed exosomes from the graft may enter the recipient and be captured by the host's APCs. These "cross-dressed" APCs may then be presented to recipient T cells.

The APCs that process donor MHC molecules migrate to the draining lymph node and activate T cells. The paracortical regions of lymph nodes draining a graft therefore contain many dividing lymphocytes. The number of these cells is greatest about 6 days after grafting and declines rapidly once the graft has been rejected. In addition to these signs of an active T-cell response, germinal center formation occurs in the cortex, and plasma cells accumulate in the medulla, indicating that antibody formation is also occurring. In a conventional immune response, only one cell in 10^5–10^6 T cells can respond to a specific antigen. In graft rejection, however, up to 10% of the T cells will respond since these cells have low activation thresholds for foreign MHC molecules.

The activated Th1 cells produce interleukin-2 (IL-2) and interferon-γ (IFN-γ), which turn on both NK cells and cytotoxic T cells. The NK cells produce more IFN-γ and tumor necrosis factor–α (TNF-α) that activates macrophages and additional NK cells. The cytotoxic T cells recognize the foreign peptides bound to recipient MHC class I molecules and kill any target cell they encounter. Donor MHC class II molecules trigger an immune response in two ways. First, because they are foreign proteins, they are processed as endogenous antigens. Second, they may directly bind to recipient T-cell receptors and trigger cytotoxicity. IL-2 and IFN-γ not only promote cytotoxic T-cell activity but also enhance the expression of MHC molecules on the cells of the graft. During allograft rejection, therefore, MHC expression is increased, and the graft becomes an even more attractive target for cytotoxic T cells.

Although cytotoxic T cells are of major importance in acute allograft rejection, antibodies, eosinophils, NK cells, and macrophages also play a significant role in hyperacute and chronic rejection (Fig. 35.5). Hyperacute rejection occurs when the recipient has preexisting antibodies to graft MHC or blood groups. These bind to graft vascular

endothelial cells, activate complement by the classical pathway, and so cause endothelial cell lysis. The damaged endothelial cells trigger platelet activation as well as generating multiple chemokines and cytokines. These also attract leukocytes, and the damage results in thrombosis and infarction. AntiMHC antibodies also play a major role in secondary rejection since they can activate the classical complement pathway and mediate antibody-dependent cytotoxic cell activity.

Graft Destruction

Once activated, cytotoxic T cells bind and destroy vascular endothelium and other accessible cells through caspase-mediated apoptosis. As a result, hemorrhage, platelet aggregation, thrombosis, and stoppage of blood flow occur. The grafted tissue dies because of the failure of its blood supply. CD4+ T cells that enter the graft may release cytotoxic cytokines such as TNF-α. This also triggers apoptosis in endothelial cells. Invading cytotoxic T cells can also cross the basement membrane and kill renal tubular cells. Activated macrophages releasing pro-inflammatory cytokines impair graft function and intensify T cell–mediated rejection (Kyles et al., 2002).

PREVENTION OF ALLOGRAFT REJECTION

In preventing allograft rejection, the transplantation surgeon seeks to induce the minimal level of immunosuppression to prevent rejection while not making the recipient more susceptible than necessary to infection. Dogs mount very strong allograft responses, and kidney allografts are rejected in 6–14 days in untreated animals. Unrelated dogs with renal allografts show about 50% 1-year survival when treated with azathioprine, prednisolone, and cyclosporine (Mathews et al., 2000). Survival is considerably enhanced by a simultaneous bone marrow allograft from the donor animal or by treatment with rabbit anti-dog thymocyte serum. In practice, median survival times of 8 months can be achieved, with some animals surviving for longer than 5 years. This, however, varies greatly between transplant centers and much depends on appropriate selection of recipients (Finco et al., 1985). Dogs have significant perioperative mortality. Thromboembolic complications are common, and many experience recurrent acute infections, especially

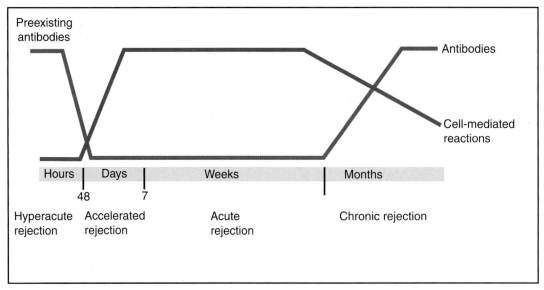

Fig. 35.5 Role of antibodies and cell-mediated immunity in different allograft rejection syndromes.

respiratory tract infections with *Bordetella bronchiseptica* as well as urinary tract infections. Newer immunosuppressive agents such as leflunomide show promise of improving the prognosis for canine renal allografting (see Chapter 42; Hopper et al., 2012).

Cats that receive renal allografts without immunosuppression die in 8–34 days. (Katayama and McAnulty, 2002). Immunosuppressive therapy in cats involves the use of prednisolone and cyclosporine possibly supplemented with ketoconazole. (The ketoconazole suppresses cyclosporine metabolism in the liver and so prolongs its half-life.) The therapy can begin 2 days before surgery so that cyclosporine levels are optimal when the graft is introduced. 6-month survival of treated cats ranges from 59% to 70%, whereas 3-year survival ranges from 40% to 50%. The longest survival time reported for cats receiving renal allografts is 8 years. These figures are gradually improving as experience grows (Gregory et al., 1992). Long-term complications include acute or chronic rejection and opportunistic infections (Infection is the second most important cause of death or euthanasia after acute rejection.) (Wormser et al., 2016). Acute rejection can occur at any time, especially if cyclosporine levels fall below the therapeutic range. Chronic allograft rejection (graft vascular disease) due to progressive arterial arteriosclerosis may cause ischemic graft destruction. It is not responsive to immunosuppressive therapy.

In some circumstances, such as when a dog has maintained functioning renal allografts for several years, immunosuppressive therapy may be reduced gradually and eventually discontinued as graft acceptance becomes complete. It is probable that the immunosuppressive drugs gradually eliminate antigen-sensitive cells. Once their numbers are sufficiently low, the large mass of grafted tissue may be sufficient to establish and maintain immune tolerance.

It is possible to induce long-term immune tolerance to canine kidney allografts by first administering donor hematopoietic cells to the recipient. These donor bone marrow cells can survive as a result of treatment with a combination of low-dose total-body irradiation and a short course of immunosuppression. As a result, the recipient becomes a hematopoietic chimera and thus effectively tolerant of donor cells. A kidney allograft from the same donor will survive indefinitely in these chimeras. Interestingly, this tolerance does not extend to skin allografts—they are rejected (Kuhr et al., 2007).

SKIN ALLOGRAFTS

Although the mechanisms of rejection are similar among different tissues, minor differences are observed in the process. For example, if a skin graft is placed on an animal, it takes several days for blood vessels and lymphatic connections to be established between the graft and the host. Only when these connections are made can host cells enter the graft and commence the rejection process. The first sign of rejection is a transient neutrophil accumulation around the blood vessels at the base of the graft. This is followed by infiltration with mononuclear cells that eventually extends throughout the grafted skin. The first signs of tissue damage are observed in the capillaries of the graft, whose endothelium is destroyed. As a result, the blood clots, blood flow stops, and tissue death follows. The presence of Langerhans cells in the epidermis significantly enhances the antigenicity of skin allografts. In a secondary reaction, host blood vessels usually do not have time to grow into a skin graft since a destructive mononuclear cell and neutrophil infiltration rapidly develop in the graft bed.

LIVER ALLOGRAFTS

It was originally reported that a high percentage of liver allografts between outbred pigs were accepted without immunosuppression. However, these pigs were not genetically defined, and the degree of MHC mismatching was unclear. When liver allografts are made between genetically defined miniature pigs with known MHC differences, it is found that their rejection rate is similar to that observed with kidney or skin allografts. Liver graft rejection in dogs tends to occur fairly slowly. This slow liver allograft rejection appears to be due to the production of indoleamine 2,3-dioxygenase (IDO) by hepatocytes. IDO destroys the amino acid tryptophan (see Chapter 21). Since tryptophan is essential for Th1 responses, its absence within the grafted liver is highly immunosuppressive (Munn et al., 1998).

CARDIAC ALLOGRAFTS

Acute rejection of canine heart allografts is associated with massive lymphocytic infiltration and myocyte damage leading to rapid graft destruction. If, however, the rejection process is slowed for some reason, the pathological process in the chronically rejected organ changes. In these cases, T cells and macrophages release a chemokine cascade that activates vascular smooth muscle and endothelial cells. The resulting smooth muscle cell growth and inflammation lead to obliteration of the blood vessel lumen and eventually cardiac failure. This graft arteriosclerosis (or graft vascular disease) results from the growth-stimulating effects of both T cell–derived cytokines and antibodies. A similar lesion is seen in renal allografts undergoing chronic rejection (Shumak et al., 1970).

CORNEAL ALLOGRAFTS

Certain areas of the body, such as the anterior chamber of the eye, the cornea, the thymus, the testes, and the brain, are immune-privileged sites. As a result, grafts made into these sites may not be rejected. In humans, for example, 90% of first-time corneal allografts survive without tissue typing or immunosuppressive drugs. These sites are privileged because the body rigorously controls inflammation in these critical tissues. Several mechanisms are involved in this. They have an impermeable blood-tissue barrier, lack dendritic cells, contain suppressor cells, express low levels of MHC class I and II molecules, and may contain high levels of immunosuppressive molecules such as IDO, transforming growth factor-β, neuropeptides, and complement inhibitors. Molecules found in normal aqueous humor can block NK cell lysis, inhibit neutrophil activation by CD95L, suppress nitric oxide production by activated macrophages, and interfere with alternative complement activation. The eyes and testes are also unique in that they express very high levels of CD95L (Fas ligand). As a result, any CD95+ T cells that enter these organs may bind to CD95L and be killed by apoptosis. The testes and epididymis contain a population of Treg cells that also maintain local tolerance to sperm antigens. In their absence autoimmune orchitis develops.

BONE ALLOGRAFTS

Bone cortical allografts are used to repair severe diaphyseal fractures as well as to reconstruct defects created by the resection of tumors. Immunological rejection of bone allografts is rarely a problem, probably because of the absence of soft tissues in the graft. Unfortunately, long-term bone allografts have a high incidence of mechanical failure because the graft is resorbed before it is replaced. Joints may be successfully transplanted in horses provided that such joints have been previously frozen.

BONE MARROW ALLOGRAFTS

High-dose, total-body irradiation may be administered to dogs to completely destroy tumors such as leukemias. Unfortunately, such treatment also destroys bone marrow stem cells, and these must be replaced by a bone marrow allograft (Harris et al., 1986). The new hematopoietic stem cells restore bone marrow function (Fig. 35.6). The recipient dog must first be conditioned by total-body irradiation or chemotherapy with cyclophosphamide. This creates space for the growing transplanted cells, reduces the intensity of the rejection process, and, in leukemic animals, destroys all tumor cells. Marrow is aspirated from the long bones of the donor and administered intravenously to the recipient. Hematopoietic stem cells migrate from the blood to colonize the bone marrow. An optimal dose is about 2×10^8 allogeneic bone marrow cells per kilogram of body weight for matched recipients. The success of this procedure is relatively low, ranging from 20% in untreated mismatched canine marrow allografts to 90% using treated matched allografts. In successfully engrafted dogs, it takes about 30 days for the granulocytes to return to normal, but the lymphocytes take

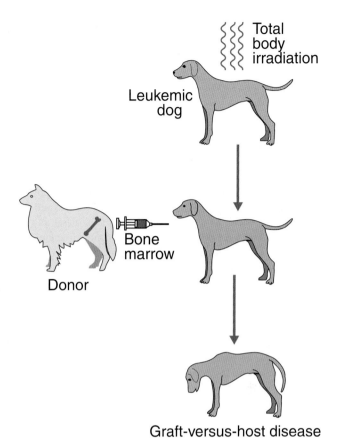

Fig. 35.6 Induction of graft-versus-host disease in dogs that have received a bone marrow allograft.

about 200 days to recover. Marrow survival is not generally enhanced by treatment with single immunosuppressive agents, but combinations such as mycophenolate mofetil plus cyclosporine or methotrexate plus cyclosporine can result in the development of stable canine bone marrow chimeras. As pointed out above, these chimeras will accept renal allografts from the donor animal.

Graft-Versus-Host Disease

If healthy lymphocytes are injected into the skin of an allogeneic recipient, they will attack the host cells and cause local inflammation. Provided the recipient has a functioning immune system, this graft-versus-host (GVH) reaction is not serious because the recipient can destroy the foreign lymphocytes and thus terminate the reaction. If, however, the recipient cannot reject the grafted lymphocytes because it has been immunosuppressed or is otherwise immunodeficient, the grafted cells may cause uncontrolled destruction of the host's tissues and, eventually, death. Thus GVH disease occurs in bone marrow allograft recipients who have been effectively immunosuppressed by total-body irradiation or cyclophosphamide treatment.

The lesions generated in GVH disease depend on the MHC differences between donor and recipient. When they differ only in the MHC class I molecules, the disease is mainly caused by cytotoxic T cells attacking the nucleated cells of the host. This leads to a wasting syndrome characterized by bone marrow destruction leading to pancytopenia, aplastic anemia, loss of recipient T and B cells, and hypogammaglobulinemia. Th17 and NK cells also participate in this process, while Tregs are lost. Lymphocytes infiltrate the intestine, skin, and liver and secrete TNF-α, IL-1, and IL-6, causing inflammation, mucosal destruction and diarrhea, skin and mouth ulcers, liver destruction, and jaundice.

If donor and recipient differ in their MHC II, both graft and host CD4$^+$ T helper cells may be stimulated. In these cases, the production of Th2-derived cytokines may lead to immunostimulation, autoantibody formation, and even a syndrome resembling systemic lupus erythematosus and polyarthritis (see Chapter 39). This is called autoimmune GVH disease.

In practice, pure class I or class II disparities rarely occur naturally. Thus, in dogs, GVH disease can either be an acute disease, causing death within 4 weeks of transplantation or prolonged and chronic. The major target organs are the skin, liver, gastrointestinal tract, and lymphoid system. The first clinical signs are exudative ear lesions, scleral injection, hyperkeratosis, alopecia, skin atrophy, and generalized erythema seen by 10 days (Fig. 35.7). Jaundice and diarrhea frequently occur, as does inflammation of the nasal and oral mucous membranes. An antiglobulin-positive hemolytic anemia may also develop. The immunosuppressive drug methotrexate, together with monoclonal antilymphocyte antibodies, may be used to suppress GVH disease.

The intestinal microbiota also influence the severity of GVH disease—at least in mice. Thus, bone marrow recipient mice that developed GVHD had a dramatic loss of bacterial diversity and a different composition compared to control mice. The changes were associated with an increase in Lactobacilli and a decrease in Clostridia. It may be that the reduction in disease severity is a result of the Lactobacilli preventing an increase in Enterococci. Similar changes in the gut commensal microflora occur in humans receiving bone marrow allografts (Lei et al., 2016).

It is of interest to note that bone marrow transplantation in cats that previously received immunosuppressive irradiation or cyclosporine is a very successful procedure and that GVH disease is not a major problem in this species.

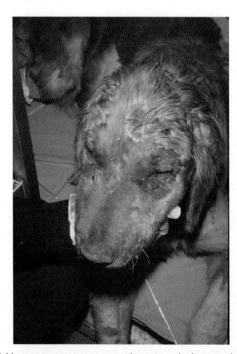

Fig. 35.7 Very severe cutaneous erythematous lesions on the face of a dog suffering from graft-versus-host disease as a result of a bone marrow allograft. From Harris, C.K., Beck, E.R., Gasper, P.W., 1986. Bone marrow transplantation in the dog. Compend. Contin. Educ. Pract. Vet. 8, 337–344.

XENOGRAFTS

Although humans currently receive organs from dead human donors, the demand for organ grafts greatly exceeds the supply. It is possible that xenografting from nonhuman species would eliminate this shortage. Unfortunately, xenografts are usually rejected within a few hours. The pathology of hyperacute xenograft rejection includes extensive hemorrhage and thrombosis brought about by massive destruction of vascular endothelial cells. This allows blood cells to escape while exposing the underlying basement membrane to platelets.

Concordant xenografts are those between two closely related species, such as a chimpanzee and a human. In these cases, rejection is largely mediated by cellular responses. In discordant xenografts (those between unrelated mammals, such as from a pig to a human), rejection is mediated largely by humoral mechanisms. In practice, concordant human xenografting from other primates, such as chimpanzees or baboons, is impractical because of the difficulty in providing large numbers of donor animals.

Pigs, however, may be more practical sources of organs. They breed rapidly, they can be genetically manipulated, and their organs are of an appropriate size (Pabst, 2020). Unfortunately, pig organs trigger a severe discordant xenograft rejection response mediated by natural anticarbohydrate antibodies. Humans and Old-World monkeys lack the enzyme α1,3-galactosyltransferase and therefore do not make carbohydrates or glycoproteins with the α1,3-galactosyl linkage (Gal α1–3 Gal). Because humans are exposed to this structure on many bacteria, we make high levels of antibodies to the Gal α1–3 Gal epitope. Indeed, more than 2% of total human IgM and IgG consists of antibodies to this epitope. The αGal epitope, on the other hand, is found in pig glycoproteins. If a pig organ is grafted into a human, these antibodies bind the graft cells, activate the classical complement pathway, and lyse them.

It is possible to clone pigs that lack α-1,3-galactosyl-transferase. This is the enzyme that generates Gal epitopes. (The genes were knocked out in cultured pig fibroblasts. The fibroblast nuclei were then transferred to pig ova, and the ova were inserted within sow's uteruses.) Gal epitopes were completely eliminated from their cell membranes (Bao et al., 2014). These pigs have been used as temporary human kidney donors in a small number of cases with encouraging results (Pierson, 2022).

A second mechanism that contributes to hyperacute rejection is activation of the alternate complement pathway as a result of the failure of human complement factor H to prevent assembly of the alternate C3 convertase on the surface of pig cells. A third mechanism results from the species-specific activity of complement control proteins. Thus, the natural inhibitors of pig complement, such as CD46, CD55, and CD59 cannot control the activation of human complement.

Transgenic pigs have been produced that express human complement inhibitors on their cells and do not trigger hyperacute rejection on grafting. Should, however, the xenograft survive attack by these natural antibodies and complement, it is still susceptible to delayed attack from induced antibodies and from cell-mediated cytotoxicity mediated through NK cells and monocytes. Many barriers are yet to be overcome if pig organs are ever to be routinely used as human organ transplants.

One other point relevant to xenografting is that donor animals may carry viruses that could cause disease in a severely immunosuppressed recipient or, even worse; recombine with human viruses to create new and potentially hazardous pathogens (Brown et al., 1998). These xenograft-derived infections (xenozoonoses) are of special concern if primates are used as organ donors. Primates are known to carry viruses such as simian immunodeficiency virus and herpesvirus B that can infect humans. Pigs possess an endogenous retrovirus that has the ability to infect some human cell lines in tissue culture, although it is not known to cause human disease (Fishman, 2022). However, it has proved possible using CRISPR technology to inactivate the retrovirus polymerase gene and so produce piglets that lack activated retroviruses (Denner, 2017).

ALLOGRAFTS AND PREGNANCY

Sperm

Allogeneic sperm can successfully and repeatedly penetrate the female reproductive tract without provoking graft rejection. One reason for this is that seminal plasma is immunosuppressive (Lenicov et al., 2012). Sperm exposed to this fluid are nonimmunogenic, even after washing. Prostatic fluid, one of the immunosuppressive components of seminal plasma, also inhibits complement-mediated hemolysis. Seminal plasma promotes the expansion of Treg cells that subsequently migrate to the endometrium and promote tolerance to paternal alloantigens. Not only does seminal plasma cause the recruitment of monocytes to the vaginal wall, but it also modulates the development of monocyte-derived dendritic cells and directs them to differentiate into a regulatory subset. These regulatory cells may promote fertility by inducing tolerance to paternal alloantigens, but they may also increase susceptibility to infectious agents. Nevertheless, occasional cases of infertility resulting from the production of antisperm antibodies in the uterus and vagina do occur.

Pregnancy

When mammals became viviparous about 200 million years ago, and the fetus developed inside its mother's uterus, a significant immunological problem had to be overcome. The fetus could not be rejected like an allograft even, though it possessed paternal MHC molecules. In a normal pregnancy, the fetus establishes and maintains itself despite MHC incompatibility. Yet, the uterus is not a privileged site since grafts from other tissues, such as skin, implanted in the uterine wall are readily rejected. Likewise, a mother may make antibodies against fetal blood group antigens, and these can destroy fetal red blood cells either in utero, as in primates, or following ingestion of colostrum, as occurs in other mammals (see Chapter 24). Nevertheless, fetal allograft rejection does not occur (Ander et al., 2019). Thus pregnancy can be considered a state of acquired immunological tolerance of the mother to her fetus (Durgam et al., 2022).

The survival of the fetus and its trophoblast is contrived by the combined activities of many different immunoregulatory mechanisms acting at the maternal-fetal interface (Fig. 35.8).

The initial steps in pregnancy include implantation of the fertilized ovum in the uterine wall and its acceptance by the mother's immune system. This implantation is regulated by communication between the conceptus and the uterus. This involves hormones such as progesterone and interferons, especially IFN-τ and IFN-γ (see Chapter 28). No polymorphic MHC molecules are expressed on preimplantation embryos or oocytes. Likewise, polymorphic MHC class Ia or class II molecules are not expressed on the cell layer of the trophoblast in contact with

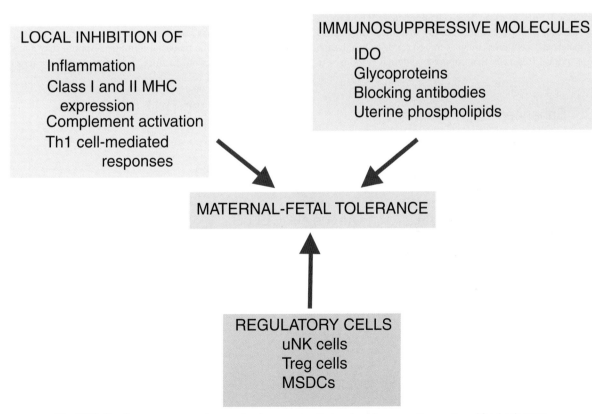

Fig. 35.8 The immunosuppressive mechanisms and cells involved in generating maternal-fetal tolerance. These include localized immunosuppressive functions. The presence of regulatory cells, most notably uterine natural killer cells (uNK cells) and regulatory T cells (Treg cells), as well as locally immunosuppressive molecules such as indolamine 2,3-dioxygenase (IDO). *MDSC,* Myeloid-derived suppressor cells; *MHC,* major histocompatibility complex; *Th1 cell,* type 1 T helper.

maternal tissues. Cytokines that usually enhance MHC expression, such as IFN-γ, have no effect on trophoblast cells. The absence of classical MHC molecules should make trophoblast cells susceptible to attack by NK cells. This is prevented, however, by their expression of the nonpolymorphic MHC class Ib molecules HLA-C, HLA-G, and HLA-E. These molecules inhibit NK cell cytotoxicity, while the NK cells control invasion of the uterine wall by the trophoblast. Thus there is a balance between MHC class Ib expression on the trophoblast and NK cells in the uterine wall that together regulates trophoblast growth and invasion. Bovine classical MHC class I molecules are not expressed on the trophoblast before day 120 gestation. Equine trophoblast cells also appear to have reduced class I expression (Matson and Caron, 2014).

NK cells predominate in the placenta, especially early in pregnancy (Stas et al., 2020). Over time, their numbers gradually decline and are replaced by T cells that predominate at term. These NK cells belong to a distinct uterine subtype called uNK cells. uNK cells, also called endometrial gland cells, have been described in rodents, dogs, pigs, and horses. They are not usually cytotoxic. These NK cells also promote immune tolerance by suppressing Th17 cells (Fig. 35.9).

In the hemochorial placenta found in humans and other primates, uNK cells release angiogenic factors that remodel the spiral arteries located within the uterus to increase their diameter and thus increase placental blood flow as the fetus grows. If they fail to do this, the blood flow to the fetus may be insufficient and can result in preeclampsia or miscarriage (Valencia-Ortega et al., 2020; Wallace et al., 2015).

Treg cells also play an important role in preventing fetal rejection. Estrogen treatment and pregnancy both induce FoxP3 expression, as does seminal plasma, and so promote Treg functions. Trophoblast cells also secrete IDO, which blocks Th1 and Th17 responses and promotes apoptosis of cytotoxic T cells. Inhibitors of IDO permit maternal rejection of allogeneic fetuses in mice. Treg cells upregulate IDO expression in dendritic cells (Durr and Kindler, 2013). In humans, substantial numbers of maternal T cells cross the placenta to reside in fetal lymph nodes. These induce Treg cells that suppress maternal responses to

paternal antigens probably through IL-10 production, while at the same time suppressing production of Th1, Th2, and Th17 cells. Treg cells also release the antiinflammatory nucleotidases CD73 and CD39. These hydrolyze ATP and ADP to adenosine, a potent antiinflammatory agent.

Galectins regulate immune responses by binding to cell surface carbohydrates (glycans). One subfamily of these galectins is specifically expressed in the placenta of primates, especially in the syncytiotrophoblast, the placental layer that contacts the fetal cells. These galectins induce apoptosis in T cells. Thus, they serve as local immunosuppressive agents (Clark, 2014). The trophoblast cells of the human fetal placenta also induce M2 macrophages that produce IL-10 (Than et al., 2009).

Although these mechanisms minimize maternal sensitization by allogeneic fetal cells, cytotoxic T cells or antibodies do develop during pregnancy. For example, in pregnant mares, placental cells invade the uterine wall to form structures called endometrial cups under the influence of IL-22 (Brosnahan et al., 2012). These in turn stimulate a strong immune response against paternal MHC antigens around day 60 of gestation. As a result, the cups are surrounded by large numbers of CD4+ and CD8+ T cells, macrophages, and plasma cells. This eventually leads to degeneration of the endometrial cups around 120 days of pregnancy. Despite these responses, the pregnancy is unaffected. It is possible that these are Th2 and Treg responses dominated by IL-10 production that do not threaten the pregnancy rather than Th1 and Th17 responses that may lead to fetal rejection (Lunn et al., 1997).

Up to 90% of pregnant mares make antibodies to foal MHC class I molecules. Similar antibodies develop in multiparous sheep and cattle. In some mouse strains, up to 95% of pregnant animals make antibodies against fetal MHC molecules. Up to 40% of women make antibodies to fetal MHC molecules after giving birth. The presence of these antibodies has no adverse effect on the course of the pregnancy. On the contrary, the maternal immune response may actually stimulate placental function. In mice, hybrid placentas are larger than the

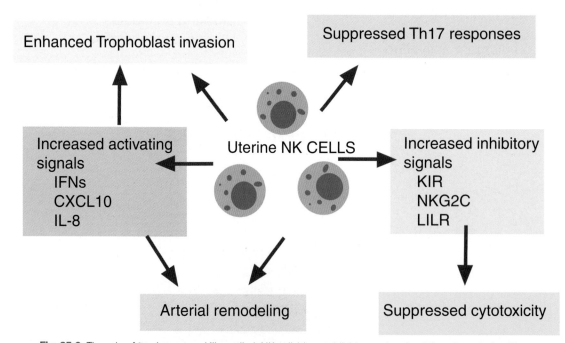

Fig. 35.9 The role of uterine nature killer cells (uNK cells) is establishing and maintaining placentation. Thus, while they are less cytotoxic than their circulating populations, they can contribute both to trophoblast invasion as well as spiral artery remodeling. *CXCL10*, Chemokine interferon-γ inducible protein 10 kDa; *IFNs*, interferons; *IL-8*, interleukin-8; *KIR*, killer-cell immunoglobulin–like receptor; *LILR*, leukocyte immunoglobulin–like receptors; *Th17*, T helper 17 cells.

placentas of inbred animals, and females tolerant to paternal antigens have smaller placentas than intolerant females. Other studies show that mothers sensitized to paternal MHC molecules have better fetal survival. This may be due to the stimulatory effect of IL-3 and granulocyte-macrophage colony-stimulating factor from maternal T cells on trophoblast growth.

Some antibodies made by the mother against fetal antigens may coat placental cells, preventing their destruction by maternal T cells. These blocking antibodies can be eluted from the placenta and shown to suppress other cell-mediated immune reactions against paternal antigens, such as graft rejection. Absence of these blocking antibodies accounts for some cases of recurrent abortion in women. Nevertheless, it can also be shown that totally immunodeficient mice can have successful pregnancies.

The fetus does not depend entirely on maternal mechanisms for its protection. The placenta is a source of many immunosuppressive factors, including estradiol and progesterone, and possibly also chorionic gonadotropin. In addition, some pregnancy-associated glycoproteins, including α_2-macroglobulin, and α-fetoprotein, the major protein in fetal serum, have immunosuppressive properties. Amniotic fluid is rich in immunosuppressive phospholipids.

In mammals, unique interferons (IFN-ω in humans, horses, and dogs; IFN-τ in ruminants; and IFN-γ and IFN-δ in pigs) from the embryonic trophoblast act as signaling proteins between the embryo and mother during early development. These interferons may also inhibit lymphocyte activities.

Despite the previous discussion, if the antigenic differences between the mother and her fetus are very great, then pregnancy may not go to completion. Studies on xenogeneic hybridization of two different mouse species show that the embryos develop until mid-gestation and are then attacked and destroyed by maternal lymphocytes. Similarly, donkey embryos transferred to horse mares may be destroyed by large numbers of maternal lymphocytes.

Mild immunosuppression is a consistent feature of late pregnancy and the early postpartum period. Pregnant animals may have minor deficiencies in cell-mediated immune reactivity to nonfetal antigens. Dairy cows experience a periparturient depression in neutrophil function and reduced T-cell cytotoxicity and cytokine production (Aleri et al., 2016). This suppression appears to be due to multiple causes, including the stress of parturition, the production of glucocorticoids, the loss of immunoglobulins into colostrum, and a negative energy balance. In mares, blood lymphocyte responses to mitogens drop from 4 weeks before to 5 weeks after parturition. NK cell activity in pigs drops at the end of gestation to reach a low point 2–3 weeks after parturition. Ewes in late pregnancy may show a reduction of some immunoglobulin classes, such as IgG1. This may be due to alterations in helper T-cell function or, more plausibly, to diversion of the IgG1 into the mammary gland to produce colostrum. This suppression may be significant in parasitized animals, in which the immune response barely controls the parasite. Similarly, immunosuppression may permit *Demodex* mite populations to rise in pregnant or lactating bitches and aid in the transmission of mites to their puppies.

Parturition can be considered to be mediated in part by a sterile inflammatory response following invasion of the uterus by large numbers of leukocytes, especially macrophages, neutrophils, and T cells, late in pregnancy. These cells release a mixture of cytokines, proteases (especially collagenases), prostanoids, and chemokines. The cytokines stimulate uterine stromal cells to amplify the process; and the collagenases remodel collagen, weakening fetal membranes, softening the cervix, and increasing the contractility of the myometrium. All this leads to fetal expulsion. After delivery, the uterus involutes as most of the leukocytes leave or are destroyed.

It is of interest to note that in cattle, there is a clear association between retention of the placenta and its MHC class I haplotype. MHC class I compatibility between a mother and her calf increases the risk of a retained placenta, whereas MHC class II compatibility has no effect. It has been suggested that the expulsion of the placenta after birth may be due, at least in part, to an allograft response (Joosten et al., 1991).

REFERENCES

Alegre, M.L., Lakkis, F.G., Morelli, A.E., 2016. Antigen presentation in transplantation. Trends Immunol. 37, 831–843.

Aleri, J.W., Hine, B.C., Pyman, M.F., Mansell, P.D., et al., 2016. Periparturient immunosuppression and strategies to improve dairy cow health during the periparturient period. Res. Vet. Sci. 108, 8–17.

Ander, S.E., Diamond, M.S., Coyne, C.B., 2019. Immune responses at the maternal-fetal interface. Sci. Immunol. 4, eaat6114.

Bao, L., Chen, H.D., Jong, U.M., Rim, C.H., et al., 2014. Generation of GGTA1 biallelic knockout pigs via zinc-finger nucleases and somatic cell nuclear transfer. Sci. China Life Sci. 57, 263–268.

Brosnahan, M.M., Miller, D.C., Adams, M., Antczak, D.F., 2012. IL-22 is expressed by the invasive trophoblast of the equine (*Equus caballus*) chorionic girdle. J. Immunol. 188, 4181–4187.

Brown, J., Matthews, A.L., Sandstrom, P.A., Chapman, L.E., 1998. Xenotransplantation and the risk of retroviral zoonosis. Trends Microbiol. 6, 411–415.

Clark, G.F., 2014. The role of glycans in immune evasion: the human fetoembryonic defense system hypothesis revisited. Mol. Hum. Reprod. 20, 185–199.

Denner, J., 2017. Paving the path toward porcine organs for transplantation. N. Engl. J. Med. 377 (19), 1891–1893.

Durgam, S.S., Alegre, M.-L., Chong, A.S., 2022. Toward an understandingof allogeneic conflict in pregnancy and transplantation. J. Exp. Med. 219 (5), e20211493.

Durr, S., Kindler, V., 2013. Implication of indolamine 2,3 dioxygenase in the tolerance towards fetuses, tumors, and allografts. J. Leuko. Biol. 93, 681–687.

Finco, D.R., Rawlings, C.A., Barsanti, J.A., Crowell, W.A., 1985. Kidney graft survival in transfused and non-transfused Beagle dogs. Am. J. Vet. Res. 46, 2327–2331.

Fishman, J.A., 2022. Risks of infectious disease in xenotransplantation. New Engl. J. Med. 387, 2258–2267.

Gregory, C.R., Gourley, I.M., Kochin, E.J., Broaddus, T.W., 1992. Renal transplantation for treatment of end-stage renal failure in cats. J. Am. Vet. Med. Assoc. 201, 285–291.

Harris, C.K., Beck, E.R., Gasper, P.W., 1986. Bone marrow transplantation in the dog. Compend. Contin. Educ. Pract. Vet. 8, 337–345.

Hopper, K., Mehl, M.L., Kass, P.H., Kyles, A., Gregory, C.R., 2012. Outcome after renal transplantation in 26 dogs. Vet. Surg. 41, 316–327.

Joosten, I., Sanders, M.F., Hensen, E.J., 1991. Involvement of major histocompatibility complex class I compatibility between dam and calf in the aetiology of bovine retained placenta. Anim. Gen. 22, 455–463.

Katayama, M., McAnulty, J.F., 2002. Renal transplantation in cats: techniques, complications, and immunosuppression. Compend. Contin. Educ. Pract. Vet. 24, 874–882.

Kenmochi, T., Mullen, Y., Miyamoto, M., Stein, E., 1994. Swine as an allotransplantation model. Vet. Immunol. Immunopathol. 43, 177–183.

Krensky, A.M., Weiss, A., Crabtree, G., et al., 1990. T-lymphocyte-antigen interactions in transplant rejection. N. Engl. J. Med. 312, 510–517.

Kuhr, C.S., Yunusov, M., Sale, G., Loretz, C., Storb, R., 2007. Long-term tolerance to kidney allografts in a preclinical canine model. Transplantation 84 (4), 545–547.

Kyles, A.E., Gregory, C.R., Griffey, S.M., et al., 2002. Evaluation of the clinical and histologic features of renal allograft rejection in cats. Vet. Surg. 31, 49–56.

Lenicov, F.R., Rodrigues, C.R., Sabatte, J., Cabrini, M., et al., 2012. Semen promotes the differentiation of tolerogenic dendritic cells. J. Immunol. 189, 4777–4786.

Lei, Y.M., Chen, L., Wang, Y., Stefka, A.T., et al., 2016. The composition of the microbiota modulates allograft rejection. J. Clin. Invest. 126, 2736–2744.

Lunn, P., Vagnoni, K.E., Ginther, O.J., 1997. The equine immune response to endometrial cups. J. Reprod. Immunol. 34, 203–216.

Matson, B.C., Caron, K.M., 2014. Uterine natural killer cells as modulators of the maternal-fetal vasculature. Int. J. Dev. Biol. 58, 199–204.

Mathews, K.A., Holmberg, D.L., Miller, C.W., 2000. Kidney transplantation in dogs with naturally occurring end-stage renal disease. J. Am. Anim. Hosp. Assoc. 36, 294–301.

Munn, D.H., Zhou, M., Attwood, J.T., et al., 1998. Prevention of allogeneic fetal rejection by tryptophan catabolism. Science 281, 1191–1193.

Nankivell, B.J., Alexander, S.I., 2010. Rejection of the kidney allograft. N. Engl. J. Med. 363, 1451–1462.

Pabst, R., 2020. The pig as a model for immunology research. Cell Tissue Res. 380, 287–304.

Pierson, R.N., 2022. Progress toward pig-to-human xenotransplantation. New Engl. J. Med. 386 (20), 1871–1873.

Shumak, K.H., Goldman, B.S., Silver, M.D., Bigelow, W.G., Crookston, J.H., 1970. Pathogenesis of rejection of canine cardiac allografts. Circulation 41, 98–103.

Stas, M.R., Koch, M., Stadler, M., Sawyer, S., et al., 2020. NK and T cell differentiation at the maternal-fetal interface in sows during late gestation. Front. Immunol. 11 https://doi.org/10.3389/fimmu.2020.582065.

Than, N.G., Romero, R., Goodman, M., et al., 2009. A primate subfamily of galectins expressed at the maternal-fetal interface that promote immune cell death. Proc. Natl. Acad. Sci. U. S. A. 106, 9731–9736.

Thomas, K.A., Valenzuela, N.M., Reed, E.F., 2015. The perfect storm: HLA antibodies, complement, FcγRs, and endothelium in transplant rejection. Trends Mol. Med. 21, 319–329.

Valencia-Ortega, J., Saucedo, R., Pena-Cano, M.I., Hernandez-Valencia, M., Cruz-Duran, G., 2020. Immune tolerance at the maternal-placental interface in healthy pregnancy and pre-eclampsia. J. Obstet. Gynaecol. Res. 46, 1067–1076.

Wallace, A.E., Whitley, G.S., Thilaganathan, B., Cartwright, J.E., 2015. Decidual natural killer cell receptor expression is altered in pregnancies with impaired vascular remodeling and a higher risk of pre-eclampsia. J. Leukoc. Biol. 97, 79–86.

Wormser, C., Mariano, A., Holmes, E.S., Aronson, L.R., Volk, S.W., 2016. Post-transplant malignant neoplasia associated with cyclosporine-based immunotherapy: prevalence, risk factors and survival in feline renal transplant recipients. Vet. Comp. Oncol. 14 (4), e126–e234.

36

Tumor Immunology and Immunotherapy

CHAPTER OUTLINE

Normal cellular functions depend on the regulation of cell division. When cells multiply, it is essential that they do so only as and when required. Unfortunately, as a result of mutations triggered by chemicals, radiation, or viruses, cells may break free of these constraints. A cell that is proliferating in an uncontrolled fashion will give rise to a growing clone of cells that eventually develops into a tumor. If these cells remain clustered together at a single site, the tumor is said to be benign. Benign tumors can usually be removed by surgery. In some cases, however, tumor cells break off from the main tumor mass and are carried by the blood or lymph to distant sites where they lodge and continue to grow. This form of tumor is said to be malignant. The secondary tumors that arise in these distant sites are called metastases. Surgical treatment of malignant tumors may be very difficult because it may be impossible to remove all metastases. Malignant tumors are classified according to their tissue of origin. Tumors arising from epithelial cells are called carcinomas; those arising from mesenchymal cells, such as muscle, lymphoid, or connective tissue cells, are called sarcomas. A leukemia is a tumor derived from hematopoietic stem cells.

The essential difference between a normal cell and a cancer cell is a loss of control of cell growth as a result of multiple mutations. These mutations may also result in cancer cells expressing abnormal proteins. These abnormal proteins may be recognized by T cells and trigger a cytotoxic T-cell response.

TUMORS AS ALLOGRAFTS?

When organ transplantation became a common procedure as a result of the development of potent immunosuppressive drugs, it was found that patients with prolonged graft survival were also more likely to develop certain cancers than nonimmunosuppressed individuals. It was, therefore, suggested that the immune system was responsible for the prevention of cancer. For example, tumors developed in 22% of cats received cyclosporine to prevent renal allograft rejection, and about half of these were B cell lymphomas. Immunosuppressed cats were six times more likely to develop cancer than normal cats (Wormser et al., 2016) . From this suggestion, the concept of immune surveillance emerged. This theory proposes that cell mutation is a common event. When mutation occurs, the protein coded by the mutated gene is altered. This alteration may make the protein antigenic. The recognition of these new antigens by cytotoxic T cells results in the elimination of any abnormal cells. Theory suggests that cancer would only result if cancer cells somehow evaded destruction by T cells.

This immune surveillance theory is only part of the story. Common human cancers, such as those of the lung or breast, do not develop more frequently in immunodeficient individuals. Likewise, nude (nu/nu) mice, although T cell-deficient, are no more susceptible than normal mice to chemically induced or spontaneous tumors (see Chapter 40). Many tumor antigens induce tolerance in a manner similar to that of

BOX 36.1 The Role of the Microbiota in Cancer Surveillance

When cancer patients are treated with modern immunotherapy, some respond much more effectively than others. One reason for these differences is attributed to their microbiota. Anticancer immune T cells are shaped by the microbiota. This may be due to cross-reactivity between microbial and tumor antigens, or microbial products stimulating PRRs that then influence the type and intensity of immune responses. Thus, the effectiveness of anti-CTLA-4 therapy in mice depends upon the presence of *Bacteroides fragilis* in their intestine. Anti-PD-1 therapy was more effective in the presence of Bifidobacterium. Some investigators have developed a "cancer hygiene hypothesis" suggesting that recent increases in the prevalence of some cancers may be due to dysbiosis or under-exposure to certain bacterial species.

From Zitvogel, L., Ayyoub, M., Routy, B., Kroemer, G., 2016. Microbiome and anticancer immunosurveillance. Cell 165, 276–287.

normal self-antigens. Thus, it is clear that the immune system does not distinguish between all cancer cells and normal, healthy cells (Box 36.1).

Notwithstanding this, there are situations in which the immune system can recognize and kill cancer cells (Zamora et al., 2018). For example, some immunodeficient mouse strains, which are "cleaner" subjects than nude mice, show an increased prevalence of spontaneous cancer. (Nude mice have some persistent T and B-cell function and intact innate defenses.) These include recombinase-activating gene (*RAG*) knockout mice that cannot produce functional T or B cells and *STAT-1* knockout mice that are unresponsive to interferon-γ (IFN-γ). *RAG* knockout mice suffer from an increased prevalence of spontaneous tumors of the intestinal epithelium, whereas *RAG/STAT-1* knockout mice develop mammary cancers.

Most humans who develop "spontaneous" cancer have a normal immune system. Immunosuppressed individuals, such as allograft recipients and AIDS victims, develop a different spectrum of cancers from that of the general population. The only cancers for which they are at greater risk are lymphoid tumors and those caused by viruses, such as Kaposi's sarcoma. Immunosuppressed humans are no more likely than the general population to develop common cancers, such as those of breast, lung, or colon. The situation is the same in animals. For example, in a study of 111 cats that received kidney allografts, 25 of these developed cancer. The most common tumor was a lymphoma that developed in 14 cats. All the lymphomas were mid- to high-grade large B-cell lymphomas. This is also the most common type of tumor in human transplant recipients (Wormser et al., 2016).

Tumor Neoantigens

Cancer cells develop as a result of multiple mutations. These mutations may generate molecules that are unique to the cancer cells (tumor-specific antigens) or, more commonly, abnormal or unusual molecules (tumor-associated antigens). To distinguish between normal and cancer cells, host T cells must recognize these new antigens. Five major types of tumor antigen have been identified. First, there are differentiation antigens associated with specific stages in the development of a cell type. For example, some cancer cells express the products of developmental genes that are turned off in adult cells and are only expressed early in an individual's development. These proteins are called oncofetal antigens. Examples include tumors of the gastrointestinal tract that produce a glycoprotein called carcinoembryonic antigen (CEA; also called CD66e), normally found only in the fetal intestine. The presence of CEA in serum may indicate the presence of a colon or rectal adenocarcinoma. α-Fetoprotein produced by hepatoma cells is normally expressed only in the fetal liver. Likewise, squamous cell carcinoma cells may possess antigens normally restricted to fetal liver and skin. These oncofetal antigens are usually poor immunogens and do not provoke protective immunity. However, their detection may be useful for diagnosis and for monitoring the progress of a tumor.

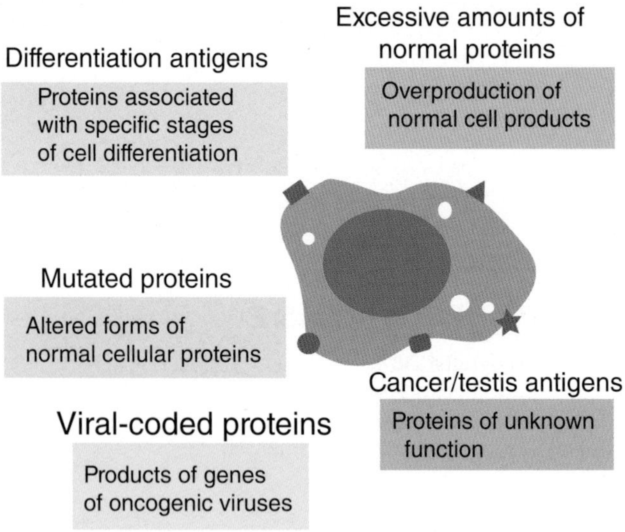

Fig. 36.1 Some of the great variety of new antigens that may appear on the surface of tumor cells and provoke an immune response.

Second, there are mutated forms of normal cellular proteins. For example, melanoma cells may express the products of mutated oncogenes on their surface (Fig. 36.1). Some tumor antigens are recognized because they are abnormally glycosylated. Chemically induced tumors may express surface antigens unique to the tumor and not to the inducing chemical. Because carcinogenic chemicals can produce many different mutations, tumors induced by a single chemical in different animals may be antigenically different. Even within a single chemically induced tumor mass, distinct antigenic subpopulations of cells exist. As a result, immunity to one chemically induced tumor does not prevent growth of a second tumor caused by the same chemical.

Third, normal proteins are produced in excessive amounts. A good example is the production of prostate-specific antigen (PSA) by prostate carcinomas of humans. PSA is exclusively produced by the prostate epithelium. Increased blood levels of this protein indicate excessive prostate activity. One cause of this is the growth of a carcinoma.

Fourth, cancer/testis (CT) antigens are a group of tumor antigens only expressed in the testes and in various malignancies. Their function is unknown.

Fifth, tumors caused by viruses may express antigens characteristic of the inducing virus. These antigens, although coded for by a viral genome, are not part of a virion. Examples include the FOCMA antigens found on the neoplastic lymphoid cells of cats infected with feline leukemia virus and Marek's cancer-specific antigens found on Marek's disease tumor cells in chickens. (Both of these are virus-induced, naturally occurring, T-cell tumors).

Studies on these mutations and the neoantigens they generate suggest that they are not widely shared but are tumor specific. Their production also differs between tumor types. Thus, neoantigen expression is very high in melanomas, lung, stomach, and colorectal tumors, and low in many leukemias. The vast majority of mutations do not however, generate antigens that can be recognized by T cells.

Inflammation and Cancer

The tumor microenvironment often determines the development and fate of cancer cells. Cancer cells can communicate with nearby cells especially fibroblasts and inflammatory cells. As a result, the survival of cancer cells is determined in part, by the presence of inflammation. Chronic inflammatory diseases increase the risk for developing many types of cancer; conversely, the use of nonsteroidal antiinflammatory drugs reduces tumor susceptibility (Fig. 36.2; Mantovani et al., 2008). Mutations in oncogenes such as *ras* and *myc* are closely linked to the inflammatory pathways. Inflammatory cytokines, chemokines, and cells are present in the microenvironment of early tumors and influence metastasis and survival time. Inflammatory cytokines, such as tumor necrosis factor–α (TNF-α), and macrophages are often required for tumor development and spread (Hagemann et al., 2007).

Cancer cells exploit signals from their microenvironment. Stromal cells such as fibroblasts, macrophages, and endothelial cells can generate IL-6, a cytokine that promotes tumor growth and angiogenesis. Inflammatory cells such as macrophages, mast cells, and TILs can promote tumor growth by remodeling tissues, stimulating angiogenesis, and suppressing immune responses. For example, the presence of tumor-associated macrophages is associated with more aggressive types of mammary tumors in dogs (Monteiro et al., 2018). As a result, more than half of the mass of a tumor may consist of supporting cells, including fibroblasts, macrophages, and vascular endothelial cells. Cancers cannot spread and metastasize without the support of these cells (Li et al., 2005).

If a metastasizing tumor does not invade lymphoid organs, it may escape immune surveillance. On the other hand, tumors that invade lymph nodes can be divided into strongly and weakly immunogenic types. Strongly immunogenic tumors elicit a T-cell response following processing by dendritic cells. Weakly immunogenic tumors tend to grow as walled-off nodules that may not be processed in sufficient amounts to trigger their destruction. These are the most common tumors in humans. Tumors that fail to generate inflammation may simply be ignored by the immune system.

CELLULAR DEFENSES

Natural Killer Cells

NK cells can detect and kill some cancer cells. They use two major types of receptors: First, receptors that can respond to the absence of MHC class I molecules on a cell surface by killing these abnormal cells; and second, receptors that can recognize stress-induced proteins on cell surfaces and, as a result, will kill stressed cells. Thus NK cells effectively kill two types of cellular targets: cells that fail to express MHC class I molecules and cells that express stress-related proteins. Both conditions commonly apply to cancer cells. As a result, NK cells play a significant role in the destruction of many tumors.

Cytotoxic T Cells

T cells also have the potential to destroy cancer cells. They possess receptors that can recognize antigen-MHC complexes expressed on all nucleated cells. The immense diversity of the T-cell antigen receptor repertoire enables them to identify and respond to new antigens made by cancer cells.

Until recently, evidence that T cells could control tumor growth came only from mice and human melanomas. For example, T-cell stimulation by IL-2 benefited a subset of melanoma patients. Subsequent studies with the checkpoint inhibitor ipilimumab, which interferes with T-cell cytotoxic T lymphocyte–associated protein–4 (CTLA-4), also showed great benefit to melanoma patients. Infusion of TILs, some of which are cytotoxic, may also benefit some melanoma patients.

Tumor-infiltrating CD8+ cytotoxic T cells are found in many cancers. Their presence tends to be associated with a better prognosis. Some success has been achieved in humans by isolating these cells from excised tumors and growing them in tissue culture. These cultured cells are then transfused into the patient and may induce remission. Similar results may be obtained with lymphokine-activated T-killer (T-LAK) cells. T-LAK cells are generated by taking the patient's peripheral blood lymphocytes, activating them in vitro with interleukin-2, and then returning them intravenously to the patient. This procedure has been shown to be effective in some dogs (Fig. 36.3).

The products of mutated genes or abnormally expressed cellular proteins may be processed and presented to T cells. As a result, lymphocytes from some tumor-bearing animals may kill cancer cells

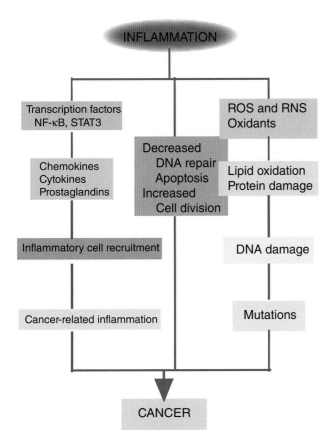

Fig. 36.2 The mechanisms by which inflammation can promote tumor formation. *DNA,* Deoxyribonucleic acid; *NF-kB,* nuclear factor kappa–B; *ROS,* reactive oxygen species; *RNS,* reactive nitrogen species; *STAT,* signal transducer and activator of transcription.

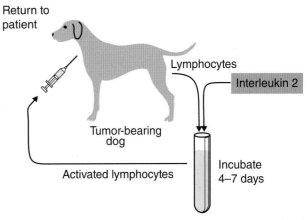

Fig. 36.3 The production of lymphokine-activated killer cells. By incubation of blood lymphocytes in the presence of interleukin-2 for 4–7 days.

cultured in vitro. For example, a protein called cyclin B1 that regulates mitosis is barely expressed in normal cells but overexpressed in many tumors, where it can stimulate T-cell cytotoxicity. Implicit in this is the fact that these T cells must recognize some peptides presented by the MHC I of malignant cells. These antigens may be normal cellular proteins to which tolerance is weak or alternatively, they may be neoantigens—peptides that are not present in normal animals but are created by tumor-specific mutations.

Macrophages

Solid tumors may be infiltrated by macrophages attracted by pro-inflammatory cytokines and prostaglandins. M2 macrophages may promote cancer cell proliferation and metastasis by releasing growth factors such as TGF-β, PDGF, and FGF. These M2 macrophages may also suppress T and NK cell responses, promote angiogenesis, and enhance cancer cell infiltration. Conversely, M1 macrophages may secrete cytotoxic molecules, including potent oxidants. Nonspecific activation of macrophages by bacillus Calmette-Guérin (BCG) or *Propionibacterium acnes* results in enhanced production of IL-1 or TNF-α and subsequent enhancement of helper T-cell and NK cell activity. IL-1 has a cytostatic effect on some tumors, and TNF-α may have potent antitumor activity. Unfortunately, malignant tumors may inhibit macrophage activation, and tumor-associated macrophages are usually of the M2 phenotype. This may be due to IL-10 produced by Treg cells or to factors such as monocyte chemotactic protein (MCP-1 or CCL2) secreted by the cancer cells themselves. These M2 macrophages may suppress T and NK cell responses, promote angiogenesis, and enhance cancer cell infiltration.

Antibody-Mediated Immunity

Antibodies to cancer cells are found in many tumor-bearing animals; for instance, about 50% of dogs with lymphosarcomas have antitumor antibodies. These antibodies may, together with complement, lyse free cancer cells within the bloodstream. Antibodies are, however, not usually effective in destroying solid cancers.

FAILURE OF IMMUNITY TO CANCER CELLS

The fact that tumors are so readily induced and are relatively common testifies to the inadequacies of the immunological protective mechanisms. Studies of tumor-bearing animals have indicated several mechanisms by which immune systems fail to reject tumors.

Cancer Cell Selection

Cancer cells do not usually become malignant in a single step. Rather, they gradually go from normal to benign to malignant in a process called tumor progression. The process occurs through a series of mutations that switch genes on and off. These mutations do not necessarily alter the immunogenicity of cancer cells or do so in small steps. Thus, their immunogenicity may not change until the cells are irreversibly committed to malignancy.

There are two selection mechanisms by which developing cancer cells can evade the host's immune response and thus enhance their own survival. One is "sneaking through," the process by which malignant cells may not trigger an immune response until the tumor has reached a size at which it cannot be controlled by the host. Thus, in experimental tumors, small numbers of cancer cells may grow after subcutaneous inoculation, although large numbers may not. It may be that the cancer cells may not reach lymph nodes and trigger an immune response until the tumor burden is too large to be controlled. Even a very small tumor may contain an enormous number of cells. For example, a 10-mm tumor contains about 10^9 cells.

The second mechanism involves "immunoediting" cancers. Thus the immune system may indeed eliminate some cancer cells, especially those that express neoantigens and trigger T-cell cytotoxicity. If, however, mutations are subtle and their immunogenicity is low, some cancer cells may escape T-cell destruction. These variants may then grow to produce clinical cancers.

Immunoediting consists of three phases: elimination, equilibrium, and escape. Immune elimination usually occurs early in tumor growth at a time when the tumor is small. If effective, the tumor cells are wiped out. If, however, some tumor cells can avoid destruction, the response moves into the equilibrium phase, where the tumor becomes established while immunological attack continues. There is ongoing elimination of some cancer cells, but variants continue to emerge that can survive, persist, and grow. Thus, there is a balance between tumor elimination and tumor growth. Eventually, however, ongoing selection for cancer cells with minimal immunogenicity permits the tumor to escape. The surviving cancer cells are resistant to immunological attack. Tumors are often in the escape phase when first diagnosed, so that, clinical cases usually fail to mount effective immune responses.

Immunosuppression

It is commonly observed that tumor-bearing animals are immunosuppressed (Fig. 36.4). This is most clearly seen in animals with lymphoid tumors. For example, B-cell tumors tend to suppress antibody formation, whereas T-cell tumors suppress cell-mediated immune responses and NK cell activity. However, it may also be observed in dogs with mammary carcinomas. This immunosuppression can include defects in antigen recognition, in costimulation, and in cytokine production. Immunosuppression in animals with chemically induced tumors is due in part to production of immunosuppressive molecules such as prostaglandin-E_2 by tumor cells or tumor-associated macrophages. The presence of actively growing cancer cells also represents a severe protein drain on an animal. This protein loss may be immunosuppressive.

Some tumor-derived molecules may redirect immune functions so that they promote tumor growth. Thus tumor-derived IL-4, IL-6, IL-10, TGF-β, prostaglandin-E_2, and macrophage colony-stimulating factor can deactivate or suppress the activation of both M1 macrophages and Th1 cells. The TGF-β can convert antitumor effector cells into Treg cells. Many tumors produce indolamine 2,3-dioxygenase (IDO), a potent immunosuppressive agent and a suppressor of NK cell function (see Chapter 21).

Studies on the immune environment of canine melanomas have also demonstrated evidence of localized immunosuppression. Thus their expression IDO is associated with increased risk of death as is the increased presence of the Treg transcription factor, FoxP3. CTLA-4 gene and protein expression are also negative prognostic factors (Porcellato et al., 2021). Interferon-induced signaling is impaired in many patients with cancer. Once tumors have effectively immunosuppressed their host, they readily enter the escape phase during which their growth is uncontrolled.

T-Cell Dysfunction

Within the tumor microenvironment, numerous factors may act together to suppress T-cell function. A combination of hypoxia, nutrient shortage, acidic pH, suppressive cytokines such as TGF-β and IL-10, lipids like PGE_2, suppress the activities of tumor-infiltrating T cells. T-cell cytotoxicity may be blocked by upregulating PD-L1 expression as a result of hypoxia, by IDO production suppressing T-cell functions, or by excessive Treg activity. Cytotoxic T cells must be able to contact cancer cells to kill them. Tumor-derived angiogenic factors such as vascular endothelial growth factor (VEGF) and endothelin-1 can block the expression of the endothelial cell adhesion molecules so that T cells

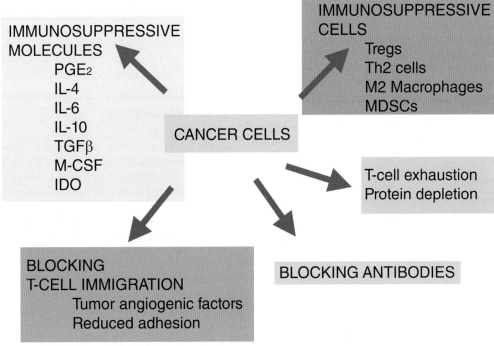

Fig. 36.4 Some of the mechanisms by which cancer cells induce immunosuppression. *IDO,* Indolamine 2,3-dioxygenase; *IL,* interleukin; *M-CSF,* M-colony-stimulating factor; *MDSCs,* myeloid-derived suppressor cells; *PGE2,* prostaglandin-E$_2$; *TGF-β,* transforming growth factor–β; *Tregs,* regulatory T cells.

may be unable to leave blood vessels. Tumor vascular endothelium may express immunosuppressive molecules such as IDO and PGE$_2$. Tumor endothelium can also express ligands such as TRAIL that may kill T cells as they cross the vascular endothelium (see Chapter 21).

CD95 Ligand

CD95 ligand (CD95L) is normally expressed on cytotoxic T cells and NK cells. When it binds to the death receptor CD95 on target cells, it triggers their apoptosis. CD95L has also been detected on some leukemic T cells and NK cells, colon adenocarcinoma cells, melanomas, and hepatocellular carcinomas. Since cytotoxic T cells may also express CD95, cytotoxicity may work in reverse and the CD95L+ tumor cells may kill the T cells. At the same time, these cancer cells may downregulate their own CD95 so that they become resistant to cell-mediated cytotoxicity. Some cancer cells such as those in lung carcinomas may secrete decoy receptors for CD95L. These decoy receptors bind CD95L and so prevent it from binding to CD95. Cancer cells that down-regulate CD95 while producing decoy receptors may be resistant to T-cell cytotoxicity.

Regulatory Cells

Much of the immunosuppression that develops in tumor-bearing individuals is due to regulatory cells. These may be CD8+ Treg cells, IL-10-secreting Th2 cells, M2 macrophages, or even Breg cells. Enhanced regulatory cell activity can be detected in many tumor-bearing animals. Thus, in normal dogs, FoxP3+ Treg cells constitute about 5% of blood T cells and 10% of lymph node T cells. In tumor-bearing dogs, however, they may constitute as many as 7.5% in blood and 17% in tumor-draining lymph nodes. Dogs with osteosarcomas have elevated Treg and fewer CD8 cells in blood, lymph nodes, and tumors. The CD8/Treg ratio is significantly lower in tumor-bearing dogs, and dogs with the greatest decrease have a shorter survival time. Treg numbers also rise in dogs with mammary carcinomas.

Myeloid-Derived Suppressor Cells

Myeloid-derived suppressor cells (MDSCs) are immature myeloid cells that normally develop into macrophages, granulocytes, and dendritic cells. They are generated by soluble factors from cancer cells and are attracted by chemokines or hypoxia to the tumors. Once inside tumors, MDSCs suppress cytotoxic T-cell responses by expressing the inhibitory surface marker PD-L1, and by secreting immunosuppressive mediators such as arginase, IL-10, TGFβ, reactive oxygen species, nitric oxide, and peroxynitrite. Peroxynitrite causes nitrate addition to TCRs and thus inactivates them. MDSCs also produce arginase that impairs T-cell function by reducing expression of CD3ζ. Some MDSCs promote the production of Treg cells. MDSCs may also enhance cancer cell survival by promoting the switch from M1 to M2 cells.

MDSCs have been identified in tumor-bearing dogs where they suppress lymphocyte proliferation. For example, immunosuppression has been well documented in dogs with mammary carcinomas. Affected dogs had normal numbers of T cells but the proportion of Treg cells was increased as were the number of MDSCs. These cells increased significantly in late-stage disease and in dogs with confirmed metastases.

Blocking Antibodies

Passively administered serum from some tumor-bearing animals may permit the tumors in recipient animals to grow even faster, a phenomenon called enhancement. This serum may also inhibit T-cell cytotoxicity. Many tumors release soluble antigens into the bloodstream, and these may bind to cytotoxic T cells, saturate their antigen receptors and block their ability to bind to target cells. Alternatively, enhancement may be due to blocking antibodies. These are noncomplement-activating, antitumor antibodies that can mask tumor antigens on cell surfaces and so protect them from attack by cytotoxic T cells.

TUMOR IMMUNOTHERAPY

For many years, immunologists have attempted to treat cancers by means of immunotherapy. Initially, progress was distressingly slow. Successes were limited to rare cancers and even when immunotherapy worked, results were unpredictable and inconsistent. That has now changed. Vaccines against cancers are still at an early stage in their development but new techniques involving both passive and active immunotherapy have begun to yield exciting results. Progress has not been confined to human cancers. Encouraging results are increasingly being obtained in the treatment of cancers in our domestic animals (Bergman, 2018).

Active Immunotherapy

In active immunotherapy, the patient's own immune system is stimulated to respond to the tumor. In passive immunotherapy, immune cells or their products are administered.

Several approaches have been used in attempts to cure or modify tumor growth through immunotherapy. The simplest is to stimulate the immune system nonspecifically (Fig. 36.5). Any improvement in an animal's immune abilities will tend to enhance its resistance to tumors, although a cure may be expected only if the tumor mass is small or is surgically excised. The most widely used immune stimulant is the attenuated strain of *Mycobacterium bovis*, BCG. This organism activates macrophages and stimulates cytokine release, thus promoting T-cell activity. It may be given systemically or injected directly into the tumor mass. Most positive results from the use of BCG have come from studies on human patients with melanomas or bladder cancer. Direct injection of BCG into skin melanomas may cause regression, not only of the injected lesion but also, occasionally, of uninjected skin metastases. However, visceral metastases usually remain unaffected. BCG enhances survival or remission in some leukemias, and its direct intravesicular application in human bladder cancer gives response rates of up to 70%. However, BCG can cause severe lesions at the site of injection and, occasionally, systemic hypersensitivity (Finocchiaro et al., 2009).

The immune response modifier Imiquimod (Aldara), has been widely used to treat many skin cancers, most notably equine sarcoids (Hollis, 2022). This drug activates TLR7 and as a result stimulates cells

to secrete IFN-α, TNF-α, and IL-6. These cytokines activate Langerhans cells as well as inducing local innate immune responses. Imiquimod also activates the opioid growth factor receptor which has antiproliferative effects. It also appears to activate NK cells, macrophages, and B cells (Miller et al., 1999). It has been used to treat warts, as well as basal cell and squamous cell carcinomas in humans, dogs, and cats with mixed results (Gill et al., 2008).

Passive Immunotherapy
Cytokine Therapy

Many attempts have been made to treat human cancer patients by administering individual cytokines but with limited success. Interferons, for example, are effective only against selected tumors. Thus 70%–90% of patients with hairy cell leukemia treated with IFN-α show complete or partial remission. On the other hand, administration of IL-2 to melanoma and renal cell cancer patients induces partial or complete remission in only 15%–20% of cases. Low doses of recombinant human IL-2 when injected locally into papillomas or carcinomas of the vulva in cattle induced remissions in 83% of treated animals. Some complete regressions were observed. IL-2 therapy produced 63% complete remissions in cattle with ocular squamous cell carcinomas (Hill et al., 1994).

Adoptive Cell Transfer

In humans, tumors have been surgically removed from cancer-bearing patients; then the lymphocytes within these tumors were cultured in the presence of IL-2 for 4–6 weeks so that their numbers grow significantly. These tumor-infiltrating lymphocytes (TILs) recognize and infiltrate only the tumors from which they come. Returned with IL-2 to the donor patients, they have produced remissions in about one-third of patients. The most encouraging results have been obtained in patients with melanomas and some leukemias.

Limited success has been obtained in treating melanomas in gray horses by immunotherapy. For example, administration of a plasmid expressing IL-13 directly into metastases produced significant regression in 60% of cases and appeared to be safe. In dogs with melanomas, plasmids containing DNA coding for the herpesvirus thymidine kinase suicide gene were able to sensitize transfected cells to ganciclovir (Ganciclovir is a potent antiherpesvirus drug). The treatment induced substantial regression. A similar therapy given in association with a subcutaneous autologous killed cancer vaccine appeared to work well in a horse.

Monoclonal Antibodies

A major advance in cancer immunotherapy has been the development of bioengineered monoclonal antibodies directed against specific tumor cell antigens or against molecules that promote tumor growth. There are now more than 75 FDA approved, monoclonal antibodies used in the treatment of human cancers. For example, in 1987 the FDA approved rituximab, a monoclonal antibody directed against the B-cell surface antigen CD20. Rituximab has revolutionized the treatment of B-cell lymphomas in humans. The anti-CD20 binds to the malignant B cells and triggers their apoptosis. Canine B cells also express CD20 although canine monoclonal anti-CD20 does not appear to cause B-cell tumor apoptosis. Canine CD20 is structurally sufficiently different from the human molecule so that Rituximab will not bind it. Caninized monoclonal antibodies against canine CD20 have been developed and some deplete B cells.

Initially, these monoclonal antibodies were derived exclusively from mice. However, as monoclonal antibody technology has improved, it has proved possible to "humanize" the murine antibodies by attaching the mouse antigen-binding region to a human immunoglobulin

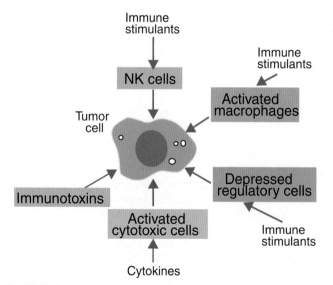

Fig. 36.5 The major cell types that participate in tumor cell destruction and methods of stimulating that activity. *NK cells*, Natural killer cells.

backbone. A similar process can produce "caninized" monoclonal anti-bodies for use in dogs. These monoclonal antibodies can be directed against the cancer cells in order to destroy them through the process of antibody-dependent cellular cytotoxicity. Alternatively, monoclonal antibodies may be used to block growth-promoting factors or their receptors, or they may enhance the activity of immune cells.

Encouraging results in treating canine B-cell lymphomas have been obtained by a method that combines administration of anti-CD20 with blockade of CD47. (CD47 is expressed on tumor cells and acts as a checkpoint regulator by inhibiting their phagocytosis by macro-phages.) The anti-CD20 kills the tumor cells while the blockade of CD47 ensures their removal.

Bevacizumab is a humanized monoclonal antibody directed against vascular epithelial growth factor. VEGF promotes angiogenesis, blood vessel growth. The monoclonal antibody inhibits the growth of cancers by preventing the development of their blood supply. Preliminary stud-ies suggest that this product may be effective in treating some canine sarcomas.

For optimal results, monoclonal antibody therapy must often be supplemented by other treatments such as chemotherapy. They are rarely sufficient by themselves to cause complete remissions (O'Connor and Wilson-Robles, 2014).

Immune Checkpoint Therapy

Recent encouraging advances in the treatment of some human cancers have resulted from the use of monoclonal antibodies that prevent T-cell inhibition by checkpoint molecules (Fig. 36.6). Checkpoint molecules are T-cell surface receptors and their ligands that normally suppress T-cell proliferation and cytotoxicity (Waldman et al., 2020).

The most important defense pathway against tumors uses cyto-toxic, CD8+ T cells. They can kill cancer cells, provided that the T cells can recognize the cancer cell neoantigens and respond accordingly. However, these T cells are readily exhausted by prolonged, low-level immune stimulation. Once exhausted, these T cells take on an immu-nosuppressive function. They persist within the tumor microenviron-ment and suppress nearby effector T cells. Exhausted CD8+ T cells express high levels of two inhibitory checkpoint molecules called pro-grammed cell death protein (PD-1) and CTLA-4. These proteins nor-mally prevent excessive T-cell cytotoxicity. Their increased expression has been detected in exhausted T cells from many human tumors and is associated with increased tumor aggressiveness. This has also been associated with metastasis and poor prognosis in malignant canine mammary gland tumors (Ariyarathna et al., 2020).

PD-1

PD-1 is a receptor expressed on effector T cells. When stimulated by its ligands (PD-1L and PD-2L), it suppresses T-cell functions. Signaling through PD-1 normally prevents T cells from generating cytotoxic sig-nals and damaging surrounding tissues. It suppresses T-cell cytotox-icity and triggers T-cell apoptosis. Thus, if cancer cells produce PD-1 ligands, they will not be attacked by cytotoxic T cells. Additionally, some cancer cells induce PD-1 expression on activated T cells. This also results in a loss of T-cell function and eventual T-cell "exhaustion" (Boussiotis, 2016).

Blockade of PD-1 or PD-1L binding by monoclonal antibodies therefore results in recovery of T-cell cytotoxic activity and a renewed antitumor response. Treatment with anti-PD-1 or anti-PD-1L mono-clonal antibodies has produced dramatic and prolonged remissions in humans with melanomas, renal cell carcinomas, and non-small cell lung cancers. For example, in patients with metastatic melanoma, those treated with checkpoint therapy have a 50% survival rate at 3 years compared to 12% survival in patients receiving chemotherapy alone.

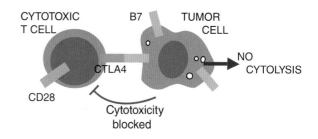
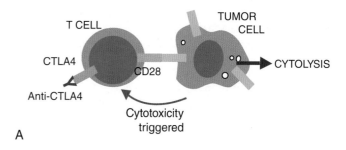
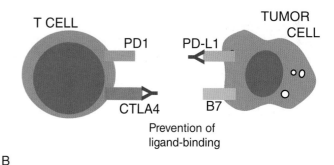

Fig. 36.6 The principles of immune checkpoint therapy. (A) cytotoxic T lymphocyte–associated protein–4 (CTLA-4) is an inhibitory receptor expressed on T cells. Its ligand is B7 expressed on tumor cells. Blocking of P CTLA-4 by antibodies permits cytotoxic T cells to exercise their full activity against the tumor cells. (B) Alternatively (or additionally), programmed cell death protein (PD-1) blocks tumor cell apoptosis by binding to its ligand programmed death ligand (PD-L1). Blockage of this interaction allows cytotoxicity and apoptosis to proceed.

PD-1-activating monoclonal antibodies have recently demonstrated success in the treatment of human rheumatoid arthritis.

Cytotoxic T Lymphocyte–Associated Protein–4

A second T-cell inhibitory receptor is CTLA-4. CTLA-4 is expressed on T-cell surfaces following their activation (see Chapter 15). Its ligands are CD80 and CD86 expressed on antigen-presenting cells. Like PD-1, its role is to prevent uncontrolled T-cell activation. Ligands acting through CTLA-4 deliver suppressive signals to the T cells and inhibit their activa-tion. Conversely, if CTLA-4 signaling is blocked, then T-cell responses will recover. CTLA-4 blockade in tumor-bearing animals therefore results in a significant increase in T cell–mediated tumor cytotoxicity and the development of new antitumor T cells. Studies on humans have shown that administration of a monoclonal antibody against CTLA-4 (Ipilimumab) results in a significant increase in T-cell antitumor activity and dramatic remissions in many (but not all) patients (Fig. 36.6).

Checkpoint inhibitors have achieved remarkable success in the treatment of metastatic melanomas, kidney and lung tumors, and hematologic cancers (Teng et al., 2016). A combination of anti-PD-1 and anti-CTLA-4 appears to be exceptionally effective in permitting T-cell cytotoxicity to proceed, which results in long-term remissions. Unfortunately, not all cancers respond to checkpoint inhibitors. In some patients, T cells may be irreversibly exhausted or so exhausted that their function may only be restored temporarily and the disease relapses after an early response.

Checkpoint inhibitors can also be used in combination with other chemotherapeutic agents such as tyrosine kinase inhibitors or therapeutic vaccines (Sharma et al., 2023). Unfortunately, checkpoint therapy is not without its problems. The activation of suppressed T cells can trigger autoimmunity or immune responses against the commensal microbiota (Hu et al., 2022).

Many canine tumors, such as mastocytomas, melanomas, renal cell carcinomas, and B-cell lymphomas, are infiltrated by T cells that overexpress PD-1-L and CTLA-4. These tumors are therefore potential targets for checkpoint therapy (Ambrosius et al., 2018). Monoclonal antibodies have been made against canine PD-1 and PD-1L. Both molecules are present on activated canine T cells, while PD-1L is expressed on canine dendritic cells. When treated with either anti-PD-1 alone or a combination of anti-PD-1 and anti-PD-1L in vitro, T-cell production of interferon γ, is significantly increased. These results are of immediate relevance to the treatment of tumors in dogs (Hartley et al., 2017).

Antibody Therapy

Some successes have been achieved by the use of monoclonal antibodies against tumor antigens. Monoclonal antibodies can be used to destroy tumors, either when given alone or when complexed with highly cytotoxic drugs or potent radioisotopes, which they carry directly to the tumor cells. One of the first such monoclonal antibodies to be produced was directed against canine T cells (CL/MAb231) and produced encouraging results when used to manage lymphomas in dogs. It apparently works by inducing ADCC and complement-mediated lysis. Monoclonal antibodies against lymphomas in dogs are currently undergoing clinical trials. Other potential animal tumor targets include CD47 in B-cell lymphomas, epithelial cell growth factor receptor in mammary carcinomas, and CEA for colon carcinomas (Rue et al., 2015). Unfortunately, the number of available monoclonal antibodies available for cancer treatment in dogs is very much less than those in humans (Klingemann, 2018).

Immunoprevention

In contrast to the techniques described previously, most of which have met with only limited success, there are established successful techniques for vaccination against tumor viruses. These include effective vaccines against hepatitis B and human papillomavirus, the causes of hepatocellular carcinoma and cervical cancer, respectively. The most important of these in veterinary medicine are the vaccines against feline leukemia. These vaccines usually contain high concentrations of the major viral antigens, and immunity is almost entirely directed against viral glycoproteins. Other important vaccines are those directed against Marek's disease, a T-cell tumor in chickens caused by a herpesvirus. The immune response evoked by these vaccines has two components. First, humoral and cell-mediated responses act directly on the virus to reduce the quantity available to infect cells. Second, an immune response is provoked against virus antigens expressed on the surface of tumor cells. Both the antiviral and antitumor immune responses act synergistically to protect the birds.

ACTIVE IMMUNIZATION

Therapeutic vaccination against cancer is a very active research area, and many promising cancer vaccines are under development. These include adjuvanted purified antigens, DNA vaccines, vector-based vaccines, tumor cell vaccines, and dendritic cell vaccines.

Tumor vaccines trigger adaptive immunity against tumor-associated antigens administered in such a way that they stimulate a potent cytotoxic T-cell response while overcoming tumor-mediated immunosuppression. They have the great advantage that they can circumvent the resistance of tumor cells to cytotoxic drugs. Additionally, they are highly specific, have low toxicity, and have a long-lasting effect as a result of memory responses.

These tumor-associated antigens belong to two broad categories. There are tumor-specific shared antigens expressed on more than one type of tumor cell, and they may also be expressed in normal tissues. The other category includes unique molecules expressed by cancer cells as a result of mutations resulting from carcinogen exposure. These tumor antigens can be obtained from either autologous sources (the cancerous animal itself) or from allogeneic sources (other animals). They can include whole cell lysates or purified tumor peptides or even defined tumor cell antigens.

Many different approaches have been tested, including proteins, peptides, cell extracts, and whole tumor cells. It is also possible to make DNA vaccines expressing the genes encoding specific tumor antigens. These can be delivered directly as DNA-plasmids or inserted into appropriate recombinant viral or bacterial vectors. In theory, injected tumor antigens should induce both memory and effector T cells. As a result, immunity should persist and control tumor growth indefinitely.

Many attempts have been made to produce tumor vaccines for animals. Thus, a canine lymphoma vaccine was first investigated in the 1980s. These early attempts used whole cell vaccines consisting of irradiated or lysed tumor cells together with an adjuvant. These early vaccines were, however, poorly defined, and it was difficult to produce a standardized product.

The lack of success of these early vaccines may also have resulted from immunosuppressive mechanisms acting within the tumor microenvironment, as well as the activation of regulatory T cells and the blocking of activation signals. As described above, these suppressive signals are mediated by checkpoint molecules such as CTLA-4, PD-1, and its ligand, PD-1L. Other checkpoint molecules that are potential targets for monoclonal antibody therapy include lymphocyte activation protein 3 found on both CD4 and CD8 T cells and NK cells; T-cell immunoglobulin and mucin domain-containing–3 (TIM-3) found on T cells; T-cell immunoreceptor with Ig and ITIM domains (TIGIT) also found on lymphocytes; and the NK cell inhibitory receptor NKG2A. Checkpoint therapy is still in its infancy, and results should steadily improve as experience is gained (Box 36.2).

Telomerase Vaccine

The telomerase reverse transcriptase (TERT) is a subcomponent of the enzyme telomerase. Telomerase ensures that telomeres (the ends of chromosomes) do not shorten each time a cell divides. It is expressed at a very low level in normal cells but is highly expressed in neoplastic cells, where it confers immortality. TERT is usually absent from normal dog tissues. Thus TERT represents a valid target for cancer immunotherapy. A current experimental vaccine consists of an adenovirus-vectored recombinant expressing TERT that is introduced into dogs by DNA electroporation. The vaccine appears to increase overall survival time in dogs with B-cell lymphoma that also received standard chemotherapy when compared to dogs that received chemotherapy alone (Peruzzi et al., 2010; Gavazza et al., 2013).

Canine Oral Melanoma

Oral melanomas in dogs have a poor prognosis because of their invasiveness and ability to metastasize. In untreated dogs with

By applying cellular genetic engineering techniques to cultured T cells, it has been possible to generate cytotoxic T cells with receptors directed specifically against selected tumor cell surface antigens. Thus, these T cells expressed engineered receptors specific for a target antigen such as CD19 or CD20. The first-generation CARs were relatively simple, consisting of an antibody V domain linked to a T-cell intracellular signaling module. Early clinical trials of these Chimeric Antigen Receptor (CAR) T cells targeting CD19 on B-cell malignancies such as acute lymphocytic leukemia and non-Hodgkin's lymphoma demonstrated favorable results. It is possible to control both the receptor specificity and avidity and remove the need for MHC recognition of the target cells. CAR T-cell therapy currently has US Food and Drug Administration approval for use in diffuse large B-cell lymphoma and acute lymphoblastic leukemia, mantle cell lymphoma, and multiple myeloma. CAR T-cell immunotherapies are also being developed for autoimmune diseases and viral infections. Although antimalignancy results of this therapy have been game changing, they do not come without cost. Various off-target effects are frequently observed, including cytokine-related toxicity that can cause severe morbidity and mortality. They often cease working as a result of T-cell exhaustion, anergy, and immunosuppression. Among the most significant complications of this therapy include infection and its sequelae related to the multifactorial immune suppression affecting this patient group.

CAR T-cell therapy has yet to be applied to animal tumors.

From June, C.H., O'Connor, R.S., Kawalekar, O.U., et al., 2018. CAR T cell immunotherapy for human cancer. Science 359, 1361–1365.

oral malignant melanoma, the median time to death is 2 months. Melanomas are uniquely immunogenic tumors, and it has been possible to make an antimelanoma DNA vaccine (Oncept, Boehringer Ingleheim). It has been approved for the treatment of stage II and III canine oral melanoma. This vaccine contains an *Escherichia coli* plasmid engineered to express the gene encoding human tyrosinase. Once inside a cell nucleus, the DNA plasmid transcribes and translates the tyrosinase gene and, as result, cells produce this enzyme within the recipient. Tyrosinase catalyzes the hydroxylation of tyrosine to dihydroxyphenylalanine, a key step in melanin production. This human tyrosinase is only 85% homologous to the canine protein. This difference is such that vaccinated dogs will mount immune responses against the human protein. However, this immune response also induces both antibodies and cytotoxic T cells against the dog's own melanoma cells, and results in their destruction (Verganti et al., 2016).

In a prospective clinical trial with 58 dogs, use of this melanoma vaccine significantly increased survival times. In one retrospective study, vaccinated dogs had a median survival time of 355 days. In another retrospective study, 8 of 13 dogs showed a clinical response, and three dogs with oral malignant melanoma survived for 171, 178, and 288 days from diagnosis. The initial four-dose series is given once every two weeks using a needle-free transdermal device. The vaccine is well tolerated with no significant adverse effects (Atherton et al., 2016). The vaccine is safe, and some individual dogs clearly benefit from its use. However, published reports on its efficacy have described mixed results (Pellin, 2022).

Osteosarcomas

Osteosarcomas are the commonest primary bone tumors in dogs. Conventional treatment consists of surgical amputation and aggressive chemotherapy. Despite this, metastasis is common. A canine osteosarcoma vaccine, Live Listeria Vector (AT-104) has been granted a conditional license (Aratana Therapeutics, Advaxis Inc.). This vaccine uses attenuated *Listeria monocytogenes* as a vector to carry a plasmid

expressing a human tumor antigen called HER2/neu into macrophages. HER2/neu is a tyrosine kinase receptor overexpressed on many aggressive carcinomas and sarcomas. When injected into an animal, the bacteria are rapidly phagocytosed. However, Listeria is a facultative intracellular bacterium and so can enter and survive within the cytosol of macrophages. It normally uses a pore-forming lysin called listeriolysin O (LLO) to escape from the phagosome into the cytosol. The plasmids expressing the genes for HER2/neu fused with a truncated form of LLO, transcribe and translate the chimeric antigen. This is carried to the cytosol, where the fusion protein is processed as an endogenous antigen (see Chapter 11) and enters the MHC class I presenting pathway. As a result, the HER2/neu is recognized by both CD4+ and CD8+ T cells and induces a potent T cell–mediated cytotoxic response. When this recombinant Listeria was administered intravenously in conjunction with amputation and chemotherapy, the median survival time of dogs with osteosarcomas was doubled when compared to amputation and chemotherapy alone. As a result, a large extended field study is currently underway.

Autologous Tumor Vaccines

It is, of course, possible to simply excise part of a tumor and prepare an inactivated vaccine to be injected back into the patient. The best example of this approach is the production of autogenous vaccines against bovine fibropapillomas. These papillomas may develop on the teats or other inconvenient sites on cattle. They are caused by members of a large family of bovine papillomaviruses. Vaccines are available that can be used for both prevention and treatment, but success depends on the specific papillomavirus involved. There are several ways to make these vaccines. For example, the papillomas can be surgically excised, and small pieces can be stored in 10% buffered formalin. After cleaning, selected pieces are suspended in saline and homogenized. A preservative or antibiotics are then added to inhibit bacterial growth. After filtration, more formalin may be added to ensure viral inactivation. The vaccine is administered subcutaneously in three doses at one-week intervals. This vaccination is often quite effective for the treatment of small warts (Terziev et al., 2015).

SOME SELECTED TUMORS

Feline Injection-Site Sarcomas

When cats are vaccinated, any inflammation at the injection site usually resolves rapidly and completely. In some cats, however, sarcomas develop at these sites many months or years after vaccination (Fig. 36.7). These tumors are mainly fibrosarcomas, malignant histiocytomas, or osteosarcomas. Less common forms include rhabdomyosarcomas, hemangiosarcomas, chondrosarcomas, liposarcomas, and lymphosarcomas (Martano et al., 2011). These tumors are highly invasive. Successful treatment requires a combination of radical surgical excision and adjunctive therapy, including radiation, immunotherapy (such as IL-2 treatment), and chemotherapy, but recurrence is common (Srivastav et al., 2012).

Injection site tumors were first noticed in the 1980s following the introduction of potent, inactivated, adjuvanted vaccines such as those directed against rabies and feline leukemia. Cats receiving FeLV vaccine were 5.5 times more likely to develop a sarcoma at the injection site than cats that had not received a vaccine. There was a twofold increase in risk with rabies vaccination. However, the risk was not enormously high. It has been calculated that 1–3.6 sarcomas develop per 10,000 vaccinated cats in the United States. The risk increases with the number of doses of vaccine administered: a 50% increase following one dose, a 127% increase following two doses, and a 175% increase following

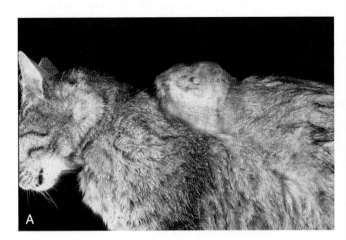
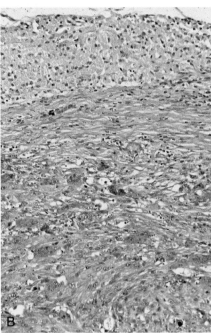

Fig. 36.7 (A) A postvaccinal sarcoma in a cat. Note its position over the scapular groove, a convenient site for subcutaneous vaccination in cats. (B) A histological section of a postvaccinal sarcoma. This is a fibrosarcoma with the characteristic interwoven bundles of spindle cells (H&E stain). Courtesy Dr. MJ Hendrick.

three or four vaccines given simultaneously. Vaccine-associated sarcomas tend to occur in younger animals and are larger and more aggressive than sarcomas arising at other sites. They metastasize in 25%–70% of cases. In one study, injection site sarcomas developed on average 26 months after rabies vaccination and 11 months after FeLV vaccination. Global, web-based surveys suggest a somewhat lower prevalence of sarcomas (0.63 sarcomas/10,000 cats or 0.32 sarcomas/10,000 doses of all vaccines, or one sarcoma from 31,000 doses administered). It must therefore be pointed out that the chances of developing a sarcoma are considerably smaller than the disease risks incurred by unvaccinated cats. In addition to rabies and FeLV vaccines, sarcomas have also been associated with the use of vaccines against feline panleukopenia, feline herpesvirus, and feline calicivirus. Similar vaccination-related injection site sarcomas have been reported (rarely) in ferrets, dogs, and a horse (Kannegieter et al., 2010).

The pathogenesis of these sarcomas is unclear. When first reported, it was assumed that tumor development resulted from the presence of potent adjuvants. Tumor development has however also been associated with the use of nonadjuvanted vaccines and even with injection of substances other than vaccines, including penicillin, glucocorticoids, lufenuron, cisplatin, and meloxicam, as well as the presence of persistent suture material, a retained surgical swab, or implanted microchips. There is no evidence that feline sarcoma virus, feline immunodeficiency virus, or feline leukemia viruses cause these tumors (Buracco et al., 2002).

Chronic, prolonged irritation leads to an increase in local stem cells and the possibility that some may mutate (Wong and Reiter, 2011). During chronic inflammation, macrophages secrete growth factors and angiogenic factors that enhance cell growth. These factors upregulate NF-κB activity in affected tissues. Oxidants released from activated macrophages may act as carcinogens, especially in rapidly dividing cells. Although the mechanisms are unclear, NF-κB promotes both malignant transformation and metastases and may inhibit apoptosis of premalignant cells (Coussens and Werb, 2002).

Fibroblasts proliferate at sites of chronic inflammation and wound healing. In some of these fibroblasts, the *sis* oncogene may be activated, whereas in others, there are mutations in the gene coding for the tumor suppressor factor *p53*. The *sis* oncogene codes for the platelet-derived growth factor (PDGF) receptor, and vaccine-associated sarcomas have been shown to express both PDGF and its receptor. In contrast, nonvaccine-associated tumors and normal cat lymphocytes are PDGF negative. It has been suggested, therefore, that lymphocytes within the vaccine-associated sarcomas secrete PDGF, which then serves as a growth factor for the fibroblasts. This combination of abnormalities could result in the loss of growth control in the fibroblasts engaged in the chronic inflammatory process.

The tumor suppressor gene *p53* codes for a nuclear protein that regulates the cell cycle. Wild-type *p53* increases in response to cell damage. This delays the cells progress through the cell cycle and permits DNA repair before the cell divides. If the cell is severely damaged, *p53* triggers apoptosis and prevents cellular damage from being transmitted to the next generation. Damaged cells in which *p53* is absent or mutated can continue to divide, giving rise to abnormal and possibly malignant cells. As many as 60% of injection site sarcomas may express mutated *p53*. It is also apparent that they contain many cells with broken DNA strands.

Notwithstanding the above, there is no evidence to prove that injecting less irritating products can reduce the incidence of sarcomas. No specific brands of vaccine, no specific manufacturers, and no other vaccination-associated factors have been associated with an increased prevalence of sarcomas in cats.

To assess the risks of tumors developing at vaccination sites, it has been recommended that vaccines be administered at standardized sites on cats. For example, current recommendations are to inject rabies vaccine into the right pelvic limb and FeLV vaccine into the left pelvic limb ("rabies, right; leukemia, left"). The interscapular region should be avoided. Vaccines should be administered as distally as possible to permit amputation if required. The site of vaccine administration and the product used should be recorded for each vaccine to help in assessing risk factors. Clients should be instructed to monitor injection sites for swellings or lumps so that any developing tumors are detected and excised as early as possible.

Canine Transmissible Venereal Sarcoma

Tumors may, under some circumstances, act in a manner similar to infectious agents. Two examples of this are canine transmissible venereal sarcoma and Devil facial tumor disease.

Transmissible venereal sarcoma is a naturally occurring lymphocytic/plasmacytic cancer transmitted between dogs during copulation. It is associated with an insertion in the *C-MYC* oncogene. It therefore usually grows around the external genitalia. It may also develop around the oronasal region as a result of dogs licking themselves. It results from transplantation of neoplastic cells. (In effect, the cancer cells act as infectious agents). To colonize a new host, these cells must establish themselves in allogeneic hosts. This is not always successful, and after an initial 1–3-month growth phase, the tumor eventually enters a stationary phase and then regresses and is eliminated. Nevertheless, lethal metastases may occur in up to 7% of puppies and immunosuppressed dogs. The tumor persists in the face of an allograft response as a result of multiple somatic mutations. When growing aggressively, these cancer cells fail to express β_2-microglobulin, and as a result, MHC class I antigens are not assembled on the cell surface. They also secrete the immunosuppressive cytokine, transforming growth factor-β; Exposed dogs, whether or not they develop progressive tumors, develop antibodies to tumor cells. Thirty to forty percent of cells in the regressive phase express MHC classes I and II. These regressing cells also express IL-6 and IFN-γ and hence counteract the TGF-β while restoring NK cell functionality. Dogs whose cancers regress also develop cytotoxic T cells. If recipient dogs are immunosuppressed, the tendency to malignant growth is enhanced. The tumor cells appear to secrete a cytotoxic factor that kills B cells. Genetic analysis of these tumor cells suggests that they originated from a clone of myeloid cells that arose in a wolf or East Asian dog about 11,000 years ago (Faro and de Oliveira, 2023).

Devil Facial Tumor Disease

The large carnivorous marsupial, the Tasmanian devil (*Sarcophilus harrissii*), is on the brink of extinction as a result of devil facial tumor disease, a transmissible cancer. This disease first appeared in the 1996 and has spread across Tasmania. It has reduced some devil populations by as much as 90% (Pye et al., 2016b). Tumor cells are transmitted when devils bite each other around the face, a common behavior. The tumor cells grow and form a large mass that is eventually lethal (Fig. 36.8). Almost every devil "infected" with these tumor cells dies of cancer. Although devils have a functioning immune system, their limited MHC diversity prevents them from recognizing the tumor cells as foreign. (The tumor cells appear to have originated from Schwann cells from a female devil in the early 1990s but are continuing to evolve).

Facial tumor cells do not express surface MHC class I due to downregulation of their β2-microglobulin and TAP genes. This downregulation is a result of epigenetic deacetylation of histones. Thus, there is no histocompatibility barrier to tumor growth. Although devils have functioning NK cells, these cannot kill the tumor cells for unknown reasons. MHC expression can be restored by exposing facial tumor cells to recombinant devil IFN-γ and subsequent activation of the MHC class II transactivator, a critical transcription factor. Blood mononuclear cells activated by mitogens in vitro can also kill devil tumor cells (Brown et al., 2016). Encouraging results have been obtained by vaccinating animals with killed adjuvanted tumor cells. It also appears that resistance to the DFT1 strain of cancer is emerging in some wild populations. Thus, transmission has slowed, and mortality is reduced.

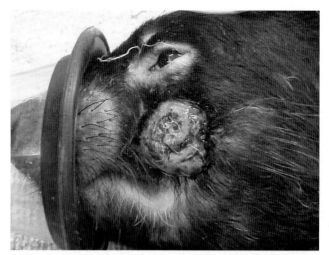

Fig. 36.8 A Tasmanian devil with facial tumor disease. Courtesy Dr. David Phalen.

A second, genetically distinct facial tumor variant (DFT2) has also been recognized in devils (Pye et al., 2016a). It originated in a male devil and shows a preference for male hosts. Unfortunately, it mutates more rapidly and is thus a major threat to the surviving devils.

Swine Melanomas

The Sinclair melanoma-bearing swine is an inbred line that spontaneously develops melanomas (Misfeldt and Grimm, 1994). Most such tumors are benign and regress spontaneously. However, some are malignant and lethal. The tumor regression seen in most of these pigs is immunologically mediated. The tumors are invaded by macrophages, and at the same time, the animals generate non-MHC-restricted cytotoxic CD4−, CD8−, and γ/δ+ T cells. Pigs with regressing melanomas possess an expanded population of CD8hi T cells (Cizkova et al., 2018). Recovering pigs may also produce antibodies against melanoma antigens.

VIRUS-INDUCED TUMORS

Equine Sarcoids

Sarcoids are the commonest skin cancers in horses. They are locally aggressive fibroblastic tumors associated with abortive infection by bovine papillomavirus types 1 and 2. They are persistent and often recur following surgery. Nevertheless, they may be amenable to immunotherapy. Sarcoids are characteristically infiltrated by CD8+ and CD4+ T cells. If BCG vaccine is infiltrated into the tissues between the tumor and normal skin, regression occurs in about two-thirds of cases. Related immunostimulants, such as Mycobacterial cell walls, have also been used to treat this tumor. They possess the advantage of not rendering an animal tuberculin positive. The rate of regression depends on the size of the tumor (surgical debulking is required to remove most of the tumor mass), and multiple treatments are usually necessary for a complete cure. The immune response modifier Imiquimod has both antiviral and antitumor activities. It has been used to treat sarcoids topically with encouraging results (Nogueira et al., 2006). Sarcoids are also responsive to other immunostimulants such as killed *P. acnes* and the antiviral drug acyclovir (Hollis, 2022).

Ocular Squamous Cell Carcinomas

Ocular squamous cell carcinoma is a common and economically important cancer of cattle that responds to immunotherapy. One successful treatment involves inoculation of affected animals with a phenol-saline extract of allogeneic carcinoma cells. This suggests that these cells possess tumor-associated antigens. Indeed, sera from affected cattle can react with tumor cells (but not normal cells) obtained from the eyes of other cattle. It is also of interest to note that sera from some cattle with ocular squamous cell carcinoma also react with equine sarcoid and bovine papilloma cells, implying that all three may have a common cause.

LYMPHOID TUMORS

Adaptive immunity requires that lymphocytes stimulated by exposure to antigen respond by division and differentiation. Much of the complexity of the immune system is due to the need to control this response. A failure may result in uncontrolled lymphoid cell proliferation and the development of lymphoid tumors. The surveillance theory was originally proposed when it was observed that immunosuppressed animals and humans had an increased prevalence of cancers. However, an unusually high proportion of these are of lymphoid origin. Therefore, it is likely that some of the lymphoid tumors that develop in immunosuppressed individuals result from a failure of immunological regulation rather than from a failure of surveillance.

Normal immune responses, whether antibody- or cell-mediated, involve a burst of rapid proliferation in lymphocytes. This burst of proliferation must be carefully controlled (see Chapter 18). Although uncontrolled lymphocyte function may induce autoimmunity, uncontrolled lymphocyte proliferation may result in the development of a lymphoma or lymphosarcoma. It is no accident that animals with autoimmune disease are more likely than normal animals to develop lymphoid cell tumors (Table 36.1).

Several important viruses stimulate nonspecific lymphocyte proliferation. These include the maedi-visna virus, the Aleutian disease parvovirus, and the herpesvirus responsible for malignant catarrhal fever (MCF). MCF is a fatal lymphoproliferative disease of cattle and sheep characterized by lymphadenopathy with widespread tissue accumulations of lymphocytes. Lymphocytes from MCF-infected animals show prolonged growth in tissue culture.

Bovine Lymphosarcoma

Lymphosarcomas are the most common cancers of cattle in the United States. They occur in two main forms: an enzootic form and a sporadic form. The enzootic form is caused by bovine leukemia virus (BLV), a deltaretrovirus. BLV is spread by contaminated instruments, by vaccines containing blood, by biting flies, or by calves who may be infected in utero. It has recently been detected in human blood and breast tissue (Buehring et al., 2019). In the United States, about 84% of dairy operations are infected with BLV based on testing of bulk milk samples. About 60%–65% of infected cattle are clinically normal, 30%–40% develop a persistent lymphocytosis (PL), and less than 5% develop lymphosarcomas. The primary target of the virus is the MHCII+, IgM+, and CD5+ B cell. The virus integrates randomly into the cellular genome. Early in infection, the proportion of B cells in peripheral blood increases before there is a significant increase in the number of blood lymphocytes. Eventually, some infected animals develop a PL with lymphocyte counts in the range of 20,000–80,000/μL. Not all BLV-infected cattle develop PL, although 95% of cattle with this condition are infected with BLV. These lymphocytes may be enlarged, CD5+, express increased levels of IgM, and have altered glycosylation. Cells in PL are not malignant and can occasionally return to the normal state. BLV becomes stably integrated into these B cells. About 1%–5% of BLV-infected cattle develop a multicentric lymphosarcoma between 1 and 8 years after infection. Susceptibility to cancer development differs among species. Sheep are very sensitive, cattle have intermediate sensitivity, and goats are the least sensitive. Animals that develop these cancers die within 3–6 months.

BLV is essential for neoplastic transformation but not for the continued growth of cancer cells. The mechanism by which BLV initiates tumor development is unclear since there is no rearrangement of any known oncogenes. A viral gene called *Tax* appears to initiate tumorigenesis. *Tax* encodes a transactivating protein that can turn on many different cellular genes and that deregulates many different regulatory pathways, rather than a single key pathway. Animals with advanced clinical bovine leukosis may be immunosuppressed as a result of the presence in their serum of a suppressor factor. This suppression is reflected by reduced numbers of T cells, less responsive B cells, lowered serum IgM and IgG2 responses, and reduced responses to many vaccines. Circulating Foxp3+ Treg numbers are also increased. Occasionally, the neoplastic cells in bovine leukosis may be sufficiently differentiated to secrete immunoglobulin as in myelomas. The cells in the sporadic form of bovine leukosis are predominantly T cells, but some originating from pre-B cells have also been identified.

Lymphomas in Other Species

In sheep, lymphomas are divided fairly evenly between T and B cells, and about 15% are unclassifiable (null cells). Some of these may be due

TABLE 36.1	Immunosuppressive Effects of Lymphoid Tumors			
Tumor	Cell Type	Evidence for Immunosuppression	Mechanisms
Feline leukemia	T cell	Lymphopenia Prolonged skin grafts Increased susceptibility to infection Lack of response to mitogens	Suppressive viral protein, p15E Suppressor cells
Marek's disease	T cell	Lack of response to mitogens Depressed cell-mediated cytotoxicity Depressed IgG production	Suppressor macrophages
Avian lymphoid leucosis	B cell	Increased susceptibility to infection	Suppressor lymphocytes
Bovine leucosis	B cell	Depressed serum IgM	Soluble suppressor factor
Myeloma	B cell	Increased susceptibility to infection	Soluble tumor-cell factor Negative feedback
Canine malignant lymphoma	B cell	Predisposition to infection associated with autoimmune disorders	Unknown
Equine lymphosarcoma	T cell	Increased susceptibility to infection	Tumor of suppressor cells

to BLV infection. A B-cell lymphoma inherited as an autosomal recessive condition is recognized in swine.

Equine lymphomas are predominantly T-cell in origin although some equine B-cell lymphomas are T-cell rich. Horses with lymphosarcomas are commonly immunosuppressed. This usually involves T cells, but B-cell function may also be impaired. Equine B-cell neoplasms generally cause a monoclonal gammopathy. A case of a horse with a lymphosarcoma with suppressor cell activity has been described. The animal presented with signs of immunodeficiency and was found to be deficient in IgM. Equine T-cell lymphomas have been associated with immune-mediated anemia and thrombocytopenia.

Lymphomas account for 5%–7% of canine malignancies. There is no evidence to suggest that these tumors are virus induced. They may be classified according to their apparent site of origin (e.g., multicentric, alimentary, zonal, or anterior mediastinal) or alternatively, by their cell type (e.g., histiocytic, lymphocytic, lymphoblastic, or plasmacytic) or by their clinical course (acute or chronic) (Box 36.3).

T-cell lymphomas/leukemias account for about 30% of lymphoproliferative tumors in dogs. These T-cell lymphomas are quite heterogeneous, and while they are usually aggressive, some, such as T-zone lymphomas, are slowly growing. Immunophenotyping can be useful in classifying these T-cell lymphomas. CD4$^+$ is the commonest subtype. T-zone lymphomas are CD45$^-$. Aggressive T-cell lymphomas may be CD45$^+$. Cutaneous CD3$^+$T-cell lymphomas (mycosis fungoides) are common in old dogs. Eighty percent are CD8$^+$, whereas the remainder are double-negative. Most (70%) have γ/δ TCRs, especially if the tumor is confined to the epidermis.

Chronic lymphoid leukemia (CLL) is the most frequent form of canine leukemia. It is characterized by the presence of large numbers of mature lymphocytes in the blood. Animals may be asymptomatic, and the course of the disease is slow. About 70% of these cases involve CD3$^+$T cells, and most are large granular lymphocytes (LGLs). Of these LGLs, about 65% are α/β T cells, and the remainder are γ/δ T cells. The non-LGL T-cell CLL cases usually involve α/β T cells.

CD21$^+$ and CD79a$^+$ malignant B cells account for about 30% of canine CLL cases. B-cell CLL is overrepresented in small-breed dogs. Chronic myeloid leukemias are extremely rare in dogs. Acute leukemias, which are also less common in dogs, may be of B-cell origin (20%) or myeloid origin (70%). The rest of these acute leukemias are difficult to classify and are considered undifferentiated. Many of these tumor cells, both myeloid and lymphoid, express CD34. The prognosis of these acute leukemias is usually very poor. Low levels of MHC class II expression on canine B-cell lymphomas carry a poor prognosis. In many cases of canine lymphoma, affected dogs produce antibodies against crude tumor antigens. These antigens are not found on normal lymphoid cells.

BOX 36.3 Lymphomas Differ Greatly among Dog Breeds

When dog lymphoid tumors are phenotyped, significant differences are seen among breeds. For example, in Irish Wolfhounds, 100% of lymphoid tumors are of T-cell origin. In Golden Retrievers, 54% of lymphoid tumors are from T cells, and the other 46% are from B cells. In Cocker Spaniels, only 6.8% are from T cells, whereas 93.2% are of B-cell origin. These differences, however, are shared among related dog breeds. For example, among Toy breeds, 68% of lymphoid tumors are of T-cell origin, whereas only 34% of Terrier lymphomas are T cells. Sex and neutering do not influence this distribution.

From Modiano, J.F., Breen, M., Burnett, R.C., et al., 2005. Distinct B-cell and T-cell lymphoproliferative disease prevalence among dog breeds indicates heritable risk. Cancer Res. 65, 5654–5661.

REFERENCES

Ambrosius, L.A., Dhawan, D., Ramos-Vara, J.A., Ruple, A., Knapp, D.W., Childress, M.O., 2018. Quantification and prognostic value of programmed cell death ligand-1 expression in dogs with diffuse large B-cell lymphoma. AJVR 79, 643–649.

Ariyarathna, H., Thomson, N.A., Aberdein, D., Perrott, M.R., Munday, J.S., 2020. Increased programmed death ligand (PD-L1) and cytotoxic T-lymphocyte antigen-4 (CTLA-4) expression is associated with metastasis and poor prognosis in malignant canine mammary gland tumours. Vet. Immunol. Immunopathol. 230. https://doi.org/10.1016/j.vetimm.2020.110142

Atherton, M.J., Morris, J.S., Mcdermott, M.R., Lichty, B.D., 2016. Cancer immunology and canine malignant melanoma: a comparative review. Vet. Immunol. Immunopathol. 169, 15–26.

Bergman, P.J., 2018. Veterinary oncology immunotherapies. Vet. Clin. Small Anim. 48, 257–277.

Boussiotis, V.A., 2016. Molecular and biochemical aspects of the PD-1 checkpoint pathway. N. Engl. J. Med. 375, 1767–1778.

Brown, G.K., Tovar, C., Cooray, A.A., Kreiss, A., et al., 2016. Mitogen-activated Tasmanian devil blood mononuclear cells kill devil facial tumour disease cells. Immunol. Cell Biol. 94, 673–679.

Buehring, G.C., DeLaney, A., Shen, H., Chu, D.L., et al., 2019. Bovine leukemia virus discovered in human blood. BMC Infect. Dis. https://doi.org/10.1186/s12879-019-3891-9

Buracco, P., Martano, M., Morello, E., Ratto, A., 2002. Vaccine-associated-like fibrosarcoma at the site of a deep nonabsorbable suture in a cat. Vet. J. 163, 105–107.

Cizkova, J., Sinkorova, Z., Strnaova, K., Cervinova, M., et al., 2018. The role of αβ T cells in spontaneous regression of melanoma tumors in swine. Dev. Comp. Immunol. https://doi.org/10.1016/j.dci.2018.10.001.

Coussens, L.M., Werb, Z., 2002. Inflammation and cancer. Nature 420, 860–867.

Faro, T.A.S., de Oliveira, E.H.C., 2023. Canine transmissible venereal tumor—from general to molecular characteristics: a review. Anim. Genet. 54, 82–89.

Finocchiaro, L.M., Riveros, M.D., Glikin, G.C., 2009. Cytokine-enhanced vaccine and suicide gene therapy as adjuvant treatments of metastatic melanoma in a horse. Vet. Rec. 164, 278–279.

Gavazza, A., Lubas, G., Fridman, A., Peruzzi, D., et al., 2013. Safety and efficacy of a genetic vaccine targeting telomerase plus chemotherapy for the therapy of canine B-cell lymphoma. Human Gene. Therap. 24, 728–738.

Gill, V.L., Bergman, P.J., Baer, K.E., Craft, D., Leung, C., 2008. Use of imiquimod 5% cream (Aldara) in cats with multicentric squamous cell carcinoma in situ: 12 cases (2002-2005). Vet. Comp. Oncol. 6 (1), 55–64.

Hagemann, T., Balkwill, F., Lawrence, T., 2007. Inflammation and cancer: a double-edged sword. Cancer Cell 12, 300–301.

Hartley, G., Faulhaber, E., Caldwell, A., Coy, J., et al., 2017. Immune regulation of canine tumour and macrophage PD-L1 expression. Vet. Comp. Oncol. 15 (2), 534–549.

Hill, F.W.G., Klein, W.R., Hoyer, M.J., et al., 1994. Antitumor effect of locally injected low doses of recombinant human interleukin-2 in bovine vulval papilloma and carcinoma. Vet. Immunol. Immunopathol. 41, 19–29.

Hollis, A.R., 2022. Management of equine sarcoids. Vet. J. https://doi.org/10.1016/j.tvjl.2022.105926

Hu, Z.I., Link, V.M., Lima-Junior, D.S., Delaleu, J., et al., 2022. Immune checkpoint inhibitors unleash pathogenic immune responses against the microbiota. Proc. Natl. Acad. Sci. 119 (26). https://doi.org/10.1073/pnas.2200348119.

Kannegieter, N.J., Schaaf, K.L., Lovell, D.K., et al., 2010. Myofibroblastic fibrosarcoma with multifocal osseous metaplasia at the site of equine influenza vaccination. Aust. Vet. J. 88, 132–136.

Klingemann, H., 2018. Immunotherapy for dogs: running behind humans. Front. Immunol. https://doi.org/10.3389/fimmu.2018.00133.

Li, Q., Withoff, S., Verma, I.M., 2005. Inflammation-associated cancer: NF-kappaB is the lynchpin. Trends Immunol. 26, 318–325.

Mantovani, A., Allavena, P., Sica, A., Balkwill, F., 2008. Cancer-related inflammation. Nature 454, 436-444

Martano, M., Morello, E., Buracco, P., 2011. Feline injection-site sarcoma: past, present and future perspectives. Vet. J. 188, 136–141.

Miller, R.L., Gerster, J.F., Owens, M.L., Slade, H.B., Tomai, M.A., 1999. Imiquimod applied topically: a novel immune response modifier and new class of drug. Int. J. Immunopharmacol. 21 (1), 1–14.

Misfeldt, M.L., Grimm, D.R., 1994. Sinclair miniature swine: an animal model of human melanoma. Vet. Immunol. Immunopathol. 43, 167–175.

Monteiro, L.N., Rodrigues, M.A., Gomes, D.A., Salgado, B.S., Cassali, G.D., 2018. Tumour-associated macrophages: relation with progression and invasiveness, and assessment of M1/M2 macrophages in canine mammary tumours. Vet. J. 234, 119–125.

Nogueira, S.A.F., Torres, S.M.F., Malone, E.D., Diaz, S.F., et al., 2006. Efficacy of imiquimod 5% cream in the treatment of equine sarcoids: a pilot study. Vet. Dermatol. 17 (4), 259–265.

O'Connor, C.M., Wilson-Robles, H., 2014. Developing T cell cancer immunotherapy in the dog with lymphoma. ILAR J. 55, 169–181.

Pellin, M.A., 2022. The use of oncept melanoma vaccine in veterinary patients: a review of the literature. Vet. Sci. https://doi.org/10.3390/vetsci9110597.

Peruzzi, D., Gavazza, A., Mesiti, G., Lubas, G., Scarselli, E., et al., 2010. A vaccine targeting telomerase enhances survival of dogs affected by B-cell lymphoma. Mol. Therap. 18, 1559–1567.

Porcellato, I., Brachelente, C., Cappelli, K., Menchetti, L., et al., 2021. FoxP3, CTLA-4, and IDO in canine melanocytic tumors. Vet. Pathol. 58 (1), 42–52.

Pye, R.J., Pemberton, D., Tovar, C., Tubio, J.M., et al., 2016a. A second transmissible cancer in Tasmanian devils. Proc. Natl. Acad. Sci. U.S.A. 113, 374–379.

Pye, R.J., Woods, G.M., Kreiss, A., 2016b. Devil facial tumor disease. Vet. Pathol. 53, 726–736.

Rue, S.M., Eckelman, B.P., Efe, J.A., Bloink, K., Deverux, Q.L., et al., 2015. Identification of a candidate therapeutic antibody for treatment of canine B-cell lymphoma. Vet. Immunol. Immunopathol. 164, 148–159.

Sharma, P., Goswami, S., Raychaudhuri, D., Siddiqui, B.A., et al., 2023. Immune checkpoint therapy-current perspectives and future directions. Cell 186, 1652–1669.

Srivastav, A., Kass, P.H., Mcgill, L.D., Farver, T.B., Kent, M.S., 2012. Comparative vaccine-specific and other injectable-specific risks of injection-site sarcomas in cats. J. Am. Vet. Med. Assoc. 241, 595–602.

Teng, M.W., Khanna, R., Smyth, M.J., 2016. Checkpoint immunotherapy: picking a winner. Cancer Discov. 6, 818–820.

Terziev, G., Roydev, R., Kalkanov, I., Borissov, I., Dinev, I., 2015. Papillomatosis in heifers. Comparative studies on surgical excision and autogenous vaccine therapies. Traka J. Sci. 13, 274–279.

Verganti, S., Berlato, D., Blackwood, L., Amores-Fuster, I., Polton, G.A., 2016. Use of oncept melanoma vaccine in 69 canine oral malignant melanomas in the UK. J. Small Anim. Pract. 58, 10–16.

Waldman, A.D., Fritz, J.M., Lenardo, M.J., 2020. A guide to cancer immunotherapy: from T cell basic science to clinical practice. Nat. Rev. Immunol. 20, 651–668.

Wong, S.Y., Reiter, J.F., 2011. Wounding mobilizes hair follicle stem cells to form tumors. Proc. Natl. Acad. Sci. U.S.A. 108, 4093–4098.

Wormser, C., Mariano, A., Holmes, E.S., Aronson, L.R., Volk, S.W., 2016. Post-transplant malignant neoplasia associated with cyclosporine-based immunotherapy: prevalence, risk factors and survival in feline renal transplant recipients. Vet. Comp. Oncol. 14 (4), e126–e134.

Zamora, A.E., Crawford, J.C., Thomas, P.G., 2018. Hitting the target: how T cells detect and eliminate tumors. J. Immunol. 200, 392–399.

37

Autoimmune Diseases and the Loss of Tolerance

Autoimmune diseases are relatively common. They occur in about 5% of humans and probably in a similar proportion of dogs and cats. Most result from the emergence of clones of "rogue" lymphocytes directed against normal body components. The fact that they tend to develop late in life suggests that these diseases, like cancer, are probably the result of accumulated random mutations. Thus, while one mutation alone may be insufficient to permit an autoimmune response, multiple mutations may collectively permit self-reactive lymphocytes to develop (Goodnow, 2007). Given the ubiquity of microbial and environmental antigens, lymphocytes are under constant pressure to proliferate. The presence of a constant supply of self-antigens is especially significant. Much of the complexity of the immune system results from the need to prevent inappropriate lymphocyte proliferation.

Lymphocyte responses are regulated by many different mechanisms. These include negative selection within the thymus, the requirement for multiple costimulatory signals, the need for lymphocyte cooperation, and the activities of regulatory cell populations. These regulatory mechanisms are effective so that the development of self-reactive rogue clones does not occur suddenly. It takes multiple individual defects, acting collectively, to cause the eventual loss of control of specific lymphocyte proliferation (Theofilopoulos et al., 2017).

By evolving antigen receptor systems that can bind to as many microbial antigens as possible, vertebrates also developed the potential for self-destruction. The random generation of antigen-binding receptors ensures that many lymphocytes are produced with receptors that can bind self-antigens. It has been estimated that as many as 50% of newly produced T cells and B cells may have receptors able to bind normal body components with high affinity. These self-reactive cells are usually rigorously suppressed. Many additional factors influence susceptibility to autoimmunity. These include sex and age, genetic background, the microbiota, and virus infections. We also know that the development of autoantibodies is a relatively common event that, by itself, does not inevitably lead to autoimmune disease. Indeed, some autoantibodies serve a physiological function.

Because we do not know precisely what triggers most autoimmune diseases in animals, this chapter reviews some of the many predisposing factors that have been identified, as well as the mechanisms by which autoimmunity causes tissue damage and disease. As with other immune functions, both B and T cells can mediate autoimmunity. Thus some autoimmune diseases are mediated by autoantibodies alone. In others, the damage may be mediated by self-reactive T cells alone or by some combination of autoantibodies and T cells. It is also important to point out that inappropriate innate immune responses may also occur, resulting in the development of severe inflammatory diseases (Tizard, 2023).

INDUCTION OF AUTOIMMUNITY

Autoimmune diseases appear to develop spontaneously, and predisposing causes are rarely obvious. Nevertheless, they fall into two major categories: they can result from a normal immune response to an unusual or abnormal antigen, or they can result from an abnormal immune response to a normal antigen (Fig. 37.1). The second category is probably the most common. In these cases, the mechanisms that normally prevent the development of self-responsive T and B cells fail. Many different environmental factors and genes contribute to this failure, and the failure may not always be complete. Autoimmune diseases may result from an aberrant response to a single specific antigen; alternatively, they may be due to a defect in the regulation of innate immune mechanisms as well as B- or T-cell functions. They may be triggered by infections and are, in effect, collateral damage from the defensive immune responses (Sfriso et al., 2009).

Normal Immune Responses

Many autoimmune responses simply reflect a normal immune response to an antigen that has been previously hidden or result from cross-reactivity between an infectious agent and normal body components. Many of these naturally occurring autoantibodies play a role in immune regulation. They are usually low-titer, low-affinity IgM or IgG antibodies directed against hidden or intracellular proteins, protein fragments, or even damaged proteins (Bach, 2002).

Cryptic Antigens

Many autoimmune responses are triggered when nontolerant T cells meet previously hidden autoantigens. After all, T cells can only be

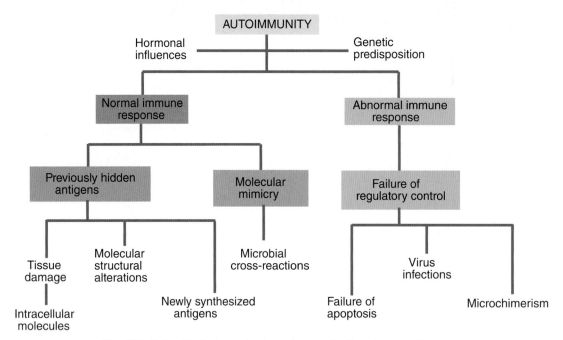

Fig. 37.1 A simplified scheme for the pathogenesis of autoimmune diseases.

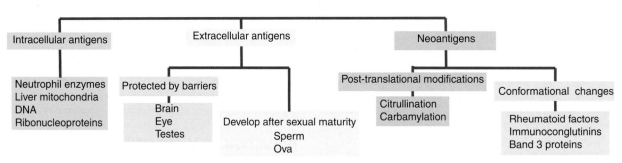

Fig. 37.2 Sources of the many different autoantigens that can be implicated in autoimmune diseases. *DNA,* Deoxyribonucleic acid.

made tolerant to autoantigens if they interact with them. While thymic epithelial cells can present them with many self-antigens, it is impossible to expose developing T cells to every normal protein. As a result, there are many autoantigens that do not induce tolerance simply because they remain hidden within cells or tissues (Lutz et al., 2009).

For example, many autoantigens are found in places where they never encounter circulating lymphocytes. In the testes, new antigens may only appear at puberty, long after the T-cell system has developed tolerance to other autoantigens. The blood-testes barrier normally keeps them apart. Trauma to the testes may permit these proteins to reach the bloodstream, encounter antigen-sensitive cells, and stimulate an immune response. Antigens may also be found hidden within cells. For example, after a heart attack, autoantibodies may be produced against the mitochondria of cardiac muscle cells. In chronic hepatitis in dogs, animals develop antibodies to liver membrane proteins. In diseases such as trypanosomiasis or tuberculosis, in which widespread tissue damage occurs, many different autoantibodies appear in the serum.

Although the control of the immune system requires that self-reactive cells be eliminated through central or peripheral tolerance, one should not assume that all autoimmune responses are bad or even cause disease. Some autoimmune responses have physiological functions. For example, red blood cells must be removed from the bloodstream once they reach the end of their lifespan. This process is accomplished

by autoantibodies. As red cells age, an anion transport protein called CD233 (or band 3 protein) is gradually oxidized, and a new epitope is generated. This new epitope is recognized by IgG autoantibodies. These autoantibodies bind only to aged red cells and trigger their phagocytosis by splenic macrophages. CD233 is found in many different cell types, and it may be that its exposure to aged cells and their subsequent removal is a major cell elimination pathway (Fig. 37.2).

Antigens Generated by Conformational Changes

The production of some autoantibodies may also be triggered by the development of new, unique, epitopes on normal proteins. Two such examples are the rheumatoid factors (RFs) and the immunoconglutinins (IKs, after the German spelling).

RFs are autoantibodies directed against other immunoglobulins. When an antibody binds to an antigen, the shape of the immunoglobulin molecule changes in such a way that new epitopes are exposed on its Fc region. These new epitopes may trigger an immune response and RF formation. RFs are produced in diseases in which large amounts of immune complexes are generated. These include the autoimmune disease of joints called rheumatoid arthritis and systemic lupus erythematosus (SLE), in which B cells respond to many different autoantigens.

IKs are autoantibodies directed against epitopes on the complement components C2, C4, and especially C3. The epitopes that stimulate IK formation are exposed when these complement components are activated. The level of IKs found in serum reflects the amount of complement activation; this, in turn, is a measure of the antigenic stimulation to which an animal is subjected. IK levels are thus nonspecific indicators of the prevalence of infectious disease within an animal population. Their physiological role is unclear, but they probably enhance complement-mediated opsonization.

ABNORMAL IMMUNE RESPONSES

Failure of Regulatory Control

A sustained autoimmune response is necessary for disease to develop. This may result from a failure of the normal control mechanisms of the immune system and can be demonstrated simply by injecting mice with rat red blood cells. Following such an injection, mice not only make antibodies to the rat cells but also develop a transient autoimmune response to their own red blood cells. This autoimmune response is rapidly controlled by regulatory cells and lasts for only a few days. If, however, regulatory cell activity in these mice is impaired, as occurs in New Zealand Black (NZB) mice, for example, these autoantibodies will persist to cause mouse red blood cell destruction and anemia (Fig. 37.3; Khatlani et al., 2003). It is clear that Treg defects like this contribute to the pathogenesis of many autoimmune diseases (Zhang et al., 2020).

Autoimmune diseases are commonly associated with lymphoid tumors. For example, myasthenia gravis, an autoimmune disease targeting neuromuscular junctions, is associated with the presence of a thymoma in dogs. In humans, there is a fourfold increase in the incidence of rheumatoid arthritis in patients with malignant lymphoid tumors, and there is evidence for a similar association in other mammals. Since many lymphoid tumors result from a failure in immunological control mechanisms, a simultaneous failure in self-tolerance

may also occur. Alternatively, some lymphoid tumors may consist of cells producing autoantibodies. It is also possible that some lymphoid tumors, such as myelomas, may eventually develop as a result of prolonged stimulation of the immune system by autoantigens.

Potentially harmful, self-reactive lymphocytes are normally destroyed in the thymus by apoptosis triggered through the CD95 (Fas) pathway (see Chapter 19). Defects in CD95 or its, ligand CD154 (CD95L), can result in the development of autoimmunity by permitting abnormal T cells to survive. This is seen in the *lpr* strain of mice. These animals have a mutation that alters the structure of the intracellular domain of CD95 and so blocks its functions. A mutation (called *gld*) in CD95L has a similar effect. Both *lpr* and *gld* mice develop multiple autoimmune lesions accompanied by lymphoproliferation. A mutation in the *fas* gene resulting in an autoimmune lymphoproliferative syndrome has also been recorded in British shorthair cats (Aberdein et al., 2017).

The autoimmune regulator (*aire*) gene regulates T-cell development and permits thymic epithelial cells to express multiple self-antigens (see Chapter 13; Passos et al., 2017). T cells that respond to these self-antigens are eliminated. As a result, humans with a defective *aire* gene develop autoimmune disease involving multiple endocrine organs and the skin (Proekt et al., 2017). It should also be pointed out that negative selection within the thymus is critical, but it does not eliminate every self-reactive T cell.

Infection-Induced Autoimmunity

Autoimmune diseases may be triggered by infectious agents. Given, however, that infections are very common and autoimmune diseases are fairly rare, they clearly cannot account for the entire autoimmune process. For example, mice infected with certain reoviruses develop an autoimmune polyendocrine disease characterized by diabetes mellitus and retarded growth. These reovirus-infected mice make autoantibodies

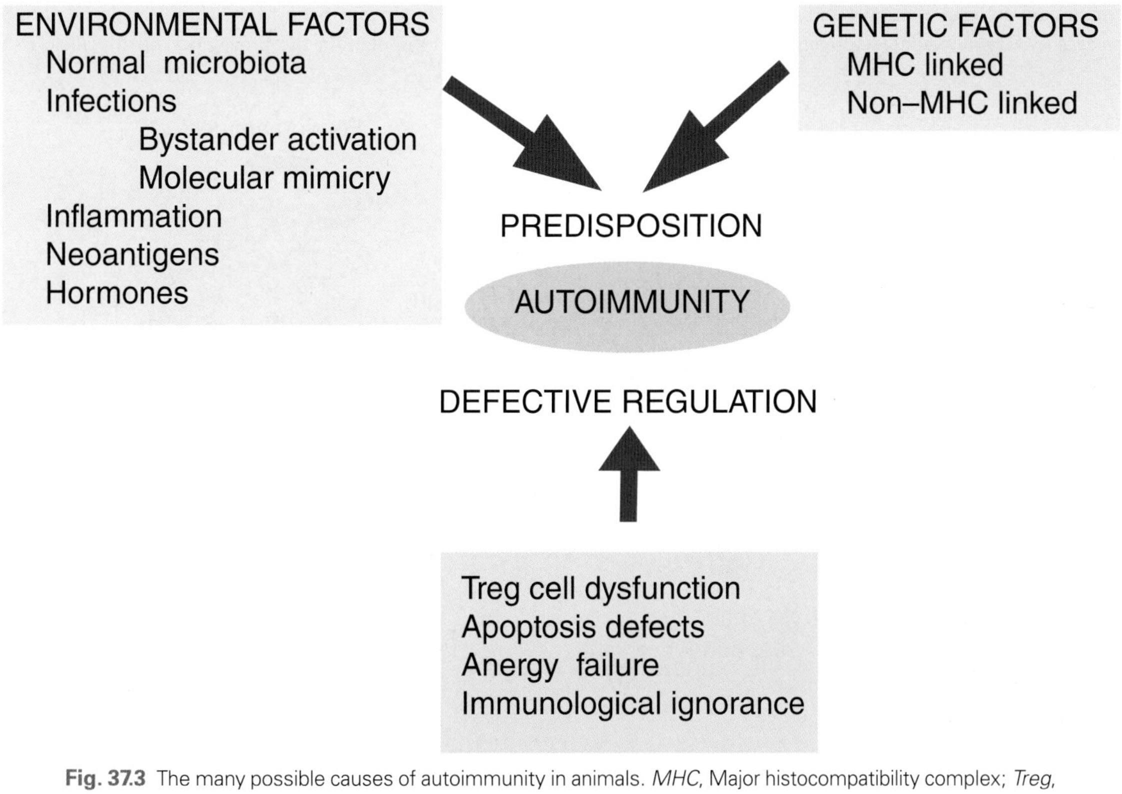

Fig. 37.3 The many possible causes of autoimmunity in animals. *MHC,* Major histocompatibility complex; *Treg,* regulatory T cells.

against normal pituitary, pancreas, gastric mucosa, nuclei, glucagon, growth hormone, and insulin. Likewise, in NZB mice, persistent infection with a type C retrovirus leads to the production of autoantibodies against nucleic acids and red blood cells. Bacteria such as *Streptococcus pyogenes*, *Borrelia burgdorferi*, and *Leptospira interrogans* may trigger autoimmune heart disease, arthritis, and uveitis, respectively. The protozoan parasite *Trypanosoma cruzi* triggers an autoimmune cardiomyopathy. SARS-CoV-2 infection, the cause of COVID-19, triggers the production of antiphospholipid autoantibodies.

The situation with spontaneous autoimmune disease is less clear. Many attempts have been made to isolate viruses from patients with autoimmune disease, but with mixed results. For example, SLE of dogs and humans has been associated with either a type C retrovirus or paramyxovirus infection. Small quantities of the Epstein-Barr virus genome can be found in the salivary glands of humans with Sjögren's syndrome. Moreover, epidemiological evidence points to some form of a viral trigger for human autoimmune diseases such as multiple sclerosis, rheumatoid arthritis, and insulin-dependent diabetes mellitus. Just how viruses can induce autoimmunity is unclear, but three major mechanisms are recognized, molecular mimicry, epitope spreading, and bystander activation.

Molecular Mimicry

Molecular mimicry is a term used to describe the sharing of epitopes between an infectious agent and an autoantigen (Fig. 37.4). B cells may be triggered by a foreign epitope that happens to cross-react with an autoantigen (Oldstone, 1998). However, they will only respond to this epitope if they also receive T-cell help. If nearby Th cells also recognize these microbial epitopes as foreign, they may trigger a B-cell response and the production of autoantibodies. Once a B-cell response is triggered in this way, the infectious agent may be removed while the autoimmune response continues—a "hit-and-run" process (Ercolini and Miller, 2009). Some of these cross-reacting antigens (termed mimotopes) may come from the intestinal microbiota (Ruff et al., 2019).

Many examples of molecular mimicry are now recognized. For example, the parasite *T. cruzi* contains antigens that cross-react with

mammalian neurons and cardiac muscle. Dogs infected with *T. cruzi* make autoantibodies that can cause nervous system and heart disease. Molecular mimicry also causes the heart lesions of rheumatic fever in children. Antibodies to the cell wall M-protein of group A streptococci cross-react with cardiac myosin. Children infected with certain strains of group A streptococci produce antimyocardial antibodies and develop heart disease. Some strains of streptococci may cause acute glomerulonephritis in children as a result of the production of antibodies cross-reacting with glomerular basement membranes (Cunningham, 2019). Other examples of molecular mimicry include the Epstein-Barr virus DNA polymerase, which cross-reacts with myelin basic protein and may be involved in the pathogenesis of multiple sclerosis, and the poliovirus capsid protein VP2, which cross-reacts with the acetylcholine receptor and may induce myasthenia gravis (Rojas et al., 2018).

The integrin CD11a/18 (LFA-1) shares an antigenic determinant with the outer surface protein of the Lyme disease bacterium, *B. burgdorferi*. Patients infected with this organism mount an initial immune response that may then develop into autoimmunity. In about 10% of humans with Lyme arthritis, antibiotics fail to resolve the arthritis, suggesting that, once triggered, the autoimmune process can proceed in the absence of the bacterium.

Antibodies against microbial heat shock proteins are found in the serum of humans and rats with rheumatoid arthritis, ankylosing spondylitis, and SLE. Injection of killed *Mycobacterium tuberculosis* in Freund's complete adjuvant can cause arthritis in rats, and T cells from these animals can transfer arthritis to normal syngeneic recipients. These T cells are responding to HSP 60, a mycobacterial heat shock protein (see Chapter 27). It has been suggested that molecular mimicry between microbial and mammalian HSP 60 may be important in initiating rheumatoid arthritis.

Ankylosing spondylitis is an autoimmune arthritis of humans that affects the sacroiliac joints, spine, and peripheral joints. Patients also develop acute anterior uveitis (inflammation of the iris and neighboring structures in the eye). More than 95% of humans with ankylosing spondylitis possess the MHC class I allele HLA-B27, whereas in the normal population, the prevalence of this allele is less than 8%.

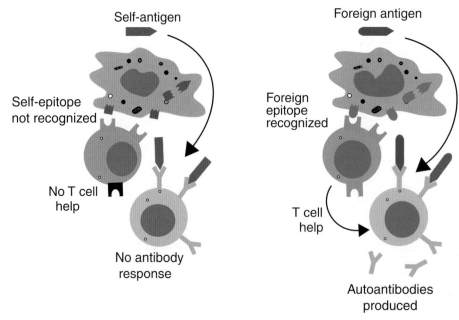

Fig. 37.4 Cross-reactions with foreign antigens (molecular mimicry) may be sufficient to trigger a helper T-cell population that will promote an autoimmune response by B cells. A helper effect triggered by a foreign antigen may inadvertently permit an autoimmune response to occur.

The disease results from molecular mimicry between the hypervariable region of HLA-B27 and antigens found in *Klebsiella pneumoniae*. *K. pneumoniae* is found more frequently than normal in the intestine of patients with active ankylosing spondylitis and uveitis, and patients with active disease have elevated levels of IgA against *Klebsiella* in their sera. Cloning of B27 into mice and subsequent infection of these animals with *K. pneumoniae* causes an acute spondylitis. HLA-B27-associated ankylosing spondylitis has been described in gorillas. Up to 20% of wild gorillas may have spondylitis, and the disease has also been described in a gibbon, in baboons, and in rhesus macaques.

In porcine enzootic pneumonia caused by *Mycoplasma hyopneumoniae*, antibodies to the mycoplasma cross-react with pig lungs. In contagious bovine pleuropneumonia, there is cross-reactivity between *Mycoplasma mycoides* antigens and normal bovine lung. There is a clear causal relationship between *L. interrogans* infection, antigenic cross-reactivity, and the development of periodic ophthalmia, the leading cause of blindness in horses (see Chapter 38).

Epitope Spreading

In some cases, autoimmunity seems to result from a normal immune response against a foreign antigen that subsequently "spreads" to recognize self-antigens. When an immune response is initiated, the initial immune response is directed against a single epitope on the inciting antigen. However, as receptor editing continues, T- and B-cell receptors diversify by somatic mutation, and receptors begin to be directed against additional epitopes. At first, they will react with other epitopes on the same protein. Eventually, however, receptors may be able to bind to epitopes on autoantigens. Epitope spreading has been demonstrated in diseases such as thyrotoxicosis and diabetes mellitus.

Bystander Activation

When viruses destroy cells, previously hidden antigens may be released. These may activate nearby lymphocytes that had not been directly involved in the antiviral response. Additionally, T cells might, in responding to an antigen, produce a mixture of cytokines, such as tumor necrosis factors, that can activate nearby cells and trigger an autoimmune response. Pathogens may trigger inappropriate lymphocyte proliferation by acting through pattern-recognition receptors to generate costimulatory molecules and proinflammatory mediators. These cytokines may activate previously quiescent T cells. As a result, nearby T cells may be triggered to attack autoantigens that they previously ignored (Fig. 37.5).

PREDISPOSING FACTORS

Genetic Predisposition

Although viruses or other infectious agents may trigger autoimmunity, it is clear that not all infected individuals develop autoimmune disease. This is because genetic factors are key determinants of disease susceptibility. Genome-wide association studies have identified hundreds of loci that harbor risk factors for autoimmune diseases. Many of these are shared by multiple diseases. It is clear from these studies, however, that the associations so far identified do not account for all genetic effects, and the effect at any individual locus is very small (Zenewicz et al., 2010).

The genes most commonly associated with naturally occurring autoimmune diseases are those in the MHC (Inshaw et al., 2018). MHC molecules regulate the presentation of processed epitopes. In theory, therefore, they determine resistance or susceptibility to many diseases.

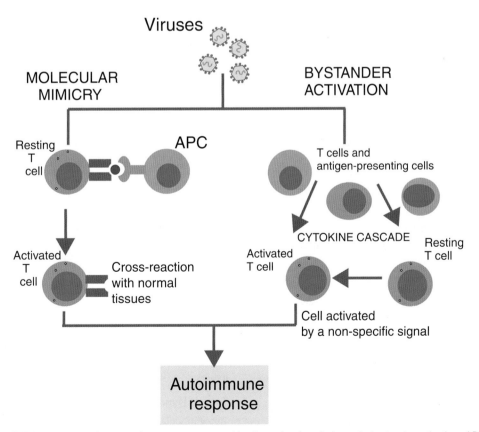

Fig. 37.5 Viruses may trigger autoimmune responses either by molecular mimicry or by bystander activation. *APC*, Antigen-presenting cells.

In practice, there is selection for MHC genes that permit a strong response to most common infectious pathogens (Kennedy et al., 2006a, 2006b). Studies of humans have shown that almost all autoimmune diseases are linked to multiple MHC loci (Holder et al., 2015). Presumably, an essential prerequisite for any autoimmune disease is that the autoantigen is appropriately processed and presented to a helper T cell by an MHC molecule. Thus the structure of the MHC antigen-binding groove determines whether or not a specific autoantigen can trigger an immune response. Some MHC alleles appear to protect against autoimmunity, and any predisposition to autoimmunity may be the result of the net effect of both enhancing and protective genes. In addition, most autoimmune diseases are associated with multiple MHC alleles (Box 37.1).

Dogs are the species in which veterinarians encounter most autoimmune diseases. Most current dog breeds have been developed as a result of aggressive phenotypic selection, in many cases resulting in inbreeding and a lack of genetic diversity (Gough et al., 2018). This has had two effects. First, it has permitted deleterious autosomal recessive genes to be expressed, as is seen in the increased prevalence of immunological disorders. Second, it has resulted in a loss of MHC polymorphism. For example, DRB1*04 is found in most Boxers, DRB1*2401 may be restricted to Akitas, DRB1*01 predominates in West Highland White Terriers, DQA*0203 is restricted to Dobermans, there is a high prevalence of DQA*0102 in Irish Wolfhounds and Chows, and DRB1*0101 is common in Irish Setters. These limited haplotypes ensure that the dogs in these breeds will respond to an unusually narrow range of antigens, thus making such dogs more susceptible to immunologic diseases (Jokinen et al., 2011).

Autoimmunity is encountered in some dog breeds more commonly than in others (Wiles et al., 2017). Old English sheepdogs are unusually prone to develop autoimmune blood diseases (Gershony et al., 2019). Certain autoimmune diseases, such as hypothyroidism, have familial associations. In dogs, there are several recognized associations between autoimmunity and MHC alleles. Diabetes mellitus is associated with DLA-A3, -A7, -A10, and -B4; antinuclear antibody production is associated with DLA-12; SLE is associated with DLA-A7; and autoimmune polyarthritis is associated with certain C4 alleles. Possession of an allele of DLA-79 (DLA-79*001:02) is associated with multiple immune-mediated diseases (hemolytic anemia, thrombocytopenia, polyarthritis, and atopic dermatitis) (Friedenberg et al., 2016).

Intestinal Microbiota

It is now well accepted that the intestinal microbiota both contribute to local host defenses and modulate systemic immune responses (Ochoa-Reparaz et al., 2009). Nutrients and microbial components are continually released into the body, where they influence immune cell function. In critically ill animals, breakdown of the intestinal epithelium and mucosal barriers may permit excessive leakage of bacterial components into the body (Van Praet et al., 2015). Conversely, depletion of the gut microbiome, especially as a result of antibiotic treatment, may make the mucosal defenses vulnerable and perhaps reduce the priming of the systemic immune responses. Because the gut microbiota influences the development of immunological tolerance, dysbiosis also affects the development of autoimmune diseases (see Chapter 22; Miyauchi et al., 2023).

Nonobese diabetic (NOD) mice develop spontaneous IDDM associated with infiltration of the pancreatic islets by lymphocytes. Their disease resembles human type 1 diabetes. The development of diabetes in these mice is influenced by their microbiota. Thus conventional NOD mice that lack MyD88 protein (MyD88 is the adaptor molecule for the toll-like receptors) do not develop diabetes, whereas totally germ-free MyD88⁻ NOD mice do. If commensal bacteria are fed to these germ-free mice, their diabetes will be less severe. Somehow the interaction of the intestinal microbiota with the immune system influences the predisposition of these mice to develop diabetes (Chervonsky, 2013).

Alterations in the intestinal microbiota also influence autoimmune diseases such as rheumatoid arthritis, systemic lupus, ankylosing spondylitis, insulin-dependent diabetes mellitus, and experimental autoimmune encephalitis (see Chapter 39; Huang et al., 2019; Rogers, 2015; Jeffrey et al., 2017). In some mouse arthritis models, changes in the gut microbiota due to antibiotic treatment can exacerbate the disease. Antinuclear antibody production in mice is also influenced by the microbiota, especially by increased colonization with segmented filamentous bacteria. The hygiene hypothesis appears to apply strongly to the development of autoimmune diseases in domestic pets, as demonstrated by their increasing prevalence (Bach, 2017; Wu et al., 2010).

MECHANISMS OF TISSUE DAMAGE IN AUTOIMMUNITY

Autoimmune disease results when tissues are damaged by autoreactive T cells or antibodies. This damage is a result of hypersensitivity reactions. However, multiple mechanisms may act together in any such disease, and their contributions may vary over time.

Type I Hypersensitivity

Milk allergy in cattle is an autoimmune disease in which a milk protein (α-casein), normally found only in the udder, gains access to the general circulation and stimulates an autoimmune response. This happens when milking is delayed and intramammary pressure forces the α-casein into the circulation. For unknown reasons, this triggers a Th2 response, and IgE autoantibodies are produced. As a result, affected cows may develop acute anaphylaxis if they are not milked regularly and casein reaches their bloodstream. (see Chapter 31). A similar condition is seen occasionally in mares. Although antibodies to milk proteins are commonly found in human serum after rapid weaning, type I hypersensitivity is not a usual sequel (Campbell, 1970).

Type II Hypersensitivity

Autoantibodies may cause target cell lysis with the assistance of complement or cytotoxic cells. Thus autoantibodies directed against red blood cells cause autoimmune hemolytic anemia; if directed against platelets, thrombocytopenia will occur; and if directed against thyroid cells, thyroiditis will result. In one form of this process in humans, autoantibodies against thyroid-stimulating hormone (TSH) receptors on thyroid cells stimulate thyroid activity rather than its destruction. Cell surface receptors are common targets of autoimmune attack. In addition to the TSH receptor, autoantibodies attack the acetylcholine receptor in myasthenia gravis and the insulin receptor in some forms of diabetes. Autoantibodies to β-adrenoceptors (see Chapter 31) have been detected in some patients with asthma. By blocking β-receptors, these antibodies make the airways highly irritable, and affected individuals develop severe asthma.

Type III Hypersensitivity

Autoantibodies form immune complexes with autoantigens, and if produced in large quantities, these complexes are deposited in tissues where they cause inflammation. This is most significant in SLE, a disease in which many different autoantibodies are produced. Immune complexes deposited in glomeruli provoke a membranoproliferative glomerulonephritis (see Chapter 33). Similarly, in rheumatoid arthritis, immune complexes are deposited in synovial membranes and trigger local inflammation resulting in the development of severe arthritis.

Type IV Hypersensitivity

Many autoimmune diseases are mediated by T cells. Cytotoxic T cells can attack brain cells to cause demyelination in experimental allergic encephalitis and multiple sclerosis. Insulin-dependent diabetes mellitus may be due to a T cell–mediated attack because the diseased pancreatic islets are infiltrated by lymphocytes. Lymphocytes from diabetics may be cytotoxic for pancreatic islet cells in vitro. Although cytotoxic T cells can kill cells directly, some cytokines may also cause tissue damage. For example, TNF-α upregulates cell adhesion molecules, including selectins, facilitating migration of neutrophils into the lesions.

REFERENCES

Aberdein, D., Munday, J.S., Gandolfi, B., Dittmer, K.E., et al., 2017. A FAS-ligand variant associated with autoimmune lymphoproliferative syndrome in cats. Mamm. Genome. 28, 47–55.

Bach, J.F., 2002. The effect of infections on susceptibility to autoimmune and allergic diseases. N. Engl. J. Med. 347, 911–918.

Bach, J.-F., 2017. The hygiene hypothesis in autoimmunity: the role of pathogens and commensals. Nat. Rev. Immunol. https://doi.org/10.1038/nri.2017.111.

Campbell, S.G., 1970. Milk allergy, an autoallergic disease of cattle. Cornell Vet. 60, 684–721.

Chervonsky, A.V., 2013. Microbiota and autoimmunity. Cold Spring Harb. Perspect. Biol. 5, a007294.

Cunningham, M.W., 2019. Molecular mimicry, autoimmunity and infection: the cross-reactive antigens of group A Streptococci and their sequelae. Microbiol. Spectr. https://doi.org/10.1128/microbiolspec GPP3-0045-2018.

Ercolini, A.M., Miller, S.D., 2009. The role of infections in autoimmune disease. Clin. Exp. Immunol. 155, 1–15.

Friedenberg, S.G., Buhrman, G., Chdid, L., Olby, N.J., et al., 2016. Evaluation of a DLA-79 allele associated with multiple immune-mediated diseases in dogs. Immunogenetics 68, 205–217.

Gershony, L.C., Belanger, J.M., Short, A.D., Le, M., et al., 2019. DLA class II risk haplotypes for autoimmune diseases in the bearded collie offer insight to autoimmunity signatures across dog breeds. Canine Genet. Epidemiol. https://doi.org/10.1186/s40575-019-0070-7.

Goodnow, C.C., 2007. Multistep pathogenesis of autoimmune disease. Cell 136, 25–35.

Gough, A., Thomas, A., O'Neill, D., 2018. Breed Predispositions to Disease in Dogs and Cats, third ed. Wiley Blackwell, Hoboken, NJ.

Holder, Al, Kennedy, L.J., Ollier, W.E.R., Catchpole, B., 2015. Breed differences in development of anti-insulin antibodies in diabetic dogs and investigation of the role of dog leukocyte antigen (DLA) genes. Vet. Immunol. Immunopathol. 167, 130–138.

Huang, C., Yi, X., Long, H., Zhang, G., et al., 2019. Disordered cutaneous microbiota in systemic lupus erythematosus. J. Autoimmun. https://doi.org/10.1016/j.jaut.2019.102391.

Inshaw, J.R.J., Cutler, A.J., Burren, O.S., Stefana, M.I., Todd, J.A., 2018. Approaches and advances in the genetic causes of autoimmune disease and their implications. Nat. Immunol. 19, 674–684.

Jeffrey, N., Barker, A.K., Alcott, C.J., Levine, J.M., et al., 2017. The association of specific constituents of the fecal microbiota with immune-mediated brain disease in dogs. PLOS One. https://doi.org/10.1371/journal.pone.0170589.

Jokinen, P., Rusanen, E.M., Kennedy, L.J., Lohi, H., 2011. MHC class II risk haplotype with canine chronic superficial keratitis in German Shepherd dogs. Vet. Immunol. Immunopathol. 140, 37–41.

Kennedy, L.J., Davison, L.J., Barnes, A., Short, A.D., et al., 2006a. Identification of susceptibility and protective major histocompatibility complex haplotypes in canine diabetes mellitus. Tissue Antigens 68, 467–476.

Kennedy, L.J., Davison, L.J., Barnes, A., Short, A.D., et al., 2006b. Identification of susceptibility and protective major histocompatibility complex haplotypes in canine diabetes mellitus. Tissue Antigens 68, 467–476.

Khatlani, T.S., Ma, Z., Okuda, M., Inokuma, H., Onishi, T., 2003. Autoantibodies against T-cell costimulatory molecules are produced in canine autoimmune diseases. J. Immunother. 26, 12–20.

Lutz, H.U., Binder, C.J., Kaveri, S., 2009. Naturally occurring auto-antibodies in homeostasis and disease. Trends Immunol. 30, 43–51.

Miyauchi, E., Shimokawa, C., Steimle, A., Desai, M.S., Ohno, H., 2023. The impact of the gut microbiota on extra-intestinal autoimmune diseases. Nat. Rev. Immunol. 23, 9–23.

Ochoa-Reparaz, J., Mielcarz, D.W., Ditrio, L.E., et al., 2009. Role of gut commensal microflora in the development of experimental autoimmune encephalomyelitis. J. Immunol. 183, 6041–6050.

Oldstone, M.B.A., 1998. Molecular mimicry and immune-mediated diseases. FASEB J. 12, 1255–1265.

Passos, G.A., Speck-Hernandez, C.A., Assis, F., Mendes-da-Cruz, D.A., 2017. Update on AIRE and thymic negative selection. Immunology 153, 10–20.

Proekt, I., Miller, C.N., Lionakis, M.S., Anderson, M.S., 2017. Insights into immune tolerance from AIRE deficiency. Curr. Opin. Immunol. 49, 71–78.

Rogers, G.B., 2015. Germs and joints: the contribution of the human microbiome to rheumatoid arthritis. Nat. Med. 21, 839–841.

Rojas, M., Restrepo-Jiminez, P., Monsalve, D.M., Pacheco, Y., et al., 2018. Molecular mimicry and autoimmunity. J. Autoimm. 95, 100–123.

Ruff, W.E., Dehner, C., Kim, W.J., Pagovich, O., et al., 2019. Pathogenic autoreactive T and B cells cross-react with mimotopes expressed by a common human gut commensal to trigger autoimmunity. Cell Host Microbe 26, 100–113.

Sfriso, P., Ghirardello, A., Botsios, C., et al., 2009. Infections and autoimmunity: the multifaceted relationship. J. Leukoc. Biol. 87, 385–395.

Tizard, I.R., 2023. Autoimmune Diseases in Domestic Animals. Elsevier, St. Louis, MO, ISBN 978-0-323-84813-8

Theofilopoulos, A.N., Kono, D.H., Baccala, R., 2017. The multiple pathways to autoimmunity. Nat. Immunol. 18, 716–724.

Van Praet, J.T., Donovan, E., Vanassche, I., Drennan, M.B., et al., 2015. Commensal microbiota influence systemic autoimmune responses. EMBO J. 34, 466–474.

Wiles, B.M., Llewellyn, A.M., Evans, K.M., O'Neill, D.G., Lewis, T.W., 2017. Large-scale survey to estimate the prevalence of disorders for 192 Kennel Club registered breeds. Canine Genet. Epidemiol. https://doi.org/10.1186/s40575-017-0047-3.

Wu, H.J., Ivanov, I.I., Darce, J., et al., 2010. Gut-residing segmented filamentous bacteria drive autoimmune arthritis via T helper 17 cells. Immunity 32, 815–827.

Zenewicz, L.A., Abraham, C., Flavell, R.A., Cho, J.H., 2010. Unraveling the genetics of autoimmunity. Cell 140, 791–797.

Zhang, X., Olsen, N., Zheng, S.G., 2020. The progress and prospect for regulatory T cells in autoimmune diseases. J. Autoimmun. https://doi.org/10.1016/j.jaut.2020.102461.

38

Selected Organ-Specific Autoimmune Diseases

CHAPTER OUTLINE

Animals, especially dogs, suffer from over 60 recognized autoimmune diseases. These diseases vary greatly in their pathogenesis. They form a continuum that ranges from "pure" autoinflammatory diseases at one end characterized by a loss of control of innate immune mechanisms to "pure" autoimmune diseases at the other extreme. Most immune-mediated diseases, however, fall between these two extremes.

Autoimmune diseases that mainly affect a single organ or tissue usually result from a "rogue" clone of B cells mounting an abnormal response to a small number of self-antigens and do not necessarily reflect loss of control of the immune system as a whole. All tissues of the body are potentially susceptible to this form of immunological attack. Nevertheless, autoimmune diseases directed against endocrine organs, skin, blood, reproductive and nervous systems, tend to be most common. Their prevalence in dogs depends to a great extent on the breed of an animal as well as its age (Tizard, 2023).

AUTOIMMUNE ENDOCRINE DISEASES

Although dogs develop autoimmune endocrine diseases, they differ from humans insofar as these tend to be targeted at single organs rather than involving multiple endocrine glands. Occasionally, a dog may experience two or more autoimmune endocrine disorders simultaneously (autoimmune polyglandular syndrome), usually affecting the thyroid and adrenals, but this is uncommon.

Lymphocytic Thyroiditis

Dogs, humans, and chickens suffer from autoimmune thyroiditis. In humans, this results from the production of autoantibodies against thyroglobulin or thyroid peroxidase. These antibodies may also react

with triiodothyronine (T_3) or thyroxin (T_4). Many dogs develop thyroiditis in the absence of these autoantibodies, and cell-mediated type 1 responses are believed to be responsible for thyroid destruction (Happ, 1995). Several dog breeds are predisposed to autoimmune thyroiditis, and relatives of affected animals may have antithyroid antibodies although clinically normal. A familial form of hypothyroidism has been demonstrated in Beagles and Great Danes. Dogs from high-risk breeds, such as Dobermans, tend to develop the disease when young, whereas dogs from low-risk breeds tend to develop it when older. Unfortunately, by the time the disease is diagnosed, the dog may already have bred. Affected thyroids are infiltrated with plasma cells and lymphocytes, and germinal center formation may occur (Fig. 38.1). The invading lymphocytes cause epithelial cell destruction through antibody-dependent cell–mediated cytotoxicity (ADCC) and T-cell cytotoxicity (Miller et al., 2015).

Disease onset is slow and insidious. Clinical signs appear after about 75% of the thyroid is destroyed. These signs are those of hypothyroidism; that is, the animals are fat and inactive and show patchy hair loss. The most common problems are a dry, dull, coarse coat; scaling; hypotrichosis; slow hair regrowth; hyperpigmentation; myxedema; and pyoderma. Tests of thyroid function, such as a radioimmunoassay for plasma T_4 or T_3, will confirm the existence of hypothyroidism. A thyroid-stimulating hormone (TSH) response test is more useful because it can confirm the inability of the affected thyroid to respond. (Plasma T_4 levels are measured before and after injection of TSH.) To confirm autoimmune thyroiditis, a biopsy must show the characteristic lymphocytic infiltration. Antithyroid antibodies must be detected in serum using an enzyme-linked immunosorbent assay, immunoblot, or an indirect fluorescent antibody test (see Chapter 43). There is often a

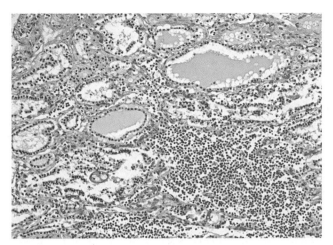

Fig. 38.1 A lymphocytic nodule in the thyroid of a dog suffering from auto-immune thyroiditis. Original magnification ×100. Courtesy Dr. G. Stoica.

poor correlation between antithyroid antibody titers and disease sever-ity, reflecting the importance of cell-mediated processes in this species. Management of affected animals involves replacement therapy with sodium levothyroxine.

Hyperthyroidism

Hyperthyroidism is a disease seen in old cats. Autoantibodies to thy-roid peroxidase have been demonstrated in almost one-third of cases of feline hyperthyroidism, and about 10% of these animals also pos-sess antinuclear antibodies. Lymphocytic infiltration is also observed in about one-third of cases. It is probable that these are secondary to the disease process and not its cause.

Lymphocytic Parathyroiditis

Dogs and cats can develop an autoimmune hypoparathyroiditis. Affected animals usually have a history of neurological or neuromus-cular disease, especially seizures. On investigation, animals are pro-foundly hypocalcemic, and serum parathormone levels are severely reduced. Normal parathyroid tissue is infiltrated by lymphocytes and plasma cells. Once hypocalcemic tetany is controlled, these animals may be treated by oral vitamin D and calcium administration. It would be logical to administer immunosuppressive therapy.

Autoimmune Diabetes Mellitus

Canine diabetes mellitus is a heterogeneous syndrome, and most cases have an unknown etiology. Some are probably immunologically medi-ated. The canine disease is associated with pancreatic islet atrophy and a loss of β cells. In some cases, the islets may be infiltrated by lym-phocytes, and the dogs may make autoantibodies to canine proinsulin. Experimentally, it has been shown that circulating mononuclear cells from some diabetic dogs can suppress insulin production by cultured mouse islet cells. Additionally, serum from some diabetic dogs may lyse these islet cells in the presence of complement. When diabetic dog serum was tested for antibodies against cultured β cells by immuno-fluorescence, 9 of 23 dogs showed strongly positive reactions, and an additional 3 showed a weak reaction. Only 1 of 15 normal dogs gave a positive response.

Humans with juvenile-onset (type 1) diabetes make autoantibodies against the 67-kDa isoform of glutamic acid decarboxylase (GAD65) and/or insulinoma antigen-2 (IA-2). Some diabetic dogs also possess these autoantibodies. Thus, four of the 30 diabetic dogs had autoanti-bodies to GAD65, and three had autoantibodies to IA-2. Two had auto-antibodies to both antigens (Davidson et al., 2008).

Certain DLA haplotypes are more prevalent in the breeds such as the Samoyed, Tibetan Terrier, and Cairn Terrier that have a high risk of developing diabetes. However, these haplotypes are not uncommon in other breeds. A predisposition to neonatal diabetes mellitus has also been observed in Keeshonds, where it appears to be controlled by a single autosomal recessive gene. Boxers, in contrast, rarely get this disease. Genes that may influence the development of canine diabetes include MHC class II genes, genes encoding the CTLA4 promoter, and those for interferon-γ (IFN-γ), interleukin-12 (IL-12), IL-4, and IL-10 (Catchpole et al., 2013; Short et al., 2009; Tsai et al., 2013).

Diabetes mellitus is rare in cattle, sheep, pigs, and horses. Affected animals have atrophied and reduced numbers of pancreatic islets with partial or complete loss of β cells. Lymphocytes commonly infiltrate the remaining islets.

Autoimmune Adrenalitis

Dogs may suffer from lymphocyte-mediated destruction of the adrenal cortex. Affected animals present with depression, weak pulse, brady-cardia, abdominal pain, vomiting, diarrhea, dehydration, and hypo-thermia. As a result of excessive sodium and chloride loss, animals develop hypovolemia and acidosis, leading to circulatory shock, hyper-kalemia, and cardiac arrhythmias. Blood corticosteroid levels are low in these animals. This disease has been observed in association with hypothyroidism.

A syndrome has been described in Italian greyhounds that resem-bles autoimmune polyendocrine syndrome type 2 in humans (Pedersen et al., 2012). This is not a random collection of unlinked diseases but a syndrome with a common etiology but diverse clinical manifestations. The autoimmunity involves mainly the adrenals, thyroid, pancreas, and gonads, as well as the skin. It tends to occur in females at mid-life (Cartwright et al., 2016).

AUTOIMMUNE REPRODUCTIVE DISEASES

If the testes are damaged so that hidden antigens are released, an auto-immune response may cause orchitis. Autoantibodies to sperm may also be detected in some animals following injury to the testes or long-standing obstruction of the seminiferous ducts. For example, dogs infected with *Brucella canis* develop chronic epididymitis and become sensitized to sperm antigens carried to the circulation after phagocy-tosis by macrophages. These sperm antigens stimulate the production of IgG or IgA autoantibodies. The autoantibodies can agglutinate and immobilize sperm, causing infertility.

In stallions and cows, antisperm autoantibodies may be associated with reduced fertility or infertility. In certain lines of black mink, 20%–30% of older males are infertile as a result of high levels of antisperm antibodies. The animals develop a monocytic orchitis, and immune complexes are deposited along the basal lamina of the seminiferous tubules.

Dermatologists recognize an autoimmune dermatitis in intact female dogs that develops as a result of hypersensitivity to endogenous progesterone or estrogens. The disease presents as a bilaterally sym-metrical intense pruritus, erythema, and papular eruption. Its develop-ment usually coincides with estrus or pseudopregnancy.

Production-enhancing vaccines are designed to interfere with nor-mal hormone production and reproductive behavior by inducing an autoimmune response. Thus, a vaccine designed to neutralize pro-duction of GnRH effectively lowers testosterone levels. This results in improved meat quality, faster growth, and reduced aggression by bulls. These vaccines are also used to reduce aggressive behavior in boars, and block the production of androstenone, the lipophilic steroid that contributes to boar taint, the offensive odor associated with cooked boar meat. In horses, a similar vaccine may be used to control estrus and estrus-related misbehavior. Sheep immunized with polyandroalbumin (androstenedione-7-carboxyethyl thioester linked to human serum albumin) have about 23% more lambs than untreated sheep. The ewes are given two doses of this vaccine before mating. It is believed that the vaccine induces autoantibodies that reduce serum androstenedione levels.

Vaccines may be used as contraceptives. If dogs are immunized with bovine or ovine luteinizing hormone (LH), the autoantibodies produced may neutralize their own LH. Similarly, it is possible to produce autoantibodies that neutralize gonadotrophin-releasing hormone (GnRH). GnRH controls the pituitary release of follicle-stimulating hormone and LH. As a result, the reproductive cycle is abolished in females, and testicular, epididymal, and prostatic atrophy occur in males. Antibodies prevent the GnRH from binding to its receptor. Thus, vaccination can be used to control inappropriate sexual behavior in both stallions and mares.

In mares, the reduction in GnRH leads to a decline in estrogen levels, so that behavioral estrus ceases. If given to young stallions, the anti-GnRH antibodies decrease testosterone, libido, sperm production, and sperm quality. GonaCon is a GnRH vaccine used as a contraceptive and inhibitor of sexual behavior in wild horses and burros. Other experimental immunocontraceptive vaccines have also been directed against prostaglandin $F_{2\alpha}$, reproductive steroids, the LH receptor, and zona pellucida protein.

AUTOIMMUNE EYE DISEASES

Equine Recurrent Uveitis

The most common cause of blindness in horses is recurrent uveitis (or periodic ophthalmia). Affected horses suffer repeated episodes of intraocular inflammation, mainly involving the anterior uveal tract. In acute cases, they develop painful blepharospasm, lacrimation, corneal changes such as edema, and vascularization and photophobia. Some horses develop a posterior uveitis, including vitritis and retinitis, resulting in photoreceptor destruction. Each attack gets progressively more severe and gradually spreads to involve other eye tissues until complete blindness results. The eye lesions are infiltrated with CD4+Th1 cells and neutrophils, with extensive fibrin and C3 deposition. Th17 cells may be responsible for chronic disease. The major autoantigen implicated is the interphotoreceptor retinoid-binding protein with subsequent epitope spreading to the retinal S-protein and other autoantigens including recoverin and cellular retinaldehyde-binding protein (Romeike et al., 1998).

Affected horses may also make autoantibodies against a protein found on the inner leaflet of the outer membrane of *Leptospira interrogans* called LruC. The titer of these antibodies tends to rise during a flare-up of the lesion and fall while in remission. If horses are immunized with either equine cornea or certain serovars of killed *L. interrogans*, they will develop corneal opacity 10 days later at the time when antibodies appear in the bloodstream. Partial antigenic cross-reactivity exists between equine corneas and these *L. interrogans* serovars, and some cases may be due to molecular mimicry of *L. interrogans* LruC (Verma et al., 2012). Other cases may be associated with *Borrelia burgdorferi* infection or with the nematode *Onchocerca cervicalis*. Systemic and topical corticosteroid therapy is required to bring the inflammation under control, although the disease usually recurs. Encouraging results have been obtained by using slow-release cyclosporine implants (Malalana et al., 2015).

Appaloosa horses are predisposed to developing equine recurrent uveitis. Three single nucleotide polymorphisms are significantly correlated with the development of this disease in this breed. One is on chromosome 1, and the other two are associated with the equine MHC region (ELA) (Fritz et al., 2014).

Uveodermatological Syndrome

Uveodermatological syndrome is a sporadic disease of dogs. A similar disease, Vogt-Koyanagi-Harada syndrome, occurs in humans. In humans, Vogt-Koyanagi-Harada syndrome is believed to be a result of an autoimmune response against melanocytes. In dogs, no consistent immunological abnormalities have been observed.

Affected dogs develop uveitis and skin depigmentation with whitening of the hair (poliosis) and skin (vitiligo). The eye lesions develop first and most animals present with sudden blindness or chronic uveitis. The early lesions vary from a severe panuveitis to a bilateral anterior uveitis. Some dogs may have detached retinas, and there may be progressive depigmentation of the retina and iris. Depigmentation of the hair and skin gradually follows the onset of eye lesions. Some cases may be generalized, involving the eyelids, nasal planum, lips, scrotum, and footpads (Fig. 38.2). These depigmented areas may become ulcerated and crusted. There is a diffuse infiltration of the uveal tract with lymphocytes, plasma cells, and macrophages. Many of the macrophages contain ingested melanin. The skin lesions consist of a mononuclear (macrophages, giant cells, lymphocytes, and plasma cells) infiltration of the dermal-epidermal junction (Fig. 38.3). The amount of melanin in the epidermis and hair follicles is greatly reduced.

AUTOIMMUNE NEUROLOGICAL DISEASE

An autoimmune brain disease known as experimental allergic encephalomyelitis can be induced by immunizing laboratory mice with brain tissue emulsified in Freund's complete adjuvant. The mice develop focal encephalitis and myelitis, possibly with paralysis. Their brain lesions consist of vasculitis, mononuclear cell infiltration, perivascular demyelination, and axon damage. Antibodies to brain tissue can be detected in the serum of these animals, although the lesion itself is a result of a cell-mediated response.

A similar encephalitis used to occur following the administration of rabies vaccines containing brain tissue to humans. For this reason, the use of adult brain tissue was stopped, and suckling mouse brain tissue obtained prior to myelination was substituted. Post-distemper demyelinating leukoencephalopathy in dogs may also be of autoimmune origin, although the production of antimyelin antibodies appears to be

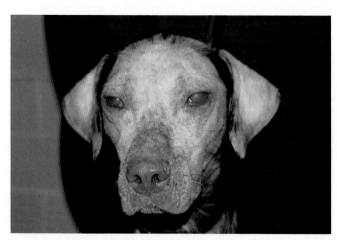

Fig. 38.2 A case of uveodermatological syndrome. Note ocular clouding, alopecia, and depigmentation of the nasal planum. Courtesy Drs. Robert Kennis, Joan Dziezc, and Larry Wadsworth.

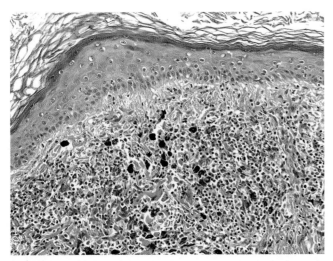

Fig. 38.3 A histological section of skin from a canine case of uveodermatological syndrome. Note the major lymphocyte infiltration associated with the skin melanocytes. It is the destruction of these melanocytes that leads to depigmentation. Courtesy Dr. Joanne Mansell.

common response to central nervous tissue damage, regardless of its cause.

Equine Polyneuritis

Equine polyneuritis (neuritis of the cauda equina) is an uncommon disease affecting the sacral and coccygeal nerves. Affected horses develop hyperesthesia, followed by progressive paralysis of the tail, rectum, and bladder and localized anesthesia in the same region. The disease may also be associated with facial and trigeminal paralysis. A chronic granulomatous inflammation develops in the region of the extradural nerve roots, so that affected nerves are thickened and discolored. There is a loss of myelinated axons; infiltration by macrophages, lymphocytes, giant cells, and plasma cells; and deposition of fibrous material in the perineurium. In severe cases, the nerve trunks may be almost totally destroyed. Affected horses have circulating antibodies to a peripheral myelin protein called P2. Although equine polyneuritis may be an autoimmune disease, equine adenovirus-1 has been isolated from its lesions, so the cause is complex. Because of the severe nerve damage, immunosuppressive or antiinflammatory therapy is rarely successful.

Canine Polyneuritis

Canine polyneuritis or "Coonhound paralysis" affects dogs following a bite or scratch from a raccoon. It presents as an ascending symmetrical flaccid paralysis with mild sensory impairment. The bitten limb is usually affected first, but the disease is progressive and will worsen for 10–12 days following the bite. In severe cases, the dog may develop quadriplegia and lose the ability to swallow, bark, or breathe. The disease is, however, self-limiting, and if respiration is not impaired, the prognosis is good. Dogs usually recover completely. Affected nerves show demyelination and axonal degeneration with macrophage infiltration. An acute polyneuritis similar to coonhound paralysis has also been described following vaccination of dogs with rabies or other vaccines. Coonhound paralysis and postvaccinal polyneuritis both closely resemble Guillain-Barré syndrome in humans. This syndrome may follow upper respiratory tract infection, gastrointestinal disease, or even vaccination. It is mediated by autoantibodies against peripheral nerve glycolipids. Veterinarians treating canine polyneuritis have traditionally administered corticosteroids, but their effectiveness is unclear.

Meningitis of Unknown Origin

Three somewhat similar inflammatory diseases of the canine central nervous system are recognized. These are necrotizing meningoencephalitis (NME), necrotizing leukoencephalitis (NLE), and granulomatous meningoencephalomyelitis (GME) (Talarico and Schatzberg, 2010). Collectively, they are classified as Meningitis of Unknown Origin (MUO). MUO appears to be immunologically mediated. Canine NME is an inflammatory disease of unknown etiology that has been described in several toy breeds such as Pugs (young females), Papillons, Shih Tzu, Maltese Terriers, Pekinese, and Chihuahuas (Cooper et al., 2014; Higgins et al., 2008). The necrotic lesions are multifocal and asymmetrical, restricted to the gray and white matter in the cerebra, and are accompanied by a severe meningitis. Macrophages predominate in the lesions, but both scattered T cells and dendritic cells are also present, whereas B cells are restricted to the meninges. Dogs with NME make autoantibodies to glial fibrillary acidic protein (Uchida et al., 2016).

NLE has been reported in Yorkshire terriers and French bulldogs. It is similar to NME, but the necrotic foci are found predominantly in the white matter of the forebrain and brainstem (Spitzbarth et al., 2010). These foci are characterized by cavitation, necrosis, demyelination, and perivascular cuffing. The primary infiltrating cells are T cells. Some investigators consider NLE to be a variant of NME.

The third form of canine MUO, GME, may account for a quarter of canine central nervous system diseases. GME is characterized by the formation of multifocal granulomas around blood vessels in the cerebellum and brainstem. T cells and macrophages predominate in the lesions. GME may be disseminated, focal or ocular. The prognosis is poor, although aggressive treatment with corticosteroids may be beneficial. IFNγ and IL-17 are elevated in NME and GME. The IL-17 in GME appears to be produced by macrophages rather than T cells (Spitzbarth et al., 2012).

Steroid-Responsive Meningitis-Arteritis

Steroid-responsive meningitis-arteritis (SRMA) is a vasculitis characterized by inflammation of the meningeal arteries resulting in cervical meningitis (Tipold and Schatzberg, 2010). This disease is characterized by increased IgA production, an acute-phase response, and the development of a necrotizing vasculitis (Schwartz et al., 2011). Several cytokines play a role in this process. IL-6 and vascular endothelial growth factor are significantly increased in cerebrospinal fluid. The changes in IL-6 levels may promote Th17 cell differentiation. The CSF in acute cases of SRMA contains high IgA and CXCL8 levels and mature neutrophils. Serum IgA, C-reactive protein, and α_2-macroglobulin are also elevated. T-cell production of IL-2 and IFN-γ is depressed, whereas Th2 production of IL-4 is enhanced and probably accounts for the increased IgA production (Maiolini et al., 2013). About 30% of these dogs have a positive lupus erythematosus (LE) cell test but no detectable antinuclear antibodies (see Chapter 39). In chronic cases, the CSF contains predominantly mononuclear cells. On necropsy, the spinal meningeal arteries show fibrinoid degeneration, intimal or medial necrosis, and hyalinization and are infiltrated with lymphocytes, plasma cells, macrophages, and a few neutrophils. Complete obliteration of the blood vessel lumina may occur, whereas rupture and thrombosis of inflamed vessels may lead to hemorrhage, compression, and infarction.

AUTOIMMUNE SKIN DISEASES

Many autoimmune skin diseases are recognized. These diseases may affect hair follicles, keratinocytes, or the skin basement membrane. Hair follicle disease can lead to alopecia. Diseases involving keratinocytes or basement membranes result in cell separation within the skin and the consequent development of blisters or vesicles (Fig. 38.4). As a result, dermatologists use the terms *pemphigus* or *pemphigoid* to describe them, after the Greek word *pemphix* meaning "blister."

Alopecia Areata

Alopecia areata is immune-mediated hair loss. It has been reported in humans, other primates, dogs, cats, horses, and cattle. In dogs, it is a rare disease. The alopecia starts locally, often on the head, but may spread to involve the entire body. It is often symmetrical. The hair follicles are infiltrated with CD4[+] and CD8[+] T cells and Langerhans cells. IgG autoantibodies are directed against cells in the lower hair follicles. C3 or IgM may also be present. This immune attack is directed against a protein called trichohyalin located in the inner root sheath of hair follicles. Alopecia areata responds to corticosteroid treatment, but spontaneous hair regrowth also occurs. Other autoimmune diseases that lead to hair loss include pseudopelade. It differs from alopecia areata in the precise location of the inflammatory infiltrate within the hair follicles. Likewise, some cases of pemphigus vulgaris (see later) may also be restricted to hair follicles (Olivry et al., 1996).

Blistering Skin Diseases

Blistering skin diseases have been described in humans, dogs, horses, and cats (Winfield et al., 2013). Known as the pemphigus complex, they are classified according to the location of the lesions within the epidermis. Some lesions develop deep within the epidermis. For example, the most severe form (although very rare) is called pemphigus vulgaris. In this disease, bullae (blisters) develop around mucocutaneous junctions, especially the nose, lips, eyes, prepuce, and anus, on the tongue and the inner surface of the ear. These bullae rupture easily, leaving weeping, shallow ulcers that may become secondarily infected. Histological examination shows separation of the skin cells (acantholysis) in the suprabasal region of the lower epidermis (Fig. 38.5). The acantholysis results when autoantibodies destroy the desmosomes that bind skin cells together. In pemphigus vulgaris, the autoantigen is a desmosomal protein called desmoglein-3. Binding of antibodies to desmoglein-3 activates the proto-oncogene *c-myc* and leads to keratinocyte proliferation. As a result, the keratinocytes above the lesion proliferate and fail to express adhesion proteins, so they separate from each other. Eventually, this leads to acantholysis and bulla formation.

Pemphigus foliaceus (PF) is the commonest autoimmune skin disease of dogs. It is a blistering disease in which the lesions develop superficially in the epidermis (Fig. 38.6). As a result, it is a milder disease than pemphigus vulgaris. It has been described in humans, dogs, cats, goats, and horses. The bullae are not confined to mucocutaneous junctions or the muzzle. Histology reveals that the bullae develop in the subcorneal region of the epidermis. These bullae are very fragile, rupture easily, and therefore rarely persist. IgG is the dominant serum

autoantibody (Bizikova et al., 2014b). In dogs, the major autoantigen is a desmosome protein called desmocollin-1 (Bizikova et al., 2012). Some cases of canine PF result from the use of antibiotics such as trimethoprim-sulfadiazine, oxacillin, cephalexin, and ampicillin, as well as some topical flea control products. They appear to result from the binding of drug thiol groups to cell membranes.

A mild variant of PF is pemphigus erythematosus. The lesions in this disease tend to be confined to the face and ears and are very similar to those of systemic lupus erythematosus (SLE). Indeed, some dogs with pemphigus erythematosus may have antinuclear antibodies in their serum. Panepidermal pustular pemphigus (pemphigus vegetans) is another rare and mild variant of PF in which papillomatous proliferation of the base of the bullae occurs on healing.

A fifth form of pemphigus, called paraneoplastic pemphigus, has been recorded in a dog. It develops in association with lymphoid or solid tumors. It resembles pemphigus vulgaris, but multiple autoantibodies against skin antigens are present.

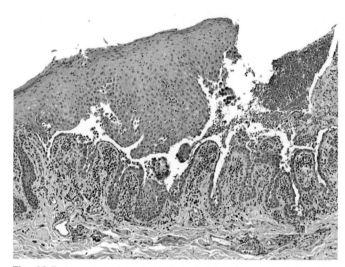

Fig. 38.5 A section of an oral lesion of pemphigus vulgaris in a dog. Note the cleft formation at the base of the epidermis accompanied by extensive cellular infiltration. Courtesy Dr. Joanne Mansell.

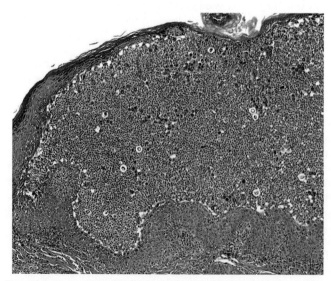

Fig. 38.6 A section from a case of canine pemphigus foliaceus. Note the subcorneal location of the cell-filled vesicle. Courtesy Dr. Joanne Mansell.

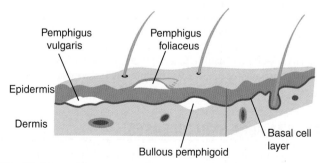

Fig. 38.4 The differential histology of the autoimmune skin diseases. Note the location of the vesicle in relation to the epidermis.

Use of a topical ectoparasiticide containing fipronil, amitraz, and S-methoprene has been associated with the development of an acantholytic pustular dermatitis resembling PF. One or two applications were sufficient to induce disease. Antikeratinocyte IgG was detected in the epidermis of 8 of 19 cases, while serum antikeratinocyte IgG was detected in 10 of 14 cases. Eleven of 14 dogs had detectable antibodies to desmocollin-1. Thus the lesions closely resembled naturally occurring PF (Bizikova et al., 2014a).

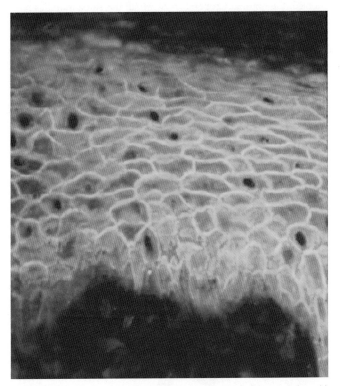

Fig. 38.7 Direct immunofluorescence of a section of normal dog skin that has been incubated in serum from a dog with pemphigus vulgaris. The intercellular cement is stained. Courtesy Dr. K. Credille.

Direct immunofluorescent examination of pemphigus lesions reveals immunoglobulins deposited on the intercellular cement in a typical "chicken-wire" pattern (Fig. 38.7).

It is important to differentiate among the forms of pemphigus for prognostic reasons. Pemphigus vulgaris has a poor prognosis; treatment tends to be unsatisfactory, and the lesions are persistent. In contrast, PF is milder, and the results of treatment may be more satisfactory. As with other autoimmune diseases, these diseases often recur when treatment is stopped.

Skin Basement Membrane Diseases

A second set of blistering diseases is associated with the development of autoantibodies against the skin basement membrane. As a result, affected dogs develop subepidermal bullae. Several such diseases have been identified in dogs and other domestic animals. They include bullous pemphigoid, linear IgA dermatosis, and epidermolysis bullosa acquisita (Bizikova et al., 2023).

Bullous Pemphigoid

Bullous pemphigoid is a rare skin disease that resembles pemphigus vulgaris. Collies, Shetland Sheepdogs, and Dobermans appear to be predisposed to it. It has also been described in humans, pigs, horses, and cats. Multiple bullae develop around mucocutaneous junctions and in the groin and axillae. However, the disease differs from pemphigus vulgaris in that the bullae develop in the subepidermis (and are therefore less likely to rupture). They tend to be filled with fibrin as well as mononuclear cells or eosinophils, and they heal spontaneously. Bullous pemphigoid results from the development of autoantibodies against type XVII collagen. This molecule is a component of hemidesmosomes, the structures that attach basal keratinocytes to the basement membrane (Fig. 38.8). The presence of IgG on the basement membrane may be demonstrated by immunofluorescence, which reveals intense linear staining. The prognosis of bullous pemphigoid is usually poor, but mild cases may recover after treatment with corticosteroids. Some dogs may develop a bullous pemphigoid-like disease mediated by autoantibodies against the basement membrane protein laminin-5 (Olivry et al., 2010).

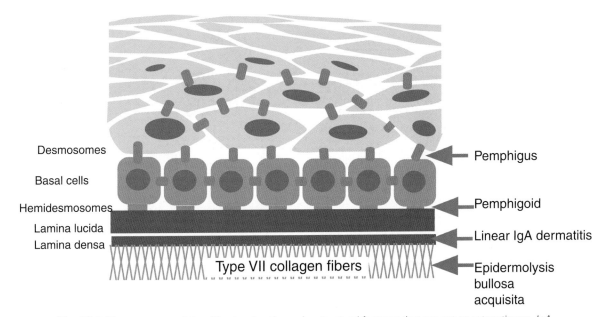

Fig. 38.8 The structures of the skin showing the major structural features that can act as autoantigens. *IgA,* Immunoglobulin A.

Linear Immunoglobulin A Dermatosis

Another group of canine skin diseases is characterized by the deposition of IgA in the lamina lucida of the skin basement membrane. One such disease, called dermatitis herpetiformis, has been recorded in a Beagle, whereas a linear IgA dermatosis has been recorded in Dachshunds. Both diseases present with pruritic, pustular, and papular lesions, resembling pyoderma, with eosinophil-filled subepidermal bullae. The target autoantigen has been identified as a processed extracellular form of collagen XVII. The drug dapsone has been recommended as the specific treatment for these diseases.

Epidermolysis Bullosa Acquisita

A generalized skin disease characterized by severe subepidermal blistering and ulcerative lesions has been identified in dogs, especially young Great Danes (Olivry et al., 1998). The bullae originate from erythematous areas on the skin and rapidly progress to ulcers. Dogs develop generalized urticaria, oral ulceration, and eventually cutaneous sloughing. A localized variant of the disease has been observed in German short-haired pointers. The dermis and epidermis separate, and neutrophils accumulate within the superficial dermis. The neutrophil infiltration may eventually result in microabscess formation. Secondary changes include deep ulceration, necrosis, and bacterial infection. Affected animals develop IgA and IgG autoantibodies against the anchoring fibrils of the lower basement membrane. These autoantibodies are specific for type VII collagen and distinctly different from those responsible for bullous pemphigoid. Another subset of canine subepidermal blistering diseases results from the production of IgG autoantibodies against the basement membrane component, laminin-332. The skin blistering and ulceration in these cases are associated with microscopic subepidermal vesiculation (Olivry et al., 2010).

Relapsing Polychondritis

Autoimmunity against type II cartilage has been described in humans and in cats. The animals present with bilateral curling of the ears and ocular changes. Their cartilage is infiltrated with plasma cells and lymphocytes. A similar proliferative and necrotizing otitis in kittens is associated with CD3+ T cells found in close approximation to apoptotic keratinocytes, suggesting that some form of T cell–mediated cytotoxicity is occurring.

AUTOIMMUNE BLOOD DISEASES

Immune-Mediated Hemolytic Anemias

Autoantibodies to red blood cell antigens cause their destruction and result in immune-mediated hemolytic anemia (IMHA). These hemolytic anemias are well recognized in humans and dogs and have been recorded in cattle, horses, mice, rabbits, and raccoons, as well as birds. They are an uncommon cause of anemia in cats.

Affected dogs are anemic. Thus pallor, weakness, and lethargy are accompanied by fever, icterus, and hepatosplenomegaly. The anemia may be associated with tachycardia, anorexia, vomiting, or diarrhea. Clinical signs are contingent on the mechanism of red cell destruction. This destruction may result from intravascular hemolysis (destruction within the bloodstream) mediated by complement or, much more commonly, by extravascular hemolysis (removal of antibody-coated red cells by the macrophages of the spleen and liver) (Fig. 38.9). In dogs, the disease occurs more often in females. The average age of onset is about 4–5 years. There is a genetic predisposition to IMHA in Cocker Spaniels and Miniature Schnauzers. The "causes" of IMHA are unknown, although some cases may be attributable to alterations in red cell surface antigens induced by drugs or viruses. In dogs, the

autoantibodies are primarily directed against red cell glycophorins, the cytoskeletal protein spectrin, and the membrane anion exchange protein CD233 (band 3). About one-third of IMHA cases are associated with other immunological abnormalities such as systemic lupus (see Chapter 39) or autoimmune thrombocytopenia (AITP) or with the presence of lymphoid and other tumors. Its onset may be associated with obvious stress such as vaccination (see Chapter 26), anaplasmosis, viral disease, or hormonal imbalances as in pregnancy or pyometra.

IMHAs in dogs are classified according to the antibody class involved, the optimal temperature at which the autoantibodies react, and the nature of the hemolytic process (Table 38.1; Warman et al., 2008).

Class I: Caused by IgG autoantibodies that agglutinate red cells at body temperature. The agglutination may be seen when a drop of blood is placed on a glass slide. Both IgG and IgM antibodies are involved. Since IgG does not activate complement efficiently, the red cells are mainly destroyed by phagocytosis in the spleen. In very severe cases, a blood smear may show erythrophagocytosis by neutrophils and monocytes.

Class II: IgM antibodies activate complement and destroy red cells by intravascular hemolysis. This results in hemoglobinemia, hemoglobinuria, icterus, and very severe anemia. Affected dogs are anemic, weak, and possibly jaundiced. Kupffer cells in the liver or macrophages in lymph nodes preferentially remove red cells with complement on their surface, so these animals develop hepatomegaly and lymphadenopathy.

Class III: Most cases of IMHA in dogs and cats are mediated by IgG1 and IgG4 antibodies, which bind to red cells at 37°C but do not activate complement or agglutinate the red cells. IgG antibodies can only form short bridges (15–25 nm) between cells. As a result, they cannot counteract the zeta potential of the red cells and will not cause direct agglutination. (In contrast, IgM antibodies form

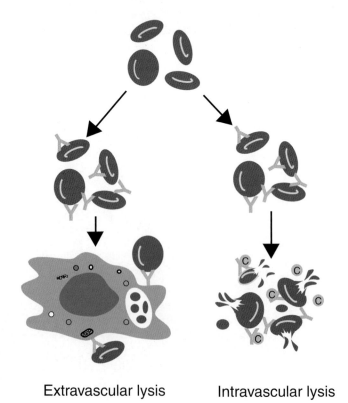

Extravascular lysis   Intravascular lysis

Fig. 38.9 The basic differences between intravascular and extravascular hemolysis.

TABLE 38.1 Classification of Canine Immune–Mediated Hemolytic Anemias

Class	Predominant Antibody	Activity	Optimal Temperature (°C)	Site of Red Cell Removal	Clinical Effect
I	G $\gg$ M	Agglutinin	37	Spleen	Intravascular agglutination
II	M	Hemolysin	37	Liver	Intravascular hemolysin
III	G	Incomplete	37	Spleen	Anemia
IV	M	Agglutinin	4	Liver	Cyanosis and infarction of extremities
V	M	Incomplete	4	Liver	Anemia

long bridges [30–50 nm] and can agglutinate cells despite their zeta potential.) Affected red cells are opsonized and removed by splenic macrophages. Splenomegaly is a consistent feature of class III disease.

Class IV: Some IgM antibodies cannot agglutinate red cells at body temperature but can only do so when the blood is chilled. These antibodies are called cold agglutinins. They can be detected by cooling blood to between 10°C and 4°C, at which point clumping occurs. The agglutination is reversed on rewarming. As blood circulates through the extremities (tail, toes, ears, and so forth) of affected animals, it may be cooled sufficiently to permit red cell agglutination within capillaries. This can lead to vascular stasis, blockage, tissue ischemia, and, eventually, necrosis. Affected animals may therefore present with necrotic lesions at the extremities, and anemia may not be a significant feature. As might be anticipated, this form of IMHA is most severe in the winter.

Class V: This is mediated by IgM antibodies that bind red cells when chilled to 4°C but do not agglutinate them. These antibodies can only be identified by an antiglobulin test conducted in the cold. They do not induce necrosis of extremities, but can activate complement leading to intravascular hemolysis.

Hematology reflects the severe anemia and a regenerative response by the bone marrow. Blood smears commonly show spherocytes, which result from red cells losing part of their cell membrane because of partial phagocytosis. They appear as small, round red cells that lack a central pale area. The number of spherocytes in blood is a measure of the intensity of red cell destruction.

To diagnose IMHA associated with the presence of nonagglutinating or incomplete antibodies (classes II, III, and V), it is necessary to use a direct antiglobulin test (see Chapter 43). The red cells of the affected animal are collected in anticoagulant, washed free of serum, and incubated in an antiglobulin serum. The best antiglobulin for this purpose is a polyclonal one with activity against IgM, IgG, and complement. Red cells coated with autoantibody or complement will be cross-linked and agglutinated by the antiglobulin. Occasionally, IgM may have a low affinity for the red cells, so it elutes, leaving only complement on their surface.

It is important to emphasize that blood samples for immunological testing should be collected before immunosuppressive therapy begins. It is also important to note that in the cat, most cases of antiglobulin-positive hemolytic anemia are secondary to feline leukemia virus or *Mycoplasma haemofelis (Haemobartonella felis)* infections. The disease in cats has a more favorable prognosis than in dogs. Dogs with IMHA have increased concentrations of C-reactive protein and α-1 acid glycoprotein, and decreased serum albumin. This acute-phase response normalizes rapidly with disease stabilization (Mitchell et al., 2009).

Treatment of IMHA involves prevention of further hemolysis, treatment of hypoxia, prevention of thromboembolism, and aggressive supportive care. The major cause of death is thromboembolic disease (Wells et al., 2009). Low-dose aspirin or heparin may reduce the risk of thromboembolism. Splenectomy should only be considered when more conservative therapy has failed and may help cases of refractory class III disease.

Secondary immune-mediated anemias occur in horses following infection with *Streptococcus fecalis*, in sheep following leptospirosis, in cats with mycoplasmosis (hemobartonellosis), in dogs with babesiosis, and in pigs with eperythrozoonosis. In these cases, IgM cold agglutinins clump red cells from normal animals of the same species when chilled. Antibodies to hemoglobin are found in the serum of cattle severely infected with *Arcanobacterium pyogenes*, perhaps as a result of bacterial hemolysis. IMHA also occurs in horses suffering from lymphosarcomas and melanomas.

Immune Suppression of Hematopoiesis

In humans, dogs, and cats, autoantibodies directed against erythroid stem cells may cause red cell aplasia. Autoantibodies to myeloid stem cells may provoke an immune neutropenia. In dogs, primary red cell aplasia has been associated with an IgG that inhibits erythroid stem cell differentiation. It appears to be especially common in Labrador Retrievers (Stokol et al., 2000). Autoantibodies to myeloid stem cells may also provoke an immune neutropenia. Diagnosis is based largely on excluding other causes of the neutropenia together with a favorable response to steroid and immunosuppressive therapy. These diseases can only be diagnosed by careful hematological analysis and by demonstration of autoantibodies by immunofluorescence on bone marrow smears. These tests are not easy and have not been validated in domestic species. Affected animals may benefit from high doses of corticosteroids or immunosuppressive therapy. Immune-mediated bone marrow aplasia is rare in cats and usually only affects erythrocyte progenitors. It has been recorded in a ferret. An immune-mediated, vaccine-induced neonatal pancytopenia has been reported in cattle (see Chapter 32).

Autoimmune Thrombocytopenia

AITP due to an immune attack on platelets has been reported in horses, dogs, and, rarely, cats (Mackin, 1995). Affected animals usually present with multiple petechiae in the skin, gingiva, other mucous membranes, and conjunctiva. Epistaxis, melena, and hematuria may occur. The predominant cause of death in these dogs is severe gastrointestinal hemorrhage. Antibodies against platelet antigens cause extravascular destruction of opsonized platelets in the spleen. As a result, affected animals have unusually low platelet counts and a prolonged bleeding time. The disease is commonly observed in association with IMHA and SLE (Goggs et al., 2008).

In dogs, the average age of onset is 6 years. Predisposed breeds include Airedales, Dobermans, Old English Sheepdogs, Cocker Spaniels, and Poodles. Antibodies to platelets may be measured by direct immunofluorescence on bone marrow aspirates looking for positive staining on megakaryocytes. However, an alternative test is one that measures the release of factor III from platelets after exposure to autoantibodies. This may be performed by incubating platelet-rich plasma with a globulin fraction of the serum under test and estimating the amount of procoagulant activity released. In about 75% of cases, the antibodies are of the IgG class. Most cases of AITP in cats are probably secondary to feline leukemia virus infection.

AUTOIMMUNE MUSCLE DISEASES

Animals suffer from several different immune-mediated inflammatory muscle diseases.

Myasthenia Gravis

Myasthenia gravis is a disease of skeletal muscle characterized by abnormal fatigue and weakness after mild exercise. It occurs in humans, dogs, and cats (Bell et al., 2012). Myasthenia gravis results from a failure of transmission of nerve impulses across the motor endplate of striated muscle as a result of a deficiency of acetylcholine receptors (Fig. 38.10). In Jack Russell Terriers, Springer Spaniels, and Fox Terriers, an inherited deficiency of these receptors occurs. This congenital form is therefore a disease of very young dogs.

In adult dogs, however, the acetylcholine receptor deficiency is due to autoimmune attack. IgG autoantibodies accelerate the degradation of the receptors, block their acetylcholine-binding sites, and trigger complement-mediated damage. As a result, the number of functional acetylcholine receptors drops significantly. Dogs may also make autoantibodies against titin, an intracellular muscle protein, and the ryanodine receptor, a Ca^{2+} release channel in striated muscle.

In normal muscles the binding of acetylcholine to its receptor opens a sodium channel to produce a localized endplate potential. If the amplitude of the endplate potential is sufficient, this will generate an action potential and trigger muscle contraction. In myasthenic junctions, however, the endplate potentials fail to trigger action potentials in many muscle fibers. This is manifested as muscle weakness. Repeating the stimulus leads to a progressive increase in weakness as transmission failure occurs at more and more neuromuscular junctions since the amount of acetylcholine released from a nerve terminal usually declines after the first few impulses.

The disease may develop in any dog, but certain breeds are predisposed to it. German Shepherds, Golden Retrievers, Labradors, and Dachshunds appear to develop more severe diseases. Rottweilers appear to be at low risk. In cats, there is a predisposition in Abyssinians and related Somalis (Hague et al., 2015). It has been recorded in ferrets (Couturier et al., 2009).

In some animals, the thymus may show medullary hyperplasia, germinal center formation, or even a thymoma, and surgical thymectomy may result in clinical improvement. About 3% of dog cases and up to 52% of cat cases are associated with the presence of a mediastinal mass, most frequently a thymoma.

Dogs may present with a history of difficulty swallowing, regurgitation, labored breathing, and generalized muscle weakness. Megaesophagus is common. Clinically, different diseases may be recognized. Thus, focal myasthenia gravis is characterized by megaesophagus and facial paralysis without limb muscle weakness; generalized myasthenia gravis cases develop limb muscle weakness associated with facial paralysis and megaesophagus; and acute fulminating myasthenia gravis develops when the disease rapidly leads to quadriplegia and respiratory difficulty. Almost 60% of cases are generalized or fulminating. Without treatment, about half of affected dogs die, whereas the others may show spontaneous remissions. Aspiration pneumonia is the main cause of death in myasthenic dogs.

Administration of a short-acting anticholinesterase drug such as edrophonium chloride (Tensilon) leads to a rapid gain in muscle strength. The anticholinesterase, by permitting the acetylcholine to accumulate at the neuromuscular junction, enables the remaining receptors to be stimulated more effectively. Dogs with transient myasthenia gravis may be supported temporarily with long-acting anticholinesterase drugs such as pyridostigmine bromide or neostigmine methyl sulfate. Dogs with progressive disease that show no signs of remission may benefit from immunosuppression.

Polymyositis

A generalized immune-mediated myositis occurs in large dogs such as German Shepherds, Boxers, and retrievers. Vizslas suffer from a breed-specific inflammatory myopathy (Tauro et al., 2015). In all these cases, the animals show progressive muscle weakness not associated with exercise intolerance. Changes in laryngeal muscle function lead to a change in the voice. Megaesophagus may lead to dysphagia and,

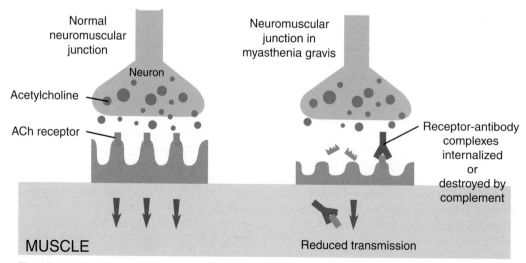

Fig. 38.10 The pathogenesis of myasthenia gravis. Destruction of acetylcholine receptors prevents effective neuromuscular transmission. Blockage of cholinesterase activity by anticholinesterase drugs permits acetylcholine to accumulate, which enhances neuromuscular transmission.

if severe, can result in aspiration pneumonia. Affected animals may develop a shifting lameness. Animals may be febrile and develop leukocytosis and eosinophilia. Biopsies show muscle fiber degeneration, necrosis, and vacuolation, and affected muscles may be infiltrated by CD8+ lymphocytes and plasma cells. About 50% of affected dogs have antinuclear antibodies or antibodies to sarcolemma, or both. Corticosteroids are the treatment of choice (Hankel et al., 2006).

A similar immune-mediated myositis has been recorded in Quarter horses and related breeds. It causes rapid atrophy of the gluteal and epaxial muscles. The affected muscles are infiltrated with macrophages and CD4+ T cells with lesser numbers of CD8+ T cells and B cells. It too may be treatable with corticosteroids. MHC classes I and II are expressed on the sarcolemma of some myofibers of affected horses but not in normal horses.

Autoimmune Masticatory Myositis

Dogs may develop a focal myositis confined to the muscles of mastication. The major autoantigen is masticatory myosin-binding protein-C found only in masticatory muscle fibers. Animals present with pain and atrophy or swelling of the jaw muscles resulting in difficulty in opening (trismus) or closing the jaw. Affected animals may also develop conjunctivitis or exophthalmos. Histology of affected muscles shows inflammatory or degenerative lesions affecting the M2 myofibrils. Myositis with lymphocytes and plasma cells predominates, and some lesions may contain many eosinophils. Myofiber atrophy, perimysial or endomysial fibrosis, and muscle fiber necrosis are consistent features. Immunoglobulins may be detected in biopsy specimens of affected muscles, and circulating antibodies to the M2 myofibrils have been demonstrated by an immunoperoxidase assay (Wu et al., 2007). Corticosteroids such as prednisone are used for treatment, but the prognosis is guarded. Cavalier King Charles Spaniels may be predisposed to this disease.

Canine Cardiomyopathy

English Cocker Spaniels may develop a cardiomyopathy with antinuclear and antimitochondrial autoantibodies and reduced serum IgA levels. It is associated with a specific complement C4 allotype (C4-4). The autoantigen has not been identified, but in humans, similar cardiomyopathies are due to autoantibodies directed against the adenine nucleotide translocator of mitochondria.

Dermatomyositis

A familial disease of dogs that resembles dermatomyositis in humans has been described in Collies and Shetland Sheepdogs. It is a complement-mediated microangiopathy in which complement-mediated vascular damage leads to muscle ischemia. The disease is inherited as an autosomal dominant involving a locus on chromosome 35, although expression is highly variable. A similar dermatomyositis-like disease has been described in other breeds such as Pembroke Welsh Corgi, Lakeland Terrier, Chow, Jack Russell Terrier, German Shepherd, and Rottweilers. Dogs develop dermatitis with a less obvious myositis. Puppies appear normal at birth, but skin lesions develop between 7 and 11 weeks of age, and myositis develops between 12 and 23 weeks. In other studies, the dermatitis developed at 3–6 months of age, and myositis was detected after the dermatitis was investigated. The dermatitis first develops on the face; subsequently, lesions may spread to the limbs and trunk, especially over bony prominences. These early lesions are erythematous and eventually lead to vesicle and pustule formation. There is diffuse hair follicle atrophy and keratinocyte degeneration that can lead to ulceration (Fig. 38.11). Once the vesicles rupture, they ulcerate and crust. Lesions occur on the bridge of the nose and around the eyes and dogs show hair loss and changes in pigmentation. The

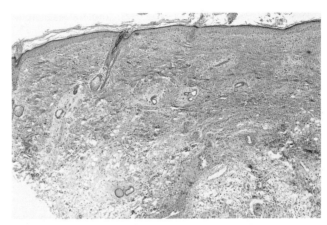

Fig. 38.11 Skin lesion in a case of canine Dermatomyositis. Note the diffuse ischemic hair follicle atrophy and multifocal basal keratinocyte degradation in the epidermis. Courtesy Dr. J. Mansell.

clinical course and severity are variable, but skin lesions usually resolve by 1 year of age.

AUTOIMMUNE HEPATITIS

Doberman Pinschers can develop an autoimmune hepatitis. The symptoms are typical of liver disease with anorexia, depression, weight loss, diarrhea, polydipsia, polyuria, icterus, and eventually ascites. The disease commonly presents between 3 and 6 years of age but may have been present subclinically for many years. On necropsy, there is intense inflammation and fibrosis around small hepatic vein branches in the liver. The lesions contain lymphocytes, plasma cells, and macrophages. The disease eventually causes progressive fibrosis and destruction of hepatocytes. About half of affected dogs develop antibodies to hepatocyte cell membranes. These antibody-positive dogs have more severe disease than dogs without antibodies. In addition, lymphocytes from about 75% of affected dogs respond to liver membrane proteins in vitro. Hepatocytes from affected dogs, but not from normal dogs, express MHC class II antigens. This MHC expression correlates with the severity of the disease, whereas corticosteroid treatment reduces both MHC expression and disease severity. It has been suggested, therefore, that the disease results from a cell-mediated attack on abnormally expressed MHC molecules or an antigen associated with them (Dyggve et al., 2010).

REFERENCES

Bell, E.T., Mansfield, C.S., James, F.E., 2012. Immune-mediated myasthenia gravis in a methimazole-treated cat. J. Small Anim. Pract. 53, 661–663.

Bizikova, P., Dean, G.A., Hashimoto, T., Olivry, T., 2012. Cloning and establishment of canine desmocollin-1 as a major autoantigen in canine pemphigus foliaceus. Vet. Immunol. Immunopathol. 149, 197–207.

Bizikova, P., Linder, K.E., Olivry, T., 2014a. Fipronil-amitraz-S-methoprene-triggered pemphigus foliaceus in 21 dogs: clinical, histological and immunological characteristics. Vet. Dermatol. 25, 103–e30.

Bizikova, P., Olivry, T., Linder, K., Rybnicek, J., 2023. Spontaneous autoimmune subepidermal blistering diseases in animals: a comprehensive review. BMC Vet. Res. https://doi.org/10.1186/s12917-023-03597-1.

Bizikova, P., Olivry, T., Mamo, L.B., Dunston, S.M., 2014b. Serum autoantibody profiles of IgA, IgE and IgM in canine pemphigus foliaceus. Vet. Dermatol. 25, 471–e75.

Cartwright, J.A., Stone, J., Rick, M., Dunning, M.D., 2016. Polyglandular endocrinopathy type II (Schmidt's syndrome) in a Dobermann pinscher. J. Small Anim. Pract. 57, 491–494. 2016

Catchpole, B., Adams, J.P., Holder, A.L., et al., 2013. Genetics of canine diabetes mellitus: are the diabetes susceptibility genes identified in humans involved in breed susceptibility to diabetes mellitus in dogs? Vet. J. 195, 139–147.

Cooper, J.J., Schatzberg, S.J., Vernau, K.M., Summers, B.A., et al., 2014. Necrotizing meningoencephalitis in atypical dog breeds: a case series and literature review. J. Vet. Intern. Med. 28, 198–203.

Couturier, J., Huynh, M., Boussarie, D., et al., 2009. Autoimmune myasthenia gravis in a ferret. J. Am. Vet. Med. Assoc. 235, 1462–1466.

Davison, L.J., Weenink, S.M., Christie, M.R., et al., 2008. Antibodies to GAD64 and IA-2 in canine diabetes mellitus,. Vet. Immunol. Immunopathol. 126, 83–90.

Dyggve, H., Kennedy, L.J., Meri, S., Spillmann, T., et al., 2010. Association of Doberman hepatitis to canine major histocompatibility complex II. Tissue Antigens 77 (1), 30–35.

Fritz, K.L., Kaese, H.J., Valberg, S.J., Hendrickson, J.A., Rendahl, A.K., et al., 2014. Genetic risk factors for insidious equine recurrent uveitis in Appaloosa horses. Anim. Genet. 45, 392–399.

Goggs, R., Boag, A.K., Chan, D.L., 2008. Concurrent immune-mediated haemolytic anaemia and severe thrombocytopenia in 21 dogs. Vet, Rec. 163, 323–327.

Hague, D.W., Humphries, H.D., Mitchell, M.A., Shelton, G.D., 2015. risk factors and outcomes in cats with acquired myasthenia gravis (2001–2012). J. Vet. Intern. Med. 29, 1307–1312.

Hankel, S., Shelton, G.D., Engvall, E., 2006. Sarcolemma-specific autoantibodies in canine inflammatory myopathy. Vet. Immunol. Immunopathol. 113, 1–10.

Happ, G.M., 1995. Thyroiditis: model canine autoimmune disease,. Adv. Vet. Sci. Comp. Med. 39, 97–129.

Higgins, R.J., Dickinson, P.J., Kube, S.A., et al., 2008. Necrotizing meningoencephalitis in five Chihuahua dogs. Vet. Pathol. 45, 336–346.

Mackin, A., 1995. Canine immune-mediated thrombocytopenia. Compend. Contin. Educ. Pract. Vet. 17, 353–362. 515–533

Malalana, F., Stylianides, A., Mcgowan, C., 2015. Equine recurrent uveitis: human and equine perspectives. Vet. J. 206, 22–29.

Maiolini, A., Otten, M., Hewicker-Trautwein, M., et al., 2013. Interleukin-6, vascular endothelial growth factor and transforming growth factor β1 in canine steroid responsive meningitis-arteritis. BMC Vet. Res. 9, 23–28.

Miller, J., Popiel, J., Chelmonska-Soyta, A., 2015. Humoral and cellular immune response in canine hypothyroidism. J. Comp. Pathol. 153, 28–37.

Mitchell, K.D., Kruth, S.A., Wood, R.D., Jefferson, B., 2009. Serum acute phase protein concentrations in dogs with autoimmune hemolytic anemia. J. Vet. Intern. Med. 23, 585–591.

Olivry, T., Bizikova, P., Dunston, S.M., et al., 2010. Clinical and immunological heterogeneity of canine subepidermal blistering dermatoses with anti-laminin-332 (laminin-5) auto-antibodies. Vet. Dermatol. 21, 345–357.

Olivry, T., Fine, J.-D., Dunston, S.M., et al., 1998. Canine epidermolysis bullosa acquisita: circulating autoantibodies target the amino terminal noncollagenous (NC1) domain of collagen VII in anchoring fibrils. Vet. Dermatol. 9, 19–31.

Olivry, T., Moore, P.F., Naydan, D.K., et al., 1996. Antifollicular cell-mediated and humoral immunity in canine alopecia areata. Vet. Dermatol. 7, 67–79.

Pedersen, N.C., Liu, H., Greenfield, D.L., Echols, L.G., 2012. Multiple autoimmune diseases syndrome in Italian greyhounds: preliminary studies of genome-wide diversity and possible associations within the dog leukocyte antigen (DLA) complex. Vet. Immunol. Immunopathol. 145, 264–276.

Romeike, A., Brügmann, M., Drommer, W., 1998. Immunohistochemical studies in equine recurrent uveitis (ERU). Vet. Pathol. 35, 515–526.

Schwartz, M., Puff, C., Stein, V.M., et al., 2011. Pathogenetic factors for excessive IgA production: Th2-dominated immune response in canine steroid-responsive meningitis-arteritis. Vet. J. 187, 260–266.

Short, A.D., Catchpole, B., Kennedy, L.J., et al., 2009. T cell cytokine polymorphisms in canine diabetes mellitus. Vet Immunol. Immunopathol. 128, 137–146.

Stokol, T., Blue, J.T., French, T.W., 2000. Idiopathic pure red cell aplasia and nonregenerative immune-mediated anemia in dogs.: 43 cases (1988–1999). J. Am. Vet. Med. Assoc. 266 (9), 1429–1436.

Spitzbarth, I., Baumgärtner, W., Beineke, A., 2012. The role of pro- and anti-inflammatory cytokines in the pathogenesis of spontaneous canine CNS diseases. Vet. Immunol. Immunopathol. 147, 6–24.

Spitzbarth, I., Schenk, H.C., Tipold, A., Beineke, A., 2010. Immunohistochemical characterization of inflammatory and glial responses in a case of necrotizing leucoencephalitis in a French bulldog. J. Comp. Pathol. 142, 235–241.

Talarico, L.R., Schatzberg, S.J., 2010. Idiopathic granulomatous and necrotizing inflammatory disorders of the canine central nervous system: a review and future perspectives,. J. Small. Anim. Pract. 51, 138–149.

Tauro, A., Addicott, D., Foale, R.D., Bowman, C., et al., 2015. Clinical features of idiopathic inflammatory polymyopathy in the Hungarian Vizsla. BMC Vet. Res. 11, 97–103.

Tizard, I.R., 2023. Autoimmune Diseases in Domestic Animals. Elsevier, St. Louis, MO, ISBN 978-0-323-84813-8

Tipold, A., Schatzberg, S.J., 2010. An update on steroid responsive meningitis-arteritis. J. Small Anim. Pract. 51, 150–154.

Tsai, K.L., Starr-Moss, A.N., Venkataraman, G.M., Robinson, C., et al., 2013. Alleles of the major histocompatibility complex play a role in the pathogenesis of pancreatic acinar atrophy in dogs. Immunogenetics 65, 501–509.

Uchida, K., Park, E., Tsuboi, M., Chambers, J.K., Nakayama, H., 2016. Pathological and immunological features of canine necrotising meningoencephalitis and granulomatous meningoencephalitis. Vet. J. 213, 72–77.

Verma, A., Matsunaga, J., Artiushin, S., Pinne, M., et al., 2012. Antibodies to a novel leptospiral protein, LruC, in the eye fluids and sera of horses with Leptospira-associated uveitis. Clin. Vaccine Immunol. 19, 452–456.

Warman, S.M., Murray, J.K., Ridyard, A., et al., 2008. Pattern of Coombs' test reactivity has diagnostic significance in dogs with immune-mediated haemolytic anaemia. J. Small Anim. Pract. 49, 525–530.

Wells, R., Guth, A., Lappin, M., Dow, S., 2009. Anti-endothelial cell antibodies in dogs with immune-mediated hemolytic anemia and other diseases associated with high risk of thromboembolism. J. Vet. Intern. Med. 23, 295–300.

Winfield, L.D., White, S.D., Affolter, V.K., Renier, A.C., et al., 2013. Pemphigus vulgaris in a Welsh pony stallion: case report and demonstration of anti-desmoglein autoantibodies. Vet. Dermatol. 24, 269–e60.

Wu, X., Li, Z.F., Brooks, R., et al., 2007. Autoantibodies in canine masticatory muscle myositis recognize a novel myosin binding protein-C family member. J. Immunol. 179, 4939–4944.

39

Selected Immune-Mediated Inflammatory Diseases

As pointed out in the previous chapter, immune-mediated diseases can range from "pure" autoimmune diseases to diseases where a loss of control of inflammatory responses contributes to the pathogenesis. In this chapter, we describe some of the more important of these inflammatory diseases (Galeazzi et al., 2006).

Animals suffer from inflammatory diseases involving multiple organ systems. In human medicine, these have been called "rheumatic" diseases, "connective tissue" diseases, or "collagen" diseases based on outdated views on their pathogenesis. These diseases or syndromes are interrelated and have many overlapping clinical features (Fig. 39.1). One common feature is extensive and uncontrolled inflammation, and it may be useful to consider them to be caused by innate autoimmunity or "autoinflammatory diseases." Because of their similarities, it is sometimes difficult to come up with a specific clinical diagnosis.

These inflammatory diseases include systemic lupus erythematosus (SLE), rheumatoid arthritis, nonerosive forms of arthritis, vasculitis, and Sjögren syndrome. Although all these diseases have some form of autoimmune component, they do not simply result from autoantibodies causing tissue destruction. Many are associated with the presence of immune complexes and activated complement in tissues resulting in chronic inflammation. Many result from uncontrolled inflammatory cytokine production. Their initiating factors are usually unknown, but many may be triggered by infectious agents acting through toll-like receptors (TLRs). All exhibit a significant genetic predisposition, commonly with linkage to the MHC (Tizard, 2023).

SYSTEMIC LUPUS ERYTHEMATOSUS

SLE is a complex disease syndrome that has been described in humans, other primates, mice, horses, dogs, and cats. It is characterized by a broad and bewildering diversity of different signs and a wide variety of disease courses as lesions flare and recede over time. The factors that cause lupus are complex, and poorly defined (Fig. 39.2; Rekvig and Van

Der Vlag 2014). Its development is affected by environmental factors, including infectious agents, hormones, drugs, and foods, as well as the intestinal microbiota in association with the effects of many different genes. Affected animals develop multiple autoantibodies, changes in

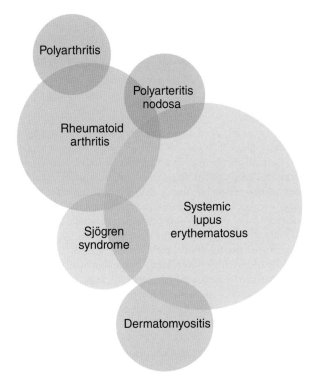

Fig. 39.1 The interrelationships among the diseases discussed in this chapter. The diagram is somewhat simplified since polyarthritis may be associated with polymyositis.

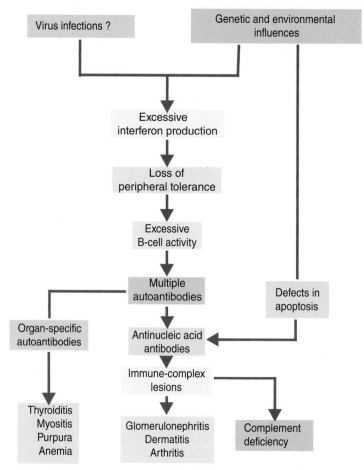

Fig. 39.2 A diagram showing a possible pathogenesis of systemic lupus erythematosus.

T-cell function, defective phagocytosis, impaired apoptosis, and multi-organ inflammation (Craft, 2011).

Pathogenesis
Genetic Factors

Lupus affects middle-aged dogs (between 2 and 12 years of age) and affects males more than females. The disease is commonly seen in Collies, German Shepherds, Nova Scotia Duck Tolling Retrievers, and Shetland Sheepdogs, but Beagles, Irish Setters, Poodles, and Afghan Hounds are also affected (Wilbe et al., 2009). Lupus (or positive lupus serology) may occur in related animals, supporting the importance of genetic factors. For example, dogs possessing the MHC class I antigen DLA-A7 are at increased risk, while those possessing DLA-A1 and B5 are at decreased risk for developing disease (Fig. 39.3; Teichner et al., 1990). When dogs with lupus are bred, the number of affected offspring is higher than can be accounted for genetically, suggesting that the disease may be vertically transmitted. A type C retrovirus has been suggested as a potential trigger of canine lupus.

B-Cell Abnormalities

B cells are central to the pathogenesis of lupus since they are the source of the autoantibodies responsible for its lesions (Lipsky, 2001). The hallmark of all forms of lupus is the development of autoantibodies against nuclear components, including nucleic acids, histones, ribonucleoproteins, and chromatin. These antinuclear antibodies (ANAs) are found in 97%–100% of dogs with lupus compared with 16%–20% of

normal control animals. Dogs mainly develop autoantibodies against histones and ribonucleoproteins. The nucleic acids that provoke ANA production probably come from three major sources; invading bacteria, neutrophil NETs, and apoptotic cells (Monestier et al., 1995).

Since mammalian and bacterial DNA have a conserved backbone, it is possible that animals with lupus may respond to bacterial infection by producing antibodies that cross-react with their own DNA. For example, the NZB/NZW mouse strain develops a lupus-like syndrome when immunized with bacterial DNA. This induces anti-DNA antibodies that form immune complexes and cause arthritis, skin rashes, and vascular disease.

When neutrophils expel NETs to capture bacteria, they release their nuclear contents. The components of these NETs are potential autoantigens and may trigger autoantibody formation. Free DNA released by bacteria or mitochondria or as a result of NETosis can bind to TLR7 and 9 and so trigger innate responses. Antibody-DNA immune complexes may also bind to TLR9 and activate B cells by triggering both their TLRs and Fc receptors. FcγR– and TLR-mediated uptake of immune complexes and nucleic acids activates plasmacytoid dendritic cells and so triggers IFN-α production. The immune responses in lupus are closely associated with IFN-α production, and the level of this cytokine correlates with disease activity. IFN-α also promotes inflammation by activating macrophages and autoreactive T cells. The production of ANAs in lupus may also result if TLR7 and TLR9, lose the ability to discriminate between microbial and self-DNA. If, at the same time, some of their B cells undergo somatic mutation that enables

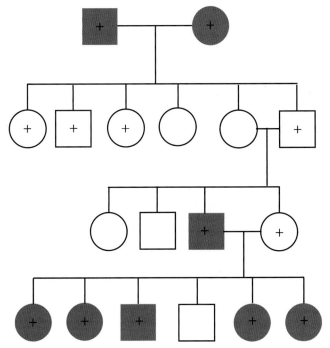

Fig. 39.3 The inheritance of canine systemic lupus erythematosus. This diagram shows four generations of a single family of dogs. Colored squares (male) or circles (female) denote those animals exhibiting clinical signs of systemic lupus; "+" denotes animals positive for antinuclear antibodies. From Teichner, M., Krumbacher, K., Doxiadis, I., et al., 1990. Systemic lupus erythematosus in dogs: association with the major histocompatibility complex class I antigen DLA-A7. Clin. Immunol. Immunopathol. 55, 225.

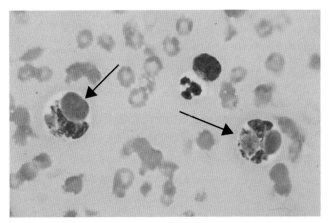

Fig. 39.4 Two lupus erythematosus cells (*arrows*) from a dog with systemic lupus erythematosus. Original magnification ×1300.

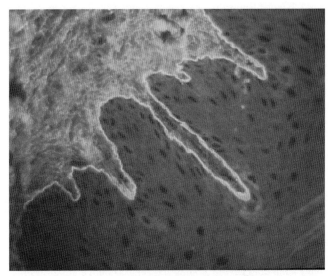

Fig. 39.5 A lupus band in a section of monkey esophagus. The indirect immunofluorescence assay shows IgG deposition on the skin basement membrane. Courtesy Dr. F.C. Heck.

their BCRs to bind self-DNA, the ingredients necessary for a profound antibody response to mammalian DNA come together.

Antinuclear antibodies can bind soluble nuclear antigens to form immune complexes that are then deposited in glomeruli, resulting in development of a membranoproliferative glomerulonephritis (MPGN) (see Chapter 33; Vinuesa and Goodnow, 2002). These immune complexes can also activate neutrophils causing them to release even more DNA and nucleoproteins through NETosis. The immune complexes may also be deposited in arteriolar walls, where they cause fibrinoid necrosis and fibrosis, or in synovia, where they provoke arthritis. ANAs bind to the nuclei of degenerating cells to produce round, or oval structures called hematoxylin bodies in the skin, kidney, lung, lymph nodes, spleen, and heart. Within the bone marrow, opsonized nuclei may be phagocytosed, giving rise to lupus erythematosus (LE) cells (Fig. 39.4).

Impaired Apoptosis

Failure of apoptosis leading to activation of autoimmune B cells and multiple autoimmune disorders is a feature of lupus. Normally, apoptotic cells are removed by macrophages without causing inflammation (see Chapter 19). Macrophages from lupus patients, however, show defective phagocytosis of apoptotic cells, which thus accumulate in tissues. The defect is most obvious in the skin of affected animals, where ultraviolet radiation damages cells and so triggers apoptotic cell death. In many dogs, lupus skin lesions may be restricted to the bridge of the nose and the area around the eyes since apoptosis is triggered by UV radiation in sunlight. Nucleic acids from these cells may activate dendritic cells and then act as autoantigens and trigger immune responses. Complement components mediate the efficient clearance of apoptotic cells, so complement deficiencies, especially C1q or C4 deficiency,

are also associated with the development of lupus-like syndromes. As described in Chapter 33, some lupus patients have a deficiency of the complement receptor CD35. As a result, immune complexes are not bound to red cells or platelets and are not removed from the circulation. These immune complexes may then be deposited in the glomeruli or in joints resulting in MPGN and arthritis.

Multiple Autoantibodies

Although ANAs are characteristic of lupus, many other autoantibodies are produced in affected animals, suggesting grossly abnormal B-cell function. Autoantibodies to red cells induce a hemolytic anemia. Antibodies to platelets induce a thrombocytopenia. Antilymphocyte antibodies may interfere with immune regulation. About 20% of dogs with lupus produce antibodies to IgG (rheumatoid factors). Antimuscle antibodies may cause myositis, and antimyocardial antibodies may provoke myocarditis or endocarditis. Antibodies to skin basement membrane cause a dermatitis characterized by changes in epidermal thickness, focal mononuclear cell infiltration, collagen degeneration, and immunoglobulin deposits at the dermoepidermal junction. These deposits form a "lupus band" (Fig. 39.5). The results of this excessive immune reactivity are also reflected in a polyclonal gammopathy, with enlargement of lymph nodes and spleen.

Affected animals show abnormalities in B-cell signaling and migration, overexpression of CD154 (CD40L), and enhanced production of interleukin-6 (IL-6) and IL-10. It is, therefore, probable that the production of multiple autoantibodies in lupus is a combined result of defective apoptosis, overstimulation of B cells, and a failure to eliminate self-reactive B cells. The diversity of autoantibodies in lupus can cause an equally great variety of clinical signs.

Canine Lupus

Dogs with systemic lupus may present with one or more signs of disease. However, the disease is progressive, so the severity of the lesions and the number of organ systems involved gradually increase in untreated cases. The most characteristic presentation is a fever accompanied by a symmetrical, nonerosive polyarthritis. Indeed, as many as 90% of dogs with lupus may develop arthritis at some stage. Other common presenting signs include renal failure (65%), skin disease (60%), lymphadenopathy or splenomegaly (50%), leukopenia (20%), hemolytic anemia (13%), and thrombocytopenia (4%). Dogs may also develop myositis (8%) or pericarditis (8%) and neurological abnormalities (1.6%). The leukopenia involves a major loss of CD8$^+$ T cells with a somewhat smaller loss of CD4$^+$ T cells, so that their CD4/CD8 ratio may climb as high as 6, compared to a normal value of about 1.7. The skin lesions are highly variable but are commonly restricted to areas exposed to sunlight. With this great variety of clinical presentations to choose from, it is not surprising that lupus is difficult to diagnose.

Several unique variants of lupus have been described in dogs. All are very rare, and many are associated with specific breeds, strongly suggesting a genetic predisposition. For example, vesicular systemic lupus is seen in Shetland Sheepdogs and Rough Collies. It is characterized by vesicular erosive and ulcerative skin lesions, subepidermal vesicles, and immunoglobulin deposition at the dermal-epidermal junction. Affected animals have antibodies against type VII collagen as well as ANAs (Jackson, 2004). Exfoliative lupus dermatitis has been described in German Short-haired Pointers (Bryden et al., 2005). Young adult dogs develop scaling and alopecia on the muzzle, pinnae, and dorsum. Some dogs may exhibit signs of pain and arthritis. Others may develop anemia and thrombocytopenia. Skin histology shows hyperkeratosis with a lymphocytic interface dermatitis similar to that seen in human lupus. IgG is deposited in the epidermal and follicular basement membranes. These dogs have circulating autoantibodies to epidermal basement membranes. Affected animals respond poorly to immunosuppressive therapy. This disease is inherited in an autosomal recessive manner.

Another lupus-related disease has been described in Gordon Setters. These dogs developed a symmetrical onychodystrophy, malformations, and loss of the claws. As a result, affected animals show lameness, severe discomfort, and acute pain. A related disease of Gordon Setters is black hair follicular dysplasia. In this disease, dogs begin to shed their black hair without normal regrowth. The remaining black hair is either short and stiff or thin and easily removed. Many affected dogs have positive ANA titers.

Mucocutaneous lupus is a form associated with skin lesion development at mucocutaneous junctions such as the perigenital and perianal areas with less involvement at perioral and periocular sites (Olivry et al., 2015). A chronic cutaneous form of lupus with bilaterally symmetrical alopecia and hyperpigmentation has been described in a Doberman.

Feline Lupus

Lupus is uncommon in cats, in which it usually presents as an antiglobulin-positive anemia. Other clinical manifestations include fever, skin disease, thrombocytopenia, polyarthritis, and renal failure. The ANA test must be interpreted with care in cats since many normal cats are ANA positive. Administration of propylthiouracil to cats with hyperthyroidism may result in the development of a syndrome resembling lupus. This may include the development of an antiglobulin-positive anemia as well as positive ANA reactions.

Equine Lupus

Systemic lupus presents as a generalized skin disease in the horse (alopecia, dermal ulceration, and crusting), usually accompanied by an antiglobulin-positive anemia. The disease is remarkable insofar as affected horses may be almost totally hairless (Fig. 39.6). Affected horses are ANA positive, although LE cell tests are equivocal in this species. Skin biopsies show basement membrane degeneration and immunoglobulin deposition typical of lupus. Affected horses may also develop glomerulonephritis, synovitis, and lymphadenopathy (Geor et al., 1990).

Diagnosis

A simple diagnostic rule for lupus may be stated as follows: Suspect lupus in an animal with multiple disorders such as those described previously and either a positive test for ANA or a positive test for LE cells (Box 39.1).

ANAs are normally demonstrated by immunofluorescence. Cultured cells or frozen sections of mouse or rat liver on a microscope slide are used as a source of antigen. Dilutions of a patient's serum are applied to this, the slide is incubated and then washed off. Binding of ANA to the cell nuclei is revealed by next incubating the tissue in a fluorescein-labeled antiserum to canine or feline immunoglobulins and then rewashing. Several different nuclear staining patterns have been described. A homogeneous staining pattern or staining of the nuclear rim is of greatest diagnostic significance, but nucleolar fluorescence is not (Fig. 39.7). Dogs with a speckled fluorescence pattern tend to have autoimmune diseases other than lupus. Some normal dogs, dogs undergoing treatment with certain drugs (griseofulvin, penicillin, sulfonamides, tetracyclines, phenytoin, and procainamide), and some dogs with liver disease or lymphosarcoma may have detectable

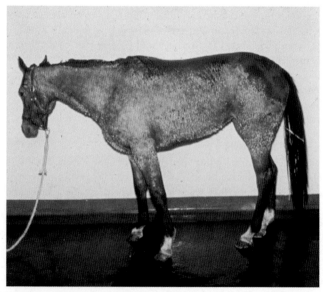

Fig. 39.6 A filly with systemic lupus erythematosus. Note the generalized alopecia and crusting. From Geor, R.J., Clark, E.G., Haines, D.M., Napier, P.G., 1990. Systemic lupus erythematosus in a filly. J. Am. Vet. Med. Assoc. 197(11), 1489–1492.

BOX 39.1 Diagnostic Criteria for Canine Systemic Lupus Erythematosus

Any two of the following must be present:

Characteristic skin lesions

Polyarthritis

Antiglobulin-positive hemolytic anemia

Thrombocytopenia

Proteinuria

And either:

A positive ANA test

Or:

A positive LE cell test

ANA, Antinuclear antibodies; *LE,* lupus erythematosus.

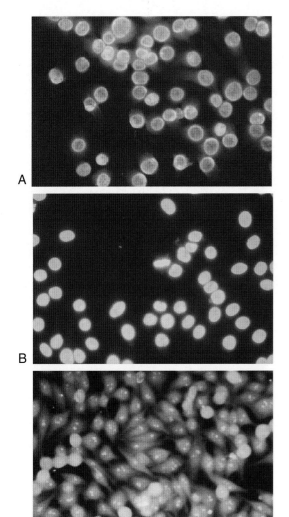

Fig. 39.7 Three positive antinuclear antibodies reactions. These are indirect fluorescent antibody reactions in which dog serum under test is layered onto a cell culture. After washing, the bound antibody is detected using a fluorescent antiglobulin. Although "rim" fluorescence (A) has traditionally been considered a positive reaction, the staining pattern obtained appears to depend in large part on the way the cells are fixed. These can, therefore, show diffuse staining (B) or nucleolar fluorescence (C). Courtesy Dr. F.C. Heck.

ANAs. ANAs are also found in dogs infected with *Bartonella vinsonii,* *Ehrlichia canis,* and *Leishmania infantum.* Dogs infected with multiple vector-borne organisms are also likely to be ANA positive (Smith et al., 2004). Thus nonspecific ANAs are present in many different neoplastic, inflammatory, and autoimmune diseases. ANA test results must, therefore, be used with caution.

LE cells, as previously mentioned, are neutrophils that have phagocytosed nuclear material from apoptotic cells (see Fig. 39.3). Their presence may be detected in the bone marrow and occasionally in buffy coat preparations from animals with lupus. It is usually necessary, however, to produce them in vitro. This can be accomplished by allowing the blood of an affected animal to clot and then incubating it at 37°C for 2 hours. During this time, normal neutrophils will phagocytose the nuclei of any apoptotic cells. Pressing it through a fine mesh then disrupts the clot, the resulting cell suspension is centrifuged, and the buffy coat is smeared, stained, and examined. LE cells are not a reliable diagnostic feature of systemic lupus in domestic animals since there is a high prevalence of both false-positive and false-negative results.

Treatment

Lupus in animals usually responds well to high doses of immunosuppressive/antiinflammatory drugs such as corticosteroids (prednisolone or prednisone), accompanied, if necessary, by cyclophosphamide, azathioprine, or chlorambucil.

DISCOID LUPUS ERYTHEMATOSUS

Discoid LE is a mild variant of SLE that occurs in two forms. The commonest form is characterized by the occurrence of facial skin lesions alone. A rarer form is generalized discoid LE (Banovic et al., 2016). There are no other pathological lesions, and ANA and LE tests are negative or weakly positive. It occurs in dogs, cats, horses, and humans. Facial discoid lupus has been described in Collies and Collie crosses, German Shepherds, Siberian Huskies, and Shetland Sheepdogs. They commonly present with nasal dermatitis with depigmentation, erythema, erosion, ulceration, scaling, and crusting. Occasionally, their feet may be affected, and some dogs may develop oral ulcers. C3, IgA, IgG, or IgM may be detected in the skin basement membrane in a typical lupus band. The skin lesions may be infiltrated with mononuclear and plasma cells. It can be treated with corticosteroids, and the prognosis is good. Since the lesions are exacerbated by sunlight, it is appropriate to use sunscreens and encourage the owner to keep the animal out of intense sunlight.

Discoid lupus in cats is characterized by a nonpruritic scaling and crusting dermatitis almost totally confined to the pinnae of the ear. There may be some ulceration and papule or pustule formation. Skin biopsy shows mononuclear infiltration of the basal cell layer with degeneration of basal cells. Direct immunofluorescence of skin sections shows a lupus band. Affected cats have negative or low ANA titers and negative LE cell tests. Treatment with corticosteroids is effective.

SJÖGREN'S SYNDROME

In this syndrome, autoimmune attack on salivary and lacrimal glands leads to conjunctival dryness (keratoconjunctivitis sicca) and mouth dryness (xerostomia). Affected animals subsequently develop gingivitis, dental caries, and excessive thirst. Sjögren's syndrome is often associated with rheumatoid arthritis, systemic lupus, polymyositis, or autoimmune thyroiditis. Affected dogs develop antibodies to nictitating membrane epithelial cells and, less consistently, to lacrimal and salivary glands or to the pancreas, and these organs may then be infiltrated with lymphocytes and other mononuclear cells. Most affected animals (90%) are hypergammaglobulinemic and have ANAs (40%) and RFs (34%). Many have other autoimmune lesions such as polyarthritis, hypothyroidism, and glomerulonephritis (Kaswan and Salisbury, 1993).

IMMUNE-MEDIATED POLYARTHRITIS

Animals develop immunologically mediated joint diseases, most of which are associated with the deposition of immunoglobulins or immune complexes within joints. Their classification is based on the presence or absence of joint erosion.

Rheumatoid Arthritis

Rheumatoid arthritis is a common, crippling disease affecting about 1% of humans. A very similar disease is seen in domestic animals, especially dogs, in which there is no obvious breed or sex predilection. Dogs with rheumatoid arthritis may present with chronic depression, anorexia, and pyrexia in addition to lameness, which tends to be most severe after rest (e.g., immediately after waking in the morning). The disease mainly affects peripheral joints, especially the carpal joints, which show symmetrical swelling and stiffness. Rheumatoid arthritis tends to be progressive and eventually leads to severe joint erosion and deformities. In advanced cases, affected joints may fuse as a result of the formation of bony ankyloses. Radiological findings are variable, but the initial swelling usually involves soft tissues only.

Pathogenesis

Rheumatoid arthritis is a disease of slow onset. It begins as a mild lymphocytic synovitis with neutrophils in the joint fluid. As the inflammation continues, the synovia swells and proliferates. Outgrowths of the proliferating synovia eventually extend into the joint cavities, where they are called pannus (Fig. 39.8; Alivernini et al., 2022). Pannus consists of fibrous vascular tissue that, as it invades the joint cavity, releases proteases that erode the articular cartilage and, ultimately, the neighboring bony structures. As the arthritis progresses, the infiltrating lymphocytes form lymphoid nodules and germinal centers within the synovia. Amyloidosis, arteritis, glomerulonephritis, and lymphatic hyperplasia are occasional complications of rheumatoid arthritis (Fig. 39.9).

It is probable that many different stimuli, especially infectious agents, trigger rheumatoid arthritis. In domestic mammals, *Mycoplasma hyorhinis*, *Erysipelothrix rhusiopathiae*, and *Borrelia burgdorferi* each produce a chronic arthritis that resembles rheumatoid arthritis. Dogs with rheumatoid arthritis have antibodies to canine distemper in their synovial fluids, antibodies that are not present in dogs with osteoarthritis. Immune complexes can be precipitated out of the synovial fluid of dogs with rheumatoid arthritis, and analysis of these complexes by Western blotting shows the presence of canine distemper virus antigens. Thus distemper virus may be detected in canine rheumatoid joints and may play a role in the pathogenesis of the disease (Bell et al., 1991).

Susceptibility to and severity of rheumatoid arthritis in humans are linked to the expression of certain MHC class II molecules (HLA-DR). This susceptibility is associated with the presence of a conserved 5-amino acid sequence located in the HLA-DRB1 antigen-binding groove and known as the "RA-shared epitope." It is interesting to note

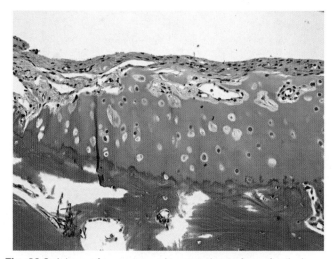

Fig. 39.8 A layer of pannus growing over the surface of articular cartilage. Notice how the underside is invading and eroding the cartilage surface. Courtesy Dr. Roy Pool.

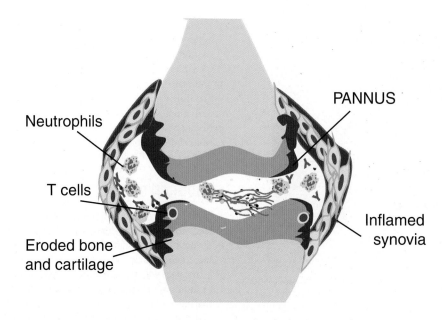

Fig. 39.9 A schematic diagram showing how joints are damaged in rheumatoid arthritis.

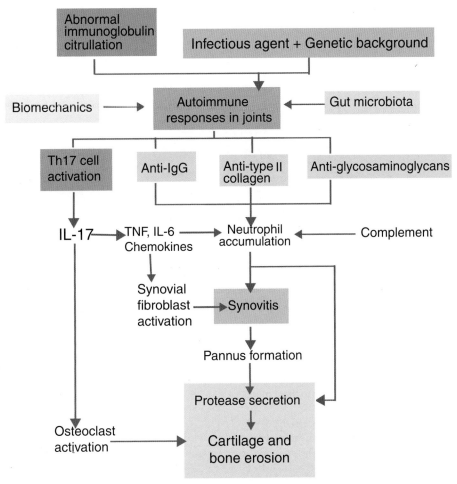

Fig. 39.10 A schematic diagram showing the possible pathogenesis of rheumatoid arthritis. *IgG*, Immunoglobulin G; *IL-6*, interleukin-6; *TH17*, T helper 17; *TNF*, tumor necrosis factor.

that this same conserved RA-shared epitope is found on canine DLA-DRB1 and is associated with susceptibility to RA in some dog breeds. Some MHC class III genes also affect susceptibility to canine RA. For example, possession of the C4 allotype C4-4 is associated with the development of autoimmune polyarthritis. Despite this, it has been estimated that non-MHC genes contribute as much as 75% of the genetic susceptibility to rheumatoid arthritis.

Although rheumatoid arthritis is generally considered an autoimmune disease, the identity of the autoantigens involved is unclear. Three that have been implicated are IgG, collagen, and citrullinated proteins. (Fig. 39.10). The development of rheumatoid factors directed against IgG is characteristic of rheumatoid arthritis. These RFs are autoantibodies directed against epitopes on the C_H2 domains of antigen-bound IgG. They can belong to any immunoglobulin class, including IgE, although IgG RFs are by far the most common. The IgG in rheumatoid arthritis patients is less glycosylated than normal IgG, and it may be that this abnormal IgG acts as an immunogen in susceptible animals. RFs are found not only in rheumatoid arthritis but also in SLE and other diseases in which extensive immune-complex formation occurs. RFs are also present in the serum and synovial fluid of some dogs with osteoarthritis (including cruciate disease), and infective arthritis.

RFs will agglutinate antibody-coated particles. In humans, latex beads coated with IgG are used for this purpose. In dogs, it is easier to make a canine antisheep-erythrocyte serum and coat sheep erythrocytes with this in a subagglutinating dose. After washing, these coated erythrocytes will agglutinate when mixed with RF-positive dog serum.

Although RFs are of diagnostic importance, their clinical significance is less clear. RFs are found in joint fluid, where their titer tends to correlate with the severity of the lesions, and the lesions themselves may be exacerbated by intra-articular inoculation of autologous immunoglobulins. Nevertheless, some dogs with rheumatoid arthritis may not have detectable RFs, and it is not uncommon to find others who have no arthritis despite the presence of RF in their serum. Thus, the measurement of RF in dogs is of doubtful specificity.

Other evidence suggests that autoantibodies to collagen may be important. Type II collagen predominates in articular cartilage and may act as an autoantigen. Autoantibodies to type II collagen can be detected in the serum and synovial fluid of dogs with rheumatoid arthritis, infective arthritis, and osteoarthritis. Horses with chronic, nonsuppurative arthritis, osteoarthritis, or traumatic arthritis develop antibodies to collagens I and II. These antibodies, as well as immune complexes, can, therefore, be found in the synovial fluid of horses with many different joint diseases (Osborne et al., 1995). An experimental disease that closely resembles rheumatoid arthritis develops in rats or sheep immunized with type II collagen. Evidence from experimental mice and some humans suggests that T cells directed against hyaluronic acid, heparin, and chondroitin sulfates may also induce an arthritis resembling rheumatoid arthritis.

It has also been suggested that rheumatoid arthritis may result from immune responses against citrullinated proteins. Citrulline is derived from arginine by the conversion of amino side chains to ketones during inflammation (Fig. 39.11). This change alters the behavior of proteins

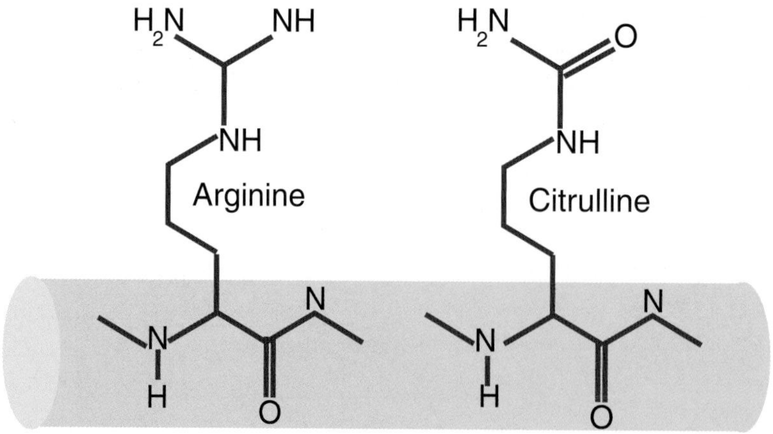

Fig. 39.11 Citrulline is generated from arginine by deimination. This occurs after a protein is translated by RNA. As a result, tolerance to citrullinated proteins can only be maintained by peripheral tolerance mechanisms.

and probably plays a role in the preparation of intracellular proteins for apoptosis. Citrullinated proteins are expressed in inflamed joints. Patients develop high levels of autoantibodies to these neoantigens before rheumatoid arthritis lesions develop, and these autoantibodies appear to be specific for this disease. They are rarely found in healthy people or in people with other diseases. It is, therefore, possible that the key initial lesion in this disease involves autoimmunity to these modified proteins (Van Gaalen et al., 2005).

Whatever the precise initiating factors, the first stage in the development of rheumatoid arthritis probably involves the unregulated activation of Th17 cells within the synovial membrane. The presence of the IL-17 activates synovial fibroblasts. Cytokines such as IL-1, IL-6, IL-22, GM-CSF, and TNF-α are produced by stromal and endothelial cells. IL-33 is released by synovial fibroblasts. Inflammatory chemokines such as CXCL8 (IL-8) also accumulate. The production of IL-17 and the escape of IL-33, together with chemokines, C5a, leukotriene B$_4$, and platelet-activating factor, results in the accumulation of neutrophils in the synovial fluid (Pei et al., 2014). Phagocytosis of immune complexes and tissue debris leads to protease escape and the release of oxidants. IL-1, IL-17, and TNF-α stimulate cartilage degradation by activating the cells that line the synovia and by stimulating the release of metalloproteases. These metalloproteases degrade the articular cartilage and ligaments (Coughlan et al., 1998). Activated platelets may enter the joint space and aggravate the process by producing more IL-1. More importantly, IL-17, TNF-α, and high mobility group box protein-1 from T cells activate bone-destroying osteoclasts. Collectively, these reactions lead to bone and cartilage erosion and the characteristic joint pathology of RA (Mills, 2023).

Circulating lymphocytes enter newly formed capillaries, emigrate into the tissues, and aggregate around the blood vessels. These infiltrating lymphocytes are primarily activated CD4$^+$ T cells. B-cell emigration into the tissues eventually leads to local RF production. The RFs form immune complexes and activate complement. Some immune complexes may precipitate within the superficial layers of the articular cartilage.

The progressive development of inflammation within synovia leads first to morning stiffness. The joints become warm as the blood flow increases, but because the inflammation is restricted to the synovia, the skin rarely becomes red. The animal may show depression and fatigue as a result of the systemic effects of IL-1 and TNF-α. If the joints develop effusions, they will be swollen. As the disease progresses, the inflamed synovia invades the cartilage, ligaments, and bone and

> ## BOX 39.2   Diagnostic Criteria for Canine Rheumatoid Arthritis
>
> - Stiffness or joint pain, especially after periods of inactivity
> - Symmetrical joint swelling, especially if multiple joints are involved
> - Sterile synovial fluid containing inflammatory cells, especially neutrophils
> - Positive rheumatoid factor test
> - Erosive polyarthritis with characteristic histology

destroys the articular cartilage while synovial lining cells, small blood vessels, and fibroblasts proliferate.

Diagnosis. Diagnosis of rheumatoid arthritis in animals is based on the criteria established for human rheumatoid arthritis. They are listed in Box 39.2. Most signs should have been present for at least 6 weeks. In addition, steps should be taken to exclude SLE (by testing for ANA) and to exclude an infectious cause for the arthritis. In practice, cytologic evaluation of synovial fluid with a protein concentration of >3.0 g/dL and a nucleated cell count of >3000 cells/mL consisting of >12% neutrophils identifies an inflammatory arthritis, especially when supported by radiographic evidence of erosion.

Treatment. Treatment of canine rheumatoid arthritis tends to be unsatisfactory, and the long-term prognosis is poor. Nonsteroidal anti-inflammatory drugs, such as aspirin, carprofen, or etodolac, have been the first choice in treating early, uncomplicated cases of rheumatoid arthritis, although their efficacy is unclear. Corticosteroids such as prednisolone should be reserved for late, severe cases in which salicylates have proved inadequate. Local steroid injections into affected joints will produce rapid relief and clinical remission. However, the joints are still subjected to stress, disease progression is not slowed, and the corticosteroids delay healing and promote articular degeneration. Their use may therefore permit articular damage to proceed unabated. Encouraging results have been obtained in humans by the aggressive use of the immunosuppressive agent methotrexate and anti-TNF monoclonal antibodies. Appropriate surgery may improve joint stability and reduce pain (Shaughnessy et al., 2016).

Nonerosive Polyarthritis

The second major group of immune-mediated arthritides consists of those in which the joint cartilage is not eroded, and the inflammatory lesion is largely confined to the joint capsule and synovia. Many resemble rheumatoid arthritis clinically but may be differentiated by their nonerosive character.

Equine Polyarthritis/Polysynovitis

Polyarthritis has been reported in foals in association with a lupus-like syndrome. Affected foals present with multiple swollen joints involving all four limbs and a persistent fever. In some cases, the synovial sheaths, including tendon sheaths and bursae, are also affected. The synovial effusions are sterile, but synovial biopsies show lymphocyte and plasma cell infiltration with some immunoglobulin deposits. The cells in the joint fluid are mainly neutrophils. These foals are negative for RF, ANA, and LE cells. Many of these animals have a lesion within the thorax, especially *Prescotella equi* pneumonia. This is classified as a type II disease (see later). It is possible that immune complexes originating in the lungs may lodge in the synovia and trigger the synovitis. The polyarthritis usually resolves as the primary lesion resolves.

An idiopathic type I immune-mediated polyarthritis has also been recorded in horses. In these cases, animals lose weight, develop an intermittent fever, and have effusions in multiple joints leading to stiffness. They have systemic signs of inflammation, including anemia, leukocytosis, hyperfibrinogenemia, and hyperglobulinemia. The synovial effusion is sterile, and immunoglobulins are present in the synovial membrane. The condition usually resolves with steroid and immunosuppressive therapy (Pusterla et al., 2006).

Canine Polyarthritis

Dogs may develop several distinct nonerosive polyarthritides, which can be divided into three major categories: arthritis associated with SLE, arthritis associated with a myositis, and idiopathic polyarthritis. Breeds predisposed to polyarthritis include German Shepherds, Irish Setters, Shetland Sheepdogs, Cocker Spaniels, and Springer Spaniels. The main clinical features are stiffness, pyrexia, anorexia, and lethargy.

Lupus Polyarthritis

Polyarthritis is a common feature of SLE. Diagnosis is contingent on making a firm diagnosis of lupus. Thus, it is necessary to show multiple-system involvement, a significant titer of serum ANAs, and immunopathological features consistent with lupus.

Polyarthritis with Polymyositis

A disease characterized by both nonerosive polyarthritis and polymyositis is recognized in young dogs. Most recorded cases have been seen in Spaniels. The animals are stiff and have painful joints, fever, lethargy, weakness, muscle atrophy, and muscle pain. They are negative for both ANA and RF. The arthritis is symmetrical, involving multiple joints. These dogs also have a symmetrical inflammatory myopathy with myalgia, atrophy, and muscle contracture. The synovial fluid contains high white cell counts, especially neutrophils. Muscle biopsies show a neutrophil or mononuclear cell infiltrate, or both, with muscle fiber atrophy and degeneration. Synovial biopsies show a neutrophil and mononuclear cell infiltration with a fibrinous exudate. IgG, IgM, and complement are deposited in the walls of the synovial vessels.

Idiopathic Polyarthritis

Most cases of canine polyarthritis fit none of the categories described previously. Although these cases are nonerosive and possess the characteristics of type III hypersensitivity, their precise etiology is unknown. They are classified into four types (Table 39.1). Type I disease is polyarthritis alone. Type II disease is a reactive arthritis associated with infections in the respiratory or urinary tract, tooth infections, or cellulitis. Type III disease is associated with the presence of gastroenteritis,

TABLE 39.1 Classification of Nonerosive Polyarthritis in Dogs

Type	Disease Associations
I	Uncomplicated polyarthritis without other disease associations
II	Polyarthritis associated with infectious lesions remote from the joints (e.g., respiratory or urinary infections)
III	Polyarthritis associated with gastrointestinal disease
IV	Polyarthritis associated with neoplastic disease remote from the joints

From Bennett, D.J., 1987. Canine idiopathic polyarthritis. Small Anim. Pract. 28, 909–928.

diarrhea, or ulcerative colitis. It is not clear whether this type of disease is truly distinguishable from type II disease. Type IV disease is associated with the presence of tumors, including seminomas and carcinomas.

An example of type I polyarthritis is the juvenile polyarthritis syndrome seen in young Akitas. These dogs have a cyclical high fever lasting 24–48 hours before resolving, and evidence of severe, incapacitating joint pain with soft tissue swelling. Radiology shows hepatosplenomegaly and lymphadenopathy. Some animals may develop meningitis or meningoencephalitis. Their erythrocytes may be antiglobulin positive. Synovial fluid shows no evidence of infection, although large numbers of neutrophils are present. Affected dogs are usually negative for RF and ANA. Pedigree analysis suggests that the disease is inherited. Some dogs respond positively to corticosteroid treatment. In refractory cases, azathioprine may also be required (Felsburg et al., 1992).

Idiopathic polyarthritis tends to be most common in male dogs, and about half of the cases are seen in young dogs between 1 and 3.5 years of age. Most affected animals show fever, anorexia, and lethargy. The animals are lame and have a history of stiffness after rest. The most commonly affected joints are the stifle, elbow, and carpus. The onset of lameness is sudden in most cases and is associated with obvious muscle atrophy. There is no significant joint erosion, although periarticular soft tissue swelling, and synovial effusions are common. Some cases may have proliferative periosteal changes. All cases are negative for RF and ANA. The joint fluid is sterile. Synovial biopsies show hypertrophy with a neutrophil or a mononuclear cell infiltration, or both. Fibrin deposits are seen in most cases, as is fibrosis. Most lesions contain IgM, IgG, and complement deposits, and some contain IgA-producing plasma cells. Some affected dogs may develop a glomerulonephritis. Animals respond well to corticosteroids.

Feline Polyarthritis

Chronic progressive polyarthritis of male cats is characterized by polyarthritis with either osteopenia or periosteal new bone formation. Periarticular erosions and eventual collapse or subchondral erosions, joint instabilities, and deformities closely resembling those of rheumatoid arthritis are also seen. Affected cats are commonly infected with feline syncytia-forming virus (FSV) or feline leukemia virus (FeLV), or both. (The prevalence of FSV in these cats is 2–4 times higher, and the prevalence of FeLV is 6–10 times higher than in normal cats.) It is described here because of suggestions that it is of immunological origin. These suggestions are based on the massive lymphocyte and plasma cell infiltration of affected joints and the presence of an immune-complex glomerulonephritis. However, affected cats are RF and ANA negative, and their serum immunoglobulin levels tend to be close to normal. Corticosteroids lessen the severity of clinical signs (Doom et al., 2008).

VILLONODULAR SYNOVITIS

Villonodular synovitis is a proliferative arthritis associated with severe pain and lameness in affected dogs. It is characterized by hypertrophy and villous proliferation of the synovial membrane accompanied by a plasma cell and lymphocyte infiltration. The stifle is most commonly affected. It is closely associated with stretching and rupture of the cruciate ligament. Its etiology is unknown, but it appears to be, at least in part, immune mediated (Mapuvire et al., 2020). The synovia of affected dogs contain B cells, IgG-positive plasma cells, and numerous MHC class II+, CD1c+ dendritic cells. Cruciate ligaments are mainly composed of type I collagen. Their rupture is associated with gradual degeneration of the ligament extracellular matrix leading to increased joint laxity. Some breeds, such as Newfoundlands, appear predisposed to the condition (Comerford et al., 2011). Autoantibodies to both type I and type II collagen are found in synovial fluid following cruciate ligament rupture, usually bound in immune complexes. They are probably secondary to tissue damage and osteoarthritis. CXCL8 (IL-8), metalloprotease, and cathepsin levels rise in joints before cruciate ligament rupture, implying that inflammation precedes rupture (Doom et al., 2008).

IMMUNE VASCULITIS

Several forms of immune-mediated vasculitis have been described in domestic animals. Some, such as equine viral arteritis, lymphocytic choriomeningitis in mice, and Aleutian disease of mink are directly mediated by viruses. Others are a result of administration of drugs such as sulfonamides or digoxin, or antigenic solutions such as serum sickness. However, many are of unknown etiology. Their precise relationships are unclear, and as a result, they have been given several different names, including canine juvenile polyarteritis, polyarteritis nodosa, and leukocytoclastic vasculitis (Fig. 39.12).

Canine juvenile polyarteritis primarily affects Beagles less than two years of age. The animals show episodes of anorexia, persistent fever of greater than 40°C, and a hunched stance with lowered head and a stiff gait, indicating severe neck pain. They may show cyclical remissions and relapses. They have a neutrophilia, elevated acute-phase proteins, elevated serum IgM and IgA, but normal IgG. Blood B cells are increased,

but their T cells are decreased. On necropsy there are few gross lesions. There may be some hemorrhage in lymph nodes. Histologically, they have systemic vasculitis and perivasculitis. In the acute disease, there is necrotizing vasculitis with fibrinoid necrosis and a massive inflammatory cell infiltration involving the small and medium-sized arteries of the heart, mediastinum, and cervical spinal cord (Fig. 39.13). Immunoglobulins are deposited in the walls of these arteries. During

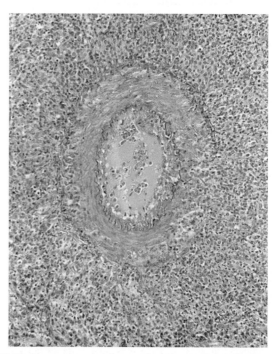

Fig. 39.13 An extramural coronary artery from a Beagle suffering from juvenile polyarteritis. This medium-sized muscular artery is characterized by medial necrosis, ruptured elastic laminae, and severe perivascular accumulations of neutrophils, lymphocytes, and macrophages. H&E stain. From Snyder, P.W., Kazacos, E.A., Scott-Moncrieff, J.C., et al., 1995. Pathologic features of naturally occurring juvenile polyarteritis in beagle dogs. Vet. Pathol. 32, 337–345.

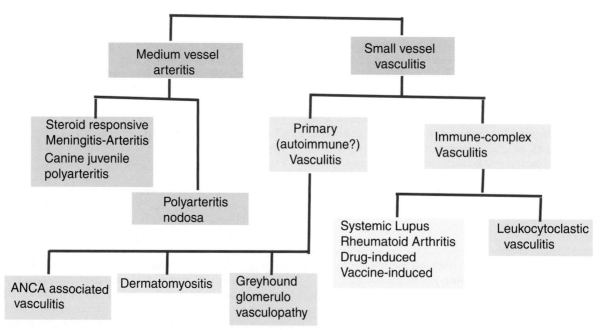

Fig. 39.12 Different forms of canine vasculitis and arteritis.

remissions, the vascular lesions consist of intimal and medial fibrosis and a mild perivasculitis, the residue of previous acute vasculitis. Chronically affected dogs may develop generalized amyloidosis.

Polyarteritis nodosa occurs sporadically in humans, pigs, dogs, and cats. It is characterized by a widespread, focal necrosis of the media of small- and medium-sized muscular arteries. The lesions are found in many organs, especially in the kidney and mesentery. Vessels in the skin are rarely involved.

On occasion, focal vascular lesions characterized by neutrophil infiltration may develop in small blood vessels throughout the body, but especially in skin. Affected dogs have mucocutaneous ulcers, bullae, edema, polyarthropathy, myopathy, anorexia, intermittent fever, and lethargy. Although called hypersensitivity vasculitis, a foreign antigen can be found in only a small proportion of cases. For this reason, a better name for this condition may be leukocytoclastic vasculitis. The cause or causes of polyarteritis nodosa and hypersensitivity vasculitis are unknown. Their histopathology suggests that they are a form of type III hypersensitivity reaction, perhaps triggered by an infectious agent and immunothrombosis. Immunosuppression with corticosteroids, together with cyclophosphamide, has given encouraging results in treating canine hypersensitivity vasculitis. Polyarteritis nodosa is usually detected as an incidental finding on necropsy, although ocular defects may present clinically if the arteries of the eye are involved.

REFERENCES

Alivernini, S., Firestein, G.S., McInnes, I.B., 2022. The pathogenesis of rheumatoid arthritis. Immunity 55, 2255–2270.

Banovic, F., Linder, K.E., Uri, M., Rossi, M.A., Olivry, T., 2016. Clinical and microscopic features of generalized discoid lupus erythematosus in dogs (10 cases). Vet. Dermatol. 27, 488–e131.

Bell, S.C., Carter, S.D., Bennett, D., 1991. Canine distemper viral antigens and antibodies in dogs with rheumatoid arthritis. Res. Vet. Sci. 50, 64–68.

Bryden, S.L., White, S.D., Dunston, S.M., et al., 2005. Clinical, histopathological and immunological characteristics of exfoliative cutaneous lupus erythematosus in 25 German short-haired pointers. Vet. Dermatol. 16, 239–252.

Comerford, E.J., Smith, K., Hayashi, K., 2011. Update on the aetiopathogenesis of canine cranial cruciate ligament disease. Vet. Comp. Orthop. Traumatol. 24, 91–98.

Coughlan, A.R., Robertson, D.H.L., Bennett, D., et al., 1998. Matrix metalloproteinases 2 and 9 in canine rheumatoid arthritis. Vet. Rec. 143, 219–223.

Craft, J.E., 2011. Dissecting the immune cell mayhem that drives lupus pathogenesis. Sci. Transl. Med. 3, 73. ps9

Doom, M., de Bruin, T., de Rooster, H., et al., 2008. Immunopathological mechanisms in dogs with rupture of the cranial cruciate ligament. Vet. Immunol. Immunopathol. 125, 143–161.

Felsburg, P.J., HogenEsch, H., Somberg, P.W., et al., 1992. Immunologic abnormalities in canine juvenile polyarteritis syndrome: a naturally occurring animal model of Kawasaki disease. Clin. Immunol. Immunopathol. 65, 110–118.

Galeazzi, M., Gasbarrini, G., Ghirardello, A., et al., 2006. Autoinflammatory syndromes. Clin. Exp. Rheumatol. 24 (Suppl. 40), S79–S85.

Geor, R.J., Clark, E.G., Haines, D.M., Napier, P.G., 1990. Systemic lupus erythematosus in a filly. J. Am. Vet. Med. Assoc. 197, 1489–1492.

Jackson, H.A., 2004. Eleven cases of vesicular cutaneous lupus erythematosus in Shetland sheepdogs and rough collies: clinical management and prognosis. Vet. Dermatol. 15, 37–41.

Kaswan, R.L., Salisbury, M.A., 1993. Canine keratoconjunctivitis sicca: etiology, clinical signs, diagnosis and treatment. Part II. Diagnosis and treatment with cyclosporine. J. Vet. Allerg. Clin. Immunol. 2, 8–12.

Lipsky, P.E., 2001. Systemic lupus erythematosus: an autoimmune disease of B cell hyperactivity. Nat. Immunol. 2, 764–766.

Mapuvire, T., Kandiwa, E., Mbiri, P., Samkange, A., et al., 2020. Chronic lymphoplasmacytic villonodular proliferative synovitis in a 10-year-old Jack Russell Terrier dog. Int. J. Vet. Sci. Med. 8 (1), 100–105.

Mills, K.H.G., 2023. IL-17 and IL-17 producing cells in protection versus pathology. Nat. Rev. Immunol 23, 38–54.

Monestier, M., Novick, K.E., Karam, E.T., et al., 1995. Autoantibodies to histone, DNA, and nucleosome antigens in canine systemic lupus erythematosus,. Clin. Exp. Immunol. 99, 37–41.

Olivry, T., Rossi, M.A., Banovic, F., Linder, K.E., 2015. Mucocutaneous lupus erythematosus in dogs (21 cases). Vet. Dermatol. 26, 256–e55. 2015.

Osborne, A.C., Carter, S.D., May, S.A., Bennett, D., 1995. Anti-collagen antibodies and immune complexes in equine joint diseases. Vet. Immunol. Immunopathol. 45, 19–30.

Pei, C., Barbour, M., Fairlie-Clarke, K.J., Allan, D., Mu, R., Jiang, H.R., 2014. Emerging role of interleukin-33 in autoimmune diseases. Immunology 141, 9–17.

Pusterla, N., Pratt, S.M., Magdesian, K.G., Carlson, G.P., 2006. Idiopathic immune-mediated polysynovitis in three horses. Vet. Rec. 159, 13–15.

Rekvig, O.P., Van Der Vlag, J., 2014. The pathogenesis and diagnosis of systemic lupus erythematosus: still not resolved. Semin. Immunopathol. 36, 301–311.

Shaughnessy, M.L., Sample, S.J., Abicht, C., Heaton, C., Muir, P., 2016. Clinical features and pathological joint changes in dogs with erosive immune-mediated polyarthritis: 13 cases (2004-2012). J. Am. Vet. Med. Assoc. 249, 1156–1164.

Smith, B.E., Tompkins, M.B., Breitschwerdt, E.R., 2004. Antinuclear antibodies can be detected in dog sera reactive to Bartonella vinsonii subsp. berkhoffii, Ehrlichia canis or Leishmania infantum antigens. J. Vet. Intern. Med. 18, 47–51.

Teichner, M., Krumbacher, K., Doxiadis, I., et al., 1990. Systemic lupus erythematosus in dogs: association to the major histocompatibility complex class I antigen DLA-A7. Clin. Immunol. Immunopathol. 55, 255–262.

Tizard, I.R., 2023. Autoimmune Diseases in Domestic Animals. Elsevier, St Louis, MO, ISBN 978-0-323-84813-8

Van Gaalen, F., Ioan-Fascinay, A., Huizinga, T.W.J., Toes, R.E.M., 2005. The devil in the details: the emerging role of anticitrulline autoimmunity in rheumatoid arthritis. J. Immunol. 175, 5575–5580.

Vinuesa, C.G., Goodnow, C.C., 2002. DNA drives autoimmunity. Nature 416, 595–598.

Wilbe, M., Jokinen, P., Hermanrud, C., et al., 2009. MHC class II polymorphism is associated with a canine SLE-related disease complex. Immunogenetics 61, 557–564.

Primary Immunodeficiency Diseases

Defects in either the innate or adaptive immune systems usually become apparent when affected animals show unusual susceptibility to infectious or parasitic diseases. Deficiencies in the immune systems may result from inherited or genetic defects (primary immunodeficiencies); or a direct result of some other cause (secondary or acquired immunodeficiencies). This chapter describes some of the primary immunodeficiencies recorded in domestic mammals.

INHERITED DEFECTS IN INNATE IMMUNITY

Inherited deficiencies in innate immunity include defects at various stages of phagocytosis as well as the complement deficiencies described previously (see Chapter 5). Phagocytic deficiency diseases are well recognized in domestic animals.

Chédiak-Higashi Syndrome

Chédiak-Higashi syndrome is an inherited disease of Hereford, Japanese Black, and Brangus cattle, Aleutian mink, "Blue smoke" Persian cats, white tigers, beige (*bg/bg*) mice, orcas, and humans (Schiflett et al., 2002). It is an autosomal recessive disease resulting from a mutation in the lysosomal trafficking regulator (*LYST*) gene encoding a protein that controls lysosomal membrane fusion. Chédiak-Higashi cattle have a missense A:T → G:C mutation that results in replacement of a histidine with an arginine residue. In

Aleutian mink, the causal mutation is a base deletion in *LYST* that causes a frame-shift leading to premature termination. These mutations produce abnormally large secretory granules in neutrophils, monocytes, eosinophils, and pigment cells (Fig. 40.1). The enlarged neutrophil granules result from the fusion of primary and secondary granules. These granules are more fragile than normal, rupturing spontaneously and causing tissue damage. Affected leukocytes have defective chemotactic responsiveness, reduced motility, and impaired intracellular killing. Cytotoxic T cells and NK cells cannot exocytose their granzyme-rich granules.

Clinically, the syndrome is associated with multiple abnormalities. In hair, the melanosomes fuse together, causing the dilution of coat color (sometimes only obvious in the newborn) and light-colored irises (pseudoalbinism). Other eye abnormalities include photophobia, and animals may develop cataracts. Their eyes have a red fundic light reflection rather than the normal yellow-green. Because of these neutrophil defects, affected animals may be more susceptible to respiratory infections and neonatal septicemia. Affected animals may show increased susceptibility to tumors and to infections such as the Aleutian disease parvovirus in mink (Anistoroaei et al., 2013). Platelets from affected animals also contain enlarged lysosomes, and as a result, affected animals may bleed excessively after surgery and develop hematomas at injection sites. Death due to acute hemorrhage is common. Chédiak-Higashi syndrome may be diagnosed by

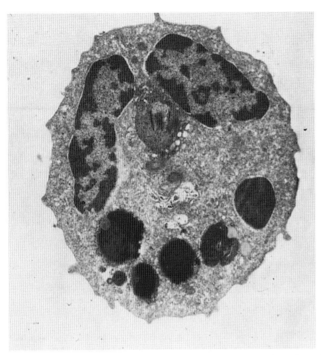

Fig. 40.1 A neutrophil from a Chédiak-Higashi syndrome calf with enlarged cytoplasmic granules. Courtesy Dr. H.W. Leopold.

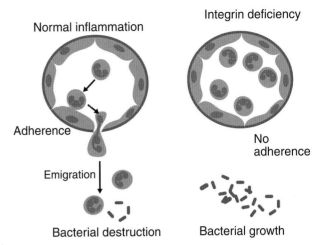

Fig. 40.2 Integrins are required to bind neutrophils firmly to blood vessel walls. This permits the neutrophils to emigrate to sites of bacterial invasion. In the absence of integrins, neutrophil emigration fails to occur. As a result, invading bacteria can grow unmolested in the tissues.

examining a stained blood smear for the presence of grossly enlarged granules within leukocytes or by examining hair shafts for enlarged melanosomes.

Pelger-Huët Anomaly

Pelger-Huët anomaly is an inherited disorder characterized by a failure of granulocyte nuclei to segment into lobes. The neutrophils therefore appear on first sight to be very immature (a left shift). The anomaly is usually detected when an animal is observed to have a persistent left shift that cannot be reconciled with its good health. Although Pelger-Huët neutrophils closely resemble band forms, their nuclear chromatin is condensed, reflecting their maturity. In humans, the anomaly is due to a mutation in the gene coding for lamin B, a nuclear membrane receptor that interacts with chromatin to determine the shape of the nucleus. Pelger-Huët anomaly has been observed in humans, Arabian horses, domestic shorthair cats, and various dog breeds such as Cocker Spaniels, Basenjis, Boston Terriers, Foxhounds, and Coonhounds (Grondin et al., 2007). In Foxhounds and Australian Shepherd dogs, the anomaly is inherited as an autosomal dominant trait. It has a minimal effect on the health of animals. Nevertheless, fewer pups are weaned from affected dogs than from unaffected ones. In addition, Pelger-Huët neutrophils are less able to emigrate from blood vessels in vivo. Their B-cell responses may also be impaired (Latimer et al., 2000).

Canine Leukocyte Adhesion Deficiency

In order for neutrophils to leave inflamed blood vessels, they must first bind to vascular endothelium. This adhesion is mediated by neutrophil integrins. In the absence of these integrins, neutrophils cannot bind to endothelial cells and so cannot leave the bloodstream (Fig. 40.2). As a result, bacteria in tissues can grow freely without fear of attack by neutrophils.

Three different forms of leukocyte adherence deficiency (LAD) are recognized. The commonest form, LAD-I results from a loss-of-function

mutation in the gene encoding the β2-integrin (CD18). LAD-II results from a defect in fucose metabolism that leads to a deficiency of the carbohydrate structure sialyl-Lewis-X and impairs neutrophil rolling. It has not been reported in dogs. LAD-III results from defective activation of β-integrins as a result of mutations in the Kindlin-3 gene. Kindlin-3 is a protein that is essential for β-integrin activation.

Canine leukocyte adhesion deficiency (CLAD) is a LAD-I disease that results from a defect in the gene encoding integrin Mac-1 (CD11b/CD18). In Mac-1-deficient dogs, neutrophils cannot respond to chemoattractants, trap complement-coated bacteria (Mac-1 is a complement receptor) or bind to endothelial cells. Affected dogs suffer recurrent infections, despite the fact that their blood neutrophil numbers are high.

CLAD has been described in Irish Setters (as well as in the related Red and White Setter breed), in which it is an autosomal recessive disease (Kijas et al., 1999). Affected animals die young as a result of recurrent severe bacterial infections (osteomyelitis, omphalophlebitis, gingivitis), lymphadenopathy, impaired pus formation, delayed wound healing, weight loss, and fever (Debenham et al., 2002). Animals have a leukocytosis (>200,000/μL), primarily a neutrophilia and eosinophilia. Although their granulocytes look normal, functional tests reveal defects in adhesion-dependent activities, including impaired adhesion to glass or plastic surfaces. They cannot ingest C3b-opsonized particles. Migration in response to chemotactic stimuli is poor. Neither CD11b nor CD18 can be detected by immunofluorescence.

The CLAD lesion results from a single missense mutation in the gene encoding the β-chain of CD18 that results in the replacement of a cysteine by a serine. The mutation disrupts a disulfide bond in CD18 and so alters its structure and function. CD11b (the α-chain) is not expressed because it must be associated with the β chain before the dimer can be expressed on the cell surface. A diagnostic PCR test for CLAD has been developed. Matched-related bone marrow allografts from normal animals have been given to CLAD dogs resulting in microchimerism and a reduction in the severity of the disease (Gu et al., 2006).

Another form of CLAD results from excessive downregulation of β2-integrin expression. This has occurred in mixed-breed dogs that presented with recurrent pyogenic infections. Their neutrophils produced significantly reduced amounts of CD18 and, hence, β2-integrin. As a result of this reduced expression, defects occur in adhesion-dependent neutrophil functions, as well as superoxide production.

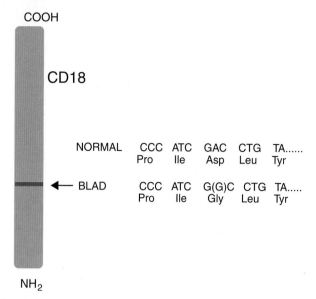

Fig. 40.3 The Bovine leukocyte adhesion deficiency (BLAD) mutation. The mutation involves replacement of a cytosine by a guanosine in the CD18 gene. As a result, an aspartic acid residue (A) is replaced by a glycine residue (G). The mutation occurs in a highly conserved region of the CD18 molecule and prevents formation of a biologically active molecule.

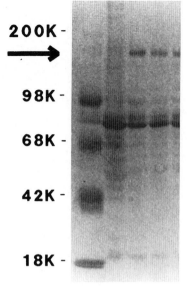

Fig. 40.4 A Western blot of bovine Mac-1. An extract has been made from the neutrophils of a Bovine leukocyte adhesion deficiency (BLAD) calf *(lane 2)* or from clinically normal calves *(lanes 3 and 4)*. The extracts have been electrophoresed and blotted onto nitrocellulose. The bands are stained to show the presence of glycoproteins. Note that CD18 *(arrow)* is absent from the lysate of neutrophils from a BLAD calf. Lane 1 shows molecular weight standards (kDa). From Kehrili Jr., M.E., Schmalstieg, F.C., Anderson, D.C., et al., 1990. Molecular definition of the bovine granulocytopathy syndrome: identification of deficiency of the Mac-1 (CD11b/CD18) glycoprotein. Am. J. Vet. Res. 51 (11), 1826–1836.

Cases of LAD-III have been reported in a German Shepherd dog and in a German Shepherd x Rottweiler cross (Hugo and Heading, 2014). The dogs developed pyrexia, persistent leukocytosis, severe periodontal disease, lameness, mucosal hemorrhage,s and poor wound healing. Because of defects in thrombocyte function, life-threatening hemorrhage was the most significant cause of death in these animals. The second case of LAD-III was shown to result from a 12-nucleotide insertion mutation in the gene encoding kindlin-3.

Bovine Leukocyte Adhesion Deficiency

Bovine leukocyte adhesion deficiency (BLAD) is an autosomal recessive trait characterized by recurrent bacterial infections, anorexia, oral ulceration, gingivitis, periodontitis, chronic pneumonia, stunted growth, delayed wound healing, peripheral lymphadenopathy, and a persistent extreme neutrophilia. It has been reported in Holstein calves. Affected calves usually die between 2 and 7 months of age. The survivors grow slowly and may develop amyloidosis. These calves have large numbers of intravascular neutrophils but very few extravascular neutrophils, even in the presence of invading bacteria.

Because T cells also use CD18 to emigrate from blood vessels, BLAD calves show poor delayed hypersensitivity responses. Their neutrophils show reduced responsiveness to chemotactic stimuli and diminished superoxide production and myeloperoxidase activity. They have increased expression of Fc receptors but decreased binding of C3b and IgM to neutrophils, implying a defect in receptor function. This is reflected by greatly reduced endocytosis and killing of *Staphylococcus aureus*.

BLAD results from a point mutation in the *CD18* gene (Fig. 40.3). An aspartic acid is replaced by a glycine, and functional CD18 is not produced. In the absence of this chain, complete integrins cannot be assembled. Neutrophils cannot attach to vascular endothelial cells or emigrate from blood vessels. Healthy heterozygotes have a single copy of the mutated gene and thus have abnormally low levels of CD18 (Fig. 40.4). Through the use of a PCR test, the presence of the altered gene can be demonstrated. In this way, it has been shown that a single bull, *Osborndale Ivanhoe*, with thousands of registered sons and daughters, was a carrier of this gene. As a result, the defective gene was widespread and common among Holstein cattle in the United States (14% of bulls, 5.8% of cows). Fortunately, carrier animals can be rapidly detected and removed from breeding programs.

Canine Cyclic Neutropenia

Canine cyclic neutropenia (Gray Collie syndrome) is an autosomal recessive disease of Border Collies. Affected dogs have diluted skin pigmentation, eye lesions, and regular cyclic fluctuations in leukocyte numbers. Their hair is a characteristic silver-gray color, and their nose is gray—a diagnostic feature. The loss of neutrophils occurs about every 11–12 days and lasts for about 3 days. It is followed by normal or elevated neutrophil counts for about 7 days. Severe neutropenia suppresses inflammation and increases their susceptibility to bacterial and fungal infections. (Their neutrophils also have reduced myeloperoxidase activity, so the disease is not entirely due to a neutrophil deficiency.) In humans, this disease results from a defect in the gene coding for neutrophil elastase, an enzyme found in azurophil granules. Affected dogs have severe enteric and respiratory infections, gingivitis, arthralgia, and lymphadenitis and rarely live beyond three years. Because platelet numbers also cycle, affected dogs may have bleeding problems, including gingival hemorrhage and epistaxis. Immunoglobulin levels rise as a result of the recurrent antigenic stimulation, but complement levels cycle in conjunction with the neutropenia. The disease begins to express itself as maternal immunity wanes. Affected puppies are weak, grow poorly, have wounds that fail to heal, and have high mortality. If they are kept alive by aggressive antibiotic therapy, chronic inflammation may lead to amyloidosis.

Treatment involves the repeated use of antibiotics to control the recurrent infections. If endotoxin is administered repeatedly, it can stimulate the bone marrow and stabilize neutrophil, reticulocyte, and platelet numbers. Lithium carbonate has a similar effect. Unfortunately, both endotoxin and lithium carbonate are toxic, and the disease recurs when the treatment is discontinued.

Trapped Neutrophil Syndrome

An autosomal recessive neutropenia has been described in Border Collies (Mason et al., 2014). This disease, called "Trapped Neutrophil Syndrome," results in recurrent bacterial osteomyelitis and gastroenteritis. Animals present with persistent fever and lameness due to lytic bone lesions. They have myeloid hyperplasia and dense accumulations of neutrophils in the marrow but few in the blood. The neutropenia apparently results from an inability of the neutrophils to escape from the bone marrow into the bloodstream. The causative mutation is a four base-pair deletion in the canine *VPS13B* gene that affects vesicular transport and protein sorting within the cell (Mizukami et al., 2013). The neutropenia renders affected dogs more susceptible to bacterial infections, and they fail to thrive. Up to 10% of Border Collies may carry the mutated gene (Zoto et al., 2022).

Other Examples of Defective Neutrophil Function

An inherited defect in neutrophil bactericidal activity has been reported in Doberman Pinschers. Affected dogs had bronchopneumonia and chronic rhinitis that developed soon after birth and persisted despite antimicrobial therapy. Although their chemotaxis and phagocytosis were apparently normal, their neutrophils were unable to kill *S. aureus*. Since these cells showed reduced reduction of nitroblue tetrazolium and superoxide production, it was suggested that they had a defect in their respiratory burst pathway.

Young Weimaraner dogs have been described as suffering from an immunodeficiency syndrome with clinical signs that include recurrent fevers, diarrhea, bronchopneumonia, pyoderma, osteomyelitis, stomatitis, and osteomyelitis. They may have a defective neutrophil respiratory burst, as shown by a depressed chemiluminescent response to phorbol ester. Their IgG levels may be significantly lower than normal and their IgM and IgA levels somewhat reduced; the other immunological parameters of these animals fall within normal ranges.

A persistent neutropenia attributable to a deficiency of granulocyte colony-stimulating factor (G-CSF) has been reported in a 3-year-old male Rottweiler. The animal had a fever due to multiple recurrent infections, especially a chronic bacterial arthritis in the presence of a persistent neutropenia. The animal was not making G-CSF. Its myeloid stem cells responded readily to additional G-CSF, suggesting that they were functionally normal. Bone marrow examination suggested that its neutrophil precursors had failed to mature (Lanevschi et al., 1999).

A myeloperoxidase deficiency has also been reported to occur in an Italian hound (Gentilini et al., 2016).

INHERITED DEFECTS IN THE ADAPTIVE IMMUNE SYSTEM

Inherited immunological defects have served to confirm the overall arrangement of the immune system, as outlined in Fig. 40.5. For example, if both the cell- and antibody-mediated immune responses are defective, it may be assumed that the genetic lesion operates at a point prior to thymic and bursal cell processing, that is, a stem cell lesion. A defect that occurs only in thymic development leads to a failure to mount cell-mediated immune responses, although antibody production may be normal. Similarly, a lesion restricted to B cells is reflected by impaired antibody responses.

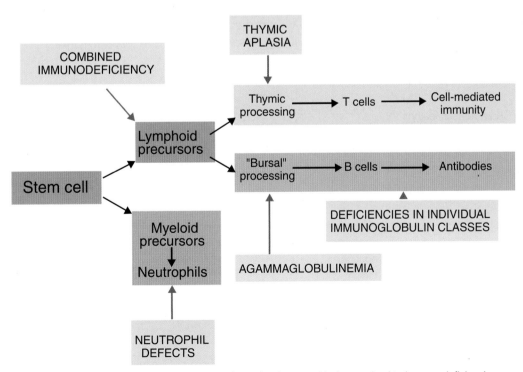

Fig. 40.5 The points in the immune system where development blocks may lead to immunodeficiencies.

IMMUNODEFICIENCIES OF HORSES

Horses are among the few domestic animals whose economic worth has permitted a thorough analysis of neonatal mortality. As a result, a significant number of primary immunodeficiency syndromes have been identified in this species (Fig. 40.6; Crisman and Scarratt, 2008).

Severe Combined Immunodeficiency

The most important congenital equine immunodeficiency is severe combined immunodeficiency (SCID). Affected foals fail to produce functional T or B cells and have very few circulating lymphocytes. If they suckle successfully, they acquire maternal immunoglobulins. Once these have declined, however, these foals cannot produce their own antibodies and eventually become agammaglobulinemic. Affected foals are therefore born healthy but begin to sicken by 2 months of age. The precise time of onset depends on the quantity of colostral antibodies absorbed. All die by 4–6 months as a result of overwhelming infection. Severe bronchopneumonia is the predominant presenting sign. Organisms that have been implicated in this bronchopneumonia include equine adenovirus, *Prescotella equi*, and *Pneumocystis* (an opportunistic fungal pathogen). The disease is manifested by a nasal discharge, coughing, dyspnea, weight loss, and fevers. Affected foals may also develop enteritis, omphalophlebitis, and many other infections. *Cryptosporidium parvum* and many different bacteria have been implicated in the enteritis.

On necropsy, the spleens of these foals lack germinal centers and periarteriolar lymphoid sheaths. Their lymph nodes lack lymphoid

follicles and germinal centers, and there are few cells in the paracortex. Their thymus may be difficult to find. Neutrophil, monocyte, and NK functions appear normal.

SCID is an autosomal recessive disease, and its occurrence therefore indicates that both parents carry the mutation. Accurate diagnosis is of great importance since the presence of the mutation significantly reduces the value of the parent animals. Thus, all suspected cases must be confirmed by postmortem examination. The clinical diagnosis of SCID requires that at least two of the following three criteria be established: (1) very low (consistently below 1000/mm³) circulating lymphocytes; (2) histology typical of SCID; that is, gross hypoplasia of the primary and secondary lymphoid organs; and (3) an absence of IgM from presuckle serum. (The normal equine fetus synthesizes small amounts of IgM. As a result, IgM in normal newborn foals is about 160 µg/mL. If the foal successfully suckles, it will obtain immunoglobulins of all isotypes from the mare's colostrum. However, the half-life of IgM is only about 6 days, so maternal IgM will disappear within a few days of birth. Thus, a normal foal will always have some IgM in its serum, but a SCID foal will have none.)

Pathogenesis

When B- and T-cell antigen receptors are generated, large segments of DNA are excised so that *V, D,* and *J* gene segments can be rejoined (Chapter 18). Several enzymes are involved in this recombination process. Some cut the DNA strands, and others join them. Studies on SCID foals show that there is a defect in the large multicomponent enzyme that rejoins the cut ends. The specific defect lies in the gene

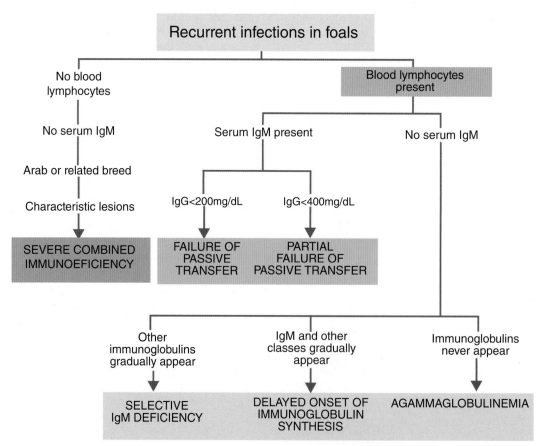

Fig. 40.6 The differential diagnosis of the equine immune deficiencies. *IgG,* immunoglobulin G; *IgM,* immunoglobulin M.

coding for the catalytic subunit of an enzyme called DNA-dependent protein kinase (DNA-PK$_{cs}$) (Fig. 40.7; Shin et al., 1997). In the mutant *DNA-PK$_{cs}$* gene, a loss of five nucleotides results in a frame-shift, premature termination of the peptide chain, and a deletion of 967 amino acids from the C-terminus of the molecule, including its entire kinase domain (Fig. 40.8). Functional *DNA-PK$_{cs}$* is totally absent from affected foals. Because of this deficiency, broken DNA strands cannot be rejoined, and neither T cells nor B cells can form functional V regions. In the absence of TCRs and BCRs, affected foals cannot respond to antigens. Since *DNA-PK$_{cs}$* is needed to rejoin broken strands of DNA, it also plays a key role in other DNA repair processes. Thus, the cells from SCID foals are unable to repair DNA damaged by radiation.

The presence of a mutant *CID* gene in horses can be detected by means of a PCR test. A sample of DNA is obtained from horse skin cells. A primer set designed to amplify only DNA containing the 5-base pair deletion and another set designed to amplify only the normal gene sequence are used to determine whether the mutant gene is present. This test has demonstrated that the frequency of the *CID* gene in Arabian horses is 8.4%. Based on this, it would be expected that 0.18%

of Arabian foals would be homozygous for the trait and hence clinically affected. Pedigree analysis suggests that the SCID trait was introduced to the United States by a single stallion in the 1920s (Bernoco and Bailey, 1998).

Immunoglobulin Deficiencies

Primary agammaglobulinemia is a rare disease of foals. Affected animals have no identifiable B cells (cells with surface immunoglobulins) and have very low serum immunoglobulin levels. Their lymphoid tissues contain no primary follicles, germinal centers, or plasma cells. Nevertheless, their blood lymphocytes can respond to mitogens. Intradermal inoculation of phytohemagglutinin induces a typical type IV delayed hypersensitivity reaction. Affected foals experience recurrent bacterial infections but may survive for up to 18 months. The disease should be suspected in a foal having a normal lymphocyte count but lacking both IgM and IgG. It may be confirmed by showing normal responses to T-cell mitogens and an absence of B cells.

Selective IgM deficiencies have been described in foals. Serum IgM levels in these animals are at least two standard deviations below normal, but IgG and IgA levels and B-cell numbers are normal. In most cases, foals develop septicemia or recurrent respiratory tract infections, often involving *Klebsiella pneumoniae* or *P. equi*, and die by 10 months. Some affected foals live longer and respond to therapy but fail to grow, have recurrent respiratory infections, and usually die by 24 months. Most affected foals have been Arabians or Quarter Horses, suggesting that the disease has a genetic basis. IgM deficiency has also been described in adult horses over 2 years of age. In many cases, such horses also have a lymphoreticular neoplasm.

A single case of IgG deficiency has been described in a 3-month-old foal with salmonellosis. The animal had normal IgA and IgM but no germinal centers, lymphoid follicles, splenic follicles, or periarteriolar lymphoid sheaths. Its serum IgG was also extremely low.

Between 2 and 3 months of age, some foals experience a transient hypogammaglobulinemia as a result of a delayed onset of immunoglobulin synthesis. These animals may suffer recurrent infections during the period when their immunoglobulin levels are low. Lymphocyte numbers and responsiveness remain normal at this time.

Common Variable Immunodeficiency

Common variable immunodeficiency is the second most common primary immunodeficiency syndrome in humans (after selective IgA deficiency.) It is a heterogeneous group of sporadic diseases all characterized by a late-onset B-cell lymphopenia. It is often accompanied by microbial dysbiosis, autoimmunity, or lymphoid malignancies. A similar syndrome occurs in horses where four genes, *E2A, PAX5, CD19,*

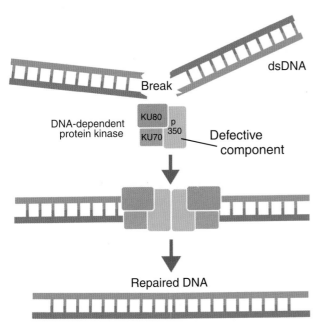

Fig. 40.7 The defect in DNA-dependent protein kinase (DNA-PK) that prevents DNA repair in severe combined immunodeficiency foals.

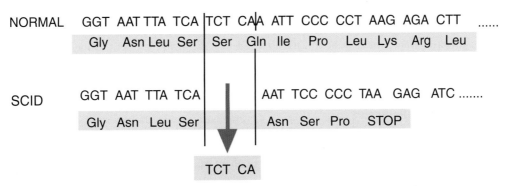

Fig. 40.8 The gene deletion in the equine DNA-dependent protein kinase gene that leads to premature termination of the molecule. *SCID*, Severe combined immunodeficiency.

and *IGD*, have significantly reduced expression (Flaminio et al., 2002). Immunohistochemistry has confirmed the absence of PAX5 in the bone marrow of these horses. PAX5 and the other molecules are transcription factors that regulate the early differentiation of B cells. Their B-cell development seems to be blocked at the transition to pro-B cells. Mutations in genes coding for tumor necrosis factor receptors and other costimulatory molecules also result in loss of helper T-cell function.

Cases of common variable immunodeficiency have been recorded in horses. Although they resemble primary immunodeficiencies in their sporadic nature and severity, they usually occur in animals over three years of age. Typically, these horses present with recurrent infections that are not responsive to treatment. Bacterial meningitis may be a consistent feature (Pellegrini-Masini et al., 2005). Their serum contains only trace levels of IgG and IgM, no detectable IgG3, and very low IgA levels (Tallmadge et al., 2012b). Sometimes individual IgG subclasses are deficient, whereas IgA levels are normal. T-cell numbers are normal, but B cells are undetectable, and there is no response to the B-cell mitogen lipopolysaccharide. On necropsy, there are no B cells in lymphoid organs, blood, or bone marrow. Some horses may develop severe liver disease, a feature also seen in humans. It is suspected that these individuals have an underlying defect that is only expressed when the immune system is stressed by infection. Other cases have included horses between 2 and 5 years old with a selective IgM deficiency. Many develop a concurrent lymphosarcoma, and they may have excessive regulatory T-cell function.

Foal Immunodeficiency Syndrome

This primary immunodeficiency syndrome was first described in the highly inbred Fell and Dales pony breeds but can occur in any horse breed. It presents as a B-cell immunodeficiency accompanied by a profound anemia (Scholes et al., 1998). Affected foals appear normal at birth but fail to thrive. Their hematocrit and B-cell numbers decline over 4–12 weeks until clinical disease develops (Thomas et al., 2003). Affected animals lack germinal centers and plasma cells. Their B-cell numbers decline to less than 10% of normal and serum immunoglobulin levels drop rapidly once maternal antibodies are catabolized. The loss of these immunoglobulins coincides with the development of clinical disease. T-cell numbers remain within the normal range. Animals develop severe respiratory disease caused by opportunistic pathogens such as adenoviruses and diarrhea caused by cryptosporidium. At the same time, they develop a profound progressive, nonregenerative anemia that alone may be sufficient to cause death. Foals inevitably die or are euthanized by 1–3 months of age (Fox-Clipsham et al., 2009; Gardner et al., 2006).

The syndrome is inherited as an autosomal recessive disease. It results from a mutation in the gene coding for the sodium/myoinositol cotransporter (*SLC5A3*). (The mutation switches a single amino acid from proline to leucine and is homozygous in affected foals.). This protein controls cellular osmotic regulation and is required for lymphoid cell survival and erythropoiesis. A PCR-based test is available that can be used to determine whether a foal carries the mutant gene. Carrier rates are about 40% for Fell ponies and 20% for Dales ponies (Tallmadge et al., 2012a). The disease prevalence has been markedly reduced as carrier breeding has been avoided, although the carrier rate remains relatively high as might be expected within such a small breeding population (Carter et al., 2013).

Prevalence of Equine Immunodeficiencies

The most important immunodeficiency in foals is not inherited but results from a failure to absorb sufficient colostral antibodies from the mare (see Chapter 24). This failure of passive transfer may affect up to 10% of all foals. SCID occurs in 2%–3% of Arab foals and is 10 times more common than selective IgM deficiency. Selective IgM deficiency is, in turn, 10 times more common than agammaglobulinemia.

IMMUNODEFICIENCIES OF CATTLE

Severe Combined Immunodeficiency

A combined immunodeficiency has been recorded in an Angus calf. The animal was apparently normal when born and suckled normally. It became ill, however, at 6 weeks of age, when it developed pneumonia and diarrhea. The animal was lymphopenic and severely hypogammaglobulinemic. It had undetectable IgM and IgA and a low level of IgG, which was believed to be due to residual maternal antibodies. The animal died within a week with systemic candidiasis. It had a hypoplastic thymus consisting of epithelial cells but no thymocytes. It had no detectable lymph nodes, and its hypoplastic spleen had no lymphocytes within its periarteriolar lymphoid sheaths. The syndrome thus closely resembled equine SCID.

Selective Immunoglobulin Deficiencies

An IgG2 deficiency has been reported in Red Danish cattle. Thus, in a survey, 1 out of 417 healthy cattle tested was completely deficient in this immunoglobulin subclass. However, in cattle suffering from pyogenic infections, 13 out of 93 animals were deficient. As a result, they appear to have an increased susceptibility to pneumonia and gangrenous mastitis. An additional 15% may also have low IgG2 levels, although this does not appear to cause any ill effects.

This condition is not restricted to the Red Danish breed. For example, a transient hypogammaglobulinemia resulting in an IgG2 deficiency has been associated with a delayed onset of immunoglobulin synthesis in a Holstein heifer. The affected heifer also had transient low levels of IgG1 and IgA as well as subnormal IgM concentrations. The animal died as a consequence of chronic respiratory disease. Likewise, a delayed onset of immunoglobulin synthesis resulting in a transient hypogammaglobulinemia has been recorded in a Simmental heifer.

Hereditary Parakeratosis

Certain Black Pied Danish and Friesian cattle carry an autosomal recessive trait of thymic and lymphocytic hypoplasia (trait A-46). Affected calves are born healthy, but by 4–8 weeks they begin to experience severe skin infections. If untreated, they die within a few weeks, and none survive for longer than 4 months. Affected calves have exanthema, hair loss on the legs, and parakeratosis around the mouth and eyes. There is depletion of lymphocytes in the intestine and atrophy of the thymus, spleen, and lymph nodes. These animals are T-cell deficient and have depressed cell-mediated immunity but normal antibody responses. Thus, they mount a normal antibody response to tetanus toxoid but respond poorly to dinitrochlorobenzene or tuberculin, both of which induce cell-mediated reactions. If these calves are treated with oral zinc oxide or zinc sulfate, they recover the ability to mount normal cell-mediated responses. If, however, the zinc supplementation is stopped, the animals will relapse within a few weeks. It is probable that these animals have a reduced ability to absorb zinc from the intestine. Zinc is an essential component of the thymic hormone thymulin (see Chapter 13) and is therefore required for a normal T-cell response.

Thymic Aplasia

When the thymuses of stillborn or weak Japanese Black calves were examined, many were very small and difficult to identify. Histology showed a reduction in thymocyte numbers. This ranged from a total absence to a lack of thymocytes and Hassall's corpuscles in the medulla. About half the calves also showed a loss of lymphocytes in the white pulp. This syndrome appears to result from growth retardation in utero perhaps resulting from maternal malnutrition or placental insufficiency (Takasu et al., 2008).

Cases of congenital thymic aplasia with or without an absence of hair have been described in Black Danish, German Holstein, and Holstein-Israeli calves. The hairless cases resemble the "nude" mutation seen in mice and cats (Usta et al., 2016). The thymus in these cases consists of loose connective tissue containing very few scattered lymphocytes. In one case, it weighed 36 g compared to 250–400 g in normal calves. These calves totally lack T cells and die as a result of diarrhea and/or pneumonia within 3–6 weeks after birth.

IMMUNODEFICIENCIES OF PIGS

Porcine SCID

A SCID has been recognized in inbred Yorkshire pigs. The piglets appeared normal while suckling but were gradually overcome by opportunistic infections resulting in reduced growth, skin lesions, and respiratory distress. They did not survive beyond 60 days. They suffered from pneumonitis, serositis, and dermatitis. Affected pigs were small with a rough hair coat. The thymus was not visible while lymph nodes and ileal Peyer's patches were small and inconspicuous. Lymph nodes, tonsils, Peyer's patches, and spleen had reduced lymphocyte numbers and no lymphoid follicles. CD3+ T cells were few in lymph nodes and absent from the spleen and bloodstream. The animals lacked both T and B cells in the bloodstream but had normal numbers of NK cells and neutrophils. They did not produce antibodies in response to PRRSV infection. There was no sex predilection. Subsequent matings of the parents of these pigs produced approximately 22% of affected piglets per litter confirming that this was a primary immunodeficiency (Perryman, 2004).

Further studies on these SCID pigs demonstrated two spontaneous mutations. Both occurred in the *Artemis* gene. One mutation (H12) occurred in the splice donor site of exon 8. As a result, exon 8 was deleted resulting in a nonfunctional protein. The second mutation (H16) was a point mutation in exon 10. This resulted in a frame-shift and a stop codon was generated so that the protein was truncated. The phenotype of these two mutations was indistinguishable (Waide et al., 2015). *Artemis* encodes a small nuclear endonuclease that plays an essential role in V(D)J recombination. (The DNA between the V and D genes is excised, and the two ends bind together to form a hairpin [Fig. 40.9]. *Artemis* then cleaves the hairpin at variable sites so that with nucleotide deletion and addition, when the ends are rejoined, there are changes in the amino acid sequences in this area.) Thus it plays a key role in generating diversity in both immunoglobulins and T cells. It also makes cells more sensitive to radiation-induced chromosome damage (Powell et al., 2016).

It has also proved possible to artificially generate SCID pigs by knocking out the genes encoding the recombinases RAG1 and RAG2. The genes were first knocked out in porcine fetal fibroblasts, and then their nuclei were used for somatic cell nuclear transfer. Of the experimental piglets, most lacked just a single RAG gene, but several were born with biallelic mutations. These pigs had hypoplastic lymphoid organs, were unable to rearrange their V(D)J genes and had arrested B- and T-cell development (Huang et al., 2014).

IMMUNODEFICIENCIES OF DOGS

The nature of dog breeding and the establishment of multiple breeds with limited genetic diversity have resulted in the development of numerous inherited canine diseases. Many of these are primary immunodeficiencies restricted to specific breeds. Few have been investigated thoroughly and the responsible genes have not been identified.

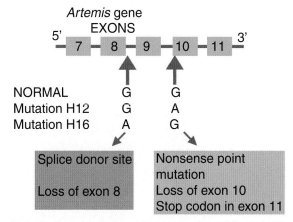

Fig. 40.9 The two identified mutations in the *Artemis* gene that lead to severe combined immunodeficiency in pigs.

Combined Immunodeficiencies

A SCID resulting from a defect in the catalytic subunit of the DNA-PK$_{cs}$ has been identified in Jack Russell Terriers. From a single breeding pair of terriers, 12 of 32 siblings died from opportunistic infections between 8 and 14 weeks of age. These animals showed a SCID phenotype with lymphopenia, agammaglobulinemia, and thymic and lymphoid aplasia. The disease was an autosomal recessive condition. It resulted from a point mutation, leading to stop codon formation and premature termination of the peptide chain. Affected dogs showed severely diminished expression of DNA-PK$_{cs}$. As in equine and porcine SCID, the defect blocks gene splicing during *V(D)J* recombination in TCR and immunoglobulin variable regions. The carrier frequency of this gene is 1.1% (Meek et al., 2001).

An X-linked SCID has also been recorded in Basset Hounds and Cardigan Welsh Corgis. The disease is characterized by stunted growth, increased susceptibility to infections, and absence of lymph nodes. Clinically, animals are healthy during the immediate neonatal period as a result of maternal antibodies. However, by 6–8 weeks, as the levels of maternal antibodies decline, the animals begin to develop infections. At first, these are relatively mild, such as superficial pyoderma and otitis media. Eventually, they become more severe, and untreated animals die of pneumonia, enteritis, or sepsis by 4 months of age. Common infections include canine distemper, generalized staphylococcal infections, adenoviral and parvoviral disease, and cryptosporidiosis. This is an X-linked immunodeficiency since breeding of a carrier female to a normal sire results in approximately half the males in each litter being affected and all the females being phenotypically normal.

Affected dogs are lymphopenic (~1000/μL). Their CD4:CD8 ratio is, however, approximately 15:1, compared with normal dogs that have a ratio of 1.7:1, indicating a major drop in CD8+ cell numbers. Their absolute number of T cells is less than 20% of normal. The dogs have normal numbers of B cells. The few lymphocytes in the blood are unresponsive to mitogens. The puppies have normal IgM levels but very low, or no, IgG and IgA. These dogs do not make antibodies against antigens such as tetanus toxoid.

On necropsy, the thymus of affected dogs is approximately 10% of the normal weight and lacks a defined cortex (Fig. 40.10). Their lymph nodes and tonsils are very small and dysplastic and may be very difficult to find. When present, the nodes are disorganized and contain very few small lymphocytes. Their spleens contain large periarteriolar lymphoid nodules with occasional small lymphocytes and few plasma cells. The bone marrow in these dogs appears normal.

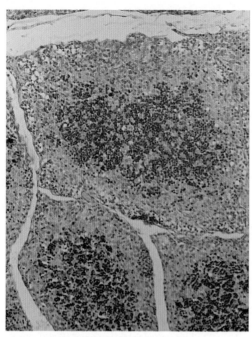

Fig. 40.10 Photomicrograph of the thymus of a basset hound with X-linked immunodeficiency. Note the lack of a defined cortex and the scattered foci of dark-staining lymphocytes (H&E stain). From Snyder, P.W., Kazacos, E.A., Felsburg, P.J., 1993. Histologic characterization of the thymus in canine X-linked severe combined immunodeficiency. Clin. Immunol. Immunopathol. 67, 55–67.

The disease results from a mutation in the gene coding for the common γc chain of the IL-2R *(IL-2Rγ)*. The same chain is also a component of the IL-4, IL-7, IL-9, and IL-15 receptors.

In affected Basset Hounds, a loss of four bases in the γc gene causes a frame-shift. As a result, a stop codon is generated. Thus, instead of the complete protein, only a small peptide is produced, and no functional protein is made. A second SCID mutation has been described in Cardigan Welsh Corgis. In these animals, a single cytosine residue is inserted into the γc gene so that a stop codon is generated before the transmembrane domain, resulting in a failure to synthesize the complete chain (Fig. 40.11). As a result, this peptide is not expressed on the cell surface. In both cases, the mutation does not interfere with IL-2 production, but the lymphocytes of these animals are unresponsive to IL-2. In the absence of a functioning IL-2 receptor, mature T cells will can not develop (Henthorn et al., 1994).

Experimentally, affected dogs may be treated by bone marrow allografts. It is interesting to note, however, that SCID dogs kept alive by stem cell allografts began to age prematurely by 2–3 years (Meek et al., 2009). They developed intestinal malabsorption and neural cell tumors. Presumably the absence of *DNA-PK*$_{cs}$ prevents the repair of other cells, leading to premature aging (Ding et al., 2002).

A SCID has been reported to occur in Frisian Water Dogs as a result of a nonsense mutation in *RAG1* leading to defective V(D)J recombination and thus a failure to make effective immunoglobulins and T-cell antigen receptors. It is inherited as an autosomal recessive disease. Affected pups die between eight and twelve weeks of age as a result of recurrent infections and neurologic disease. Blood lymphocytes accounted for less than 1% of blood leukocytes. IgM, IgG, and IgA are undetectable (Verfuurden et al., 2011).

Common Variable Immunodeficiency

Common variable immunodeficiency has been documented in Miniature Dachshunds and a Pomeranian. In the case of the

Dachshunds, seven animals under one year of age developed Pneumocystis pneumonia. Investigation showed that the animals were deficient in IgG, IgM, and IgA. Their lymphocytes failed to respond to the mitogens phytohemagglutinin or pokeweed. B cells were absent from their lymphoid organs (Lobetti, 2000). The Pomeranian was 20 months-old when it developed Pneumocystis pneumonia and demodectic mange. Its IgG and IgA levels were low. It showed severe lymphoid depletion in the spleen and other lymphoid organs. Its lymphoid follicles contained mainly T cells with a few B cells. Thus, in both cases, the defects appeared to primarily affect B cells (Kanemoto et al., 2015).

Selective IgM Deficiency

A selective IgM deficiency has been reported in two related Doberman Pinschers. One animal was asymptomatic, whereas the other had a chronic mucopurulent nasal discharge and bronchopneumonia. Both of these animals had high IgA, low IgG, and very low IgM. They experienced only a chronic nasal discharge, so the clinical significance of this deficiency is in doubt.

Selective IgA Deficiency

IgA deficiencies are the most common primary immune deficiency disorder in both humans and dogs. They tend to be insidious and associated with an increased level of mucosal infections and allergic diseases. They occur with a high prevalence in several breeds of dogs (Ellis, 2019). German Shepherd dogs, Golden Retrievers, Labrador Retrievers, and Shar-Peis are especially predisposed to a range of infectious disorders, including mycoses, anal furunculosis, deep pyoderma, and small intestinal bacterial overgrowth. This suggests that they have deficiencies in mucosal immunity.

Genome-wide association studies in susceptible breeds have identified 35 genomic loci associated with low IgA levels. In German Shepherd dogs, three genes (*KIRREL3, SERPINA9*, and *SLIT1*) have been associated with low IgA levels. *SLIT1* is expressed in the bone marrow and plays a key role in B-cell development. *SERPINA9* is also expressed on developing B cells and plasma cells Olsson et al., 2015). Consistent with this is the observation that German Shepherd dogs in the United Kingdom have normal IgM and IgG levels but significantly reduced levels of IgA (~80 mg/dL, as opposed to 170 mg/dL in control dogs) (Littler et al., 2006). Likewise, dogs of this breed have significantly lower concentrations of IgA in their tears compared with other breeds. However, they have normal numbers of IgA-producing plasma cells, implying that the deficiency may be due to defective synthesis or secretion of IgA. Some German Shepherds may have significantly reduced median IgA levels in feces compared with control dogs of other breeds. Many have IgA concentrations below the 95% confidence limit of the control population, and some lack detectable fecal IgA. Their fecal IgG and albumin levels also tend to be higher than in control dogs. Other breeds with a significant proportion (>10%) of dogs with low IgA include Hovawarts, Norwegian Elkhounds, Nova Scotia Duck Tolling Retrievers, Bull Terriers, Golden Retrievers, and Labrador Retrievers (Box 40.1; Olsson et al., 2015).

Shar-Pei puppies with recurrent cough, nasal discharge, conjunctivitis, and pneumonia, as well as demodicosis and *Microsporum canis* infections, have been identified as having a selective IgA deficiency (<15 mg/dL). Likewise, abnormally low IgA concentrations are found in a high percentage of clinically normal Shar-Peis. Atopic disease is common in these dogs, a feature also seen in IgA-deficient humans. In German Shepherd dogs, low IgA levels are also associated with the development of canine atopic dermatitis as well as pancreatic acinar atrophy.

A primary IgA deficiency has been described in inbred Beagles. The dogs had a history of parainfluenza and endemic kennel cough due to *Bordetella bronchiseptica*. Despite vaccination, these animals

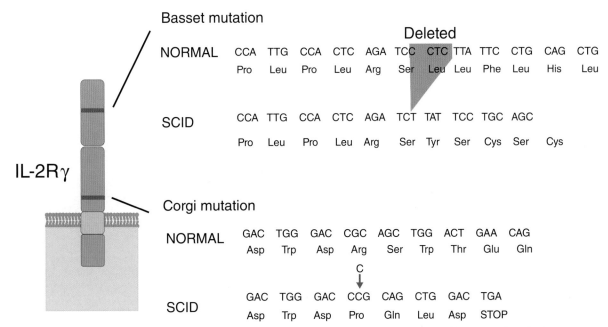

Fig. 40.11 The two defined canine X-linked severe combined immunodeficiency (SCID) mutations in the *IL-2Rγ* gene. In the Corgi mutation, the insertion of a single cytosine residue into the gene leads to the generation of a stop codon and premature termination of peptide synthesis. In the Basset mutation, deletion of four bases causes a frame-shift mutation and also leads to the generation of a stop codon (not shown). Data from Henthorn, P.S., Somberg, R.L., Fimiani, V.M., et al., 1994. IL-2R gamma gene microdeletion demonstrates that canine X-linked severe combined immunodeficiency is a homologue of the human disease. Genomics 23, 69–74; and from Somberg, R.L., Pullen, R.P., Casal, M.L., et al., 1995. A single nucleotide insertion in the canine interleukin-2 receptor gamma chain results in X-linked severe combined immunodeficiency disease. Vet. Immunol. Immunopathol. 47, 203–214.

BOX 40.1   IgA Deficiency in Wolves

IgA concentrations have been measured in the serum of 163 free-ranging and captive wolves in Scandinavia as well as from 33 Canadian wolves. The median IgA concentration for Scandinavian wolves was 0.054 g/L. The median value for Canadian wolves was 0.18 g/L. The median values in dogs range from 0.15 to 0.3 g/L depending on the breed. Thus, relative to dogs and Canadian wolves, Scandinavian wolves are IgA deficient. Up to 60% of Scandinavian wolves had IgA levels as low as high-risk dog breeds such as Shar-Peis. Whether this difference in serum levels is clinically significant, and whether the difference extends to IgA levels on body surfaces or in secretions such as milk is unclear.

Frankowiack, M., Olsson, M., Cluff, H.D., Evans, A.L., et al., 2015. IgA deficiency in wolves from Canada and Scandinavia. Dev. Comp. Immunol. 50, 26–28; Frankowiack, M., Hellman, L., Zhao, Y., Arnemo, J.M., Lin, M., et al., 2013. IgA deficiency in wolves. Dev. Comp. Immunol. 40, 180–184.

continued to experience recurrent respiratory tract infections and otitis. Immunoelectrophoresis and radial immunodiffusion showed normal serum IgG and IgM levels but very little IgA (<5 mg/dL). Phenotypically normal parent dogs also had very low IgA levels. Four affected dogs had circulating anti-IgA antibodies. Their T and B lymphocyte numbers and lymphocyte responses to mitogens were normal, as was their response to tetanus toxoid. They had a normal number of plasma cells secreting IgG and IgM but no plasma cells secreting IgA. When two affected animals were mated, four out of five pups in the litter were IgA deficient. The disease was not sex linked. An inherited rhinitis/bronchopneumonia syndrome has been identified in Irish Wolfhounds and is also presumed to result from an IgA deficiency.

Other Immunoglobulin Deficiencies

A transient hypogammaglobulinemia has been seen in two puppies from a litter of Spitz puppies that experienced recurrent upper respiratory tract infections between 8 and 16 weeks of age. These dogs had normal T-cell numbers and mitogen responses. They had low immunoglobulin levels and low antibody titers to vaccine antigens at 16 weeks. The puppies responded very weakly to tetanus toxoid when it was administered at 4 months. By 6 months, however, their immunoglobulins had risen to normal levels, and the puppies had regained their health. It is believed that these puppies experienced a delayed onset of immunoglobulin synthesis. Symptomatic treatment is sufficient to support these animals until their immune system becomes functional.

Cavalier King Charles Spaniels with *Pneumocystis* pneumonia had IgG concentrations that were significantly lower in affected dogs (median, 3.2 mg/mL) than in breed- and age-matched control dogs (median, 8.5 mg/mL). IgM levels, in contrast, were significantly higher in the affected dogs. IgA levels were within the normal range. Lymphocyte counts in affected dogs were normal or high. This may well be an IgG-deficiency syndrome (Hagiwara et al., 2001; Watson et al., 2006).

Pneumocystis pneumonia has been observed repeatedly in Miniature Dachshunds. The affected animals are usually less than 1 year old and appear to be immunodeficient. Serum electrophoresis shows a marked reduction in IgM, IgG, and IgA. In addition, lymphocyte responses to both phytohemagglutinin and pokeweed mitogens are severely depressed. There is a reduction in B-cell numbers. Although the *Pneumocystis* pneumonia responds to aggressive therapy, these animals rarely do well and die young.

T-Cell Deficiencies

A family of inbred Weimaraners has been reported as having immunodeficiency and dwarfism. The animals appeared normal at birth, but at 6–7 weeks they developed a wasting syndrome characterized by emaciation and lethargy. The puppies began to experience recurrent infections that eventually killed them. On necropsy, their thymuses were atrophied and lacked a cortex. These animals had normal immunoglobulin levels, their helper cell activity was unimpaired, and their secondary lymphoid organs appeared normal. Their lymphocytes were unresponsive to mitogens. Growth hormone treatment caused thymic cortical regeneration and a dramatic clinical improvement. However, growth hormone did not restore lymphocyte responsiveness to mitogens. The disease was almost certainly due to a deficiency of growth hormone as a result of a lesion in the hypothalamus, which confirms that the thymus requires growth hormone to function.

Lethal acrodermatitis has been identified in Bull Terriers (McEwan, 2001). This is a complex immunodeficiency syndrome associated with growth retardation, skin lesions (acrodermatitis, chronic pyoderma, and paronychia), diarrhea, recurrent pneumonia, and abnormal behavior. The puppies were weak at birth and did not nurse well. Some showed a lighter pigmentation than their littermates. When weaned, they had difficulty eating and failed to grow. Small, crusted lesions developed between the digits, and a pustular dermatitis developed around the eyes and mouth at 6–10 weeks. The lesions developed into a severe pyoderma. Fungi such as *Malassezia* and *Candida* were readily isolated from the lesions. Diarrhea developed early in the disease, and respiratory tract infections were common. The puppies became depressed and sluggish and died by 15 months of age, with a median survival of 7 months. They had a neutrophilia, normal IgG and IgM levels but significantly lower IgA levels, and hypercholesterolemia. Plasma zinc levels were unusually low. They showed depressed lymphocyte mitogen responses. On necropsy there was a severe loss of T cells, that the puppies lacked a thymus, and the lymph nodes and spleen were very small. The disease is inherited as an autosomal recessive disease, and the parents of affected puppies could be traced to one common ancestor. Because of its similarities to trait A-46 of cattle, these dogs were treated with oral zinc. Very high doses resulted in some clinical improvement, but this could not be sustained.

German Shepherd pyoderma is, as its name implies, a chronic skin disease that occurs in middle-aged German Shepherd dogs and is associated with infection with coagulase-positive staphylococci. These cases do not respond well to antibiotic therapy, and they are believed to reflect some form of underlying genetic or immunological defect. Although affected dogs appeared to mount normal humoral responses, limited studies have shown reduced lymphocyte responses to mitogens, an imbalance of lymphocyte subsets (CD4 cells are depressed, CD8 cells are increased), and a decline in the level of CD21+ B cells. (The complement receptor CD21 plays a role in B-cell activation.) When the number of CD3+ T cells and B cells were examined in normal dog skin and in the skin of dogs with pyoderma, it was found that the B-cell numbers were similar but that the number of T cells infiltrating the lesions in German shepherds was significantly reduced, suggesting that T-cell dysfunction may play a role in the pathogenesis of pyoderma in this breed.

Uncharacterized Immunodeficiencies

The veterinary literature contains several reports of dogs with severe recurrent infections caused by organisms that are not normally considered to be highly pathogenic. Prototothecosis, an algal infection caused by *Prototheca* spp., has been recorded in immunodeficient dogs. One-third of the cases have been in collies, suggesting an inherited predisposition. Weimaraners are unusually susceptible to some systemic

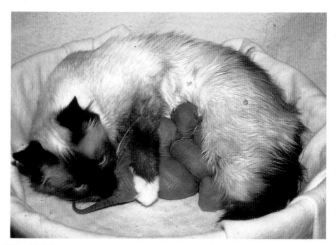

Fig. 40.12 Kittens born with an autosomal recessive form of congenital hypotrichosis with thymic aplasia-nude kittens. From Casal, M.L., Straumann, U., Sigg, C., et al., 1994. Congenital hypotrichosis with thymic aplasia in nine Birman kittens. J. Am. Anim. Hosp. Assoc. 30, 600–602. Courtesy Dr. Margret L Casal.

bacterial infections; German Shepherds are susceptible to generalized systemic *Aspergillus* infections, whereas some Rottweiler and Doberman families are unusually susceptible to parvovirus infection. None of these have been shown to be due to primary immunodeficiencies, and all require further investigation.

IMMUNODEFICIENCIES OF CATS

Hypotrichosis with Thymic Aplasia

The nude mouse has long been accepted as an important model of immunodeficiency. Nude mice are a strain of hairless mice that fail to develop a functional thymus. This condition has also been described in rats, guinea pigs, and calves. A similar mutation has been described in Birman kittens. These kittens were born without any body hair (Fig. 40.12). On necropsy, they also had no thymus and had depletion of lymphocytes in the paracortex of lymph nodes, spleen, and Peyer's patches. Thus they were effectively T-cell deficient. Analysis of the pedigree suggested that the disease was inherited in an autosomal recessive manner (Casal et al., 1994).

IMMUNODEFICIENCIES OF MICE

Many different genetic mutations have been shown to impair immunity in mice. Some of these mutant mice are widely employed for research investigating basic immunologic mechanisms.

Nude Mice

The best-known mouse model of immunodeficiency is the nude mouse. Nude mice are a strain of hairless mice whose thymic epithelial cells are nonfunctional as a result of a defect in the gene encoding the transcription factor FoxN1. Because their thymic epithelial cells fail to function, the primitive thymus in nude mice develops into cysts with walls of immature epithelial cells that do not produce mature T cells. These mice possess a limited number of immature T cells and B cells, so a few lymphocytes may be found in peripheral blood. Normal thymus grafts, by restoring epithelial cell function, permit the T cells of nude mice to mature and develop immune competence. Nude mice are deficient in conventional cell-mediated immune responses, as reflected by prolonged allograft survival and a lack of responses to T-cell mitogens. Their IgG and IgA levels are also depressed, presumably because of a loss of helper T cells.

Although nude mice show enhanced susceptibility to virus-induced tumors, they fail to develop more than the normal level of spontaneous tumors. This observation was, for many years, a major objection to the immunological surveillance theory because if T cells destroy tumors, T-cell-deficient animals should have an increased incidence of cancer. However, nude mice possess normal numbers of NK cells, which may protect them in the absence of T cells.

Severe Combined Immunodeficient Mice

SCID mice have very low numbers of B cells and T cells because of a mutation that affects the differentiation of lymphoid stem cells. Development of B cells is halted before expression of cytoplasmic or cell membrane immunoglobulins. T-cell development is also arrested at a very early stage, and those lymphocytes that do reach the bloodstream are CD4−, CD8−. They have no immunoglobulins and are unable to mount cell-mediated immune responses. SCID mice survive relatively well for about a year in specific-pathogen-free facilities but eventually die of *Pneumocystis* pneumonia. The defects in SCID mice result from an inability to rearrange their BCR or TCR V region genes correctly. Several different mutations in the DNA joining enzymes have been identified. As a result, the cells cannot produce functional receptors, and no functional T or B cells are produced. As in SCID horses, the mouse *scid* mutations also increase sensitivity to ionizing radiation since these animals are unable to repair DNA damage. About 15% of SCID mice are "leaky"; they have low levels of immunoglobulins of limited heterogeneity and can reject allografts. Antigen-presenting cells, myeloid and erythroid cells, and NK cells are normal in SCID mice.

Motheaten Mice

Motheaten mice have defective dendritic cell and neutrophil function as a result of a mutation in a protein-tyrosine phosphatase gene, SHP1. Their name comes from their appearance. Within a few days of birth, neutrophils invade their hair follicles and cause patchy loss of pigment. The deletion in neutrophils results in enhanced integrin signaling leading to cutaneous and lung inflammation. The deletion in dendritic cells is due to exaggerated MyD88-dependent signaling and results in severe autoimmunity. They produce excessive quantities of immunoglobulins and develop autoimmune disease. Mice that are *me/me* have a short lifespan and usually die as a result of lung damage. The B-cell hyperactivity may be due to excessive production of some B cell–stimulating cytokines.

X-Linked Immunodeficient Mice

Xid mice have a recessive, X-linked B-cell defect. The mutation affects a cytoplasmic tyrosine kinase. As a result, B cells cannot respond to certain T-independent carbohydrate antigens. They lack certain B-cell subsets. Mice that are *bg/nu/xid* are severely immunosuppressed since they lack T, B, and NK cells. Lightly irradiated *bg/nu/xid* mice can accept human bone marrow xenografts.

IMMUNODEFICIENCIES OF HUMANS

Many different immunodeficiency syndromes have been reported in humans. It is anticipated that investigators will eventually succeed in identifying most of these syndromes in domestic animals as well.

The most important phagocytic deficiency syndrome of humans is chronic granulomatous disease. This has not yet been reported as occurring in domestic animals, although it undoubtedly does. Children affected with chronic granulomatous disease have recurrent infections characterized by the development of septic granulomas in lymph nodes, lungs, bones, and skin. The neutrophils of these children are less capable than normal cells of destroying organisms such as staphylococci and coliforms. Their specific lesion is a defect in one of the subcomponents of the NADPH oxidase (NOX) complex. At least 40 such mutations have been identified.

Infants may also suffer from several different forms of combined immunodeficiency. The most severe is reticular dysgenesis, which results from a defect in the development of both myeloid and lymphoid stem cells. Other combined immunodeficiencies result from defects in the development of both T and B lymphoid stem cells. Some of these CID cases are due to a deficiency of the enzyme adenosine deaminase. In other cases, there is a defect in the genes coding for interleukin-2 (IL-2) or IL-7 receptors, for recombinase-activating gene proteins, for CD25, for the CD3γ chain, or for MHC class I or class II molecules. The standard treatment for all these diseases is a stem cell allograft.

T-Cell Deficiencies

The DiGeorge anomaly results from a failure of the third and fourth thymic pouches to develop. In consequence, no thymic epithelial tissue develops, and few cells populate the T-dependent areas of the secondary lymphoid tissues. Since these infants have no functional T cells, they can neither mount a delayed hypersensitivity reaction nor reject allografts. The importance of T cells in protection against viruses is emphasized by the observation that infants with the DiGeorge anomaly generally die of virus infections but remain resistant to bacteria.

B-Cell Deficiencies

The most severe of the human B-cell deficiencies, called Bruton-type agammaglobulinemia, is an X-linked recessive disease that affects early B-cell development. Affected infants are devoid of all immunoglobulin classes. They experience recurrent infections due to bacteria such as pneumococci, staphylococci, and streptococci but are usually resistant to viral, fungal, and protozoan infections. The disease results from a mutation in a receptor tyrosine kinase. Inherited deficiencies of individual immunoglobulin classes have also been recorded in humans. As might be anticipated, there are many possible combinations of deficiencies in IgG, IgM, IgA, and IgE, and a tendency to give each a specific name leads to confusion. One of the most important of these is Wiskott-Aldrich syndrome. In this disease, a selective IgM deficiency is associated with multiple infections, eczema, and thrombocytopenia. Another such syndrome is ataxia-telangiectasia, in which serum IgA and IgE levels are extremely low or absent and cerebellar and cutaneous abnormalities exist. Affected children, lacking an effective surface immune system, have recurrent bacterial respiratory tract infections. Ataxia-telangiectasia results from a defect in DNA repair mechanisms. In another disease called hyper-IgM syndrome, a defect in the CD40 ligand leads to a defect in late B-cell development and a failure in the IgM class switch, so that affected individuals have high levels of IgM but very low (or absent) IgG and IgA. Patients suffer from recurrent respiratory tract infections. The most common human primary immunodeficiency is an IgA deficiency that affects 1 in 600 Caucasians. Some of these individuals are asymptomatic; others suffer from an increased frequency of respiratory and gastrointestinal infections. The genetic defect appears to lie within the MHC complex.

REFERENCES

Anistoroaei, R., Krogh, A.K., Christensen, K., 2013. A frameshift mutation in the *LYST* gene is responsible for the Aleutian color and the associated Chediak-Higashi syndrome in American mink. Anim. Genet. 44, 178–183.

Bernoco, D., Bailey, E., 1998. Frequency of the SCID gene among Arabian horses in the USA. Anim. Genet. 29, 41–42.

Carter, S.D., Fox-Clipsham, L.Y., Christley, R., Swinburne, J., 2013. Foal immunodeficiency syndrome: carrier testing has markedly reduced disease incidence. Vet. Rec. 172 (15), 398.

Casal, M.L., Straumann, U., Sigg, C., et al., 1994. Congenital hypotrichosis with thymic aplasia in nine Birman kittens. J. Am. Anim. Hosp Assoc. 30, 600–602.

Crisman, M.V., Scarratt, W.K., 2008. Immunodeficiency disorders in horses. Vet. Clin. Equine. 24, 299–310.

Debenham, S.L., Millington, A., Kijas, J., et al., 2002. Canine leucocyte adhesion of deficiency in Irish red and white setters. J. Small Anim. Pract. 43, 74–75.

Ding, Q., Bramble, L., Yuzbasiyan-Gurkan, V., et al., 2002. DNA-PKcs mutations in dogs and horses: allele frequency and association with neoplasia. Gene 283, 263–269.

Ellis, J.A., 2019. Canine IgA and IgA deficiency: implications for immunization against respiratory pathogens. Can. Vet. J. 60, 1305–1311.

Flaminio, M.J.B., LaCombe, V., Kohn, C.W., Antczak, D.F., 2002. Common variable immunodeficiency in a horse. J. Am. Vet. Med. Assoc. 221, 1296–1302.

Fox-Clipsham, L., Swinburne, J.E., Papoula-Pereira, R.I., et al., 2009. Immunodeficiency/anemia syndrome in a Dales pony. Vet. Rec. 165, 289–290.

Gardner, R.B., Hart, K.A., Stokol, T., et al., 2006. Fell pony syndrome in a pony in North America. J. Vet. Intern. Med. 20, 198–203.

Gentilini, F., Zambon, E., Mancini, D., Turba, M.E., 2016. A nonsense mutation in the myeloperoxidase gene is responsible for hereditary myeloperoxidase deficiency in an Italian hound dog. Anim. Genet. 2016 (47), 632–633.

Grondin, T.M., DeWitt, S.F., Keeton, K.S., 2007. Pelger-Huët anomaly in an Arabian horse. Vet. Clin. Pathol. 36, 306–310.

Gu, Y.-C., Bauer, T.R., Sokolic, R.A., Hai, M., 2006. Conversion of the severe to the moderate disease phenotype with donor leukocyte microchimerism in canine leukocyte adherence deficiency. Bone Marrow Transplant. 37, 607–614.

Hagiwara, Y., Fujiwara, S., Takai, H., et al., 2001. *Pneumocystis carinii* pneumonia in a Cavalier King Charles Spaniel. J. Vet. Med. Sci. 63, 349–351.

Henthorn, P.S., Somberg, R.L., Fimani, V.M., et al., 1994. IL-2Rγ gene microdeletion demonstrates that canine X-linked severe combined immunodeficiency is a homologue of the human disease. Genomics 23, 69–74.

Huang, J., Guo, X., Fan, N., Song, J., et al., 2014. RAG1/2 knockout pigs with severe combined immunodeficiency. J. Immunol. 193, 1496–1503.

Hugo, T.B., Heading, K.L., 2014. Leukocyte adhesion deficiency III in a mixed-breed dog. J. Aust. Vet. Med. Assoc. 92, 299–302.

Kanemoto, H., Morikawa, R., Chambers, J.K., Kasahara, K., et al., 2015. Common variable immunodeficiency in a Pomeranian with *Pneumocystis carinii* pneumonia. J Vet. Med. Sci. 77 (6), 715–719.

Kijas, J.M.H., Bauer Jr, T.R., Gäfvert, S., et al., 1999. A missense mutation in the β-2 integrin gene *(ITGB2)* causes canine leukocyte adhesion deficiency. Genomics 61, 101–107.

Lanevschi, A., Daminet, S., Niemeyer, G.P., Lothrop, C.D., 1999. Granulocyte colony-stimulating factor deficiency in a Rottweiler with chronic idiopathic neutropenia. J. Vet. Intern. Med. 13, 72–75.

Latimer, K.S., Campagnoli, R.P., Danilenko, D.M., 2000. Pelger-Huet anomaly in Australian shepherds: 87 cases (1991–1997). Comp. Haematol. Int. 10, 9–13.

Littler, R.M., Batt, R.M., Lloyd, D.H., 2006. Total and relative deficiency of mucosal IgA in German Shepherd dogs demonstrated by fecal analysis. Vet. Rec. 158, 334–341.

Lobetti, R., 2000. Common variable immunodeficiency in miniature dachshunds affected with *Pneumocystis carinii* pneumonia. J. Vet. Diagn. Invest. 12 (1), 39–45.

Mason, S.L., Jepson, R., Maltman, M., Batchelor, D.J., 2014. Presentation and management of trapped neutrophil syndrome (TNS) in UK Border collies. J. Small Anim. Pract. 55, 57–60.

McEwan, N.A., 2001. Malassezia and Candida infections in bull terriers with lethal acrodermatitis. J. Small Anim. Pract. 42, 291–297.

Meek, K., Jutkowitz, A., Allen, L., et al., 2009. SCID dogs: similar transplant potential but distinct intra-uterine growth defects and premature replicative senescence compared to SCID mice. J. Immunol. 183, 2529–2536.

Meek, K., Kienker, L., Dallas, C., et al., 2001. SCID in Jack Russell terriers: a new animal model of DNA-PKcs deficiency. J. Immunol. 167, 2142–2150.

Mizukami, K., Yabuki, A., Kawamichi, T., Chang, H.S., et al., 2013. Real-time PCR genotyping assay for canine trapped neutrophil syndrome and high frequency of the mutant allele in Border collies. Vet. J. 195, 260–261,.

Olsson M, Tengvall K, Frankowiak M, Kierczak M, et al. Genome-wide analyses suggest mechanisms involving early B-cell development in canine IgA deficiency. *PlosOne*, 2015. https://org.doi:10.1371/journal.pone.0133844.

Pellegrini-Masini, A., Bentz, A.I., Johns, I.C., et al., 2005. Common variable immunodeficiency in three horses with presumptive bacterial meningitis. J. Am. Vet. Med. Assoc. 227, 114–122.

Perryman, L.E., 2004. Molecular pathology of severe combined immunodeficiency in mice, horses, and pigs. Vet. Pathol. 41, 95–100.

Powell, E.J., Cunnick, J.E., Knetter, S.M., Loving, C.L., et al., 2016. NK cells are intrinsically functional in pigs with severe combined immunodeficiency (SCID) caused by spontaneous mutations in the Artemis gene. Vet. Immunol. Immunopathol. 175, 1–6.

Scholes, S.F.E., Holliman, A., May, P.D.F., Holmes, M.A., 1998. A syndrome of anaemia, immunodeficiency and peripheral ganglionopathy in Fell pony foals. Vet. Rec. 142, 128–134.

Shiflett, S.L., Kaplan, J., Ward, D.M., 2002. Chédiak-Higashi syndrome: a rare disorder of lysosomes and lysosome related organelles. Pigment Cell Res. 15, 251–257.

Shin, E.K., Perryman, L.E., Meek, K., 1997. A kinase-negative mutation of DNA-PKcs in equine SCID results in defective coding and signal joint formation,. J. Immunol. 158, 3565–3569.

Tallmadge, R.L., Stokol, T., Gould-Earley, M.J., Earley, 2012a. Fell Pony syndrome: characterization of developmental hematopoiesis failure and associated gene expression profiles. Clin. Vaccine Immunol. 19, 1054–1064.

Tallmadge, R.L., Such, K.A., K., Miller, K.C., Bu, M., et al., 2012b. Expression of essential B cell development genes in horses with common variable immunodeficiency. Mol. Immunol. 51, 169–176.

Takasu, M., Shirota, K., Ohba, Y., Nishii, N., et al., 2008. Thymic hypoplasia in Japanese Black calves with stillbirth/perinatal weak calf syndrome. J. Vet. Med. Sci. 70 (11), 1173–1177.

Thomas, G.W., Bell, S.C., Phythian, C., et al., 2003. Aid to the antemortem diagnosis of Fell pony foal syndrome by the analysis of B lymphocytes. Vet. Rec. 152, 618–621.

Usta, Z., Jacobsen, B., Kuiper, H., Haas, L., Distl, O., 2016. Congenital hypotrichosis with thymus hypoplasia in a female German Holstein calf. Harran Univ. Ver. Fak. Derg. 5 (2), 173–176.

Verfuurden, B., Wempe, F., Reinink, P., van Kooten, P.J.S., et al., 2011. Severe combined immunodeficiency in Frisian water dogs caused by a *RAG1* mutation. Genes Immun. 12, 310–313.

Waide, E.H., Dekkers, J.C., Ross, J.W., Rowland, R.R., et al., 2015. Not all SCID pigs are created equally: two independent mutations in the artemis gene cause SCID in pigs. J. Immunol. 195, 3171–3179.

Watson, P.J., Wotton, P., Eastwood, J., et al., 2006. Immunoglobulin deficiency in Cavalier King Charles Spaniels with *Pneumocystis pneumonia*. J. Vet. Intern. Med. 20, 523–527.

Zoto, A., Stecklein, C., Scott, M.A., Bauer, T.R., 2022. Multiorgan neutrophilic infiltration in a Border Collie with "trapped" neutrophil syndrome. J. Vet. Intern. Med. 36, 2170–2176.

41

Secondary Immunological Defects

CHAPTER OUTLINE

The immune system, like any body system, is liable to destruction and dysfunction as a result of attacks by pathogenic and environmental agents. Among the most important of these agents are microorganisms, especially viruses, environmental toxins, stress of various types, malnutrition, and the progressive deterioration of old age. Infectious agents are a common cause of secondary immunodeficiencies. Bacteria, fungi, and viruses will survive and grow much more successfully if they can suppress the body's immune defenses (Sykes, 2010).

VIRUS-INDUCED IMMUNOSUPPRESSION

Viruses that attack the immune system may be divided into those that affect primary lymphoid tissues and those that affect secondary lymphoid tissues. Both types of viruses can cause immunodeficiencies. For example, in chickens, infectious bursal disease virus (IBDV) destroys lymphocytes in the bursa of Fabricius. IBDV is not completely specific for bursal cells; it also destroys cells in the spleen and thymus. These tissues usually recover, whereas the bursa atrophies. The resulting immunosuppression, as might be predicted, is most severe in young chicks infected soon after hatching, at a time when the bursa is actively engaged in generating B cells.

Canine Distemper

One of the most important viruses that destroys secondary lymphoid organs is canine distemper (Beineke et al., 2009). Canine distemper virus (CDV), almost certainly originated as a dog-specific mutant of the human measles virus. Although it can multiply in many different cell types, CDV has a predilection for lymphocytes, epithelia, and nervous tissues. It invades target cells via its hemagglutinin. This binds to two cellular receptors SLAM (signaling lymphocyte activation molecule) (CD150) and nectin 2—both of which are required for viral invasion. These molecules are expressed on activated B and T cells as well as on dendritic cells and macrophages (Henning et al., 2001). CDV is carried by macrophages from its initial invasion sites in the respiratory tract to the bloodstream, where it kills both T and B cells, resulting in a lymphopenia. Subsequently, it invades the thymus, spleen, lymph nodes, mucosal lymphoid tissues, and bone marrow, where it destroys yet more cells (von Messling et al., 2004). Infected cells shed from these lymphoid organs enable the virus to reach epithelial tissues and the brain. CDV infection triggers lymphocyte and macrophage apoptosis and so produces profound immunosuppression. It also suppresses production of interleukin-1 (IL-1) and IL-2. As a result, lymphocyte responses to mitogens are depressed, immunoglobulin levels fall, and skin allograft rejection is suppressed. Additionally, the virus acts on dendritic cells to downregulate MHC expression and the production of costimulatory cytokines while enhancing IL-10 production, thus effectively blocking antigen presentation (Qeska et al., 2014).

This immunosuppression accounts, in large part, for the clinical signs of canine distemper. For example, many infected dogs develop *Pneumocystis* pneumonia. (*Pneumocystis canis* is a fungal commensal that occurs in the lungs. It does not cause disease in immunocompetent animals but produces a severe pneumonia in immunosuppressed animals. The development of *Pneumocystis* pneumonia is evidence of a significant immunodeficiency.) If virulent distemper virus infects germ-free dogs, they develop a relatively mild disease, presumably because secondary infection does not occur (Rendon-Marin et al., 2019; Danesi et al., 2022).

Loss or functional exhaustion of lymphocytes is common in many virus infections since viral survival and persistence may require immunosuppression (Fig. 41.1). Thus lymphopenia occurs in feline panleukopenia, canine parvovirus-2 infection, feline leukemia, and African swine fever. Bovine virus diarrhea virus (BVDV) causes destruction of both B and T cells. As in canine distemper, surviving B cells fail to make immunoglobulins and respond poorly to mitogens. Destruction of Peyer's patches by BVDV causes intestinal ulceration and leads to secondary bacterial invasion of the intestinal mucosa.

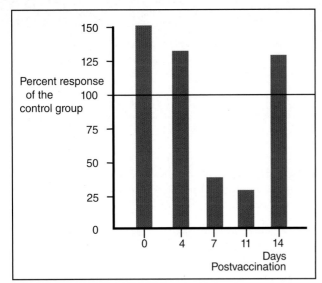

Fig. 41.1 The immunosuppressive effect of viruses. The effect of administering a mixed vaccine (containing canine distemper, canine adenovirus, canine parainfluenza, canine parvovirus-2, and leptospira) on the response of a puppy's lymphocytes to the mitogen phytohemagglutinin. Control levels were 100%. From Phillips, T.R., Jensen, J.L., Rubino, M.J., et al., 1989. Effects of vaccines on the canine immune system. Can. J. Vet. Res. 53, 154–160.

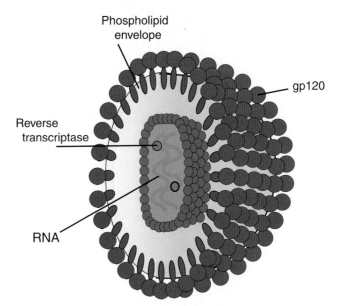

Fig. 41.2 The structure of a typical retrovirus such as feline leukemia virus or feline lentivirus. *RNA*, Ribonucleic acid.

Herpesviruses are also immunosuppressive. For example, equine herpesvirus–1 causes a drop in T-cell numbers and depresses cell-mediated responses in foals. Bovine herpesvirus–1 (BHV-1) also causes a drop in T-cell numbers and their responses to mitogens. Although BHV-1 stimulates bovine alveolar macrophages, thus increasing expression of MHC class II and promoting phagocytosis, it also depresses macrophage-mediated cytotoxicity and IL-1 synthesis. Parainfluenzavirus-3 and infectious bovine rhinotracheitis viruses have long been known to interfere with alveolar macrophage functions. They inhibit phagosome-lysosome fusion paving the way for secondary infections with *Mannheimia hemolytica* in calves. Porcine reproductive and respiratory syndrome (PRRS) virus kills alveolar macrophages and predisposes affected pigs to severe enzootic pneumonia. It also kills dendritic cells, a feature that may account for the ability of the PRRS virus to persist in pigs for up to 6 months.

The results of virus-induced lymphoid tissue destruction or exhaustion are usually obvious. Animals become lymphopenic and have reduced lymphocyte responses to mitogens. For example, responses to phytohemagglutinin are depressed in influenza, canine distemper, Marek's disease, Newcastle disease, feline leukemia, bovine virus diarrhea, and lymphocytic choriomeningitis. Destruction of lymphoid tissues may also result in hypogammaglobulinemia or a reduced response to vaccines. Thymic atrophy and lymphopenia are common manifestations of many virus infections, and before any primary immunodeficiency syndrome is diagnosed, steps must be taken to exclude the possibility that it is, in fact, secondary to a virus infection.

Primate Retroviruses

More than 40 lentiviruses related to HIV have been isolated from non-human primates, especially African species. SIV_{cpz} from a chimpanzee (*Pan troglodytes*), is the ancestor of HIV-1. All these viruses selectively destroy CD4$^+$ T cells. They initially stimulate a strong but ineffective immune response. Viral replication continues and eventually causes an immunodeficiency syndrome similar to human AIDS. The infection is believed to be transmitted sexually. Clinical disease progresses slowly, but the animals eventually develop lymphadenopathy, severe weight loss, chronic diarrhea, lymphomas, neurological lesions, and opportunistic infections by organisms such as *Pneumocystis*, *Mycobacterium avium-intracellulare*, *Candida albicans*, and *Cryptosporidium parvum*. The virus invades both T cells and macrophages using two cellular receptors, CD4 and the chemokine receptors CCR5 or CXCR4. About 25% of infected animals do not mount a significant response to SIV and die within 3–5 months from severe SIV encephalitis. Spontaneous recovery does not occur (Lackner and Veazey, 2007).

CAT RETROVIRUSES

Feline leukemia virus (FeLV) and Feline Immunodeficiency virus (FIV) are both retroviruses. FIV causes an acquired immunodeficiency syndrome, neurologic disease, and some tumors. It is not itself highly pathogenic and FIV-infected cats may live for many years. FeLV is more pathogenic and causes diverse clinical diseases, including lymphomas, bone marrow suppression leading to anemia, and immunosuppression. Effective vaccines have significantly reduced the prevalence of FeLV.

Feline Leukemia

FeLV is an oncogenic retrovirus that causes both proliferative and degenerative diseases in cats (Fig. 41.2).

FeLV is shed in saliva and nasal secretions and is thus transmitted between cats by grooming. Once FeLV infects a cat, it first grows in the lymphoid tissues of the pharynx and tonsils. This is followed by a transient viremia as it spreads throughout the body and invades the other lymphoid organs. A mild lymphopenia and neutropenia occur 1–2 weeks after infection.

Cats probably have the highest prevalence of lymphoid tumors of any domestic mammal. FeLV causes most of these tumors. These include lymphosarcomas, reticulum-cell sarcomas, erythroleukemias, and granulocytic leukemias. FeLV lymphosarcomas are usually of T-cell origin, although FeLV grows in many cell types and is not restricted to lymphoid tissues. Some alimentary lymphomas may be of B-cell origin. The proportion of virus-positive tumors ranges from 100% of myeloid leukemias to 30% of alimentary lymphomas. In young cats, FeLV-induced tumors are mainly of T-cell origin. In older cats, they originate from both T and B cells.

FeLV develops T-cell tropic variants (FeLV-T) as a result of mutations in viral gp70. These variants can replicate to high numbers in T cells. FeLV-T is fusion-defective and enters T cells using, as a cofactor, a truncated envelope protein called FeLIX encoded by an endogenous FeLV ("FeLV Infectivity X-essory protein"). FeLIX binds to Pit1, a phosphate transporter protein, leading to membrane fusion.

The lymphopenia in FeLV-T-infected cats results from a loss of CD4+ T cells. CD8+ T cells may also drop in the early stages of the disease so that the CD4:CD8 ratio may initially remain within normal limits. (The CD4:CD8 ratio in normal cats ranges from about 0.4–3.5, with a median value of about 1.9.) CD8+ T-cell numbers eventually recover while the CD4:CD8 ratio then drops. B-cell numbers may also be depressed, but this depends on the severity of secondary infections. In cats without secondary infection, lymphoid atrophy is associated with loss of cells from the paracortex of lymph nodes. Changes in the spleen are less marked but may result in shrinkage of the entire white pulp. As a result of T-cell loss, FeLV-infected cats have depressed cell-mediated immunity. This depression is also due to the effects of p15e, the immunosuppressive envelope protein of FeLV, which is produced in very large quantities by dying cells. p15e suppresses the responses of cats to Feline Oncornavirus Cell Membrane Antigen (FOCMA) and to lymphocyte mitogens and blocks the responses of T cells to IL-2. As a result, FeLV-infected cats may carry skin allografts for about twice as long as normal cats (24 days compared with 12). Bone marrow stem cells are also inhibited by p15e, preventing production of erythroid cells and resulting in a nonregenerative anemia. In contrast to the severe T-cell dysfunction, B-cell functions in FeLV-infected cats are only mildly impaired.

Kittens infected with FeLV-T develop a wasting syndrome associated with thymic atrophy and recurrent infections. Depending on the severity of these secondary infections, the syndrome may be associated with either lymphoid atrophy or lymphoid hyperplasia. In adult cats, this syndrome is characterized by progressive weight loss and lymphoid hyperplasia followed by severe lymphoid depletion, and chronic diarrhea. The immunosuppression also predisposes viremic cats to secondary infections such as feline infectious peritonitis, mycoplasmosis, toxoplasmosis, septicemia, and fungal infections. Widespread vaccination has significantly reduced the prevalence of this disease in the United States.

FOCMA

As described earlier, a unique protein, called FOCMA, is expressed on FeLV-infected cells. It is encoded by endogenous retroviral genes within the cat genome. It is not expressed on normal cells but rather on cells infected with FeLV or FeSV. It was originally believed that the presence of FOCMA on a cell membrane identified the cell as an FeLV-induced tumor cell. Of those cats that fail to make neutralizing antibodies to FeLV and remain viremic, about 80% develop antitumor activity by making antibodies against FOCMA. A cat that makes antibodies to FOCMA can usually destroy virus-induced tumor cells. A direct immunofluorescent test on a buffy coat smear using antibodies to group-specific antigen can detect cell-associated antigen and hence intracellular viremia (Fig. 41.3).

Feline Immunodeficiency Virus

FIV is an enveloped, single-stranded RNA virus belonging to the lentivirus subgroup of retroviruses (Fig. 41.4). It is differentiated from FeLV (a γ-retrovirus) by the biochemical requirements of its reverse transcriptase. FIV is spread by territorial, free-roaming male cats through aggressive biting. As a result, it occurs predominantly in old male cats that spend a lot of time outdoors.

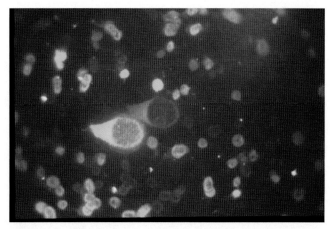

Fig. 41.3 A positive indirect immunofluorescence assay for Feline leukemia virus in a peripheral blood smear. Courtesy Dr. F.C. Heck.

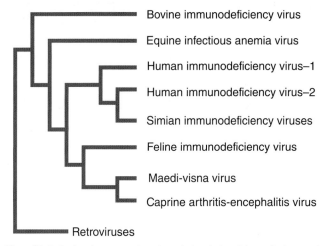

Fig. 41.4 A dendrogram showing the relationships of the major lentiviruses.

FIV replicates in CD4+ and CD8+ T cells, B cells, megakaryocytes, neuronal cells, and macrophages. Some strains only replicate well in lymphocytes, whereas others replicate in both lymphocytes and macrophages. Primary targets of FIV infection are the lymphocytes. However, as infection persists, the virus increasingly affects macrophages. In clinically ill cats with a high viral load, macrophages are the major sites of viral replication. FIV-infected cats have fewer neutrophils, a lower proportion of T cells, and a higher proportion of B cells compared to uninfected animals.

FIV binds specifically to CD134 expressed on a subset of CD4+ T cells. This binding, in conjunction with binding to the α-chemokine receptor CXCR4 (CD184), is required for FIV to infect a cell. Most naturally infected cats suffer a critical loss of CD4+ T cells (Fig. 41.5). This loss is due to destruction of infected cells, decreased production, and premature apoptosis. The surviving CD4+ cells may have reduced responses to mitogens.

FIV cats may show a shift away from a Th1 cytokine production pattern. They may also show an increase in CD8+ T cells. As a result, the CD4:CD8 ratio of FIV-infected cats may drop to less than one. Affected cats show decreased IL-2 and IL-12 production as well as increased IL-10. Thus the rise in the IL-10:IL-12 ratio is especially immunosuppressive (Miller et al., 2013).

During the acute phase of FIV, Treg cells are infected and activated by the virus. The virus induces both Foxp3 and membrane-bound TGF-β production. The TGF-β converts Th1 cells into Treg cells. The

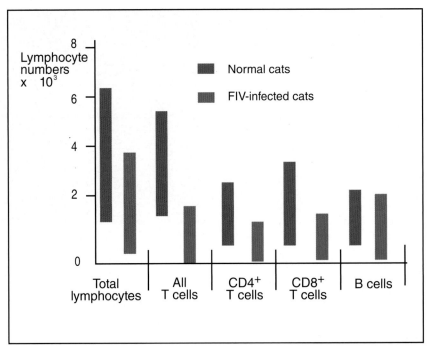

Fig. 41.5 The numbers of cells in different lymphocyte populations (pan T, CD4, CD8, B cells) for 11 normal cats and 11 cats infected with feline immunodeficiency virus. From Novotney, C., English, R.V., Housman. J., et al., 1990. Lymphocyte population changes in cats naturally infected with feline immunodeficiency virus. AIDS. 4, 1213–1218.

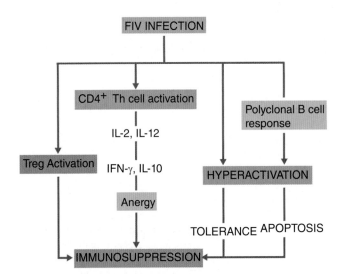

Fig. 41.6 The major immunosuppressive pathways activated in feline immunodeficiency virus (FIV) infections. *IFN-γ*, Interferon-γ; *IL-12*, interleukin-12; *Tregs*, regulatory T cells.

Treg cells also suppress CD8+ T-cell responses by inducing cell cycle arrest. The Treg cells induce their targets to produce Foxp3, which then binds to the IL-2 promoter and effectively inhibits IL-2 production and effector cell function. This Treg activation severely limits the development of an effective antiviral response.

The lymphopenia that develops in both FeLV and FIV infections is due to a loss of T cells (Fig. 41.6). CD4+ T cells are depressed in both, but the depression is much greater in FIV-infected animals. FIV-infected cats show a rapid drop in T-cell numbers, whereas their B cells are unaffected. Their CD8+ T cells recover, but their CD4+

T cells fail to do so. Within 6 months of FIV infection, there is a measurable drop in CD4+ T cells. Their response to thymus-dependent and -independent antigens initially remains unchanged. By 2–3 years after the onset of infection, however, the drop in CD4+ T cells continues, and their response to thymus-dependent antigens is profoundly depressed, while the response to thymus-independent antigens is unchanged. FIV-infected cats may have normal numbers of CD8+ T cells and B cells and normal levels of IgM and IgA. Indeed, more than 25% of FIV-infected cats may be hypergammaglobulinemic as a result of polyclonal B-cell activation. Affected cats may also deposit immune complexes in their renal glomeruli (Elder et al., 2008).

Bovine Retroviruses

Bovine immunodeficiency virus (BIV) is a lentivirus originally isolated from a cow with lymphosarcoma. The BIV-infected animal developed lymph node hyperplasia, lymphocytosis, central nervous system lesions, loss of weight, and weakness. When used to infect experimental calves, the animals develop transient lymphocytosis, lymphadenopathy, and a nonsuppurative meningoencephalitis. BIV infection may also cause minor changes in the response of lymphocytes to mitogens and may suppress some neutrophil functions, such as antibody-dependent cell-mediated cytotoxicity. BIV can also infect sheep. In this species, experimental infection is associated with an increase in CD2+ and CD4+ T cells, as well as in the CD4:CD8 ratio, between 6 and 8 months after inoculation. The sheep showed no signs of illness by 1 year after inoculation and appeared to have normal immune function.

Canine Retroviruses

Several different retroviruses have been isolated from dogs. Some appear to be lentiviruses, although the existence of a "canine immunodeficiency virus" has not been established. For example, a lentivirus has been isolated from the mononuclear cells of a leukemic German Shepherd dog. This virus does not appear to be closely related to the other major lentiviruses. On inoculation into newborn Beagles, it caused pronounced lymphadenopathy.

A lentivirus has also been isolated from a dog with hemorrhagic gastroenteritis. This animal developed a lymphopenia and agammaglobulinemia with lymphoid and bone marrow hypoplasia. The virus could grow in canine lymphocytes and thymocytes; it had a magnesium-dependent reverse transcriptase. The virus was present in bone marrow, intestine, and lymph nodes. It caused reduced synthesis of, and reduced responsiveness to IL-2, and it was cytotoxic for lymphocytes.

A C-type retrovirus has also been isolated from a dog. This animal suffered from anemia, neutropenia, lymphopenia, and thrombocytopenia, as well as depressed humoral and T-cell-mediated immune responses. On necropsy, the dog showed depletion of lymphoid organs and bone marrow hypoplasia. Yet it also had plasma cell infiltrates in many organs as well as multiple secondary infections.

Circoviruses

Porcine circovirus-2 (PCV2) is associated with the development of postweaning multisystemic wasting syndrome (PMWS). PMWS is an acquired immunodeficiency syndrome of piglets characterized by wasting, lymphadenopathy, and respiratory disease with occasional pallor, jaundice, and diarrhea. Some affected piglets have profound lymphocyte depletion, initially involving CD4+, CD8+, and double-positive T cells. T-cell areas in tonsils and lymph nodes are depleted, and there is an absence of follicles in the cortex. Some pigs develop a necrotizing lymphadenitis as a result of hypertrophy and hyperplasia of their high endothelial venules, leading to thrombosis and necrosis. IgM-positive B-cell numbers are also reduced in more chronic cases. Infected piglets suffer from diverse secondary and opportunistic infections. Although PCV2 is the most likely causative agent, it has proved difficult to reproduce the disease consistently, and other factors, including environment, and other infectious agents are also involved.

OTHER SECONDARY IMMUNODEFICIENCIES

Microbial and Parasite Infections

Immunosuppression generally accompanies infestation with *Toxoplasma* or trypanosomes, helminths such as *Trichinella spiralis*, arthropods such as *Demodex*, and bacteria such as *M. hemolytica*, the actinobacilli, and some streptococci (see Chapters 27 and 29). Bacteria such as *Bordetella bronchiseptica* can paralyze respiratory cilia, while *Anaplasma phagocytophilum* can suppress neutrophil functions (Sykes, 2010).

Toxin-Induced Immunosuppression

Many environmental toxins such as polychlorinated biphenyls, polybrominated biphenyls, dieldrin, iodine, lead, cadmium, methyl mercury, and DDT are immunosuppressive. $CdCl_2$ and $HgCl_2$ both inhibit phagocytosis by bovine leukocytes at very low concentrations. Higher concentrations are required to inhibit NK cell function and cell proliferation.

Mycotoxins are important immunosuppressants in cattle, pigs, or poultry fed moldy grain. The most prevalent of these are derived from *Fusarium* species. These include the trichothecenes (T-2 toxin and deoxynivalenol) and the fumonisins. When deoxynivalenol is administered to pregnant sows, it results in low levels of colostral IgA and reduced IgA and IgG in their piglets. It can also significantly reduce the response of pigs to some vaccines. Deoxynivalenol causes immunosuppression, greater susceptibility to mastitis in dairy cattle, and high somatic cell counts in milk. T-2 toxin depresses the response of calf lymphocytes to mitogens and decreases the chemotactic

response of neutrophils. T-2 toxin also reduces IgM, IgA, and C3 levels in cattle. Trichothecenes are also immunosuppressive in pigs and birds. Fumonisin B1 inhibits division of both T and B cells in piglets, increases interferon-γ (IFN-γ) production while suppressing IL-4 production, and increases susceptibility to *Escherichia coli* infections.

Aflatoxins from *Aspergillus* species increase the susceptibility of chickens to *Salmonella* as a result of depressed phagocytosis. They also increase the susceptibility of dairy cattle to mastitis. They depress piglet growth and suppress immune responses to *Mycoplasma*. Toxin-induced immunosuppression may be especially important in wild carnivores situated at the top of the food chain. A good example of this is seen in seals feeding on environmentally contaminated fish. These seals show depressed responses to vaccines, impaired mitogenic responses, lowered delayed hypersensitivity responses, and reduced NK cell numbers. This immunosuppression also decreases their resistance to phocine morbillivirus.

Malnutrition

It has long been recognized that famine and disease are closely associated, and we tend to assume that malnutrition leads to increased susceptibility to infection. The effects of malnutrition on immune functions are, however, complex. Malnutrition includes not only deficiencies but also excesses or imbalances of individual nutrients.

In general, severe nutritional deficiencies reduce T-cell function and therefore impair cell-mediated responses, at the same time sparing B-cell function and humoral immunity. Thus starvation rapidly induces thymic atrophy. The number of circulating T cells drops, and cells are lost from the T-cell areas of secondary lymphoid organs. Delayed hypersensitivity reactions are reduced, allograft rejection is delayed, and IFN-γ production is impaired. Protein starvation selectively suppresses Th2 responses such as IL-4 and IgE production, leading to increased susceptibility to parasites (Bastien et al., 2015).

Severe starvation has little effect on B-cell functions. The B-cell areas in lymphoid tissues and the number of circulating B cells remain largely unchanged. Serum immunoglobulin levels remain normal or even rise. Secretory IgA levels commonly drop, but secretory IgE may rise, suggesting abnormal immunoregulation. Starvation, however, depresses complement levels and impairs neutrophil and macrophage chemotaxis, the respiratory burst, release of lysosomal enzymes, and microbicidal activity.

Obesity

Adipose tissue was long considered a resting tissue where fat reserves were stored until needed. We now know, however, that adipose tissue plays an active role in both innate and adaptive immunity. The major cell types found in adipose tissue are adipocytes and macrophages. Both produce multiple cytokines. For example, adipocytes produce two cytokines (also called adipokines); leptin and adiponectin. Leptin levels increase in the obese, and this suppresses appetite. Adiponectin, in contrast, counteracts the activities of leptin, and its level drops in the obese. Leptin levels are elevated in obese dogs, and adiponectin levels are elevated in lean dogs. Serotonin also controls appetite. Its levels are higher in lean dogs, and it may play a role in controlling appetite. All three molecules, leptin, adiponectin, and serotonin influence the immune system (Park et al., 2014).

Leptin is a 16-kDa protein produced by adipocytes. While first described as an antiobesity hormone, it also influences both innate and adaptive immunity and promotes inflammatory responses. It binds to receptors in the hypothalamus and suppresses the appetite. The amount of leptin in blood is proportional to the amount of fat in the body. The fatter an animal, therefore, the more leptin is produced, and appetite is correspondingly suppressed. Conversely, caloric restriction

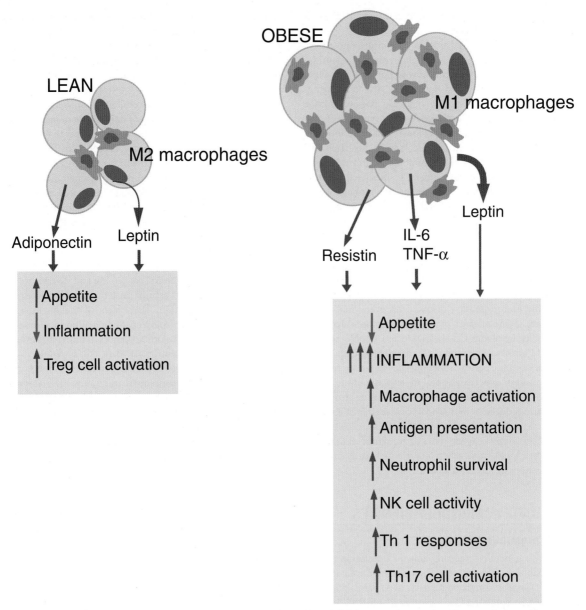

Fig. 41.7 Obese adipose tissue is rich in classically activated (M1) macrophages that, in association with large quantities of leptin, generate pro-inflammatory cytokines, resulting in enhanced inflammation throughout the body. Lean adipose tissue, in contrast, contains small numbers of alternatively activated (M2) macrophages and produces little leptin, tending to suppress inflammatory reactions. Adiponectin contributes to this antiinflammatory effect, whereas resistin is proinflammatory. *IL-6,* Interleukin-6; *NK cell,* nature killer cell; *TNF-α,* tumor necrosis factor–α; *Th1,* Type 1 T helper; *Treg,* regulatory T cells.

and weight loss lead to a loss of adipocytes, a drop in leptin levels, and an increase in appetite (Fig. 41.7). Breed-specific differences in leptin levels occur in dogs. The significance of this is unknown. In cats, leptin levels rise after spaying, which may account for the weight gain commonly observed in these animals. In mares, leptin levels in colostrum are two to three times those in blood, and it has been suggested, that leptin may be required for intestinal development in foals (Naylor and Petri, 2016).

Adipose tissue in lean humans contains about 10% macrophages, whereas in the obese, it may contain 50% macrophages. The adipose tissue macrophages found in obese individuals are M1 cells activated by leptin. Leptin increases their tumor necrosis factor–α (TNF-α), IL-6, and IL-1 production and upregulates MHC class II expression. This increased IL-6 production also promotes Th17-mediated inflammatory responses. Leptin also enhances Th17 responses by upregulating the transcription factor RORγt and suppressing Treg differentiation.

In obese animals, this widespread macrophage activation predisposes to inflammatory diseases such as atherosclerosis, arthritis, type 2 IDDM, and autoimmunity, as well as cancer (German et al., 2010). There is thus a clear link between obesity and chronic low-grade inflammation. Given the increasing obesity of pets as well as some of the effects of rapid growth in food animals, veterinarians would be well advised to take this link into account.

Leptin also enhances NK cell development and activation. It promotes Th1 cell production of IFN-γ, TNF-α, and leptin itself, thus generating an autocrine feedback loop. In lean animals where leptin levels are low, macrophage activation is suppressed, inflammatory responses are reduced, and there is a shift from Th1 to Th2 responses while increasing Treg cells.

Adiponectin, a 28 kDa protein, counteracts the activities of leptin (German, 2012). Its concentration is inversely related to body weight, and it has strong anti-inflammatory activity. In lean animals, it decreases production of IL-8, IFN-γ, IL-6, and TNF-α while increasing the production of IL-1RA and IL-10. It induces maturation and activation of dendritic cells. As a result, it reduces Th1 and Th17 responses. Adiponectin also regulates glucose and fatty acid metabolism. In obesity, adiponectin production drops, and adipose tissue macrophages then produce a hormone called resistin that increases insulin resistance leading to diabetes (Nguyen, 2020).

Mineral and Vitamin Deficiencies

Several trace elements are required for optimal functioning of the immune system. The most important are zinc, copper, selenium, and iron. Deficiencies of any of these are immunosuppressive. Zinc is especially critical to the proper functioning of the immune system since it acts as an ionic signaling messenger to promote T-cell activation. Zinc-deficient pigs have reduced thymus weight, depressed cytotoxic T-cell activity, depressed B-cell activity, depressed NK cell activity, and decreased antibody production. If pregnant animals are deprived of zinc, their offspring are immunosuppressed. Neutrophils from zinc-deficient animals have reduced chemotaxis and phagocytosis. Mild zinc supplementation may promote immunity. On the other hand, because many bacteria utilize zinc, the body also sequesters it to limit its availability during infections.

Copper deficiencies are also immunosuppressive. Thus a copper deficiency reduces neutrophil numbers and function by depressing superoxide production. It also reduces lymphocyte responsiveness to mitogens; reduces T, B, and NK cell numbers; and enhances mast cell histamine release. Selenium deficiency depresses the function of most immune cells, reducing neutrophil, T and NK cell responses, and IgM production. Supplementation with selenium upregulates the expression of IL-2R and prevents oxidative damage to immune cells. Iron deficiency is immunosuppressive for cell-mediated responses. However, the effects of this on resistance to infection are complex since many pathogens require iron to replicate (see Chapter 8). A magnesium deficiency also reduces immunoglobulin levels.

Three vitamins, A, D, and E are critical for proper immune function (Mora et al., 2008). If a pregnant animal is vitamin A deficient, the lymphoid tissue development in its fetus is impaired. Deficiencies of vitamin A reduce lymphocyte proliferation, NK cell activity, and cytokine

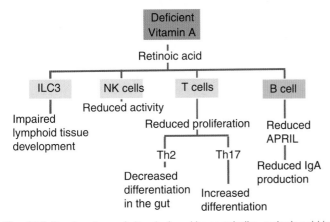

Fig. 41.8 The functions of vitamin A and its metabolite, retinoic acid in immunity. *IgA,* Immunoglobin; *ILC3,* group 3 innate lymphoid cells; *NK cells,* nature killer cells; *Th2,* T helper 2 cells.

and immunoglobulin production (Fig. 41.8). Some vitamin A metabolites, such as retinoic acid, enhance T-cell proliferation and cytotoxicity. Retinoic acid is especially important in promoting Th2 and dendritic cell differentiation in the intestine and in the homing of IgA-positive B cells to mucosal surfaces. It also maintains Treg and ILC3 levels in the intestinal mucosa and thus regulates tolerance to food antigens (see Chapter 23).

A prenatal vitamin A deficiency affects the responses of piglets to rotavirus vaccine. Deficient piglets shed the virus at 350% of the level of vitamin A-sufficient piglets. Only 25% of the deficient piglets were protected as compared to 100% of the sufficient piglets. Deficient piglets had fewer IgG-secreting cells in the ileum and fewer IgA-secreting cells in the duodenum. Intestinal IgA titers were 11-fold less than in vitamin A–sufficient animals. Deficient animals did, however, have higher levels of IL-8 and IFN-γ than sufficient piglets (Chattha et al., 2013).

Calves fed a low vitamin A diet and immunized with an inactivated bovine coronavirus vaccine had reduced IgG1 antibody levels against bovine coronavirus suggesting that Th2 responses may be impaired in these animals (Jee et al., 2013).

Vitamin E is a major antioxidant in cell membranes and is important in regulating the oxidants produced by phagocytic cells. Vitamin E deficiency depresses immunoglobulin levels through its effects on Treg cells and decreases lymphocyte responses to mitogens. Animals deficient in vitamin E also show reduced IL-2 and transferrin receptor expression and depressed phagocytic function. Vitamin E is one of the few vitamins for which supplementation has been shown to enhance immune responses and disease resistance (Finch and Turner, 1996). The importance of vitamin E for proper functioning of the immune system has been seen in an inbred population of donkeys whose foals were dying from overwhelming bacterial infections at 3–5 months of age (Verdonck et al., 2007). Investigations revealed that these foals were agammaglobulinemic but also lacked detectable vitamin E in their serum. Vitamin E supplementation by injection caused an immediate clinical improvement, and within two months, immunoglobulin levels were within normal limits. It was suggested that affected foals lacked a vitamin E transport protein. All subsequent foals in this herd received supplemental vitamin E and remained healthy. Supplemental vitamin E given to cats appeared to enhance T-cell responsiveness to mitogens and leukocyte phagocytic activity (O'Brien et al., 2015).

When *Mycobacterium tuberculosis* interacts with toll-like receptor 1 or TLR2 on macrophages, it upregulates many different genes and enhances their antimicrobial activity. One such gene is that encoding the vitamin D receptor (Fig. 41.9). This receptor is present on most immune system cells, including neutrophils, macrophages, and T cells. The binding of vitamin D to its receptor on T cells downregulates IFN-γ and IL-2 expression and promotes Th2 responses. It also promotes Treg cell differentiation in the skin. Binding to the receptor on macrophages, in contrast, promotes their activation and the production of cathelicidin and β-defensin-2 (Corripio-Miyar et al., 2017). It is no coincidence that resistance to tuberculosis and other respiratory diseases is directly related to serum vitamin D levels and that humans with a deficiency of vitamin D have significantly decreased resistance to this infection (Colotta et al., 2017). It has been suggested that mice use nitric oxide rather than vitamin D as an intermediate in innate signaling because they are nocturnal, whereas humans acquire vitamin D from sunlight on exposed skin. It is unclear whether similar mechanisms operate in domestic mammals. Vitamin D levels decline with age. Th2 cytokines such as IL-13 enhance vitamin D-mediated expression of cathelicidins in bronchial epithelial cells (White, 2008).

Taurine (2-aminoethanesulfonic acid) is an essential amino acid in cats. Deficiencies can result in a neutropenia, although mononuclear cell numbers may rise. The neutrophils of taurine-deficient cats show decreased respiratory burst activity and phagocytosis. Although these

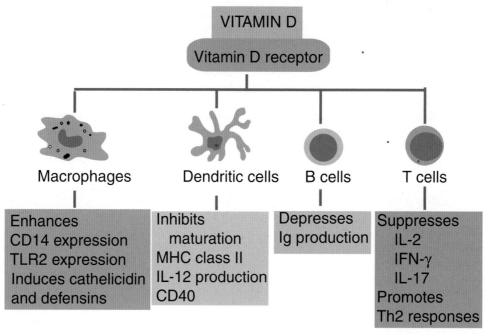

Fig. 41.9 The importance of vitamin D in immunity. Note that vitamin D is a potent stimulator of innate immunity by enhancing production of antimicrobial peptides. It is, however, somewhat suppressive of adaptive immune responses. *IFN-γ*, Interferon-γ; *IL-2*, interleukin-2; *MHC*, major histocompatibility complex; *Th2*, T helper 2 cells; *TLR2*, toll-like receptor 2.

cats may show a hypergammaglobulinemia, germinal centers shrink, suggesting a loss of B-cell activity.

The effects of malnutrition may be reflected in altered resistance to infectious diseases. Because bacteria can readily survive and multiply in body tissues despite malnutrition of the host, starvation commonly increases the severity of bacterial infections such as pneumonia. Viruses, in contrast, require healthy host cells in which to grow. Malnutrition, by rendering host cells unhealthy, may therefore increase resistance to viruses. Overnutrition can also influence susceptibility to viruses. For example, overfed dogs show an increased susceptibility to canine distemper and canine adenovirus–1.

Exercise and Immunity

Regular moderate exercise boosts immune function. For example, increased antibody responses are observed in mice that get moderate exercise, compared with unexercised control mice. Exercise also raises blood neutrophil counts, enhances NK cell activity, promotes lymphocyte responses to mitogens, and increases blood levels of IL-1, IL-6, and TNF-α (Rogers et al., 2008). Although mild exercise is good for immune function, high-intensity exercise, prolonged exhaustive exercise, or over-training may induce a functional immunodeficiency. In horses, blood lymphocytes show a decreased proliferative response for up to 16 hours after a race. Acute exercise in the unfit animal can be especially stressful. Unfit horses subjected to strenuous exercise showed significantly raised steroid levels, resulting in reduced lymphocyte responses to mitogens or influenza virus antigens and reduced neutrophil chemotactic responsiveness and chemoluminescence (a measure of respiratory burst activity) (Fig. 41.10). These animals show a decline in their CD4:CD8 ratio as well as in both the number and activity of their NK cells. The age of an animal may moderate the effect of exercise on immune responses. For example, strenuous exercise significantly reduces lymphocyte proliferative responses in young horses yet has much less effect on older animals. This resistance of older horses to exercise-induced immunosuppression may be due to their reduced steroid production.

The complex effects of extreme exercise on the immune system are well seen in dogs undergoing long endurance sled races (The Ididarod). The proportion of dogs with low total globulin immediately after racing was significantly greater than before racing. In some of these dogs, it remained low for 4 months after the race. IgG was also lower after racing than before racing. Likewise, serum IgM and IgE were higher before racing, although IgA was higher after racing. These changes in immunoglobulins might well affect resistance to infectious diseases. There is also evidence of increased inflammation in these dogs after racing (McKenzie et al., 2010).

Stress

Stress has profound effects on the immune system (Fig. 21.14; Padgett and Glaser, 2003). Small bouts of stress are believed to enhance immune responses, but prolonged stress is detrimental. One obvious example is shipping fever. This is a complex pneumonia of cattle caused by several viral respiratory pathogens with secondary infection by *Mannheimia haemolytica*. It develops in cattle that have been transported in confined spaces for long distances (and hence, many hours) with minimal feed and water, usually after rapid weaning and castration. The stress involved in the shipping process is sufficient to make these cattle highly susceptible to pneumonia. Stress depresses T-cell responses, NK cell activity, IL-2 production, and expression of IL-2R on lymphocytes. Reduction in stress can have a reverse effect. In studies investigating innate responses among calm and temperamental Brahman bulls, it was found that calm bulls had elevated neutrophil L-selectin expression and increased neutrophil phagocytic and oxidative burst activity when compared to temperamental bulls, 48 hour posttransportation. By 96 hours, neutrophil phagocytosis, oxidative burst, and cell adhesion molecule expression were enhanced in all bulls, but the effects were most pronounced in calm bulls.

Stress can be due to something as simple as early weaning, which reduces IL-2 production in piglets. Stress in pregnant sows, results in immunosuppression of their offspring. Thus confinement stress late in pregnancy results in the birth of piglets with T and B cells that have a

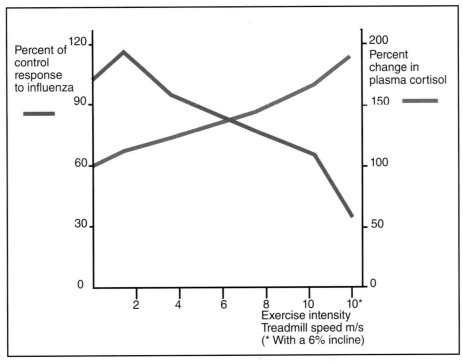

Fig. 41.10 Although a moderate amount of exercise is good for the immune system, excessive exercise causes severe stress that can be immunosuppressive. In this example, six thoroughbred horses were subjected to a treadmill-based exercise challenge of various intensities (speed and incline). Blood samples were assayed for plasma cortisol levels by radioimmunoassay, and influenza virus–specific lymphocyte proliferation was assayed by thymidine incorporation. A clear relationship exists among exercise intensity, the stress response, and immune responsiveness. From data kindly provided by Drs. S.G. Kamerling, P.A. Melrose, D.D. French, and D.W. Horohov.

reduced ability to respond to mitogens. Both morbidity and mortality are increased in piglets from stressed sows.

A different form of stress may result from mammalian social structures. A dominance hierarchy regulates many mammalian populations. Depending on the way the hierarchy is established, some members may be highly stressed. Animals of high rank will be stressed if it requires constant fighting to maintain dominance. This occurs, for example, in wild dogs, lemurs, and mongooses. In hierarchies in which dominant members rule through psychological intimidation, such as in mice, rats, and many monkeys, low-ranking individuals may be stressed and immunosuppressed. If new individuals are introduced into a group, or a dominant animal loses its position, stresses occur as a result of the reorganization. In pigs, it has been shown that there is a relationship between social status and disease susceptibility. For example, morbidity and mortality among pigs challenged with pseudorabies virus were highest among subordinate animals. Dominant pigs had lymphocytes that were more responsive to virus antigens. This, of course, makes sense from an evolutionary point of view in that the least reproductively fit animals were more likely to die of disease, but it is difficult to separate cause and effect in this phenomenon. Were subordinate animals immunosuppressed because they were under stress as a result of their lowly status? Alternatively, could it be that those animals with a highly effective immune system were healthier and thus better able to reach high social status within the population? Certainly, high levels of social stress are found in confined, crowded animal populations. Social subordination in rhesus monkeys, results in changes in gene expression that are biased towards inflammation including genes associated with lymphocyte proliferation, innate immunity and cytokine responsiveness. In stressed subordinate monkeys, TLR4 signaling predominantly used the MyD88-NF-κB pathway, while in dominant monkeys it used the TRIF-IFN pathway (see Chapter 3).

When the behavior of pigs is examined, they can be divided into two groups: aggressive animals that tend to fight other animals and then may flee rapidly, and passive animals that tend to cope with stress by withdrawing gradually from stressful situations. Aggressive pigs had higher in vitro and in vivo cell-mediated immune responses but lower humoral responses than passive animals (Hessing et al., 1994). This suggests that there were differences in their relative Th1 and Th2 responses. However, when these animals were stressed, the aggressive ones showed a much greater drop in these responses than the passive animals. Differences in the way animals cope with stress are thus reflected in differences in immune reactivity (Hessing et al., 1994).

Heat stress in cattle activates the hypothalamic-pituitary-adrenal axis and increases blood glucocorticoid levels thus suppressing the production of cytokines such as IL-4, -5, -6, -12, IFN-γ, and TNF-α, resulting in severe immunosuppression (Bagath et al., 2019).

The stress effect is mediated by two major pathways. One involves the autonomic nervous system acting through its neurotransmitters adrenaline, noradrenaline, and acetylcholine, and the other is the hypothalamic-pituitary-adrenal cortical axis producing glucocorticoids. Stress signals the brain to activate these pathways (see Chapter 21).

Transportation stress is well recognized as predisposing to the development of respiratory disease in horses. One major reason for the impairment of respiratory defenses in transported horses is prolonged head elevation. With the head held high, mucociliary clearance is significantly reduced. Over time, this elevation permits the accumulation of bacteria, particulates, and inflammatory exudates in the trachea. After 24 hours of head elevation, significant pulmonary inflammation develops. It takes about 12 hours of free head movement for this inflammation to decline to normal levels.

It is well recognized that 70%–80% of young racehorses beginning training commonly develop airway inflammation (see Chapter 33). This appears to result, in part, from an induced immunodeficiency. It appears that exercise induces a reduction in the phagocytic ability of equine alveolar macrophages as well as a reduced response to TLR ligands. Analysis of bronchoalveolar cells shows alterations in the expression of the genes associated with airway immunity (Karagianni et al., 2022).

Stress may result in immunodeficiencies. For example, it is possible to provoke a combined immunodeficiency syndrome by chilling newborn puppies for 5–10 days. Diverse stressors such as rapid weaning, sleep deprivation, general anesthesia, prolonged transportation, and overcrowding are all effective immunosuppressants.

Post-traumatic Immune Deficiency

Trauma and tissue destruction initiate a response triggered by alarmins such as HMGB1, as well as enzymes escaping from damaged cells. Inflammasomes are generated, inflammatory cytokines are released, and macrophages are activated (Stoecklein et al., 2012). Th1 cell activity is suppressed, while Th2 responses may be enhanced. This suppressive effect on Th1 responses may be mediated, by activated Treg cells and macrophages. Large amounts of IL-10 and other immunosuppressive cytokines are produced. Corticosteroids, prostaglandins from damaged tissues, and a small glycoprotein called suppressive active peptide, which appears in serum following a burn or blunt trauma, all have immunosuppressive properties. The deficiency develops within minutes or hours and recovers as wounds heal. It affects T cell, macrophage, and neutrophil function, but B-cell function appears to be normal. As a result, delayed hypersensitivity reactions, allograft rejection, and T-dependent antibody responses are all impaired. IL-2 and IL-2R production are reduced. CD8+ T cells are increased in injured individuals, suggesting that regulatory cell function may be enhanced. Macrophages lose antigen-presenting ability as they express decreased

levels of MHC class II. Neutrophil and macrophage phagocytosis and respiratory burst activities are both impaired. Although surgery may result in some suppression of lymphocyte responses to mitogens, evidence suggests that routine surgery has no significant effect on the response of healthy animals to vaccination (Ozkan et al., 1988).

OLD AGE

As animals age, their immune systems change. In general, aging is associated with a decline in cell-mediated immunity and an increase in innate immunity, especially chronic inflammation. Thus, as the immune system ages, a phenomenon called immunosenescence results (Candore et al., 2006; Fig. 41.11).

Lymphoid Organs

Thymic involution is the most obvious of these age-related changes. As a result, T-cell numbers drop over time while memory cells accumulate. There is also a progressive shift in the helper T-cell balance from Th1 to Th2 responses associated with a decline in IL-2 production (Schumaker et al., 2021). Ileal Peyer's patches involute after sexual maturity in dogs. Old dogs also have a reduced splenic white pulp. Lymph node changes vary depending on their location but include cortical atrophy and medullary fibrosis. The bone marrow is relatively unaffected by old age, and an aged bone marrow can reconstitute the body as well as a young one can.

Innate Immunity

The aging process appears to differ between individuals and possibly species. Some animals experience increased inflammation, whereas others show a decrease. This may be related to age. Day has reported that aged cats increase their production of proinflammatory cytokines, but this has not been reported in dogs (Day, 2010).

In those species where inflammation increases, aging is associated with a progressive increase in a chronic low-grade inflammation—a process called inflammaging. This is a result of the gradual

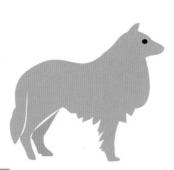

REDUCED IMMUNITY
Respiratory burst
Chemotaxis
NO production
T-cell numbers
T-cell proliferation
NK cell functions

SKIN
REDUCED
Neutrophil recruitment
DTH responses
Wound healing
Langerhans cells

RESPIRATORY TRACT
INCREASED
Inflammatory responses
Infections

BLOOD VESSELS
INCREASED
IL-6 production
Atherosclerosis

ADIPOSE TISSUE
INCREASED
Metabolic syndrome
Insulin resistance

Fig. 41.11 The changes in the immune system that occur with aging. *DTH*, Delayed-type hypersensitivity; *IL-6*, interleukin-6; *NK cells*, natural killer cells.

accumulation of damaged or dying cells and organelles over time. These dying cells generate senescence-associated DAMPs that act through TLR2 and IL-1β to activate the NF-κB pathway. This in turn results in chronic activation of the innate immune system. This chronic activation eventually leads to changes in the phenotype of cells, such as macrophages. These cells develop what is known as the senescence-associated secretory phenotype (SASP). These SASP macrophages produce increased quantities of TNF-α, IL-6, matrix metalloproteases, and monocyte chemoattractant protein. As a result, pro-inflammatory cytokine levels in the bloodstream gradually increase over time.

In those species and individuals where inflammation appears to decrease with age, macrophage numbers decline, and they express lower levels of TLRs. Aging is associated with impaired TLR signaling. When stimulated with TLR ligands, these aged macrophages secrete reduced amounts of IL-6 and TNF-α. Aged macrophages also mount reduced responses to activators such as IFN-γ and produce less nitric oxide. For example, aged horses have decreased monocyte counts and plasma myeloperoxidase (Miller et al., 2021). They produced more TNF-α and less IL-17—Perhaps this is a compensatory response.

Neutrophils from the aged have an impaired ability to produce a respiratory burst and generate reactive nitrogen species. As a result, they are less able than cells from the young to kill ingested bacteria. For example, Beagles over 8 years of age show decreased neutrophil phagocytosis and a marked decline in their ability to kill bacteria such as *Lactococcus lactis*.

Generation of SASP macrophages is the main driver of age-related inflammation. At low levels, these cells may be protective, but as the levels of proinflammatory cytokines increase, they eventually provoke the development of many of the chronic diseases of aging, such as heart disease, neurodegeneration, and arthritis. In some respects, therefore, inflammaging can be considered a manifestation of innate autoimmunity (Kale et al., 2020; Adams et al., 2009). Eliminating these SASP macrophages can delay age-related tissue dysfunction and potentially increase lifespan (Baker et al., 2016).

Adaptive Immunity
Cell-mediated, and humoral immune responses also decline with advancing age. This is characterized by decreased responsiveness to antigenic stimulation (Candore et al., 2006).

T Cells
The greatest impact aging has on the immune system is the decline in the numbers of CD4+ T cells. In addition, the lymphocyte population of the aged changes from a naïve population to a memory cell population. T cells from aged animals lose their ability to progress through the cell cycle. As a result, early events in the T-cell response to antigens, such as activation of protein kinase C and the rise in intracellular calcium, are impaired. Even after expressing IL-2 receptors and being exposed to IL-2, aged T cells may not respond effectively to antigens. Analysis shows that some aged T cells continue to produce normal amounts of IL-2, but many do not. Thus aged T-cell populations appear to be mixtures of fully functional and impaired cells.

Blood lymphocyte numbers decline significantly with age (Blount et al., 2005). Aged dogs and cats have reduced CD4+ T-cell numbers and increased CD8+ numbers leading to a reduction in the CD4:CD8 ratio (Day, 2010). Their response to mitogens declines as does the intensity of cutaneous delayed hypersensitivity responses. In dogs, there is reduced T-cell diversity with increasing age (Holder, et al., 2018). γ/δ T cells tend to accumulate with age in adipose tissue and produce IL-17, which controls both Treg cells and also the maintenance of core body temperature (Papotto and Silva-Santos, 2018). IL-10-producing Tfh cells also accumulate with age and so mediate age-related immunosuppression (Almanan et al., 2020).

The numbers of Th17 cells have been assessed over time in dogs, and it has been found that their numbers increase with age, a finding compatible with the concept of inflammaging. Thus, in dogs under 1 year of age, the proportion of IL-17+ T cells averaged 1.52%, while in dogs 6 years of age or older, they averaged 7.49% (Akiyama et al., 2019).

Cats between 10 and 14 years of age also have lower leukocyte counts than cats between 2 and 5 years of age (Campbell et al., 2004). Absolute numbers of T cells, B cells, and NK cells are also lower in aged animals. The relative percentages of lymphocytes and CD4+ T cells decrease, whereas the percentage of granulocytes and CD8+ T cells increases (Nikolich-Zugich, 2018). As a result, there is a decline in the CD4:CD8 ratio (Hogg et al., 2011).

In old horses (>20 years), there is a significant decrease in the proportion of CD8+ T cells and a rise in the CD4:CD8 ratio compared with young animals. Horses older than 20 years of age have reduced lymphocyte responses to mitogens, and this deficiency cannot be overcome by exposure to additional IL-2 (Horohov et al., 2002; Herbst et al., 2022).

B Cells
Somatic mutation in immunoglobulin V region genes ceases in old animals, so antibody affinity tends to be lower than in young animals. Nevertheless, immunoglobulin concentrations do not decline in old age. Old dogs show little decline in antibody responses, although old horses have reduced antibody responses to influenza vaccination. Serum levels of IgM increase with age, but there is no obvious effect on IgG or C-reactive protein levels. Levels of IgA and heat shock protein also increase (Alexander et al., 2018; Day, 2010).

Consequences
Aging leads to increased susceptibility to certain viral infections, including herpesviruses. This increased susceptibility of aged mice results from increased production of IL-17. This, in turn, leads to increased neutrophil recruitment and enhanced tissue damage. These mice also show a coincident decrease in IFN-γ production leading to a failure to control viral replication. Both of these changes are necessary to account for the increased lethality of herpesviruses in aged mice. A similar imbalance could explain the recurrence of shingles caused by Herpes simplex virus in elderly humans.

Although aged animals may mount poorer primary responses to vaccines, their memory responses tend to remain unaffected. Elderly animals generally have persistent protective antibody levels and do respond to revaccination by increasing antibody titers. There is, however, a difference with novel antigens. A study of dogs receiving rabies vaccine for the first time showed that a significant decrease in antibody titers and a corresponding increase in vaccine failures occurred in older dogs (HogenEsch and Tompson, 2010).

Feeding a low-calorie diet has been shown to extend the lifespan of dogs. Prolonged calorie restriction in dogs retarded age-related declines in lymphoproliferative responses, in absolute numbers of lymphocytes, and in the CD4+ and CD8+ T-cell subsets. This may result from low circulating leptin levels. Calorie restriction appears to have no effect on neutrophil phagocytic activity, antibody production, or NK activity.

OTHER IMMUNODEFICIENCIES
Immunodeficiencies can result from a wide variety of insults to the body. For example, immunoglobulin synthesis is generally reduced in individuals with absolute protein loss (patients with the nephrotic syndrome, heavily parasitized or tumor-bearing individuals, and patients who have experienced severe burns or trauma). Physical destruction

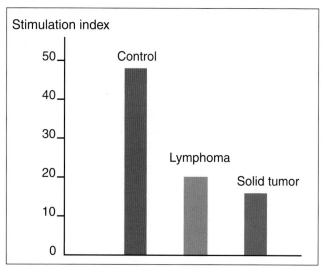

Fig. 41.12 Immunosuppression in dogs with lymphomas or solid tumors compared with normal control dogs. The stimulation index is a measure of the response of lymphocytes to the mitogenic lectin phytohemagglutinin. Data taken from Weiden, P.L., Storb, R., Kolb, H.J., et al., 1974. Immune reactivity in dogs with spontaneous malignancy. J. Natl. Cancer Inst. 53, 1049–1056.

of lymphoid tissues can result in immunodeficiencies. For example, loss of lymphoid tissue leading to immunosuppression may occur in tumor-bearing animals, especially if the tumors themselves are lymphoid in origin (Fig. 41.12). Adult horses with chronic diarrhea are immunosuppressed, as reflected by reduced IgA and reduced lymphocyte responses to mitogens. Some endocrine diseases, such as thyrotoxicosis and diabetes mellitus, may also result in immunosuppression.

REFERENCES

Adams, A.A., Katepalli, M.P., Kohler, K., et al., 2009. Effect of body condition, body weight and adiposity on inflammatory cytokine responses in old horses. Vet. Immunol. Immunopathol. 127, 286–294.

Akiyama, S., Asahina, R., Ohta, H., Tsukui, T., et al., 2019. Th17 cells increase during maturation in peripheral blood of healthy dogs. Vet. Immunol. Immunopathol. 209, 17–21.

Alexander, J.E., Colyer, A., Haydock, R.M., Hayek, M., Park, J., 2018. Understanding how dogs age; Longitudinal analysis of markers of inflammation, immune function and oxidative stress. J. Gerontol. A Biol. Sci. Med. Sci. 73 (6), 720–728.

Almanan, M., Raynor, J., Ogunsulire, I., Malyshkina, A., et al., 2020. IL-10-producing Tfh cells accumulate with age and link inflammation with age-related immunosuppression. Sci. Adv. 6 (31), eabb0806.

Bagath, M., Krishman, G., Devaraj, C., Rashamol, V.P., et al., 2019. The impact of heat stress on the immune system in dairy cattle: a review. Res. Vet. Sci. 126, 94–102.

Baker, D.J., Childs, B.G., Durik, M., Wijers, M.E., et al., 2016. Naturally occurring p16lnk4a-positive cells shorten healthy lifespan. Nature 530, 184–189.

Bastien, B.C., Patil, A., Satyaraj, E., 2015. The impact of weight loss on circulating cytokines in Beagle dogs. Vet. Immunol. Immunopathol. 163, 174–182.

Beineke, A., Puff, C., Seehusen, F., Baumgärtner, W., 2009. Pathogenesis and immunopathology of systemic and nervous canine distemper. Vet. Immunol. Immunopathol. 127, 1–18.

Blount, D.G., Pritchard, D.L., Heaton, P.R., 2005. Age-related alterations in immune parameters in Labrador retriever dogs. Vet. Immunol. Immunopathol. 108, 399–407.

Campbell, D.J., Rawlings, J.M., Koelsch, S., et al., 2004. Age-related differences in parameters of feline immune status. Vet. Immunol. Immunopathol. 100, 73–80.

Candore, G., Colonna-Romano, G., Balistreri, C.R., Di Carlo, D., et al., 2006. Biology of longevity: the role of the innate immune system. Rejuvenation Res. 9 (1), 143–148.

Chattha, K.S., Kandasamy, S., Vlasova, A.N., Saif, L.J., 2013. Vitamin A deficiency impairs adaptive B and T cell responses to a prototype monovalent attenuated human rotavirus vaccine and virulent human rotavirus challenge in a gnotobiotic piglet model. PLoS One 8, e82966.

Colotta, F., Jansson, B., Bonelli, F., 2017. Modulation of inflammatory and immune responses by vitamin D. J. Autoimmunity 85, 78–97.

Corripio-Miyar, Y., Mellanby, R.J., Morrison, K., McNeilly, T.N., 2017. 1m25-dihydroxyvitamin D3 modulates the phenotype and function of monocyte derived dendritic cells in cattle. BMC Vet. Res. https://doi.org/10.1186/s12917-017-1309-8

Danesi, P., Petini, M., Falcaro, C., Bertola, M., et al., 2022. *Pneumocystis* colonization in dogs is as in humans. Int. J. Environ. Res. Public Health. https://doi.org/10.3390/ijerph19063192.

Day, M.J., 2010. Ageing, immunosenescence and inflammaging in the dog and cat. J. Comp. Pathol. 142, S60–S69.

Elder, J.H., Sundstrom, M., de Rozieres, S., et al., 2008. Molecular mechanisms of FIV infection. Vet. Immunol. Immunopathol. 123, 3–13.

Finch, J.M., Turner, R.J., 1996. Effects of selenium and vitamin E on the immune responses of domestic animals. Res. Vet. Sci. 60, 97–106.

German, A.J., Ryan, V.H., German, A.C., et al., 2010. Obesity, its associated disorders and the role of inflammatory adipokines in companion animals. Vet. J. 185, 4–9.

German, A.J., 2012. Barking up the wrong tree: what's the deal with obesity, adiponectin and inflammation in dogs? Vet. J. 194, 272–273.

Henning, G., Kraft, M.S., Derfuss, T., Pirzer, R., et al., 2001. Signaling lymphocyte activation molecule (SLAM) regulates cellular cytotoxicity. Eur. J. Immunol. 31, 2741–2750.

Herbst, A.C., Reedy, S.E., Page, A.E., Horohov, D.W., Adams, A.A., 2022. Effect of aging on monocyte phagocytic and inflammatory functions, and on the ex vivo inflammatory response to lipopolysaccharide in horses. Vet. Immunol. Immunopathol. https://doi.org/10.1016/j.vetimm.2022.110459.

Hessing, M.J.C., Hagelsø, A.M., Schouten, W.G.P., Wiepkema, P.R., Van Beek, J.A.M., 1994. Individual behavioral and physiological strategies in pigs. Physiol. Behav. 55 (1), 39–46.

HogenEsch, H., Tompson, S., 2010. Effect of ageing on the immune response of dogs to vaccines. J. Comp. Pathol. 142, S74–S77.

Hogg, A.E., Parsons, K., Taylor, G., et al., 2011. Characterization of age-related changes in bovine CD8+ T-cells. Vet. Immunol. Immunopathol. 140, 47–54.

Holder, A., Mirczuk, S.M., Fowkes, R.C., Palmer, D.B., 2018. Perturbations of the T cell receptor repertoire occurs with increasing age in dogs,. Dev. Comp. Immunol. 79, 150–157.

Horohov, D.W., Kydd, J.H., Hannant, D., 2002. The effect of aging on T cell responses in the horse. Dev. Comp. Immunol. 26, 121–128.

Jee, J., Hoet, A.E., Azevedo, M.P., et al., 2013. Effects of dietary vitamin A content on antibody responses of feedlot calves inoculated intramuscularly with an inactivated bovine coronavirus vaccine. Am. J. Vet. Res. 74, 1353–1362.

Kale, A., Sharma, A., Stolzing, A., Desprez, P.-Y., et al., 2020. Role of immune cells in the removal of deleterious senescent cells. BMC Immun. Ageing. https://doi.org/10.1186/s12979-020-00187-9.

Karagianni, A.E., Kurian, D., Cillán-Garcia, E., Eaton, S.L., et al., 2022. Training associated alterations in equine respiratory immunity using a multiomics comparative approach. Sci. Reps. 12, 427. https://doi.org/10.1038/s41598-021-04137-3.

Lackner, A.A., Veazey, R.S., 2007. Current concepts in AIDS pathogenesis: insights from the SIV/Macaque model. Adv. Rev. Med. 58, 461–476.

McKenzie, E., Lupfer, C., Banse, H., et al., 2010. Hypogammaglobulinemia in racing Alaskan sled dogs. J. Vet. Intern. Med. 24, 179–184.

Miller, A.B., Loynachan, A.T., Barker, V.D., Adams, A.A., 2021. Investigation of innate immune function in adult and geriatric horses. Vet. Immunol. Immunopathol. 235 https://doi.org/10.1016/j.vetimm.2021.110207.

Miller, M.M., Fogle, J.E., Tompkins, M.B., 2013. Infection with feline immunodeficiency virus directly activates CD4+ CD25+ T regulatory cells. J. Virol. 87, 9373–9378.

Mora, J.R., Iwata, M., von Andrian, U.H., 2008. Vitamin effects on the immune system: vitamins A and D take centre stage. Nat. Rev. Immunol. 8, 685–698.

Naylor, C., Petri JR., W.A., 2016. Leptin regulation of immune responses. Trends Mol. Med. 22, 88–98. 2016.

Nguyen, T.M.D., 2020. Adiponectin: role in physiology and pathophysiology. Int. J. Prev. Med. 11, 136–144.

Nikolich-Zugich, J., 2018. The twilight of immunity: emerging concepts in aging of the immune system. Nat. Immunol. 19, 10–19.

O'Brien, T., Thomas, D.G., Morel, P.C.H., Rutherfurd-Marwick, K.J., 2015. Moderate dietary supplementation with vitamin E enhances lymphocyte functionality in the adult cat. Res. Vet. Sci. 99, 63–69.

Ozkan, A.N., Hoyt, D.B., Tompkins, S., Ninnemann, J.L., Sullivan, J.R., 1988. Immunosuppressive effects of a trauma-induced suppressor active peptide. J. Trauma 28 (5), 589–592.

Padgett, D.A., Glaser, R., 2003. How stress influences the immune response. Trends Immunol. 24 (8), 444–448.

Papotto, P.H., Silva-Santos, B., 2018. Got my γδ17T cells to keep me warm. Nat. Immunol. 19, 426–434.

Park, H.J., Lee, S.E., Oh, J.H., Seo, K.W., Song, K.H., 2014. Leptin, adiponectin and serotonin levels in lean and obese dogs. BMC Vet. Res. 10, 113–121.

Qeska, V., Barthel, Y., Herder, V., Stein, V.M., et al., 2014. Canine distemper virus infection leads to an inhibitory phenotype of monocyte-derived dendritic cells in vitro with reduced expression of co-stimulatory molecules and increased interleukin-10 transcription. PLosOne 9 (4), e96121. https://doi.org/10.1371/journal.pone.0096121.

Rendon-Marin, S., Budaszewski, R.F., Canal, C.W., Ruiz-Saemz, J., 2019. Tropism and molecular pathogenesis of Canine distemper virus. Virol. J. https://doi.org/10.1186/s12985-019-1136-6.

Rogers, C.J., Zaharoff, D.A., Hance, K.W., et al., 2008. Exercise enhances vaccine-induced antigen-specific T cell responses. Vaccine 26, 5407–5415.

Schumacher, B., Pothof, J., Vijg, J., Hoeijmakers, J.H., 2021. The central role of DNA damage in the aging process. Nature 592, 695–703.

Stoecklein, V.M., Osuka, A., Lederer, J.A., 2012. Trauma equals danger-damage control by the immune system. J. Leukoc. Biol. 92, 539–551.

Sykes, J.E., 2010. Immunodeficiencies caused by infectious diseases. Vet. Clin. Small Anim. 40, 409–423.

Verdonck, F., Merlevede, I., Goddeeris, B.M., et al., 2007. Vitamin E deficiency and decreased immunoglobulin concentrations in a population of donkeys. Vet. Rec. 160, 232–233.

von Messling, V., Milosevic, D., Cattaneo, R., 2004. Tropism illuminated: lymphocyte-based pathways blazed by lethal morbillivirus through the host immune system. Proc. Natl. Acad. Sci. U.S.A. 101, 14216–14221.

White, J.H., 2008. Vitamin D signaling, infectious diseases and regulation of innate immunity. Infect Immun. 76, 3837–3843.

42

Drugs and Other Agents That Affect the Immune System

CHAPTER OUTLINE

Many clinical situations exist in which it is desirable to either stimulate or suppress the innate or adaptive immune systems. Many different drugs and techniques are available to do this. Indeed, this area of immunology is a discipline called immunopharmacology.

SUPPRESSION OF THE IMMUNE SYSTEM

Immunosuppression is indicated for the treatment of immune-mediated diseases, including allergies and autoimmunity. The methods available for suppressing adaptive immune responses may be classified into two main groups. Older techniques generally involved treatment that, by inhibiting all cell division, reduced the response of T and B cells to antigens. This approach is crude and dangerous since other rapidly proliferating cell populations, such as intestinal epithelium and hematopoietic stem cells, are also prevented from dividing with potentially disastrous consequences. Alternatively, it is now possible to selectively eliminate specific immune cell populations by the use of monoclonal antibodies or by the use of highly selective immunosuppressive drugs (Whitley and Day, 2011).

NONSPECIFIC IMMUNOSUPPRESSION

Radiation

Electromagnetic radiation is immunosuppressive because it prevents cell division. It affects cells by several different mechanisms. The simplest of these is through ionizing rays hitting an essential, unique molecule, such as DNA, within the cell. A loss of even one nucleotide results in a permanent mutation of a gene, with potentially lethal effects on the progeny of the affected cell. Radiation also causes ionization of water and the formation of reactive free oxygen and hydroxyl radicals within the cell. The hydroxyl radicals react with dissolved oxygen to form toxic peroxides that destroy DNA and inhibit cell division. Although radiation is of some use in prolonging graft survival in experimental animals, especially laboratory rodents, the amount of radiation required for effective prolongation of graft survival in dogs is so high that it is often lethal.

GLUCOCORTICOSTEROIDS

Until recently, the only medications proven to ameliorate severe immune-mediated inflammatory diseases were the glucocorticosteroids—powerful, broad-spectrum antiinflammatory drugs. As a result, they are the most widely employed antiinflammatory agents, and their prolonged use is often necessary for the treatment of autoimmune diseases. Corticosteroids are able to suppress both immunologic and inflammatory responses. They also work rapidly. Unfortunately, their use is complicated by their diverse and serious adverse effects.

Corticosteroids affect many different cell types. They are lipid soluble and, as a result, can pass through cell membranes directly into cells, where they bind to receptors in the cytosol. The natural corticosteroid, cortisol (hydrocortisone) binds to two different receptors, a glucocorticoid receptor and a mineralocorticoid receptor. Most therapeutic corticosteroids, however, are designed so that they do not bind the mineralocorticoid receptor. The glucocorticoid receptor is found in most body cells and mediates the antiinflammatory responses (Box 42.1). Some therapeutic glucocorticoids do not themselves bind

BOX 42.1 Effects of Corticosteroids on the Immune System

Neutrophils
Neutrophilia
Depressed chemotaxis
Depressed margination
Depressed phagocytosis
Depressed ADCC
Depressed bactericidal activity
Stabilization of membranes
Inhibition of phospholipase A_2

Macrophages
Depressed chemotaxis
Depressed phagocytosis
Depressed bactericidal activity
Depressed IL-1 and IL-6 production
Depressed antigen processing

Lymphocytes
Depressed proliferation
Depressed T-cell responses
Impaired T cell–mediated cytotoxicity
Depressed IL-2 production
Depressed lymphokine production

Immunoglobulins
Minimal decrease

Complement
No effect

directly to glucocorticoid receptors but, when given orally, are converted to active derivatives. Thus cortisone is converted to cortisol and prednisone is converted to prednisolone.

Unbound glucocorticoid receptors are found free in the cytosol, but once they bind a glucocorticoid, the complexes are rapidly transported to the cell nucleus where they bind to DNA and regulate gene transcription. There are at least eight different forms of glucocorticoid receptor, and it is likely that each has a slightly different biological function. Once they bind to DNA, the glucocorticoid receptor complexes trigger two different gene transcription processes: transactivation and transrepression (Hardy et al., 2020).

Transactivation

In transactivation, the steroid-receptor complex binds to specific DNA sequences called glucocorticoid response elements (GREs) and activates gene transcription. To add complexity to the process, the complexes may bind to different GREs in different cell types or at different stages in cell development.

Among the most important targets of glucocorticoids is the NF-κB pathway. They stimulate the synthesis of IκBs, the inhibitors of the key regulator of gene transcription, NF-κB (Fig. 42.1). In a resting cell, NF-κB is inactive since its nuclear binding site is masked by IκB. When a lymphocyte is activated by antigens or cytokines, signals from its receptors cause the two molecules to dissociate, the IκB is degraded, and the released NF-κB can then move into the nucleus, where it activates the genes involved in inflammation and immunity. Glucocorticosteroids, however, stimulate the synthesis of excess IκB. As a result, its levels remain high and continue to suppress NF-κB-mediated processes, including cytokine synthesis and T-cell responses.

Transrepression

Steroid-receptor complexes may also bind to some specific gene enhancers and prevent them from binding to DNA. As a result, this interferes with downstream proinflammatory signaling pathways. They may also bind to "negative" GREs that can inhibit gene transcription.

Corticosteroids suppress both the innate and adaptive immune systems: For example, they suppress leukocyte production and circulation and modulate the activities of inflammatory mediators, thus suppressing innate responses. They influence the effector mechanisms of lymphocytes and promote regulatory T-cell (Treg) responses, and suppress adaptive immunity as well (Rhen and Cidlowski, 2005).

Effects on Leukocytes

The effects of corticosteroids on blood leukocytes vary among species. In horses, the number of circulating eosinophils, basophils, and lymphocytes declines within a few hours of corticosteroid administration as a result of increased sequestration in the bone marrow. Blood neutrophil counts, on the other hand, increase as a result of decreased adherence to vascular endothelium and reduced emigration into inflamed tissues. Neutrophil, monocyte, and eosinophil chemotaxis are suppressed by corticosteroids. Corticosteroids suppress the cytotoxic and phagocytic abilities of neutrophils in some species, but in others, such as the horse, they have no discernible effect (Slack et al., 2000). They may also block neutrophil nitric oxide synthase and so prevent the production of antibacterial nitric oxide. Macrophage production of prostaglandins and proinflammatory cytokines such as IL-1, as well as antigen processing, are reduced in some species. Steroid-treated macrophages also tend to assume an M2 phenotype and release anti-inflammatory cytokines. Glucocorticoids also decrease dendritic cell cytokine production and suppress antigen presentation.

In humans, glucocorticoids inhibit eosinophil production of IL-1, TNF-α, and IL-4 as well as IL-3, IL-5, and GM-CSF. As a result, they inhibit eosinophil migration. They reduce eosinophil lifespans by enhancing their apoptosis. They cause a rapid and profound fall in the number of circulating eosinophils and decrease the recruitment of eosinophils to sites of allergic inflammation.

Effects on Lymphocytes

Glucocorticoid suppression of Th1-mediated inflammation is their most obvious therapeutic benefit. They inhibit the ability of Th1 cells to produce IL-1, IL-6, IL-8, IL-12, IFN-γ and TNF-α. Corticosteroids also upregulate the expression of the IL-1 receptor, CD121b. This is a decoy receptor that binds active IL-1 but does not generate a signal, thus blocking IL-1 functions. Conversely, glucocorticoids upregulate the production of IL-4, IL-10, and IL-13 by Th2 cells (Elenkov, 2004). As a result, they force a change in the Th1/Th2 balance. They also act on Th17 cells to suppress their differentiation and cytokine production. Steroids act on cytotoxic T cells to inhibit their effector functions and cytokine release while promoting their apoptosis.

Glucocorticoids act through JAK-STAT signaling pathways to reduce the production of IL-5, IL-9, and IL-13 by innate lymphoid cells. Conversely, IL-10 production may be upregulated.

In addition to suppressing Th1 responses, glucocorticoids increase Treg numbers. They do this in part by upregulating FoxP3 expression as well as by modulating the cytokine mixture within the T-cell environment. In the absence of FoxP3+ Treg cells, glucocorticoids are ineffective.

The effects of corticosteroids on antibody responses are variable and depend on both timing and dose. In general, B cells tend to be corticosteroid resistant, and enormous doses are usually required to decrease BCR signaling and suppress antibody synthesis.

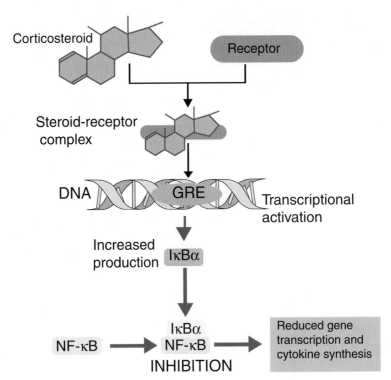

Fig. 42.1 A schematic diagram showing the mode of action of corticosteroids. Normally, signal transduction and cytokine synthesis occur when the transcription factor nuclear factor kappa B (NF-κB) dissociates from its inhibitor IκBα. The released inhibitor of nuclear factor kappa B (IκBα) is rapidly degraded. Corticosteroids stimulate the synthesis of excessive amounts of IκBα, which binds to NF-κB and continues to prevent its activation. *DNA,* Deoxyribonucleic acid; *GRE,* glucocorticoid response elements.

Other Effects

Glucocorticoids enhance the production of lipocortin, which inhibits phospholipase A_2 and so interrupts arachidonic acid metabolism. This, in turn, inhibits leukotriene synthesis. They also inhibit cyclooxygenase (COX-2) gene transcription and so block prostaglandin synthesis as well.

Synthetic corticosteroids act on small blood vessels to suppress acute inflammation by preventing increased vascular permeability and vasodilation and thus prevent edema formation and fibrin deposition. In the later stages of inflammation, they inhibit capillary and fibroblast proliferation and enhance collagen breakdown. As a result, corticosteroids also delay wound and fracture healing.

Adverse Effects

While highly effective, glucocorticoid treatment is not without significant risks. The wide distribution of glucocorticoid receptors in many different cell types makes adverse events inevitable. Most importantly, they have the potential to supply the body's corticosteroid needs, suppress the pituitary-adrenal axis, and induce Cushing syndrome—iatrogenic hyperadrenocorticism. Side effects include polyuria, increased thirst, and appetite leading to obesity. They also cause cutaneous and muscle atrophy with alopecia and delayed wound healing. In addition, by suppressing inflammation and phagocytosis, corticosteroids can render animals susceptible to secondary infections. For example, they predispose dogs to bacterial urinary tract and fungal infections as well as demodicosis and toxoplasmosis in cats.

Because these adverse events are generally a result of prolonged high doses, oral glucocorticoids are best used for short-term palliative treatments such as the suppression of acute disease. Animals receiving long-term treatment should be examined regularly to monitor for adverse effects. Once a satisfactory clinical response has been induced, the dose of corticosteroids should be gradually reduced to enable the adrenal cortex to resume its normal functions. This is usually achieved by lengthening the dose interval and then decreasing the dose (Bizikova and Olivry 2015).

CYTOTOXIC DRUGS

Cytotoxic drugs inhibit cell division by blocking nucleic acid synthesis and activity. The major cytotoxic drugs currently in use are alkylating agents, folic acid antagonists, and DNA synthesis inhibitors.

Alkylating Agents

Alkylating agents cross-link DNA helices, preventing their separation, and thus block cell division. The most important of these is cyclophosphamide (Fig. 42.2). Cyclophosphamide is toxic for resting and dividing cells, especially for dividing immunocompetent cells. It impairs both B- and T-cell responses, especially the primary immune response. It blocks mitogen- and antigen-induced cell division and the production of IFN-γ. It prevents B cells from renewing their antigen receptors. Early in therapy, cyclophosphamide tends to destroy more B cells than T cells. In long-term therapy, it affects both cell populations. It also suppresses macrophage function. Cyclophosphamide may be administered parenterally or orally and is inactive until biotransformed by hepatic microsomal enzymes to active metabolites in the liver. It has a half-life of about 6 hours and is largely excreted through the kidney. It is of interest to note that corticosteroids enhance the metabolism of cyclophosphamide and so reduce its potency. The main toxic effect of cyclophosphamide is bone marrow suppression, leading to leukopenia with a predisposition to infection. Other adverse effects may include thrombocytopenia, anemia, and bladder damage. As a result, it may cause a hemorrhagic cystitis.

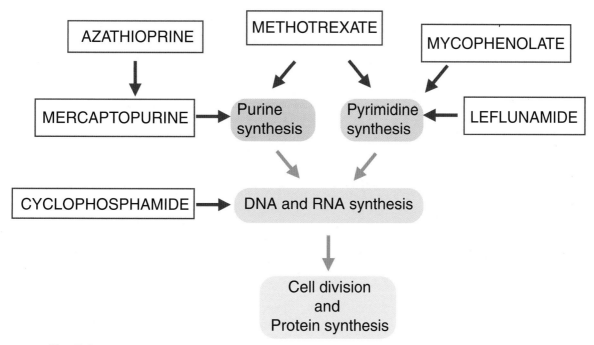

Fig. 42.2 The targets of some commonly employed immunosuppressive drugs. *DNA*, Deoxyribonucleic acid; *RNA*, ribonucleic acid.

Cytarabine

Cytarabine also called cytosine arabinoside, is an antimetabolite that acts by blocking the actions of DNA polymerase. It is therefore an effective inhibitor of lymphocyte division and a potent immunosuppressant, and it is widely used for the treatment of leukemias. It can cross the blood-brain barrier and has been used in combination with prednisolone to treat successfully inflammatory nervous system diseases such as meningitis of unknown origin and steroid-responsive meningitis-arteritis in dogs (Lowrie et al., 2016).

Folic Acid Antagonists

Methotrexate is a folic acid antagonist that has two mechanisms of action. Acting directly, it binds to dihydrofolate reductase and blocks the synthesis of tetrahydrofolate, inhibiting the synthesis of both pyrimidines and purines. As a result, it interferes with DNA synthesis. This blocks B-cell division so that it can also suppress antibody formation. Methotrexate also acts indirectly on the intestinal microbiota to alter its composition in such a way that Th1 and Th17 cell activation are minimized. Low doses of methotrexate are used for the treatment of systemic lupus, rheumatoid arthritis, vasculitis, and inflammatory bowel disease in humans. Much higher doses are used for cancer chemotherapy (Nayak et al., 2021).

DNA Synthesis Inhibitors
Azathioprine

Azathioprine is a nucleoside analog that suppresses purine synthesis and hence lymphocyte activation and mitosis. It is a prodrug that is oxidized by thiopurine methyltransferase in the liver to two active metabolites, 6-mercaptopurine and 6-thioinosinic acid. These metabolites inhibit both DNA and RNA synthesis. T and B cells are especially susceptible to this effect since they lack a salvage pathway that can repair purine biosynthesis. Thus, azathioprine affects rapidly dividing cells, such as T cells responding to an antigen. Azathioprine can suppress both primary and secondary antibody responses if given after antigen exposure. Azathioprine also has significant antiinflammatory activity since it inhibits the production of macrophages. It has no effect on the synthesis of cytokines or immunoglobulins but tends to suppress T cell–mediated responses to a greater extent than B-cell responses. There are breed-related variations in azathioprine metabolism in dogs that may also influence its effectiveness and toxicity. Azathioprine should not be used in cats since they have low levels of the enzyme thiopurine methyltransferase that breaks down 6-mercaptopurine.

SELECTIVE IMMUNOSUPPRESSANTS
Calcineurin Inhibitors

Perhaps the single most important step in the development of routine, successful organ allografting has been the development of very potent but selective immunosuppressive agents. Of these, cyclosporine has been by far the most successful. Cyclosporine (also called ciclosporin) is a polypeptide derived from the soil fungus, *Tolypocladium inflatum*. This fungus yields several natural forms of cyclosporine, of which the most important is cyclosporin A, a circular peptide of 11 amino acids (Fig. 42.3). As a result, cyclosporine has two surfaces that allow it to bind two proteins simultaneously. When it enters the T-cell cytosol, one surface binds to an intracellular receptor called cytophilin, whereas the other binds and blocks the intracellular transmitter calcineurin, a serine-threonine phosphatase (Fig. 42.4).

Cyclosporine therefore blocks cyclophilin-calcineurin interactions and, as a result, interferes with many NF-AT-mediated T-cell functions such as the production of IL-2, IL-3, IL-4, GM-CSF, TNF-α, and IFN-γ. The primary effect of cyclosporine treatment is therefore the blocking of helper T-cell responses.

Cyclosporine also has indirect suppressive effects on macrophages, B cells, and natural killer cells. It inhibits degranulation of neutrophils, eosinophils, and mast cells and suppresses eicosanoid formation. It reduces eosinophil survival, degranulation, and cytokine production. Thus, cyclosporine prevents inflammation by inhibiting the functions of many of the participating cells. In many respects, it has similar

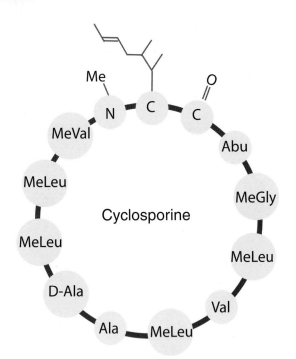

Fig. 42.3 The structure of the immunosuppressive drug cyclosporine. *Abu*, Aminobutyric acid.

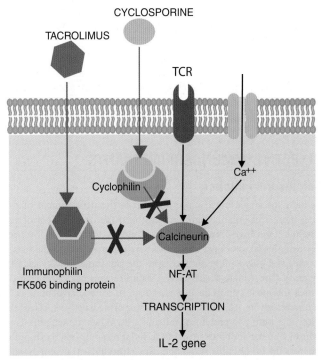

Fig. 42.4 The mode of action of cyclosporine and tacrolimus. Both prevent activation of the signaling molecule calcineurin. As a result, the transcription factor nuclear factor of activated T cells (NF-AT) is inhibited, and activation of genes such as those for interleukin-2 (IL-2) production is prevented. *TCR*, T-cell antigen receptor.

effects to glucocorticoids. Cyclosporine simply interferes with different cell signaling pathways.

Because cyclosporine inhibits IFN-γ production by activated T cells, it blocks MHC class I expression on allografts. Since corticosteroids

have a similar effect, the combination of corticosteroids and cyclosporine is especially potent and can enhance allograft survival while leaving other immune functions intact. This is a significant advantage over other older immunosuppressants. The use of cyclosporine has made tissue transplantation a routinely successful and safe procedure. In cats that received renal allografts from unrelated blood group-compatible donors and were treated with cyclosporine and prednisolone, mean survival was greater than 12 months. Cyclosporine is also effective in treating a variety of immunologically mediated dermatologic diseases and appears to have a wide safety margin in dogs (Fellman et al., 2011; Archer et al., 2014; Koch et al., 2018; Palmeiro, 2013).

Tacrolimus

Tacrolimus is a macrolide antibiotic produced by the fungus *Streptomyces tsukubaensis*. It also interferes with the NF-AT pathway by preventing an activating molecule, immunophilin, from binding to calcineurin in a manner similar to cyclosporine. It therefore inhibits the production of IL-2, IL-3, IL-4, IL-5, IFN-γ, and TNF-α. Tacrolimus is a much more potent immunosuppressant than cyclosporine. It downregulates cytokine production by mast cells, basophils, eosinophils, keratinocytes, and Langerhans cells. Topically, it has been used to treat cutaneous lupus erythematosus, pemphigus foliaceus, and pemphigus erythematosus. A related macrolide antibiotic calcineurin inhibitor, pimecrolimus, has been shown to be safe and effective when used in the form of oil-based eye drops to treat keratoconjunctivitis sicca in dogs (Fig. 42.4). It is also superior to cyclosporine in preventing or reversing allograft and xenograft rejection in humans and can prevent graft vascular disease (see Chapter 35).

Target of Rapamycin Inhibitors

The macrolide antibiotic rapamycin (sirolimus) and the related molecule everolimus specifically inhibit a serine kinase known as mechanistic target of rapamycin (mTOR). mTOR plays a critical role in regulating T-cell activation by integrating the signals received from specific antigen, costimulatory receptors, and cytokines and directing the T-cell differentiation into effector, regulatory, or memory pathways (Fig. 42.5; Janes and Fruman, 2009). mTOR also acts in nondividing macrophages and dendritic cells by associating with MyD88, activating IFN regulatory factors, and inhibiting caspase-1. Rapamycin acts on macrophages and dendritic cells, enhancing IL-12 and nitric oxide production but inhibiting IL-10. This, in turn, promotes Th1- or Th17-mediated inflammation. Rapamycin inhibits B- and T-cell proliferation by blocking stimulatory signals from IL-2, IL-4, and IL-6. It enhances Treg cell production and promotes tolerance.

Mycophenolate Mofetil

Mycophenolate mofetil is a prodrug that is metabolized to mycophenolic acid. This inhibits inosine-5'-monophosphate dehydrogenase found in activated but not resting lymphocytes. This causes the depletion of guanosine nucleotides, which prevents synthesis of DNA. It therefore blocks both B- and T-cell proliferation, T-cell differentiation, antibody formation, and dendritic cell maturation. It may also be antifibrotic. Oral mycophenolate has been reported to be effective in controlling canine diseases such as immune-mediated thrombocytopenia and hemolytic anemia, meningoencephalitis, polymyositis, acquired myasthenia gravis, pemphigus foliaceus, and pemphigus vulgaris, as well as systemic histiocytosis (Cummings and Rizzo, 2017).

Leflunomide

Leflunomide is a synthetic isoxazole derivative that is metabolized to its active metabolite malononitrilamide and selectively inhibits pyrimidine synthesis. As a result, it blocks DNA and RNA synthesis and

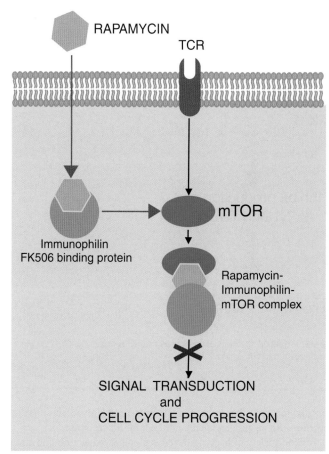

Fig. 42.5 The mode of action of rapamycin. This drug blocks activation of mTOR (mechanistic target of rapamycin). As a result, numerous cell functions are blocked, including gene activation pathways and cell cycle progression. *mTOR*, Mechanistic target of rapamycin; *TCR*, T-cell antigen receptor.

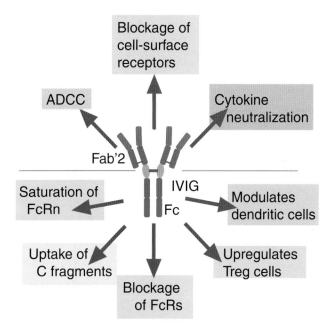

Fig. 42.6 Some of the many postulated activities mediated by Intravenous Immunoglobulins (IVIG). In addition, the Sialyl groups bind to SIGN and trigger immunomodulatory pathways. *ADCC*, Antibody-dependent cell–mediated cytotoxicity; *FcRn*, Fc receptor of the neonate; *Treg cells*, regulatory T cells.

inhibits lymphocyte division. Leflunomide suppresses T and B cells that lack a pyrimidine salvage pathway. It also inhibits several tyrosine kinases. Given orally, it has been used to treat several canine autoimmune and inflammatory diseases, especially in cases refractory to corticosteroid treatment or where corticosteroids are contraindicated (Sato et al., 2017).

Pentoxifylline

Phosphodiesterases are enzymes with multiple functions. Most importantly, they stimulate cell signaling. Pentoxifylline (PTX) is a widely employed competitive phosphodiesterase inhibitor that can reverse this. It also inhibits the NF-κB pathway. As a result, PTX decreases the production of IL-1, IL-6, TNF-α, and leukotrienes. It therefore acts as antiinflammatory agent. PTX also facilitates blood flow by decreasing blood viscosity and the flexibility of red blood cells so that they suffer less damage when passing through small blood vessels. Given orally, it is safe and moderately effective in reducing the severity of some autoimmune diseases, especially those mediated by T cells (Ji et al., 2004).

Intravenous Immunoglobulin Therapy

Although immunoglobulin replacement is appropriate for animals with antibody deficiencies, intravenous immunoglobulin (IVIG) therapy is immunosuppressive and antiinflammatory (Gelfand, 2012). Human IVIG has been used to treat autoimmune and inflammatory diseases

in domestic animals (Bianco et al., 2009). This is a pooled IgG preparation derived from a large number of healthy donors. Administered intravenously, its beneficial effects are probably mediated by IgG molecules with sialic acid on their Fc region. These bind to the integrin DC-SIGN on myeloid cells. This, in turn, stimulates IL-33 production that then promotes IL-4 production which in turn upregulates the inhibitory receptor FcγR2b on effector macrophages and dendritic cells. This then inhibits the activities of autoantibodies. In addition, administration of IVIG has been shown to increase the production of transforming growth factor-β and IL-10 by Treg cells (Fig. 42.6). In dogs, it may act by saturating Fc receptors such as CD16 and CD32 on monocytes. IVIG may also interfere with Fas-mediated apoptosis (Kessel et al., 2007).

When administered to dogs, IVIG causes a mild thrombocytopenia, leucopenia, increased total plasma protein, increases in fibrin degradation products, thrombin-antithrombin complexes, and C-reactive protein. In effect, it enhances blood coagulation and some inflammatory responses. It also binds to canine monocytes and lymphocytes (CD4+T, CD8+T, and B) and inhibits phagocytosis by monocytes. IVIG has been used to successfully treat immune-mediated hemolytic anemia, thrombocytopenia, and pemphigus, as well as severe cutaneous drug reactions such as erythema multiforme and Stevens-Johnson syndrome (see Chapter 34). Most authors report positive clinical responses with minimal adverse reactions. However, the number of such reports is small and more controlled trials of IVIG use in animal diseases are urgently required.

ITCH INHIBITORS

Oclacitinib

The synthetic JAK inhibitor, oclacitinib maleate (Apoquel) blocks signal transduction by the cell receptor kinases, JAK1 and JAK3. These are components of the receptors for IL-31, IL-2, IL-4, IL-6, and IL-13.

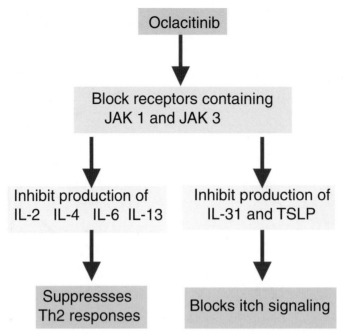

Fig. 42.7 The consequences of oclacitinilib blocking signal transmission through Janus Kinase (JAK) receptors. *IL-2*, Interleukin-2; *Th2*, T helper 2 cells; *TSLP*, thymic stromal lymphopoietin.

The IL-31R is expressed on NP3 prurinergic neurons, where it triggers the itch sensation. IL-4R and IL-13R are found on the other NP neurons, where they enhance neuronal responsiveness to multiple other pruritogens. As a result, oclacitinib can inhibit not only Th2 responses but, more importantly, the severe chronic pruritus associated with atopic dermatitis. It has been approved for use in dogs over twelve months of age for control of IL-31-mediated pruritus associated with allergic skin diseases. Oclacitinib is also an effective treatment for cutaneous lupus erythematosus (Harvey et al., 2023; Fig. 42.7).

Fatty Acids

Inflammation is mediated by many different molecules, including lipids such as the leukotrienes and prostaglandins. Certain polyunsaturated fatty acids are the precursors of these prostanoids and so can regulate their production (Venter et al., 2019). Omega-6 fatty acids such as arachidonic acid tend to be proinflammatory, whereas omega-3 fatty acids such as eicosapentaenoic acid and docosahexaenoic acid tend to have antiinflammatory effects since they suppress eicosanoid production (Miyata and Arita, 2015). The omega-3 fatty acids also promote production of resolvins and protectins. These fatty acids suppress NF-κB signaling and inhibit the production of IL-1 and TNF-β. They tend to be immunosuppressive as well, suppressing B cell and helper T cell activities in cat skin. They do not appear to influence NK-cells, IL-2 responses, delayed hypersensitivity, or immunoglobulin levels. The feeding of oils containing omega-3 fatty acids such as fish oil, evening primrose oil, or flaxseed oil may therefore reduce skin inflammation and be of clinical benefit in the treatment of allergic skin diseases, especially atopic dermatitis (Rutherfurd-Marwick et al., 2013; Bauer et al., 2011; Hall et al., 2004; Lenox and Bauer, 2013).

STIMULATION OF THE IMMUNE SYSTEM

There are many situations in veterinary medicine in which it is desirable to enhance innate or adaptive immunity, for example, increasing resistance to infection and treating immunosuppressive disorders. In contrast to adjuvants, immunostimulants need not be administered together with an antigen to enhance an immune response.

A wide variety of bacteria have been employed as immunostimulants. These act as sources of pathogen-associated molecular patterns and stimulate one or more TLRs. As a result, they activate macrophages and dendritic cells and stimulate cytokine synthesis. The most potent of these cytokine synthesis enhancers is bacille Calmette-Guérin (BCG), the live attenuated vaccine strain of *Mycobacterium bovis*. BCG generally enhances B and T cell–mediated responses, phagocytosis, allograft rejection, and resistance to infection. Unfortunately, whole BCG induces tuberculin hypersensitivity in treated animals and is therefore unacceptable for use in livestock. Purified cell wall fractions of BCG have been developed. These have been used to treat equine sarcoid tumors, equine endometritis, bovine colibacillosis, and ocular squamous cell carcinoma. They are also of benefit in the treatment of upper respiratory tract infections in horses. One of their active constituents is trehalose dimycolate, which promotes nonspecific immunity against several bacterial infections and may provoke regression of some experimental tumors. Another is muramyl dipeptide (MDP), a simple mycobacterial glycopeptide that enhances antibody production, stimulates polyclonal activation of lymphocytes, and activates macrophages. Because MDP is rapidly excreted in the urine, its biological activity is enhanced by its incorporation into liposomes. Polymerization and conjugation with glycopeptides or synthetic antigens can also enhance the immunostimulating effects of MDP. MDP prolongs survival time and decreases metastases in dogs with osteosarcoma.

Killed anaerobic corynebacteria, such as *Propionibacterium acnes*, also promote antibody formation. These bacteria stimulate cytokine synthesis through TLRs. *P. acnes* has a complex activity since it stimulates macrophages and the antibody response to thymus-dependent antigens, but it has a variable effect on the response to thymus-independent antigens. Killed *P. acnes* has been used in the treatment of staphylococcal pyoderma, malignant oral melanoma in dogs, feline leukemia, and respiratory disease in horses (Paillot, 2013). Other bacterial components, such as staphylococcal cell walls (especially staphylococcal phage lysate), some streptococcal components, and components of *Bordetella pertussis*, *Brucella abortus*, *Bacillus subtilis*, and *Klebsiella pneumoniae*, also have immunostimulating activity.

Immunomodulators have never been widely employed in veterinary medicine, largely because of the biological variability of the results obtained by their use. *Parapoxvirus ovis* (orf), mycobacterial cell wall fractions, and killed *P. acnes* have, however, been employed in equine medicine. They improve immune defenses nonspecifically and provide support for other antimicrobial therapy. While they do not appear to protect against respiratory infection, they may reduce respiratory disease severity, reduce the frequency of complications, and accelerate recovery.

Certain complex carbohydrates derived from yeasts, namely, zymosan, glucans, aminated polyglucose, and lentinans, can also activate macrophages. These may function as adjuvants and potentiate resistance to infectious agents. Fish such as trout, salmon, and catfish appear to respond especially well to these immunostimulants when incorporated into the diet. As a result, immunostimulation by complex carbohydrates, especially glucans, is routine in aquaculture.

CYTOKINES AND MONOCLONAL ANTIBODIES

Antilymphocytic Serum

Allograft rejection can be minimized by reducing T-cell numbers through administration of an antiserum specific for T lymphocytes produced in rabbits or horses. Thus, polyclonal antilymphocytic serum (ALS) suppresses the cell-mediated immune response and leaves the humoral immune response relatively intact. In practice, ALS is of variable efficiency and specificity and may cause severe side effects as a result of global immunosuppression. ALS-treated mice have been shown to accept rat xenografts, whereas clinical use of ALS in humans has not been universally accepted as useful.

Monoclonal Antibodies

The first humanized monoclonal antibody Omalizumab, sold under the name of Xolair, is directed against the constant domains of the IgE molecule. It effectively blocks IgE from binding to its high-affinity receptor on mast cells and basophils. It downregulates IgE production by B cells. As a result, allergic responses are blocked, and mast cells and basophils will not degranulate. It is widely used for severe persistent allergic asthma and chronic urticaria in humans (Box 42.2).

Omalizumab was just the beginning. In the search for allergy treatments and the prevention of graft rejection, monoclonal antibodies have been developed against all the major cytokines and/or their receptors.

As a result of issues with polyclonal antibodies, much more specific mouse monoclonal antibodies have been produced. The first to be employed was monoclonal antiCD3. AntiCD3 is directed only against T cells and is effective in reversing allograft rejection in humans. An even more specific monoclonal antibody is antiCD25. This binds to the α chain of the IL-2 receptor and so prevents lymphocyte activation. AntiCD25 helps prevent acute renal allograft rejection and, since it does not cause T-cell depletion, has fewer adverse effects and results in fewer opportunistic infections than crude ALS.

Monoclonal antibodies against canine CD4 and CD8 have been used to control rejection of canine renal allografts. They are very effective, even with highly mismatched mongrel dogs. Both antiCD4 and antiCD8 must be used together, and their immunosuppressive effect lasts for about 10 days. (The dogs eventually develop neutralizing antibodies against these mouse antibodies.) These are especially effective in combination with cyclosporine.

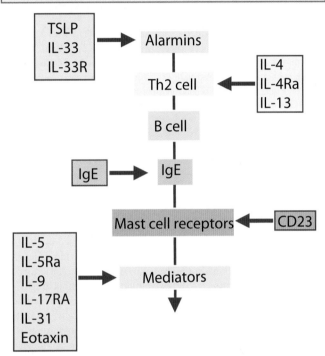

Fig. 42.8 Current and proposed monoclonal antibody therapy is primarily directed against certain key cytokines or their receptors that participate in the T helper 2 cells (Th2) response pathway (Red rectangles). While few are currently available for use in domestic species, the remarkable successes of many of these treatments are ensuring that this is changing rapidly. *IgE*, Immunoglobin E; *IL-4*, interleukin-4; *IL-5Ra*, interleukin 5 receptor subunit alpha; *TSLP*, thymic stromal lymphopoietin.

Anticytokine Antibodies

In some diseases, especially those due to excessive immune function, it may be beneficial to neutralize excessive cytokine activity using monoclonal antibodies against a cytokine or against its receptor (Fig. 42.8). Monoclonal antibodies directed against these targets are widely employed in humans. The original monoclonal antibodies were of mouse origin and, as a result, had a short half-life and were relatively ineffective. Subsequently, these antibodies have been "humanized," and their effectiveness has increased significantly. Thus anti-TNFR (Enbrel) and anti-TNFα (Humira) have been used to treat rheumatoid arthritis. Monoclonal antibodies against the checkpoint molecules CTLA4 and PD-1 are being used for cancer treatment with remarkable success (see Chapter 36; Beirao et al., 2016; Box 42.3).

Anti-IL-31

Anti-IL-31 (Lokivetmab) is marketed for the relief of itch in canine atopic dermatitis (Ozdemir, 2015). As noted, interleukin-31 is the

BOX 42.3 **Monoclonal Antibodies for Animals**

One of the first monoclonal antibodies licensed for use in domestic animals is a felinized anti–nerve growth factor (NGF) called Frunevetmab (Solensia). It is designed to treat severe pain in cats caused by chronic osteoarthritis. It consists of a monoclonal antibody designed to antagonize nerve growth factor (NGF), a molecule involved in pain regulation. It is administered by subcutaneous inoculation once a month.

A caninized monoclonal antibody against NGF (bedinvetmab) (Librela™ Zoetis) has also been approved by the FDA for the control of pain use in dogs with osteoarthritis. It is administered by injection once monthly and significantly improves the quality of life of arthritic dogs. It has been widely used in Europe (Gruen et al., 2021).

The USDA has also given provisional approval of a monoclonal antibody designed for the treatment of canine parvovirus produced by ELANCO Animal Health. This is a chimeric immunoglobulin made by combining a dog constant region with a rat variable region. It can be given to puppies as young as 6 weeks of age. A single intravenous dose of this antibody resulted in significantly faster recovery times as well as reducing mortality.

From Gruen, M.E., Myers, J.A., Tena, J.-K.S., Becskei, C., et al., 2021. Frunevetmab, a felinized anti-nerve growth factor monoclonal antibody, for the treatment of pain from osteoarthritis in cats. J. Vet. Intern. Med. 35, 2752–2762.

major cause of the severe itching observed in atopic dermatitis in dogs. The production of IL-31 in affected skin can be inhibited by the JAK inhibitor oclacitinib. It can also be neutralized by the administration of a caninized monoclonal antibody, Lokivetmab (Cytopoint), directed specifically against canine IL-31. Lokivetmab binds to circulating IL-31 and thus prevents its binding to the IL-31 receptor. In double-blind, placebo-controlled trials, a single dose has provided relief from itch, prevention of flares, and a reduction in disease severity in dogs with chronic AD. It has a prolonged duration of action, it is administered subcutaneously every 4–8 weeks as needed. It appears to be safe and effective (Michels et al., 2016).

Cytokines

The successful use of monoclonal antibodies against cytokines and tumor cells may be contrasted with the disappointing effects of administering cytokines to animals. Since purified cytokines produced by recombinant DNA techniques are available, it has been assumed that the amount of these molecules in a sick animal is rate-limiting and that administering additional cytokines in pure form will somehow promote disease resistance or healing. It has also been assumed that by administering a single new cytokine, one will not trigger mechanisms that will regulate its activity or even neutralize its effects. None of these assumptions may be valid. The major cytokines (IL-1, IL-2, IL-12, colony-stimulating factors, and the IFNs) have all been tested on animals in vivo. Unfortunately, the administration of these cytokines has usually had minimal effects on disease processes and has been accompanied by significant adverse effects.

For example, administration of interferons should inhibit virus replication as well as stimulate cellular functions such as macrophage activity, thereby promoting disease resistance. This has proved to be an oversimplification. High doses of interferons are very toxic and cause severe fever, malaise, and appetite loss. They inhibit hematopoiesis and cause thrombocytopenia and granulocytopenia. They can also cause liver, kidney, and neural toxicity. In addition, these IFNs seem to be relatively poor antiviral agents when used in this way.

Recombinant human IFN-α has been used to treat rhinopneumonitis caused by bovine herpesvirus–1 (BHV-1) and rotavirus-induced diarrhea in calves (Akiyama et al., 1993). Recombinant bovine interferons (rBoIFN-α or rBoIFN-γ) have also been used to treat BHV-1, *Mannheimia hemolytica*, *Histophilus somni*, vesicular stomatitis, coliform mastitis, brucellosis, and salmonellosis in calves and transmissible gastroenteritis in piglets. Recombinant porcine IFN-γ has been used on *Actinobacillus pleuropneumoniae* infections in pigs. Porcine IFN-α is a powerful adjuvant for foot-and-mouth disease vaccine in swine. Both human and bovine IFN-α have been used for the treatment of feline leukemia. Recombinant feline IFN-ω has also been tested in feline leukemia virus and feline immunodeficiency virus infections. In almost all cases, high-dose IFN treatment of infectious diseases has produced some positive responses. Recombinant feline IFN-ω has also been used to successfully treat feline parvoviral enteritis. These are not impressive, however, and the treatments may have adverse effects, such as fever, inappetence, and malaise. Large-scale clinical trials are needed (Mueller and Hartmann, 2021).

A modified form of granulocyte colony-stimulating factor (pegbovigrastim, Elanco) has been used to elevate neutrophil numbers in dairy cattle around the time of parturition. It is given by injection just before and after calving. This is effective in decreasing the prevalence of mastitis in these animals. This G-CSF molecule is "pegylated", that is, linked to the hydrophilic polymer polyethylene glycol (PEG). This modification significantly increases its half-life and stability.

Recombinant IL-2 has been administered to pigs at the same time that they were vaccinated against *A. pleuropneumoniae* or pseudorabies, and to calves vaccinated against BHV-1. Although it enhances immunity, IL-2 is very toxic. It causes severe side effects, including malaise, a capillary leak syndrome, diarrhea, and fever. It is interesting to note, however, that relatively low doses of rHuIL-2, when injected directly into papillomas or carcinomas of the vulva in cattle, induced tumor regression in more than 80% of cases, and some complete remissions were observed. With this exception, clinical trials employing purified cytokines have generally produced disappointing results.

REFERENCES

Akiyama, K., Sugii, S., Hirota, Y., 1993. A clinical trial of recombinant bovine interferon α1 for the control of bovine respiratory disease in calves. J. Vet. Med. Sci 53, 449–452.

Archer, T.M., Boothe, D.M., Langston, V.C., et al., 2014. Oral cyclosporine treatment in dogs: a review of the literature. J. Vet. Intern. Med. 28, 1–20.

Bauer, J.E., 2011. Therapeutic use of fish oils in companion animals. J. Am. Vet. Med. Assoc. 239, 1441–1451. 2011

Beirao, B.C., Raposo, T., Jain, S., Hupp, T., Argyle, D.J., 2016. Challenges and opportunities for monoclonal antibody therapy in veterinary oncology. Vet. J. 218, 40–50.

Bianco, D., Armstrong, P.J., Washabau, R.J., 2009. A prospective, randomized, double blinded, placebo-controlled study of human intravenous immunoglobulin for the acute management of presumptive primary immune-mediated thrombocytopenia in dogs. J. Vet. Intern. Med. 23, 1071–1078.

Bizikova, P., Olivry, T., 2015. Oral glucocorticoid pulse therapy for induction of treatment of canine pemphigus foliaceus—a comparative study. Vet. Dermatol. 26, 534–e77.

Cummings, F.O., Rizzo, S.A., 2017. Treatment of presumptive primary immune-mediated thrombocytopenia with mycophenolate mofetil versus cyclosporine in dogs. J. Small Anim. Pract. 58, 96–102.

Elenkov, E.J., 2004. Glucocorticoids and the Th1/Th2 balance. Ann. N. Y. Acad. Sci. 1024, 138–146.

Fellman, C.L., Stokes, J.V., Archer, T.M., et al., 2011. Cyclosporine A affects the in vitro expression of T cell activation-related molecules and cytokines in dogs. Vet. Immunol. Immunopathol. 140, 175–180.

Gelfand, E.W., 2012. Intravenous immune globulin in autoimmune and inflammatory diseases. N. Engl. J. Med. 367, 2015–2025.

Gruen, M.E., Myers, J.A., Tena, J.-K.S., Becskei, C., et al., 2021. Frunevetmab, a felinized anti-nerve growth factor monoclonal antibody, for the treatment of pain from osteoarthritis in cats. J. Vet. Intern. Med. 35, 2752–2762.

Hall, J.A., Van Saun, R.J., Tornquist, S.J., Gradin, J.L., Pearson, E.G., Wander, R.C., 2004. Effect of type of dietary polyunsaturated fatty acid supplement (Corn oil or fish oil) on immune responses in healthy horses. J. Vet. Intern. Med. 18, 880–886.

Hardy, R.S., Raza, K., Cooper, M.S., 2020. Therapeutic glucocorticoids: mechanisms of action in rheumatic diseases. Nat. Rev. Immunol. 16, 133–144.

Harvey, R.G., Olivri, A., Lima, T., Olivry, T., 2023. Effective treatment of canine chronic cutaneous lupus erythematosus variants with oclacitinib: seven cases. Vet. Dermatol. 34, 53–58.

Janes, M.R., Fruman, D.A., 2009. Immune regulation by Rapamycin: moving beyond T cells. Sci. Signl. 2, 65–68.

Ji, Q., Zhang, L., Jia, H., Yang, J., Xu, J., 2004. Pentoxifylline inhibits endotoxin-induced NF-kappa-B activation and associated production of proinflammatory cytokines. Ann. Clin. Lab Sci. 34, 427–436.

Kessel, A., Ammuri, H., Peri, R., et al., 2007. Intravenous immunoglobulin therapy affects T regulatory cells by increasing their suppressive function. J. Immunol. 179, 5571–5575.

Koch, S.N., Torres, S.M., Diaz, S., Gilbert, S., Rendahl, A., 2018. Subcutaneous administration of ciclosporin in 11 allergic cats—a pilot open-label uncontrolled clinical trial. Vet. Dermatol. 29, 107–e43.

Lenox, C.E., Bauer, J.E., 2013. Potential adverse effects of omega-3 fatty acids in dogs and cats. J. Vet. Intern. Med. 27, 217–226.

Lowrie, M., Thomson, S., Smith, P., Garosi, L., 2016. Effect of a constant rate infusion of cytosine arabinoside on mortality in dogs with meningoencephalitis of unknown origin. Vet. J. 213, 1–5.

Michels, G.M., Ramsey, D.S., Walsh, K.F., et al., 2016. A blinded randomized, placebo controlled, dose determination trial of Lokivetmab (ZTS-00103289), a caninized, anti-canine IL-31 monoclonal antibody in client owned dogs with atopic dermatitis. Vet. Dermatol. 27, 478–e129.

Mueller, R.S., Hartmann, K., 2021. Interferon therapies in small animals. Vet. J. 2371 https://doi.org/10.1016/j.tvjl.2021.105648

Miyata, J., Arita, M., 2015. Role of omega-3 fatty acids and their metabolites in asthma and allergic diseases. Allergol. Int. 64, 27–34.

Nayak, R.R., Alexander, M., Deshpande, I., et al., 2021. Methotrexate impacts conserved pathways in diverse human gut bacteria leading to decreased host immune activation. Cell Host Microbe 29, 362–377.

Ozdemir, C., 2015. Monoclonal antibodies in allergy: updated applications and promising trials. Recent Pat. Inflamm. Allergy Drug Disc. 9, 54–65.

Paillot, R., 2013. A systematic review of the immune-modulators *Parapoxvirus ovis* and *Propionibacterium acnes* for the prevention of respiratory disease and other infections in the horse. Vet. Immunol. Immunopathol. 153, 1–9.

Palmeiro, B.S., 2013. Cyclosporine in veterinary dermatology. Vet. Clin. North Am. Small Anim. Pract. 43, 153–171.

Rhen, T., Cidlowski, J.A., 2005. Anti-inflammatory action of glucocorticoids: new mechanisms for old drugs. N. Engl. J. Med. 353, 1711–1723.

Rutherfurd-Markwick, K.J., Hendriks, W.H., Morel, P.C.H., Thomas, D.G., 2013. The potential for enhancement of immunity in cats by dietary supplementation. Vet. Immunol. Immunopathol. 152, 333–340.

Sato, M., Veir, J.K., Legare, M., Lappin, M.R., 2017. A retrospective study on the safety and efficacy of Leflunomide in dogs. J. Vet. Intern. Med. 31, 1502–1507.

Slack, J., Risdahl, J.M., Valberg, S.J., et al., 2000. Effects of dexamethasone on development of immunoglobulin G subclass responses following vaccination of horses. Am. J. Vet. Res. 61, 1530–1531.

Venter, C., Meyer, R.W., Nwaru, B.I., et al., 2019. EAACI position paper: influence of dietary fatty acids on asthma, food allergy, and atopic dermatitis. Allergy 74, 1429–1444.

Whitley, N.T., Day, M.J., 2011. Immunomodulatory drugs and their application to the management of canine immune-mediated disease. J. Small Anim. Pract. 52 (2), 70–85.

43

Immunodiagnostic Methods

CHAPTER OUTLINE

The exquisite specificity of antibody-mediated immune responses may be exploited in two general ways to assist in disease diagnosis. First, specific antibodies may be used to detect or identify an antigen of interest. These antigens may be associated with an infectious agent or can simply be molecules that need to be located or measured. Second, by detecting specific antibodies in serum, it is possible to determine whether an animal has been exposed to an infectious agent. This may establish a diagnosis or determine the degree of exposure of the population to that agent. The measurement of antigen-antibody interactions for diagnostic purposes is called serology (Carter and Moojen, 1981).

Serological techniques can be classified into three broad categories. Primary binding tests directly measure the binding of antigen to its antibody (Table 43.1). Secondary binding tests measure the results of this antigen-antibody interaction in vitro. These tests are usually less sensitive than primary binding tests but may be simpler and require less complex technology. The third category, in vivo tests, measure the actual protective effect of antibodies in living animals.

For many years, available immunologic assays largely consisted of the technically simple secondary binding tests such as immunodiffusion and immunoelectrophoresis, tube or slide agglutination tests, virus neutralization and hemagglutination inhibition assays, and complement fixation tests. In recent years, diagnostic technology has advanced significantly. There has been a switch to primary binding tests and rapid diagnostic kits, especially in well-equipped laboratories and in societies that can afford them. These are usually much more specific, rapid, and require less trained labor to perform than older tests. However, the older assays that are relatively cheap and require a minimal of equipment are still widely employed in developing countries.

REAGENTS USED IN SEROLOGICAL TESTS

Serum

The most common source of antibodies is serum obtained from clotted blood. Serum may be stored frozen and tested when convenient. If necessary, the serum can be depleted of complement activity by heating to 56°C for 30 minutes. Plasma may also be used in these assays, but the results obtained may be affected by the anticoagulant employed.

Antiglobulins

Immunoglobulins are antigenic when injected into an animal of a different species. For example, purified dog immunoglobulins can be injected into rabbits. The rabbits respond by making specific antibodies called antiglobulins. Depending on the purity of the injected immunoglobulin, it is possible to make nonspecific antiglobulins against immunoglobulins of all classes, or very specific antiglobulins directed against single classes. Antiglobulins are essential reagents in many immunological tests.

TABLE 43.1 Smallest Amount of Antibody Protein Detectable by Selected Immunological Tests	
Tests	**Protein (μg/mL)**
Primary Binding Tests	
ELISA	0.0005
Competitive radioimmunoassay	0.00005
Secondary Binding Tests	
Gel precipitation	30
Ring precipitation	18
Bacterial agglutination	0.05
Passive hemagglutination	0.01
Hemagglutination inhibition	0.005
Complement fixation	0.05
Virus neutralization	0.00005
Bactericidal activity	0.00005
Antitoxin neutralization	0.06
In Vivo Test	
Passive cutaneous anaphylaxis	0.02

ELISA, Enzyme-linked immunosorbent assay.

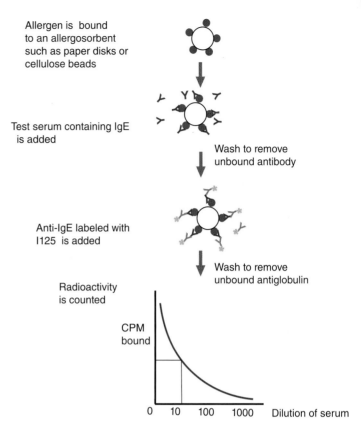

Fig. 43.1 The principle of competitive radioimmunoassay. Unlabeled antigen in the test solution displaces labeled antigen from immune complexes. The amount of labeled antigen released will be proportional to the amount of unlabeled antigen added. *CPM,* Counts per minute; *IgE,* immunoglobulin E.

Monoclonal Antibodies

Hybridoma-derived monoclonal antibodies are pure and specific, can be used as standard chemical reagents, and can be obtained in almost unlimited amounts (see Chapter 16). As a result, monoclonal antibodies frequently replace conventional antiserum as reagents in commercial immunodiagnostic tests.

Specific Antibodies

When detecting antigens in tissues or body fluids, the first steps may involve the use of a specific antibody against the antigen of interest. Although these antibodies are usually made by immunizing goats or rabbits, there is a growing interest in using chicken IgY antibodies in serologic tests. Birds may react very strongly against mammalian antigens. Chickens produce large amounts of IgY antibodies that are concentrated in the egg yolk. It may be much more convenient to harvest large amounts of antibody from egg yolks than to have to bleed animals repeatedly. Antiglobulins may then be used to detect the bound-specific IgY.

PRIMARY BINDING TESTS

Primary binding tests are performed by allowing antigen and antibody to combine and then measuring the immune complexes formed. To measure these reactions, one of the reactants must be labeled. Radioisotopes, fluorescent dyes, plastic beads, colloidal metals, and enzymes have all been used as labels in these tests.

Radioimmunoassays

Assays that use radioisotope labels have the advantage of being incredibly sensitive. On the other hand, isotope detection systems are expensive. This expense, combined with the hazards of radioactivity and the need to dispose of radioactive material in a safe manner, has ensured that radioimmunoassays are only used when highly sensitive assays are required to detect small amounts of antigens such as performance-enhancing drugs.

Competitive immunoassays are based on the principle that unlabeled antigen will displace radiolabeled antigen from immune complexes

(Fig. 43.1). The antigen (or drug) is labeled with a radioactive isotope such as tritium (H^3), carbon-14, or iodine-125. When radiolabeled antigen is mixed with its specific antibody, the two combine to form immune complexes that can be precipitated out of solution. Any radioactivity remaining in the supernatant fluid is due to the presence of unbound antigen. If unlabeled antigen is added to the mixture before adding the antibody, it will compete with the labeled antigen for antibody-binding sites. As a result, some labeled antigen will be unable to bind, and the amount of radioactivity in the supernatant will increase. If a standard curve is first constructed based on the use of known amounts of unlabeled antigen, the amount of antigen in a test sample may be measured by reference to this standard curve (Cripps et al., 1985).

Immunofluorescence Assays

Fluorescent dyes are commonly employed as labels in primary binding tests, the most important being fluorescein isothiocyanate (FITC). FITC is a yellow compound that can be chemically linked to proteins, such as antibodies, without affecting their function. When radiated with invisible ultraviolet or blue light at 290 and 145 nm, FITC re-emits visible green light at 525 nm. This green light can be readily seen under a fluorescent microscope. FITC-labeled antibodies are used in both direct and indirect fluorescent antibody tests.

Direct Fluorescent Antibody Tests

Direct fluorescent antibody tests are used to identify the presence of an antigen in a tissue sample. Antibody directed against a specific antigen, such as a bacterium or virus, is first labeled with FITC. A tissue section or smear suspected of containing the organism is fixed to a glass slide, incubated with the labeled antiserum, and then washed to remove any unbound antibody (Fig. 43.2). When examined by dark field illumination under a microscope with an ultraviolet light source, any organisms that bind the labeled antibody will fluoresce brightly. This test can identify the presence of small numbers of bacteria in a sample. For example, it can be used to detect *Mycobacterium avium* subspecies *paratuberculosis* in feces, or to detect bacteria such as *Dichelobacter nodosus*, *Listeria monocytogenes*, or clostridia in diseased tissues (Fig. 43.3).

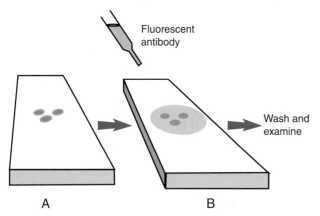

Fig. 43.2 The direct fluorescent antibody assay. This technique is used to detect antigen by means of fluorescein isothiocyanate-labeled antibody. The antigens are first applied to slide A. A fluorescent antibody solution is then applied to coat them (slide B).

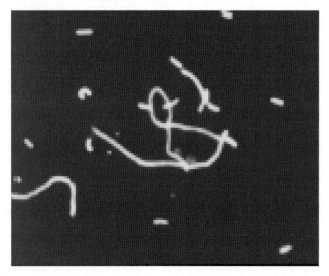

Fig. 43.3 Direct immunofluorescence of a smear of *Clostridium septicum* (see also Figs. 22.9 and 38.3). Courtesy Dr. John Huff.

It may also be employed to detect viruses in tissue culture or in tissues from infected animals. Examples include the detection of rabies virus in the brains of infected animals or feline leukemia virus in infected cat leukocytes (see Fig. 41.3).

Indirect Fluorescent Antibody Tests

Indirect fluorescent antibody tests are used to measure antibodies in serum or to identify specific antigens in tissues or cell cultures. When measuring antibody levels, the antigen is employed as a tissue smear, section, or cell culture on a slide or coverslip. This is incubated in serum suspected of containing antibodies to that antigen. The serum is then washed off, leaving any specific antibodies bound to the antigen (Fig. 43.4). These bound antibodies may then be visualized by incubating the smear in FITC-labeled antiglobulin. When the unbound labeled antiglobulin is removed by washing and the slide is examined, the presence of fluorescence indicates that antibody was present in the test serum. The quantity of antibody in the test serum may be estimated by testing increasing dilutions of serum on different antigen preparations.

The indirect fluorescent antibody test has two advantages over the direct technique. Since several labeled antiglobulin molecules can bind to each antibody molecule, the fluorescence will be considerably brighter than in the direct test. Similarly, by using antiglobulins specific for each immunoglobulin class, the class of the bound antibody may also be determined.

Particle Concentration Fluorescence Immunoassays

Immunofluorescence assays can be automated and quantitated by means of particle immunoassays (Fig. 43.5). For example, antigen-coated, sub-micrometer polystyrene particles (beads) can be mixed with test serum. After incubation, the particles are recovered by vacuum filtration, washed to remove unbound antibody, and exposed to a fluorescent antiglobulin. After filtering the suspension again and washing to remove unbound antiglobulin, the particle suspension can be placed in a spectrofluorometer and the intensity of particle-bound fluorescence measured. This provides a measure of the level of antibodies in the test serum. A very useful variation on this is the competitive assay used as a rapid test for antibodies to *Brucella abortus* in cattle. In this case, *Brucella* antigen–coated polystyrene particles are mixed with a standard amount of fluorescent anti-*Brucella* serum and the serum under test. If positive, the unlabeled test serum blocks the binding of fluorescent antibodies to the particles. The more antibodies in the test serum, the greater is the inhibition of fluorescent antibody binding.

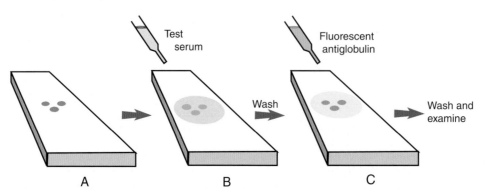

Fig. 43.4 The indirect fluorescent antibody test may be used to detect either antigen or antibody. The antigen, (A) in a section, smear, or culture, will bind antibody from the test serum (B). After washing the slide, any bound antibody may be detected by incubation in a fluorescein labeled antiglobulin solution (C).

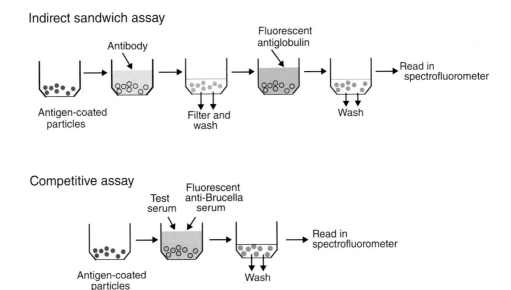

Fig. 43.5 The principle of the particle concentration fluorescence immunoassay.

Immunoenzyme Assays

Among the most widely employed immunoassays in veterinary medicine are the enzyme-linked immunosorbent assays (ELISAs). As with other primary binding tests, ELISAs may be used to detect and measure either antibodies or antigens. They have good sensitivity and specificity and can be performed in many different formats ranging from individual animal testing to automated high-throughput screening of large numbers of samples. Unlike fluorescent antibody tests, they do not require specialized equipment to read the results.

Microwell Enzyme-Linked Immunosorbent Assay Tests

The most common form of ELISA is used to detect and measure specific antibodies. In order to perform this assay, it is usual to use microwells in polystyrene plates (the commonly used plate uses 96 wells). The wells are first filled with an antigen solution (Fig. 43.6). Proteins bind firmly to polystyrene surfaces, so after unbound antigen is removed by vigorous washing, the wells remain coated with a layer of antigen. These coated plates can be stored until required. The serum under test is added to each well. Any antibodies in the serum will bind to the antigen layer. After incubation and washing to remove unbound antibody, the presence of bound antibodies can be detected by adding a solution containing an antiglobulin chemically linked to an enzyme. This labeled antiglobulin binds to the antibody and, following incubation and washing, can be detected and measured by adding a solution containing the enzyme substrate. The enzyme and substrate are selected to ensure that a colored product develops in the tube. The intensity of the color that develops is therefore proportional to the amount of enzyme-linked antiglobulin that is bound, which in turn is proportional to the amount of antibody present in the serum under test. The color intensity may be estimated visually or by spectrophotometry.

One modification of this technique is the antibody sandwich ELISA, which can be used to detect and measure a specific antigen (Fig. 43.7). The wells in polystyrene plates are coated with specific antibody (capture antibody) before testing. To conduct the test, the antigen solution to be tested is added to each well. The capture antibody will bind any antigen present in the test solution. This step is followed, after washing, by adding specific antibody, which also binds the antigen

(the detection antibody). After washing to remove unbound antibody, enzyme-labeled antiglobulin, and substrate are added, as described for the indirect technique. (It is important that the capture antibody and the detection antibody are from a different species and that a species-specific antiglobulin is used for visualization of the detection antibody. This will avoid false-positive results caused by binding of the antiglobulin to the capture antibody). The intensity of the color reaction is directly related to the amount of bound antigen. Because these tests involve the formation of antibody-antigen-antibody layers, they are called sandwich ELISAs. They can be used, for example, to detect feline leukemia virus in cat blood.

Another common modification of this technique is the labeled-antigen ELISA used to detect antibodies. This is favored in manufactured diagnostic kits. The antigen is bound to the microwells before testing (Fig. 43.8). The serum to be tested is added, followed, after washing, by labeled antigen. Any serum antibodies present will bind the labeled antigen to the microwell where it can be measured.

A competitive ELISA can be used to measure hapten molecules or viral antigens (Fig. 43.9). In this technique, each microwell is coated with specific antibody before testing. In a single reaction, the test sample and enzyme-labeled antigen are placed in the well where the antigens compete for the antibody-binding sites. The amount of labeled antigen bound to the microwell is inversely related to the concentration of antigen in the test sample. This technique is faster than other ELISA techniques. It can be made very sensitive if the sample antigen is permitted to react with the antibody before the labeled antigen is added.

Western Blotting

One solution to the problem of identifying protein antigens in a complex mixture is by using a technique called Western blotting. This is a three-stage primary binding test (Fig. 43.10). Stage 1 involves electrophoresis of the protein mixture on a gel so that each component is resolved into a single band. Stage 2 involves blotting or transfer of these protein bands to an immobilizing nitrocellulose membrane. This is accomplished by placing the membrane on top of the gel and sandwiching the two between sponges saturated with buffer. The membrane-gel

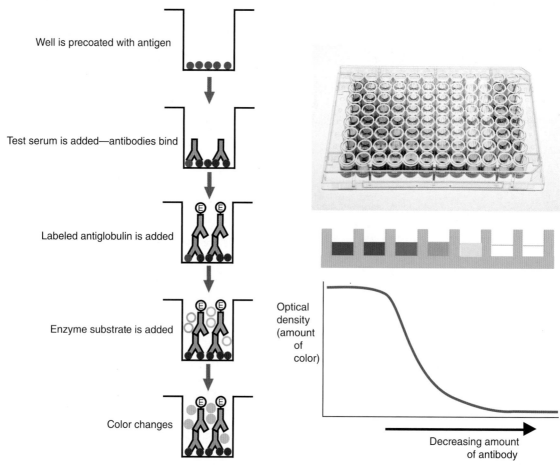

Fig. 43.6 (A) The indirect enzyme-linked immunosorbent assay (ELISA) technique. (B) Antigen is bound to the wells in a styrene plate. The presence of bound antibody is detected by means of an enzyme-labeled antiglobulin. Addition of the enzyme substrate results in a color change proportional to the amount of bound antibody. The color intensity can be estimated visually or read in an ELISA reader (a specially adapted spectrophotometer).

sandwich is supported between rigid plastic sheets and placed in a buffer reservoir, and an electrical current is passed between the sponges. The protein bands are transferred from the gel to the membrane without loss of resolution.

The third stage involves visualization of transferred antigens by means of an enzyme immunoassay or radioimmunoassay. When an enzyme immunoassay is employed, the membrane is first incubated in specific antiserum. After the membrane has been washed, an enzyme-labeled antiglobulin solution is added. When this is removed by washing, substrate is added, and a color develops in the bands where the antibody has bound to antigen. When an isotope-labeled antiglobulin is used, any labeled bands must be identified by darkening of a photographic emulsion applied to the strip; an autoradiograph. Western blotting is used to identify the important antigens in complex microorganisms or parasites (Fig. 43.11; Boto et al., 1984).

A variant form of the Western blot is the dot blot. This can be used to detect the presence of specific antibodies in the serum of vaccinated animals. In the first step, an antigen solution is filtered through a nitrocellulose membrane so that its proteins bind to the membrane. This coated membrane can be used in the form of a sheet or even as a dipstick. The presence of antibodies in a test serum can be determined by first passing the test serum through the membrane, washing the membrane to remove unbound antibodies and then applying enzyme-labeled antiglobulin in sequence. After exposure to enzyme substrate, the presence of a stained dot is a positive reaction. (Use of nasal washings as a source of the antigen, such as when trying to detect respiratory viruses, is called a snot-blot!) These tests can produce very rapid results and so can be used as "point of care" screening assays (Egerer et al., 2022).

It is possible to put "dots" of many different monoclonal antibodies on a single sheet of nitrocellulose. They may then be exposed to a complex labeled-antigen mixture, such as a cell protein extract, and after washing and development, the relative concentrations of many different antigens can be visualized. This is known as an antibody microarray (Fig. 43.12).

Alternatively, antigen dots, such as those from a virus, may be printed onto nitrocellulose membranes. Sequential addition and washing of the test serum, an enzyme-labeled antiglobulin, and substrate will result in the development of a colored dot on the substrate. The intensity of the dot is proportional to the amount of antiviral antibody in the test sample. It is used, for example, to measure antibody levels in dogs following vaccination. If multiple antigen dots plus control dots are printed in an array on a glass slide or nitrocellulose, many assays can be conducted simultaneously using very small sample volumes. These can be measured using array scanners. This is called a multiantigen print immunoassay.

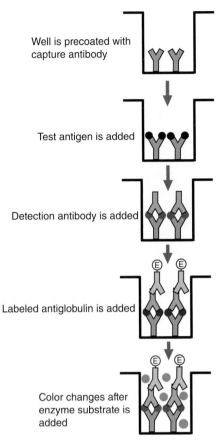

Fig. 43.7 The antibody sandwich enzyme-linked immunosorbent assay. Antigen is bound to the plate by means of an antibody. The presence of that bound antigen is detected by sequential addition of a second antibody and an enzyme-labeled antiglobulin. Addition of the enzyme substrate leads to a color change proportional to the amount of bound antigen.

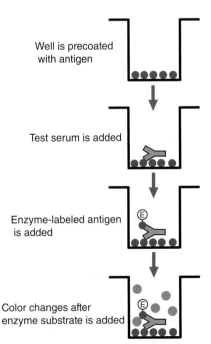

Fig. 43.8 The labeled antigen enzyme-linked immunosorbent assay. The serum under test is added to an antigen-coated plate. Bound antibodies are then detected by an enzyme-labeled antigen.

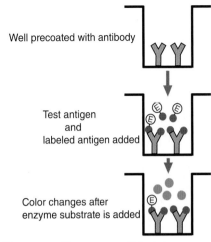

Fig. 43.9 The competitive enzyme-linked immunosorbent assay. Labeled and unlabeled antigens compete for binding to antibody. Addition of the enzyme substrate leads to a color change inversely proportional to the amount of test antigen bound.

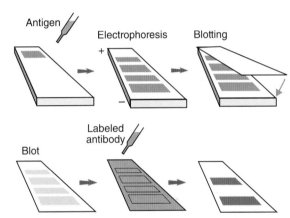

Fig. 43.10 The Western blotting technique. Serum is separated by electrophoresis and blotted onto nitrocellulose paper; the antigen bands are revealed by use of specific antibody and an enzyme- or isotope-labeled antiglobulin. The blotting stage may be a passive transfer, or an electric potential may be used to accelerate the blotting process.

ELISAs can be used to test fluids other than blood. For example, saliva or tears can be tested for the presence of feline leukemia virus. In most cases, these are simply modified versions of the serum ELISA tests. However, in one such test, a hard plastic swab with antibody to feline leukemia virus bound to the tip is rubbed throughout the cat's mouth. The antibodies on the swab are protected by a sugar coating that is removed by soaking before the test. The antibody on the swab will bind any viral antigen in the saliva. The swab is then inserted into a tube containing enzyme-labeled monoclonal antibodies against feline leukemia virus antigens. After washing, the swab is placed in a solution of the enzyme substrate and the color change noted. This technique is much less sensitive than testing blood directly but is very convenient.

Immunohistochemistry

Enzymes conjugated to immunoglobulins or antiglobulins can be used to locate specific antigens in tissue sections. Horseradish peroxidase is the most widely employed label. The tests are performed in a manner similar to the immunofluorescence tests. In the direct immunoperoxidase test, the tissue section is treated with the enzyme-labeled antibody.

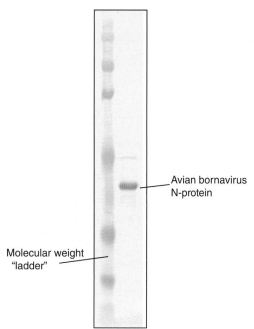

Fig. 43.11 A Western blot assay. In this example, the serum of a bird was tested for the presence of antibodies to avian bornavirus N-protein. Proteins from a culture of avian bornavirus were first separated by electrophoresis. The electrophoresed material was then blotted onto nitrocellulose paper. Serum from the bird to be tested was allowed to react with the viral proteins and unbound antibodies removed by washing. Finally, the presence of bound antibodies was revealed using an enzyme-labeled antiglobulin followed by enzyme substrate. The N-protein is revealed as a colored band of the correct size. The stained bands on the left are markers of defined molecular weights. Courtesy Dr. I. Villanueva.

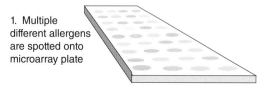

1. Multiple different allergens are spotted onto microarray plate

2. Test serum added and then washed off

3. Biotin-labeled antiglobulin added and then washed off

4. Fluorescent strepavidin is used to detect any bound biotin

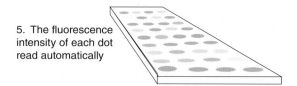

5. The fluorescence intensity of each dot read automatically

Fig. 43.12 The principle of an antibody microarray. Serum can be tested for reactivity to hundreds of different allergens at one time. Allergen spots are applied automatically to the plate in a defined pattern. For example, it is usual for the allergen spots to be applied in triplicate. Both positive and negative control spots must also be present. Either colored or fluorescent-labeled antiglobulins may be used to detect any bound immunoglobulin E. The plates are read automatically by a plate reader.

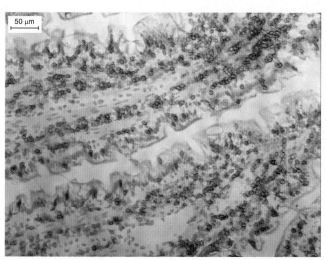

Fig. 43.13 The immunoperoxidase technique showing the presence of α/β T cells in the lamina propria and epithelium of canine duodenum. Cells binding the monoclonal antibody are exposed to peroxidase-labeled specific antiglobulin. The presence of the peroxidase is revealed as a brown deposit. From German, A.J., Hall, E.J., Moore, P.F., et al., 1999. The distribution of lymphocytes expressing alpha/beta and gamma/delta T-cell receptors, and the expression of mucosal addressin cell adhesion molecule-1 in the canine intestine. J. Comp. Pathol. 121, 249–263.

After washing, the tissue is incubated in a solution of the appropriate enzyme substrate. Bound antibody is detected by the development of a brown color at the site of antibody binding (Fig. 43.13). In the indirect test, bound antibody is detected by means of a labeled antiglobulin. This technique has an advantage over immunofluorescence techniques in that the tissue can be examined by conventional light microscopy and can be stained so that structural relationships are easier to see (Bradley et al., 1990).

ELISpot Assays

As described in Chapter 34, It is possible to use a variation of a sandwich ELISA assay to identify cytokine-secreting cells (see Fig. 34.11). In the enzyme-linked immunospot (ELISpot) assay, a monoclonal or polyclonal antibody directed against the antigen of interest coats the bottom of plastic tissue culture wells. Stimulated cells are pipetted into the wells. If the cells secrete the antigen of interest, it will bind to the capture antibodies. Once the culture period is completed, cells and unbound material are washed away. A biotinylated detection antibody is then added. After incubation and washing, alkaline-phosphatase conjugated avidin is then added. After another wash and addition of the enzyme substrate a pattern of colored spots develops that correspond to the location of each antigen-secreting cell. These spots can be counted, and the frequency of specific antigen-producing cells can be determined. This assay can also be used to quantitate cytokine production or to identify cytotoxic cells by detecting granzyme or perforin production. The assay has a sensitivity as low as one cell in 100,000. Depending on the antigen analyzed, this assay is between 20 and 200 times more sensitive than a conventional ELISA (Lefevre et al., 2009).

Multiplex Immunoassays

While ELISA assays can conventionally measure only a single analyte, the use of colored bead-based substrates permits many different immunoassays to be performed and analyzed simultaneously on a single sample. These multiplex immunoassays are available in several different formats depending on the manufacturer and whether they are designed to detect antibodies, antigens, oligonucleotides, enzyme substrates, or specific receptors (Whelan et al., 2008).

For example, in order to detect specific antigens. Multiple sets of beads are internally colored with a specific mixture of fluorescent dyes. These mixtures are designed so that each set of beads can be readily differentiated. Then, each set is coated with a different specific antibody and the beads mixed together. The bead mixture is first added to the solution under test, such as serum. As a result, some of the beads in the mixture will capture the specific antigen being assayed. The bead mixture is then washed and mixed with fluorescent-labeled, antigen-specific, reporter antibodies. These form a labeled antibody-antigen-antibody sandwich on the bead surface. A commonly used label is the fluorescent dye phycoerythrin conjugated to streptavidin. This binds specifically to biotinylated antibodies. (Avidin and biotin bind each other strongly and specifically.) After washing, the bead suspension is then passed through a dual laser flow-based detection instrument—essentially a specialized flow cytometer. One laser identifies the color of the bead (and thus which antigen is being detected), while the other measures the intensity of the reporter fluorescence (and hence the amount of bound antigen). High-speed digital processors can record the signals from each bead and with appropriate software translate the results into usable data (Wilchek and Bayer, 1984).

In an alternative to flow-based assays, labeled magnetic beads can be employed. After reacting with their specific reagents, the beads can be captured in such a way that they form a monolayer on a metal surface. When the layer of beads is illuminated with two sources of light of specific wavelengths, they will fluoresce. Light of one wavelength can identify the antigen on each bead, while the other can determine its amount. These automated assays can simultaneously and rapidly detect and quantitate many different analytes from a single biological sample (Wood et al., 2011).

Chemiluminescence Assays

Chemiluminescence assays are highly sensitive alternatives to conventional enzyme-based assays (Dudley, 1990). Their basic principle is the same, but instead of a label that changes color, they use a label that emits light when exposed to its substrate. This light can be detected and measured in a luminometer. These assays not only have a very high sensitivity, good specificity, and a much wider dynamic range than simple colorimetric ELISAs but they are also easier to measure. As a result, they are employed in a wide range of diagnostic applications (Cinquanta et al., 2017).

Two different types of chemical reaction are commonly employed in chemiluminescence assays. In the direct method, the reactant, such as antigen, antibody, or antiglobulin, is labeled with a chemical that can emit light. Examples include acridinium or ruthenium esters, which, when exposed to sodium hydroxide, emit a flash of light. The light emitted by these reactants is of significantly greater intensity than that emitted by other reactions.

A second, indirect, method uses enzymes as reactant labels. Reactions can be measured by using a substrate that emits light when acted on by the enzyme. For example, luminol (3-aminophthal hydrazide) emits a flash of light when it reacts with oxidized horseradish peroxidase. Thus the peroxidase is used as the label, and the luminol substrate is added later. The reaction results in the emission of light flashes at a wavelength of 425 nm. Luminol, when used with the correct enhancers (substituted phenols, naphthols, or aromatic amines), gives bright and stable light emission.

Another similar system uses alkaline phosphatase as the enzyme and adamantane-1,2-dioxetane aryl phosphate (AMPPD) as the substrate. When the phosphate is cleaved off the AMPPD molecule, a flash

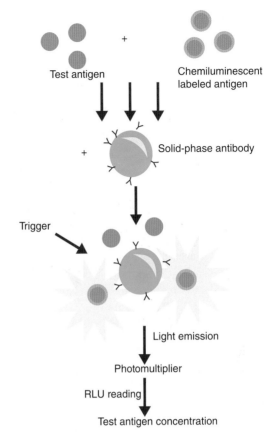

Fig. 43.14 The principle of a competitive binding assay using a chemiluminescent label. A fixed amount of labeled antigen is first mixed with the test sample. To the mixture is then added specific antibody bound to a solid substrate, in this case latex particles. After the reaction, the particles are washed and exposed to the exciting chemicals. The emitted light is detected and measured by relative light units (RLU). The greater the amount of antigen in the test sample, the less labeled antigen will bind. The test may be quantitated by reference to a standard curve.

of light is emitted at a wavelength of 470 nm. Enhancers, such as ferrocyanide or metallic ions, may be added to boost light emission. These assays are incredibly sensitive and can detect up to a mol^{-16} per liter of the label.

Chemiluminescence assays are employed in competitive ELISA tests (Fig. 43.14). For example, they can be used to measure the thyroid hormone T_4. The response is measured in "Relative Light Units." This may then be converted into absolute units (μg/dl) by comparison to a standard curve. Another such test can be used to measure specific IgE levels against a panel of multiple allergens, for example, food allergens or respiratory allergens, and can be fully automated—the multiple allergen simultaneous test (MAST). Rather than being restricted to 96 well plates, these MAST assays can be applied to immunoblots or even to allergen-impregnated threads. Chemiluminescence assays are good alternatives to radioimmunoassays and have largely replaced them in many diagnostic laboratories.

Disposable Immunoassay Devices

Recent years have seen the development of simple immunoassays that can be employed animal-side and provide diagnostic results within a few minutes. These assays simply provide all necessary reagents in excess, and the sample under test becomes the limiting feature. Most

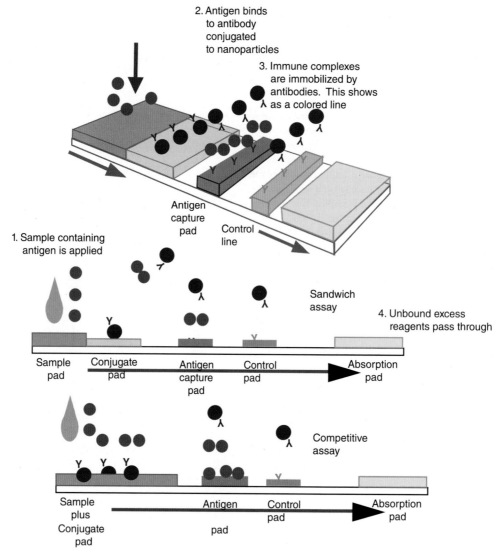

Fig. 43.15 The principle of an immunochromatography assay. These have been widely employed as rapid tests for the presence of COVID-19 in humans.

disposable devices use this form of assay because the use of excess reagents makes the accurate metering of the sample unnecessary. Examples include the widely employed immunochromatography assays (Fig. 43.15; McVicker et al., 2002).

Immunochromatography

Immunochromatography assays are simple devices that are used to simply detect the presence or absence of a target antigen, such as a viral antigen. They are simple, fast, and easy to read. In their simplest form, they involve allowing a solution containing antigen (such as infected serum, saliva, or nasal washes) to flow laterally through a porous strip by capillary action. As the solution passes through the strip, it first passes through a pad, where it meets and solubilizes dried labeled specific antibody. Any antigen present is captured and forms immune complexes. This antibody may be labeled with either colloidal gold (pink color) or colloidal selenium (blue color). Any immune complexes in the fluid are then carried through a detection zone containing immobilized antibody against the antigen. Here any immune complexes are captured, and as a result, a pink or blue line or dot develops in the detection zone

in a positive test (Fig. 43.16). Finally, the fluid flows into an absorption pad that acts as a sink at the end of the strip and prevents fluid backflow. Drops of buffer may be added to speed the flow of antigen solution. All these components are mounted on a backing card.

This simple procedure permits multiple samples to be analyzed in a one-step procedure. A positive control band can be developed as well, and the use of an effective prefilter can permit the use of whole blood. Lateral flow assays are used for the detection of heartworm or feline leukemia antigens. Similar assays may be used to detect many different viruses, such as rota- or parvoviruses, and bacteria, such as salmonella or tuberculosis. Results are available within minutes. Many home COVID-19 tests use this technology.

Competitive Assays

In a variant assay, the antigen solution can be dropped onto a pad containing labeled antibody. This is followed by wash buffer that drives the immune complexes through the pad to a second pad containing immobilized antigen. If antigen is present in the test solution, it will bind the antibodies and prevent them from binding in the test pad.

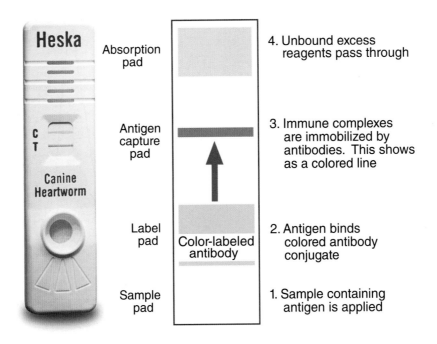

Fig. 43.16 Immunochromatography. A sample containing antigen flows through a porous strip, and positive reactions are shown by the appearance of a colored band. Courtesy Heska Inc.

Thus, in a positive test, no line or a weak line will appear. This is followed by a control pad containing immobilized antiglobulin. Excess reagents flow through to the absorption pad. This type of assay is best suited to detecting low-molecular-weight compounds that cannot bind two antibodies simultaneously.

SNAP® Assays

The SNAP® assay is a variant immunochromatography assay with each step performed in a timed sequence within a plastic device. It is rapid and specific and can easily be employed animal-side. More than 20 different commercial kits are available to detect both antigens and antibodies against diverse pathogens. In order to detect specific antigen, an enzyme-labeled antibody conjugate is first mixed with the test serum, plasma, or whole blood in a tube. The mixture is added to the sample well on the device. The mixture flows through a matrix and is allowed to interact with test as well as positive and negative control dots printed on a matrix. The test dot contains antigen-specific antibodies that will bind any antigen-antibody conjugate within the test sample. This takes about 60 seconds. The device is then "activated" releasing stored wash buffer and enzyme substrate solution that also wash over the test and control dots. Unbound conjugate is washed away. The substrate binds to any bound conjugate. As a result, color develops in the appropriate dots within 10 minutes. This assay can also be used to detect specific antibodies by using dots of immobilized antigen and enzyme-conjugated antigen (O'Connor, 2015). If required, this assay can also be made semiquantitative by measuring the intensity of the blue-colored dot.

ANTIBODY LABELS

Although radioisotopes and enzymes are commonly used as labels for primary binding tests, both have disadvantages. For example, radioactive isotopes may have a short half-life, are potentially hazardous, and require expensive detection devices. Enzymes, though stable and relatively cheap, are large molecules that may inhibit antibody activity or lose enzymatic activity in the process of being bound to antiglobulin. One alternative is to use the small molecule biotin and its specific binding protein avidin. Biotin can bind to proteins without affecting their biological activity. Avidin binds very strongly and specifically to biotin and may be conjugated with enzymes.

The most popular enzymes used in ELISAs include alkaline phosphatase, horseradish peroxidase, and β-galactosidase. Colored dyes linked to antibodies have been used in dipstick assays. Reagents linked to ferritin or colloidal gold may be used to identify the location of antigens in cells examined by electron microscopy because such labels are electron dense. As described above, colloidal gold and colloidal selenium are colored and may be used as labels in immunochromatography tests.

FLOW CYTOMETRY

Flow cytometry is an automated technique that rapidly scans single cells and is able to count and sort them. Cells are passed through a capillary tube in single file. A laser beam is directed through the cell stream, and the effects of each cell on the light beam are measured. The scatter of the light beam in a forward direction can be used to give a measure of a cell's size. The light scattered to the side gives a measure of a cell's surface roughness and internal complexity. A combination of these two parameters can be used to identify all the leukocytes in a blood sample (Smith et al., 1994).

Flow cytometry can, however, be use for more complex studies by using specific cell surface markers. Thus, cell surface antigens can be

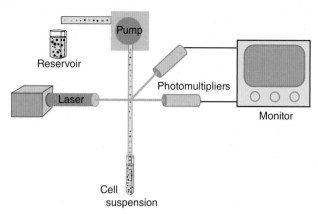

Fig. 43.17 A simplified view of the mechanism of action of the flow cytometer.

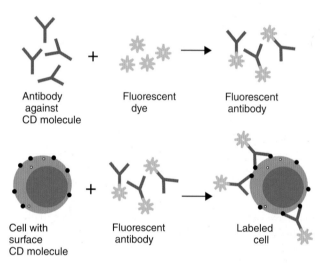

Fig. 43.18 How an immunoglobulin bound to a fluorescent dye can be used to identify cell surface antigenic molecules in a flow cytometer.

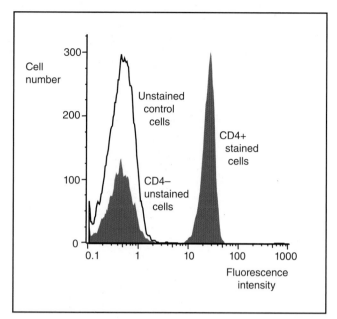

Fig. 43.19 A typical flow cytometer readout from labeling a cell population with antiequine CD4. The intensity of fluorescent labeling increases from left to right. Thus, unlabeled control cells form the unshaded left peak. When a mixture of CD4+ and CD4− cells is examined, it forms two distinct peaks (*shaded area*). The left peak consists of unlabeled (CD4−) cells. The right peak consists of labeled (CD4+) cells. The area under each peak is a measure of the size of each cell subpopulation. Courtesy Dr. R.R. Smith III.

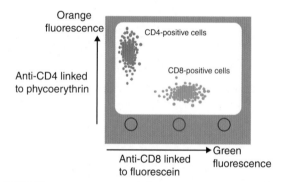

Fig. 43.20 The pattern seen on a flow cytometer screen when analyzing lymphocyte populations stained with two different fluorescence-conjugated antibodies. It is usual to label one population with a green dye and the second population with a red or orange dye.

labeled with specific antibodies conjugated to fluorescent dyes. The cell suspension is then passed through a capillary tube in single file. The labeled cells pass one-by-one through a laser beam that excites the dye molecules. The emission spectra of these dyes are recorded, and the markers on each individual cell are identified. Flow cytometry can be used to quantify the numbers and size of each specific cell type and subpopulation in the mixture. It can also be used to sort specific cell populations for future studies. The cells are not harmed by passage through the laser beam (Figs. 43.17–43.20). By using antibodies labeled with different colored fluorescent dyes, the expression of multiple cell surface antigens can be analyzed simultaneously. It is possible to use the flow cytometer to follow sequential changes in the phenotype of mixed-cell populations. Flow cytometry can even be used to measure cell activation by using labels that specifically bind the phosphorylated state of the target protein. The main limitation of flow cytometry is that even the most sophisticated machines are limited to measuring fewer than 20 markers at any one time.

SECONDARY BINDING TESTS

Many of the earliest immunodiagnostic tests relied on secondary phenomena. Thus, reactions between antigens and antibodies in solution are commonly followed by a secondary reaction. If antibodies combine with soluble antigens, the resulting immune complexes may precipitate out. Antibodies binding to a suspension of particulate antigens (e.g., bacteria or red blood cells) may make them clump or agglutinate. If an antibody can activate the classical complement pathway and the antigen is on a cell surface, cell lysis may result. These reactions are employed in many different serological assays.

Precipitation Tests

If a solution of a soluble antigen is mixed with a strong antiserum, the mixture becomes cloudy within a few minutes, and then flocculent; eventually, a precipitate settles to the bottom of the tube. This precipitate consists of antigen-antibody complexes. If increasing amounts of soluble antigen are mixed with a constant amount of antibody, the amount of precipitate that develops is determined by the relative

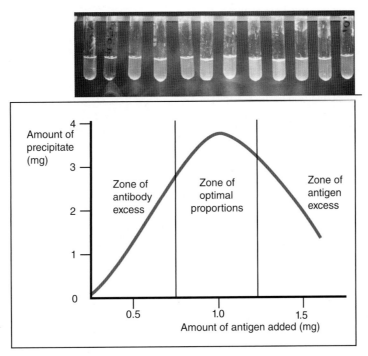

Fig. 43.21 The effect of mixing increasing amounts of antigen (bovine serum) with a constant amount of antibody (rabbit antiserum). The tube with the greatest amount of precipitate is the one in which the ratio of antigen to antibody is optimal. A quantitative precipitation curve of this test shows this effect graphically.

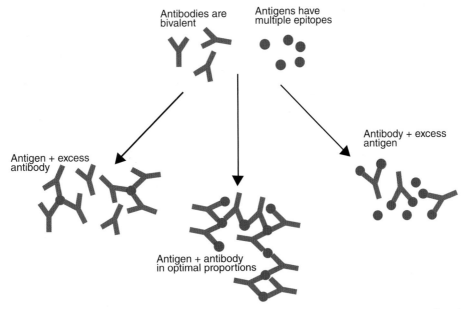

Fig. 43.22 The mechanism of immunoprecipitation. In both antigen and antibody excess, small, soluble, immune complexes are produced. However, at optimal proportions, large insoluble complexes are generated.

proportions of the reactants. No obvious precipitate is formed at low antigen concentrations. As the amount of antigen increases, larger quantities of precipitate form until the amount is maximal. However, with the addition of yet more antigen, the amount of precipitate gradually diminishes, until none is present in tubes containing a large excess of antigen (Fig. 43.21). Equine IgG3 antibodies behave in a somewhat different fashion, producing a distinct flocculation over a very narrow range of antigen concentrations.

In the first stage of these reactions, only a little antigen is complexed to antibody, so little precipitate is deposited. In the tubes where most precipitation occurs, both antigen and antibody are completely complexed, and neither can be detected in the supernatant fluid. This is called the equivalence zone, and the ratio of antibody to antigen is optimal. When antigen is added to excess, a precipitate does not form, although small soluble immune complexes are present and free antigen may be detected in the supernatant fluid.

This pattern of precipitation results from the fact that antibodies are bivalent and therefore can cross-link only two epitopes at a time, but complex antigens are generally multivalent, possessing many epitopes (Fig. 43.22). Where there is excess antibody, each antigen molecule is covered with antibody molecules, preventing cross-linkage and thus precipitation. When the reactants are in optimal proportions, the ratio of antigen to antibody is such that cross-linking, and lattice formation are extensive. As this lattice grows, it becomes insoluble and eventually precipitates. In mixtures in which antigen is in excess, each antibody molecule binds two antigen molecules. Further cross-linkage is impossible, and since these complexes are small and soluble, no precipitation occurs. Mononuclear phagocytes are most efficient at binding and removing complexes formed at optimal proportions and in antibody excess. Small immune complexes formed in antigen excess are poorly removed by phagocytic cells but are deposited in vessel walls and in glomeruli, where they may cause type III hypersensitivity reactions (see Chapter 33).

Immunodiffusion

One simple method of demonstrating precipitation is immunodiffusion or gel diffusion. Round wells, about 5 mm in diameter and about 1 cm apart, are cut in a layer of clear agar. One well is then filled with soluble antigen and the other with antiserum; the reactants diffuse out radially. Where the reactants meet in optimal proportions, an opaque white line of precipitated immune-complex forms.

If the solutions used contain multiple antigens and antibodies, the components are unlikely to reach optimal proportions in exactly the same position. Consequently, a separate line of precipitate is produced for each interacting set of antigens and antibodies. This test can be used to determine the relationship between antigens. If two antigen wells and one antibody well are set up as in Fig. 43.23, lines will form between each antigen well and the antibody well. If these two lines join, the two antigens are probably identical. If the lines cross, the two antigens are completely different. If the lines merge with spur formation, a partial identity exists, indicating that one antigen possesses epitopes absent in the other. The Coggins test is a gel-diffusion method used to detect antibodies against equine infectious anemia (EIA) virus in horse serum. In this test, an extract of infected horse spleen or a cell culture viral antigen reacts with the serum of the horse under test in agar gel, and the development of a line of precipitate constitutes a positive reaction. A similar test is used to identify cattle infected with bovine leukemia virus. Immunodiffusion assays are, however, insensitive and, as a result, are subject to numerous false-negative results. ELISA tests are significantly more sensitive. Thus, the combination of ELISA plus immunodiffusion resulted in the detection of 17% more positive cases of EIA. These false-negative results would ensure that EIA cannot be eradicated if testing were based on the Coggins test alone (Issel et al., 2012).

Radial Immunodiffusion

If an antigen solution diffuses into agar in which specific antiserum has been incorporated, a ring of precipitate will form around the antigen well. The area of this ring is proportional to the amount of antigen in the well. A standard curve may therefore be constructed using known amounts of antigen (Fig. 43.24). Unknown solutions of antigen can then be accurately assayed by comparing the ring diameters from unknowns with the standard curve. This test is used to measure serum immunoglobulin levels in newborn foals (see Chapter 24) and in cases of suspected immunodeficiency.

If, instead of being permitted to passively diffuse into agar-containing antiserum as in the radial immunodiffusion technique, the antigen is driven into the antiserum agar by electrophoresis, the ring of precipitation around each well becomes deformed into a rocket shape. The length of the rocket is proportional to the amount of antigen placed in each well. This technique is called rocket electrophoresis.

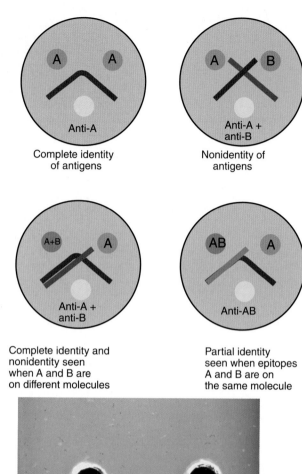

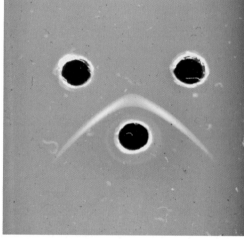

Fig. 43.23 Precipitation in agar gel. Antigen and antibody diffusing from their respective wells precipitate immune complexes in a region where optimal proportions are achieved. In this example, the antigen is identical in both top wells. As a result, the precipitation lines fuse to show complete identity B. The gel-diffusion technique to determine the relationship of two antigens.

Immunoelectrophoresis and Related Techniques

Although conventional gel-diffusion techniques give a separate precipitation line for each antigen-antibody system in a mixture, it is often difficult to resolve all the components in a very complex mixture. One way to improve the resolution of the system is to first separate the antigen mixture by electrophoresis before undertaking immunodiffusion. This technique is called immunoelectrophoresis and is used to identify proteins in body fluids (Fig. 43.25).

Immunoelectrophoresis involves the electrophoresis of serum in agar gel in one direction. A trough is then cut in the agar parallel to

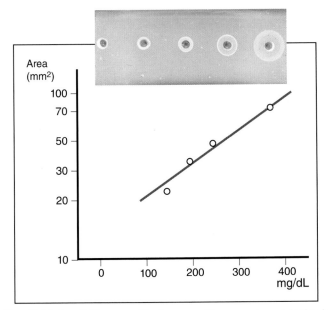

Fig. 43.24 A radial immunodiffusion assay. The area of precipitation is proportional to the concentration of antigen. In this case antiserum to bovine immunoglobulin A (IgA) is incorporated in the agar and is used to measure bovine serum IgA levels.

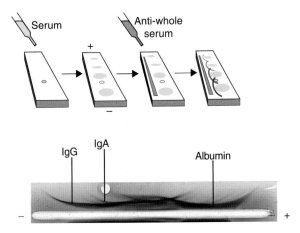

Fig. 43.25 The technique of immunoelectrophoresis (see text for details). Immunoelectrophoresis of pig serum showing the lines of precipitation produced by some of the major serum proteins (see also Fig. 16.23). *IgA,* Immunoglobulin.

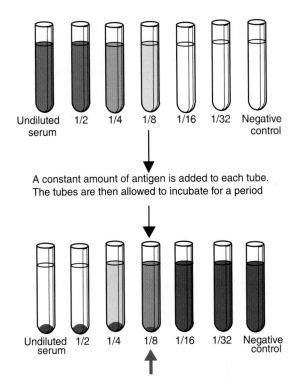

Fig. 43.26 The principle of antibody titration. Serum is first diluted in a series of tubes. A constant amount of antigen is then added to each tube, and the tubes are incubated. At the end of the incubation period, the last tube in which a reaction has occurred is identified. In this example, agglutination has occurred in all tubes up to a serum dilution of 1:8. The agglutination titer of the serum is said to be 8.

this line of separated proteins. Antiserum against the whole serum is placed in this trough and allowed to diffuse laterally. When the diffusing antibodies encounter antigen, curved lines of precipitate are formed. One arc of precipitation forms for each of the constituents in the antigen mixture. This technique can resolve the proteins of normal serum into 25–40 distinct precipitation lines. This technique has been used to identify the absence of a normal serum protein, as in animals with a congenital deficiency of some complement components. It is also used to detect the presence of excessive amounts of an individual component, as in animals with a myeloma (Fig. 16.21).

Titration of Antibodies

Although the simple detection of antibodies or antigen is sufficient for many purposes, it is usually desirable to quantitate the reaction. One way of measuring specific antibody levels is by titration. The

serum under test is diluted in a series of decreasing concentrations (Fig. 43.26). Each dilution is then tested for activity. The reciprocal of the highest dilution giving a positive reaction, called the titer (or titre), provides an estimate of the amount of antibody in that serum.

Agglutination

Because antibodies are bivalent, they can cross-link particulate antigens such as bacteria or foreign red cells, resulting in their clumping or agglutination. Antibodies differ in their ability to cause agglutination; for example, IgM antibodies are more efficient than IgG antibodies (Table 43.2). If excess antibody is added to a suspension of antigenic particles, then, just as in the precipitation reaction, each particle may be so coated by antibody that agglutination is inhibited. This lack of reactivity at high concentrations of antibody is termed a prozone. Another cause of prozone formation is the presence of antibodies that cannot cause agglutination. These nonagglutinating antibodies are also called (incorrectly!) "incomplete" antibodies. The reason for their lack of agglutinating activity is not completely understood; one possibility is that the epitopes with which they react lie deep within the surface coat of the particle, so deep that cross-linking cannot occur. An alternative suggestion is that they are capable of only restricted movement in their hinge region, causing them to be functionally monovalent (see Chapter 17).

Antiglobulin Tests

If it is necessary to test for the presence of nonagglutinating antibodies on the surface of particles such as bacteria or erythrocytes, a direct antiglobulin test may be used. The washed particles may be mixed with an antiglobulin, and if antibodies are present on their surface,

TABLE 43.2 Role of Specific Immunoglobulin Classes in Serological Assays

Property	IgG	IgM	IgA	Equine IgG3
Agglutination	+	+++	+	−
Complement activation	+	+++	−	−
Precipitation	+++	+	±	±
Time of appearance (days)	3–7	2–5	3–7	3–7
Time to peak titer (days)	7–21	5–14	7–21	7–21

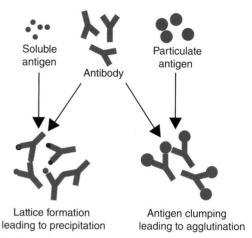

Fig. 43.28 The relationship between precipitation and agglutination. This is essentially a consequence of the size of the antigenic particle. Large particles agglutinate. Small particles and soluble molecules precipitate.

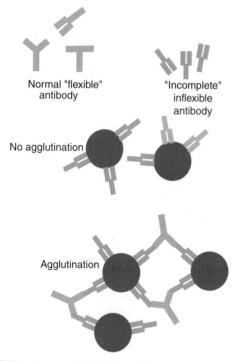

Fig. 43.27 The direct antiglobulin test. The presence of the antiglobulin is required to agglutinate particles coated with nonagglutinating antibody.

agglutination will occur (Fig. 43.27). This is sometimes called the Coombs' test after the veterinarian who invented it.

Instead of using 96-well plates for direct agglutination tests, it is possible to use gel-based antiglobulin tests (Pieck et al., 2012). These use whole blood samples rather than washed and resuspended red cells. The blood sample is layered into a tube containing a viscous gel matrix impregnated with a rabbit antiglobulin specific for the species to be tested. The tubes are gently centrifuged for a defined time. In a positive test the clumped red cells cannot penetrate the gel and hence layer at the top of the tube. If the test is negative, the individual red cells can pass through the gel and pellet at the bottom of the tube (see Fig. 32.5). Matrix gel agglutination is also used for blood typing in dogs and cats. It relies on performing the agglutination test on top of a viscous gel layer containing specific antibody.

Passive Agglutination Tests

Since agglutination is a much more sensitive technique than precipitation, it is sometimes useful to convert a precipitating system to an

agglutinating one (Fig. 43.28). This may be done by chemically linking soluble antigen to inert particles such as erythrocytes or latex beads. Erythrocytes are among the best particles for this purpose, and tests that employ coated erythrocytes are called passive hemagglutination tests. Sensitized microspheres of polystyrene or latex are also commonly used in qualitative agglutination tests because of their uniformity and stability (Molina-Bolivar et al., 2005). Recent advances have developed particles with polystyrene cores covered by thin shells of reactive chemicals. The cores have a well-defined size that can be colored so that they can be used in nephelometric assays. For example, the shells may consist of a polystyrene/polymethacrylate/ copolymer that allows covalent protein binding (Kapmeyer et al., 1988).

Viral Hemagglutination and Its Inhibition

Some viruses can bind and agglutinate red blood cells. This virus-induced hemagglutination may assist in characterizing an unknown virus. Inhibition of viral hemagglutination by antibody can then be used either as a method of identifying a specific virus or to measure antibody levels in serum. Hemagglutinating organisms include orthomyxoviruses and paramyxoviruses, alphaviruses, flaviviruses, and bunyaviruses, as well as some adenoviruses, reoviruses, parvoviruses, and coronaviruses. They also include some mycoplasma, such as *Mycoplasma gallisepticum*.

Complement Fixation Tests

The activation of the classical complement pathway by antibody bound to antigen results in the generation of terminal complement complexes that can disrupt cell membranes. If the antibody binds red cells, these will be ruptured, and hemolysis occurs. This phenomenon can be used to measure serum antibody levels in a test called the complement fixation test.

Complement is a normal constituent of all fresh serum, but the complement in fresh, unheated guinea pig serum is the most efficient in hemolytic tests. Serum used as a source of complement for serological applications should be stored frozen in small volumes. Once thawed, it should be used promptly. It should not be repeatedly frozen and thawed.

The complement fixation test is performed in two parts. First, antigen and antibodies (the serum under test deprived of its complement by heating at 56°C) are mixed and incubated in the presence of

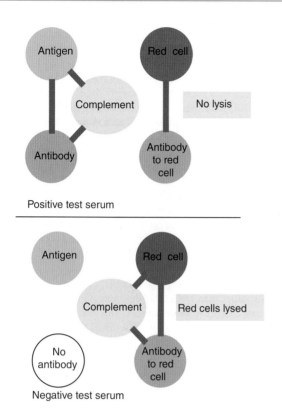

Fig. 43.29 The principle of the complement fixation test. Complement, if fixed by antigen and antibody, is unavailable to lyse the target cells in the indicator system. In the absence of antibody, the complement remains unfixed and is available to lyse the indicator system. (Modified from Roitt, I., 1971. Essential Immunology. Blackwell Science, Oxford.)

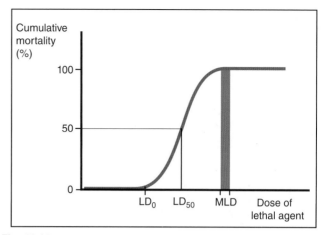

Fig. 43.30 A cumulative mortality curve showing how the lethal dose-50 (LD_{50}) provides a more accurate estimate of the lethal effects of a toxin than either the LD_0 or the median lethal dose (MLD).

normal guinea pig serum as a source of complement. After the antigen-antibody-complement mixture reacts, the amount of free complement remaining in the mixture is then measured by adding an indicator system consisting of antibody-coated sheep red cells. Lysis of these cells (seen as the development of a transparent red solution) is a negative result because it indicates that antibody was absent from the serum under test and that the complement was not consumed (or fixed) (Fig. 43.29). Absence of lysis (seen as a cloudy red cell suspension), indicating that complement was consumed, is a positive result. It is usual to titrate the serum being tested so that, if antibodies are present in that serum, as it is diluted, the reaction in each tube will change from no lysis (positive) to lysis (negative). The titer is the highest dilution of serum in which no more than 50% of the red cells are lysed.

Cytotoxicity Tests

Complement may cause membrane damage, not only to erythrocytes but also to nucleated cells and to protozoa. Antibodies against cell surface antigens may thus be measured by reacting target cells with antibody and complement and estimating the resulting cell death. This form of assay has been employed to type cells by determining which major histocompatibility complex class I molecules they are expressing.

ASSAYS IN LIVING SYSTEMS

If an organism or antigen possesses biological activity, antibodies can be measured by their ability to neutralize this activity. Activities that may be neutralized include hemolysis of erythrocytes, lysis of nucleated cells, and disease or death in animals. Reactions such as these are subject to a high degree of variability because they tend to change gradually over a wide range of doses of organism or antigen. For this reason, results obtained from a single positive or negative neutralization test are usually of little use. For example, 0.003 mg of tetanus toxin may kill some mice in a test group, but about five times that dose is required to kill all mice in the same group. In addition, if an attempt is made to assess the lowest dose of tetanus toxin that will kill all the animals in a group (the minimal lethal dose), it is found to be highly variable. It is equally difficult to estimate with precision the highest dose of toxin that will just fail to kill all test animals. The most exact method of measuring the lethal effects of a toxin has been to estimate the dose that will just kill 50% of a group of test animals (Fig. 43.30). In practice, it is usually not possible to arrive at this 50% end point by direct experimentation. For this reason, it is usually necessary to calculate it by plotting the results against the dose of toxin given and arriving at the 50% end point by calculation.

In the example cited in the previous paragraph, the lethality of the toxin can be estimated by measuring the dose required to kill 50% of a group of experimental animals. This lethal dose is called the LD_{50}. Similarly, the dose of complement that just hemolyzes 50% of a red cell suspension is called the CH_{50}. The dose of organisms that infect 50% of animals is the ID_{50}, and the dose that just infects 50% of tissue cultures is the $TCID_{50}$.

Neutralization Tests

Neutralization tests estimate the ability of antibody to neutralize the biological activity of antigen when mixed with it in vitro. These tests may be used to identify bacterial toxins such as *Clostridium perfringens* α-toxin or staphylococcal α-toxin. Viruses may be prevented from infecting cells after specific antibody has combined with and blocked their critical attachment sites. This reaction is the basis of the virus neutralization tests that are employed either for the identification of unknown viruses or for the measurement of specific antiviral antibody. Virus neutralization tests are highly specific and extremely sensitive. Thus, antiserum to coliphage T4 will neutralize phage-induced lysis of *Escherichia coli* because antibodies can block the receptor on the phage tail, thus preventing its attachment to a bacterium. A single antibody molecule is sufficient to cause this, and a phage neutralization test may therefore detect as little as 0.00005 mg of antibody.

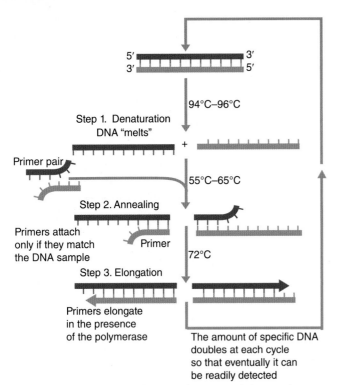

Fig. 43.31 The principle of the polymerase chain reaction test. Essentially by performing a cycle of reactions repeatedly, it is possible to produce large amounts of Deoxyribonucleic acid (DNA) coding for the gene of interest. Once produced in sufficient amounts, this DNA can be detected by electrophoresis.

Protection Tests

A protection test is a form of neutralization test carried out entirely in vivo. The protective properties of a specific antiserum are measured by administering it in increasing dilutions to a group of test animals, which may then be challenged with a standard dose of pathogenic organisms or toxin. Although protection tests provide a direct measure of the therapeutic efficacy of an antiserum, they are also subject to great experimental variation because of differences among animals. Animals differ in their susceptibility to infection and in a number of other factors, such as the rate of absorption of antiserum, the level of activity of the mononuclear phagocyte system, and the half-life of the passively administered immunoglobulin. As in neutralization tests, meaningful results can be obtained only if large numbers of animals are employed and if the challenge dose is carefully standardized. It is usual to use a dose of organisms or toxin containing a known number of LD_{50} or ID_{50}. Similarly, the protective effect of an antiserum may be expressed as a PD_{50}, the dose required to protect 50% of a group of animals.

MOLECULAR METHODS

Although immunological assays have historically provided the most sensitive assays for diagnostic purposes, modern molecular techniques have proved to be even more sensitive and specific. The detection of the nucleic acid of an infectious agent through polymerase chain reactions (PCRs) is often superior to immunological methods (Fig. 43.31). This method is based on the ability of very small quantities of nucleic acid to be amplified in a highly specific manner so that they can be readily detected. Thus, for example, small amounts of viral DNA may be present in a tissue sample. If the sample is heated, the paired DNA

strands will separate into two single strands. If the nucleotide sequence of this DNA is known, specific primers (oligonucleotides of single-stranded DNA) can be added to the sample, where they bind the viral DNA and act as a template for new DNA synthesis. These primers are selected so that they are complementary to the 3′ ends of the sequence to be amplified. Thus, these primers will bind to the ends of the sample DNA, a process called annealing. By adding an enzyme called DNA polymerase, new complementary strands of DNA are then assembled on the primers. The cycle can then be repeated: heating → primer annealing → new DNA assembly. Each cycle doubles the amount of specific DNA present, so in theory, 30 such cycles should result in the production of 2^{30} copies of the original DNA sample. Once cycling is completed, the products can be examined by gel electrophoresis and the characteristic DNA bands can be identified. If necessary, the bands may be sequenced to provide assurance that the correct DNA has been amplified.

As might be anticipated many different variations of the basic PCR process have been developed. For example, if the nucleic acid of interest is RNA rather than DNA (e.g., detecting an RNA virus), a reverse-transcriptase PCR may be performed. This simply involves the initial conversion of the viral RNA to DNA using a reverse transcriptase, before beginning the PCR cycle.

Real-time PCR simply measures the amplification of the DNA of interest as it is amplified (in real-time). The current methods measure fluorescence-resonance energy transfer to quantitate the amplification of a specific DNA of interest. As the cycles proceed, the amount of fluorescence gradually increases and can be plotted as a curve. With this test, it is possible to measure the initial copy number, and it is less susceptible to contamination errors.

PCR assays are not only useful in detecting the presence of trace amounts of viral nucleic acid in tissues. They can also be used to amplify specific genes from within an animal's own DNA. For example, if the primers are correctly selected, they can be used to amplify normal or abnormal genes. Thus, PCR can identify SCID foals or cattle with leukocyte adherence deficiency (see Chapter 40).

DIAGNOSTIC APPLICATIONS

The presence of antibodies to a specific organism in an animal's serum indicates previous exposure to an epitope present on that organism. It does not, however, prove that infection exists or that any concurrent disease is actually caused by the organism in question. For example, the fact that the sera of most healthy horses contain antibodies to *Salmonella typhimurium* does not prove that most horses are suffering from clinical salmonellosis. The presence of antibodies to an organism in a single serum sample is rarely of diagnostic significance. Only if at least two samples are taken 1–3 weeks apart and show at least a four-fold rise in titer can a diagnosis be made. This should be done only in conjunction with careful clinical assessment.

A second feature that must be considered in the interpretation of serological tests is the possibility of errors. Technical errors are usually prevented by incorporation of appropriate controls into the test system. Other errors, however, are largely unavoidable. For example, if test results are obtained from a known diseased population and from a known disease-free population, it will be rare to find that the results obtained separate perfectly. Much more commonly, the test results overlap, and the test cannot distinguish normal from diseased with 100% accuracy (Fig. 43.32). As a result, irrespective of the selected cut-off point, there will be some correct results and some incorrect ones. There will be four types of result: true-positive and true-negative results and false-positive and false-negative results. A test in which a large proportion of the positive results are true is considered to be specific, whereas

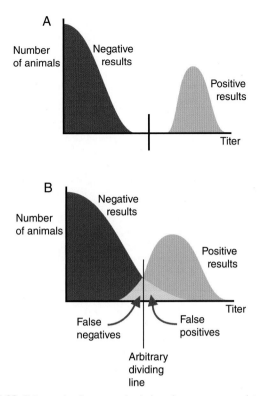

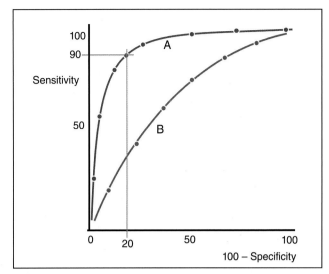

Fig. 43.33 An receiver operating characteristic curve plots a test sensitivity against 100-specificity for an entire range of cut-off points (e.g., different optical density values in an Enzyme-linked Immunosorbent Assay test). In a good test, specificity and sensitivity approach 100%, and the appropriate cut-off value may be very obvious. Thus in test A, the best cut-off point would give a sensitivity of 90% and a specificity of 80%. Unfortunately, this is not always the case (B).

Fig. 43.32 Schematic diagrams depicting the errors associated with immunological tests. The top diagram (A) depicts an ideal test in which there is no ambiguity in interpreting test results. The bottom diagram (B) depicts a more typical test in which an arbitrary line must be used to separate positive from negative results. By moving this dividing line, the relative proportions of false-positive and false-negative results may be changed.

one that correctly identifies the true-negative responses is considered sensitive. A perfect test would be highly sensitive and highly specific. In ideal tests, it would be desirable for the criteria used in interpreting the test results to be so obvious and absolute that each test would be absolutely sensitive and specific. Unfortunately, such ideal tests are uncommon. In general, the level of test errors can be adjusted by the criterion used to differentiate positive from negative reactions. If this cut-off point is adjusted downward so that the criterion for a positive test is made less strict, the number of false-positive results will increase, but there will also be a decrease in the number of false-negative results. In practice, therefore, highly sensitive tests tend to be relatively nonspecific, and highly specific tests are generally insensitive. The establishment of the cut-off point in reading test results and, from this, the sensitivity and specificity of a test are determined both by the requirements of the test procedure and by the significance of false-positive and false-negative reactions (Gerstman and Cappucci, 1986).

The sensitivity and specificity of any test can be calculated using the number of true-positive (a), false-positive (c), true-negative (d), and false-negative (b) results. The sensitivity of a test is the probability that a test result will be positive when the disease is present (true-positive rate) will be $a/(a + b)$. The specificity of a test is the probability that a test will be negative when the disease is absent (the negative rate will be $d/(c + d)$). Because of the reciprocal nature of sensitivity and specificity (one goes up as the other goes down), it is possible to plot this graphically using a Receiver Operating Characteristic (ROC) curve (Fig. 43.33). In this procedure, the test sensitivity is plotted as a function of 100 minus the specificity for multiple different cut-off points. Each point on the

ROC curve thus represents sensitivity/specificity for a given cut-off point. A test with perfect discrimination will thus have a ROC plot that passes through the upper left corner (100% sensitivity and 100% specificity). In less-than-perfect tests, an investigator can determine the optimal cut-off point by selecting the point on the curve closest to the upper left corner. The area under the curve also provides a measure of how well the test separates the two populations being tested. An area of 1 represents a perfect test, whereas an area of 0.5 represents a test whose results do not differ from random and hence is useless. ROC curve analysis is very useful in determining the best way to interpret a serological test, especially assays such as ELISAs, in which quantitative results are obtained, but whose significance is not immediately apparent. Tests with high sensitivity are needed if it is essential that no positive cases be missed, as in disease eradication programs. Tests with high specificity are needed if the false-positive results would have inappropriate consequences, such as requiring unnecessary animal euthanasia.

As has been evident from the discussions earlier in this chapter, the advantages and disadvantages of each immunodiagnostic test vary according to the requirements of the investigator, the nature of the antigen employed, and the complexity, sensitivity, and specificity of each method. In general, the selection of a diagnostic test represents a compromise among its sensitivity, its specificity, and its complexity. The latter includes the number of steps involved, the time involved, the degree of technical expertise required, its cost, and the nature of the equipment needed to conduct the test. Although precise guidelines cannot be drawn, it is usually most appropriate to use the most sensitive and specific test that can be satisfactorily performed with the available technical assistance and equipment at the lowest cost in the shortest possible time.

REFERENCES

Boto, W.M.O., Powers, K.G., Levy, D.A., 1984. Antigens of *Dirofilaria immitis* which are immunogenic in the canine host: detection by immuno-staining of protein blots with the antibodies of occult dogs. J. Immunol. 133, 975–980.

Bradley, G.A., Calderwood Mays, M.B., 1990. Immunoperoxidase staining for the detection of autoantibodies in canine autoimmune skin disease: comparison of immunofluorescence results. Vet. Immunol. Immunopathol. 26, 105–113.

Carter, G.R., Moojen, V., 1981. A summary of serologic tests used to detect common infectious diseases of animals. Vet. Med/Small Anim. Clin. 76, 1725–1730.

Cinquanta, L., Fontana, D.E., Bizzaro, N., 2017. Chemiluminescent antibody technology: what does it change in autoantibody detection? Auto Immun. Highlights. https://doi.org/10.1007/s13317-017-0097-2

Cripps, A.W., Husband, A.J., Scicchitano, R., Sheldrake, R.F., 1985. Quantitation of sheep IgG_1, IgA and IgM and albumin by radioimmunoassay. Vet. Immunol. Immunopathol. 8, 137–147.

Dudley, R.F., 1990. Chemiluminescence immunoassay: an alternative to RIA. Lab. Med. 21 (4), 216–222.

Egerer, A., Schaefer, Z., Larson, L., 2022. A point-of-care dot blot ELISA assay for detection of protective antibody against canine adenovirus, canine parvovirus and canine distemper virus is diagnostically accurate. J. Am. Vet. Med. Assoc. https://doi.org/10.2460/javma.22.05.0224

Gerstman, B.B., Cappucci, D.T., 1986. Evaluating the reliability of diagnostic test results. J. Am. Vet. Med. Assoc. 188, 248–251.

Kapmeyer, W.H., Pauly, H.-E., Tuengler, P., 1988. Automated nephelometric immunoassays with novel shell/core particles. J. Clin. Lab. Anal. 2, 76–83.

Lefevre, E.A., Carr, B.V., Prentice, H., Charleston, B., 2009. A quantitative assessment of primary and secondary immune responses in cattle using a B cell ELISPOT assay. Vet. Res. 40, 3–12.

Issel, C.J., Scicluna, M.T., Cook, S.J., Cook, R.F., Caprioli, A., Ricci, I., et al., 2012. Challenges and proposed solutions for more accurate serological diagnosis of equine infectious anaemia. Vet. Rec. https://doi.org/10.1136/vr.100735

McVicker, J.K., Rouse, G.C., Fowler, M.A., et al., 2002. Evaluation of a lateral-flow immunoassay for use in monitoring passive transfer of immunoglobulins in calves. Am. J. Vet. Res. 63, 247–250.

Molina-Bolivar, J.A., Galisteo-Gonzalez, F., 2005. Latex Immunoagglutination assays. J. Macromol. Sci. https://doi.org/10.1081/MC.200045819

O'Connor, T.P., 2015. SNAP assay technology. Top. Companion Anim. Med. 30, 132–138.

Pieck, C.J., Teske, E., van Leeuwen, M.W., Day, M.J., 2012. Good agreement of conventional and gel-based direct agglutination test in immune-mediated hemolytic anemia. Acta Vet. Scand. https://doi.org/10.1186/1751-0147-54-10

Smith, H.E., Jacobs, R.M., Smith, C., 1994. Flow cytometric analysis of ovine peripheral blood lymphocytes. Can J. Vet. Res. 58, 152–155.

Whelan, C., Shuralev, E., O'Keeffe, G., et al., 2008. Multiplex immunoassay for serological diagnosis of *Mycobacterium bovis* infection in cattle. Clin. Vaccine Immunol. 15, 1834–1838.

Wilchek, M., Bayer, E.A., 1984. The avidin-biotin complex in immunology. Immunol. Today 5, 39–43.

Wood, B.A., O'Halloran, K.P., Vandewoude, S., 2011. development and validation of a multiplex microsphere-based assay for detection of domestic cat (*Felis catus*) cytokines. Clin. Vaccine Immunol. 18, 387–392.

Selected CD Molecules

Note: Of the 371 currently recognized cell surface CD molecules, many have no known function or do not play a significant role in immunity. Most are glycoproteins. This list summarizes the features of only the most important.

CD1 A family of major histocompatibility complex (MHC) class I–like molecules that are antigen-presenting molecules for lipids and glycolipids. Found on thymocytes, macrophages, dendritic cells, NKT (natural killer T) cells, and some B cells.

CD2 Also called LFA-2, this is a cell adhesion molecule whose ligands are CD58 (nonrodents) and CD48 (rodents only). It is found on T cells and some B cells.

CD3 A collective designation for the signal-transducing molecules of the T-cell receptor (TCR). They are found only on T cells.

CD4 A receptor for MHC class II molecules that plays a key role in the recognition of processed antigens by helper T cells. It is expressed on helper T cells, thymocytes, and monocytes.

CD5 A receptor for CD72. It is found on T cells and a subpopulation of B cells in most species, including mice and humans, but not on B cells in rats or dogs.

CD8 This dimeric glycoprotein is a receptor for MHC class I molecules that plays a key role in the recognition of endogenous antigens. It is expressed on cytotoxic T cells.

CD11 Also called LFA-1, this is an integrin α chain found on leukocytes. Three forms are known: 11a, 11b, and 11c. They bind leukocytes to the vascular endothelium.

CD14 This is the receptor for lipopolysaccharide-binding protein and therefore regulates the biological activities of this molecule. It is expressed on macrophages and granulocytes.

CD15 A complex carbohydrate also called Lewis-X. Its sialylated form, sialyl Lewis^x is expressed on NK cells. Its ligand is the selectin CD62. It is found on many cells, especially granulocytes.

CD16 Also called FcγRIII, this is a low-affinity receptor for IgG and CD4. It is found on NK cells, granulocytes, and macrophages.

CD18 This is the integrin β1 chain found on all leukocytes. It is associated with the various forms of CD11. A mutation in the *CD18* gene is responsible for leukocyte adherence deficiency in calves.

CD19 A protein that associates with CD21 and plays a key role in regulating the B-cell response to antigen. It is expressed on B cells and their precursors but not on plasma cells. It is also expressed on dendritic cells.

CD20. A protein found on all B cells. A monoclonal antibody to CD20 is used to treat B-cell lymphomas in dogs.

CD21 A complement receptor also called CR2. Its several ligands include CD23 and C3d. It regulates B-cell responses in association with CD19. CD21 is found on B cells, some T cells, and dendritic cells.

CD22 Also called Siglec-2, it is a B-cell inhibitory receptor and a receptor for soluble IgM.

CD23 A receptor for IgE also called FcεRII. In its soluble form it regulates the production of IgE. It can also regulate B-cell responses by binding to CD21. It is found mainly on mature B cells.

CD25 The α chain of the interleukin 2 (IL-2) receptor. CD25 associates with the IL-2Rβ chain (CD122). It is expressed on activated T cells, B cells, and monocytes. CD25 expression is a feature of regulatory T cells.

CD28 The ligand for both CD80 and CD86 that plays a key role in T-cell costimulation. It is also expressed on activated B cells and other antigen-presenting cells. CD28 delivers an activating signal to T cells as opposed to CD152, which delivers a suppressive signal.

CD29 A β$_1$ integrin expressed on leukocytes and platelets. In conjunction with its α chain (one of the forms of CD49), it binds these cells to extracellular matrix proteins.

CD31 Mediates adhesion between cells that express CD31 (e.g., leukocytes to endothelial cells) (CD31 binds CD31 on the apposing cell). It regulates the phagocytosis of dead and dying cells.

CD32 A medium-affinity IgG receptor also called FcγRII, different forms of which are expressed on macrophages, granulocytes, and B cells.

CD35 This is the receptor for the complement components C3b and C4b, so it is also called CR1. It is expressed on granulocytes, monocytes, B cells, NK cells, and primate erythrocytes.

CD36 A pattern-recognition receptor that binds many different ligands, especially lipids. CD36 on intestinal γ/δ T cells binds bacterial lipoteichoic acids and helps trigger innate responses. Found on many different cell types.

CD40 A member of the tumor necrosis factor (TNF) receptor superfamily. Binding to its ligand CD40L (CD154) on activated helper T cells is essential for a successful antibody response and class switching. It is expressed in all antigen-presenting cells.

CD43 Also called sialophorin or leukosialin, this glycoprotein serves as an antiadhesive molecule on leukocytes. It is expressed on T cells as well as granulocytes, macrophages, NK cells, platelets, and activated B cells.

CD44 A receptor for hyaluronic acid that mediates the binding of cells to high endothelial venules. It is expressed in large amounts on T and B cells, monocytes, granulocytes, and many other cells.

CD45 A family of tyrosine phosphatases, some of which are required for signaling through the TCR. Multiple isoforms of CD45 are generated by alternative splicing of three exons. They are found on all cells of hematopoietic origin except red cells.

CD46 Also called membrane cofactor protein. CD46 is a receptor for C3b and C4b. Once bound, these complement components are destroyed by factor I. It is expressed on T cells, B cells, monocytes, granulocytes, NK cells, platelets, fibroblasts, endothelial cells, and epithelial cells, but not on red cells.

CD48 A GPI-linked glycoprotein that is a ligand for CD2 and CD247 in rodents. It is expressed on all blood lymphocytes.

CD49 A family of integrin α-chains associated with the CD29 β-chain. They are expressed in various forms on leukocytes, platelets, and epithelial cells. Also called very-late antigens (VLAs), their ligands are extracellular matrix proteins.

CD50 ICAM-3, the ligand for DC-SIGN (CD209) on dendritic cells. It is expressed on T cells.

CD54 Also called ICAM-1, this glycoprotein is the ligand for the CD11a/CD18 and CD11b/CD18 integrins. It is expressed on a wide variety of cells, most notably vascular endothelial cells.

CD55 Also called decay accelerating factor, this glycoprotein blocks the assembly of C3 convertase and accelerates its disassembly. It thus protects normal cells against attack by complement. It is broadly distributed on many cell types.

CD56 An adhesion molecule expressed on NK cells and nerve cells.

CD58 Also called LFA-3, this is a glycoprotein found on most cells, where it is a ligand for CD2.

CD59 A glycoprotein also called protectin, acts as an inhibitor of the terminal complement pathway by binding to C8 and C9 and blocking the assembly of the terminal complement complex. It is expressed on leukocytes, vascular endothelium, and epithelial cells.

CD62 The selectins (S-lectins) bind to carbohydrate structures such as CD15s (sialyl Lewis^x) on neutrophils. CD62E is E-selectin, CD62L is L-selectin, and CD62P is P-selectin. They are expressed on platelets, lymphocytes, and endothelial cells.

CD64 Also called FcγRI, this high-affinity IgG receptor plays a key role in antibody-dependent cellular cytotoxicity. It is expressed on monocytes and interferon-γ-stimulated granulocytes.

CD66e Also called carcinoembryonic antigen, this glycoprotein is expressed in large quantities by malignant intestinal cells. Its detection is, therefore, diagnostic of intestinal malignancy in humans.

CD71 A transferrin receptor expressed on activated leukocytes. It is required by dividing cells to import iron. It may also act as a selective IgA receptor.

CD72 Found on B cells (but not plasma cells) and is a ligand for CD5. It may participate in an alternative pathway of B-cell and T-cell activation.

CD74 Also called the γ or invariant chain, this protein associates with intracellular MHC class II molecules. Found in all MHC class II–positive cells. It is believed to prevent the premature binding of endogenous peptides.

CD79 CD79a is an alternative name for the BCR signal-transducing peptide, Ig-α, and CD79b is another name for Ig-β.

CD80 Also called B7-1, this is a high-affinity receptor for CD28 and CD152 (CTLA-4). The interaction of CD80 with its ligands is crucial to stimulating T-cell responses to antigen-presenting cells.

CD85 A family of leukocyte Ig-like receptors that bind MHC class I molecules. They are expressed on macrophages, dendritic cells, and B cells.

CD86 Related to CD80 and also called B7-2, this costimulatory receptor is expressed on antigen-presenting macrophages, activated B cells, and dendritic cells. Its ligands are CD28 and CD152 (CTLA-4) on T cells.

CD88 The C5a receptor found on granulocytes, macrophages, and mast cells.

CD89 This IgA receptor (FcαRI) is expressed on granulocytes, monocytes, and some subpopulations of T and B cells.

CD93 The C1q receptor. Found on monocytes and neutrophils, but not on lymphocytes. It modulates phagocytosis of apoptotic cells.

CD94 An NK cell receptor that associates with NKG2D and binds target cell MHC class I molecules.

CD95 Otherwise known as Fas, this is a receptor for the Fas ligand (CD95L or CD178) and a signaling component of an important cell death pathway. It is found on myeloid and T cells and plays a key role in the elimination of self-reactive T cells.

CD102 Also called ICAM-2, a glycoprotein expressed on vascular endothelial cells, resting lymphocytes, and monocytes but not neutrophils. It is the ligand for integrin.

CD106 Also called VCAM-1, a glycoprotein expressed on endothelial cells. It is the ligand for CD49d/CD29 (VLA-4).

CD120a and **b** Two TNF receptors (TNFR-I [CD120a] and TNFR-II [CD120b]). TNFR-I is expressed on epithelial cells, whereas TNFR-II is more highly expressed on myeloid cells.

CD121 Two IL-1 receptors, IL-1RI and IL-1RII, expressed on thymocytes, fibroblasts, keratinocytes, endothelial cells (type I), and macrophages and B cells (type II).

CD131 The common β chain of the IL-3 (with CD123), IL-5 (with CD125), and GM-CSF (with CD123) receptors.

CD132 The common γ chain of IL-2 (with CD25 and CD122), IL-4 (with CD124), IL-7 (with CD127), IL-9 (with CD129), and IL-15 receptors.

CD134 A member of the TNF receptor family that serves as the cell-binding receptor of feline immunodeficiency virus.

CD142 Tissue factor, a key initiator of blood clotting and mediator of DIC.

CD150 Also called SLAM (signaling lymphocyte activation molecule). The receptor for canine distemper virus expressed on T and B cells as well as dendritic cells and macrophages.

CD152 Also known as CTLA-4, this is the ligand for CD80 and CD86 and acts as a suppressor of T-cell activation by competing with CD28. It is expressed on CD4+T cells.

CD154 A member of the TNF family. Since it serves as the ligand for CD40, it is also called CD40L. Found on activated Th cells, it plays a key role in T-cell activation by cross-linking with CD40 on antigen-presenting cells.

CD158 Killer cell immunoglobulin-like receptors (KIRs). A family of MHC class I receptors expressed on NK cells. They play a key role in NK cell activation in primates and cattle.

CD169 Siglec 1 or sialoadhesin, a macrophage lectin-like adhesion molecule.

CD178 Also called Fas ligand (CD95L). A member of the TNF superfamily, and a key molecule in the induction of cell death by apoptosis.

CD206 The mannose-binding receptor found on mature macrophages and immature dendritic cells.

CD207 Langerin, a C-type lectin receptor on dendritic cells.

CD209 DC-SIGN found on a subset of dendritic cells. This molecule permits transient binding between T cells and dendritic cells. It is a C-type lectin whose ligand is ICAM-3 (CD50).

CD233 An erythrocyte membrane protein that functions as an anion (chloride and bicarbonate) exchanger. Also called band 3 protein. It plays a major role in the removal of aged cells.

CD240 The Rhesus blood group antigens found in humans and some primates.

CD247 The T-cell antigen receptor zeta (ζ) chain.

CD256 APRIL, a B-cell–stimulating cytokine from macrophages and dendritic cells.

CD257 BAFF, a B-cell–stimulating cytokine expressed by B cells, macrophages, and dendritic cells. It is active in a cell-bound form or as a soluble fragment.

CD295 The leptin receptor.

CD314 NKG2D, the NK cell receptor for the cellular stress proteins MICA and MICB.

CD335 Also called NKp46. A member of the KIR family and an important receptor expressed on NK cells.

CD369 Dectin-1. A C-type lectin important in antifungal immunity.

Some Selected Cytokines

Adiponectin. A glycoprotein secreted exclusively by adipocytes (an "adipokine"). It has antiinflammatory activities since it inhibits macrophage development and the production of tumor necrosis factor-α (TNF-α). Adiponectin regulates both glucose and lipid metabolism (Chapter 41).

APRIL (A proliferation-inducing ligand). A member of the TNF superfamily produced by monocyte, dendritic cells, T cells, and enterocytes. It stimulates the proliferation of B cells and inhibits B-cell apoptosis (Chapter 16).

BAFF (B-cell–activating factor). A member of the TNF superfamily produced by T cells, macrophages, dendritic cells, and neutrophils. It is expressed on the surfaces of producing cells but can be cleaved off to act as a soluble cytokine. Like APRIL it is an essential survival factor for B cells (Chapter 16).

Eotaxins. A family of CC chemokines that selectively attract eosinophils and mobilize these cells from the bone marrow (Chapter 30).

Granulocyte colony–stimulating factor. A growth factor produced by macrophages, endothelial cells, and fibroblasts. It regulates the maturation of granulocyte progenitors into neutrophils. The term *colony-stimulating factor* refers to its ability to promote the growth of bone marrow stem cell "colonies" in tissue culture (Chapter 6).

Granulocyte-monocyte colony–stimulating factor. It is produced by T cells, macrophages, fibroblasts, and endothelial cells. It is the major regulator of granulocyte and macrophage stem cells. It induces phagocytosis, superoxide production, and cellular cytotoxicity by neutrophils (Chapter 6).

High-mobility group box 1 (HMGB1) is a chromatin-binding protein that is either actively secreted by inflammatory cells, such as macrophages, or escapes from necrotic cells. HMGB1 acts through TLRs to promote macrophage cytokine release, thereby enhancing inflammation. It has bactericidal activity and is a potent pyrogen (Chapter 8).

Interferon-αs are a large protein family with many different isoforms. They are produced in large quantities by plasmacytic dendritic cells and in much smaller amounts by lymphocytes, monocytes, and macrophages. They have significant antiviral activity. They activate natural killer (NK) cells and stimulate the differentiation of monocytes into dendritic cells, as well as the maturation and activity of dendritic cells. Interferon alpha (IFN-α) also drives certain γ/δ T-cell responses (Chapter 28).

Interferon-β is a type I interferon produced by most nucleated cells and is coded for by a single gene in most mammals. It is produced in response to viral infections and has similar properties to IFN-α (Chapter 28).

Interferon-γ, a type II interferon, is a glycoprotein produced by CD4$^+$ Th1 cells, some CD8$^+$ T cells, and NK cells. IFN-γ acts on B cells, T cells, NK cells, and macrophages and is the key mediator of cell-mediated immune responses (Fig. 15.16).

Interferon-λ is a collective name for three type III interferons: IL-28A, IL-28B, and IL-29. All are distantly related to IL-10. They use a unique receptor system to trigger antiviral defenses.

Interleukin 1 Proinflammatory cytokines produced by macrophages, dendritic cells, T cells, B cells, NK cells, vascular endothelium, fibroblasts, and keratinocytes. The two most important forms of IL-1 (α and β) act on Th2 cells, B cells, NK cells, neutrophils, eosinophils, dendritic cells, fibroblasts, endothelial cells, and hepatocytes (Fig. 3.1).

Interleukin 2 is an immunoregulatory cytokine produced by Th1 and NK cells. Its targets are T cells, B cells, and NK cells. IL-2 activates helper and cytotoxic T cells and NK cells. IL-2 stimulates T-cell proliferation and cytotoxicity (Fig. 15.17).

Interleukin 3 is produced by activated T cells, NK cells, eosinophils, and mast cells. It stimulates the growth and maturation of bone marrow stem cells for eosinophils, neutrophils, and monocytes.

Interleukin 4 is produced by activated Th2 cells, mast cells, and basophils. It regulates the activities of B cells, T cells, macrophages, endothelial cells, fibroblasts, and mast cells. IL-4 stimulates the growth and differentiation of B cells and promotes type 2 immune responses (Fig. 15.19).

Interleukin 5 is a growth factor produced by activated Th2 cells, mast cells, and eosinophils. In humans, it promotes eosinophil production.

Interleukin 6 is produced by activated macrophages, T and B cells, mast cells, vascular endothelial cells, fibroblasts, keratinocytes, and mesangial cells. It acts on T cells, B cells, hepatocytes, and bone marrow stromal cells, as well as the brain where it induces a fever (Chapter 8).

Interleukin 7 is a growth factor produced by bone marrow and thymic stromal cells. It generates lymphoid stem cells. Its major role, however, is to control lymphocyte function by regulating V(D)J recombination in both B and T cells.

Interleukin 8 is a proinflammatory chemokine (CXCL8). Like other chemokines it is a relatively small (8.4-kDa) protein produced by macrophages and endothelial cells. IL-8 attracts and activates neutrophils (Fig. 3.5).

Interleukin 9 is a growth factor produced by Th2 cells activated by IL-2 (Th9 cells). It promotes the growth of helper T cells and mast cells. It also potentiates the effects of IL-4 on IgE production and thus plays an important role in allergic diseases. It is also produced by ILC2 cells and mast cells.

Interleukin 10 is an immunosuppressive and antiinflammatory cytokine. It suppresses the activities of T cells, NK cells, and macrophages. IL-10 is mainly produced by T cells, especially Treg cells but also by M2 macrophages, NK cells, and some dendritic cells. Its targets are Th1 cells, B cells, macrophages, NK cells, and mast cells (Fig. 21.12).

Interleukin 11 is a growth factor produced by bone marrow stromal cells, epithelial cells, and fibroblasts. It stimulates B-cell growth in association with IL-6.

Interleukin 12 is an immunoregulatory cytokine produced by monocytes and macrophages, dendritic cells, B cells, and keratinocytes. IL-12 acts on Th1 cells and NK cells to stimulate IFN-γ production and type 1 responses (Chapter 15).

Interleukin 13 is an immunoregulatory cytokine produced by activated Th2 cells, cytotoxic T cells, NK cells, mast cells, and dendritic cells. It has biological activities similar to those of IL-4 since they share a common receptor α chain (CD213) (Chapter 15).

Interleukin 14 is produced by T cells. It is a B-cell growth factor that inhibits immunoglobulin secretion and selectively expands some B-cell subpopulations.

Interleukin 15 is produced by activated macrophages, dendritic cells, endothelial cells, and fibroblasts. It shares many biological activities with IL-2. IL-15 acts as a T-cell, B-cell, and NK-cell growth factor. IL-15 is essential for the prolonged survival of memory T cells (Chapter 15).

Interleukin 16 is produced by CD8$^+$ T cells, eosinophils, dendritic cells, and mast cells. Its receptor is CD4 through which IL-16 regulates CD4$^+$ T-cell recruitment and activation.

Interleukin 17 is a family of at least six proteins (IL17A-F) produced by Th17 helper cells and other innate immune cells. IL-17 stimulates macrophages and endothelial cells to secrete proinflammatory cytokines and chemokines, leading to the recruitment and activation of neutrophils. Members of the IL-17 family play a key role in the development of acute inflammation, in autoimmune diseases, and in cancer (Fig. 15.21).

Interleukin 18 is an IL-1 family member produced by epithelial cells as well as macrophages and monocytes. It is an inflammatory mediator. In addition, IL-18 activates Th1 cells and NK cells to promote the production of IFN-γ, TNF-α, IL-1, CD95L, and several chemokines (Chapter 3).

Interleukin 19 is a member of the IL-10 family produced by B cells and activated monocytes. It is a proinflammatory cytokine that acts on monocytes to stimulate the production of IL-1, IL-6, and TNF-α.

Interleukin 20 is a regulatory cytokine and a member of the IL-10 family. It is produced by monocytes and keratinocytes and acts as a hematopoietic growth factor.

Interleukin 21 is produced by activated Th2 cells and is structurally related to IL-2 and IL-15. It promotes the differentiation of B cells into plasma cells and memory B cells. It regulates NK-, B-, and T-cell function.

Interleukin 22 is a member of the IL-10 family produced by activated Th17 cells, NK cells, and mast cells. It suppresses IL-4 production by Th2 cells and induces acute-phase protein production in the liver. It acts on B cells to promote lymphoid tissue development (Chapter 21). It appears to be especially important in promoting epithelial barrier functions such as wound healing.

Interleukin 23. IL-23 is produced by activated macrophages, dendritic cells, and γ/δ T cells. It stimulates Th17 cells to produce IL-17 and IL-22 (Chapter 21).

Interleukin 24 is a member of the IL-10 family produced by activated monocytes and Th2 cells. It stimulates apoptosis in many tumor cell lines and stimulates acute-phase responses in hepatocytes.

Interleukin 25 is a member of the IL-17 family produced by Th2 cells and mast cells and is also called IL-17E. It plays an important role in intestinal immunity, where it promotes Th2 and Tuft cell cytokine responses and resistance to helminths (Chapter 29).

Interleukin 26 is a member of the IL-10 family produced by activated T cells (especially Th17 cells), memory cells, and NK cells. It induces the proliferation of keratinocytes and T cells. It has direct antimicrobial activity against many gram-negative bacteria. Horses do not possess IL-26.

Interleukin 27 is expressed by activated monocytes and dendritic cells. IL-27 suppresses the activation of all three helper T-cell subsets and prevents neutrophil activation. It suppresses mast cell activation and induces T-cell production of IL-10. It thus serves a major antiinflammatory role (Chapter 21).

Interleukin 28 Type III interferons produced by virus-infected cells. They are also called IFN-λ2 (IL-28A) and IFN-λ3 (IL-28B). They share a common three-dimensional structure with IL-10 but have limited sequence similarity (Chapter 28).

Interleukin 29 (IFN-λ1). Another type III interferon. It is closely related to IL-28A and IL-28B.

Interleukin 30 is produced by antigen-presenting cells. IL-30 acts on naive CD4 T cells and synergizes strongly with IL-12 to promote IFN-γ production by Th1 cells.

Interleukin 31 is produced by activated Th2 cells and is related to IL-6. Its receptor is expressed on keratinocytes and induced on monocytes by IFN-γ. It plays an important role in allergic dermatitis (Chapter 31). A monoclonal antibody against IL-31 prevents itch in dogs with atopic dermatitis.

Interleukin 32 is produced by activated lymphocytes, NK cells, dendritic cells, and endothelial cells. It induces monocytes to develop into macrophages and enhances macrophage production of the proinflammatory cytokines, TNF-α, IL-1β, IL-6, and IL-8. It has significant antiviral activity.

Interleukin 33 is a proinflammatory member of the IL-1 family that is found within the cell nucleus. It is secreted by epithelial and endothelial cells as well as released by injured cells. Its targets include Th2 cells, ILC2 cells, basophils, and mast cells. It drives the production of IL-4, IL-5, and IL-13 by Th2 cells, ILC2 cells, and mast cells. IL-33 plays a major role in type 2 immune responses (Chapters 30 and 31) (Fig. 30.12).

Interleukin 34 is expressed in spleen, liver, heart, brain, and lungs. It is a growth factor that acts through the macrophage colony–stimulating factor receptor to promote monocyte maturation, as well as the development and maintenance of Langerhans cells and microglia. It promotes B-cell proliferation.

Interleukin 35 is produced by B cells. It stimulates the growth of Treg cells while suppressing Th17 cells. It thus has antiinflammatory effects and regulates immune responses in infectious and autoimmune diseases.

Interleukin 36 consists of a family of three IL-1-like cytokines (IL-36α, IL-36β, and IL-36γ) that signal through a common receptor. They are highly expressed in epithelial tissues such as the skin, lung, and intestine, as well as in macrophages. They act on keratinocytes and immune cells to trigger inflammation.

Interleukin 37 is an antiinflammatory member of the IL-1 family produced by monocytes and myeloid dendritic cells. It suppresses the production of IL-17 by inhibiting NF-κB and some protein kinases, such as mTOR.

Interleukin 38 is a member of the IL-36 family expressed in the spleen, skin, thymus, heart, and tonsils. It binds to the IL-36 receptor and acts as a receptor antagonist. It has been implicated in cardiovascular and autoimmune diseases.

Interleukin 39 is a member of the IL-12 family. It is a heterodimeric protein that mediates inflammation in lupus-like mice by promoting neutrophil expansion and differentiation.

Interleukin 40 is produced by activated B cells. It plays a role in the development of the intestinal lymphoid tissues.

Interleukin 41 is thought to have an immunoregulatory function and is highly expressed in the synovium of humans with psoriatic arthritis as well as skin and mucosa.

Leptin A protein produced by adipocytes that suppresses appetite by signaling through a receptor in the hypothalamus. It has a proinflammatory effect by promoting dendritic cell activation and Th1 responses (Chapter 41).

Macrophage colony–stimulating factor is a growth factor produced by lymphocytes, macrophages, fibroblasts, epithelial cells, and endothelial cells. It acts on monocyte stem cells to induce their proliferation and differentiation and promote macrophage cytotoxicity.

Macrophage migration inhibitory factor (MIF) is a protein produced by macrophages and T cells. It acts on macrophages to prevent their random migration, hence its name. It also activates lymphocytes. MIF promotes the production of the proinflammatory mediators TNF-α and IFN-γ.

Thymic stromal lymphopoietin is a member of the IL-2 family that activates antigen-presenting cells, resulting in the release of monocyte chemoattractants. It is produced by fibroblasts, enterocytes, epithelial cells, mast cells, keratinocytes, and Th2 cells. It promotes mast cell production of Th2 cytokines. It is also a potent pruritogen causing severe itching (Chapter 31).

Transforming growth factor-β (TGF-β) is a family of five signaling proteins. They are produced by platelets, activated macrophages, neutrophils, B cells, and T cells and act on T and B cells, dendritic cells, macrophages, neutrophils, and fibroblasts. The TGF-βs inhibit T- and B-cell proliferation and macrophage function and are immunosuppressive (Fig. 21.13).

Tumor necrosis factor-α (TNF-α) is a proinflammatory cytokine produced by macrophages, mast cells, T cells, endothelial cells, B cells, adipocytes, and fibroblasts. It is toxic to many tumor cells. TNF-α is the primary inducer of inflammation (Fig. 3.3).

Tumor necrosis factor-β (TNF-β) is produced by activated T and B cells and has similar properties to TNF-α. It is either secreted in a soluble form or forms a heterodimer with lymphotoxin-β in the T-cell membrane. TNF-β kills tumor cells and activates neutrophils, macrophages, endothelial cells, and B cells (Chapter 3).

Immunologists and cell biologists are incorrigible users of acronyms. While convenient, abbreviations can readily overwhelm students and newcomers to the subject. Here are some that have been widely employed in this book.

ACD	allergic contact dermatitis
ADCC	antibody-dependent cell-mediated cytotoxicity
AhR	aryl hydrocarbon receptor
AITP	autoimmune thrombocytopenia
ANA	anti-nuclear antibody
APC	antigen-presenting cell
APP	acute-phase protein
APRIL	a proliferation-inducing ligand
ATP	adenosine triphosphate
BAFF	B cell–activating factor
BALT	bronchus-associated lymphoid tissue
BCG	bacillus Calmette-Guérin (*Mycobacterium bovis*)
BCR	B-cell (antigen) receptor
BLAD	bovine leukocyte adherence deficiency
BLV	bovine leukemia virus
BoLA	bovine leukocyte antigen
C	complement
CAM	cell adhesion molecule
CBH	cutaneous basophil hypersensitivity
CD	cluster of differentiation
cDC	classical dendritic cell
CDR	complementarity-determining region
cGAS	cyclic GMP-AMP synthase
CID	combined immunodeficiency
CLL	chronic lymphoid leukemia
cM	centimorgans, a unit of genetic distance
CTL	cytotoxic T-cell or C-type lectin
Con A	concanavalin A
CR	complement receptor
CRP	C-reactive protein
CSF	colony-stimulating factor (or cerebrospinal fluid)
CTLA-4	cytotoxic T-lymphocyte associated (protein)–4
CXCL	a chemokine
DAF	decay accelerating factor
DAG	diacylglycerol
DAMP	damage-associated molecular pattern
DC	dendritic cell
DC-SIGN	dendritic cell specific-ICAM-grabbing nonintegrin
DIC	Disseminated intravascular coagulation
dsRNA	double-stranded RNA
DTH	delayed-type hypersensitivity
EAE	experimental allergic encephalitis
EAN	experimental allergic neuritis
ELISA	enzyme-linked immunosorbent assay
EPO	eosinophil peroxidase

Fab	antigen-binding fragment
FACS	fluorescence-activated cell sorter
Fc	crystallizable fragment (of immunoglobulin)
FcR	immunoglobulin (Fc) receptor
FeLV	feline leukemia virus
FoxP3	Forkhead box P3
FPT	failure of passive transfer
FH	factor H
FIP	feline infectious peritonitis
FITC	fluorescein isothiocyanate
FIV	feline immunodeficiency virus
GALT	gut-associated lymphoid tissue
GM-CSF	granulocyte-macrophage colony-stimulating factor
GPI	glycosyl-phosphatidylinositol
GTP	guanosine triphosphate
GVH	graft-versus-host (disease)
HDN	hemolytic disease of the newborn
HEV	high endothelial venule
HI	hemagglutination inhibition (test)
HIV	human immunodeficiency virus
HLA	human leukocyte antigen
HMGB1	high-mobility group box protein–1
HSC	hematopoietic stem cell
HSP	heat shock protein
ICAM	intercellular adhesion molecule
IDDM	insulin-dependent diabetes mellitus
IDO	indoleamine 2,3-dioxygenase
IEL	intraepithelial lymphocyte
IFA	indirect fluorescence assay
IFN	interferon
Ig	immunoglobulin
IGH	immunoglobulin heavy chain (locus)
IK	immunoconglutinin
IL	interleukin
ILC	innate lymphoid cell
IMHA	immune-mediated hemolytic anemia
ISCOM	immune-stimulating complex
ISG	immune serum globulin
ITAM	immunoreceptor tyrosine-based activation motif
IU	international unit
IVIG	intravenous (human) immunoglobulins
J	joining
JAK	janus tyrosine kinase
kb	kilobases, a measure of gene size
kDa	kilodalton
KIR	killer immunoglobulin–like receptor
LAD	leukocyte adherence deficiency
LAK	lymphokine-activated killer (cells)

LD$_{50}$	lethal dose 50
LE	lupus erythematosus
LFA	leucocyte function–associated antigen
LGL	large granular lymphocyte
lpr	lymphoproliferation
LPS	lipopolysaccharide
LT	lymphotoxin (or leukotriene)
β_2M	β_2-microglobulin
MAb	monoclonal antibody
MAMP	microbial-associated molecular pattern
MAP	major acute-phase protein
MAPK	mitogen-activated protein kinase
MBL	mannose-binding lectin
MCP	monocyte chemoattractant protein, male chauvinist pig
M-CSF	macrophage colony-stimulating factor
MDGF	macrophage-derived growth factor
MHC	major histocompatibility complex
MIP	macrophage inflammatory protein
MLD	minimal lethal dose
MLR	mixed lymphocyte reaction
MLV	modified live virus
MPGN	membranoproliferative glomerulonephritis
mTOR	mechanistic target of rapamycin
NET	neutrophil extracellular trap
NF-κB	nuclear factor-κB
NK	natural killer (cell)
NKT	natural killer T (cell)
NLR	NOD-like receptor
NOD	nucleotide-binding oligomerization domain
NOS	nitric oxide synthase
NOX	NADPH oxidase
NS	natural suppressor (cell)
PAF	platelet-activating factor
PAMP	pathogen-associated molecular pattern
PCA	passive cutaneous anaphylaxis
PCR	polymerase chain reaction
PD-1	programed death–1
pDC	plasmacytoid dendritic cell
PF	protective fraction
PFC	plaque-forming cell
PG	prostaglandin
PHA	phytohemagglutinin
pIgR	receptor for polymeric immunoglobulin
PKC	protein kinase C

PPD	purified protein derivative of tuberculin
PRM(R)	pattern-recognition molecule (receptor)
PTX	pentraxin
PWM	pokeweed mitogen
R	receptor (e.g., IL-2R)
RA	receptor antagonist
RAST	radioallergosorbent test
RF	rheumatoid factor
RIA	radioimmunoassay
RIG	retinoic acid–inducible gene
RLR	retinoic acid–inducible gene-like receptor
ROS	reactive oxygen species
RNS	reactive nitrogen species
S19	strain 19 *Brucella abortus* vaccine
SAA	serum amyloid A (protein)
SAP	serum amyloid P
SCFA	short-chain fatty acid
SCID	severe combined immunodeficiency
SID	single intradermal test
SIRS	systemic inflammatory response syndrome
SLA	swine leukocyte antigen
SLAM	signaling lymphocyte activation molecule
SLE	systemic lupus erythematosus
SMAC	supramolecular activation cluster
ssRNA	single-stranded RNA
STAT	signal transducers and activators of transcription
STING	stimulator of interferon genes
TAP	transporter for antigen processing
TCC	terminal complement complex
TCID$_{50}$	tissue culture infective dose 50
TCR	T-cell (antigen) receptor
TdT	terminal deoxynucleotidyl transferase
TGF	transforming growth factor
Th cell	helper T cell
TIL	tumor-infiltrating lymphocytes
TLR	toll-like receptor
TK	thymidine kinase
TNF	tumor necrosis factor
TSLP	thymic stromal lymphopoietin
Treg	regulatory T (cell)
WC	workshop cluster
ZAP	zeta-associated protein

GLOSSARY

Actinobacteria   A major phylum of gram-positive bacteria with a high guanosine + cytosine content. They include important pathogens, such as *Mycobacteria*, *Corynebacteria*, and *Prescottella*.

Activated macrophage   A macrophage in a state of polarized metabolic and functional activity.

Active immunity/immunization   Immunity produced as a result of administration of an antigen, thus triggering an immune response.

Acute inflammation   Rapidly developing inflammation of recent onset. It is characterized by increased blood flow and tissue infiltration by neutrophils.

Acute-phase proteins   Proteins, synthesized by the liver and other tissues, whose level in serum rises rapidly in response to acute inflammation and tissue damage.

Adaptive immunity   Specific immunity that develops in response to stimulation by antigens.

Adjuvant   Any substance that, when given with a vaccine, enhances the immune response to that vaccine.

Affinity   The strength of binding between two molecules, such as an antigen and antibody. Usually expressed as an association constant (K_a).

Affinity maturation   The progressive increase in antibody affinity for antigen that occurs during the course of an immune response as a result of somatic mutation in B-cell *V* genes.

Agammaglobulinemia   The absence of γ-globulins in blood.

Agglutination   The clumping of particulate antigens by antibody.

Alarmins   Molecules released by dead or damaged tissues trigger innate immune responses, especially inflammation. See also Damage-associated molecular patterns.

Albumin   The major plasma/serum protein largely responsible for maintaining plasma osmotic pressure.

Alleles   Different forms of a gene that occupy the same polymorphic locus.

Allergens   Antigens that provoke allergic reactions. Usually type I hypersensitivity responses.

Allergic contact dermatitis   An inflammatory skin reaction mediated by T cells responding to reactive chemicals bound to skin cells.

Allergy   A type I hypersensitivity reaction initiated by IgE-mediated mast cell degranulation.

Allograft   An organ graft between two genetically dissimilar animals of the same species.

Allotype   Antigenic and structural differences between the proteins of different individuals of the same species as a result of transcription of different alleles.

Alternative complement pathway   The complement pathway triggered by the activation of C3 by the presence of an activating surface.

Amyloid   An extracellular, amorphous, waxy protein deposited in the tissues of individuals with a chronic inflammation or a myeloma. It consists of misfolded, insoluble protein fibers.

Anamnestic response   A secondary immune response.

Anaphylatoxins   Complement-derived peptides that stimulate mast cell degranulation and smooth muscle contraction.

Anaphylaxis   A severe, life-threatening systemic type-1 hypersensitivity reaction.

Anergy   The failure of a sensitized animal to respond to an antigen—a form of immunological tolerance.

Antibiotic   A chemical compound, usually obtained from microorganisms, that can prevent growth or kill bacteria. Do not confuse this with antibody.

Antibody   An immunoglobulin molecule made by an appropriately stimulated B cell following exposure to an antigen, which can combine specifically with that antigen.

Antibody-dependent cellular cytotoxicity (ADCC)   The killing of antibody-coated target cells by cytotoxic cells through their surface Fc receptors.

Antigen   Any foreign substance that can bind to specific lymphocyte receptors and so induce an adaptive immune response.

Antigen-presenting cells   Cells that can ingest, process, and present antigen peptides to T cells. These cells express major histocompatibility complex (MHC) class I or class II molecules on their surface. This forms a complex with these peptides that can activate T-cell antigen receptors.

Antigen processing   The series of events that degrade foreign proteins into short peptides that bind to MHC molecules that can be recognized by T cells with appropriate T-cell receptors (TCRs).

Antigen-sensitive cells   Cells that can bind and respond to a specific antigen.

Antigenic determinant   See Epitope.

Antigenic variation   The progressive changes in surface antigens exhibited by viruses, parasites, and some bacteria to evade immune destruction.

Antigenicity   The ability of a molecule to be recognized by an antibody or lymphocyte.

Antiglobulin   An antibody made against an immunoglobulin, usually by injecting the purified immunoglobulin into an animal of another species.

Antiglobulin test   A method for detecting the presence of nonagglutinating antibody on the surface of a particle.

Antiserum   Serum that contains specific antibodies. Synonymous with immune globulin.

Antitoxin   Antiserum directed against a bacterial toxin and used for passive immunization.

Apoptosis   The controlled self-destruction of a cell; one form of programmed cell death.

Arthus reaction   A local inflammatory response due to a type III hypersensitivity reaction; it is induced by the injection of antigen into the skin of an immunized animal.

Asthma   A hypersensitivity disease characterized by a reduction in airway diameter, leading to difficulty in breathing (dyspnea). There are many possible causes but type I hypersensitivity to aeroallergens is most common.

Atopy   A genetic predisposition to become sensitized and produce IgE antibodies in response to common environmental allergens.

Attenuation   The reduction of virulence of a pathogen.

Autoantibodies   Antibodies directed against normal body components.

Autoantigen   A normal body component that acts as an antigen.

Autograft   A tissue or organ graft made between two sites within the same animal.

Autoimmune disease   Disease caused by an immune response against antigens from an individual's own tissues.

Autoimmunity   An immune response against normal body components.

Autophagy   A process of cellular self-digestion by which cells can ingest and destroy intracellular microbes or damaged organelles.

B lymphocytes (B cells)   Lymphocytes that have undergone development within the avian bursa of Fabricius or its mammalian equivalent. They are responsible for antibody production.

Bacille Calmette-Guérin (BCG) vaccine   An attenuated strain of *Mycobacterium bovis*. This may be used as a specific vaccine or as a nonspecific immune stimulator.

Bacterin   A vaccine containing killed bacteria.

Basophil   A polymorphonuclear leukocyte that contains granules that bind basic dyes such as hematoxylin. It participates in type I hypersensitivity reactions.

BCG   See Bacille Calmette-Guérin (BCG) vaccine.

Bence-Jones protein   Immunoglobulin light chains found in the urine of animals with myelomas. They precipitate out of solution when the urine is warmed and redissolve at higher temperatures.

Benign tumor   A tumor that does not spread from its site of origin.

Blast cells   Cells just prior to undergoing mitosis. As a result, they have large amounts of cytoplasm.

Blocking antibody   A noncytotoxic, noncomplement-activating antibody that, by coating cells, may protect them against immune destruction.

Blood groups   Antigens expressed on the surface of red blood cells. Their presence and expression are inherited.

Bursectomy   Surgical removal of the bursa of Fabricius.

C-terminus   The end of a peptide chain with a free carboxy (COO-) group.

C3 convertases   Enzymes that can cleave native C3 into C3a and C3b fragments.

Capsid The protein coat around a virus.

Carrier An immunogenic macromolecule to which a hapten may be bound, making the hapten immunogenic.

Cascade reactions A linked series of enzyme reactions in which the products of one reaction catalyze a second reaction, and so forth.

Cell-mediated cytotoxicity The killing of target cells induced by contact with cytotoxic T cells, natural killer (NK) cells, or macrophages.

Cell-mediated immunity A form of immune response mediated by T lymphocytes and macrophages; it can be conferred on an animal by adoptive transfer of these cells.

Chemokine A family of proinflammatory and chemotactic cytokines with a characteristic sequence of cysteine residues. They regulate the migration of leukocytes to the sites of inflammation.

Chemotaxis The directed migration of cells under the influence of a chemical concentration gradient.

Chimera An animal that contains cells from two or more genetically different individuals.

Chromosome translocation A form of mutation in which portions of two chromosomes switch position.

Chronic inflammation Slowly developing or persistent inflammation characterized by tissue infiltration with macrophages and fibroblasts.

Class The five major forms of immunoglobulin molecules common to all members of a species (see Isotype). Each class uses a different set of heavy chain genes.

Class switch The change in immunoglobulin class that occurs during the course of an immune response as a result of a change in heavy chain gene use.

Classical complement pathway The complement pathway triggered by activation of C1 by antibodies coating a microbial or cell surface.

Clonal deletion The elimination of self-reactive T-cell clones in the thymus.

Clonal selection The proliferation of specific lymphocyte clones in response to a specific epitope. The response is triggered through antigen-binding receptors.

Clone The progeny of a single cell.

Clonotype A clone of B cells with identical antigen receptors and thus the ability to bind a single epitope.

Cluster of differentiation (CD) A set of monoclonal antibodies that recognize a single protein on a cell surface. A CD antigen is by extension; therefore a defined protein on the surface of a cell.

Collectins A family of carbohydrate-binding lectins that depend on calcium for their adhesion.

Colostrum The secretion that accumulates in the mammary gland in the last weeks of pregnancy. It is very rich in immunoglobulins and so transfers immunity to a suckling newborn animal.

Combined immunodeficiency A deficiency in both the T cell– and B cell–mediated components of the immune system.

Complement A group of serum and cell surface proteins activated by factors such as the combination of antigen and antibody and results in the generation of enzyme cascades that have a variety of biological consequences, including chemotaxis, cell lysis, and opsonization.

Complosome The active complement components found within cells.

Commensal Species that live together and share resources.

Complementarity-determining region Those areas within the variable regions of antibodies and T-cell antigen receptors that bind to antigen and so determine the molecule's antigen-binding specificity. Synonymous with hypervariable region.

Concanavalin A (Con A) A lectin extracted from the Jack bean that makes T cells divide.

Conglutinin A bovine mannose-binding protein that also binds to C3b and acts as an opsonin.

Constant domains Structural domains with little sequence variability found in antibodies and TCRs.

Constant region The portion of immunoglobulin and TCR peptide chains with a conserved structure that consists of a relatively constant sequence of amino acids.

Convertase A protease that acts on a protein to cause its activation.

Cortex The distinct outer region of an organ such as the thymus, cerebrum, or lymph node.

Corticosteroids Steroid hormones released from the adrenal cortex that have profound effects on the immune system. Some corticosteroids may be synthetic in origin.

Costimulators Molecules required to stimulate an antigen-sensitive cell simultaneously with antigen to trigger an effective immune response.

Cross-reaction The reaction of an antibody or an antigen receptor directed against one specific antigen with a second antigen. This occurs because the two antigens possess structural features in common.

Cutaneous basophil hypersensitivity A form of delayed hypersensitivity reaction in skin associated with an extensive basophil infiltration.

Cytokine storm The pathological effects induced by the uncontrolled activation of T cells, and as a result, the unregulated and excessive production of many different cytokines.

Cytokines Proteins that mediate cellular interactions and regulate cell growth and secretion. As a result, they control most aspects of the immune systems.

Cytolysis Lysis of cells by immune processes.

Cytotoxic T cell A lymphocyte that can bind to target cells and kill it by inducing apoptosis.

Damage-associated molecular patterns (DAMPs) Conserved molecules derived from damaged cells and diseased tissues that trigger inflammation.

Delayed hypersensitivity A T cell–mediated inflammatory reaction in the skin, so called because it takes 24 to 48 hours to reach maximum intensity.

Dendritic cells Specialized antigen-processing cells. They possess long cytoplasmic processes (dendrites), and their primary role is to function as antigen-trapping and antigen-presenting cells.

Desensitization The prevention of allergic reactions through the use of multiple injections or oral administration of an allergen.

Disseminated intravascular coagulation Inappropriate activation of the clotting cascade within the blood vascular system.

Domain Discrete structural units from which protein molecules are constructed.

Dysbiosis A disturbance or imbalance in the types and numbers of species in the normal intestinal, respiratory, or skin microbiota.

Effector cell A cell that is able to "effect" an immune response. These cells include cytotoxic T cells and NK cells.

Eicosanoids A family of lipids that include prostaglandins and leukotrienes and play a key role in inflammation and allergic diseases.

Electrophoresis The separation of the proteins in a complex mixture by subjecting them to an electrical potential on a substrate such as a gel or paper. Each protein migrates at a rate determined by its isoelectric point.

ELISA Enzyme-linked immunosorbent assay. A serologic test that uses enzyme-linked antiglobulins and substrate bound to an inert surface to measure antigens or antibodies.

Endocytosis The intake of extracellular substances by cells.

Endogenous antigen Foreign antigen synthesized within body cells. Examples include newly formed virus proteins.

Endosomes Intracellular vesicles formed by endocytosis.

Endothelium The cells that line blood vessels and lymphatics.

Endotoxins Toxic lipopolysaccharide components of gram-negative bacterial cell walls.

Enhancement Improved survival of grafts or cancer cells mediated by blocking antibodies.

Eosinophil A polymorphonuclear leukocyte containing characteristic granules that stain intensely with the acid dye eosin.

Eosinophilia Increased numbers of eosinophils in the blood.

Epithelioid cells Macrophages that accumulate around a tubercle and resemble epithelial cells in histological sections.

Epitope A site on the surface of an antigen that is recognized by an antigen receptor. As a result, immune responses are directed against specific epitopes. Synonymous with antigenic determinant.

Erythema Redness due to inflammation.

Exocytosis The release of material from a cell by the fusion of cytoplasmic vesicles with the outer cell membrane.

Exogenous antigen A foreign antigen that originates at a source outside the body, for example, bacterial antigens.

Exon An expressed region within a gene that is transcribed into mRNA.

Exotoxins Soluble protein toxins, usually produced by gram-positive bacteria, that have a specific toxic effect.

Fab fragment   The antigen-binding fragment of a partially digested antibody. It consists of a light chain bound to the *N*-terminal half of a heavy chain.

Facultative intracellular organism   An organism that can, if necessary, grow within cells.

Fc receptor   A cell surface receptor that specifically binds antibody molecules through their Fc region.

Fc region   A part of an immunoglobulin molecule consisting of the C-terminal halves of heavy chains. It is responsible for the biological activities of the molecule.

Firmicutes   A bacterial phylum consisting mainly of gram-positive bacteria characterized by having a low G + C ratio. They include important bacteria such as *Clostridia*, *Listeria*, *Erysipelothrix*, and *Bacillus*.

Fluorescent antibody   An antibody chemically linked to a fluorescent dye.

Framework regions   The parts of a variable region of immunoglobulins and TCRs that have a relatively constant amino acid sequence and so form a structure on which the hypervariable complementarity-determining regions may be constructed.

G-proteins   Guanosine triphosphate–binding proteins that act as signal transducers for many cell surface receptors.

Gamma-globulins (γ-globulins)   Serum proteins that migrate in the gamma band toward the cathode on electrophoresis. They contain most of the immunoglobulins.

Gammopathies   Abnormal increases in γ-globulin levels.

Gel diffusion   An immunoprecipitation technique that involves letting antigen and antibody interact and precipitate in a clear gel such as agar.

Gene complex   A cluster of related genes occupying a restricted area of a chromosome.

Gene conversion   The exchange of blocks of DNA between different genes.

Gene segment   Another term for exon. It tends to be used to denote the exons that code for immunoglobulin and TCR V, D, and J regions.

Germinal center   A structural characteristic of many lymphoid organs in which rapidly dividing B cells form a pale-staining spherical mass surrounded by a zone of dark-staining cells. This is the site where somatic mutation occurs and memory cells are generated.

Glomerulonephritis   Pathological lesions in the glomeruli of the kidney.

Glycoprotein   A protein that contains carbohydrate side chains.

Graft-versus-host disease   Disease caused by an attack of transplanted lymphocytes (usually in the form of a bone marrow allograft) on the cells of a histoincompatible and immunodeficient recipient.

Granulocyte   A myeloid cell family containing prominent cytoplasmic granules. They include neutrophils, eosinophils, and basophils.

Granuloma   A chronic inflammatory lesion characterized by mononuclear cell infiltration and extensive fibrosis.

Granzymes   A family of proteases found in the granules of cytotoxic T cells.

Growth factors   Molecules that promote cell growth.

Haplotype   The complete set of linked alleles within a gene complex. They are inherited as a group and determine a specific phenotype.

Hapten   A small molecule that cannot initiate an immune response unless first bound to an immunogenic carrier molecule.

Heat shock proteins   Proteins synthesized by cells in response to many different physiological stresses including increased temperature.

Helper T cells   A subpopulation of T cells that promote immune responses by providing required costimulation from cytokines and costimulatory receptors.

Hemagglutination   The agglutination of red blood cells.

Hematopoietic organ   An organ in which blood cells are produced.

Hemolysin   An antibody that can lyse red blood cells in the presence of complement.

Hemolytic disease   Disease occurring as a result of destruction of red blood cells by antibodies transferred to the young animal from its mother.

Herd immunity   Immunity conferred on a population as a whole as a result of the presence of immune individuals within that population.

Heterodimer   A molecule constructed by linking two different peptide chains.

Heterophile antibodies   Antibodies that react with epitopes found on a wide variety of unrelated molecules.

High endothelial venule   A specialized blood vessel lined with high epithelium found in the paracortex of lymph nodes and other lymphoid organs.

Hinge region   The region between the first and second constant domains in some immunoglobulin molecules with an amino acid sequence that permits them to bend freely.

Histiocytes   Tissue macrophages.

Histocompatibility molecules   Cell membrane proteins that trigger graft rejection. The most important are required to present antigen to antigen-sensitive cells.

Homodimer   A molecule consisting of paired identical peptide chains.

Homology   The degree of sequence similarity between two genes (nucleotide sequences) or two proteins (amino acid sequences).

Humoral immunity   An immune response mediated by antibodies.

Hybridoma   A cultured cell line that produces monoclonal antibodies formed by the fusion of a myeloma cell with a normal antibody-producing cell.

Hypersensitivity   Clinical disease or lesions in a sensitized animal initiated by exposure to an antigen at a dose tolerated by normal individuals.

Hypervariable regions   Areas within immunoglobulin or TCR variable regions where the greatest variations in amino acid sequence and chain conformation occur and which therefore bind antigens.

Hypogammaglobulinemia   Low levels of γ-globulins in blood.

Immediate hypersensitivity   The hypersensitivity reaction mediated by IgE and mast cells. Otherwise known as type I hypersensitivity. It usually occurs within minutes of encountering an allergen.

Immune complex   Another term for antigen-antibody complexes.

Immune elimination   The removal of an antigen from the body by circulating antibodies and phagocytic cells.

Immune exclusion   The prevention of absorption of antigens into the body through epithelial surfaces by binding to immunoglobulin A.

Immune globulin   An antibody preparation containing specific antibodies against a pathogen or toxin and used for passive immunization.

Immune paralysis   Tolerance induced by very high doses of antigen.

Immune response genes   MHC class II genes, so called because they regulate the ability of an animal to respond to specific antigens.

Immune surveillance   The concept that lymphocytes survey the body for cancerous or abnormal cells and then eliminate them.

Immune synapse   An organized molecular structure that forms when receptors cluster in the area of contact between a T cell and an antigen-presenting cell or a target cell.

Immunity   The state of resistance to an infectious agent.

Immunization   The administration of an antigen to an individual to confer immunity.

Immunoconglutinins   Physiological autoantibodies directed against activated complement components.

Immunodiffusion   Another name for the gel diffusion technique.

Immunodominant   The epitopes on a molecule that provoke the most intense immune responses.

Immunoelectrophoresis   A procedure involving electrophoresis in gel followed by immunoprecipitation; it is used to identify the proteins in a complex solution such as serum.

Immunofluorescence   Serologic tests that make use of antibodies conjugated to a fluorescent dye to identify antigens or measure antibodies.

Immunogenetics   The portion of immunology that deals with the direct effects of genes on the immune system.

Immunogenicity   The ability of a molecule to elicit an immune response.

Immunoglobulin   A glycoprotein with antibody activity.

Immunoglobulin superfamily   A family of proteins that are constructed using immunoglobulin domains.

Immunological paralysis   A form of immune tolerance in which an ongoing immune response is inhibited by the presence of large amounts of antigen.

Immunoperoxidase   A serologic test that makes use of antibodies chemically conjugated to the enzyme peroxidase.

Immunosuppression   Inhibition of the immune system by drugs or other processes.

Inactivated vaccine   A vaccine containing an agent that has been treated in such a way that it can no longer replicate in the host.

Incomplete antibody   An antibody that can bind to a particulate antigen but cannot make it agglutinate.

Inflammasome   A multiprotein complex that forms in sentinel cells in response to triggering certain pattern-recognition receptors and the synthesis of inflammatory cytokines.

Inflammation   The innate response of tissues to injury or invasion. It involves both vascular and cellular changes. These responses eliminate microbial invaders and initiate repair.

Innate immunity   Immunity present in all animals that need not be induced by prior exposure to an infectious agent. It is mediated by proteins encoded in the germline.

Innate lymphoid cells (ILCs)   A family of lymphocytes present in all normal animals. They do not express antigen-specific receptors. However, they produce multiple cytokines, act as helper cells, and some (NK cells) are cytotoxic.

Inoculation   Administration of a vaccine by injection or scratching.

Integrins   A family of adhesion proteins found on cell membranes that bind either to ligands on the surface of other cells or to connective tissue proteins such as fibronectin or collagen.

Interchain bond   A bond between two different peptide chains. Usually formed by a disulfide linkage between two cysteine residues.

Interferons   Cytokines that interfere with viral replication. Some interferons also play an important role in the regulation of immunity.

Interleukins   Cytokines that act as growth and differentiation factors for the cells of the immune system.

Intrachain bond   A bond between two cysteine residues on a single peptide chain. Because disulfide bonds are short, its effect is to produce a fold in the peptide chain.

Intraepithelial lymphocytes   Lymphocytes, mainly T cells, located among the epithelial cells lining the intestinal and respiratory tracts.

Intron   A sequence of nucleotides inserted within a gene that separates exons and is not usually transcribed into mRNA.

Isoform   Different molecular forms of a protein that are generated by differential processing of RNA transcripts of a single gene.

Isograft   A graft between two genetically identical animals.

Isotype   Closely related proteins that arise as a result of gene duplication. They are found in all animals of a species. Thus the classes and subclasses of immunoglobulins are actually isotypes.

Isotype switching   The change in immunoglobulin class that occurs during the course of the immune response as a result of heavy chain gene switching.

J chain   A short peptide that joins units in the polymeric immunoglobulins IgM and IgA.

Joining (J) gene segment   A short gene segment that is located 3′ to the *V* gene segments in immunoglobulin and TCR *V* genes and codes for part of the variable region.

K antigens   Capsular antigens of gram-negative bacteria.

Killer cell   See Cytotoxic T cell and NK cell.

Kinins   Vasoactive peptides produced in injured or inflamed tissue.

Kupffer cells   Macrophages lining the sinusoids of the liver.

Langerhans cells   A population of specialized dendritic cells found in the skin. They are effective antigen-presenting cells.

Lectin   A protein that can bind specifically to a carbohydrate. Some lectins of plant origin can also induce lymphocytes to divide.

Leukemia   A cancer consisting of white cells that proliferate within the bloodstream.

Leukocytes   White blood cells. This general term covers all the nucleated cells of blood.

Leukopenia   The absence of leukocytes.

Leukotrienes   Lipid mediators derived from arachidonic acid by the actions of 5-lipoxygenase and responsible for potent proinflammatory responses.

Ligand   A generic term for the molecules that bind specifically to a receptor.

Linkage disequilibrium   A situation in which paired genes are found in a population at an unexpectedly high frequency when compared with the frequency of the individual genes.

Locus   The location of a gene on a chromosome.

Looping out   A method of excising a segment of intervening DNA (intron) to join two gene segments (exons).

Lymph   The clear tissue fluid that flows through lymphatic vessels.

Lymphadenopathy   Literally, "disease of lymph nodes." In practice it is used to describe enlarged lymph nodes.

Lymphoblast   A dividing lymphocyte.

Lymphocyte   A small mononuclear cell with a round nucleus containing densely packed chromatin found in blood and lymphoid tissues. Most have only a thin rim of cytoplasm. They recognize foreign antigens through specialized receptors.

Lymphocyte trapping   The blocking of lymphocyte migration within a lymph node as a result of the node's response to antigen.

Lymphokine-activated killer (LAK) cells   Lymphocytes activated by exposure to cytokines such as interleukin 2 in vitro.

Lymphokines   Cytokines secreted by lymphocytes.

Lymphopenia   Abnormally low numbers of lymphocytes in blood.

Lymphosome   The area of tissues drained by lymphatics that converge on a single lymph node.

Lymphotoxins   Cytotoxic cytokines secreted by lymphocytes.

Lysosomal enzymes   The complex mixture of enzymes, many of which are proteases, found within lysosomes.

Lysosomes   Cytoplasmic organelles found within phagocytic cells that contain a complex mixture of potent proteases.

Lysozyme   An enzyme present in tears, saliva, and neutrophils. It digests carbohydrates in the cell walls of gram-positive bacteria.

Macrophages   Large phagocytic cells containing a single rounded nucleus.

Major histocompatibility complex   The genomic region that contains the genes for the major histocompatibility molecules, as well as for some complement components and related proteins.

Malignant tumors   Tumors whose cells tend to invade normal tissues, break away, and spread by lymphatics or the bloodstream to distant tissue sites.

Maternal antibodies   Antibodies that originate in the mother but enter the bloodstream of her offspring either by transport across the placenta as in primates or by adsorption of ingested colostrum in other mammals.

Medulla   The region in the center of lymphoid organs such as the thymus or lymph nodes.

Memory cells   A population of long-lived lymphocytes formed in response to antigen. On subsequent exposure to that antigen, they mount a faster and stronger immune response.

Memory response   The enhanced immune response that is triggered as a result of exposing a primed animal to antigen.

Mesangial cells   Modified smooth muscle cells found within a glomerulus.

MHC molecules   Proteins encoded by genes located in the major histocompatibility complex.

MHC restriction   The requirement that a helper T cell can only recognize an antigen presented in close association with an MHC molecule.

Microbiota   The collective term for the microbial populations that colonize body surfaces.

Microglia   Resident macrophages within the brain.

Mitogen   Any substance that makes cells divide.

Modified live virus (MLV)   A virus whose virulence has been reduced so that it can replicate in the host but cannot cause disease in normal animals.

Molecular mimicry   Molecules from infectious agents whose structure closely resembles molecules found in their host. In this way the invaders may be able to trigger autoimmunity.

Monoclonal antibody   Antibody derived from a single clone of cells and hence chemically homogeneous.

Monoclonal gammopathy   The appearance in the serum of a high level of a monoclonal immunoglobulin. This is usually associated with the presence of a myeloma.

Monocytes   Immature macrophages circulating in the bloodstream.

Mononuclear cells   Leukocytes with a single rounded nucleus; for example, lymphocytes and macrophages.

Mononuclear-phagocytic system   The cells that belong to the macrophage family.

Myeloid system   The granulocytes and their precursors. These precursor cells are found in the spleen and bone marrow.

Myeloma   A plasma cell tumor.

Myeloma protein   The immunoglobulin secreted by myeloma cells.

***N*-terminus**   The end of a peptide chain with a free amino (NH_2) group.

Natural antibodies   Antibodies against foreign antigens found in serum in the absence of known antigenic stimulation.

Natural killer cells Large granular lymphocytes that are found in normal, unsensitized animals and that can recognize and kill abnormal cells such as tumor- and virus-infected cells.

Necrosis Cell death due to pathological causes. If programmed it is called necroptosis.

Negative feedback A control mechanism whereby the products of a reaction act to suppress their own production.

Negative selection The killing of self-reactive immature T cells. A key mechanism in the prevention of autoimmunity.

Neutralization Blockage of the growth of an organism or the toxicity of a toxin by antibody.

Neutropenia Low numbers of neutrophils in blood.

Neutrophilia High numbers of neutrophils in blood.

Neutrophils Polymorphonuclear neutrophil granulocytes.

NK cells Natural killer cells.

Noncovalent bonds Low-affinity chemical bonds that reversibly link chemical groups on peptide chains.

Nucleocapsid The key structural component of a virus consisting of the viral nucleic acid enclosed within its protective capsid coat.

Nude mice A mutant strain of athymic hairless mice.

O antigens Somatic antigens of gram-negative bacteria.

Obligate intracellular parasite An organism such as a virus that cannot grow outside the cells.

Oncofetal antigens Antigens found on fetal and tumor cells.

Oncogene A gene whose protein product plays a key role in cell division. As a result, its uncontrolled production may lead to excessive cell growth and tumor formation.

Oncogenic virus A virus that causes cancer.

Ontogeny The embryonic development of an organ or animal.

Opportunistic pathogen An organism that, although unable to cause disease in a healthy individual, may invade and cause disease in an individual whose immunological defenses are impaired.

Opsonin A molecule that facilitates phagocytosis by coating foreign antigenic particles.

Optimal proportions The ratio of reactants that generates the largest immune complexes when antigens and antibodies combine.

Orthologous Genes that have a conserved structure and are clearly descended from a common ancestral gene.

Paracortex The region located between the cortex and medulla of lymph nodes where T cells predominate.

Paralogous Genes or gene clusters that, although descended from a single ancestral gene, have diverged significantly following the original duplication.

Passive agglutination The agglutination of inert particles by antibody directed against antigen bound to their surface.

Passive immunization Protection of one individual conferred by administration of immunoglobulins produced in another individual.

Pathobiont A member of the normal microbiota that has the ability to become a pathogen if circumstances permit.

Pathogen-associated molecular patterns (PAMPs) Conserved molecular structures widely distributed among pathogenic microbes that, when recognized by sentinel cells, can trigger inflammation.

Pattern-recognition receptors (PRRs) Cellular receptors that can recognize conserved microbial structures. PRRs include toll-like receptors, among others.

Perforins A family of proteins made by T cells and NK cells that, when polymerized, can form tubular structures and insert themselves into target cell membranes to cause cell lysis.

Phagocytes Leukocytes whose prime function is to eat foreign particles, especially bacteria. They include macrophages and related cells, neutrophils, and eosinophils.

Phagocytosis The ability of some cells to ingest foreign particles. Literally, "eating by cells."

Phagolysosome A structure produced in a phagocytic cell by the fusion of a phagosome and lysosomes following phagocytosis.

Phagosome The cytoplasmic vesicle in a phagocytic cell that encloses an ingested organism.

Phenogroup A set of blood group alleles that are consistently inherited as a group.

Phytohemagglutinin (PHA) A lectin derived from the red kidney bean that is a potent T-cell mitogen.

Pinocytosis The endocytosis of small fluid droplets—drinking by cells.

Plasma The clear fluid that forms the liquid phase of blood.

Plasma cell A fully differentiated B cell capable of synthesizing and secreting large amounts of antibody.

Point mutation A mutation resulting from an alteration in a single nucleotide in a gene.

Polyclonal gammopathies An increased level of immunoglobulins of many different specificities in serum originating from the activation of many different B-cell clones.

Polymorphism Inherited structural differences among proteins generated by multiple alternative alleles at a single locus.

Polymorphonuclear neutrophil granulocytes Blood leukocytes possessing neutrophilic cytoplasmic granules and an irregular lobed nucleus.

Positive selection Enhanced proliferation of cells within the thymus that can respond optimally to foreign antigens.

Precipitation The clumping of soluble antigen molecules by antibody to reproduce a visible precipitate.

Premunition A form of immunity seen in some parasitic diseases that depends on the continued presence of the parasite in the host.

Prevalence The number of cases of a disease.

Primary binding tests Serological assays that directly detect the binding of antigen and antibody.

Primary immune response The immune response resulting from an individual's first encounter with an antigen.

Primary immunodeficiencies Inherited immunodeficiency diseases.

Primary lymphoid organ An organ that serves as a source of lymphocytes or in which lymphocytes mature.

Primary pathogen An organism that can cause disease without first suppressing an individual's immune defenses.

Privileged sites Locations within the body where foreign grafts are not rejected. A good example is the cornea of the eye.

Prostanoids A class of lipid mediators derived from arachidonic acid produced by the actions of the enzyme cyclooxygenase. They include prostaglandins, thromboxanes, and prostacyclin.

Protein kinase An enzyme that phosphorylates proteins.

Proteasome A large tubular multienzyme structure found in the cytosol. They act on ubiquinated cellular proteins to cleave them into small fragments.

Prozone Inhibition of agglutination by the presence of high concentrations of antibody.

Pseudogenes DNA sequences that resemble functional genes but, as a result of mutations, cannot be transcribed.

Pyrexia Fever

Pyroninophilic Stained by the dye pyronin. This stain preferentially binds to RNA, so a cell whose cytoplasm stains intensely with pyronin is rich in ribosomes and is therefore probably a protein-synthesizing cell.

Pyroptosis An inflammatory form of programmed cell death.

Radioimmunoassay An immunological test that requires the use of an isotope-labeled reagent.

Reaginic antibody An antibody of the IgE class that mediates type I hypersensitivity.

Recombinant vaccine A vaccine that contains pure antigen prepared by recombinant DNA techniques.

Respiratory burst The rapid increase in metabolic activity that occurs in phagocytic cells while particles are being ingested.

Reticuloendothelial system All the cells in the body that take up circulating colloidal dyes. Many are macrophages. This term is best avoided because it is not a true body system.

Retrovirus An RNA virus that employs the enzyme reverse transcriptase to transcribe its RNA into DNA.

Reverse transcriptase An enzyme that reversely transcribes RNA to DNA. It is found in retroviruses such as Feline immunodeficiency virus.

Rheumatoid factor An autoantibody directed against epitopes on immunoglobulin Fc regions. Classically found in the blood of patients with rheumatoid arthritis.

Sarcoma   A tumor arising from cells of mesodermal origin.

Secondary binding tests   Serological tests that detect the consequences of antigen-antibody binding, such as agglutination and precipitation.

Secondary immune response   An enhanced adaptive immune response that results from second or subsequent exposure to an antigen.

Secondary immunodeficiencies   Immunodeficiency diseases resulting from a known, noninherited cause.

Secondary infections   Infections by organisms that can invade only a host whose defenses are first weakened or destroyed by other infectious agents or toxins.

Secondary lymphoid organ   A lymphoid organ containing mature lymphocytes whose function is to trap and respond to foreign antigens.

Secretory component   A protein produced by mucosal epithelial cells; it functions as an IgA receptor and protects IgA against proteases in the intestine.

Selectin   A family of cell surface adhesion proteins that bind cells to glycoproteins on vascular endothelium.

Self-cure   The elimination of intestinal worms by a localized type I hypersensitivity reaction in the intestinal tract.

Septic shock   A severe disease condition that results from the massive release of cytokines such as tumor necrosis factor alpha as a result of infection.

Seroconversion   The appearance of antibodies in blood indicating the onset of an infection.

Serology   The science of antibody detection in serum or other body fluids.

Serum   The clear, yellow fluid that is expressed when blood has clotted and the clot contracts.

Serum sickness   A type III hypersensitivity response to the administration of foreign proteins as a result of the development of immune complexes in the bloodstream.

Signal transduction   The transmission of a signal through a receptor to a cell by means of a series of linked reactions.

Somatic antigens   Antigens associated with bacterial bodies.

Somatic mutation   Mutations that occur in somatic rather than germline cells. In immunology, this refers to the extensive mutations that occur in the *V* genes of B cells during the development of an antibody response.

Specificity   A term that describes the ability of a test to give true-positive reactions.

Stem cell   A cell that can maintain itself and also serve as a source of many different differentiated cell lines.

Stimulation index   A measure of the extent to which a cell population is stimulated to divide by an antigen or a mitogen.

Subclass   Different immunoglobulin isotypes closely related within a specific class.

Substrate modulation   A method of controlling enzyme activity seen in the complement system by which a protein cannot be cleaved by a protease until it first binds to another protein.

Superantigen   A molecule that, as a result of its ability to bind to certain TCR variable regions, can cause T cells to divide.

Superfamily   A grouping of protein molecules that share common structures. For example, the members of the immunoglobulin superfamily all contain characteristic immunoglobulin domains.

Symbiosis   The relation between species that live together.

Synapse   The area of contact between cells. Within the synapse, cell surface molecules are arranged in a well-defined pattern designed to optimize signaling between the cells.

Syndrome   A group of clinical signs that together are characteristic of a specific disease.

Syngeneic (isogeneic)   Genetically identical.

T lymphocyte   A lymphocyte that has matured within the thymus and is responsible for mediating cell-mediated immune responses. T cells are characterized by the presence of characteristic antigen receptors and their associated CD3 complex.

T-cell receptor (TCR)   The antigen-binding receptors of T lymphocytes.

Terminal complement complex   A multimolecular structure formed by polymeric C9 that generates pores in target cell membranes, leading to osmotic lysis and cell death.

Tertiary binding tests   Serological tests that measure the protective ability of an antibody in living animals.

Thetis cell   A specialized dendritic cell found in the intestinal tract that mediates food tolerance.

Thoracic duct   The major lymphatic vessel that collects the lymph that drains from the posterior of the body.

Thymectomy   Surgical removal of the thymus.

Thymocytes   Developing lymphocytes in the thymus.

Thymus-independent antigen   An antigen that can activate B cells and trigger an antibody response without help from T cells.

Titer   The reciprocal of the highest dilution of a serum that gives a reaction in an immunological test.

Titration   The measurement of the level of specific antibodies in a serum, achieved by testing increasing dilutions of the serum for antibody activity.

Tolerance   A state of specific unresponsiveness to an antigen induced by prior exposure to that antigen.

Tolerogen   An antigen that induces tolerance.

Toxic shock   A disease resulting from exposure to large amounts of staphylococcal superantigen.

Toxoid   Nontoxic derivatives of chemically treated toxins used as vaccines.

Transcription   The conversion of a DNA nucleotide sequence into an RNA nucleotide sequence by complementary base-pairing.

Transcription factors   Specialized proteins that regulate gene activity by binding to the promoter region of genes. They thus turn gene transcription on or off.

Transduction   The conversion of a signal from one form to another.

Translation   The conversion of the RNA nucleotide sequence into an amino acid sequence in a ribosome.

Transporter protein   Proteins that bind fragments of endogenous antigen and carry them to newly assembled MHC class I molecules in the endoplasmic reticulum.

Tubercle   A persistent granulomatous inflammatory response to the presence of mycobacteria in the tissues.

Tuberculin   An extract of tubercle bacilli used in a diagnostic skin test for tuberculosis.

Tumor necrosis factors   Macrophage and lymphocyte-derived cytokines that regulate many aspects of innate and adaptive immunity. They can exert a direct toxic effect on neoplastic cells.

Type 1 immune responses   Cell-mediated immune responses mediated by Th1 cells.

Type 2 immune responses   Immune responses mediated by Th2 cells, ILC2 cells, M2 macrophages, and type 2 cytokines. They involve antibody production and protect against helminths and toxins.

Tyrosine kinases   Enzymes that phosphorylate tyrosine residues in proteins. They play a key role in signal transduction.

Urticaria   Inflammatory and edematous skin reactions due to allergic mechanisms and associated with intense itching.

Vaccination   The administration of an antigen (vaccine) to stimulate a protective immune response against an infectious agent. The term is synonymous with immunization.

Vaccine   A suspension of living or inactivated organisms used to induce an adaptive immune response and hence confer immunity.

Variable region   That part of the immunoglobulin or TCR peptide chains in which the amino acid sequence shows significant variation among molecules.

Vasculitis   Inflammation of blood vessel walls.

Vasoactive molecules   Molecules that cause changes in local blood flow such as those observed during inflammation.

Virion   A virus particle.

Virulence   The ability of an organism to cause disease.

Xenograft   A graft between two animals of different species.

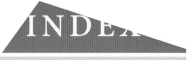

age numbers followed by *f* indicate figures, *t* indicate tables, and *b* indicate boxes.